James J. Nora, M.D.
University of Colorado Medical Center
4200 East Ninth Avenue
Denver, Colorado 80220

Heritable disorders of connective tissue

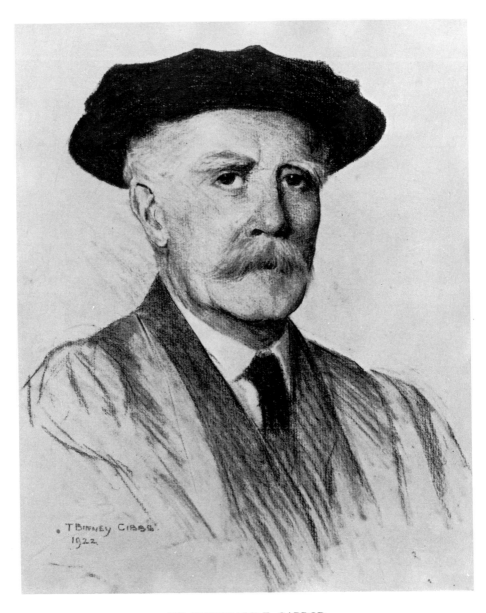

SIR ARCHIBALD E. GARROD

*Author of Inborn Errors of Metabolism (1909, 1923) and Successor
to Osler as Regius Professor of Medicine at Oxford*

*(From a previously unpublished crayon drawing made in 1922. Reproduced here through
the kindness of Sir Archibald's daughter, Miss Dorothy A. E. Garrod.)*

Heritable disorders of connective tissue

Victor A. McKusick, M.D.

Professor of Medicine, The Johns Hopkins University School of Medicine;
Physician, The Johns Hopkins Hospital,
Baltimore

FOURTH EDITION

With 1099 illustrations and 2 color plates

The C. V. Mosby Company
Saint Louis　1972

Dedicated to the memory of

Sir Archibald E. Garrod (1857-1936)

and

*to all who believe, as he did, that the
clinical investigation of hereditary
disorders can shed light
on normal developmental and
biochemical mechanisms*

Preface

Heritable disorders of connective tissue are generalized defects involving primarily one element of connective tissue—collagen, elastin, or mucopolysaccharide—and transmissible in a simple Mendelian manner.

Probably the first disorder to be interpreted as a generalized disorder of connective tissue was osteogenesis imperfecta. In 1920 Bauer[2] and in 1952 Follis[5] discussed this disorder in essentially the terms just stated. In 1931 Weve,[8] in calling the Marfan syndrome "dystrophia mesodermalis congenita, typus Marfanis," also recognized the nature of the condition. In 1955 I[7] introduced the designation *heritable disorders of connective tissue* for the class of disorders that included, in addition to those mentioned, the Ehlers-Danlos syndrome, pseudoxanthoma elasticum, and gargoylism, which Brante[4] had characterized in 1952 as a disorder of mucopolysaccharide metabolism. "Heritable disorders of connective tissue," like Garrod's[6] "inborn errors of metabolism," has gained wide currency. The term "heritable," although essentially synonymous with "genetic" and "inherited," may have the advantage that in the case at hand the disorder, although capable of hereditary transmission in the same or other patients, is not in that instance inherited, having arisen instead by new mutation.

It has been seventeen years since some of the material in this monograph was first published as a series of articles in the *Journal of Chronic Diseases*. The continued interest in the heritable disorders of connective tissue and their continued importance to clinical medicine and the biology of connective tissue are notable. In the interval, understanding of these diseases from both the clinical and the biologic points of view has increased appreciably. The collagen molecule has become more familiar in its physicochemical details, although it has far to go to match that paragon of protein molecules—hemoglobin. Characterization of the nature and metabolism of mucopolysaccharides has also advanced.

In connection with the Marfan syndrome, surgical treatment of the aortic complications is entirely a development of the last seventeen years. An exciting discovery is that an inborn error of metabolism (homocystinuria) is responsible for a clinical picture which, because of ectopia lentis and vascular disease, simulates the Marfan syndrome. The vascular complications of the Ehlers-Danlos syndrome have become better appreciated. The existence of a recessive form of osteogenesis imperfecta now seems certain. Evidence for involvement primarily of the elastic fiber in pseudoxanthoma elasticum has forced revision of the view held seventeen years ago. Furthermore, the recessive inheritance and histopathologic features, as well as the experience with homocystinuria, suggest that an inborn error of metabolism should be sought. The example of homocystinuria also suggests that alkaptonuria deserves classification as a heritable disorder of connective tissue. Increased understanding of cutis laxa and of the Weill-Marchesani syndrome justify separate chapters in the present edition.

Nosology has advanced farthest in relation to the mucopolysaccharidoses. Whereas in 1955 the nature of gargoylism as a mucopolysaccharidosis was recognized on histochemical grounds and two genetic forms—the autosomal recessive and the X-linked—were distinguished, characterization of the mucopolysacchariduria and identification of several other distinct varieties are developments of the 1960's.

It is especially the generalist—the *general practitioner* and the *internist* and the *pediatrician* without particular subspecialization—to whom the problems related to the several syndromes discussed here are of importance and to whom this book is addressed. He is in the best position to size up the total situation in the individual patient and relate it to the family background, with which he is most likely to have firsthand familiarity. He can best evaluate what may be excessive loose-jointedness and "ganglingness" or mild pectus excavatum, pigeon breast, kyphoscoliosis, and flatfeet. In the light of the general manifestations and the family background he can best appraise the significance of internal medical manifestations, which may be integral parts of a generalized syndrome.

Asboe-Hansen[1] has made the following cogent comment: "Connective tissue connects the numerous branches of medical science. Without connective tissue, medicine would come to pieces, even non-viable pieces, just like the cells of the human body."

The ubiquity of connective tissue is responsible for its unifying influence on medicine, referred to in the statement quoted from Asboe-Hansen. Furthermore, its ubiquity is responsible for the fact that concern with the problems of generalized and hereditary disorders of connective tissue extends also to many divisions of medical science and practice.

The *ophthalmologist* sees grave changes in the eyes in pseudoxanthoma elasticum, in the Marfan and Weill-Marchesani syndromes, and in homocystinuria and sees less serious, yet significant, alterations in osteogenesis imperfecta, the Ehlers-Danlos syndrome, and the mucopolysaccharidoses.

The *otologist* sees the patients with certain of the mucopolysaccharidoses, those with osteogenesis imperfecta, and rarely those with the Marfan syndrome.

The *orthopedist* is concerned with cases of osteogenesis imperfecta, the Ehlers-Danlos syndrome, mucopolysaccharidoses (e.g., Morquio syndrome), and sometimes the Marfan syndrome. Patients with fibrodysplasia ossificans progressiva are frequently seen by him.

The *general surgeon* repairs the hernias of the patient with the Marfan syndrome, the Ehlers-Danlos syndrome, osteogenesis imperfecta, or the Hurler syndrome.

The *hematologist* is consulted for the bruisability in the Ehlers-Danlos syndrome, for the tendency to multiple hemorrhages in patients with pseudoxanthoma elasticum, and for the multiple venous and arterial thromboses in homocystinuria.

The *gastroenterologist* is likely to encounter a case of pseudoxanthoma elasticum if he treats a sizable group of patients with gastrointestinal hemorrhage.

Increasingly the *cardiologist* is finding the Marfan syndrome of greater importance among the "causes" of aortic regurgitation and of dissecting aneurysm of the aorta than he had previously realized. In the Hurler syndrome and other mucopolysaccharidoses the cardiac involvement may bring the patient to medical attention and is frequently the cause of death at an early age. Among cases of *peripheral vascular disease,* pseudoxanthoma elasticum or homocystinuria occasionally figures as the etiologic factor.

Aside from the cardiovascular manifestations, the *chest physician* will be interested in the occurrence of cystic disease of the lung in the Marfan syndrome and of rupture of the lung with pneumothorax or mediastinal emphysema in the Marfan syndrome and in the Ehlers-Danlos syndrome.

The *dermatologist* treats patients with pseudoxanthoma elasticum and the Ehlers-Danlos syndrome.

The *plastic surgeon* is called in to provide cosmetic relief for the unsightly changes in the skin of the neck in pseudoxanthoma elasticum and of the face in cutis laxa.

The *dentist* sees abnormalities, especially in osteogenesis imperfecta and the mucopolysaccharidoses.

The *rheumatologist,* interested in connective tissues in general, is likely to see in these heritable disorders of connective tissue, derangements in purer culture and more easily analyzed form than in the acquired disorders of connective tissue such as the arthritides. Specifically, the rheumatologist may be consulted for the repeated hydrarthroses that may accompany the loose-jointedness of the Ehlers-Danlos syndrome, for the stiff joints of the mucopolysaccharidoses, and for the arthritis of alkaptonuria.

The *endocrinologist* is frequently consulted by the parents of a child with the Marfan syndrome or the Hurler syndrome and by the patient with osteogenesis imperfecta or fibrodysplasia ossificans progressiva, the incorrect supposition being that an endocrinopathy is present.

By reason of their hereditary nature, all these conditions are of interest to the *medical geneticist.*

The *pathologist,* of course, must be familiar with them, and the *radiologist* will find in every one of these syndromes diagnostic features that can be revealed by his rays.

For the *medical student* (in either the narrow sense or in the broad sense under which everyone in medicine should qualify) the disorders discussed in this book and other syndromes are important ingredients of the curriculum. They force the student to muster all his knowledge of anatomy, biochemistry, physiology, developmental biology, and genetics to account for the phenomena he observes.

Obviously, one objective of this book and of the clinical investigations on which it is based is a synthesis of the scattered information about several conditions which have in common the facts that they are (1) generalized disorders of connective tissue and (2) heritable, even if not inherited in the individual instance. To my knowledge, only Bauer and Bode[3] have previously attempted such a synthesis.

A second objective has been to see what justification could be found for a favorite, although (witness the following quotation from Harvey as well as the dedication) far from original, notion of mine: that clinical investigation of pathologic states is as legitimate a method as any other for studying biology. Specifically, the hereditary syndromes are tools for study of the normal situation—in this case for the elucidation of connective tissue. When the clinician compares his methods as biologic tools with the electron microscope, analytical chemistry, tissue culture, and others, he tends to get an inferiority complex. I will leave it to the reader to judge whether the clinical researches, which are reported here but which are in only small part my own, demonstrate that the clinician can take his place with the so-called "pure scientists" in the group now trying to fit together the varishaped pieces of the intricate jigsaw puzzle that is connective tissue.

*Nature is nowhere accustomed more openly to display her secret mysteries than in cases where she shows traces of her workings apart from the beaten path; nor is there any better way to advance the proper practice of medicine than to give our minds to the discovery of the usual law of Nature by careful investigation of cases of rarer forms of disease. For it has been found, in almost all things, that what they contain of useful or applicable nature is hardly perceived unless we are deprived of them, or they become deranged in some way.**

*From a letter written by William Harvey in 1657, six weeks before his death. Quoted by Garrod, Sir Archibald: The lessons of rare maladies, Lancet 1:1055, 1928. Also see translation of *The Circulation of the Blood* and other writings of Harvey by K. J. Franklin, Everyman's Library, New York, 1963.

Victor A. McKusick

REFERENCES

1. Asboe-Hansen, G., editor: Connective tissue in health and disease, Copenhagen, 1954, Ejnar Munksgaards Forlag.
2. Bauer, K. H.: Über Osteogenesis imperfecta, Dtsch. Z. Chir. 154:166, 1920.
3. Bauer, K. H., and Bode, W.: Erbpathologie der Stützgewebe beim Menschen. In Handbuch der Erbpathologie, vol. 3, Berlin, 1940, Julius Springer.
4. Brante, G.: Gargoylism—a mucopolysaccharidosis, Scand. J. Clin. Lab. Invest. 4:43, 1952.
5. Follis, R. H., Jr.: Osteogenesis imperfecta congenita: a connective tissue diathesis, J. Pediat. 41:713, 1952.
6. Garrod, A.: The lessons of rare maladies, Lancet 1:1055, 1928.
7. McKusick, V. A.: The cardiovascular aspects of Marfan's syndrome: a heritable disorder of connective tissue, Circulation 11:321, 1955.
8. Weve, H. J. M.: Über Arachnodaktylie (Dystrophia mesodermalis congenita, Typus Marfan), Arch. Augenheilk. 104:1, 1931.

Acknowledgments

The original investigations referred to in this book were supported in part by a grant from the Daland Fund of the American Philosophical Society held at Philadelphia for Promoting Useful Knowledge and in part by grants-in-aid from the National Institutes of Health, Public Health Service.

The late Dr. Joseph Earle Moore encouraged these studies, by wise suggestions improved their published form, and in general made this book possible.

To the late Dr. Richard H. Follis, Jr., I owe the largest debt of conceptual nature; his concept of osteogenesis imperfecta as a generalized unitary defect of connective tissue probably catalyzed my own thinking along these lines.

It would be impossible to name all the individuals who have assisted in accumulating the data presented. Nor can I list all the persons whose thoughts have influenced mine during the course of analyzing these disorders.

To my fellow members of the Galton-Garrod Society, founded at The Johns Hopkins University in the early 1950's by several of us who share an interest in human genetics, I am indebted for the pleasure and profit of many stimulating exchanges of ideas. Among others, Dr. Barton Childs, Dr. Bentley Glass, and Dr. Abraham Lilienfeld have been especially helpful to me.

The course in biophysical and biochemical cytology conducted by Professor F. O. Schmitt, Dr. Jerome Gross, and colleagues at the Massachusetts Institute of Technology, June, 1955, was of great assistance in the preparation of the brief survey of the biology of normal connective tissue. In recent years Dr. Karl A. Piez and Dr. George R. Martin, as well as others of the National Institutes of Health, have continued my education in this area.

The editors and publishers of *American Journal of Human Genetics, Bulletin of The Johns Hopkins Hospital, Circulation, Bulletin of the New York Academy of Medicine, Medicine,* and *Annals of Internal Medicine* kindly permitted reuse of illustrative material.

The annual conferences on The Clinical Delineation of Birth Defects held here at Johns Hopkins beginning in 1968 have provided valuable information that has been used in this fourth edition. I am grateful to many participants and to the National Foundation–March of Dimes, which provided financial support and published the proceedings, for permission to reuse illustrative and other material here.

In recent years several of my research fellows have contributed importantly to the study of several of the heritable disorders of connective tissue. Deserving particular mention are Drs. Roswell Eldridge, Richard M. Goodman, W. Bryan Hanley, Irene E. Hussels, R. Neil Schimke, Charles I. Scott, and David Wise. Dr. A. E. Maumenee and several members of his staff at the Wilmer Ophthalmological Institute, past and present, particularly Drs. Harold E. Cross, James P. Gills, Jr., Morton F. Goldberg, Howard A. Naquin,† David Paton, Gunter K. von Noorden, and George Weinstein, have contributed in many ways to the study of these disorders of connective tissue, almost all of which seem to have ocular manifestations. I owe a particular debt to Dr. John P. Dorst, Professor of Radiology here at Johns Hopkins, for a long, stimulating, and productive collaboration in the study of skeletal disorders and for specific assistance in the analysis of radiologic aspects of the entities discussed here.

Conversations with Dr. Karl Meyer, formerly of Columbia University, have been stimulating and informative. Dr. David Kaplan, Downstate Medical Center, Brooklyn, and Dr. Elizabeth F. Neufeld, National Institutes of Health, Bethesda, contributed significantly to the biochemical study of the mucopolysaccharidoses, and Dr. B. Shannon Danes, New York Hospital, New York, to their cytologic study. Numerous colleagues at other institutions deserve acknowledgments for their assistance to me: Drs. Robert J. Gorlin (Minneapolis), Leonard O. Langer (Minneapolis), John S. O'Brien (La Jolla, California), William B. Reed (Burbank, California), Jürgen W. Spranger (Kiel, Germany), and many others.

The late Dr. Ernst Oppenheimer, in preparing the German translation of the first edition, made several worthwhile suggestions that were incorporated in subsequent editions.

I am indebted to Professor Charles E. Dent, London, for directing my attention specifically to the simulation of the Marfan syndrome by homocystinuria. Dr. Robert A. Milch gave valuable assistance in the original preparation of the chapter on alkaptonuria and has been a constant source of stimulation and insight.

To the many others who directly or indirectly contributed to this book I extend my grateful appreciation. Essential to the successful pursuit of a study such as this, which is partly retrospective and which concerns disorders of relatively infrequent occurrence, are the careful recording of information by many individuals over a long period of time and its careful preservation in the archives of our hospitals and other institutions. I am deeply grateful for the contributions of many members of the staff of The Johns Hopkins Hospital over a period of many years.

---

†Died September 21, 1972.

Contents

xiii

Color plates

1 · The clinical behavior of hereditary syndromes, with a précis of medical genetics

We must analyse, and seek to interpret partnerships in disease.
JONATHAN HUTCHINSON*

Many of the inherited ailments of man have importance far out of proportion to their numerical significance because of the light they shed on normal mechanisms. Such has been shown to be the case with the hereditary disorders of connective tissue. This consideration, together with the increasing recognition of internal medical ramifications of these diseases, prompted this survey, first undertaken twenty years ago, and its continuation since that time.

Terms

Most of the disorders discussed here present clinically as combinations of clinical manifestations, or syndromes.† (The manifestations in each of the principal heritable disorders of connective tissue are outlined in Table 15-1.) Meaning literally a "running together," the term syndrome is legitimately applied to any consistent combination of two or more clinical manifestations. The term has no necessary etiologic connotations; specifically a syndrome need not be gene-determined. In the minds of many, *syndrome* and *disease* are distinguishable terms, the latter referring to a specific etiopathogenetic entity and the former to a combination of manifestations that may have diverse causes. For example, it might be argued that now that the specific defect involving the enzyme hypoxanthine-guanine-phosphoribosyltransferase (HGPRT) has been identified in the Lesch-Nyhan syndrome, it should be termed the Lesch-Nyhan *disease*. In this discussion, however, *syndrome* will be used in a specific sense—to signify a distinct etiopathologic entity, the diverse manifestations of which result from a single primary cause.

The use of the term syndrome in the specific sense need not, and should not, becloud the issue of genetic heterogeneity. Cases that might legitimately be called

---

*From Hutchinson, J.: Arch. Surg. 4:361, 1893.
†It has been claimed[25] that the correct pronunciation of this word is "syndrŏmē," not "syndroam."

instances of the Hurler syndrome by satisfying the main criteria described by Hurler are now known to be examples of a distinct entity and are assigned a different name. Some patients who show features of the Marfan syndrome have a distinct inborn error of metabolism, homocystinuria. Such cases are called by the more specific designation, leaving "the Marfan syndrome" as a label for those cases which thus far seem to represent a large homogeneous residual group, of which the precise basic defect is not yet known.

The term *heritable* was selected for the title of this book (rather than inherited or hereditary) to convey the sense that in a given individual the gene and/or the disease, although transmissibile to offspring, may not have been inherited but rather may have arisen by mutation. The terms *inherited, genetic, hereditary,* and *familial* are essentially synonymous with *heritable* but have particular shades of meaning. Mongolism is a genetic disorder, since it results from a change in the genetic material. It is also heritable but is usually not inherited from a parent. *Familial* is a loose term that can refer to concentration of a given trait in families for reasons other than genetic ones.

Congenital and *hereditary* (and cognate terms of the latter, listed above) are not synonymous. Congenital means simply "present at birth"; it has no etiologic connotations. A disorder may be congenital and not hereditary, or, conversely, may be hereditary and not congenital. Thalidomide embryopathy is congenital but not hereditary. Pseudoxanthoma elasticum is hereditary but not congenital. *Connatal* is synonymous with *congenital.*

Abiotrophy is a term suggested in the early years of this century by Gowers[8] for neurologic disorders in which a particular tissue or cell class is capable of function for only a limited time because of an innate weakness. Friedreich's ataxia and Huntington's chorea are examples. The abiotrophies are not congenital although they are hereditary. The changes in the aorta in the Marfan syndrome; in the skin, eye, and blood vessels in pseudoxanthoma elasticum; and in the joints in alkaptonuria are of abiotrophic nature. Abiotrophy, as a term, means no more than the late onset of degenerative changes. In using the term one should not deceive himself that he understands the nature of the basic defect.

Pleiotropic (meaning loosely "many effects") is a term applied to those single genes which are responsible for multiple manifestations. Although the gene may have many phenotypic effects, the primary action of the gene is unitary. *Polyphenic* is a useful term synonymous with pleiotropic.

Chromosomes

Biologically inherited human characteristics, both normal and pathologic, are determined by genes carried on the chromosomes. These number 46 in normal

---

Fig. 1-1. Metaphase plate, **A,** and karyotype, **B,** of the normal male. **A,** The chromosome set of a single lymphocyte undergoing cell division. **B,** The chromosomes have been arranged in a karyotype according to descending length. The 46 chromosomes in the male occur in 22 pairs of similar (i.e., homologous) chromosomes, plus the sex chromosomes X and Y. In the female the sex chromosomes are homologous; that is, there are two X chromosomes. (New methods for staining the chromosomes, e.g., with fluorochromes and with Giemsa stain at pH 9, reveal banding detail that permits separate identification of each chromosome and recognition of small abnormalities.)

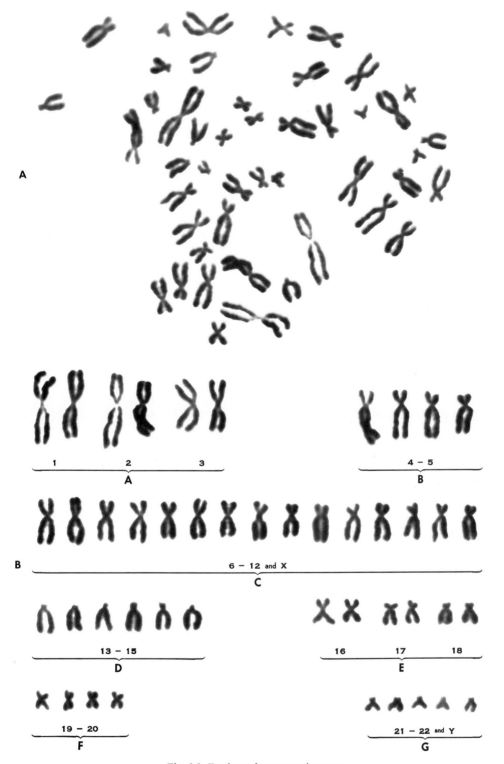

Fig. 1-1. For legend see opposite page.

man (Fig. 1-1): 22 pairs of autosomes (nonsex chromosomes) and the pair of sex chromosomes—two X's in the female, an X and a Y in the male. With few exceptions (such as the Hunter syndrome), the mutant genes that determine ("cause," if you will) the heritable disorders of connective tissue are carried on one of the 22 pairs of autosomes. Which autosome carries a particular gene (e.g., that for the Marfan syndrome) is not yet known. Information on specific chromosomal localization of specific genes is thus far scanty,[19] although it is known, for example, that the Duffy blood group locus is on chromosome 1[6] and that a haptoglobin locus is on chromosome 16.

Categories of genetic disease

In considering the role of genetic factors in disease, it is useful to consider disease in three main categories:

1. *Single-gene disorders.* Many diseases are determined by a single mutant gene in single or double dose. That a single gene is responsible is indicated by the characteristic Mendelian pedigree patterns. Most Mendelian disorders are individually rare, but there are many of them,[14] so that this first category represents a significant body of disease. Most heritable disorders of connective tissue discussed in this monograph fall into this category.

2. *Multifactorial disorders.* Some diseases that "run in families" do not show simple pedigree patterns. Multiple genetic and exogenous (environmental) factors appear to collaborate in etiology and pathogenesis. This category includes common disorders such as congenital hip dysplasia and degenerative osteoarthritis.

3. *Chromosomal aberrations.* Relatively gross abnormalities of the chromosomes can be recognized with the light microscope by means of techniques of study developed in the last fifteen years or so. These include abnormalities of chromosome number, e.g., trisomy 21 mongolism (Down's syndrome), and of chromosome structure, e.g., deleted short arm of chromosome 5 in the *cri du chat* syndrome. Because many genes are involved in an aberration identifiable by our relatively crude methods, complex malformations are usually the result. In most instances these chromosome aberrations are not inherited, in the usual sense of that word, yet they are abnormalities of the genetic material, the chromosomes, and therefore represent one category of genetic disease.

Pedigree patterns[3,13]

As indicated above, the autosomes in both sexes and the X chromosome in the female occur in pairs. The genes that are at the same locus on a pair of chromosomes are called alleles. Any person has two alleles at a given locus. If they are identical, the person is said to be homozygous; if different, he or she is said to be heterozygous. The male with only one X chromosome is said to be hemizygous with respect to genes on that chromosome.

Each of the disorders for main discussion is determined by a single mutant gene in either single (heterozygous) state, e.g., the dominant conditions, or in double (homozygous) state, e.g., the recessive conditions. Some are determined by genes on an autosome, i.e., are autosomal and at least one is determined by a gene on the X chromosome; that is, the disorder is sex-linked, or, more precisely, X-linked.

Rare monomeric genetic disorders such as these show characteristic pedigree patterns depending on whether the disorder is autosomal dominant, autosomal recessive, or X-linked recessive.

For rare *autosomal dominant traits,** the affected person is almost always heterozygous and is likely to be married to an unaffected person. Since the affected person is equally likely to give the "normal" chromosome as to give the homologous chromosome carrying the mutant gene to a particular child, the chance of an offspring's being affected is 50%. Furthermore, since the mutant gene is carried by one of the nonsex chromosomes, both males and females are affected and can transmit it to both their sons and their daughters. (See Fig. 1-2A.)

As a generalization, dominant traits are less severe than recessive ones. In part, an evolutionary or selective reason for this observation can be offered. A dominant lethal, that is, a dominant mutation that determines a grave disorder precluding reproduction, will promptly disappear. On the other hand, a recessive mutation, even if in homozygous state it prevents reproduction, can gain wide dissemination in heterozygous carriers.

A biochemical explanation is also possible for the greater severity of recessive traits. One might expect a greater derangement when both genes specifying a particular protein, let us say an enzyme, are of mutant type than if only one is mutant.

Although, like most generalizations, this one is not always true, dominantly inherited traits tend to be structural anomalies, such as brachydactyly, whereas recessively inherited traits tend to be inborn errors of metabolism, e.g., enzyme defects. The distinction is well illustrated by the two types of hereditary methemoglobinemia. All have cyanosis as the phenotypic characteristic. Some cases are due to a defect in an enzyme of the red blood cell; this type is inherited as an autosomal recessive. Others have an aberrant amino acid sequence of hemoglobin; this type is inherited as an autosomal dominant.

Among the children of two individuals who are both heterozygous for a dominantly inherited trait, the genotypic expectations are precisely those described by Mendel: one fourth homozygous, affected; two fourths heterozygous, affected; and one fourth homozygous, normal. The homozygous state of few dominant traits has been observed. In some disorders that are relatively mild in the heterozygous individual, the homozygous state is lethal. Severe abnormality leading to early death has been observed, for example, in offspring of parents who both have the Marfan syndrome (p. 153) or who both are achondroplastic dwarfs (p. 757). Probably few traits are completely dominant, that is, have the same phenotype in heterozygotes and homozygotes.

Another characteristic of dominant traits is wide variability in severity, or "expressivity" (p. 117). Sometimes the expressivity is so much reduced that the presence of the gene cannot be recognized, at least by methods currently available. When this is the case, the trait or the gene is said to be "nonpenetrant." Sometimes in pedigrees of families with a dominant trait, so-called "skipped gen-

---

*Because of the experience with sickle cell anemia (a homozygous state) and sickle cell trait (the corresponding heterozygous state), the word *trait* tends to suggest to clinicians the heterozygous carrier state of any recessive disorder. The geneticist, however, uses the term synonymously with *character* or *characteristic,* to refer to any phenotype.

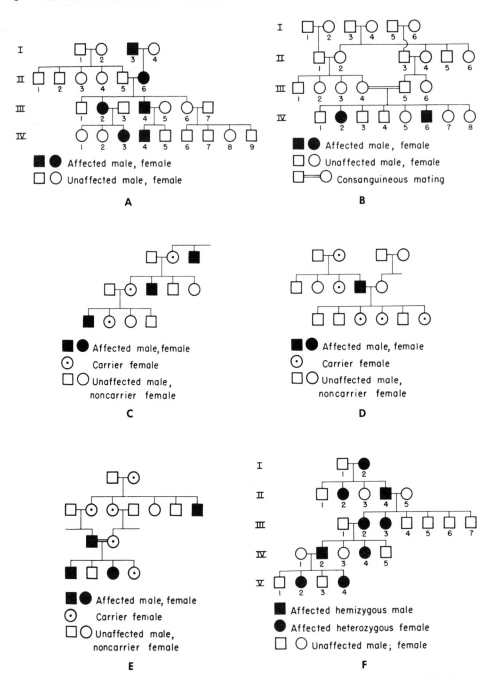

Fig. 1-2. Idealized pedigree pattern. **A,** The pattern of a rare autosomal dominant disorder. **B,** The pattern of a rare autosomal recessive disorder. **C, D,** and **E,** The pattern of an X-linked recessive disorder. In **D** the fact that all daughters of an affected male are carriers and all sons are normal is indicated. In **E** the offspring of the mating of an affected male with a carrier female are represented. The affected son is not an exception to the rule of "no male-to-male transmission," since the gene came from the carrier mother. **F,** The pattern of an X-linked dominant trait. Although the families with affected mother suggest autosomal dominant inheritance, all daughters of affected males are affected and all sons of affected males are normal.

erations" occur. In the "skipped" individual, expressivity is so low that the presence of the gene is not recognizable. Closer study of persons who clearly transmitted the trait from grandparent to grandchild sometimes shows mild but definite manifestations.

Another phenomenon based largely on the wide variability of dominant traits is "anticipation": the given hereditary disorder manifests itself earlier, is more severe, and leads to earlier death in each successive generation or at least in one generation than in the one just preceding it. This has been purported for myotonic dystrophy. It is clear, however, that anticipation is the result of biases of ascertainment. Obviously, the affected persons in generation I who have children are those at the milder end of a bell-shaped distribution curve for severity. On the other hand, *their* affected children, in generation II, are likely to cover more nearly the whole range of severity. On the average, then, generation II is likely to be more severely affected than generation I by any gauge, such as age of onset, degree of incapacitation, or age at death. Another source of bias leading to the artifactual phenomenon of anticipation is the following: the parent-child sets used in the calculations are often selected through the children who, the more severely they are affected, are the more likely to come to attention. *Anticipation has no genuine biologic basis.*

Autosomal recessive disorders (Fig. 1-2B) likewise occur with equal frequency in males and in females. When the condition is rare, almost all the affected individuals have normal parents, but both are heterozygotes. *Autosomal recessive inheritance is inheritance from both parents.* Since related individuals are more likely to be heterozygous for the same mutant gene, consanguineous matings, e.g., of first cousins, have a higher probability of producing offspring affected by a recessive disorder. Viewed in another way, a greater proportion of the parental matings in families affected by recessive traits are likely to be consanguineous than is true generally. The rarer the recessive condition, the higher is the proportion of consanguineous parental matings. For the more frequent autosomal recessive disorders (cystic fibrosis of the pancreas may be an example), there is little or no more consanguinity among the parents than expected by chance. In the case of a very rare recessive disorder, the occurrence of parental consanguinity may be of a very first clue to the fact that the trait is genetic.

Among the offspring of two heterozygous parents, one fourth of males and females are expected to be homozygous and affected. However, in human genetics, sibships with both parents heterozygous are generally ascertained only through the occurrence in them of at least one affected member. Since there is usually no way to recognize those matings of two appropriately heterozygous parents who are so fortunate as to escape having affected children, a collection of sibships containing at least one affected child is a biased sample. In the ascertained families, more than the expected one fourth are affected. Obviously in ascertainable one-sib families, not 25% but 100% of the children are affected. It can be shown that in a collection of two-sib families that can be ascertained because at least one of the two children is affected, 57%, not 25%, are affected; and so on. Methods of correcting for the "bias of ascertainment" have been developed. Their use in testing the recessive hypothesis is illustrated for alkaptonuria (p. 466) and for homocystinuria (p. 252).

The study of inbred groups such as the Old Order Amish is useful for

Table 1-1. Proportion of ascertainable sibships with only one sib (the proband) affected with a rare recessive disorder

S*	Proportion	S	Proportion
1	100%	7	36%
2	87%	8	30%
3	73%	9	24%
4	62%	10	20%
5	52%	11	16%
6	43%	12	13%

*Sibship size.

identification of autosomal recessive disorders because homozygosity is "brought out" by the inbreeding.[16] All of us carry a few genes in heterozygous state that would cause serious abnormality in the homozygous state. That our children are no more often affected than they are can be credited to the fact that as a rule we do not marry close relatives. Table 1-1 indicates another reason for increased "visibility" of recessive disorders in inbred groups such as the Amish—large family size, which increases the chance that more than just one child in a given family will be affected. It was this combination of circumstances which permitted identification of the "new" skeletal dysplasia, cartilage-hair hypoplasia (Chapter 13), which occurs, of course, in non-Amish but had previously escaped recognition as a distinct entity.

If an individual affected by a recessive trait marries a heterozygous carrier of the same recessive gene, one half of the offspring, on the average, will be affected, and a pedigree pattern superficially resembling that of a dominant trait results. Previously, it was thought that two genetic forms of alkaptonuria (Chapter 9) exist—one inherited as an autosomal recessive and one as an autosomal dominant. However, closer investigation revealed that the apparently dominant form was the same disease as the clearly recessive one. Because of inbreeding, homozygous affected individuals frequently mated with heterozygous carriers, and a quasidominant pedigree pattern resulted.

As originally defined by Mendel* and as used most accurately, the terms *dominant* and *recessive* refer to the character, trait, or phenotype—not to the gene. (For convenience, the geneticist often speaks of a "recessive gene" or a "dominant gene," especially in population genetics. But this is merely a variety of shorthand; he says "recessive gene," for example, to avoid saying "a gene that produces particular phenotypic effects only when present in homozygous state.")

---

*In 1866, Mendel wrote, "Henceforth . . . those characters which are transmitted entire, or almost unchanged in the hybridization, and therefore in themselves constitute the characters of the hybrid, are termed the *dominant,* and those which become latent in the process *recessive*" [italics mine]. Recall that Mendel was hybridizing pure lines, which were either homozygous dominant or homozygous recessive at any given locus. The hybrid, or F_1, generation was heterozygous. If the word *heterozygote* is substituted for *hybrid* the definition is precisely the one currently used. The terms refer to characters, not genes. That part of the definition saying "almost unchanged in the hybridization" allows for phenotypic differences in the dominant character in the homozygote as compared with the heterozygote.

Confusion arises if one fails to remember that dominance and recessivity are attributes of the phenotype, not of the gene. Of two related characters, one may be dominant and the other recessive, depending on the acuteness of the methods for defining phenotype. An illustration: the phenotype sickle cell anemia is recessive, since the homozygous state of the gene is required. Sickling, however, is a dominant phenotype, since the gene in heterozygous state is expressed. By electrophoresis of the blood of heterozygotes, both hemoglobin S and hemoglobin A are demonstrated, so at this level of study the phenotypes are codominant.

X-linked inheritance. Like autosomal traits, those which are determined by genes on the X chromosome may be either dominant or recessive. At least the female with 2 X chromosomes may be either heterozygous or homozygous for a given mutant gene, and in the female the trait can demonstrate either recessive or dominant behavior. But the male with a single X chromosome can have only one genetic constitution—the hemizygous; regardless of the behavior of the gene in the female, whether recessive or dominant, it is always expressed in the male.

The critical characteristic of X-linked inheritance, both dominant and recessive, is the *absence of male-to-male, i.e. father-to-son, transmission.* This is a necessary result of the fact that the X chromosome of the male is transmitted to none of his sons, although it passes to each daughter.

The pedigree pattern of an autosomal dominant trait tends to be a vertical one, which the trait passed from generation to generation. That of an autosomal recessive trait tends to be a horizontal one, with affected persons confined to a single generation. The pedigree pattern of a rare *X-linked recessive character* (Fig. 1-2C) tends to be an oblique one, since the affection is one almost exclusively of males and is transmitted to the sons of their normal carrier sisters. Bateson likened this pattern to the knight's move in chess. Often, tracing of X-linked recessive characters through many generations is difficult because the patronymic of affected persons usually changes with each generation.

Among the children of a male affected by an X-linked recessive trait (Fig. 1-2D), all sons are unaffected and all daughters are carriers, provided that the mother is not affected and is not a heterozygous carrier. Father-to-son transmission of X-linked traits cannot occur.

If an affected male marries a carrier female—and for rare conditions this is more likely to occur in a consanguineous marriage, as shown in Fig. 1-2E—half the daughters will be homozygous and affected and the others will be carriers. Half the sons are expected to be affected. This is not a true exception to the rule of no male-to-male transmission because the mutant gene came from the carrier mother.

In some instances it is impossible by pedigree pattern alone to distinguish between an X-linked recessive trait and an autosomal dominant male-limited trait. In both modes of inheritance, the trait occurs only in males and is transmitted by females who do not show it. Prime examples are the testicular feminization syndrome[15] and the Reifenstein syndrome,[2] both of which are forms of familial male pseudohermaphroditism resulting apparently from a defect in testicular hormonogenesis. Testes must be present for the disorder to be expressed. The female cannot show the disorder even if she possesses the appropriate genotype. The main way to distinguish X-linked recessive and autosomal dominant inheritance is by the findings in the progeny of affected males. If

X-linked, the trait will be transmitted to none of his sons by an affected male. The progency test is not available in the genetic analysis of the two examples cited because affected males are sterile. The test is also not available in X-linked recessive conditions which, although not affecting the reproductive capacity directly, are of such a nature that affected males do not survive to reproduce. The X-linked mucopolysaccharidosis, the Hunter syndrome, is such a condition (Chapter 11). Formally, from pedigree pattern alone, either X-linked recessive or autosomal dominant male-limited inheritance is possible. Favoring X-linked inheritance are the facts (1) that there is no plausible reason that the disorder should not be expressed in the female and (2) that this appears to be an enzyme disorder which in the overwhelming proportion occurs only in homozygous persons or in the hemizygous male.

The Lyon principle (formerly, the Lyon hypothesis) is important in connection with X-linked inheritance and provides a method for proving X-linked recessive inheritance in situations, such as the Hunter syndrome, in which affected males do not reproduce. As diagrammed in Fig. 1-3, the Lyon principle is that in the XX female one X chromosome in each cell becomes genetically inactive at an early stage of embryogenesis. The genetically inactive X chromosome is the one that constitutes the Barr body, or sex chromatin, a chromatin mass that lies just under the nuclear membrane of cells of the females (with the exception of the germ cells, which do not participate in the process called lyonization). It is a random matter which X chromosome—the one from her father (X^P) or the one from her mother (X^M)—is inactivated in a given cell, but once lyonization has occurred in a given cell, all cells descendant from that cell have the same X chromosome active or inactive. Thus the female is a mosaic of two classes of cells, those with X^M active and those with X^P active. If the female is heterozygous for the Hunter syndrome (a "carrier"), those cells

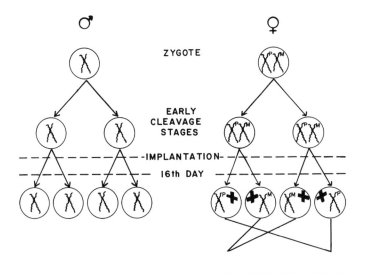

Fig. 1-3. The Lyon principle.

which have the mutant-bearing X chromosome as the active one will be abnormal (like all cells in the affected male), whereas those cells with the X chromosome bearing the normal allele active will be perfectly normal. As reviewed in Chapter 11, it is possible to clone two classes of cells from Hunter heterozygotes.

Another consequence of the Lyon principle is that the phenotype of heterozygous females varies widely. The proportion of relevant anlage cells that opt for the mutant-bearing X chromosome as the active one can vary from 0% to 100%, although the largest number of heterozygous females will have about 50% of cells of mutant type. If the number of anlage cells present at the time of lyonization is small, the chance is increased that some heterozygotes will have a majority with the mutant X chromosome active. Such females will be so-called manifesting heterozygotes. This phenomenon has been observed in glucose-6-phosphate dehydrogenase deficiency and in hemophilia.

In *X-linked dominant inheritance* (Fig. 1-2F), both females and males are affected, and both males and females transmit the disorder to their offspring, just as in autosomal dominant inheritance. Superficially, the pedigree patterns in the two types of inheritance are similar, but there is a critical difference. In X-linked dominant inheritance, although the affected female transmits the trait to half her sons and half her daughters, the affected male transmits it to *none* of his sons and to *all* of his daughters. One of the best-studied X-linked dominant traits is vitamin D—resistant rickets, or hypophosphatemic rickets. The skeletal defect alone gives a pedigree pattern that tends to be inconclusive. However, whene hypophosphatemia is used as the trait for analysis, the inheritance becomes clear. *All* the daughters and *none* of the sons of affected males are affected.

With a rare X-linked dominant trait, such as hypophosphatemic rickets, about twice as many females are affected as males—a clue to the mode of inheritance when one is investigating the matter for the first time. Furthermore, the disorder tends to vary in severity much more in females than in males. This is because of the statistical variation in the proportion of relevant anlage cells that have the mutant-bearing X chromosome as the active one. On the other hand, all cells of the affected male have a mutant-bearing X chromosome genetically active, it being the only one present.

Some rare X-linked dominant traits are so severe in the hemizygous affected male that he does not survive to birth but is lost as an abortion. The pedigree characteristics are that the disorder occurs only in females, that it may be transmitted from mother to daughter, and that a deficiency of males and excess of abortions occur in the offspring of affected females. No heritable disorder of connective tissue shows this pattern, which is, however, well established for focal dermal hypoplasia, orofaciodigital (OFD) syndrome, and incontinentia pigmenti.

The following disorders, listed here according to mode of inheritance, are discussed later:

Autosomal dominant

  Marfan syndrome
  Ehlers-Danlos syndrome
  Cutis laxa (one form)
  Osteogenesis imperfecta
  Fibrodysplasia ossificans progressiva

Autosomal dominant—cont'd

Osteopoikilosis
Achondroplasia
Hypochondroplasia
Osteopetrosis, benign type
Cleidocranial dysplasia
Multiple cartilaginous exostoses
Dyschondrosteosis (Léri)

Autosomal recessive

Homocystinuria
Ehlers-Danlos syndrome (at least one form)
Cutis laxa (one form)
Osteogenesis imperfecta (one or more forms)
Alkaptonuria
Pseudoxanthoma elasticum
The mucopolysaccharidoses (except MPS II)
Diastrophic dwarfism
Metatropic dwarfism
Ellis–van Creveld syndrome
Asphyxiating thoracic dysplasia
Achondrogenesis
Cartilage-hair hypoplasia
Osteopetrosis, malignant type
Pyknodysostosis
Engelmann's disease
Weill-Marchesani syndrome

X-linked recessive

Ehlers-Danlos syndrome (one form)
Mucopolysaccharidosis II (Hunter syndrome)
Spondyloepiphyseal dysplasia, tarda type

X-linked dominant

Hereditary hypophosphatemia (vitamin D–resistant rickets)*

Conventions for the construction of pedigree charts are illustrated by the idealized examples, shown in Fig. 1-2, of the several modes of inheritance. Squares are used for males and circles for females, rather than the symbols ♂ and ♀, which are more generally used by British writers. Solidly "blacked-in" symbols indicate affected individuals and an arrow indicates the propositus (–a), or proband, the affected person who first brings the kindred to the attention of the medical geneticist.

The genetic basis of syndromes

Some congenital syndromes are nongenetic in etiology, e.g., the thalidomide syndrome and the rubella syndrome. The Marfan syndrome and Down's syndrome (mongolism) are examples of syndromes resulting from a change in the genetic material. Formally, at least four types of genetic change-producing syndromes are recognized.

1. Probably the largest number of recognized genetic syndromes result from

---

*From McKusick, V. A.: Mendelian inheritance in man: catalogs of autosomal dominant, autosomal recessive and X-linked phenotypes, ed. 3, Baltimore, 1971, The Johns Hopkins Press.

mutation in a single structural gene. The manifold features of the syndrome result from the fact that the primary gene product, enzyme or nonenzymic protein, has a rather wide role in the body's economy. All the conditions discussed here seem to fall into this class. Since search for a unitary defect is based on the premise of a one-gene–one-syndrome relationship, it is well to examine the evidence that one gene is primarily responsible for all manifestations and that, for example, two or more closely linked genes are not involved.

a. It is unlikely that several genes would undergo mutation simultaneously to reproduce these syndromes again and again with such exactitude.

b. Linkage is the location of genes on the same chromosome. Crossing-over tends to separate even closely linked genes so that with the passage of generations, a larger number of generations if the linkage is close, no particular association of the characters determined by the linked genes is observed in a given individual. *Genetic linkage produces no permanent association of characters.* It is true that for closely neighboring genes the rate of crossing-over is so low that the relatively few human generations available for study may, in any one kindred, be inadequate to demonstrate separation of the components of a given syndrome. However, in the population at large, the situation is as stated by Snyder[22]:

The occurrence of genetic linkage between the genes for two traits does not change the association for these traits in the population from what it would be if they are not linked. Stated conversely, a correlation between two traits in a free-breeding population does not indicate genetic linkage between the genes for these traits.*

Monogenic determination is given strong support when one component of a dominantly inherited syndrome is present in a grandparent and grandchild and absent in the intervening generation. The failure to appear in the parent could be accounted for by crossing-over, but reappearance in the next generation would be inexplicable.

c. The most telling argument for a single-gene mechanism for syndromes comes from the possibility of relating all manifestations of a syndrome to a single basic disturbance. In the mouse, in *Drosophila,* and in other species, including man, unitary defects have been demonstrated as the basis of hereditary syndromes. In some instances definition of the basic defect has been carried to the level of the molecule. Sickle cell anemia, which has manifold clinical features constituting a syndrome, represents an instance where definition of the basic defect has met with outstanding success. Elucidation of the basic defect at a more superficial level can still provide strong support for the one-gene–one-syndrome hypothesis. Grüneberg[9] has constructed convincing "pedigrees of causes" for complex single-gene syndromes of the mouse. In osteogenesis imperfecta, although the nature of the defect of connective tissue (probably collagen) is not known at the molecular level, no one would now seriously doubt that the bone fragility, blue sclerotics, and deafness are the result of one and the same defect of connective tissue.

---

*From Snyder, L. H.: Principles of gene distribution in human populations, Yale J. Biol. Med. **19**:817, 1947.

It is true that in the present state of our ignorance it is impossible, in the case of some syndromes, to relate all components to a unitary biochemical anomaly. For example, in the syndrome of polyposis of the small intestine and melanin spots of the buccal mucosa, lips, and digits,[11] there is no obvious common denominator. Even in such a situation, however, the other arguments listed previously make a single-gene mechanism likely.

2. Although genetic linkage is an unlikely explanation for relatively frequent genetic syndromes that have arisen on many separate occasions, some specific populations might have many cases of an unusual syndrome produced by mutation in 2 or more closely linked genes that have not yet become separated by the mechanism of crossing-over. No convincing example in man is known.

3. The operon mechanism is a special case of linkage, since by definition an operon consists of 2 or more closely linked structure genes. Mutation in an operator gene that controls the function of the structure genes comprising the operon could produce a syndrome. Again, no fully established example is it hand. The most plausible example is provided by the hemoglobin genes. The genes determining the structure of beta polypeptide chains of hemoglobin A and of delta polypeptide chains of hemoglobin A_2 are apparently adjacent and, together with an operator gene that "turns them off and on," may constitute an operon. Mutation in the operator gene may be responsible for a condition called "high fetal hemoglobin," or "hereditary persistence of fetal hemoglobin." The features of this condition, which may be considered a syndrome, are high fetal hemoglobin, low or absent hemoglobin A, and low or absent hemoglobin A_2. (The operon theory is not yet fully established.[23])

4. Chromosomal aberrations can result in syndromes, and a number of examples have been provided by the explosive development of the field of human cytogenetics since 1959. The aberration may consist of abnormalities of chromosome number or abnormalities of chromosome structure or both. The Turner syndrome (XO sex chromosome constitution) results from a deficiency of one sex chromosome. The Klinefelter syndrome (XXY sex chromosome constitution) results from an excess (by one) of sex chromosomes. The Down syndrome (mongolism) results from an excess of an autosome, namely chromosome 21, which is present in triplicate. Deletions, translocations, inversions, insertions, duplications, and isochromosomes are some of the structural abnormalities of chromosomes that can result in syndromes.

As stated earlier, the term syndrome will be used in a specific sense in this book. Medical genetics forces one to think in terms of a specific gene producing a specific disease. (In his scholarly *Nosography*[7] Knut Faber, a Copenhagen professor of medicine, assigned to Gregor Mendel a significant role in the definition of specific disease entities.) One occasionally hears statements such as "That is one of those congenital-familial affairs with which anything can occur." It should not be necessary to emphasize the direct corollary of the single-gene proposition: the clinical picture in each of these syndromes is as clear-cut and specific (with, of course, the clinical variability discussed below) as the clinical picture produced by a pathogenic microorganism. In many respects, hereditary disease differs from infectious disease only in that the etiologic agent is a mutant gene operating from within rather than a bacterium invading from without.

The virologists have rather long been aware of the basic analogies between their field and that of the geneticist.[15]

The concept of the specific nature of given entities is not inconsistent with the existence of considerable variability in each. Learning clinical medicine is, to a large extent, a matter of learning the clinical variability in individual disease entities. Medical genetics is no exception.

Mutation, equilibrium, and sporadic cases

All monomeric genetic disorders arose by genetic mutation at some time in recently or more remotely past generations. A proportion of cases of dominant disorders and of X-linked recessive disorders owe their abnormality to a mutation that occurred in the germ cells of one or the other parent. These are sporadic or nonfamilial cases. The more severe the particular dominant or X-linked trait and the more drastically it interferes with reproduction of the affected persons as a group, the higher is the proportion of cases that are new mutants. This follows directly from an assumption of genetic equilibrium. If no mutation occurred and the affected individuals reproduced less often than the average of the population, then the disorder would disappear. If, on the other hand, mutation continued—even at a low frequency—and the reproductive fitness of affected persons were not reduced, the condition would become very frequent. Genetic equilibrium can be compared to a bucket of water from which water (the genes) may be lost through a hole at the bottom (negative selection), but other genes are added from a tap at the top (mutation). At equilibrium, the loss and gain of genes balance each other.

Considerations of equilibrium and the proportion of cases that are sporadic and nonfamilial, having arisen by new mutation, are illustrated by Duchenne's pseudohypertrophic muscular dystrophy, the Hunter type of mucopolysaccharidosis (Chapter 11), and by other X-linked recessive conditions in which few if any affected males reproduce. One third of cases owe their disease to mutation affecting the X chromosome that the mother gave the affected son. In two thirds the

Table 1-2. Mutation rates

	If affected person does not reproduce ($f = 0$)	If affected person has reproductive fitness f relative to general population ($f = 1.0$)
Autosomal dominant	$\mu = \dfrac{n}{2N}$	$\mu = \dfrac{(1-f)n}{2N}$
Autosomal recessive*	$\mu = \dfrac{2n}{2N} = \dfrac{n}{N}$	$\mu = \dfrac{(1-f)n}{N}$
X-linked recessive*	$\mu = \dfrac{n}{3N}$	$\mu = \dfrac{(1-f)n}{3N}$

*It is assumed that heterozygotes have the same reproductive performance as do homozygous normal persons. It is further assumed that the level of consanguinity is negligible.

mutation occurred in a generation earlier than the mother's, and other affected males may be identified in the family.

Mutation rates are calculated on the basis of this principle of equilibrium. The mutation rate is a gametic rate. The values usually found are of the order of 1 in 100,000 gametes per generation, or, as it is more often stated, 1×10^{-6} per gamete per generation. If n is the number of affected persons and N the total number of persons in the population from which the affected are drawn, the mutation rates (μ) are as given in Table 1-2.

If the mutation rate is the same for an autosomal recessive disorder and an X-linked recessive disorder (both of which preclude reproduction by affected persons), it can be shown from the considerations implicit in Table 1-2 that the population frequency of the X-linked recessive disorder is expected to be one and one-half times that of the autosomal recessive disorder. This is discussed further in relation to the relative frequencies of the Hurler and Hunter syndromes in Chapter 11.

When one encounters a "sporadic" case (i.e., an isolated instance, with parents and all other relatives of the subject normal) of a disorder that is generally considered to be heritable or that may be heritable, the following possibilities must be considered.

1. As outlined above, the case in question may be the result of new mutation. This is possible when the condition is autosomal dominant or X-linked recessive. The possibility of fresh dominant mutation as the basis of the case at hand is strengthened if paternal age is elevated. As discussed later in connection with each disorder, the average age of fathers of sporadic, presumably new mutation, cases of the Marfan syndrome, of fibrodysplasia ossificans progressiva, and of achondroplasia is five to seven years greater than the average age of fathers generally.

2. The affected individual may have a recessive gene in homozygous state. If the parents are consanguineous, this possibility is strengthened. Since human families are small a majority of families have only one child affected by a recessive disorder. In the early stages of recognition of a "new" recessive disorder, genetic causation and specifically recessive inheritance may be missed because all cases are "sporadic," as discussed later. Table 1-1 presents information on what proportion of *ascertainable* sibships of various sizes have only one child affected. It will be noted that not until six-child families are reached does one find more than half with more than one affected sib.

3. Although no certain example can be cited in man, it is theoretically possible that the disorder requires the existence of two complementary but independently inherited dominant genes. Neither gene alone can produce abnormality. In such a case, the patient demonstrating a "sporadic case" would have derived one dominant gene from each parent.

4. Possibly the trait is in fact dominant, but the parent who is heterozygous has the disorder in such subtle form that it defies detection.

5. Theoretically, somatic mutation can account for sporadic cases, especially when the anomaly is localized. The genetic change would need to occur in the zygote or in the embryo at a rather early stage.

6. Severely affected sporadic cases could result from a chromosomal aberration.

7. The sporadic case may represent a phenocopy. Goldschmidt introduced the term *phenocopy* to signify the situation in which an environmental factor produces the same clinical disorder, the same phenotype, that occurs as a genetic derangement. As indicated on p. 468, ochronosis closely similar to that of alkaptonuria was produced by the prolonged use of carbolic acid dressings on chronic cutaneous ulcers.

Genotype, phenotype, expressivity, and penetrance

Although some of these terms have already been used, specific definition and discussion are warranted. The *genotype* is the genetic constitution of the individual, with regard either to a specific genetic locus or to the whole genome. The *phenotype* is the character or trait or the composite of characters that is capable of being observed by one means or another but may be many steps removed from the genotype. The distinction may be compared to that between character and reputation. Genotype and character are what one really is; phenotype and reputation are what one appears to be. (As stated earlier, the *karyotype* is the chromosomal constitution of the individual.)

Expressivity is the term that has been applied to the variability in phenotype produced by a given genotype and is equivalent to the grade of severity in clinical medicine. *Penetrance* is an all-or-none affair, contingent on whether the methods for studying phenotype do or do not permit identification of the specific genotype in the individual. In a group of persons with the same genotype there may be some with manifestations so mild that they do not deviate sufficiently from certain members of the "normal" group to be recognized as affected.

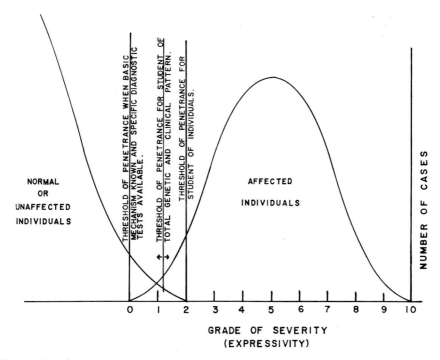

Fig. 1-4. The interrelationship of penetrance and expressivity in hereditary syndromes. (See text.) (Inspired by Dr. H. Bentley Glass.)

These cases, the instances of incomplete penetrance, or *forme fruste,* correspond to the subclinical cases of infectious diseases. The familiar bell-shaped Gaussian curve probably accurately describes the distribution of cases as to severity (expressivity). (See Fig. 1-4.) The three vertical lines of the diagram indicate various thresholds of penetrance. These lines cross the distribution curve on the side constituted by cases of lesser grades of severity. At this end also the curve is overlapped by the normal distribution curve. The majority of recognizable cases are of intermediate severity; there are some very severe cases and some very mild ones. Those affected individuals in the zone of overlap have mild manifestations which, because of their occurrence as "normal variations" in a small proportion of the normal population, cannot be recognized as abnormal when the individual is studied. For the student of the individual, then, the threshold of penetrance is at the point of overlap of the two curves. A certain number of additional cases can be recognized by the student of the total genetic and clinical picture, by one who investigates the entire family in detail. (There are risks, of course, that some unaffected individuals will be incorrectly classified as affected.) It seems probable that when the basic defect in each of these syndromes is known, and when a specific method for demonstrating the defect becomes available, all cases of each syndrome will be identifiable. At this point the

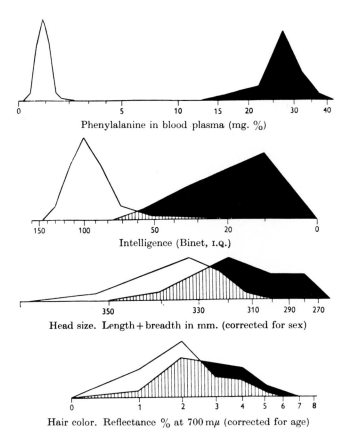

Phenylalanine in blood plasma (mg. %)

Intelligence (Binet, I.Q.)

Head size. Length + breadth in mm. (corrected for sex)

Hair color. Reflectance % at 700 mμ (corrected for age)

Fig. 1-5. The dependence of penetrance on the phenotype selected for study. (See text.) (From Penrose, L. S.: Ann. Eugen. 16:134, 1951.)

threshold of penetrance will be moved back to the limit; penetrance, an artificial concept at best, will no longer have significance for these syndromes.

Variations in expressivity and differences of penetrance, depending on what phenotype is analyzed, are well illustrated by phenylketonuria, as pointed out by Penrose.[18] (See Fig. 1-5.) If hair color or head size is taken as the phenotype for study, differentiation of affected from unaffected is poor. Intelligence is a better discriminant. The level of phenylalanine in the blood—a phenotype closely related to the basic defect, which involves the enzymatic conversion of phenylalanine to tyrosine—is by far the best discriminant.

In the case of the multifaceted syndromes of the type discussed in this book, each component may have partially independent behavior so far as penetrance and expressivity are concerned. For example, in the case of the Marfan syndrome, any one of the three major components (ocular, aortic, skeletal) may be present with little or no involvement in the other two areas. Variation in expressivity of a disorder, e.g., variation among affected members of the same family who can with confidence be assumed to have the same major gene, is due to differences in the rest of the genetic constitution of the individual and differences in the environment. The single major gene does not, of course, operate *in vacuo*. That brothers with the Marfan syndrome (Chapter 3) can show wide differences in clinical picture, with absence of eye involvement in one and full-blown manifestations in a second, for example, is not surprising since in brothers, on the average, only half the genes are identical by descent. Differences in the rest of their genetic makeup may be considerable.

Genetic disorders that interfere seriously with reproductive fitness show less variability in expressivity than do milder conditions. There is an inverse relationship, for example, between the degree of variability and the proportion of cases of a dominant trait that are the result of fresh mutation. About 15% of Marfan syndrome cases are the result of new mutation, and expressivity varies widely. About 80% of achondroplasia cases are the result of new mutation, and expressivity in this disorder varies remarkably little. When the nature of a dominant mutation is such that the heterozygote individuals reproduce only rarely, there is little opportunity for selection of modifiers favoring mild expression of the major gene.

Principles of inborn errors of metabolism

The disorder of connective tissue in alkaptonuria was adequately recognized, characterized, and analyzed from the standpoint of mechanism only after the nature of the disorder as an inborn error of metabolism had been established. Homocystinuria is a second clear example of a heritable disorder of connective tissue caused by an inborn error of metabolism. Both of these conditions are autosomal recessive; as stated earlier, this mode of inheritance should always alert one to the possibility of an inborn error of metabolism, i.e., an enzyme defect, whereas dominant inheritance is more suggestive of a structural abnormality in a nonenzymic protein. For example, the dominant inheritance of the Marfan syndrome, Ehlers-Danlos syndrome, and osteogenesis imperfecta suggests an alteration of structure of a connective tissue protein, whereas the recessive inheritance of pseudoxanthoma elasticum and the several mucopolysaccharidoses urges search for an enzyme defect.

Garrod, whose portrait appears as the frontispiece, especially appropriately

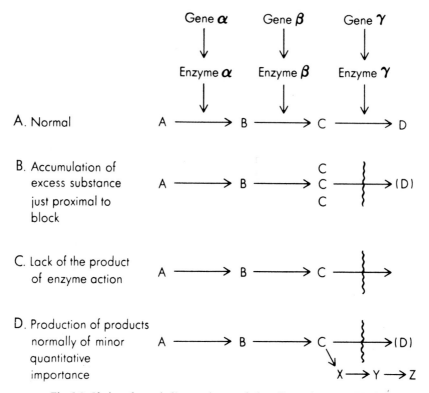

Fig. 1-6. Chains of metabolic reactions and the effects of enzyme blocks.

so with the inclusion of two inborn errors of metabolism, directed thinking along the lines of chains of metabolic reactions and blocks at specific points as a result of mutation in the gene controlling a particular enzymatic step. (As Beadle[1] pointed out in his Nobel lecture, the one-gene–one-enzyme hypothesis was implicit in Garrod's work and conclusions.)

As schematized in Fig. 1-6, there are at least three mechanisms by which a genetic enzyme block can result in the phenotypic features of an inborn error of metabolism. (1) Excess substance may accumulate proximal to the block. The connective tissue features of alkaptonuria have this basis. (2) Lack of the product of the chain of reactions may lead to the phenotypic features. Albinism, the several forms of congenital adrenal hyperplasia, and genetic defects in thyroid hormonogenesis leading to familial goiter are examples. (3) The production, through an alternative pathway, of products that normally are of minor quantitative importance may be responsible for some or all of the phenotypic features. Phenylketonuria is a case in point; some of the urinary excretory products are produced through an alternate metabolic pathway.

Yet another mechanism by which a genetic enzyme block can have pathologic consequences is a special case of point 2, above: the failure of synthesis of a product may remove a feedback control mechanism. In orotic aciduria, for example, large amounts of orotic acid are produced and result in hematuria from irritation of the urinary tract by orotic acid crystals. The relatively massive urinary excretion of orotic acid is due not only to the accumulation of same proximal to the enzyme block but also to loss of the feedback control of the first step in the pyrimidine pathway, exercised normally by the end products of the pathway.[21] In the Lesch-Nyhan syndrome, uric acid is synthesized in unprecedented excess because of loss of feedback control on the first step in purine metabolism when the enzyme hypoxanthine-guanine-phosphoribosyltransferase (HGPRT) is deficient.[20]

Defects in membrane transport systems

Several hereditary syndromes have been shown to be the result of a gene-determined defect in a membrane transport system. Cystinuria, not to be confused with homocystinuria (Chapter 4), is an example. The defect concerns transport of cystine and related amino acids (lysine, ornithine, and arginine) across the renal tubule cells. The plasma level of cystine and of the other three amino acids is normal or low. By contrast the aminoaciduria of inborn errors of metabolism such as homocystinuria is of the overflow type; the plasma level of the amino acid that accumulates proximal to a Garrodian block in intermediary metabolism is elevated or, if there is no renal threshold for the substance, unaltered.

Disorders of end-organ unresponsiveness

Several disorders, such as the testicular feminization syndrome and nephrogenic diabetes insipidus, are the result of mutations that result in loss of capacity of the end-organ to respond to a hormone—testosterone and vasopressin, respectively, in the two examples given. There appear to be several forms of midgets ("sexual ateleiosis") in which the defect is not deficiency of growth hormone but rather end-organ unresponsiveness. In one, the Laron dwarf, unresponsiveness to growth hormone has been related to failure of synthesis of sulfation factor, a mediator of the effects of growth hormone.[5] In pseudohypoparathyroidism Chase and associates[4] have demonstrated that cyclic AMP, which mediates the effects of parathormone on the kidney and on bone, is not synthesized.

The molecular basis of inherited disease

It is beyond the scope of this presentation to discuss in full the important information on (1) the chemical nature of the gene (DNA, deoxyribonucleic acid) and the manner in which genetic information is encoded therein; (2) the role of RNA (ribonucleic acid) in conveying the genetic code from the chromosome in the nucleus to the ribosomes, sites of protein synthesis in the cytoplasm; and (3) the various mechanisms by which gene action is controlled during development and differentiation.

It is relevant to mention briefly, however, the following facts:
1. The primary product of gene action is a protein.
2. The function of the gene is to specify the sequence of amino acids in a given protein (or polypeptide chain, because some proteins, e.g., hemoglobin, are made up of more than one polypeptide chain, each determined by a different gene).
3. The series of purine and pyrimidine bases in DNA are the "letters" which in various combinations of three spell the code words (or codons), each specific for a particular amino acid.

4. The codons in the gene are colinear, that is, in the same linear sequence, with the amino acids in the protein specified by that gene.

5. The protein specified by a given gene may be an enzyme, and mutation may result either in the formation of an enzyme with deficient enzymatic activity or in the failure of any enzyme at all to be formed. In either case, a disorder may result which, if the enzyme involved is concerned in intermediary metabolism, will be classed as an inborn error of metabolism.

6. On the other hand, the protein specified by the gene and formed on the cytoplasmic ribosomes may be a nonenzymic protein. Hemoglobin is an extensively studied example; collagen may be another. (The genetic control of protein synthesis is schematized in Fig. 1-7.)

It was earlier indicated that recessively inherited disorders tend to be inborn errors of metabolism and dominantly inherited disorders have been found, when the molecular defect is known, to be the result of a change in the structure (i.e., amino acid sequence) of a nonenzymic protein. This is perhaps not surprising. Because of a margin of safety with which the organism is blessed, the effects of an enzyme deficiency are likely to be evident only in the homozygote, that is, when there is none at all of the particular enzyme or when all of the enzyme is of the defective mutant type. On the other hand, when the gene-determined change involves a nonenzymic protein, such as a structural protein like collagen, the resulting change in the physical properties of the protein may be evident in the phenotype even though only part of the total protein is atypical or abnormal, as is the case in the heterozygote.

The above considerations are important as guides to the study of the basic

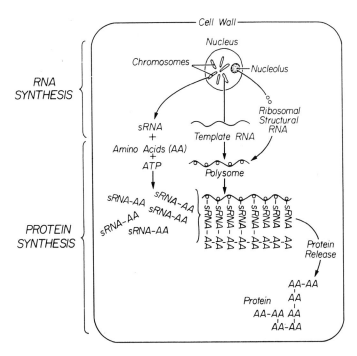

Fig. 1-7. The genetic control of protein synthesis. (Courtesy Dr. J. D. Wilson, Dallas, Texas.)

defect in each of the heritable disorders of connective tissue. In the dominant disorders—Marfan syndrome, Ehlers-Danlos syndrome, and osteogenesis imperfecta—change in a structural protein should be sought. In the recessive disorders, homocystinuria and alkaptonuria, an enzymatic defect has already been identified; such should also be sought in pseudoxanthoma elasticum, a recessive disorder. The several mucopolysaccharidoses, all recessives, are the result of a defect in one or another enzyme involved in the degradation of mucopolysaccharides.

One can imagine exceptions to the rule of thumb that recessive inheritance and enzyme defects are not to be found when a defect in a structural protein is demonstrated. The function of the enzyme may be to add a side group. For example, in collagen, lysine and proline are converted to hydroxylysine and hydroxyproline after incorporation into the amino acid chain, and galactose and glucose residues are attached to specific amino acids of collagen. (See Chapter 2.) A deficiency of one of the hydroxylases or of one of the transferases involved in these processes might lead to a heritable disorder of connective tissue, with a structural defect of the collagen molecule inherited as a recessive. Indeed, a recessive form of the Ehlers-Danlos syndrome has been found to be "caused" by deficiency of lysine hydroxylase (p. 345).

Furthermore, even if no structural abnormality is found in a given protein, the genetic defect may involve its synthesis and the disorder may behave as a dominant. In bacteria a class of "noninducible" mutations is known. In these instances the mutation occurs in a controller gene and is of such a type that the repressor substance determined by the gene fails to recognize the normal inducer substance and thus continues to repress the gene that determines the structural protein. Such a mutation behaves as a dominant.

One can imagine a type of mutation in an enzyme that would behave as a dominant[12]: a change in enzyme structure which alters its specificity so that it "attacks" a different substrate. No example of this type of mutation is known in man.

Acute intermittent porphyria is almost unique among enzyme-deficiency diseases in having clinical expression in the heterozygote. The reason is that the involved enzyme, uroporphyrinogen-I synthetase, is a bottleneck in heme synthesis. Especially when the pathway is stressed, about half the normal amount of enzyme is not adequate for the job. The intermittent character of the disease and the precipitation of attacks by factors that stress the pathway are explained by the findings.[16a] This is an exception which proves (tests) the rule of thumb.

Heterogeneity of genetic disease*

It has happened so often in medical genetics as to be considered the rule, that—when subjected to penetrating scrutiny—a condition which appears at first

---

*The concept of genetic heterogeneity was implicit in the work of Johannsen in Copenhagen in the first decade of this century leading to his introduction of the terms *genotype* and *phenotype* and was emphasized by Curt Stern in the first edition of his textbook[24] when he used the analogy of stalling of a car (the phenotype), which can have many causes (genotypes). The term *genetic heterogeneity* was used by Harry Harris[10a] in 1953 in a discussion of the several forms of cystinuria and by F. Clarke Fraser[7a] in 1956 in a discussion of pitfalls of genetic counseling.

to be homogeneous is found in fact to comprise two or more separate and distinct entities. Examples are albinism, the thalassemias, the glycogen storage diseases, intestinal polyposis, and elliptocytosis.

Heterogeneity of genetic disease is a corollary of the axiom that the phenotype is not a necessary indication of the genotype. Several different genotypes can lead to the same phenotype. This is to be expected, since many steps, each separately gene-controlled, go into the determination of most phenotypes, and mutation at any of several different steps can lead to the same end effect. The situation has been compared to the stalling of a car, which can have many causes even though the end result, or phenotype, is identical. "Genetic mimic" or "genocopy" are terms given to a genetic condition that is phenotypically similar or identical to another but has a different genetic basis. (As stated earlier, "phenocopy" is the designation given to a phenotype that is similar or identical to a genetically determined one but that is determined by exogenous factors.)

Separate entities are discerned (1) by subtle phenotypic differences, (2) by genetic differences, (3) by biochemical differences, or (4) by physiologic differences. Each of these approaches is illustrated below.

The presence or absence of corneal dystrophy is a feature distinguishing two forms of gargoylism, the autosomal recessive type described by Hurler and the X-linked recessive form described by Hunter (Chapter 11). The association of soft tissue and osseous tumors distinguishes the colonic polyposis of the Gardner syndrome from familial polyposis of the colon.

The genetic means of distinguishing separate genetic entities include demonstration of different modes of inheritance or different linkage relationships and the study of offspring produced by the marriage of two persons with a recessively inherited disorder. Spastic paraplegia, retinitis pigmentosa, and Charcot-Marie-Tooth peroneal muscular atrophy are three disorders that are inherited as autosomal dominant in some families, as autosomal recessive in others, and as X-linked recessive in yet others. Usually, in conditions with these three forms of inheritance, the autosomal recessive form is clinically most severe, the dominant form least severe, and the X-linked recessive form intermediate in severity.

Two distinct forms of elliptocytosis (ovalocytosis), both inherited as dominants, have been distinguished on the basis of linkage relationships, although no definite phenotypic differences are discernible. Linkage studies[17] indicate that one form is determined by a gene at a locus which is on the same pair of chromosomes as the locus occupied by the Rh blood group genes, whereas a second form of elliptocytosis is determined by a gene at some position far removed from the Rh locus.

In many instances, congenital deafness (deaf-mutism) can be shown to be inherited as a simple autosomal recessive. Assortative (i.e., nonrandom) mating is often practiced by deaf-mutes; deaf persons marry other deaf persons much more often than would occur on a random basis. All children of two deaf persons, each from a family with a recessive pattern of inheritance, are deaf if the two parents are homozygous at the same locus. Families fulfilling this expectation have been observed. However, in other families the two parents, both affected by phenotypically identical and recessively inherited deafness, have all normal children. The explanation is that the deaf parents are homozygous at different loci and suffer from genetically distinct forms of deafness.

Observations are available on the marriage of two individuals, both of whom appear to be identically affected by albinism. In the case of one such mating, all four children were normally pigmented. When the parents were examined closely it was concluded that the father may in fact suffer from albinoidism, a condition of pigment dilution but not absence, easily confused with albinism.

Biochemical means of differentiating phenotypically similar genetic entities are illustrated by the nonspherocytic hemolytic anemias and by certain of the mucopolysaccharidoses (Chapter 11). In the first example, it is found that any one of several different red cell enzymopathies can cause the same phenotype. In the latter example, differences in the pattern of urinary excretion of mucopolysaccharides are used to distinguish entities. A particularly nice example of the biochemical approach to genetic heterogeneity is the differentiation of two phenotypically indistinguishable forms of the Sanfilippo syndrome (MPS III) on the basis of deficiency of different enzymes involved in the degradation of the mucopolysaccharide heparan sulfate (p. 582).

The physiologic method for differentiating phenotypically similar genetic diseases is nicely demonstrated by hemophilia. Prior to about 1950 all sex-linked hemophilia was assumed to be one and the same disease, although the possibility of multiple allelism had been suggested to explain the occurrence of clinically mild and clinically severe forms. It was then discovered that the blood from some hemophilic subjects would correct the clotting defect in others. The correctability was mutual. The explanation is that the location of the defect in the chain of clotting reactions is different, and bloods from two hemophilic persons complement each other, each providing an essential clotting factor missing in the other. Thus, hemophilia A (classic hemophilia) and hemophilia B (Christmas disease) were distinguished. Although both are determined by genes on the X chromosome, the genes are known to be on different parts of the chromosome; linkage studies indicate that the hemophilia A gene is fairly close to the color blindness locus, the glucose-6-phosphate dehydrogenase locus, and the Xg blood group locus, whereas the Christmas disease gene is far removed from these loci. Thus, evidence from genetic linkage corroborates the evidence from physiologic studies.

A physiologic method for identifying heterogeneity in the mucopolysaccharidoses is the Neufeld technique of mixing fibroblasts from different patients (Chapter 11). Cross-correction of the metabolic defect or its morphologic expression indicates that the entities are different.

Phenotypic diversity caused by allelic series

Whereas genes at different loci can give rise to one and the same phenotype, as in the two forms of the Sanfilippo syndrome referred to above, different genes at the same locus (alleles) can produce a change in the same enzyme or other protein product, resulting in quite a different clinical picture. A striking example is provided by two mucopolysaccharidoses—Hurler syndrome (MPS I H) and Scheie syndrome (MPS I S). They were previously considered separate disorders because of their great difference in phenotype and called MPS I and V. Now they are known to have deficiency of the same enzyme α-L-iduronidase, and they are presumably produced by homozygosity for different genes at the iduronidase locus. (An alternative possibility, if iduronidase has two different subunits determined by different loci as does hemoglobin, is that the Hurler and Scheie syndromes are in fact nonallelic.)

In man and even more in other species there is extensive precedence for allelic series with rather wide phenotypic range. The various alleles at the beta hemoglobin locus can for example lead to phenotypes as disparate as persistent anemia with painful crises (sickle cell anemia), drug-induced anemia (Hb Zürich), methemoglobinemia (Hb M$_{Saskatoon}$), or polycythemia (Hb Chesapeake).

Yet further phenotypic diversity arises from allelic series because of the occurrence of *genetic compounds*, the situation where the individual carries two different mutant alleles. (*Double heterozygote* is a term best reserved for the condition of heterozygosity at two different loci.) Hemoglobins S and C are determined by allelic genes. The genetic compound, SC disease, is phenotypically distinct from both SS disease and CC disease. To return to the mucopolysaccharidosis example, if the Hurler syndrome (comparable to SS disease) is allelic with the Scheie syndrome (comparable to CC disease), then among the mucopolysaccharidoses patients there should be some who are Hurler/Scheie compounds. Such individuals are thought to exist (see p. 553). They have a phenotype intermediate between those of the Hurler and Scheie syndromes and have deficiency of the same enzyme, α-L-iduronidase. It is possible, of course, that these persons are homozygous for yet another allele at the iduronidase locus.

An allelic series is suspected at the MPS II locus (p. 574) because mild and severe forms of MPS II seem clearly distinguishable but have deficiency of the same corrective factor. However, since the MPS II locus is X-linked, no male can be a genetic compound.

Detection of heterozygous carriers

The detection of heterozygous carriers of recessive traits, either autosomal or X-linked, has practical importance in genetic counseling. It also has scientific importance in the establishment of mode of inheritance; e.g., discovery of a partial defect such as an intermediate level of enzyme activity in both parents of affected persons, or in the mother only, is strong support for autosomal recessive or for X-linked recessive inheritance, respectively. Furthermore, the findings in heterozygotes for X-linked traits have special genetic interest in connection with the Lyon hypothesis.

Methods for detecting heterozygotes consist mainly of (1) demonstration of an intermediate deficiency of a gene product, such as an enzyme, and (2) demonstration of less than normal functioning when a particular metabolic step is placed under stress by a so-called loading test, or tolerance test. In a number of recessively inherited inborn errors of metabolism in which the specific defective enzyme has been identified, partial deficiency of that enzyme has been demonstrated in parents. Homocystinuria (Chapter 4) is a case in point. In phenylketonuria, loading tests that use orally administered phenylalanine demonstrate increases in blood levels persisting for a longer time than usual.

Females heterozygous for X-linked recessive traits are likely to show directly or indirectly a reduced level of the particular gene product. Reduced red cell glucose-6-phosphate dehydrogenase (G6PD) activity in primaquine sensitivity or favism and reduced antihemophilic factor in hemophilia A are examples. (The elevated plasma level of creatine phosphokinase [CPK], found in about 70% of women heterozygous for Duchenne muscular dystrophy, is probably a manifestation rather far out on the phenotypic limb from the primary gene action.) In addition the considerations of the Lyon principle dictate that if the phenotype is observable at the cellular level, heterozygotes for X-linked traits are found to be a mosaic of cells with the same defect as in cells of the hemizygous affected male and cells that are perfectly "normal."

Mosaicism in heterozygotes has been demonstrated for several X-linked recessive traits in man. For example, the female who is heterozygous for X-linked ocular albinism shows a mosaic pigmentary pattern of the fundus oculi. The female heterozygous for G6PD deficiency has two classes of erythrocytes—deficient and normal. In the X-linked disorder of mucopolysaccharide metabolism, the Hunter syndrome (Chapter 11), two classes of connective tissue cells can be demonstrated in the heterozygous female.

Complex genetic predisposition

Many disorders have a tendency to run in families, but unlike those conditions with which we are concerned in this book, the pattern of familial occurrence does not suggest simple Mendelian inheritance. As stated earlier, whenever one undertakes to survey the role of genetic factors in the diseases of a given system, it is found that the entities tend to fall into two categories (exclusive of chromosomal aberrations whose effects are usually not limited to one system): (1) the relatively uncommon simply inherited one and (2) the common conditions in which genetic factors seem to play some role but environmental factors are also involved, often in a complex manner. Rheumatoid arthritis, rheumatic fever, systemic lupus erythematosus, and scleroderma (systemic sclerosis) are generally considered "connective tissue diseases," although it can be argued that they are diseases *in* but not *of* connective tissue.* In each of these, some evidence for familial aggregation is available.

The questions which the geneticist considers are different in the two categories of disease. In the rare simply inherited disorders he is interested in gene frequency, mode of inheritance, nature of the basic defect, mechanism of the phenotypic features, mutation rate, selection factors, and so forth. In the more common conditions of multifactorial causation, in which genetic factors—themselves multiple (polygenic)—may play a role, the questions are likely to be: "How important is the genotype in determining the occurrence of the disease?" and "If important, by what mechanism does the genetic constitution contribute to the development of the disease?" The methods for answering these two questions, especially the first, include study of familial aggregation, comparison of concordance rates of monozygotic and like-sex dizygotic twins, comparison of different racial groups, study of the genetics of separate components in patho-

---

*The conditions discussed in this book are the true disorders of connective tissue. I was amused by the element of truth contained in the misprint of the title of this book as cited among the references of an article: *"Veritable* Disorders of Connective Tissue" (Ann. Thorac. Surg. 2:64, 1966).

genesis, search for blood group and disease association,* and genetic study of homologous disorders in experimental animals.

Discussion of the genetics of common connective tissue disorders, such as systemic lupus erythematosus, is beyond the scope of this book.

Chromosomal aberrations

Most of the chromosomal aberrations lead to defects in several systems, and although the connective tissue system is significantly involved in several of them, a comprehensive review is beyond the scope of this presentation. A few illustrations must suffice.

Patients with the XXXY and XXXXY Klinefelter syndromes frequently have radioulnar synostosis. Patients with the XO Turner syndrome have large medial condyles of the femur and a complementary defect in the medial aspect of the proximal tibia. Coarctation of the aorta, which occurs in about 10% of patients with the Turner syndrome, might be considered a connective tissue malformation. The pelvis in patients with trisomy 21 (mongolism; Down's syndrome) is sufficiently characteristic as to aid in the diagnosis. Changes like those of chondrodystrophia calcificans congenita occur in infants with trisomy 18 (Edward's syndrome). All of these, however, are relatively minor parts of the complex malformation syndrome.

Eponyms

It is desirable to avoid eponyms whenever possible. It is preferable, at any rate, to use designations that indicate as precisely as possible the fundamental nature of the disease entity under consideration. In the present state of knowledge, however, there are good reasons to use eponyms for many syndromes. (1) Eponyms do not prejudice the search for the fundamental defect or conceal our ignorance of its nature. For the Hurler syndrome the name "lipochondrodystrophy" was used, with the erroneous notion that the basic defect is one of cellular fat metabolism. (2) Since it does not use one feature of a complex syndrome as the designation, an eponym does not convey the impression that the presence of some one specific feature is a *sine qua non* for the diagnosis or that the feature mentioned occurs exclusively as a component of the particular syndrome. "Arachnodactyly" is a poor term for the Marfan syndrome, because the fingers of many of the patients are not more spidery than those of normal persons. "Cutis hyperelastica" is a poor term for the Ehlers-Danlos syndrome, since skin abnormalities may be relatively inconspicuous in patients who for one reason or another clearly have the disorder. The pity is not that eponyms are

---

*Blood group and disease association is often confused with genetic linkage. As stated earlier, genetic linkage produces no permanent association in the population. Although the locus for the gene determining the nail-patella syndrome is on the same pair of chromosomes as that for the ABO blood group genes, a large series of unrelated patients with the nail-patella syndrome would show the same distribution of ABO blood types as the population from which they came. The fact that as a group persons with duodenal peptic ulcer show a higher frequency of blood type O than does the general population of which they are a part is due not to the location of an ulcer gene and a blood group O gene on the same chromosome but rather to a physiologic peculiarity of the type O person that renders him slightly but definitely more prone to duodenal ulcer.

employed in these diseases but rather that no phonetically satisfactory or widely accepted eponyms are available for use in connection with syndromes such as osteogenesis imperfecta and pseudoxanthoma elasticum, in which the defect and its manifestations are much broader in their localization than bone or skin, respectively.

Eponyms are merely tags. They often have no justification from the standpoint of historical priorities, since frequently either someone else had described the condition earlier or the man whose name is used eponymously did not describe the full syndrome. Largely for the latter reason, it is preferable to say *the* Marfan syndrome or *the* Hurler syndrome rather than Marfan's syndrome or Hurler's syndrome.

Role of genetics in clinical practice

Hill[10] pointed out that the practice of medicine consists of seeking the answer to three questions: What is wrong? (diagnosis), What is going to happen? (prognosis), and What can be done about it? (treatment). (It is the social and scientific responsibility of the physician to keep a fourth question always in mind: Why did it happen? On the answer depends both prevention and scientific progress.)

Medical genetics contributes to *diagnosis* through the family history and through the phenomenon of pleiotropism. Some of the pleiotropic effects of a single gene may be important external clues to the presence of a serious internal disorder; for example, the ectopia lentis of the Marfan syndrome can be a useful clue in the differential diagnosis of aortic regurgitation, and the presence of angioid streaks in the fundus oculi can be an aid in the differential diagnosis of gastrointestinal bleeding.

Prognosis ("What is going to happen?") in medical genetics concerns mainly the unborn child of parents who have had a previously affected child, or the child of a parent who is himself affected or who has an affected relative. The art and science of gauging the risk and informing and advising the consultand* are embraced in what is called *genetic counseling*.

Recognition of the carrier state is particularly useful in the case of X-linked recessive disorders. Whereas the normal but heterozygous sister of a homocystinuric patient will have affected offspring only if she marries another carrier, an unlikely possibility, the normal heterozygous sister of a patient with the Hunter syndrome has a 50% risk that any son will be affected, regardless of the genotype of her husband. Methods for heterozygote detection were outlined above.

Genetic counseling has found a strong ally in the methods for prenatal diagnosis based on amniotic fluid withdrawn at about the fourteenth week of pregnancy. In a rapidly increasing list of disorders it is now possible to recognize the affected fetus by study of the amniotic fluid itself or, more often and more reliably, by chemical or chromosomal study of cultured amniotic cells. Among the heritable disorders of connective tissue, homocystinuria and the mucopolysaccharidoses lend themselves particularly well to prenatal diagnosis. Prenatal

---

Consultand is a useful term to refer to the person seeking genetic counsel. *Patient* is often an inappropriate term, and *client* has nonprofessional, even mercenary, connotations.

diagnosis by amniocentesis is used in high-risk families, that is, those in which the parents are known to have a significant risk of affected children. By prenatal diagnosis and selective abortion, it is possible to help such parents have normal children.

Although admittedly the "short suit" of medical genetics, *treatment* is rapidly becoming more effective in the group of hereditary disorders. Modalities of therapy now include restriction of particular dietary constituents (e.g., low methionine diet in homocystinuria), administration of cofactor in pharmacologic dosage (e.g., high dosages of vitamin B_6, again in homocystinuria), surgical replacement of the defective organ or tissue (e.g., the aorta in the Marfan syndrome), attenuation of physiologic stress on the genetically defective tissue (e.g., use of propranolol in the Marfan syndrome). Enzyme replacement entered the realm of reality with the important work of Neufeld and her colleagues on the mucopolysaccharidoses (Chapter 11). Dramatic approaches to the definitive repair of the underlying genetic defect will undoubtedly be devised before the end of this century.

SUMMARY

Among the principles presented and discussed in this chapter are the following:

1. Disease tends to fall into three categories as to genetic factors in etiopathogenesis: single-gene disorders, mulifactorial disorders, and chromosomal aberrations.

2. Congenital is not synonymous with genetic.

3. Mendelizing syndromes are usually the result of pleiotropism.

4. Under the assumption of genetic equilibrium, the more an autosomal dominant or X-linked recessive interferes with reproduction, the larger is the proportion of cases which are the result of fresh mutation.

5. The average age of fathers of new mutation cases of dominant disorders is five to seven years greater than the average age of fathers generally.

6. Genetic heterogeneity (two or more fundamentally distinct entities that share approximately the same phenotype) is the rule. If a disorder is thought to be a single entity, it usually means that the disorder is not well understood.

7. Phenotypic diversity, i.e., phenotypical distinctive diseases with deficiency of the same enzyme, can result from allelic series.

8. The Lyon principle predicts that the heterozygous female has two classes of cells, a fact that can be used in heterozygote detection.

REFERENCES

1. Beadle, G. W.: Genes and chemical reactions in neurospora, Science **129:**1715, 1959.
2. Bowen, P., Lee, C. S. N., Migeon, C. J., Kaplan, N. M., McKusick, V. A., and Reifenstein, E. C., Jr.: Hereditary male pseudohermaphroditism with hypogonadism, hypospadias and gynecomastia (Reifenstein's syndrome), Ann. Intern. Med. **62:**252, 1965.
3. Carter, C. O.: An ABC of medical genetics, Boston, 1969, Little, Brown & Co.
4. Chase, L. R., Melson, G. L., and Aurbach, G. D.: Pseudohypoparathyroidism: defective excretion of 3′-5′AMP in response to parathyroid hormone, J. Clin. Invest. **48:**1832, 1969.
5. Daughaday, W. H., Laron, Z., Pertzelan, A., and Heinz, J. N.: Defective sulfation factor generation: a possible etiological link in dwarfism, Trans. Ass. Amer. Physicians **82:**129, 1969.
6. Donahue, R. P., Bias, W. B., Renwick, J. H., and McKusick, V. A.: Probable assignment

of the Duffy blood group locus to chromosome 1 in man, Proc. Nat. Acad. Sci. **61**:949, 1968.

7. Faber, K. H.: Nosography, ed. 2, New York, 1930, Paul B. Hoeber, Inc., Medical Book Department of Harper & Row, Publishers.

7a. Fraser, F. C.: Heredity counseling: the darker side, Eugen. Quart. **3**:45, 1956.

8. Gowers, W. R.: Abiotrophy, Lancet **1**:1003, 1902.

9. Grüneberg, H.: Animal genetics and medicine, New York, 1947, Paul B. Hoeber, Inc., Medical Book Department of Harper & Row, Publishers.

10. Hill, A. B. (London): Personal communication.

10a. Harris, H.: Introduction to human biochemical genetics, Cambridge, 1953, Cambridge University Press.

11. Jeghers, H., McKusick, V. A., and Katz, K. H.: Generalized intestinal polyposis and melanin spots of the oral mucosa, lips and digits, New Eng. J. Med. **241**:993, 1031, 1949.

12. Kirkman, H. N.: Dominant mutations—biochemical basis for phenotype. In Fraser, F. C., and McKusick, V. A., editors: Congenital malformations (conference at the Hague, 1969), Amsterdam, 1970, Excerpta Medica Foundation.

13. McKusick, V. A.: Human genetics, ed. 2, Englewood Cliffs, N. J., 1969, Prentice-Hall, Inc.

14. McKusick, V. A.: Mendelian inheritance in man: catalogs of autosomal dominant, autosomal recessive and X-linked phenotypes, ed. 3, Baltimore, 1971, Johns Hopkins University Press.

15. McKusick, V. A.: On the X-chromosome of man, Washington, D. C., 1964, American Institute of Biological Sciences.

16. McKusick, V. A., Hostetler, J. A., Egeland, J. A., and Eldridge, R.: The distribution of certain genes in the Old Order Amish, Sympos. Quant. Biol. **29**:99, 1964.

16a. Meyer, U. A., Strand, L. J., Doss, M., Rees, A. C., and Marver, H. S.: Intermittent acute porphyria—genetic defect in porphobilinogen metabolism, New Eng. J. Med. **286**:1277, 1972.

17. Morton, N. E.: The detection and estimation of linkage between the genes for elliptocytosis and the Rh blood type, Amer. J. Hum. Genet. **8**:80, 1956.

18. Penrose, L. S.: Measurement of pleiotropic effects in phenylketonuria, Ann. Eugen. **16**:134, 1951.

19. Renwick, J. H.: Progress in mapping the autosomes of man, Brit. Med. Bull. **25**:65, 1969.

20. Seegmiller, J. E., Rosenbloom, F. M., and Kelley, W. N.: Enzyme defect associated with a sex-linked human neurological disorder and excessive purine synthesis, Science **155**:1682, 1967.

21. Smith, L. H., Jr., Huguley, C. M., Jr., and Bain, J. A.: Hereditary orotic aciduria. In Stanbury, J. B., Wyngaarden, J. B., and Fredricksen, D. S., editors: The metabolic basis of inherited disease, ed. 2, New York, 1966, McGraw-Hill Book Co.

22. Snyder, L. H.: Principles of gene distribution in human populations, Yale J. Biol. Med. **19**:817, 1947.

23. Stent, G. S.: The operon—on its third anniversary, Science **144**:816, 1964.

24. Stern, C.: Principles of human genetics, San Francisco, 1949, W. H. Freeman & Co., Publishers.

25. Vertue, H. St. H.: Medical mispronunciation, Guy's Hosp. Gaz. **68**:237, 1954.

2 · The biology of normal connective tissue

If by some magic solution one could dissolve all the connective tissue of the body, all that would remain would be a mass of slimy epithelium, quivering muscle and frustrated nerve cells.
ARCADI*

Connective tissues, the supporting structures of the body, include cartilage, ligaments, tendons, fascia, joint capsules, the subepidermal portions (corium) of the skin, important elements of the heart valves and aorta and smaller blood vessels, and finally bone. In general, connective tissue consists of cellular and fibrous constituents embedded in the so-called ground substance. Reference is made to textbooks of histology (e.g., Fig. 45 of reference 71) for graphic presentation of the structural interrelationships of these elements.

In connection with his theory that organs are composed of a limited number of tissues, Bichat (1771-1802) distinguished fibrous tissue as one variety. About 1830 Johannes Müller (1801-1858) assigned the generally used designation "Bindegewebe." Schwann discovered the connective tissue cells.

Cellular elements

Virtually all the other endogenous elements of connective tissue are elaborated by the fibroblast, the main cellular constituent of connective tissue, or by its congeners, such as the osteoblast and the chondroblast. Sometimes the term "fibrocyte" is used and, in the older literature, "lamellar" or "fixed tissue cell." Other cellular elements include the mast cell and wandering cells such as macrophages. (The mast cell,[102] which has long been implicated in the formation of heparin, has been thought to be concerned also in the formation of hyaluronic acid.[2]) Some information has accumulated about the enzymatic processes involved in the formation and degradation of acid mucopolysaccharides.[27,44i] Also, information on the synthesis of collagen, a protein formed on the ribosomes of the fibroblast, is accumulating, as will be briefly reviewed later.

Modulation and differentiation are important features of the biology of the fibroblast. Differentiation[31] indicates a maturation of the cell with specialization

---

*Arcadi, J. A.: Bull. Hopkins Hosp. 90:334, 1952.

of function and usually increased structural complexity; with this specialization the potentiality to develop along certain lines is lost—a chrondroblast cannot, for example, develop into a fat cell even though both are descendants of a common mesenchymal cell. Modulation is the term used to indicate changes of such a type, as in a fat cell, let us say, that the fundamental nature of the cell is not lost although the functional capacity has been quantitatively altered and the structural features that permit identification of the precise species of the cell may be lost. Differentiation and modulation in the group of connective tissue cells are particularly complex matters.

The fibroblast has many metabolic potentialities, as revealed by cell-culture studies. Not only can it synthesize collagen, elastin, and mucopolysaccharide, but other enzyme systems are functional. This circumstance is fortunate for human biochemical genetics because it has permitted the elucidation of many inborn errors of metabolism. For example, enzymatic proof of homocystinuria (Chapter 4) can be obtained from cultured skin fibroblasts since normally the relevant enzyme is present in significant levels, whereas it has only very low levels of activity in fibroblasts from affected persons. Thus, with a few notable exceptions such as phenylketonuria, in which the relevant enzyme (phenylalanine hydroxylase) is not present, skin biopsy and culture of fibroblasts are a useful substitute for biopsy and culture of the liver or of other, even less accessible organs, as well as for study of the whole man.

Fibrous constituents

The fibrous constituents of connective tissue comprise two main groups: collagenous and elastic. The reticulin fiber would be classified by some as a separate category, but most consider it a member of the collagen group although its precise relationship to the classic collagen fiber is moot.

Collagen was defined by the Oxford Dictionary (1893 edition) as "that constituent of connective tissue which yields gelatin on boiling."[97a] The definition is implied by the name that comes from the Greek word for "glue" and that for "producing." The word has been used in the English language since at least 1865.

Collagen is a fibrous protein occurring in wide, straight, unbranching white bundles that possess high tensile strength and low elasticity.* Collagen fibers at times have a tensile strength as high as 100 kg./sq. cm., as high as some metals.[22] Collagen has characteristic 640 Å periodicity by small-angle x-ray diffraction and by electron microscopy. It contains two unique amino acids, hydroxyproline and hydroxylysine.[46] The former is present in relatively large amounts and, because it constitutes an unvarying proportion of collagen and is unique to collagen and elastin, is used in quantitative determination of collagen.[81] It also contains large amounts of glycine.† Aromatic and sulfur amino acids are present only in low concentration.

The biologic importance of collagen in the individual organism and in the

---

*See p. 298 for a discussion of the several definitions of elasticity. As used here, the term refers principally to extensibility.

†In 1820, by boiling gelatin with dilute sulfuric acid, Braconnet isolated glycine, which he called "sucre de gelatine" because of its sweet taste. In 1848 Berzelius suggested the term glycine for this constituent, which accounts for about one third of the amino acid structure of this protein. Hydroxyproline was discovered by Emil Fischer in 1902.

phylogenetic series is tremendous. Collagen represents approximately 30% of the total protein of the human body. In the vertebrate animal it is what cellulose is to plants.[70] As the matrix of bone[12] it was referred to as "ossein" in the older literature. Even the vitreous humor of the eye contains fibers with the properties of collagen, the so-called "vitrosin" of Gross.[41] That it is not limited to vertebrates is indicated (as merely one example) by the fact that collagen is the skeleton of the invertebrate sponge familiar in household and other usage.

The economic importance of collagen dates back to prehistory when the manufacture of leather[68] and glue was first undertaken. About A.D. 50 Pliny made reference to glue making. Isinglass, made from the swim bladder of fish such as the sturgeon, was also collagenous in nature. It was in leather manufacture that one property of collagen, thermal shrinkage (at 60° to 65° C.), was discovered and used in judging adequacy of tannage. Some of the best studies of collagen have been directly or indirectly supported by the leather industries.[37,42,109] Gustavson[42] demonstrated that thermal shrinkage is the result of breaking of cross-links in the collagen molecule. Gustavson[123q] has further suggested the intriguing possibility that *in vivo* "tanning" may be the basis of some changes seen with aging and in pathologic states.

Collagen also serves an important role in normal hemostasis. Derangement of this mechanism may be a factor in the excessive susceptibility to bruising and bleeding of the Ehlers-Danlos syndrome (p. 346). When collagen is exposed to the blood, platelets adhere to collagen fibrils and as a result undergo morphologic changes. Intraplatelet substances such as adenosine diphosphate are released and

Table 2-1. Characteristics of collagen—a partial tabulation

Category based on method of study	Characteristic features

Histologic properties[99a]	Tinctorial characteristics:
	    Acid fuchsin—bright red staining
	    Periodic acid and Schiff's reagent—faint red staining
	    Silver agents—staining poor or absent
	Dilute acids and alkalis—swelling

Electron microscopic features	640 Å periodicity
Chemical features	14% hydroxyproline by weight; hydroxylysine also a unique amino acid; low content of tyrosine, methionine, and histidine; absence of cystine and tryptophane; 1% hexosamine (associated carbohydrate)
Shrinkage characteristics	Temperature: 60° to 65° C. (shrinkage to about one third of original length) certain electrolyte solutions
Behavior toward enzymes	Attacked by pepsin at 37° C. Attacked by "collagenases" of *Clostridium histolyticum* and *Cl. welchii*[99b] Resistant to trypsin, chymotrypsin, papain
Isotope tracer studies of metabolic turnover rate	Relative metabolic inertia[79]
X-ray crystallography	Characteristic pattern(s)[7]
Immunology	Very low antigenicity of unaltered collagen,[110,126] viz., use for suture material; antigenicity primarily in α2 chain[75a]

platelet aggregation occurs.[54,55,128] The molecular basis of platelet-collagen binding has been studied.[18a] The membranes of platelets contain glucosyl and galactosyl transferases that recognize and bind the hydroxylysyl groups in collagen.

The importance of collagen in pathology will be evident to a medical audience, since the concept of "collagen vascular diseases" has seemingly gained such wide acceptance. Gut sutures are collagen derived from the serosa and submucosa of sheep and hogs. Further medical implications appear to be represented by certain of the hereditary disorders of connective tissue under discussion here.

These implications—biologic, economic, and medical—have been responsible for very extensive investigations of the nature of collagen[7,15,61,96,99] by scientists of diverse interests and perspectives. The result, in the past at least, was similar to the result of the examination of the elephant by the six blind men. However, several excellent symposia, reviews, and monographs have effected a synthesis of the diverse bits of information.[4,36,36a,44,97,111]

Collagen has a triple-stranded ropelike coiled-coil structure, as indicated particularly by x-ray diffraction (the reader is referred to the excellent nontechnical description of the principles of x-ray analysis of fiber structure by Crick and Kendrew[24]). Its rodlike shape has the dimensions of about 3000 × 15 Å. (Some of the properties of collagen are listed in Table 2-1.)

The steps in the formation of collagen fibrils are listed below. Probably most of the steps are under genetic control and are subject to derangement as a result of mutation.

1. Translation
2. Hydroxylation
3. Helix formation
4. Glycosylation
5. Secretion
6. Conversion of precursor
7. Aggregation
8. Cross-linking*

Translation. Three polypeptide chains make up the collagen molecule. The chains are of two different varieties ($\alpha1$ and $\alpha2$), suggesting that at least two cistrons are involved in determining the amino acid sequence of the molecule. In skin each collagen molecule contain two $\alpha1$ chains and one $\alpha2$ chain. The assemblage of amino acids into polypeptide chains occurs in the cytoplasm of the fibroblast (or one of its congeners such as the chondroblast or osteoblast) on clusters of ribosomal particles, polyribosomes.[65]

In a Dintzis type of experiment, it has been shown that the $\alpha1$ and $\alpha2$ chains are synthesized as single polypeptide chains by sequential addition of amino acids from the N-terminal end,[125] as in the polypeptides of hemoglobin. For both $\alpha1$ and $\alpha2$ chains, mRNA is monocistronic.[66a]

The polypeptide chains of collagen as initially synthesized are unusual only in their length and amino acid content (particularly large amounts of glycine and proline). Alterations that occur after synthesis are deviations from the familiar pattern of synthesis of other proteins. As discussed later, these alter-

---

*Modified from Piez, K. A.: Cross-linking of collagen and elastin, Ann. Rev. Biochem. 37:547, 1968.

ations include (1) hydroxylation of proline and lysine to produce hydroxyproline and hydroxylysine, (2) formation of lysine and hydroxylysine derivatives, which are precursors of covalent cross-links, and (3) glycosylation, i.e., the addition of carbohydrate moieties in glycosidic linkage to hydroxylysine. Some of these alterations show specificity for tissue and/or for time of development.

The introduction of covalent cross-links between alpha chains results in double-chain β components and triple-chain γ components. (By the conventions of collagen chemistry, the designations β and γ refer to dimers and trimers, not to different polypeptide chains, as in hemoglobin chemistry.) Two different types of alpha chains, $\alpha1$ and $\alpha2$, are found in most collagens in a ratio of 2:1. Thus the formula is $(\alpha1)_2\alpha2$.

As with all proteins, its primary structure, i.e., the sequence of amino acids in the chain, determines many of the properties of collagen. Some of its properties are consequences of the cross-linking and other processing that takes place after chain synthesis.

Sufficient data are available to indicate that a large part of the collagen molecule is composed of repeating triplets $(Gly-X-Y)_n$ where X and Y are often proline and hydroxyproline but may be any amino acid (Fig. 2-1A). Alternate regions of polar and nonpolar amino acids with side chains are responsible for the characteristic banding seen in electron micrographs of collagen fibrils. Many of the characteristic properties of collagen (Table 2-1) and its stabilization are importantly related to the occurrence of glycine as every third residue and the high content of amino acid residues that restrict rotation about bonds along the polypeptide chain.[49] Glycine has no side chain; the association of the three chains places the α-carbon atom of every third residue in the interior of the molecule in such a way that there is no room for an L-amino acid side chain. The stereochemical properties of the pyrrolidine ring of proline and hydroxyproline balance the effects of the relatively unrestricted rotation of glycine. Evolution seems to have assured a content of the amino acid for adequate stability. Together glycine and the amino acids constitute more than half the residues of the α chain. Other amino acids are present in proportions like those in other proteins, but unlike these others, all the side chains are on the exterior of the molecule, where they may serve some role in intermolecular interactions but none in stabilization of the molecule.

Analyses of fragments of polypeptide chains obtained by cleavage with cyanogen bromide (which breaks the chains at methionine residues) or with enzymes such as collagenase have led to determination of the amino acid sequence of about a seventh of the length of the collagen molecule. This approach has permitted examination of the evolutionary stability of collagen and has demonstrated genetically distinct collagens in different tissues.

The magnitude of the job of sequencing of collagen is indicated by the 2060 amino acids in the $\alpha1$ and $\alpha2$ chains when compared with the largest protein so far sequenced, γ_G-immunoglobulin, which contains 660 residues in its light and heavy chains.

The sequence of amino acids at the NH_2-end of the $\alpha2$ chain of skin collagen from several species is as given[122] in Fig. 2-1. (The positions of residues in parentheses and separated by commas were assigned on the basis of homology but represent only one possible arrangement.) Each of the three chains contains 1030

A. TYPICAL SEQUENCE

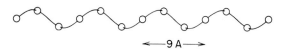

GLY - X - Y - GLY - PRO - Y - GLY - X - HYP - GLY - PRO - HYP

B. MINOR HELIX

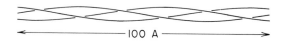

←—9 A—→

C. MAJOR (TRIPLE) HELIX

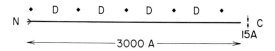

←——————— 100 A ———————→

D. MOLECULE

N ▸——————————————————————— C

⬩ D ⬩ D ⬩ D ⬩ D ⬩

15A

←———————— 3000 A ————————→

E. FIBRIL

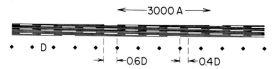

←———3000 A———→

⬩ ⬩ D ⬩ ⬩ ⬩ ⬩ ⬩ ⬩ ⬩ ⬩ ⬩

→| |←0.6D →| |←0.4D

Fig. 2-1. Structure of collagen. **A,** Glycine occurs in every third position throughout most of the polypeptide chains. Proline and hydroxyproline are abundant. X and Y represent any amino acid. **B,** Each polypeptide chain has a polyproline helical conformation. **C,** The three polypeptide chains of each collagen molecule are further coiled about one another. **D,** The NH$_2$-ends of the three chains are together at one end of the molecule. The distribution of amino acids is unique throughout the length of the molecule, but there is a pseudo repeat (D) of about 680 Å periodicity. **E,** Collagen fibrils are formed by association of molecules in such a way that regions of length D are in register. Length D corresponds to the repeats seen in electron micrographs. Each molecule extends 4.4D, and a space, or "hole," of 0.6D is left between molecules in line. (Courtesy Karl A. Piez, Bethesda, Md.)

Chick	pGlu-Met-Ser-Tyr-Gly-Tyr-Asp-Glu-Lys-Ser-Ala-Gly-	Val-Ala-Val-Pro-Gly-Pro-Met-
Rat	Gly-Tyr-Asp-Glu-Lys-Ser-Ala-Gly-	Val-Ser-Val-Pro-Gly-Pro-Met-
Rabbit	(pGlu,Met,Ser,Tyr,Gly,Tyr,Asp,Glu,Lys,Ser,Ala,Gly,	Val,Ser,Val,Pro,Gly,Pro)Met-
Calf	(pGlu,Leu,Ser,Tyr,Gly,Tyr,Asp,Glu,Lys,Ser,Thr,Gly,	Val,Ser,Ile,Pro,Gly,Pro)Met-
Baboon	(pGlu,Leu,Ser,Tyr,Gly,Tyr,Asp,Glu,Lys,Ser,Thr,Gly,Gly,Val,Ser,Ile,Pro,Gly,Pro)Met-
Human	(pGlu,Leu,Ser,Tyr,Gly,Tyr,Asp,Glu,Lys)Ser-Thr-Gly-Gly(Val,Ser,Ile,Pro,Gly,Pro)Met-
	1 5 10	15 20

Fig. 2-2. Amino acid sequences of N-terminal end of the αl chain of skin collagen from several species. The positions of residues within parentheses and separated by commas were assigned on the basis of homology. (From Traub, W., and Piez, K. A.: The chemistry and structure of collagen, Advances Protein Chem. 25:243, 1971.)

```
Chick     pGlu-Tyr-Asp-Pro-Ser-Lys-Ala-Ala-Asp-Phe-Gly-Pro-Gly-Pro-Met-Gly-Leu-Met-
Rat       pGlu-Tyr-    Ser-Asp-Lys-Gly-Val-Ser-Ala-Gly-Pro-Gly-Pro-Met(Gly,Leu)Met-
Rabbit    (pGlu,   Asp,    Gly,Lys,Gly,         Phe,Gly,Pro,Gly,Pro)Met(Gly,Leu)Met-
Calf      (pGlu,Tyr,Asp,Ser,Gly,Lys,     Ala,Asp,Phe,Gly,Glx,Gly,Pro)Met(Gly,Leu)Met-
Baboon    (pGlu,Tyr,Asp,     Gly,Lys,Gly,Val,    Leu,Gly,Pro,Gly,Pro)Met(Gly,Leu)Met-
Human     (pGlu,Tyr,Asp,     Gly,Lys,Gly,Val,    Leu,Gly,Pro,Gly,Pro)Met(Gly,Leu)Met-
            1               5                   10                  15
```

Fig. 2-3. Amino acid sequences at the N-terminal end of the $\alpha2$ chain of skin collagen from several species. The positions of residues within parentheses and separated by commas were assigned on the basis of homology and represent only one possible arrangement. Note the differences from the $\alpha1$ chain (Fig. 2-2). (From Traub, W., and Piez, K. A.: The chemistry and structure of collagen, Advances Protein Chem. **25:**243, 1971.)

```
pGlu-Met-Ser-Tyr-Gly-Tyr-Asp-Glu-Lys-Ser-Ala-Gly-Val-Ser-Val- 15
Pro-Gly-Pro-Met-Gly-Pro-Ser-Gly-Pro-Arg-Gly-Leu-Hyp-Gly-Pro-  30
Hyp-Gly-Ala-Hyp-Gly-Pro-Gln-Gly-Phe-Gln-Gly-Pro-Hyp-Gly-Glu-  45
Hyp-Gly-Glu-Hyp-Gly-Ala-Ser-Gly-Pro-Met-Gly-Pro-Arg-Gly-Pro-  60
Hyp-Gly-Pro-Hyp-Gly-Lys-Asn-Gly-Asp-Asp-Gly-Glu-Ala-Gly-Lys-  75
Pro-Gly-Arg-Hyp-Gly-Gln-Arg-Gly-Pro-Hyp-Gly-Pro-Gln-Gly-Ala-  90
Arg-Gly-Leu-Hyp-Gly-Thr-Ala-Gly-Leu-Hyp-Gly-Met-Hyl-Gly-His- 105
Arg-Gly-Phe-Ser-Gly-Leu-Asp-Gly-Ala-Lys-Gly-Asn-Thr-Gly-Pro- 120
Ala-Gly-Pro-Lys-Gly-Glu-Hyp-Gly-Ser-Hyp-Gly-Glx-Asx-Gly-Ala- 135
Hyp-Gly-Gln-Met-
```

Fig. 2-4. Amino acid sequence of 139 residues at the N-terminal end of the $\alpha1$ chain of rat skin (or tendon) collagen. The order of residues 134 to 136 was derived from the assumptions that each third amino acid is glycine and that hydroxyproline can occur only in the position preceding glycine. Many of the residues shown as hydroxyproline are proline as a result of incomplete hydroxylation. In rat skin collagen (Fig. 2-2), the first four residues are absent. (From Traub, W., and Piez, K. A.: The chemistry and structure of collagen, Advances Protein Chem. **25:**243, 1971.)

amino acids and has a molecular weight of about 95,000. With the work of Balian, Click, and Bronstein[4a] the known structure of the α_1 chain of rat skin has now been extended to a total of 234 residues from the NH_2 terminus.

The N-terminal ends of the collagen polypeptides are not helical. The first ten to fifteen residues in both $\alpha1$ and $\alpha2$ chains (Figs. 2-2 and 2-3) do not have glycine in every third position, an absolute requirement for the triple-chain helical structure of collagen. The distinctive terminal portions were recognized by Schmitt and colleagues,[110] who termed them telopeptides and suggested that their role in cross-linking and antigenicity.

In one segment of $\alpha1$ chain of calf skin collagen the sequences of residues 34 to 43 and residues 64 to 73 are both Gly-Asp-Arg-Gly-Glu-Thr-Gly-Pro-Ala-Gly.[122] This suggests that the now familiar phenomenon of DNA duplication has occurred in the evolution of the collagen genes.

The major collagen of skin, tendon, and bone is the same protein in the sense that they are derived from the same structural genes, presumably one for the $\alpha1$ chain and one for the $\alpha2$ chain. Differences in the collagens from these three tissues are a function of degree of hydroxylation, aldehyde formation for cross-linkage, and glycosylation (see below). The $\alpha1$ chain of the collagen of cartilage, on the other hand, is determined by a different structural gene. (The same is probably true of the collagen in basement membrane.) Furthermore, the collagen of cartilage has no $\alpha2$ chains. Hence if the formula of skin collagen is $(\alpha_1^I)_2\,(\alpha_2^I)$, then cartilage collagen might be represented as $(\alpha_1^{II})_3$. The fetus contains a fetal collagen of distinctive structure $(\alpha_1^{III})_3$.

Hydroxylation. Hydroxyproline and hydroxylysine are not incorporated into collagen as such but rather as proline and lysine, which are hydroxylated after these amino acids are incorporated into the peptide linkage. Hydroxylation occurs in the ribosomal-RNA—bound peptide.[65,89] A specific hydroxylase catalyzes each of these reactions. Genetic deficiency of lysine hydroxylase is known to lead to a defect in cross-linking of collagen and the clinical picture of the Ehlers-Danlos syndrome (p. 345). This is because hydroxylysine is involved in cross-linking of collagen (p. 41).

Helix formation. The minor helix of collagen has three residues per turn (Fig. 2-1B). Because it has no side chain, the presence of glycine in every third position permits supercoiling of the three polypeptide chains about a common axis in the major helix (Fig. 2-1C). Speakman[118] suggested that the polypetide chains of collagen have "terminal segments with structures which facilitate rapid association." Presumably, the extra segment is cleaved off enzymatically after the formation of the helix. These extra terminal segments, called RP ("registration peptides") by Speakman, would explain why the triple helix is assembled in minutes *in vivo* but requires days and carefully controlled conditions *in vitro,* where yields are low at best. Bellamy and Bornstein[9] found that procollagen (pre-α1 chain) has a molecular weight of about 120,000, as contrasted with the molecular weight of about 100,000 for the α chains.

Glycosylation (or glycosidation). By an enzymatic process, galactose is attached to hydroxylysine of the collagen polypeptide chains by an O-glycosidic linkage, and glucose is attached to galactose through the agency of a separate enzyme. Thus collagen is a glycoprotein. Although glucose and galactose are the major carbohydrate components, there may be others as well. In both skin and bone of man, one third of the total hydroxylysine is glycosylated; however, in skin, glucosylgalactosylhydroxylysine predominates, whereas in bone, galactosylhydroxylysine predominates.[91a]

Secretion. A collagen precursor,[9] which has a longer chain length than the alpha chains of mature collagen, is synthesized.[9,78a] The additional portion presumably serves a function of facilitating or regulating the secretion of collagen from the fibroblast and the formation of the triple helix (see above) and may inhibit intracellular fibrogenesis.

Conversion of a precursor. It appears that outside the cell at the time of fibril formation, collagen is derived from procollagen through proteolytic cleavage.[9,23a,66,118] Thus a situation probably obtains which is comparable to that of insulin synthesis, where the molecule initially synthesized is larger than the final products produced by cleavage. The portion cleaved off is made up of the "registration peptides" referred to above. A specific enzyme, procollagen peptidase, is responsible for the cleavage.[65a] In cattle, deficiency of the enzyme leads to persistence of procollagen and a serious disorder called dermatosparaxis (p. 346).

Aggregation. After extrusion of the rod-shaped, triple helical, 3000×15 Å molecules from the synthesizing fibroblasts, the molecules are assembled into cylindrical fibrils, the diameters of which are fairly uniform for a given tissue

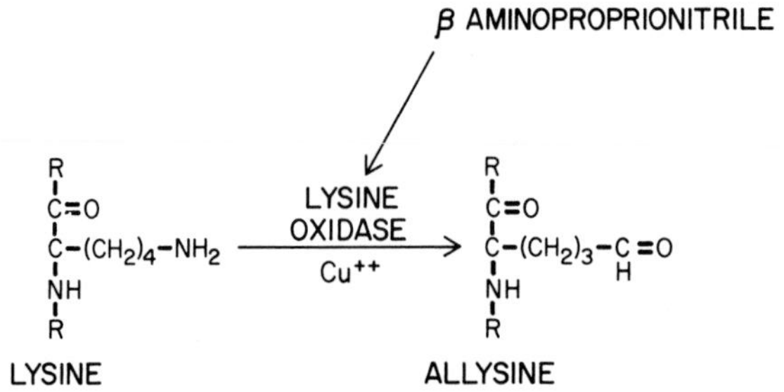

Fig. 2-5. Oxidative deamination of lysine to form allysine, which is important to the cross-linking of collagen and elastin. Hydroxylysine can be similarly changed to form hydroxyallysine. The enzyme lysine oxidase is irreversibly inhibited by β-aminoproprionitrile. R = rest of α chain of collagen.

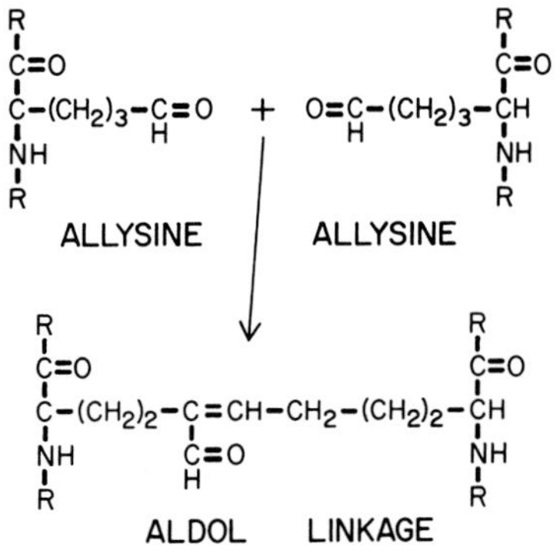

Fig. 2-6. Formation of an aldol linkage between two allysines in the cross-linking of collagen. R = rest of α chain of collagen.

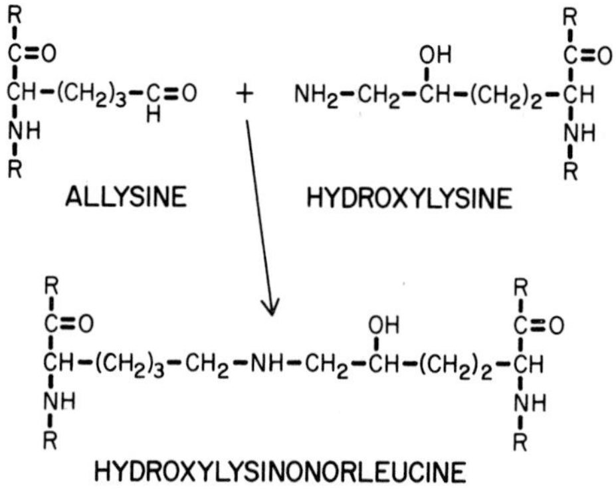

Fig. 2-7. Reduced Schiff base product of reaction of allysine and hydroxylysine in cross-linking of collagen. R = rest of collagen molecule.

or stage of development, and vary from 50 to 200 Å. Fibrils are further aggregated in ways appropriate to the particular tissue. Bundles of parallel fibrils comprise tendons, whereas stacked sheets occur in the cornea, accounting for the important transparency of that specialized tissue. Harkness[36f] and Jackson[36j] have described the various fibril-fiber arrangements observed in different tissues. Dermatan sulfate proteoglycans (p. 49) appear to be important in the aggregation process that takes place extracellularly for formation of collagen fibers.

Cross-linking.[18,90] Until the 1960's the only type of cross-linking known between polypeptide chains of protein molecules was the disulfide bond. Since collagen contains no cysteine and therefore no disulfide cross-links, some other type of bond had to be sought. It turns out that the cross-linking in collagen occurs at specific lysyl and hydroxylysyl residues near the amino end of the $\alpha 1$ and $\alpha 2$ chains (Figs. 2-2 and 2-3).

As stated above, specific lysyl or hydroxylysyl residues in collagen are enzymatically converted to aldehydes (called allysine or hydroxyallysine) by oxidative deamination (Fig. 2-5). Two allysines, or an allysine and a hydroxyallysine, undergo spontaneous aldol condensation to form cross-links between the polypeptide chains of the same or separate molecules (Fig. 2-6). The aldol product of an allysine and a hydroxyallysine is called syndesine. Alternatively, a Schiff base product can be formed, for example, between a hydroxylysine and an allysine (Fig. 2-7). (Because of the importance of hydroxylysine to cross-linking of collagen, it is not surprising that deficiency of lysine hydroxylase results in a clinical disorder in the category of the Ehlers-Danlos syndrome.) The cross-links which form can be either intramolecular (between alpha chains or the same molecule) or intermolecular (Fig. 2-8).

The N-terminal ends of the collagen polypeptides are closely aligned so that cross-links form between lysine residues 9 in $\alpha 1$ chain and 6 in $\alpha 2$ chain (Figs. 2-2 and 2-3). These lysine residues are first converted to the cross-link precursor

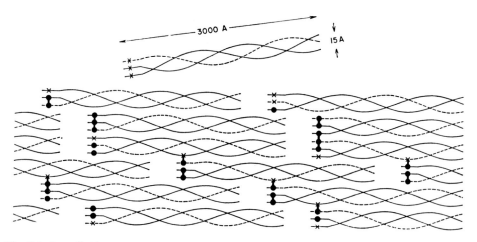

Fig. 2-8. Cross-linking of collagen, intermolecular and intramolecular. (Courtesy Karl A. Piez, Bethesda, Md.)

allysine by an enzymatic step: the oxidative deamination of the ε-amino group to form the aldehyde (Fig. 2-5). The enzyme lysyl oxidase was demonstrated by Pinnell and Martin,[91a] using as a substrate aortic elastin from chicks given β-aminopropionitrile, which inhibits this enzyme. As indicated later, the initial step in the formation of cross-links is identical in collagen and elastin. The exogenously induced disorder of connective tissue, lathyrism, affects both collagen and elastin because the toxic principle of *Lathyrus odoratus* irreversibly inhibits the enzyme common to cross-linking in both. Some heritable disorders of connective tissue may similarly have involvement of both collagen and elastin because of a gene-determined defect in some shared biochemical mechanism.

Lysyl oxidase has the cupric ion as a cofactor.[114] Copper deficiency results in deficient cross-linking of collagen and elastin. Although similar in many ways to the amine oxidase of plasma,[23] lysyl oxidase is distinctive since only it is active on elastin and collagen under physiologic conditions.[114]

In summary, although the basic properties of amino acids and polypeptide chains that have become familiar to the biochemist and geneticist from hemoglobin are evident also in collagen, biologically and probably pathologically important complexities of collagen biochemistry are evident. Alterations in the collagen molecule after translation of the genetic message contained in the structural genes include several steps showing variability in development from tissue to tissue and from time to time: degree of hydroxylation of proline and lysine, rate and degree of aldehyde formation, pattern of covalent cross-linking, proteolytic alteration at the N-terminal and C-terminal ends and possibly the amount and site of attachment of carbohydrate. Even without consideration of the influence of other elements of connective tissue, particularly acid mucopolysaccharides, it is evident that the genetic control of collagen fiber formation is complex and that failure at any one of several points can lead to disease. Some possible sites of genetic defects in collagen synthesis leading to heritable disorders of connective tissue are outlined in Table 2-2. Fig. 2-9 diagrams the steps in collagen synthesis.

Elastic fibers[104,105] are large branching refractile structures, light yellow or brown, depending on their age; with a high degree of extensibility; extreme

Table 2-2. Some possible sites of genetic defects in collagen

I	Pretranslation (shift from embryonic to adult collagen)
II	Translation (distinctive embryonic and adult skin and cartilage collagens)
III	Posttranslation

    a. *Hydroxylation* of proline, lysine*

    b. *Glycosylation* (addition of galactose, or of galactose and glucose, to selected hydroxylysine residues)

    c. *Oxidative deamination* of specific lysyl and hydroxylysyl residues to aldehydes (and subsequent aldol condensation to form intramolecular cross-links)

    d. Production of Schiff bases between molecules and subsequent *reduction*, probably enzymatic, to form stable intramolecular cross-links

    e. *Cleavage* of "registration peptide" from N-terminal end of alpha chains†

*Defect in this step demonstrated in a form of Ehlers-Danlos syndrome in man (p. 345).
†Defect at this step demonstrated in disease of cattle, dermatosparaxis (p. 346), and in a form of Ehlers-Danlos syndrome in man (p. 341).

insolubility; indestructibility in relation to heat, drastic pH changes, and enzymes; a low content of polar amino acids; and, finally, certain distinctive tinctorial characteristics. The nature of their staining by orcein and related dyes is not at all well understood; the staining bears no relationship to pH. and there is no other evidence that salt linkages are involved.[127] The property of stretching easily and rapidly, with little loss of energy in heat, and of retracting rapidly to their original dimensions when the stress is removed is popularly referred to as elasticity. Elasticity is defined in strict physical terms, however, as resistance to deformation (p. 298). In these terms, steel and glass are highly elastic materials, and elastic fibers are highly inelastic!

Elastic fibers were first described in blood vessels by Henle in 1842. In 1902 Richards and Gies[101] described the chemical properties of elastin.

Whereas collagen is present in areas where a pliant but relatively non-extensible building material is necessary (ligaments, tendons, fascia, joint capsules), elastic fibers serve important functions in areas such as the media of the aorta (where they are responsible for the compression chamber, reservoir, or *Windkessel* hemodynamic function of that structure), in the elastic cartilage of the ear, and in ligaments with large elastic components such as those of the foot and the ligamenta flava of the spine. They are important also to the function of

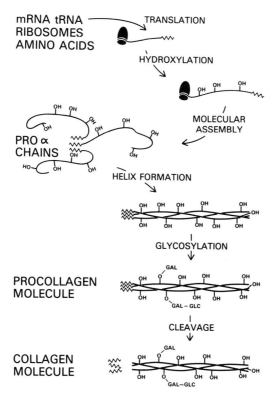

Fig. 2-9. The synthesis of collagen. (Courtesy Thomas P. Nigra, Michael L. Friedland, and George R. Martin, Bethesda, Md.)

the lung, specifically in passive recoil in expiration after the active expansion of inspiration. In ligaments the elastic fibers are cylindrical and weave among the bundles of collagen fibers. In the arterial walls the elastic fibers form concentric layers, with holes that enable the muscle cells in the media to communicate between layers. In the skin, elastic fibers are found mainly in the outermost layer of the corium. The leather industry has been a source of information on elastic fibers as well as on collagen. The outer part of the corium represents the grain layer of leather, so-called because it swells less with tanning and produces grain, which may or may not be desirable in the particular instance. Empirically, "bating"—treatment of the hides with pancreas—was practiced in order to remove the grain layer. Baló and Banga[5] subsequently found that the basis of the "bating" process is the presence of elastase in pancreas.

Electron microscopy[39] shows that elastic fibers have two components: a microfibril about 110Å in diameter and an amorphous material composed largely of an unusual protein called elastin. The microfibrillar component contains many cystine disulfide bonds (-S-S-), whereas elastin contains none. By breaking the disulfide bonds, the microfibrils can be solubilized and removed from the insoluble elastin residue.

In the embryo, elastic fibers consist mainly of microfibrils; these microfibrils have staining properties, suggesting a negative surface charge. Later in development the amorphous material begins to appear, and in the adult the elastic fibers consist predominantly of elastin.

Relatively small subunits of the amorphous elastin polymer (tropoelastin) are synthesized on ribosomes in the cytoplasm, secreted like the collagen precursor(s), and assembled extracellularly into the finished product. Elastin and microfibrils, the two components of elastic fibrils, are markedly different in amino acid composition.[32b] It is thus clear that the microfibril is not a precursor of elastin. They must be separately synthesized and must be determined by separate genes. The predominant amino acids of elastin (such as valine, alanine, glycine, and proline) are uncharged and hydrophobic, tending to render the molecule insoluble in water. Tropoelastin may have enough lysine to form a hydrophilic "shell," making the molecule soluble and facilitating its transport out of the cell.

The fibroblast synthesizes the elastin of ligaments, tendons, and skin, but a surprising finding of Ross and Klebanoff[106a] is that in arterial wall, smooth-muscle cells synthesize collagen and both components of the elastic fiber, the microfibrils and elastin. Radioactively labeled proline was used in autoradiographic studies to arrive at this conclusion.

The lack of cysteine in elastin, as in collagen, and therefore the lack of -S-S- bonds lead to a search for the nature of the cross-linking. The first clue was discovered by Partridge,[88] who, with his colleagues, found two "new" amino acids that occur uniquely in elastin and named them desmosine and isodesmosine (from the Greek word *desmos*, band) because of an apparent role in cross-linking.

It was next shown that the desmosines are tetracarboxylic, tetra-amino substituted pyridinium compounds derived from four lysyl side chains, three of which have been oxidatively deaminated prior to condensation.[1] The elastin precursor is thought to have a globular shape. The four-pronged desmosine can link together as many as four tropoelastin chains (see Fig. 2-10).

Lysyl oxidase, the enzyme responsible for oxidative deamination of lysine to

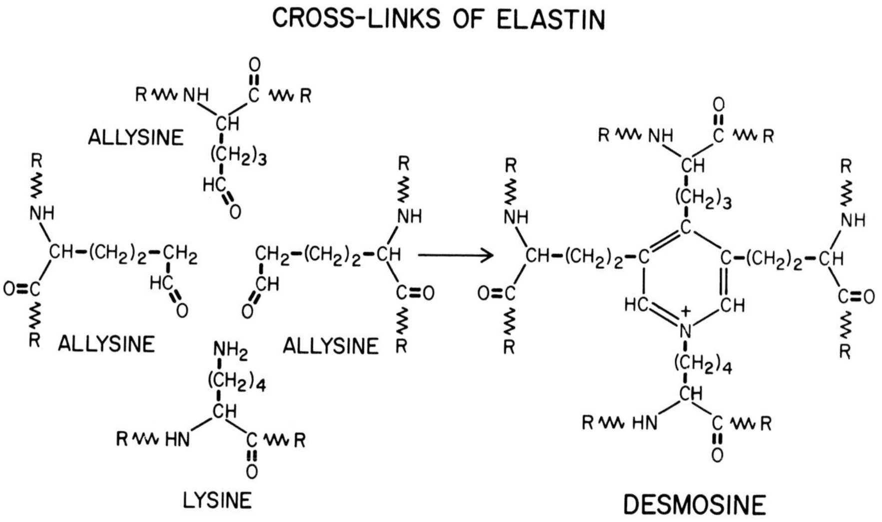

CROSS-LINKS OF ELASTIN

Fig. 2-10. Formation of desmosine cross-linkage in elastin from three allysines and a lysine. R = rest of elastin polypeptide chain.

allysine as the first step in cross-linking of both collagen and elastin, is, as mentioned earlier, a copper-containing enzyme and may require pyridoxal phosphate, although this has not been proved; both copper and pyridoxine deficiency result in defective cross-linking of collagen and elastin.[51,120] Copper deficiency in swine is accompanied by connective tissue and aortic changes which, like lathyrism, bear some similarity to those in the genetic disorder Marfan syndrome; rupture of the aorta occurs in copper deficiency also. In the aorta of copper-deficient pigs, a soluble elastin precursor lacking desmosine and isodesmosine, but rich in lysine, has been isolated.[108,117]

Much information about the chemical nature of cross-linking of collagen and elastin came from study of the defect in experimental osteolathyrism. This condition, traced to effects of β-aminonitrile in the seed of the sweet pea *Lathyrus odoratus,* has been viewed as a possible model of the Marfan syndrome because of the occurrence of both skeletal changes and rupture of the aorta (Fig. 3-74).

Lathyrogens have their effects through inhibition of the enzyme that catalyzes oxidative deamination of lysine to allysine as the first step in the formation of cross-links in collagen and elastin.[17,91a]

Other chemical agents affect performed aldehydes involved in collagen-elastin cross-links and reverse certain labile cross-links. These agents include penicillamine,[26,63,83,92] cysteamine, and other aminothiols that have the ability to extract collagen from tissues and to reduce the tensile strength of skin and tendon. This action appears to be the result of their ability to form condensation products with aldehydes. The experimental observations may have a counterpart in the connective tissue aspects of homocystinuria; homocysteine bears structural similarities to penicillamine. *Thiolism* is the term applied to these effects of sulfhydryl-containing compounds on connective tissues.

To return to elastin. After secretion of tropoelastin from the cell, the conversion of hydrophilic lysines to cross-links exposes the predominantly hydrophobic nature of the molecule so that it becomes insoluble. The microfibrils, which as noted earlier are negatively charged, interact with the positively charged tropoelastin molecules and orient them in the shape of a fiber.

Studies with radioisotope tracer methods[115] indicate what is probably an even lower level of metabolic activity than in collagen.[79] With aging there is a chemical alteration in elastin,[96,11b] including a change in the amino acid profile and an increased affinity for calcium and basophilic dyes. Formation of elastic fibers in tissue culture is observed with more difficulty than in the case of collagen fibers.[13,84,85]

Ground substance

The term ground substance is a mistranslation of that used by the early German histologists—*Grundsubstanz,* meaning "fundamental substance." Although the ground substance has long been known (in 1861 there was enough information to justify a review of the subject by Kölliker), the first step in mucopolysaccharide biochemistry was taken by Krukenberg in 1884 when he isolated a polysaccharide from cartilage with dilute sodium hydroxide. The substance he termed chondroitic acid was chondroitin-4-sulfate (chondroitin sulfate B). Since only small quantities were obtained when water was used as the solvent, Schmiedeberg deduced that in cartilage the material is bound to protein. Karl Meyer[73] proposed the term mucopolysaccharide to designate "hexosamine-containing polysaccharides of animal origin occurring either in a pure state or conjugated with protein through a salt linkage."

The most intensive investigations in this area did not come until the discovery of the "spreading factor" by Duran-Reynals and Suner Pi in 1929[28] and the studies of mucopolysaccharides of the ground substance and of hyaluronidase in the laboratory of Karl Meyer at Columbia University beginning in the early 1930's.[75]

The ground substance is the extracellular, extrafibrillar, amorphous matrix of connective tissue. It has components derived from the fibroblast, such as acid mucoprotein, acid mucopolysaccharide, and dispersed (soluble or pro-) collagen, and components not elaborated locally, such as water, ions, small organic molecules such as glucose, cell metabolites, plasma proteins, and others. It is important not to equate ground substance with acid mucoproteins and acid mucopolysaccharides, as has become a frequent practice, since on a quantitative basis, and possibly on a functional basis, some of the other constituents such as plasma proteins, soluble collagen, and neutral mucoproteins are as important. Another assumption that may be fallacious is that changes in serum mucoprotein (which is neutral) reflect changes in acid mucopolysaccharide of the ground substance; chemically the two are quite distinct.

There are several presumably distinct acid mucopolysaccharides in connective tissue (Table 2-3). All are polymers of high molecular weight and contain hexosamine and hexuronic acid moieties. Hyaluronic acid, which has been identified in synovial fluid, vitreous humor, and umbilical cord, is composed, among other moieties, of glucosamine and glucuronic acid. It is digested by hyaluronidase. Chondroitin, which has been isolated only from cornea, differs from hyaluronic acid by the replacement of glucosamine by galactosamine; its properties are similar, however. One can distinguish three chondroitin sulfates, or ChS (A, B, and C), on the basis of solubility, optical rotation, and enzymatic properties. All contain galactosamine, not glucosamine. ChS A (now preferably termed chondroitin-4-sulfate) has been demonstrated in cartilage, bone cornea, aorta, and ligamentum nuchae. ChS B (now preferably termed dermatan sulfate), in which the hexuronic acid moiety is iduronic acid, not glucuronic acid, has been isolated from skin, tendon, heart valves, ligamentum nuchae, and aorta. ChS C (now called chondroitin-6-sulfate) has been found in cartilage, umbilical cord, tendons, and nucleus pulposus. Keratosulfate (now called keratan sulfate), the only sulfate mucopolysaccharide free of uronic acid, has been isolated from cornea, where it represents about 50% of total mucopolysaccharide. Heparitin sulfate (now called heparan sulfate), which as its name indicates has chemical, physical, and other properties resembling those of heparin, has normally been found only in aorta.

Two acid mucopolysaccharides excreted in the urine in excess in the major mucopolysaccharidoses (Chapter 11) are dermatan sulfate (DS) and heparan sulfate (HS). Both are found normally in blood vessels and heart valves, and DS is an important constituent of skin (hence its designation; Table 2-3), as well as of arterial walls and heart valves. They occur as large polymers, consisting of a protein core with numerous carbohydrate branches. The carbohydrates consist of alternating units of a uronic acid and a sulfated hexosamine. In DS the repeating dimer is L-iduronic acid linked to N-acetylgalactosamine-4-sulfate, whereas in HS it is D-glucuronic acid linked to N-acetylglucosamine, which is sometimes sulfated in the 6-position or has an N-sulfate replacing the N-acetyl (Fig. 2-11). Both acid mucopolysaccharides have the polysaccharide side

Table 2-3. Acid mucopolysaccharides of connective tissue*

	Hexosamine	Hexuronic acid	Source
Nonsulfated			
Chondroitin	Galactosamine	Glucuronic	Cornea
Hyaluronic acid	Glucosamine	Glucuronic	Vitreous humor
			Synovial fluid
			Umbilical cord
Sulfated			
Keratan sulfate	Glucosamine	(Galactose)	Cornea
			Cartilage
			Nucleus pulposus
Heparan sulfate	Glucosamine	Glucuronic	Aorta
		Iduronic	
Chondroitin-4-sulfate	Galactosamine	Glucuronic	Cornea
			Cartilage
Dermatan sulfate	Galactosamine	Iduronic	Skin
			Heart
			Aorta
Chondroitin-6-sulfate	Galactosamine	Glucuronic	Cartilage
			Tendon
Heparin	Glucosamine	Glucuronic	

*The nomenclature is that given by Jeanloz,[60] who further suggests that mucopolysaccharides be called glycosaminoglycans.

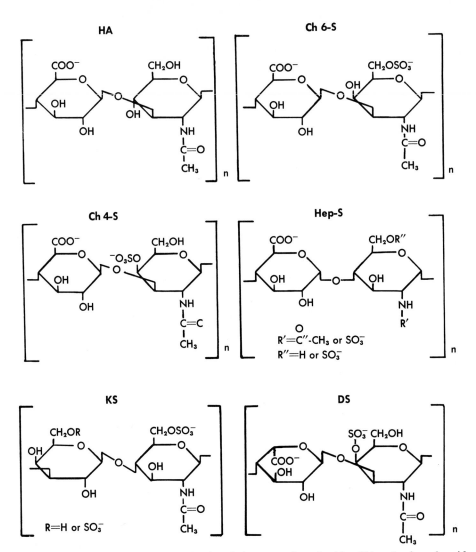

Fig. 2-11. Structure of the repeating subunits of six mucopolysaccharides. HA = hyaluronic acid. Ch6-S = chondroitin-6-sulfate (formerly chondroitin sulfate C). Ch4-S = chondroitin-4-sulfate (formerly chondroitin sulfate A). Hep-S = heparan sulfate (formerly heparitin sulfate). KS = keratan sulfate (formerly keratosulfate). DS = dermatan sulfate (formerly chondroitin sulfate B). (From Meyer, K.: Amer. J. Med. **47:**664, 1969.)

chains linked to the serine of the protein core by the sugar xylose. Two residues of galactose are linked to the xylose, followed by a residue of glucuronic acid and one of N-acetylhexosamine.[8] Then the distinctive sequences shown in Fig. 2-11 begin.

Chondroitin-4-sulfate and chondroitin-6-sulfate[78] differ only in the position of the sulfate group (Fig. 2-11). They are the most abundant of the mucopolysaccharides, occurring in both the skeletal and soft connective tissues. Genetic disturbances of the metabolism of these mucopolysaccharides have not been well elucidated (Chapter 11).

Dermatan sulfate (formerly called chondroitin sulfate B) differs from the chondroitin sulfates in that it contains iduronic acid in place of glucuronic acid, its epimer at carbon 5 (Fig. 2-11). Dermatan sulfate is, however, hybrid[32a,72]; all DS fractions contain both L-iduronic acid and D-glucuronic acid moieties.

Dermatan sulfate proteoglycans display *in vitro* a striking ability to precipitate soluble tropocollagen,[121] a property not shared by chondroitin sulfate proteoglycans. The main function of DS may be in the formation of collagen fibers.[70] The collagenosis observed in the mucopolysaccharidoses with excretion of excessive DS (MPS I, II, V, and VI) may have its basis in this property of DS.

Heparan sulfate (formerly heparitin sulfate), like dermatan sulfate, has not been identified in normal skeletal tissue or cornea. It is found mainly in blood vessels. It is excreted in large amounts as the main urinary MPS in the Sanfilippo syndrome (MPS III) and is excreted in excess along with dermatan sulfate in MPS I and II. It is the main MPS stored in the liver in the latter conditions. It is now clear that heparan sulfate has a small proportion of L-iduronic acid, the main repeating unit in dermatan sulfate. Thus, explanation is provided for the fact that deficiency of α-L-iduronidase in the Hurler syndrome (MPS I) leads to excessive urinary excretion of both DS and HS (Chapter 11).

Heterogeneity and variability in the mucopolysaccharides are very great, making chemical studies difficult. Unlike the structures of proteins, which vary almost none at all, having been synthesized under direct specification of the genetic code, the degree of sulfation and the relative proportions of other components may vary considerably. The occurrence of hybrid proteoglycans has already been noted.

Keratan sulfate[11] (KS) occurs particularly in cartilage, nucleus pulposus, and cornea, and these tissues are affected in the Morquio syndrome, in which excessive KS is excreted in the urine. As diagrammed in Fig. 2-5, galactose replaces the uronic acid.

Meyer[72] distinguishes two types of KS: KS I, found in cornea, and KS II, found in cartilage and nucleus purposus. It is clear that keratan sulfate and chondroitin sulfate are linked to the same protein core to form chondroitin sulfate–keratan sulfate proteoglycans in cartilage. Mixed proteoglycans of this type are excreted, for example, in the Morquio syndrome.[62] The proportion of KS in the mixed proteoglycans is a function of age, cartilage from older persons showing more KS.

It appears that in the synthesis of mucopolysaccharides the protein core is first manufactured in a conventional manner and that the carbohydrate chains are then added, one sugar at a time, starting with the attachment of xylose to serine. Sulfation occurs after the appropriate sugar has been linked into the growing chain. The sugars and the sulfate come from "activated" precursors: sugar nucleotides and phosphoadenosine 5'-phosphosulfate, respectively. Chain elongation and sulfation occur on the endoplasmic reticulum as the protein progresses from the polysomes, where it is synthesized, to the exterior of the cell. The incorporation of sugar and sulfate is inhibited by compounds that inhibit protein synthesis, such as puromycin and cycloheximide. This indicates that the side chains are not synthesized independently of the protein core.

Introduction of ^{35}S into the study of acid mucopolysaccharides by Dziewiatkowski[29] in 1949 has permitted insight into problems of the metabolism of these materials. Studies of mucopolysaccharide formation in microorganisms and in cell cultures have been helpful. Production of components of the ground substance in tissue culture has been observed.[14,124] In the hands of Neufeld and her colleagues, studies of fibroblasts from patients with the Hurler syndrome and other disturbances of mucopolysaccharide metabolism, particularly studies using ^{35}S, have illustrated the principle stated by William Harvey and quoted in the Preface (p. x): rare abnormalities teach us about the normal.

Study of the Hurler and Hunter syndromes, disorders of mucopolysaccharide metabolism (Chapter 11), indicates that once synthesized by fibroblasts in tissue culture, about three fourths is secreted into the medium. The remainder is diverted to a storage pool within the cell, which it can leave only by the process of degradation. In normal fibroblasts most of this mucopolysaccharide pool has a half-life of about 8 hours, whereas a minor fraction has a half-life of about 3 days. Mixing experiments[80] involving fibroblasts from different forms of mucopolysaccharidosis show that one or another heat-labile, enzymelike substance which is normally involved in degradation of mucopolysaccharides and which is found in the medium in which these cells are grown is missing or defective.

Degradation of mucopolysaccharide occurs primarily, it seems, in the lysosomes, which contain over forty known distinct acid hydrolases. The enzymes involved in mucopolysaccharide degradation are not well characterized. By the fact that degradation is defective when the enzyme is genetically deficient (Chapter 11), at least four lysosomal enzymes are known to be essential to degradation: α-L-iduronidase, heparan sulfate sulfatase, N-acetyl-α-D-glucosaminidase, and β-glucuronidase. In mammals hyaluronidase has been identified with certainty only in testis.

The amount of mucopolysaccharide turnover in the normal individual can be estimated indirectly from the amount of uronic acid that passes through the glucuronic acid cycle of the liver and kidney. This metabolic pathway probably has, as its major function, salvage of glucuronic and iduronic acids from the breakdown of mucopolysaccharides and return of their carbon skeletons to the general metabolic pool. Pentosuria is a benign Garrodian defect of the glucuronic acid cycle such that affected persons excrete in their urine an intermediate metabolite. In the adult 1 to 4 grams of uronic acid pass through this cycle daily, an amount corresponding to 3 to 12 grams of mucopolysaccharide broken down. This figure includes all mucopolysaccharides. It is not surprising that in the Hurler syndrome the excretion of DS and HS may be as high as 200 mg. daily in children.

Metachromatic staining of connective tissues, as by toluidine blue, is a function largely of mucopolysaccharides.[20,35] (Metachromasia is a term introduced by Ehrlich in 1877 to indicate the property of a tissue to stain one color when exposed to a dye of a different color.)

The importance of the ground substance is evident when one considers that it must be traversed by all materials entering and leaving the cells.[107b] The concept[25,38,61,82f] that mucopolysaccharides function like a reactive gel of the ion exchange resin group is intriguing but as yet unproved. It is at least theoretically possible that changes in the concentration or state of polymerization might modify greatly the capacity of connective tissues to bind inorganic ions and water. Hyaluronic acid, highly hygroscopic in the purified state, may be concerned in water-binding by tissues. It may also serve as a lubricant and shock absorber.

Jackson[57] has presented data which he interprets as indicating an important role of mucopolysaccharide in the organization of collagenous structures such as tendon and in giving them certain properties. Trypsin will digest gelatin but not native collagen. The characteristic shrinkage temperature of native collagen is altered by treatment directed at the matrix. The role of dermatan sulfate in collagen fibrogenesis has already been mentioned. Acid mucopolysaccharides are also important to cell-cell interactions leading to aggregation, adhesion, and so on.[88a]

As outlined in Chapter 11, genetic disturbances of mucopolysaccharide metabolism have been related to three of the acid mucopolysaccharides listed in Table 2-3: dermatan sulfate, heparan sulfate, and keratan sulfate. The excessive urinary excretion of various ones of these substances is the biochemical characteristic of six genetic disorders that have been delineated by combined clinical, genetic, and biochemical study. The methods used by Kaplan in a collaborative study of the genetic mucopolysaccharidoses were as follows. (See reference 62a for technical references.)

Mucopolysaccharides were isolated from urine by a method which, in brief, consisted of (1) removing as much salt as possible by centrifugation in the cold, (2) diluting the urine with distilled water to reduce salt concentration further, (3) adjusting the pH to 5 to 6 with glacial acetic acid, and (4) precipitating the mucopolysaccharides with cetylpyridinium chloride. The precipitate, after washing with NaCl-saturated 95% ethanol, was dissolved in acetate buffer, pH 5.5, and stirred with a chloroform—amyl alcohol mixture to extract protein and peptides. The aqueous phase was precipitated with ethanol and then redissolved in acetate buffer and stirred with a mixture of Lloyd's reagent and kaolin to remove further traces of protein. The mucopolysaccharides were then reprecipitated with ethanol. The precipitate was dissolved in distilled water and treated again with Lloyd's reagent and kaolin. The clean solution was brought to 2.5% calcium acetate—0.5N acetic acid, and appropriate alcohol fractions were made, the precipitates from which were dried and weighed.

Analyses done on the isolated materials consisted of the following: carbazol and orcinol reactions for uronic acid, anthrone reaction for neutral sugar, determination of total hexosamine, column chromatography to determine relative amounts of glucosamine and galactosamine, paper chromatography to demonstrate the presence of galactose, measurements of optical rotation, elemental sulfur analyses, and incubation with testicular hyaluronidase to demonstrate resistance or susceptibility to this enzyme.

Dermatan sulfate was identified by its low alcohol solubility, a low carbazol and high orcinol value, no anthrone value, a high negative optical rotation, resistance to digestion by testicular hyaluronidase, and the presence of galactosamine. Heparan sulfate was identified by a high carbazol and low orcinol value, no anthrone value, a high positive optical rotation, resistance to digestion by testicular hyaluronidase, and the presence of glucosamine. Keratan sulfate was identified by its high alcohol solubility, no carbazol or orcinol value, a high anthrone value, the presence of glucosamine, the demonstration of galactose by paper chromatography, and resistance to testicular hyaluronidase. Chondrotin-4-sulfate and chondroitin-6-sulfate, the major normal constituents of urine, were identified by a carbazol-to-orcinol ratio of about 3:2, no anthrone value, susceptibility to digestion by testicular hyaluronidase, and the presence of galactosamine.

Further considerations

The indications of an intimate interrelationship between the several elements of connective tissue, e.g., between collagen and elastin, and between mucopolysaccharide and collagen, are numerous. The details of these interrelationships are not yet fully known.

In addition to these general features of connective tissue, which undoubtedly assist in the understanding of the heritable disorders to be discussed, there are some specific questions about the biology of connective tissue that come to mind with study of these diseases. A few examples follow. *In the Marfan syndrome:* What does the suspensory ligament of the ocular lens have in common with the media of the aorta? What controls longitudinal growth of bone? *In pseudoxanthoma elasticum:* What is the nature of Bruch's membrane of the eye and what does it have in common with elastic fibers? *In the Ehlers-Danlos syndrome:* What is responsible for the tensile strength of the skin and for its elasticity? What is the organization of collagen bundles in ligaments, tendons, and joint capsules, and what is the relationship between this organization and the stretchability of these structures? What determines the elastic properties of the collagen and elastin molecules, and of fibers of these proteins? *In osteogenesis imperfecta:* What is the normal organization of apatite on collagen, which accounts for the important structural properties of bone, and in this disease what change in collagen has occurred to disrupt the normal collagen-apatite relationship? In disorders such as osteogenesis imperfecta and the Ehlers-Danlos syndrome, is there any abnormality of amino acid sequences[123z] of collagen comparable to the abnormalities demonstrated by Ingram[56] in the aberrant hemoglobins? In connection with the full discussion of each of the entities, what is known in answer to these questions and others will be presented. Unfortunately, much remains to be learned in all these areas.

REFERENCES

1. Anwar, R. A., and Oda, G.: The biosynthesis of desmosine and isodesmosine. II. Incorporation of specifically labeled lysine into desmosine and isodesmosine, Biochim. Biophys. Acta **133**:151, 1967.
2. Asboe-Hansen, G.: The origin of synovial mucin. Ehrlich's mast cell—a secretory element of connective tissue, Ann. Rheum. Dis. **9**:149, 1950.
3. Asboe-Hansen, G. editor: Connective tissue in health and disease, Copenhagen, 1954, Ejnar Munksgaard Forlag.
   (a) Asboe-Hansen, G.: Introduction, p. 9. (b) Robb-Smith, A. H. T.: Normal morphology and morphogenesis of connective tissue, p. 15. (c) McManus, J. F. A.: Histochemistry of connective tissue, p. 31. (d) Meyer, K.: Chemistry of ground-substance, p. 54. (e) Kulonen, E.: Chemistry of collagen, p. 70. (f) Dorfman, A.: Metabolism of mucopolysaccharides, p. 81. (g) Boström, H.: Sulphate exchange of sulpho-mucopolysaccharies, p. 97. (h) Duran-Reynals, F.: The spreading reaction, p. 103. (i) Mathews, M. B., and Dorfman, A.: Inhibition of hyaluronidase, p. 112. (j) Iversen, K.: Hormonal influence on connective tissue, p. 130. (k) Banfield, W. G.: Aging of connective tissue, p. 159. (l) Howes, E. L.: Connective tissue in wound healing, p. 159. (m) Altschuler, C. H., and Angevine, D. M.: The pathology of connective tissue, p. 178. (n) Teihum, G.: Cortisone, ascorbic acid and changes in the reticulo-endothelial system, p. 196, (o) Sprunt, D. H.: Connective tissue and infection, p. 208. (p) Cavallero, C.: Influence of hormones on infection, p. 214. (q) Simpson, W. L.: Connective tissues and cancer, p. 225. (r) Rinehart, J. F.: Histogenesis and pathogenesis of arterioclerosis, p. 239. (s) Klemperer, P.: Collagen diseases, p. 251. (t) Ragan, C.: Arthritis, p. 263. (u) Asboe-Hansen, G.: Systemic connective tissue disorders pertaining to dermatology, p. 274. (v) Godtfredsen, E.: Mesenchymal aspects in ophthalmology, p. 296. (w) Zacharias, L.: Fibroses due to injury, p. 308.
4. Balazs, E. A., editor: Chemistry and molecular biology of the intercellular matrix, New York, 1970, Academic Press, Inc.
4a. Balian, G., Click, E. M., and Bornstein, P.: Structure of rat skin collagen α_1-CB8. Amino

acid sequence of the hydroxylamine-produced fragment HA1, Biochemistry 10:4470, 1971.

5. Baló, J., and Banga, I.: The elastolytic activity of pancreatic extracts, Biochem. J. 46:384, 1950.

6. Banga, I., and Baló, J.: Elastin and elastase, Nature 171:44, 1953.

7. Bear, R. S.: The structure of collagen fibrils, Advances Protein Chem. 7:69, 1952.

8. Bella, A., Jr., and Danishefsky, I.: The dermatan sulfate–protein linkage region, J. Biol. Chem. 243:2660, 1968.

9. Bellamy, G., and Bornstein, P.: Evidence for procollagen, a biosynthetic precursor of collagen, Proc. Nat. Acad. Sci. 68:1138, 1971.

10. Bhavananden, V. P., and Meyer, K.: Studies on keratosulfates: methylation, desulfation, and acid hydrolysis studies on old human rib cartilage keratosulfate, J. Biol. Chem. 243: 1052, 1968.

11. Bhavanandan, V. P., and Meyer, K.: Studies on keratosulfates: methylation and partial acid hydrolysis of bovine corneal keratosulfate, J. Biol. Chem. 242:4352, 1967.

12. Blackett, N. M.: On the organization of collagen fibrils in bone, Biochim. Biophys, Acta 16:161, 1955.

13. Bloom, W.: Studies on fibers in tissue culture. II. The development of elastic fibers in cultures of embryonic heart and aorta, Arch. Exp. Zellforsch. 9:6, 1929.

14. Bollet, A. J., Boas, N. F., and Bunim, J. J.: Synthesis of hexosamine by connective tissue (in vitro), Science 120:348, 1954.

15. Borasky, R.: Guide to the literature on collagen, Philadelphia, 1950, Agricultural Research Administration, United States Department of Agriculture (Eastern Regional Research Laboratory).

16. Bornstein, P.: In Bondy, P. K., editor: Duncan's diseases of metabolism, Philadelphia, 1969, W. B. Saunders Co., p. 654.

17. Bornstein, P.: The cross-linking of collagen and elastin and its inhibition in osteolathyrism. Is there a relation to the aging process? Amer. J. Med. 49:429, 1970.

18. Bornstein, P., and Piez, K. A.: A biochemical study of human skin collagen and the relation between intra- and intermolecular cross-linking, J. Clin. Invest. 43:1813, 1964.

18a. Bosmann, H. B.: Platelet adhesiveness and aggregation: the collagen: glycosyl, polypeptide: N-acetylgalactosaminyl and glycoprotein: galactosyl transferases of human platelets, Biochem. Biophys, Res. Commun. 43:118, 1971.

19. Bowes, J. H., and Kenten, R. H.: Summary of published results (1900-1946) on amino acid composition of gelatin and collagen, 1947, Leather Manufacturers Research Association, pp. 1-22.

20. Braden, A. W. H.: The reactions of isolated mucopolysaccharides to several histochemical tests, Stain Techn. 30:19, 1955.

21. Campani, M.: Function of mast cells, Lancet 1:802, 1951.

22. Castor, C. W.: Approaches to the study of connective tissue, Bull. Rheum. Dis. 9:177, 1959.

23. Chou, W. S., Savage, J. E., and O'Dell, B. L.: Relation of monamine oxidase activity and collagen cross-linking in copper-deficient and control tissues, Proc. Soc. Exp. Biol. Med. 128:948, 1968.

23a. Church, R. L., Pfeiffer, S. E., and Tanzer, M. L.: Collagen biosynthesis: synthesis and secretion of a high molecular weight collagen precursor (procollagen), Proc. Nat. Acad. Sci. 68:2638, 1971.

24. Crick, F. H. C., and Kendrew, J. C.: X-ray analysis and protein structure, Advances Protein Chem. 12:133, 1957.

25. Day, T. D.: The mode of reaction of interstitial connective tissue with water, J. Physiol. (London) 109:380, 1949.

26. Deshmukh, K., and Nimni, M. E.: A defect in the intramolecular and intermolecular cross-linking of collagen caused by penicillamine. II. Functional groups involved in the interaction process, J. Biol. Chem. 244:1787, 1969.

27. Dorfman, A.: Metabolism of the mucopolysaccharides of connective tissue, Pharmacol. Rev. 7:1, 1955.

28. Duran-Reynals, F., and Suner Pi, J.: Exaltation de l'activité du staphylocoque par les extracts testiculaires, C. R. Soc. Biol. 99:1908, 1929.

29. Dziewiatkowski, D. D.: Rate of excretion of radioactive sulfur and its concentration in

some tissues of the rat after intraperitoneal administration of labeled sodium sulfate, J. Biol. Chem. **178:**197, 1949.

30. Edelman, G. M.: The covalent structure of a human gamma g-immunoglobulin. XI. Functional implications, Biochemistry **9:**3197, 1970.
31. Fawcitt, D. W.: Cell differentiation and modulation. In An introduction to cell and tissue culture, by the staff of the Tissue Culture Course, Cooperstown, N. Y. 1949–1953, Minneapolis, 1955, Burgess Publishing Co.
32. Fleischmajer, R., and Fishman, L.: Amino acid composition of human dermal collagen, Nature **205:**264, 1965.
32a. Fransson, L. A., and Rodén, L.: Structure of dermatan sulfate. II. Characterization of products obtained by hyaluronidase digestion of dermatan sulfate, J. Biol. Chem. **242:** 4170, 1967.
32b. Franzblau, C., and Lent, R. W.: Studies on the chemistry of elastin, Brookhaven Symposia in Biology, no. 21: Structure, function, and evolution in proteins, BNL50116, Brookhaven National Laboratory, 1969.
33. Gerarde, H. W., and Jones, M.: The effect of cortisone on collagen synthesis in vitro, J. Biol. Chem. **201:**553, 1953.
34. Gersh, I., and Catchpole, H. R.: The nature of ground substance of connective tissue, Perspect. Biol. Med. **3:**282, 1960.
35. Gomori, G.: The histochemistry of mucopolysaccharides, Brit. J. Exp. Path. **35:**377, 1954.
36. Gould, B. S., editor: Treatise on collagen, vol. 2, Biology of collagen, New York, 1968, Academic Press, Inc.
    Part A. (a) Ross, R.: The connective tissue fiber forming cell, p. 1. (b) Rudall, K. M.: Comparative biology and biochemistry of collagen, p. 83. (c) Gould, B.: Collagen biosynthesis, p. 139. (d) Jackson, D. S., and Bentley, J. P.: Collagen-glycosaminoglycan interactions, p. 189. (e) Prockop, D. J., and Kivirikko, K. I.: Hydroxyproline and the metabolism of collagen, p. 215. (f) Harkness, R. D.: Mechanical properties of collagenous tissues, p. 248. (g) O'Dell, D. S.: Immunology of collagen and related materials, p. 311. (h) Gould, B. S.: The role of certain vitamins in collagen formation, p. 323. (i) Dougherty, T. F., and Verliner, D. C.: The effects of hormones on connective tissue cells, p. 367.
    Part B. (j) Jackson, S. F.: The morphology of collagen, p. 1. (k) Glimcher, M. J., and Krane, S. M.: The organization and structure of bone, and the mechanism of calcification, p. 68. (l) Woessner, J. F., Jr.: Biological mechanisms of collagen resorption, p. 253. (m) Gillman, T.: On some aspects of collagen formation in localized repair and in diffuse fibrotic reactions to injury, p. 331. (n) Sinex, F. M.: The role of collagen in aging, p. 409.
36a. Grant, M. E., and Prockop, D. J.: Biosynthesis of collagen, New Eng. J. Med. **286:**194, 242, and 291, 1972.
37. Grassmann, W.: Unsere heutige Kenntnis des Kollagens, Das Leder **6:**241, 1955.
38. Gray, J.: The properties of inter-cellular matrix and its relations to electrolytes, Brit. J. Biol. **3:**167, 1926.
39. Greenlee, T. K., Jr., Ross, R., and Hartman, J. L.: The fine structure of elastic fibers, J. Cell Biol. **30:**59, 1966.
40. Gross, J., Highberger, J. H., and Schmitt, F. O.: Collagen structures considered as states of aggregation of a kinetic unit. The tropocollagen particle, Proc. Nat. Acad. Sci. **40:**679, 1954.
41. Gross, J., Matoltsy, A. G., and Cohen, C.: Vitrosin: a member of the collagen class, J. Biophys. Biochem. Cytol. **1:**215, 1955.
42. Gustavson, K. H.: The chemistry and reactivity of collagen, New York, 1956, Academic Press, Inc.
43. Hall, D. A.: The chemistry of connective tissue, Springfield, Ill., 1961, Charles C Thomas, Publisher.
44. Hall, D. A., editor: International review of connective tissue research, New York, Academic Press, Inc.
    I. (1963) (a) Branwood, A. W.: The fibroblast, p. 1. (b) Asboe-Hansen, G.: The hormonal control of connective tissue, p. 29. (c) Lowther, D. A.: Chemical aspects of collagen fibrillogenesis, p. 64. (d) Ramachandran, G. N.: Molecular structure of collagen, p. 127. (e) Loeven, W. A.: The enzymes of the elastase complex, p. 184. (f) Baló, J.: Connective tissue changes in atherosclerosis, p. 241.
    II. (1964) (g) Wood, G. C.: The precipitation of collagen fibers from solution, p. 1.

(h) Ayer, J. P.: Elastic tissue, p. 33. (i) Muir, H.: Chemistry and metabolism of connective tissue glycosaminoglycans (mucopolysaccharides), p. 101. (j) Harkness, R. D.: The physiology of the connective tissue of the reproductive tract, p. 155. (k) Glynn, L. E.: Diseases of collagen and related tissues, p. 214. (l) Verzár, F.: Aging of the collagen fiber, p. 244. (m) Delaunay, A., and Bazin, S.: Mucopolysaccharides, collagen, and nonfibrillar proteins in inflammation, p. 244.

III. (1965) (n) Fullmer, H. M.: The histochemistry of connective tissues, p. 1. (o) Schultz-Haudt, S. D.: Connective tissue and periodontal disease, p. 77. (p) Tanzer, M. L.: Experimental lathyrism, p. 91. (q) Veis, A.: The physical chemistry of gelatin, p. 113. (r) Woessner, J. F., Jr.: Acid hydrolases of connective tissue, p. 201.

IV. (1968) (s) Kirrane, J. A., and Glynn, L. E.: Immunology of collagen, p. 1. (t) Gould, B. S.: Collagen biosynthesis at the ribosomal level, p. 35. (u) Chvapil, M., and Hurych, J.: Control of collagen biosynthesis, p. 68. (v) Carnes, W. H.: Copper and connective tissue metabolism, p. 197. (w) Bailey, A. J.: Effect of ionizing radiation on connective tissue components, p. 233. (x) Eldin, H. R.: Physical properties of collagen fibers, p. 283.

45. Hall, D. A., and Jackson, D. S., editors: International review of connective tissue research, New York, 1970, Academic Press, Inc.
(a) Adams, E.: Metabolism of proline and of hydroxyproline, p. 2. (b) Kivirikko, K. I.: Urinary excretion of hydroxyproline in health and disease, p. 93. (c) Bachra, B. N.: Calcification of connective tissue, p. 165. (d) Dische, Z.: Biochemistry of connective tissue of the vertebrate eye p. 209.

46. Hamilton, P. B., and Anderson, R. A.: Hydroxyproline in proteins, J. Amer. Chem. Soc. **77**:2892, 1955.

47. Harkness, R. D.: Biological functions of collagen, Biol. Rev. **36**:399, 1961.

48. Harkness, R. D.: Marko, A. M., Muir, H. M., and Neuberger, A.: The metabolism of collagen and other proteins in the skin of rabbits, Biochem. J. **56**:558, 1954.

49. Harrington, W. F., and von Hippel, P. H.: The structure of collagen and gelatin, Advances Protein Chem. **16**:1, 1961.

50. Hass, G. M.: Elastic tissue, Arch. Path. **27**:334, 543, 1939.

51. Hill, C. H., and Kim, C. S.: The derangement of elastin synthesis in pyridoxine deficiency, Biochem. Biophys. Res. Commun. **27**:94, 1967.

52. Hlaváčková, V., and Hruoza, Z.: The role of mucopolysaccharides in the mechanism of contraction of collagen fibres in rats of various ages, Gerontologia **9**:84, 1964.

53. Hovig, T.: Aggregation of rabbit blood platelets produced in vitro by saline "extract" of tendons, Thromb. Diath. Haemorrh. **9**:248, 1963.

54. Hovig, T.: Release of a platelet-aggregating substance (adenosine diphosphate) from rabbit blood platelets induced by saline "extract" of tendons, Thromb. Diath. Haemorrh. **9**:264, 1963.

55. Hovig, T., Jørgensen, L., Packham, M. A., and Mustard, J. F.: Platelet adherence to fibrin and collagen, J. Lab. Clin. Med. **71**:29, 1968.

56. Ingram, V. M.: Gene mutations in human haemoglobin; the chemical difference between normal and sickle cell haemoglobin, Nature **180**:326, 1957.

57. Jackson, D. S.: The nature of collagen-chondroitin sulfate linkages in tendon, Biochem. J. **56**:699, 1954.

58. Jackson, D. S.: Some biochemical aspects of fibrogenesis and wound healing, New Eng. J. Med. **259**:814, 1958.

59. Jackson, S. F., and Smith, R. H.: Studies on the biosynthesis of collagen. I. The growth of fowl osteoblasts and the formation of collagen in tissue culture, J. Biophys. Biochem. Cytol. **3**:897, 1957.

60. Jeanloz, R. W.: The nomenclature of mucopolysaccharides, Ann. Rheum. Dis. **3**:233, 1960.

61. Joseph, N. R., Engel, M. B., and Catchpole, H. R.: Interaction of ions and connective tissue, Biochim. Biophys. Acta **8**:575, 1952.

62. Kaplan, D., McKusick, V. A., Trebach, S., and Lazarus, B.: Keratosulfate-chondroitin sulfate peptide from urine of patients with Morquio syndrome (mucopolysaccharidosis IV), J. Lab. Clin. Med. **71**:48, 1968.

62a. Kaplan, D.: Classification of the mucopolysaccharidoses based on the pattern of mucopolysacchariduria, Amer. J. Med. **47**:721, 1969.

63. Keiser, H. R., Henkin, R. I., Kare, M.: Reversal by copper of the lathyrogenic action of D-penicillamine, Proc. Soc. Exp. Biol. Med. **129**:516, 1968.

64. Kretsinger, R. H., Manner, G., Gould, B. S., and Rich, A.: Synthesis of collagen on poly-ribosomes, Nature 202:438, 1964.
65. Kivirikko, K. I., and Prockop, D. J.: Enzymatic hydroxylation of proline and lysine in protocollagen, Proc. Nat. Acad. Sci. 57:782, 1967.
65a. Lapière, C. M., Lenaers, A., and Kohn, L. D.: Procollagen peptidase: an enzyme excising the coordination peptides of procollagen, Proc. Nat. Acad. Sci. 68:3054, 1971.
66. Layman, D. L., McGoodwin, E. B., and Martin, G. R.: The nature of the collagen synthesized by cultured human fibroblasts, Proc. Nat. Acad. Sci. 68:454, 1971.
66a. Lazarides, E., and Lukens, L. N.: Collagen synthesis on polysomes *in vivo* and *in vitro*, Nature (N.B.) 232:37, 1971.
67. Leach, R. M., Jr.: Role of manganese in mucopolysaccharide metabolism, Fed. Proc. 30: 991, 1971.
68. McLaughlin, G. D., and Theis, E. R.: The chemistry of the leather industry, New York, 1945, Reinhold Publishing Corp.
69. Matthews, M. B.: Macromolecular evolution of corrective tissue, Biol. Rev. 42:499, 1967.
70. Mathews, M. B., and Decker, L.: The effect of acid mucopolysaccharide-proteins on fibril formation from collagen solutions, Biochem. J. 109:517, 1968.
71. Maximow, A. A., and Bloom, W.: A textbook of histology, Philadelphia, 1942, W. B. Saunders Co.
72. Meyer, K.: Biochemistry and biology of mucopolysaccharides, Amer. J. Med. 47:664, 1969.
73. Meyer, K.: The chemistry and biology of mucopolysaccharides and glycoproteins, Sympos. Quant. Biol. 6:91, 1938.
74. Meyer, K.: Nature and function of mucopolysaccharides in connective tissue. In Nachmanson, D., editor: Molecular biology, New York, 1960, Academic Press, Inc., p. 69.
75. Meyer, K., and Palmer, J. W.: The polysaccharide of the vitreous humor, J. Biol. Chem. 107:629, 1934.
75a. Michaeli, D., Martin, G. R., Kettman, J., Benjamini, E., Leung, D. Y. K., and Blatt, B. A.: Localization of antigenic determinants in the polypeptide chains of collagen, Science 166: 1522, 1969.
76. Miller, E. J., Epstein, E. H., and Piez, K. A.: Identification of three genetically distinct collagens by cyanogen bromide cleavage of insoluble human skin and cartilage collagens, Biochem. Biophys. Res. Commun. 42:1024, 1971.
76a. Miller, E. J., and Martin, G. R.: The collagen of bone, Clin. Orthop. 59:195, 1968.
77. Morrione, T. G.: The formation of collagen fibers by the action of heparin on soluble collagen, J. Exp. Med. 96:107, 1952.
78. Muir, H.: The structure and metabolism of mucopolysaccharides (glycosaminoglycans) and the problem of the mucopolysaccharidoses, Amer. J. Med. 47:673, 1969.
78a. Muller, P. K., McGoodwin, E., and Martin, G. R.: Studies on protocollagen: identification of a precursor of proto α 1, Biochem. Biophys. Res. Commun. 44:110, 1971.
79. Neuberger, A., Perrone, J. C., and Slack, H. G. B.: Relative metabolic inertia of tendon collagen in the rat, Biochem. J. 49:199, 1951.
80. Neufeld, E. F., and Fratantoni, J. C.: Inborn errors of mucopolysaccharide metabolism, Science 139:141, 1970.
81. Neuman, R. E., and Logan, M. A.: The determination of collagen and elastin in tissues, J. Biol. Chem. 186:549, 1950.
82. New York Heart Association Symposium: Connective tissue: intercellular macromolecules, Biophys. J. (supp.) 4:1964. Selected contributions: (a) Gross, J.: Organization and disorganization of collagen, p. 63. (b) Gallop, P. M.: Concerning some special structural features of the collagen molecule, p. 79. (c) Robertson, W. van B.: Metabolism of collagen in mammalian tissues, p. 93. (d) Schubert, M.: Intercellular macromolecules containing polysaccharides, p. 119. (e) Strominger, J. L.: Nucleotide intermediates in the biosynthesis of heteropolymeric polysaccharides, p. 139. (f) Dorfman, A.: Metabolism of acid mucopolysaccharides, p. 155. (g) Porter, K. A.: Cell fine structure and biosynthesis of intercellular macromolecules, p. 167. (h) Thomas, L.: The effects of papain, vitamin A, and cortisone on cartilage matrix *in vivo*, p. 207. (i) Dziewiatkowski, D. D.: Effect of hormones on the turnover of polysaccharides in connective tissue, p. 215. (j) Holtzer, H.: Control of chondrogenesis in the embryo, p. 239.
83. Nimni, M. E.: A defect in the intramolecular and intermolecular cross-linking of collagen

caused by penicillamine. I. Metabolic and functional abnormalities in soft tissues, J. Biol. Chem. **243**:1457, 1967.

83a. Nordwig, A.: Collagenolytic enzymes, Advances Enzym. **34**:155, 1971.

84. Odiette, D.: La fibre élastique dans les cultures de tissues in vitro. Étude histo-physio-pathologique, J. Physiol. Path Gén. **32**:715, 1934.

85. Odiette, D.: La fibre élastique dans les cultures de tissues in vitro (deuxième mémoire), J. Physiol. Path. Gén. **33**:475, 1935.

86. Page, R. C., and Benditt, E. P.: A molecular defect in lathyritic collagen, Proc. Soc. Exp. Biol. Med. **124**:459, 1967.

87. Page, R. C., and Benditt, E. P.: Molecular diseases of connective and vascular tissues. II. Amine oxidase inhibition by the lathyrogen, β-aminopropionitrile, Biochemistry (Wash.) **6**:1142, 1967.

88. Partridge, S. M.: Elastin, Advances Protein Chem. **17**:227, 1962.

88a. Pessac, B., and Defendi, V.: Cell aggregation: role of acid mucopolysaccharides, Science **175**:898, 1972.

89. Peterkofsky, B., and Udenfriend, S.: Conversion of proline to collagen hydroxyproline in a cell-free system from chick embryo, J. Biol. Chem. **238**:3966, 1963.

90. Piez, K. A.: Cross-linking of collagen and elastin, Ann. Rev. Biochem. **37**:547, 1968.

90a. Piez, K. A., Bethesda: Personal communication, 1971.

91. Pinnell, S. R., Fox, R., and Krane, S. M.: Human collagens: differences in glycosylated hydroxylysines in skin and bone, Biochim. Biophys. Acta **229**:119, 1971.

91a. Pinnell, S. R., and Martin, G. R.: The cross-linking of collagen and elastin: enzymatic conversion of lysine in peptide linkage to α-amino-adipic-δ-semialdehyde (allysine) by an extract from bone, Proc. Nat. Acad. Sci. **61**:708, 1968.

92. Pinnell, S. R., Martin, G. R., and Miller, E. J.: Desmosine biosynthesis: nature of inhibition of D-penicillamine, Science **161**:475, 1968.

93. Prockop, D. J.: Role of iron in the synthesis of collagen in connective tissue, Fed. Proc. **30**:984, 1971.

94. Prockop, D. J., and Kivirikko, K. I.: Relationship of hydroxyproline excretion in urine to collagen metabolism, Ann. Intern. Med. **66**:1243, 1967.

95. Quintarelli, G.: The chemical physiology of mucopolysaccharides, Boston, 1968, Little, Brown & Co.

96. Ragan, C., editor: Josiah Macy Jr. Foundation Conferences on Connective Tissues.
I. (1950) (a) Angevine, D. M.: Structure and function of normal connective tissue, p. 13. (b) Bennett, G. A.: Pathology of connective tissue; fibrinoid degeneration, p. 44. (c) Meyer, K.: Chemistry of connective tissue; polysaccharides, p. 88 (d) Perlmann, G. E.: Enzymatically modified ovalbumins, p. 101. (e) Ragan, C.: Effect of ACTH and cortisone on connective tissues, p. 137.
II. (1951). (a) Gersh, I.: Some functional considerations of ground substance of connective tissues, p. 11. (b) Lansing, A. I.: Chemical morphology of elastic fibers, p. 45. (c) Travell, J.: Pain mechanisms in connective tissues, p. 86. (d) Porter, K. R.: Repair processes in connective tissues, p. 126. (e) Morrione, T. G.: Regression of scar tissue, p. 159.
III. (1952) (a) Lillie, R. D.: Connective tissue staining, p. 11. (b) Wyckoff, R. W. G.: The fine structure of connective tissues, p. 38. (c) Robb-Smith, A. H. T.: The nature of reticulin, p. 92. (d) Fischel, E. E.: Hypersensitivity and the hyperadrenal state, p. 117.
IV. (1953) (a) Ashley, C. A., Schick, A. F., Arasimavicius, A., and Hass, G. M.: Isolation and characterization of mammalian striated myofibrils, p. 47. (b) Fell, H. B.: The effect of vitamin A on organ cultures of skeletal and other tissues, p. 142. (c) Meyer, K.: Outline of problems to be solved in the study of connective tissues, p. 185.
V. (1954) (a) Zweifach, B. W.: The exchange of materials between blood vessels and lymph. (b) Gaudino, M.: Interstitial water and connective tissues. (c) Asboe-Hansen, G.: Hormonal effects on connective tissue.

97. Ramachandran, G. N., editor: Treatise on collagen. I. Chemistry of collagen. New York, 1967, Academic Press, Inc.
(a) Eastoe, J. E.: Composition of collagen and allied proteins, p. 1. (b) Hannig, K., and Nordwig, A.: Amino acid sequences in collagen, p. 73. (c) Ramachandran, G. N.: Structure of collagen at the molecular level, p. 103. (d) Hodge, A. J.: Structure at the electron microscopic level, p. 185. (e) Piez, K. A.: Soluble collagen and the components resulting

from its denaturation, p. 207. (f) von Hippel, P. H.: Structure and stabilization of the collagen molecule in solution, p. 253. (g) Gallop, P. M., Blumenthal, O. O., and Seifter, S.: Subunits and special structural features of tropocollagen, p. 330. (h) Veis, A.: Intact collagen, p. 367. (i) Carver, J. P., and Blout, E. R.: Polypeptide models for collagen, p. 441.

98. Ramanathan, N., editor: Collagen, New York, 1962, Interscience Publishers, Inc.

99. Randall, J. T., editor: Nature and structure of collagen (symposium), New York, 1953, Academic Press, Inc.

(a) Jacobson, W.: Histological survey of the normal connective tissue and its derivatives, p. 6. (b) Robb-Smith, A. H. T.: Significance of collagenase, p. 14. (c) Cruickshank, B., and Hill, A. G. S.: Histochemical identification of a connective tissue antigen, p. 27. (d) Kramer, H., and Little, K.: Nature of reticulin, p. 33. (e) Slack, H. G. B.: Metabolism of collagen in the rat, p. 51. (f) Hoppey, F., McCrae, T. P., and Naylor, A.: X-ray crystallographic investigation of the changes with age in the structure of the human intervertebral disk, p. 65. (g) Armstrong, D. M. G.: Donnan membrane equilibrium in collagen-water systems, p. 91. (h) Robinson, C.: The hot and cold forms of gelatin, p. 96. (i) Jackson, S. F., Kelly, F. C., North, A. C. T., Randall, J. T. Seeds, W. E., Watson, M., and Wilkinson, G. R.: The byssus threads of Mytilus edulis and Pinna nobilis, p. 106. (j) Brown, G. L., Kelly, F. C., and Watson, M.: Quantitative paper chromatography of amino acids in collagen, p. 117. (k) Stack, M. V.: Properties of dentine collagen, p. 124. (l) Martin, A. V. W.: Fine structure of cartilage matrix, p. 129. (m) Jackson, S. F.: Fibrogenesis in vivo and in vitro, p. 140. (n) M'Ewen, M. B., and Pratt, M. I.: Scattering of light by collagen solutions, p. 158. (o) Brown, G. L., and Kelly, F. C.: Electrophoresis of collagen solutions, p. 169. (p) Jackson, D. S.: Chondroitin sulphate as a factor in the stability of tendon, p. 177. (q) Jackson, S. F., and Randall, J. T.: The reconstitution of collagen fibrils from solution, p. 181. (r) Consden, R.: Observations on the composition of human subcutaneous tissue, p. 196. (s) Bowes, J. H., Elliott, R. G., and Moss, J. A.: Some differences in the composition of collagen and extracted collagens and their relation to fibre formation and dispersion, p. 199. (t) Harkness, R. D., Marks, A. M., Muir, H. M., and Neuberger, A.: Precursors of skin collagen, p. 208. (u) Randall, J. T. Brown, G. L., Jackson, S. F., Kelly, F. C., North, A. C. T., Seeds, W. E., and Wilkinson, G. R.: Some physical and chemical properties of extracted skin collagen, p 213. (v) Randall, J. T.: Physical and chemical problems of fibre formation and structure, p. 232. (w) Cowan, P. M., North, A. C. T., and Randall, J. T.: High-angle x-ray diffraction of collagen fibers, p. 241. (x) Seeds, W. E.: Infra-red absorption and collagen structure, p. 250.

100. Rich, A., and Crick, F. H. C.: The molecular structure of collagen, J. Molec. Biol. **3:**483, 1961.

101. Richards, A. N., and Gies, W. J.: Chemical studies of elastin, mucoid and other proteids in elastic tissue, with some notes on ligament extractives, Amer. J. Physiol. **7:**93, 1902.

102. Riley, J. F.: Pharmacology and functions of the mast cells, Pharmacol. Rev. **7:**183, 1955.

103. Riley, J. F.: The riddle of the mast cells, Lancet **1:**841, 1954.

104. Ross, R.: The smooth muscle cell. II. Growth of smooth muscle in culture and formation of elastic fibers, J. Cell Biol. **50:**172, 1971.

105. Ross, R., and Bornstein, P.: The elastic fiber. I. The separation and partial characterization of its macromolecular components, J. Cell Biol. **40:**366, 1969.

106. Ross, R., and Bornstein, P.: Elastic fibers in the body, Sci. Amer. **224:**44, June, 1971.

106a. Ross, R., and Klebanoff, S. J.: The smooth muscle cell. I. *In vivo* synthesis of connective tissue proteins, J. Cell Biol. **50:**159, 1971.

107. Rothman, S.: Physiology and biochemistry of the skin, Chicago, 1954, University of Chicago Press.

(a) Felsher, Z.: Collagen, reticulin and elastin, chap. 17, p. 391. (b) Wells, G. C.: Connective tissue ground substance, chap. 18, p. 418.

108. Sandberg, L. B., Weissman, N., and Smith, D. W.: The purification and partial characterization of a soluble elastin-like protein from copper-deficient porcine aorta, Biochemistry **8:**2940, 1969.

109. Schmitt, F. O., Gross, J., and Highberger, J. H.: Tropocollagen and the properties of fibrosis collagen, Exp. Cell. Res. **3** (supp.):326, 1955.

110. Schmitt, F. O., Levine, L., Drake, M. P., Rubin, A. L., Pfahl, D., and Davison, P. F.: The antigenicity of tropocollagen, Proc. Nat. Acad. Sci. **51**:493, 1964.

111. Schubert, M., and Hamerman, D.: A primer on connective tissue biochemistry, Philadelphia, 1968, Lea & Febiger.

112. Seifter, S., and Gallop, P. M.: In Neurath, H., editor: The proteins, vol. 4, New York, 1966, Academic Press, Inc., p. 238.

113. Shulman, H. J., and Meyer, K.: Cellnular differentiation and the aging process in cartilaginous tissues, J. Exp. Med. **128**:1358, 1968.

114. Siegel, R. C., Pinnell, S. R., and Martin, G. R.: Cross-linking of collagen and elastin: properties of lysyl oxidase, Biochemistry **9**:4486, 1970.

115. Slack, H. G. B.: Metabolism of elastin in the adult rat, Nature **174**:512, 1955.

116. Slack, H. G. B.: Some notes on the composition and metabolism of connective tissue, Amer. J. Med. **26**:113, 1959.

117. Smith, D. W., Weissman, N., and Carnes, W. H.: Cardiovascular studies on copper-deficient swine. XII. Partial purification of a soluble protein resembling elastin, Biochem. Biophys. Res. Commun. **31**:309, 1968.

118. Speakman, P. T.: Proposed mechanism for the biological assembly of collagen triple helix, Nature **229**:241, 1971.

119. Stacy, M., and Barker, S. A.: Carbohydrates of living tissues, New York, 1962, D. Van Nostrand Co., Inc.

120. Starcher, B. C.: The effect of pyridoxine deficiency on aortic elastin biosynthesis, Proc. Soc. Exp. Biol. Med. **132**:379, 1969.

121. Toole, B. P., and Lowther, D.: Dermatan sulphate protein: isolation from and interaction with collagen, Arch. Biochem. **128**:567, 1968.

122. Traub, W., and Piez, K. A.: The chemistry and structure of collagen, Advances Protein Chem. **25**:243, 1971.

123. Tunbridge, R. E., and others, editors: Connective tissue, a symposium, Springfield, Ill., 1957, Charles C Thomas, Publisher.
   (a) Astbury, W. T.: Introduction, p. 1. (b) Asboe-Hansen, G.: On the structure and function of the mast cells, p. 12. (c) Sylvén, B.: On the topographical cystochemistry of tissue mast cells, p. 27. (d) Neuberger, A.: Observations on the presence and metabolism of plasma proteins in skin and tendon, p. 35. (e) Gross, J.: Studies on the fibrogenesis of collagen. Some properties of neutral extracts of connective tissue, p. 45. (f) Jackson, D. S.: The formation and breakdown of connective tissue, p. 62. (g) Jackson, S. F.: Structural problems associated with the formation of collagen fibrils in vivo, p. 77. (h) Meyer, K., Hoffman, P., and Linker, A.: The acid mucopolysaccharides of connective tissue, p. 86. (i) Snellman, O.: Evaluation of extraction methods for acid tissue polysaccharides, p. 97. (j) Delaunay, A., and Bazin, S.: Combinaisons in vitro collagène-mucopolysaccharides et modifications apportés à ces combinaisons par des sels et des polyosides bactériens, p. 105. (k) Gillman, T., Hathorn, M., and Penn, J.: Micro-anatomy and reactions to injury of vascular elastic membranes and associated polysaccharides, p. 120. (l) Snellman, O., Ottoson, R., and Sylvén, B.: On the nature of the metachromatic ground substance polysaccharides of healing wounds, p. 136. (m) Schwarz, W.: Morphology and differentaition of the connective tissue fibers, p. 144. (n) Grassmann, W., Hofmann, U., Kühn, K., Hörmann, H., Endres, H., and Wolf, K.: Electron microscope and chemical studies of the carbohydrate groups of collagen, p. 157. (o) van den Hooff, A.: A few remarks on connective tissues rich in mucoid, p. 172. (p) Robb-Smith, A. H. T.: What is reticulin? p. 177. (q) Gustavson, K. H.: Some new aspects of the stability and reactivity of collagens, p. 185. (r) Verzár, F.: The ageing of collagen, p. 208. (s) Partridge, S. M., Davis, H. F., and Adair, G. S.: The composition of mammalian elastin, p. 222. (t) Hall, D. A.: Chemical and enzymatic studies on elastin, p. 238. (u) Banga, I., and Baló, J.: The structure and chemical composition of connective tissue, p. 254. (v) Bowes, J. H., Elliott, R. G., and Moss, J. A.: The composition of some protein fractions isolated from bovine skin, p. 264. (w) Orekhovitch, V. N., and Shpikiter, V. O.: Procollagens as biological precursors of collagen and the physio-chemical nature of these proteins, p. 281. (x) Muir, H. M.: The structure of a chondroitin sulphate complex from cartilage, p. 294. (y) Reed, R.: The architecture of the collagen fibril, p. 299. (z) Grassmann, W., Hannig, K., Endres, H., and Riedel, A.:

amino acid sequences of collagen, p. 308. (aa) Bear, R. S., and Morgan, R. S.: The composition of bands and interbands of collagen fibrils, p. 321.

124. Vaubel, E.: The form and function of synovial cells in tissue cultures, J. Exp. Med. **58**:85, 1933.
125. Vuust, J., and Piez, K. A.: Biosynthesis of the alpha chains of collagen studied by pulse-labeling in culture, J. Biol. Chem. **245**:6201, 1970.
126. Waksman, B. H., and Mason, H. L.: The antigenicity of collagen, J. Immun. **63**:427, 1949.
127. Weiss, J.: The nature of the reaction between orcein and elastin, J. Histochem. **2**:21, 1954.
128. Zucker, M. B., and Borrelli, J.: Platelet clumping produced by connective tissue suspensions and by collagen, Proc. Soc. Exp. Biol. Med. **109**:779, 1962.

3 • The Marfan syndrome

In an era when slenderness and ectomorphy are
being equated with long life, it may be wise to
*point out an exception**

Historical survey

In 1896[351] the gross skeletal manifestations of the syndrome that bears his name† were described by Marfan,‡ who called the condition *dolichostenomelia* (long, thin extremities) (Fig. 3-2). The condition was renamed arachnodactyly by Achard§ in 1902[3]; Marfan had used the simile "pattes d'araignée," spider legs. Marfan's patient, Gabrielle P., was 5½ years old at the time of the original report[351] and 11½ years old at the time of the follow-up report by Méry and Babonneix.[369] The latter authors commented on Gabrielle's scoliosis, which was studied by the method that had been introduced by Wilhelm Röntgen in the same year as Marfan's report. Gabrielle also had fibrous contractures of the fingers, but no ocular or cardiac abnormality was noted. Méry and Babonneix[369] used the denomination "hyperchondroplasie," a term used also by Rubin[468] (in its anglicized form). In suggesting the designation hyperchondroplasia, they had the contrast with achondroplasia specifically in mind.

Salle[475] in 1912 reported necropsy observations in the case of a 2½-month-old infant who died with cardiac symptoms and showed generalized dilatation of the

---

*From Editorial: New Eng. J. Med. **256:**39, 1957.

†Beals and Hecht[31] suggest that Marfan's patient did not have the Marfan syndrome! They suggest that instead the girl suffered from the disorder that Epstein and colleagues[146] described and that Beals and Hecht refer to as contractural arachnodactyly (p. 169).

‡Antoine Bernard-Jean Marfan (1858-1942), Parisian professor of pediatrics, did much to establish pediatrics as a specialty in France and elsewhere. He was the author of several widely read textbooks and monographs on pediatric topics and editor of *Le Nourrisson* for a great many years. In addition to the syndrome under discussion here, his name is often attached to Marfan's law (that immunity to pulmonary phthisis is conferred by the healing of a local tuberculous lesion) and Marfan's subxiphoid method for aspirating fluid from the pericardial sac.[352] (For other biographic details, see references 11-13, 260; for portrait, see Fig. 3-1.)

§Parish[414] suggested that Achard's patient had a separate disorder characterized by hypognathism, arachnodactyly, and loose-jointedness limited to the hands: Achard's syndrome; see p. 169.

heart and patent foramen ovale. Changes in the mitral leaflets were found in that case.[475] In 1914 Boerger[55] first clearly related ectopia lentis to the other manifestations. As is usually the case, vague references to cases of what was certainly this syndrome can be found in medical reports antedating the definitive descriptions. For instance, Williams,[604] an ophthalmologist in Cincinnati, in 1876

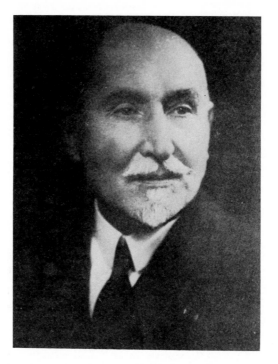

Fig. 3-1. Marfan. (Courtesy Académie de Médecine, Paris.)

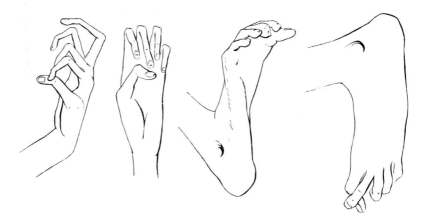

Fig. 3-2. Arachnodactyly in Marfan's case. (From Marfan, A. B.: Bull. Mém. Soc. Med. Hôp. Paris 13:220, 1896.)

described ectopia lentis in a brother and sister who were exceptionally tall and had been loose-jointed from birth. Inasmuch as both Marfan's patient and Achard's patient seem not to have had the Marfan syndrome (see footnotes), Williams' report was over thirty-five years ahead of its time—assuming that the cases of Salle and Boerger were the first valid ones.

Weve of Utrecht,[595] publishing in 1931, first clearly demonstrated the heritable nature of the syndrome and its transmission as a dominant trait. Furthermore, he conceived of this syndrome as a disorder of mesenchymal tissues and accordingly designated it *dystrophia mesodermalis congenita, typus Marfanis*.

The major cardiovascular complications, namely aortic dilatation and dissect-

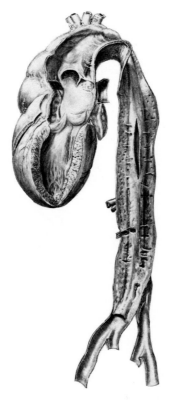

Fig. 3-3. An early reported case[331] of dissecting aneurysm in a patient who in retrospect appears to have had the Marfan syndrome. In 1909 MacCallum reported from The Johns Hopkins Hospital the case (Med. 15454; autopsy 2087) of "L. R., Negro, aged 30 . . . slender built." The man had been seen one year before death, at which time signs of aortic regurgitation were present. The patient was described in life as having a congenital umbilical hernia. A difference in the radial pulses was noted by Dr. Thomas McCrae. Dissecting aneurysm was not suspected, however, by Osler, Rufus Cole, and the other physicians who examined him. There was paralysis of the left recurrent laryngeal nerve. The mother and several brothers had died, as well as the patient's only child, who died at the age of 2 years. No definitely corroboratory features of the family history were recorded, however, and no note of ocular abnormality was made. The ascending aorta, as shown here, resembles that seen in Fig. 3-26E. Furthermore, the pronounced dilatation in the region of the sinuses of Valsalva suggests the Marfan syndrome. (From MacCallum, W. G.: Bull. Hopkins Hosp. **20**:9, 1909.)

ing aneurysm, were first clearly described in 1943 by Baer and associates[20] and by Etter and Glover,[151] respectively. Again, although earlier reports of the aortic complications can be discovered (e.g., reference 77 and Fig. 3-3), these later authors first drew attention to them and opened the way for clearer recognition of the internal medical implications of this syndrome in adults.

It is difficult to imagine a better description of the Marfan syndrome than that given by Bronson and Sutherland[77] in 1918 in the case of a 6-year-old child with aneurysm of the ascending aorta which ruptured into the pericardium. "The unusual shape of his head and ears and the looseness of his joints attracted attention early in infancy." Inguinal hernia was repaired surgically at the age of 2 years, and left diaphragmatic hernia was discovered by x-ray examination. He was always undernourished but was sensitive and mentally advanced for his age, with a quaint way of expressing himself and a "sense of humor of his own." The forehead was high and full, the palate highly arched. The ears were large and without the normal folds of the pinnae. The joints were lax, the limbs were flaillike, and the elbows showed definite subluxation. There were lordosis and pigeon breast with an increased prominence of the right side of the chest, which showed better expansion than the left side. A pulsating mass was discernible to the right of the sternum. Although no diastolic murmur was mentioned, the left ventricle was

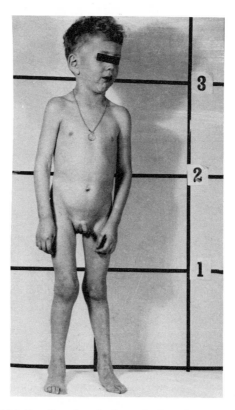

Fig. 3-4A. Photograph of M. D., affected male shown in **B** and **C**, taken in February, 1948 (3½ years of age). Dolichostenomelia is often less impressive at this age.

hypertrophied at autopsy. There was also partial coarctation proximal to the left subclavian artery. The authors presented a detailed review of reports made previous to that time; many of these cases also are reasonably clear instances of the Marfan syndrome.

Gordon[193] and Schwartz[488] have suggested that Abraham Lincoln had the Marfan syndrome.[469] Both based the impression in part on Lincoln's long extremities and statements of his contemporaries that he was unusually loose-jointed. Nathaniel Hawthorne described him as a "tall, loose-jointed figure." The Washington correspondent of the London *Times* described Lincoln as a "tall, lank, lean man, considerably over six feet in height, with stooping shoulders, long pendulous arms terminating in hands of extraordinary dimensions, which, however, were far exceeded in proportion by his feet." Lincoln's mother, Nancy Hanks, who in the opinion of Gordon had the Marfan syndrome, was of unknown paternity. (Her death is more usually attributed to "milk sickness," hypoglycemia

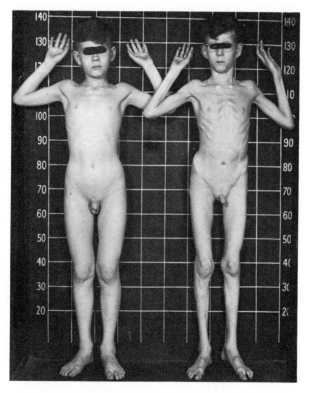

Fig. 3-4B. Brothers, one with the Marfan syndrome. The one on the left is normal, 10 years of age. M. D. (A59949), on the right, is only 8 years old. He shows ectopia lentis, contracture of the fifth fingers (Fig. 3-16*A*), heterochromia iridis (right iris, blue; left, light green), Horner's syndrome on left, lack of subcutaneous fat, high palate, scoliosis, thoracic deformity, and abnormal electroencephalogram. This is probably a sporadic case (original mutation). Contracture of the fifth fingers (clinodactyly or camptodactyly) occurred in other patients of this series (e.g., J. A. M., A65283). Photograph, May, 1953. Heterochromia iridis occasionally is found as an isolated hereditary abnormality, transmitted probably as a dominant.[83] It is sometimes due to birth injury to the cervical sympathetics.

Continued.

from milk from cows that have fed on white snakeroot.) On the other hand, Schwartz[488] believes he has evidence that Lincoln inherited the Marfan gene from his father; he has a patient named Lincoln, with seemingly typical Marfan syndrome, who is a descendant of Lincoln's grandfather. From a photograph of Lincoln, Schwartz[488a] concluded that the president had aortic regurgitation. Lincoln himself on seeing the photograph commented that the foot of the leg crossed over the other was blurred, and concluded that the blurring resulted from movement of that leg from the arterial pulse. Schwartz added the idea that the pulse was exaggerated by the hemodynamic changes of aortic valve leak.

Gordon suggested that Thomas Lincoln, who resembled his father closely and died at 18 years of age of "dropsy of the chest," had the Marfan syndrome with cardiovascular complications.

Because of the obvious general interest, the conclusions of Gordon and Schwartz found their way into the lay press. The public reaction has had interesting features. For example, in a letter-to-the-editor (*Newsweek*, June 11, 1962), one reader insisted that Lincoln could not have suffered from such a "loathsome disease." The statement reflects an unfortunate and uninformed attitude toward hereditary disease, which is no more (or less) loathsome than poliomyelitis, sar-

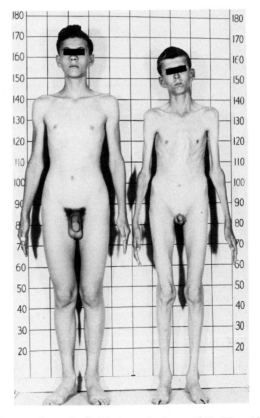

Fig. 3-4C. Same brothers as shown in **B.** Photograph, June, 1958. The older, unaffected brother has now outstripped the affected brother in height.

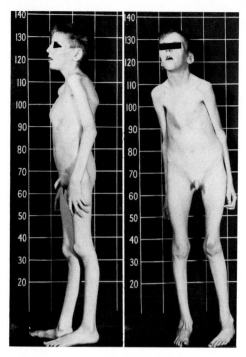

Fig. 3-5A. C. A. B. (B9912; 692938), 7 years old. Pronounced pectus carinatum. Normal mentality. Nystagmus. Bilateral ectopia lentis. "Rocker-bottom" feet. Sparse subcutaneous fat. Photograph, August, 1954.

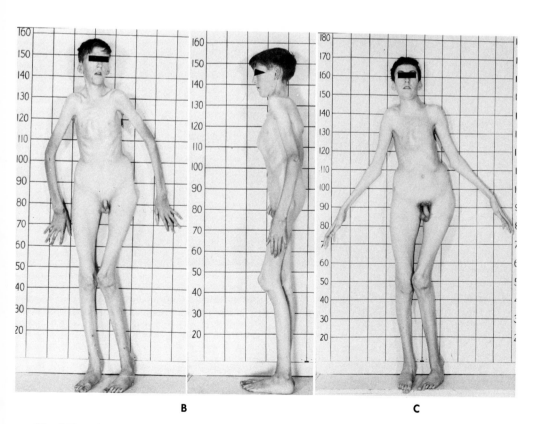

B   C

Fig. 3-5B and C. B, Same patient as shown in A. Photograph, August, 1958. C, Same patient, November, 1960.

coma, myocardial infarction, alcoholism, and cerebral arteriosclerosis, with which other Presidents have been afflicted.

"Marfan's syndrome," or better "the Marfan syndrome," is, in my opinion, the preferred designation until such time as the basic defect is known and an accurate name based thereon can be devised. (F. Parkes Weber[589] was of the same view.) Arachnodactyly is, on the one hand, not striking in some patients; on the other hand, it occurs with other developmental disorders, both acquired and genetic.

Clinical manifestations

Patients with the Marfan syndrome display abnormalities mainly in three areas: the *skeletal system* (where the hallmark is excessive length of the limbs, as well as loose-jointedness, scoliosis, and anterior chest deformity); the *eye* (where the hallmark is ectopia lentis, although myopia and retinal detachment also occur); and the *cardiovascular system* (especially a defect in the tunica media of the ascending aorta, leading to diffuse and/or dissecting aneurysm, but also a defect known as "floppy mitral valve," with mitral regurgitation). Wide variability from case to case, even in a single family, is the rule, and patients may

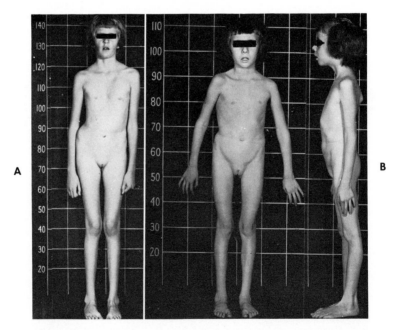

Fig. 3-6. A, M. McG. (A92675), 7 years of age. Bilateral ectopia lentis. Severe pectus excavatum. Highly intelligent. Frequent respiratory infections. Loud systolic murmur of unclear origin. The mother has the full-blown syndrome and is sightless in one eye from spontaneous retinal detachment. This child died at the age of 10 years. The clinical picture was that of mitral regurgitation with progressive cardiac enlargement. Atrial fibrillation had its onset eight months before death. The mitral valve showed three cusps and abnormally short chordae tendineae. The left atrium was huge, with thickened endocardium. Both ventricles were grossly dilated. **B,** D. W. (B8430), 4 years 2 months of age, is thought to have minimal dilatation of the ascending aorta and mitral regurgitation. Also has kyphoscoliosis and ectopia lentis. Parents appear unaffected but parental great-grandfather was 6 feet 7 inches tall.

lack some abnormalities. The patients tend to have a characteristic facial appearance. Children look wise beyond their years. (Compare Figs. 3-23, 3-29, and 3-42.)

Skeletal aspects. See Figs. 3-4B to 3-9 for the various body types encountered. Dolichomorphism characterizes the skeletal abnormality of the syndrome. The victim often suggests the subject of an El Greco painting.* The extremities are long, and characteristically the lower segment (pubis-to-sole) measurement is in excess of the upper segment (pubis-to-vertex) measurement, and the arm span is in excess of height. In general, the more distal bones of the extremities tend to demonstrate this excess length most strikingly. Arachnodactyly is the result (Fig. 3-15).

Skeletal proportions are more important than actual height. It is true that these patients are often very tall. One patient was 6 feet tall at the age of 12 years.[89] Another patient[600] was 7 feet tall. The tallest patient encountered in our

---

*Astigmatism is thought to have been the basis for El Greco's distorted representations, as in *St. Martin and the Beggar* (National Gallery, Washington, D. C.). Actually the legs are not disproportionately long in El Greco figures. Furthermore, as Medawar[305] points out, if El Greco was astigmatic, his paintings would look nonetheless normal to us, since they would have had to look normal to him.

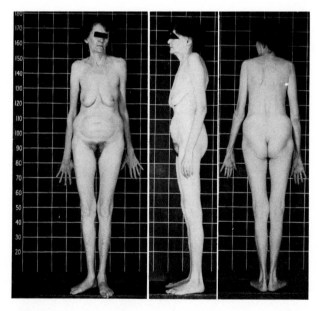

Fig. 3-7. M. P. (362804), 53 years old, one of the oldest patients with the Marfan syndrome I have had the opportunity to examine. I have in the past seen a 59-year-old man with the Marfan syndrome manifested by ectopia lentis, dolichostenomelia, and aortic aneurysm. One man with probable Marfan's syndrome was killed accidentally at the age of 82 years. He was still well preserved at that time. He was 75 inches tall and had fathered at least 2 offspring with full-blown Marfan's syndrome (see Fig. 3-53 for the x-ray film of one) and 4 probably affected individuals out of a sibship numbering 12 in all. Extensive pedigree of the Marfan syndrome. Systolic crunch (extracardiac sound) present for many years. The patient is now (1972) 71 years old.

investigation was 6 feet 7 inches. As indices of arachnodactyly it has been proposed[600] that the hand-height ratio should be greater than 11% and the foot-height ratio greater than 15%. Furthermore, it is stated that the finger, especially the middle finger, should be one and one-half times greater than the lengths of the metacarpal. Excessive length of the inferior patellar ligament has been proposed as a useful diagnostic index. There is so much overlap with the normal proportions that measurement cannot be relied on as the sole diagnostic criterion in individual cases. More significance can be attached to measurements if they are particularly abnormal or if they represent marked deviations from the measurements in certain other members of the family.

Possibly the index of most usefulness, or at least one that is as reliable as any, is the ratio of upper segment (US) to lower segment (LS). The lower segment is measured from the top of the pubic symphysis to the floor. The upper segment is derived by subtracting this value from the height. As indicated by the familiar illustration provided by Stratz in 1902 (Fig. 3-10), the legs grow relatively faster than the trunk during postnatal life. As a result, the midportion of the body moves progressively downward. The US/LS ratio is roughly 0.93 in the normal white adult, having been higher in the prepubertal period. The individual born with the "Marfan gene" tends to have an abnormally low segment ratio in infancy. Furthermore, he passes more rapidly through the sequence shown in Stratz' drawing, overshoots the mark, and ends with a segment ratio in the vicinity of 0.85.

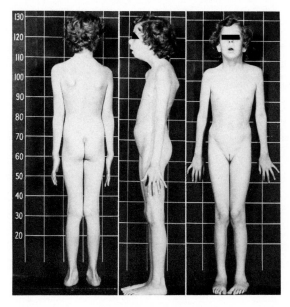

Fig. 3-8. D. L. F. (516670), 7 years of age. The ptosis was thought to be part of the general muscular hypotonia, which was so severe that amyotonia congenita was suspected when the patient was seen at the age of 4 years. Umbilical and bilateral inguinal hernias have been repaired surgically. The feet are very long, flat, and narrow. Kyphoscoliosis is evident. No ectopia lentis or ocular abnormality other than ptosis demonstrated. Intelligent. The ptosis has been corrected surgically since these photographs were taken. The patient may represent a new mutation. Possibly the bilateral ptosis is an independent mutation.

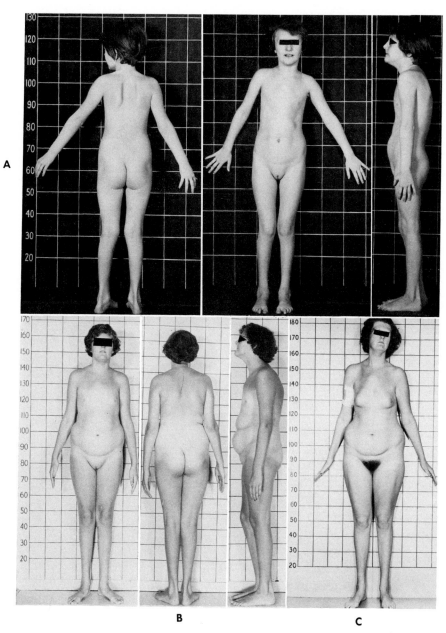

Fig. 3-9. A, J. A. L. (661948), 5 years 8 months of age. Ectopia lentis. Probably *de novo* mutation. Shown very well is the eversion of the feet with low position of the internal malleolus
("rocker bottoms"). Child bright, but highly nervous. Photograph, January, 1954. **B,** Same
patient at age 10 years. Photograph, August, 1958. Sparsity of subcutaneous fat is not demonstrated in all cases of the Marfan syndrome. **C,** Same patient at 14 years of age, November,
1962. The patient is now (1972) about 6 feet tall.

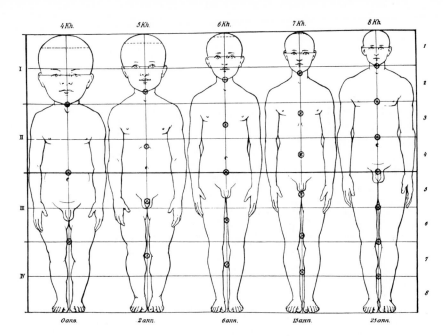

Fig. 3-10. Ordinarily the adult skeletal proportions are not attained until after puberty. There is evidence that the body proportions (as indicated by upper segment—lower segment ratio) are different now than at the turn of the century, when this diagram was made, and that the pattern differs in whites and Negroes. This diagram will require redrawing on the basis of the data presented in Fig. 3-11. (From Stratz, C. H.: Der Körper des Kindes, Stuttgart, 1902, Ferdinand Enke.)

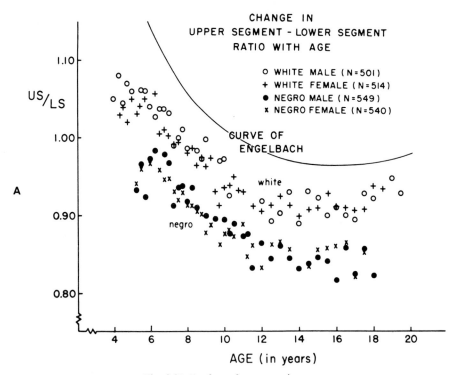

Fig. 3-11. For legend see opposite page.

Because there were no recent data on white persons and no published data whatever on Negroes, measurements of segments were made on 2100 Baltimore schoolchildren of both races and sexes. The data are presented in Fig. 3-11. They should prove useful in the evaluation and follow-up of cases of the Marfan syndrome, as well as in the study of the hemoglobinopathies, endocrinopathies, and other disorders that influence body proportions. It is planned to increase the

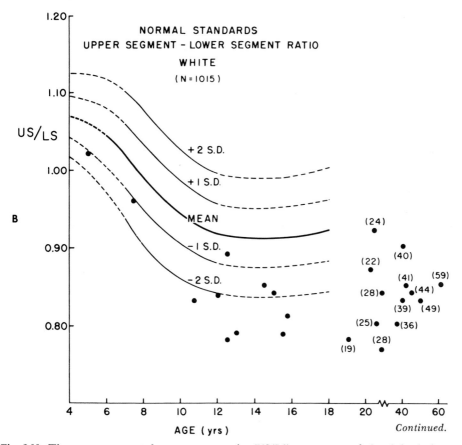

Continued.

Fig. 3-11. The upper segment—lower segment ratio (US/LS) as a gauge of the skeletal changes in the Marfan syndrome. Because of the lack of recent data on US/LS in either whites or Negroes, measurements were made in 1959 on over 2,100 Baltimore schoolchildren. In brief, the findings were as follows: (1) Engelbach's data,[144] compiled from measurements made by various observers in whites only, between about 1860 and 1928, are not presently applicable for either race, **A.** (2) At all ages there is a significantly lower US/LS in Negroes than in whites, **A.** (3) Negroes have a slightly shorter upper segment and slightly longer lower segment than do whites. As a result the US/LS is strikingly different. (4) Within both racial groups no significant sex difference in the mean US/LS or the standard deviations of the means could be demonstrated, at least in the measurements up to the age of about 15 years. This is the rationale for considering the sexes together in **B** and **C.** It will almost certainly be necessary to consider the sexes separately in presenting data now being collected on persons 15 to 30 years of age. As shown in **B** and **C,** the US/LS of most patients with the Marfan syndrome fell in the abnormally low range. Measurements on 34 patients are shown. The number in the parentheses is the age in years. (Data from V. A. McKusick, M. A. Ferguson-Smith, J. T. Leeming, and C. F. Merryman.)

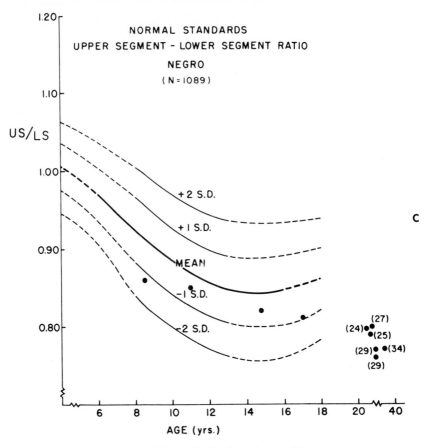

Fig. 3-11, cont'd. For legend see p. 73.

data at both ends of the age span shown in Fig. 3-11 and to extend them to about 30 years of age.

The photograph in the nude on the measured grid cannot be relied on for more than a rough estimate of body proportions. Errors in estimating the site of the pubic symphysis and parallax make for poor reproducibility and inaccuracy in checking with direct measurements.

The dip in the US/LS ratio at the stage of puberty, with subsequent slight rise, is noteworthy.[539] If puberty is delayed, the dip may be even more striking. The possibility of the Marfan syndrome was raised in the patient (E. K., 766137) shown in Fig. 3-59B. The presence of gynecomastia strengthens the impression of anomalous pubertal transition.

Sinclair and co-workers[509] suggested the metacarpal index as an objective indication of arachnodactyly. In the x-ray film of the right hand, the length (in millimeters) of the second, third, fourth, and fifth metacarpals is measured. At the exact midpoint of each shaft, the breadth is also measured, and this value is divided into the length. The figures for the four metacarpals are averaged. The metacarpal index is, then, the average ratio of length to breadth of metacarpals II to V. The data from 20 cases of the Marfan syndrome and 100 normal subjects

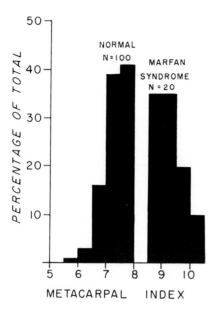

Fig. 3-12. Metacarpal index. (Data from Sinclair, R. J. G., Kitchin, A. H., and Turner, R. W. D.: Quart. J. Med. **29**:19, 1960.)

Table 3-1. Upper limits of normal for metacarpal index in adults*

	Male		Female	
	Left	**Right**	**Left**	**Right**
Mean + 2 S.D.	8.0	7.7	8.7	8.6
Mean + 3 S.D.	8.4	8.2	9.2	9.1

*From Parish, J. G.: Skeletal hand charts in inherited connective tissue disease, J. Med. Genet. **4**:227, 1967.

are plotted in Fig. 3-12. Since skeletal features alone were accepted in the diagnosis of the Marfan syndrome, some circular reasoning may have entered this study. The frequency distribution is distinctly peculiar; it suggests a continuous distribution with one class missing. Parish[415] and Eldridge[141] reported metacarpal index data. Parish[415] provided data on the upper limits of normality of the metacarpal index, as given in Table 3-1. He also gave data on the "relative slimness" —ratio of breadth to length—of normal proximal and distal phalanges. In one patient with the Marfan syndrome, more striking changes were found in the slimness index of the proximal phalanges than in the metacarpal index. Table 3-2 presents data on the metacarpal index of normal Caucasian infants 2 years old and younger.[275] Compare with these the measurements in 3 infants with the Marfan syndrome: a 6-month-old boy had an index of 7.0; a 12-month-old girl, 8.4; a 24-month-old girl, 7.4. It is doubtful that the metacarpal index is more specific than the US/LS ratio or the ratio of arm span to height. It may be useful, however, to have another objective measure of skeletal peculiarity.

Sickle cell anemia is a recognized cause of growth disturbance that can result in body proportions resembling those of the Marfan syndrome. The patient (D. M., 659463) shown in Fig. 3-59*A* is an example. The osseous hyperemia that accompanies hyperactivity of the bone marrow in the long bones may be the mechanism.

Table 3-2. Metacarpal index of 25 English boys and 25 girls during first two years*

Age (mo.)	Sex	Mean	S.D.
6	M	5.23	0.46
	F	5.60	0.37
12	M	5.30	0.41
	F	5.75	0.41
18	M	5.28	0.40
	F	5.82	0.45
24	M	5.40	0.43
	F	5.84	0.43

*From Joseph, M. C., and Meadow, S. R.: The metacarpal index of infants, Arch. Dis. Child. **44**:515, 1969.

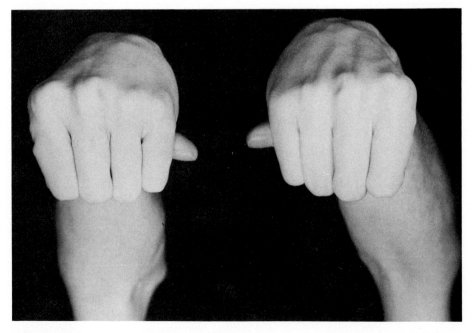

Fig. 3-13. Steinberg thumb sign in the Marfan syndrome. A combination of narrow hand, long digits, and loose-jointedness permits the thumb to extend well beyond the ulnar surface of the hand when held as shown here.

In cases of the Marfan syndrome the occurrence of kyphoscoliosis with shortening of the trunk also reduces the segment ratio; two factors, trunk shortening and extremity lengthening, are collaborating in producing the low segment ratio. However, before the age of 10 or 12 years kyphoscoliosis is in most cases not of sufficient severity to be of major significance.

The relatively narrow palm of the hand, together with a long thumb and loose-jointedness, is the basis of Steinberg's thumb sign.[528] The thumb opposed across the palm extends well beyond the ulnar margin of the hand (Fig. 3-13). Feingold[163] found the "thumb sign" positive in 1.1% of normal white children and 2.7% of normal Negro children. It was negative in children with homocystinuria (Chapter 4). The wrist sign[586] reflects both the thin wrist and the long digitis; the thumb and fifth finger, when clasped around the wrist, usually overlap appreciably in the patient with the Marfan syndrome (Fig. 3-14).

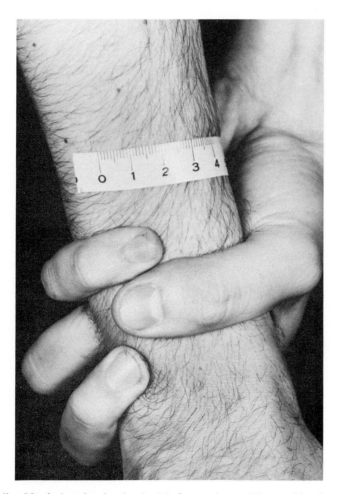

Fig. 3-14. Walker-Murdoch wrist sign in the Marfan syndrome. The combination of thin wrist and long digits results in overlap of fingers I and V when the wrist is grasped as shown here.

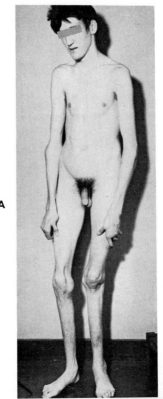

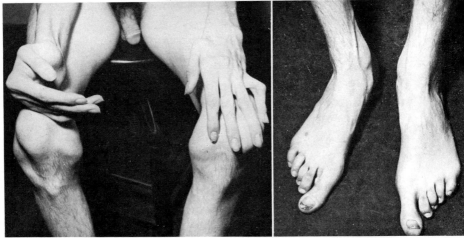

Fig. 3-15. H. W. (464314), 17 years old. Died suddenly at home eighteen months later. The patient was moderately crippled by the skeletal abnormality. Pain in the joints, especially those of the knees, seemed to be related to the loose-jointedness. A long follow-up in an orthopedic clinic. Ectopia lentis. Referred because of spontaneous retinal detachment. **A,** General view. **B,** Striking arachnodactyly with partial contractures of fingers. Children delight in doing contortions with their fingers but should not be permitted to do this, since serious damage may result. **C,** Extraordinary length of the great toes is well demonstrated. Even more pronounced excess of length of great toe shown in case illustrated by Whitfield and associates.[600]

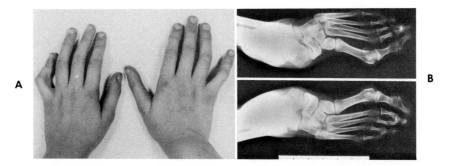

Fig. 3-16. A, Flexion deformity (camptodactyly) of fifth fingers, particularly on left. Taken at age of 38 months in M. D. (A59949), who is shown at a later age in Fig. 3-4B. Other patients in this series have shown this feature. **B,** X-ray films of feet in case with so-called "rocker bottoms," i.e., pronounced flatfoot. Patient J. M. (544088); see also Fig. 3-31.

At times the great toes are elongated out of proportion to the others (Fig. 3-15C).[6,159,393,561] This may be related to the fact that the terminal center of ossification normally appears somewhat earlier in the metatarsus of the great toe than of the others. (The long bones of the hands and feet usually grow from one terminus only or predominantly. The first metatarsal has a proximal epiphyseal junction, whereas the epiphysis is distal in the other metatarsals—another point of difference in development of the first and other toes.) Hallux valgus and contractures of the toes—hammertoes—are frequent (Fig. 3-17D). Fifth-finger camptodactyly, a frequent finding in the Marfan syndrome (e.g., Figs. 3-15B, 3-16A, and 3-19B), is a comparable abnormality. In one family, members of which are shown in Fig. 3-66, camptodactyly extending to all four fingers was present in members of several generations, and in some—e.g., the father of the proband—it was a leading feature of the Marfan syndrome. (See p. 168 for a discussion of the differential diagnosis of camptodactyly.)

The ribs participate in the excessive longitudinal growth with formation of pectus excavatum (Fig. 3-6A), "pigeon breast" (Fig. 3-5), or less symmetric varieties (Fig. 3-18A) of thoracic cage deformity. The bones of the skull and face are likewise affected, with resulting dolichocephaly, highly arched palate, long, narrow face, and prognathism. (That a palate is highly arched is a subjective statement. Methods for palate measurement are available.[295,445,457,496] The gothic palate is not specific to the Marfan syndrome. Patients with congenital or early myopathy, such as myotonic dystrophy or nemaline myopathy, have a high-arched palate. The possibility of a diagnosis of the Marfan syndrome is sometimes raised in such patients.) There may be "spurring" of the heels as a result of excessive length of the os calcis.

Redundancy and "weakness" of joint capsules, ligaments, tendons, and fascia are responsible for a large group of manifestations, including pes planus; genu recurvatum; hyperextensibility of joints; habitual dislocation of hips,[204] patella,[408] clavicles, mandible,[379] and other joints; ganglia*; hernias; synovial diverticula*;

---

*In one case,[33] a peculiar pelvic cyst communicating with the lining of the sacral canal occasioned difficulties in delivery.

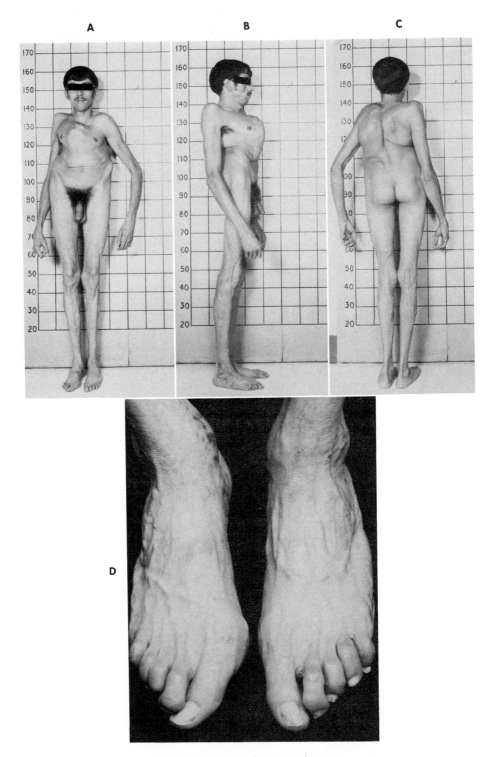

Fig. 3-17. For legend see opposite page.

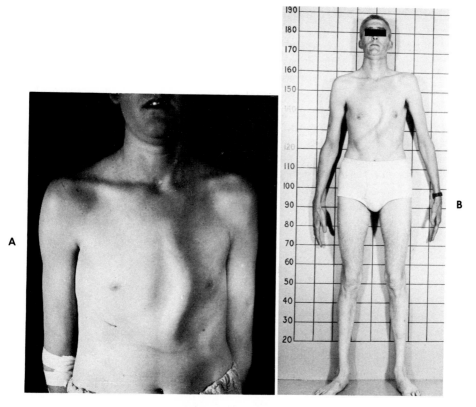

Fig. 3-18. A, Asymmetric pigeon-breast type of chest deformity in 14-year-old boy (J. S., 543026) with full Marfan's syndrome. This particular type of anterior chest deformity seems to be of frequent occurrence in the Marfan syndrome. At the age of 18 years, the patient was 73 inches tall. Incomplete right bundle branch block is present. The patient's father was 6 feet 7 inches tall, and at the age of 28 years died suddenly on a bus. He had been observed for two years for aortic regurgitation that had been considered rheumatic in origin. **B,** Same patient in 1963, age 29 years. (See reference 20 for photographs of the external appearance of this patient; also p. 356 of reference 602.)

Fig. 3-17. Severe scoliosis in the Marfan syndrome. L. Y. (J.H.H. 1399693), aged 29 years, is only 63 inches tall, with a low US/LS value, as demonstrated by the pictures, **A, B,** and **C.** He has bilateral slight upward displacement of the lenses, marked striae distensae of both thighs, bilateral varicosities of the leg veins, and pes planus, with contracture of the toes, **D,** but no heart murmur and no hernia. Respiratory function tests showed severe reduction in forced vital capacity; the CO diffusing capacity at rest was moderately reduced. The patient's older brother, R. Y. (J.H.H. 568718), died of profound heart failure and uremia secondary to the aortic and mitral regurgitation of the Marfan syndrome. A younger sister has the Marfan syndrome. The mother and the mother's father died of aortic rupture, and a maternal uncle has the Marfan syndrome.

and kyphoscoliosis. Bilateral dislocation of the hips was present at birth in the affected daughter of the girl with the Marfan syndrome shown in Fig. 3-32. Because of the loose-jointedness, the long limbs, and the thin torso, the patient is often able to touch his umbilicus with the right hand passed around the back and approaching the umbilicus from the left. The "flat feet" are often so advanced that the internal malleolus almost literally rests on the floor (Fig. 3-16B). Much less commonly a pes cavus deformity is present.[606] Kyphoscoliosis can be very severe (Fig. 3-18B). In rare instances, hemivertebra is responsible in part for spinal deformity.[326] At times, the spinal deformity has been thought to be due to Scheuermann's epiphysitis.[349] Scoliosis is likely to increase rapidly during the years of maximal vertebral growth, from 11 to 15 years of age. Early recognition of scoliosis is assisted by examining the patient in a bending-forward position. This maneuver renders asymmetry more obvious because of angulation of the ribs on one side.[458] While the deformity is still slight much can be accomplished

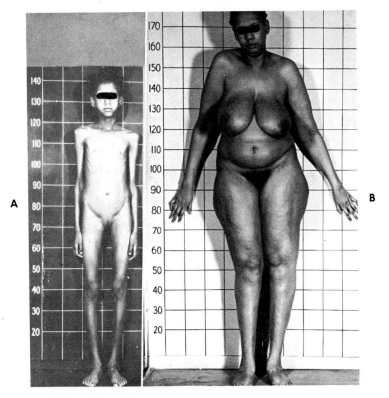

Fig. 3-19A and B. L. T. (221183), at the age of 8 years, **A,** and at age 23, **B.** At 8 years the patient is virtually the same height as M. D. (Fig. 3-4B), also 8 years old. The patient became almost completely blind from bilateral retinal detachment. With the inactivity associated therewith, she became very obese, as demonstrated in **B.** White atrophic striae appeared on the shoulders, upper arms, hips, and thighs, as has been described previously in patients with Marfan's syndrome.[589] The patient probably had rheumatic fever with carditis as a child, but no residua are detectable. She has demonstrated, in addition to ectopia lentis, accessory rudimentary sixth digit bilaterally, highly arched palate, and pupils that react poorly to mydriatics.

by means of exercises and other measures. Nelson[393] emphasizes the presence of a large spinal canal, the enlargement being in depth or width or both. Mitchell and co-workers[376] described a patient with many skeletal features of the Marfan syndrome and with a sacral arachnoid cyst and pelvic meningocele. (The lateral view of the lumbar vertebrae suggested the osteoporosis seen in homocystinuria.) Scalloping, an exaggeration of the normal slight concavity of the dorsal aspect of the vertebral bodies, has been described in the Marfan syndrome[393,605] and also in the Ehlers-Danlos syndrome (p. 83).

Sinclair[508] found complaints of musculoskeletal nature of sufficient severity "to warrant medical attendance" in 20 of 40 cases of the Marfan syndrome. Of the 20 patients, 7 had low back pain. Two of these were at first considered to have ankylosing spondylitis. In 5 cases there were joint effusions; of these, 3 had been diagnosed as tubercular, 1 as rheumatic fever, and 1 as rheumatoid arthritis. Hip joint pain was severe in 2. Metatarsalgia was prominent in 3 patients. Precocious osteoarthrosis tends to develop in patients with joint hypermobility of any cause[291] but cannot be said to be a conspicuous feature of the Marfan syndrome.

Even femoral hernias occur rather commonly in men with the Marfan syndrome, and diaphragmatic hernia has been present in some of our patients and in some of those reported.[293] Hydrocele is occasionally present (Fig. 3-29).

Muscular underdevelopment and hypotonia is a frequent[158,554] but by no means invariable feature. This feature has been so striking as to suggest a primary disorder of muscle in some instances. The converse error of diagnosis—

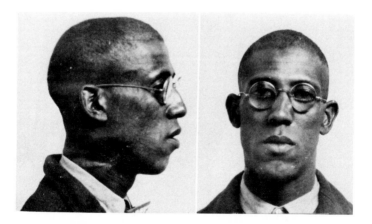

Fig. 3-19C. Prison photograph of the proposita's father (B. R.). The character of the spectacles suggests hyperopia, an unusual although occasional finding in the Marfan syndrome. He had several admissions to the Norfolk, Va., General Hospital (A46772) for hernia repair, for acute dissection of the aorta (age 38), for varicose veins, and for pain in the low back. The final hospital admission was to the St. Luke's Hospital, Newburgh, N. Y., because of severe pain up and down his back. Profound aortic regurgitation and a pulsating abdominal mass were discovered. Serologic tests for syphilis were negative. The patient died suddenly (age 39). Autopsy revealed old dissection of the aorta with recent rupture into the pericardial cavity, and tamponade. Both the father and the paternal grandfather of this man seem to have had the Marfan syndrome, making a total of four generations affected.

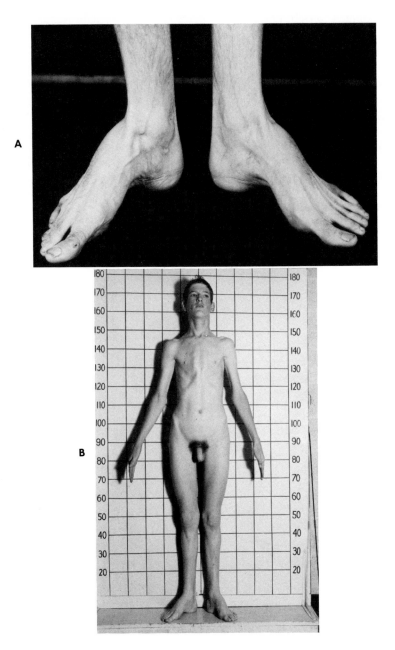

Fig. 3-20. Pes cavus in the Marfan syndrome. E. B. (J.H.H. 940374) shows pes cavus, **A,** in association with otherwise typical Marfan skeletal features, **B.** He also has ectopia lentis. The brother, J. B. (J.H.H. 940375), and the mother, I. B. (J.H.H. 221234), have the more usual flatfoot of the Marfan syndrome. The mother died of aortic complications of the Marfan syndrome.

primary muscular dystrophy called Marfan's syndrome—has occurred in isolated instances (Fig. 3-64*A* and *B*). It is probable that the muscular manifestations are secondary to the abnormality of bones and joints and to abnormality of the perimysial connective tissue and are not due to primary involvement of the muscle cell itself. This view is supported by the finding of a normal creatinine coefficient, an index of total muscle mass.[565]

Pronounced sparsity of subcutaneous fat is a striking feature of most cases (Figs. 3-4*B* and 3-5*A*) and is not easily reconciled with a fundamental defect of connective tissue. In children, it may be that the rapid growth accounts for the failure to store fat. One patient who was thin as a child has become exceedingly obese in recent years (she is now 35 years old), due in large part to inactivity associated with the blindness produced by bilateral retinal detachment (Fig. 3-19*A* and *B*). As demonstrated in Fig. 3-9*B*, others of these patients may have abundant subcutaneous fat.

Van Buchem[571] concluded that bone age is in advance of chronologic age and that the epiphyses tend to close earlier than normal. In our group of patients no marked deviation was observed, although no systematic controlled observa-

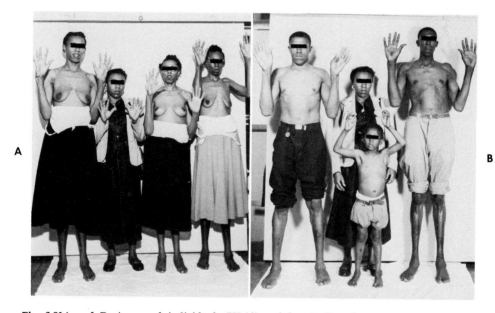

Fig. 3-21A and B. A normal individual (III-12) and her 5 sibs affected by the Marfan syndrome (III-15, III-14, III-13, III-11, and III-8). In **B** is a 4-year-old affected member (IV-13) of the next generation, son of III-8. (The numbers correspond to those used in a pedigree shown in Fig. 3-40*A*.) Individual III-11 subsequently died of bacterial endocarditis engrafted on a mitral valve probably affected by connective tissue changes of the Marfan syndrome.[335] There was chromotropic degeneration of the ascending aorta and pulmonary artery, as well as advanced congenital cystic disease of the lungs. Individual III-14 is 78 inches tall. (History numbers: 176836, 176837, 176838, 103632, 637693, 637694, 392843.) The father of the sibship (W. R., 101043) died suddenly at home at the age of 43 years, presumably of aortic rupture. He was well known as a patient with the Marfan syndrome and had been under treatment for a cardiac ailment with aortic regurgitation for about two years. (Individual III-15 of the pedigree, the adult male on the far left in **B,** died in 1956 with aortic regurgitation.)

Continued.

tions were undertaken. Certainly the excess length of the legs is not due to delayed closure of the epiphyses. The excess length is often demonstrable at birth (Fig. 3-21*I*) and throughout childhood and adolescence.

The eye.[7,245,460,542] Ectopia lentis, almost always bilateral, is the hallmark of ocular involvement in this syndrome (Fig. 3-22). The suspensory ligaments, when visualized with the slit lamp, are redundant, attenuated, and often broken. The lower ligaments are more likely to be defective, with displacement of the lens upward as the usual finding. The lens is often abnormally small[166,320,321] and spherical. Iridodonesis, tremor of the iris, is often a tip-off to the presence of dislocation of the lens. Occasionally the edge of the dislocated lens is visible through the undilated pupil, or, of course, there may be complete dislocation of the lens into the anterior chamber. To exclude minor subluxation it is necessary to dilate the pupil fully and perform a slit-lamp examination. Bowers[69] describes an in-

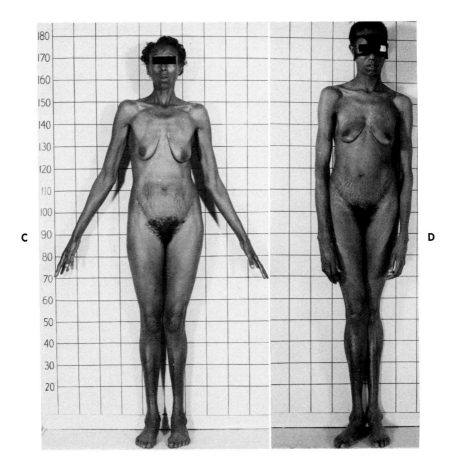

Fig. 3-21C and D. C, P. R. (103632), individual III-8 in Fig. 3-40*A*, 33 years of age. Bilateral ectopia lentis and dolichosteonomelia. The patient died at the age of 34 years. Autopsy revealed pulmonary embolus. The base of the aorta was thin-walled. An anomalous flap of the mitral valve caused mitral regurgitation. **D,** H. R. (176837), individual III-13 in Fig. 3-40*A*, 29 years of age. Bilateral ectopia lentis and dolichostenomelia.

teresting family in which members would seek the presence of dislocation by gently shaking the infant or small child while observing the eye in bright sunlight. The appearance of the dislocated lens was aptly compared to the bubble in a spirit level. When complete or almost complete detachment of the lens occurs, the patient can move the lenses about voluntarily[114] by changing the position of the head (e.g., J. B., 940375).

Jarrett[266] reviewed 166 cases of ectopia lentis admitted to this hospital. These included 24 cases of the Marfan syndrome, 2 of homocystinuria (some of the "Marfan" cases may have had this disorder instead), and 2 of the Weill-Marchesani syndrome. The most frequent cause was trauma, in 85 cases. Of the 85 traumatic cases, 27% had a positive serologic test for syphilis. A coincidence of trauma and syphilis may be merely a reflection of the social behavior of the population living in the vicinity of The Johns Hopkins Hospital.

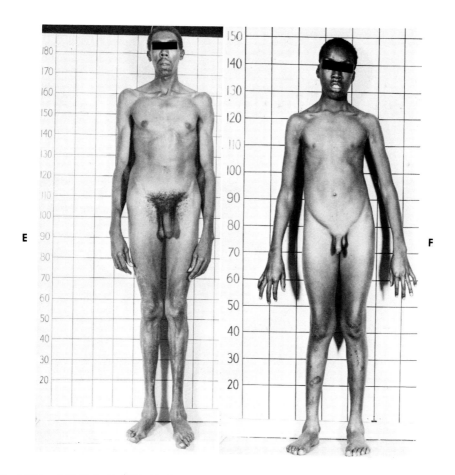

Fig. 3-21E and F. E, L. R. (176838), individual III-14 in Fig. 3-40*A*, 24 years of age. Bilateral ectopia lentis and dolichostenomelia. **F,** J. R. (637698), individual IV-8 in Fig. 3-40*A*, 11 years of age. Bilateral ectopia lentis and dolichostenomelia.

Continued.

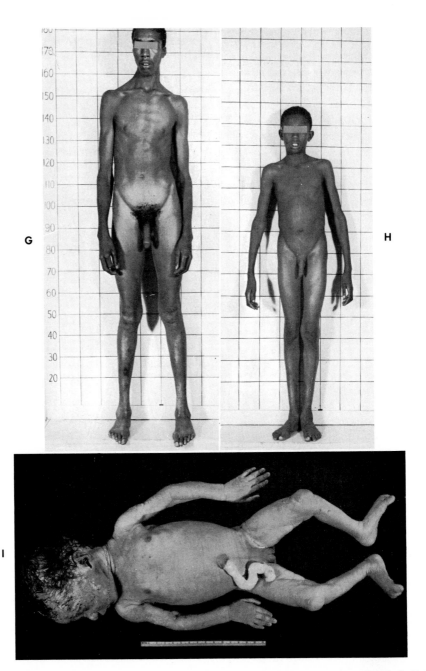

Fig. 3-21G to I. G, Same patient as shown in **F,** 15½ years of age. **H, P. R.** (637693), individual IV-13 in Fig. 3-40*A,* 9½ years of age. Bilateral ectopia lentis and dolichostenomelia. **I,** The still-born infant (autopsy 29095) of patient shown in Fig. 3-40*B.* The infant is believed to be affected. For her age (8½ months) the foot was probably long (7.25 cm. as compared with 6.5). The crown-heel measurement was 46 cm. (usual, 43.5) and the crown-anus dimension 30.5 cm. (usual, 28 cm.). See reference 325 for normal standards used in these studies. The infant showed no other abnormality on gross and histologic study, except an abnormality of pulmonary lobation of the type described in cases of the Marfan syndrome. Specifically, the aorta was grossly and histologically normal! Heldrich and Wright[241] described 2 live-born infants in whom the diagnosis was made in the neonatal period.

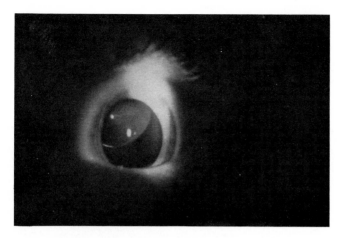

Fig. 3-22. Displacement upward and temporally of the lens in a case of the Marfan syndrome. (Courtesy Dr. Béla Varga, Eger, Hungary.)

Among Marfan patients, Jarrett[266] found 8 eyes in which retinal detachment occurred before lens extraction and only 3 in which it occurred (all within three months) after lens extraction.

At least a third of spontaneous ectopia lentis occurs as a component of the Marfan syndrome.[266] Homocystinuria and the Weill-Marchesani syndrome (discussed in Chapters 4 and 5, respectively) together account for 5% to 10% of cases. Of all patients with the Marfan syndrome, about 80% have ectopia lentis.

Heterochromia iridis was present in at least 2 patients in this series (Figs. 3-4B and 3-53).

Myopia is usually present in rather high degree. The excessive length of the eyeball appears to indicate involvement of the sclera, fundamentally a ligamentous structure, in the basic connective tissue defect. Staphyloma (protrusion of the sclera) was repaired with a scleral graft in a 5-year-old girl by Goldberg and Ryan.[187] The scleral defect occasionally has its counterpart in the cornea as keratoconus[16] or as megalocornea[533] (G. H., B50120). Megalocornea is often impressive to the unaided eye (Figs. 3-23 and 3-42P). Wachtel,[582] in an anatomic study of the eye from 4 patients with the Marfan syndrome, found enlargement of the globe and microphakia. The two factors summate in causing the myopic refractive error. The spherophakia may be the result of lack of the normal tension on the lens by the suspensory ligament.

The sclera may be impressively blue in the Marfan syndrome.[53] Clouding of the cornea occurs occasionally; this is probably not a primary element of the connective tissue disease but rather a result of the secondary iritis and glaucoma.

Spontaneous retinal detachment[385] occurs with what is probably an unusually high incidence and is a frequent complication of lens extraction. In one series,[385] 9 of 142 cases of juvenile retinal detachment had the Marfan syndrome. Retinal detachment is probably related in part to the long myopic eyeball and therefore indirectly to the connective tissue defect; that there is a more direct relationship is strongly suspected[250] because of the high incidence in the Marfan syndrome even without more than a moderate degree of myopia. The pupil is often difficult to dilate in the Marfan syndrome, and the dilator muscle appears to be hypoplastic.[478]

Ectopia lentis *per se* would probably represent relatively little impairment of vision. Severe myopia (20 diopters in Boerger's[55] case), retinal detachment, and the iritis and/or glaucoma that may result from the ectopia lentis are often re-

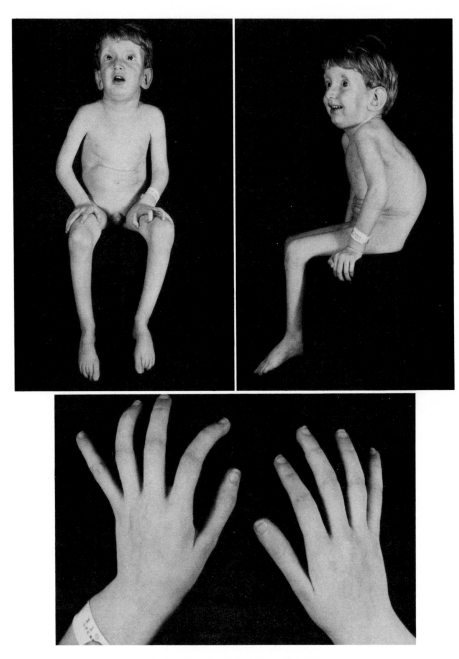

Fig. 3-23. For legend see opposite page.

sponsible for severe limitation of visual acuity or even for total blindness. The lens may become secondarily cataractous.

I was previously suspicious that estimations that only 50% to 70% of persons with clear-cut Marfan's syndrome have ectopia lentis were incorrectly low as a result of inadequate examination of the eyes and that virtually 100% would display at least minor redundancy of the suspensory ligament if subjected to maximal mydriasis and slit-lamp examination. It may be true that the first estimate above is indeed too low. However, we have now observed patients who showed advanced Marfan's disease with characteristic habitus, involvement of other members of the family, and dissection of the aorta, with autopsy demonstration of pathognomonic changes in the tunica media, who did not have ocular abnormality on careful examination. For example, in the 2 brothers shown in Fig. 3-31*A* and *B* there were characteristic changes discovered in the skeleton and aorta but no ectopia lentis. However, 3 of the 5 children of one of the men do show ectopia lentis, as well as skeletal changes. Furthermore, the older brother shown in Fig. 3-24 has no ectopia lentis although the diagnosis of Marfan syndrome is undoubted.

By gonioscopy, von Noorden and Schultz[580] detected changes in the angle of the anterior chamber of the eye, bridging pectinate strands, iris processes, irregularity and fraying of the iris root, etc. (Fig. 3-25). These findings are not specific for the Marfan syndrome, since they were found by Burian and associates[80] in a variety of conditions that may be construed as connective tissue disorders: severe idiopathic scoliosis, idiopathic genu varum, Legg-Perthes disease, slipped upper femoral epiphyses, and Osgood-Schlatter disease. When the angle changes are extreme in the Marfan syndrome, they may lead to glaucoma.[79] Contact lenses[383] have been found satisfactory by a number of patients (e.g., R. L., 864749).

Cardiovascular system.[200,335,346,504] Since most of the early autopsies in cases of this syndrome were in infants and children (who might not yet have developed the characteristic changes in the great vessels) and since interatrial septal defect was found (probably largely by coincidence) in several of the cases, this malformation and "congenital heart disease" in general came to be considered

---

Fig. 3-23. J. S. (1184635) was born in 1964. The diagnosis of the Marfan syndrome was made at birth by the pediatrician. Right inguinal hernia was detected at 2 weeks and was corrected surgically at 3 months of age. Kyphoscoliosis was first noted at 1 year. When first seen at this hospital at 20 months of age (after two episodes of congestive heart failure), he demonstrated signs of severe Marfan syndrome: striking arachnodactyly, subluxated lenses, large anterior segments of the eyes, and mitral regurgitation. Cardiac catheterization showed mild tricuspid regurgitation, dilated pulmonary artery and aortic root without regurgitation, and severe mitral regurgitation.

The father, aged 33, and the mother, aged 30 years at his birth, as well as 4 sibs, were unaffected. The child died March 4, 1968, of heart failure at the age of 4 years. Autopsy (Dr. W. E. B. Hall) showed marked generalized cardiac enlargement, changes in the tricuspid aortic and mitral valves, and a remarkably thin-walled aorta without aneurysm (indeed of reduced caliber). The tricuspid and mitral valves were thickened and puckered. The mitral orifice was reduced in size, suggesting mitral stenosis. The mitral chordae were thickened. The left atrium was markedly dilated, with thickening of the endocardium. The aortic valve had a peculiar cordlike thickening of the entire margin of one cusp and part of a second.

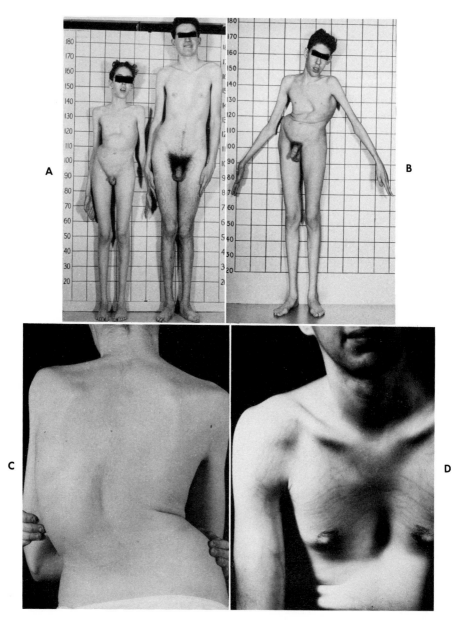

Fig. 3-24. Brothers with the Marfan syndrome (871800; 871801). **A,** The older brother (right), age 17, has no detectable ocular or intrinsic cardiovascular anomaly, although the skeletal features, especially pectus excavatum and scoliosis, are pronounced. In him the diagnosis of the Marfan syndrome could not have been made with confidence but for the facts that his younger brother (left), age 13, has ectopia lentis and even more marked skeletal abnormalities and that the father, who had similar skeletal characteristics, died at 36 years of age, of aortic regurgitation. **B,** The younger brother at age 15. **C,** Severe scoliosis in the younger brother. **D,** Striae distensae in the older brother, in infrared photograph.

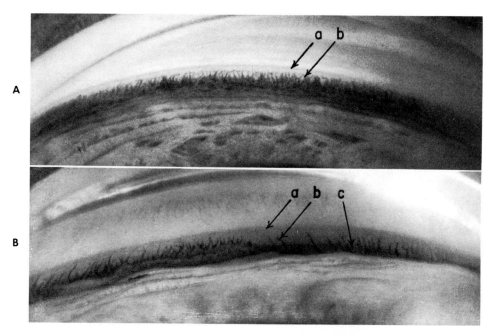

Fig. 3-25. The angle of the anterior chamber in 2 cases of the Marfan syndrome with ectopia lentis: **a,** Schwalbe's line; **b,** pectinate ligaments; **c,** ciliary body band. In both **A** and **B,** note the pectinate strands as described by von Noorden and Schultz.[580] In **B** note the irregular insertion of the peripheral iris. (Courtesy Dr. Gunter K. von Noorden, Baltimore, Md.)

the usual form of cardiovascular involvement. As more adult cases were recognized, it became apparent (1) that an inborn weakness (with subsequent degeneration) of the tunica media of the aorta and main pulmonary artery is of much greater statistical importance and is of more functional importance in the individual patient and (2) that this abnormality is an abiotrophy, not a congenital malformation. The abnormality of the tunica media may result in diffuse dilatation of the ascending aorta or pulmonary artery, in dissecting aneurysm, or in a combination of dilatation and dissection. Striking involvement of the pulmonary artery occurs[20,335,568] much less commonly than the corresponding involvement of the aorta. However, a clinical picture like that of so-called[281] "congenital idiopathic dilatation of the pulmonary artery" may occur,[90] as well as dissecting aneurysm of the pulmonary artery.[9,603] (See Figs. 3-41 and 3-48.) A yet more recent development in the nosography of the Marfan syndrome is appreciation of the importance, in terms of frequency and functional significance, of mitral regurgitation.

In the aorta, dilatation usually begins in the aortic ring* and intrapericardial portion of the ascending aorta, as suspected clinically and as demonstrated in patients dying before further progression of their disease.[327] This initial dilata-

---

*The term "aortic ring" is recognized to be inexact and difficult to define in precise anatomic terms. As used here it refers to the very base of the aorta, particularly the sinuses of Valsalva and the lines of attachment of the aortic cusps. Annuloaortic ectasia is the term used by Chapman and colleagues[92] to designate the change that occurs in the Marfan aorta.

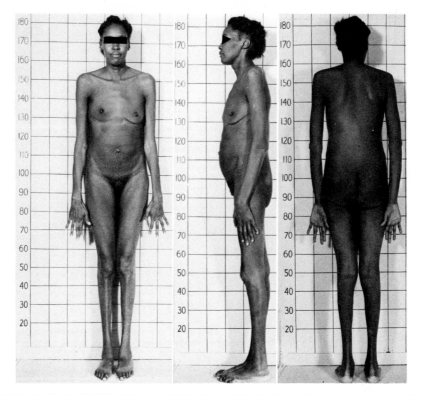

Fig. 3-26A. L. F. Y. (690823), 33 years old. Patient died of effects of severe aortic regurgitation. Autopsy revealed characteristic changes in the media of the aorta and pulmonary artery, with old dissecting aneurysm of the ascending aorta. The dissection may have occurred during pregnancy.

tion, together with stretching of the aortic cusps, may produce profound aortic regurgitation before clear roentgenologic signs of aortic dilatation[567] are present (Figs. 3-26B and 3-31 to 3-33). If syphilis, rheumatism, and bacterial endocarditis can be excluded, traumatic rupture of an aortic cusp is often suspected.[34,335] (See Fig. 3-28.)

Furthermore, a deceptive prominence of the pulmonary conus and main pulmonary artery may be produced by the dilated aortic base and may compound the confusion.[20,335,417] (Dilatation of the pulmonary artery itself contributes to the prominence.) In a case of mine (J. M., J.H.H. 544088) the aneurysm at the base of the aorta apparently caused partial obstruction of outflow from the right ventricle with the development of progressive right axis deviation, as shown by electrocardiogram. In these cases, the second heart sound in the pulmonary area may be unusually loud due to close proximity of the pulmonary artery to the anterior chest wall.

Aortic dilatation is usually progressive. The patient may be free of symptoms for five or more years after the development of aortic regurgitation, but once angina pectoris or symptoms of left ventricular failure have developed, he may live no more than two years. On the whole, the prognosis is quite similar to that

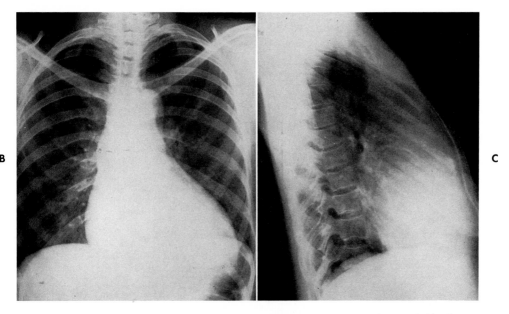

B   C

Fig. 3-26B and C. Posteroanterior and lateral views of chest in L. F. Y. It is remarkable that enlargement of the aorta is not more evident. In lateral view there is opacification behind the sternum.

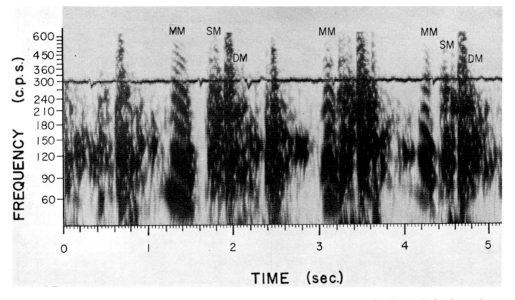

Fig. 3-26D. A spectral phonocardiogram of the sounds as recorded at the base of the heart in L. F. Y. Bigeminy was present as indicated by the electrocardiogram. There was a systolic murmur, **SM,** and a decrescendo diastolic murmur, **DM.** Near the end of the long diastolic periods that followed the extrasystoles there was a murmur, **MM,** that was strikingly musical as indicated by the conspicuous harmonics. When the bigeminy was absent and the rate higher, with short diastole, the murmur did not occur. (From McKusick, V. A., Murray, G. E., Peeler, R. G., and Webb, G. N.: Bull. Hopkins Hosp. 97:136, 1955.)

Continued.

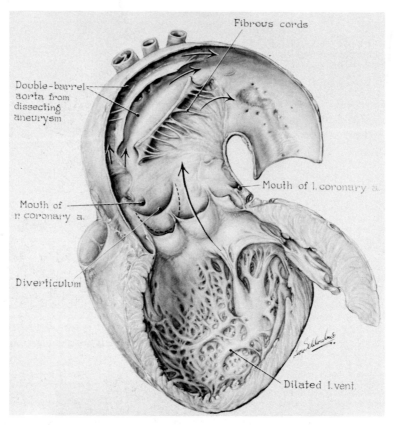

Fig. 3-26E. The autopsy specimen in patient L. F. Y. A chronic dissection of the ascending aorta is present. The patient died of heart failure. The drawing demonstrates three structures that might vibrate periodically, with production of a musical murmur as seen in **D:** (1) the fibrous cords that traverse the false channel, (2) the lip of the inner tube of the double-barrel aorta, and (3) the lip of the "diverticulum" above the sinuses of Valsalva. Why any one of these three structures should be incited in late diastole, with production of the musical murmur, is not clear. (From McKusick, V. A., Murray, G. E., Peeler, R. G., and Webb, G. M.: Bull. Hopkins Hosp. **97:**136, 1955.)

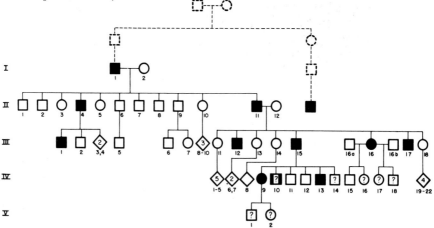

Fig. 3-27A. For legend see opposite page.

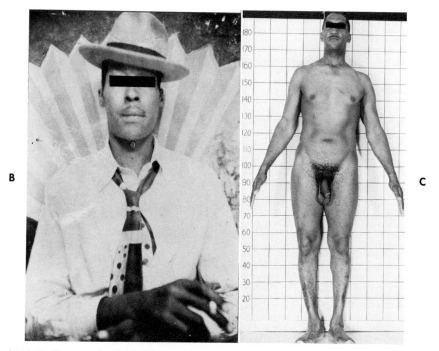

Fig. 3-27A. Pedigree of the F. kinship.

   II. 1, Charles; died of acute indigestion at age 47 years. **4,** Grant; about 6 feet 4 inches tall; died at age 35 years; 2 of his children died at 8 and 12 months, respectively. **8,** Henry; examined; unaffected.

   III. 1, James Aloysius; typical Marfan syndrome; 6 feet 4½ inches tall, size 13 shoe; ectopia lentis with secondary cataract formation; complete loss of vision from bilateral detachment of retina; early aortic diastolic murmur. **11,** Josephine; examined; unaffected. **12,** Clarence (352936); at age 32 years found to have complete detachment of right retina; left lens dislocated and cataractous; partial detachment of left retina; died at age 34 years, 18 days after onset of congestive heart failure attributed to syphilitic heart disease, because of finding of aortic regurgitation. **13,** Blanche; examined; unaffected. **15,** Theodore (see B); typical Marfan syndrome, with cardiovascular death in 1952. **16,** Leona (see Fig. 3-26A to C); typical Marfan syndrome, with autopsy confirmation of dissecting aneurysm of the aorta. **17,** James Leon (424834); ectopia lentis with severe secondary iridocyclitis and glaucoma; detachment of right retina; 75 inches tall, weight 172 pounds; kyphoscoliosis; varicocele; lax sternocleidomastoid joints, mobile patellae; flat feet; cardiomegaly with globular shape by x-ray examination; no murmurs. This individual and Theodore and Clarence, "always looked just like twins." Positive serologic test for syphilis.

   IV. 9, Mary Isabelle (844914), born 1939; definitely affected, with bilateral dislocation of lenses. **10,** James Leroy (844924), born 1940; possible slight lens dislocation. **11,** James Arthur (844925), born 1944; normal. **12,** John Edward (844922), born 1945; normal. **13,** David Theodore (844921), born 1950; definite Marfan syndrome; 38 inches tall at 30 months of age; long, peculiarly shaped head; dislocated lenses. **14,** Joseph Melvin (844923), born 1952; possibly affected.

   V. 1, James Allen (844915), born 1945; uncertain status. **2,** Mary Anne, born 1947; uncertain status.

Fig. 3-27B and C. B, Carnival snapshot of III-15 (T. F.). Arachnodactyly is evident. In his left hand he holds his spectacles. He died suddenly at the age of 33 years, two weeks after consulting a physician for exertional dyspnea. Aortic regurgitation had been discovered. An optometrist reports that he had "a decided miosis and the ophthalmoscopy showed the media to be cloudy." He was myopic. Worker as farm laborer until a few days before death. **C,** J. A. F. (816419), individual III-1 in **A,** at 33 years of age. Bilateral ectopia lentis, dolichostenomelia, and mild aortic regurgitation.

of syphilitic aortitis.[590] In fact, the similarities of the two diseases are in many respects striking. It seems to matter little whether the defect of the tunica media is produced by the spirochete from without or by the mutant gene from within.

As in syphilitic aortitis with aortic regurgitation, revision in the prognostic evaluation of aortic regurgitation in the Marfan syndrome is necessary on the

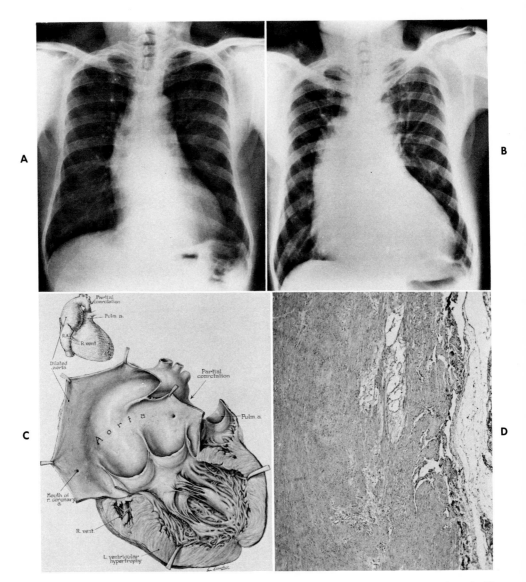

Fig. 3-28. A, Dilatation of the ascending aorta is present but is not impressive. Patient L. K. (film taken eighteen months before death). **B,** Film four months before death, same patient. **C,** Sketch of the heart and great vessels as visualized at autopsy in patient L. K. Mild coarctation was present. Dilatation limited to the ascending aorta and tremendous sacculation of the aortic cusps are conspicuous features. Note the relatively high position of the coronary ostia. **D,** Histologic section from the ascending aorta in same case.

Fig. 3-28, cont'd.

L. K. (J.H.H. 571745), a white man born in 1913, was first admitted to this hospital in May, 1951. On April 16, 1951, while riveting at an aircraft plant he noted the rather sudden onset of severe steady pain in his right chest, radiating down the right arm. This pain disappeared in a few hours, and he was essentially asymptomatic thereafter but was aware of profuse sweating, particularly of the hands and feet.

Examination revealed that the blood pressure was 195/40/0. He was a slightly built man of average height. There was alternating external strabismus, and the pupils were rather small but normally reactive. No other ocular abnormality was detected at that time. There were pronounced cardiac and peripheral signs of aortic regurgitation.

There was no history of rheumatic fever or syphilis and no laboratory or clinical evidence of syphilis or bacterial endocarditis. There was a story that in his work as a riveter the instrument which he held in front of his chest had, on several occasions, slipped, striking his chest forcefully. The possibility of traumatic rupture of an aortic cusp was considered most likely. In fact, this was considered so likely by his physicians that with their assistance the patient succeeded in making a $4,000 settlement with his employer! The history of his having been previously turned down for insurance was not elicited.

The patient was virtually asymptomatic until September, 1951, when he began to have attacks heralded by very profuse sweating and consisting of pain under the lower sternum, severe palpitation, and coughing. Rapid eating and excitement would precipitate the attacks. They occurred most often about midnight.

The patient's second admission was in May, 1952. At that time Dr. F. W. Dick first noted that the patient had iridodonesis bilaterally and that the edge of ectopic lenses could be seen with the ophthalmoscope. From the age of 10 years the patient had worn glasses for myopia, and bifocals from the age of 19 years. Examination revealed profuse sweating, even in a cool room. The lid slits were wide and there was lid lag; these were interpreted as probably being related to the effort to accommodate. (The excessive sweating was probably that frequently seen with left ventricular failure.) The head was round and the neck rather short. There was kyphosis without scoliosis. Muscular development was on the whole rather poor. The shoulders were rounded and scapulae moderately winged. His height was 5 feet 7 inches and fingertip-to-fingertip span 5 feet 11 inches. Pubic symphysis-to-heel dimension was 34 inches (over half his total height). There was syndactylism of the second and third toes bilaterally. There was a diastolic thrill at the right border of the sternum, and mediastinal dullness was increased to the right. It was then very apparent that the patient had Marfan's syndrome. Superannuated dissecting aneurysm of the aorta was considered likely.

The remainder of the patient's life was characterized by severe attacks of sweating, anginal pain, and orthopnea. At no time were there signs of right-sided failure. Comparison of early and late films are presented in **A** and **B**. The patient died Jan. 23, 1953.

At autopsy (24360) his height was determined to be 5 feet 6 inches. (There is a discrepancy among the various reported measurements.) The kyphosis was again described. The significant findings were limited to the heart, **C**, which weighed 980 grams. The increased weight was almost entirely the result of very marked left ventricular hypertrophy. The ascending aorta was the site of pronounced fusiform dilatation. The aortic valve ring was dilated to about four times the normal circumference. The sinuses of Valsalva were greatly dilated, and the aortic valve cusps themselves were relatively enormous baggy structures. The aortic dilatation stopped at the mouth of the innominate artery. Beyond the mouth of the left subclavian the aorta narrowed sharply in a typical, although only partial (about 40%), stenosis of the isthmus.

Microscopic sections of the aorta, **D**, revealed replacement of most of the media by scar tissue. There were some areas of cystic medial degeneration. Elastic tissue stains revealed marked disruption, fragmentation, and sparsity of elastic fibers.

After the death of the patient, an investigation revealed, in the records of an insurance company, information that the patient was turned down for insurance in 1944 because of aortic regurgitation. Therefore an aortic diastolic murmur had been present for at least nine years before death and for several years before symptoms of significance. It should also be noted that he had had varicose veins that required surgical treatment.

Continued.

Fig. 3-28, cont'd.

Comments. The aorta was not conspicuously dilated at the time the patient was first seen, in spite of the presence of striking aortic regurgitation. A possibly useful point may be a finding at fluoroscopy at the time of the first admission: "The lower right border of the heart in the region of the right atrium showed a marked increase in amplitude of pulsation. The pulmonary artery segment on the left side of the heart also pulsated vigorously, although the vascular markings of the lung were if anything decreased." In some of these cases the outflow tract of the right ventricle and the base of the pulmonary artery are evidently displaced forward and to the left (by the dilatation of the base of the aorta), simulating enlargement of these structures.[417] On the other side the intrapericardial portion of the aorta may be responsible for displacement and active pulsations in the right atrium.

A feature of equal diagnostic significance and of considerable genetic interest is the relative submersion of the full-blown skeletal manifestations when the Marfan mutation occurred in this pyknic stock. When first seen the patient did not impress anyone as being beyond the normal range as to habitus. Discovery of ectopic lenses resulted in the observer's being more impressed with the habitus. Comparison with his brothers and sisters would likewise have impressed the physician with the patient's abnormality. Other members of the family were about 5 feet 3 inches tall and were very heavily muscled, with short, powerful extremities and stubby fingers. The moral to the diagnostician is obvious. Although extensive studies of the families were not undertaken, several cases in the literature probably illustrate this same phenomenon.[617]

This case bears many resemblances to Case 3 of Tung and Liebow.[568] The type of aortic involvement which they illustrate is almost identical to that in **C.** Their patient, who died of aortic insufficiency at the age of 42 years, had had two herniorrhaphies and had varicose veins. Although the authors state that "no suggestion of arachnodactyly nor of any other external sign of Marfan's syndrome [was] recorded by any of several senior physicians who were concerned with the care of this man," it must be noted that he died in 1932, which was before a single case of the Marfan syndrome had been reported in the internal medical literature of this country and over ten years before the association of aortic dilatation and arachnodactyly was first clearly described.[20]

(From McKusick, V. A.: Circulation 11:321, 1955.)

---

basis of recent experience. From our own series it is now clear that the asymptomatic period may extend for appreciably more than five years. Furthermore, patients have survived five years or longer after the onset of major symptoms.

Chest pain that may have features usually associated with angina pectoris but that more often is imperfectly relieved by nitroglycerin is a rather frequent finding in the Marfan syndrome. In some patients the pain may be due to relative coronary insufficiency and may be of the same nature as the pain that occurs with aortic regurgitation, on a rheumatic basis, for example. In other cases, aneurysmal dilatation of the aorta, even before it is radiologically evident, may be the basis. Furthermore, chest pain may be striking before aortic regurgitation of hemodynamic significance develops. In one patient (A. S.) the pain was present for ten years before death occurred suddenly at the age of 35 years. In 2 other patients (R. C., 155970; A. D., 341643) chest pain was present for five and eight years, respectively, before death. Coronary ostial anomalies of apparently congenital type occur in some cases. Granting the importance of other factors in the angina pectoris of the Marfan syndrome, one cannot help but wonder if one factor may not be the pronounced dragging of the large blood-laden aortic cusps on the coronary ostia in diastole and the dilated aorta during systole. (See Fig. 3-56*B* for another instance of prolonged chest pain in the Marfan syndrome.)

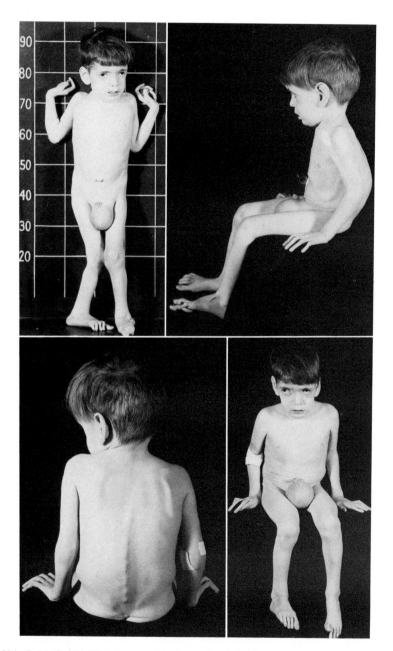

Fig. 3-29A. J. M. G. (795394), 26 months of age, has full-blown aortic regurgitation. The family history is negative. Dislocation of both lenses with striking iridodonesis, characteristically misshapen head and ears, kyphoscoliosis with "cat back" in sitting, arachnodactyly, and a large left inguinal hernia are present. (From McKusick, V. A.: Ann. Intern. Med. **49:**556, 1958.)

Continued.

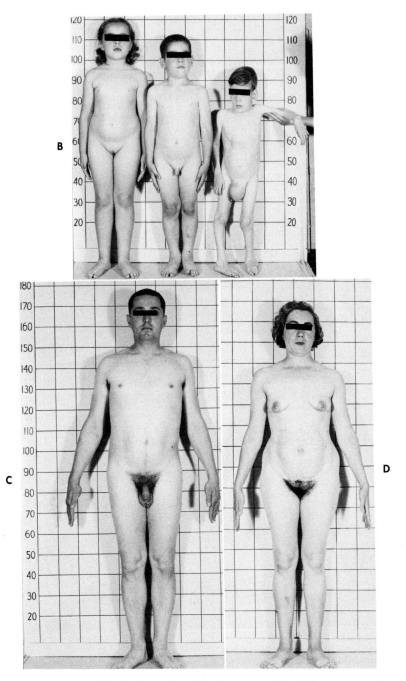

Fig. 3-29B to D. Two older children, **B**, and both parents, **C** and **D**, show no stigmata of the Marfan syndrome. The patient shown in **A** is probably the product of a new mutation. He died at the age of 3½ years. Autopsy revealed characteristic changes in the ascending aorta.

The onset of aortic dilatation may be as early as the first year or at least as late as the sixth decade. The oldest reported patient with aortic regurgitation without evident aortic dilatation was 56 years of age.[277] In one reported case,[560] dilatation of the ascending aorta with aortic regurgitation and marked left ventricular hypertrophy resulted in the death of a 10-month-old infant; in another case,[516] death occurred at 55 years. Another report[412] described 4 children varying in age from 5 to 26 months and demonstrating typical features of the Marfan syndrome, including aneurysms of the aortic sinuses of Valsalva and dilatation of the ascending aorta and main pulmonary artery. In my series the youngest patient with outspoken aortic regurgitation was 2 years old (Fig. 3-29A). The

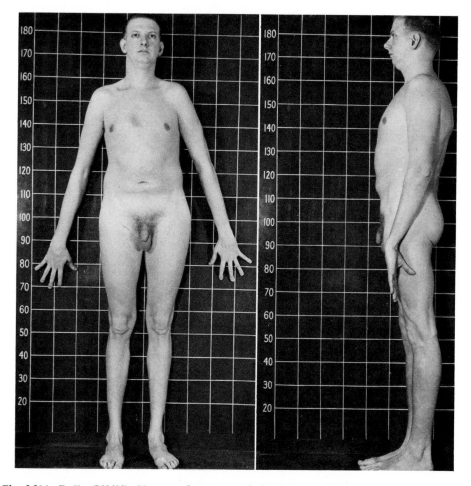

Fig. 3-30A. E. K. (760410), 26 years of age, was admitted for consideration of surgical correction of an abdominal aneurysm. The skeleton was considered to be typical of the Marfan syndrome. Both lenses were displaced upward and outward. The patient was partially deaf, but the hearing loss was of the conductive type, was largely limited to the left ear, and was readily accounted for on the basis of old otitis media. (From McKusick, V. A.: Ann. Intern. Med. 49:556, 1958.)

Continued.

oldest patient with aortic regurgitation was 59 years old (H. B., 621760). He showed no radiologic evidence of dilatation of the ascending aorta.

The dilatation is almost always confined to the ascending aorta proximal to the innominate artery. However, in Case 3 of Thomas and co-workers[553] the descending aorta was also involved. Furthermore, several instances of fusiform aneurysm of the abdominal aorta have been described.[306,358]

One of our patients (H. B., 621760), 59 years of age, had what appears by ordinary radiography to be a well-circumscribed orange-sized aneurysm of the descending thoracic aorta. Aortograms show both the thoracic and abdominal aorta to be diffusely dilated, with buckling in the lower thoracic area as well as in the abdomen, creating a false impression of saccular aneurysm at these sites.

Fig. 3-30 describes another of our cases in which cylindric aneurysm was limited to the abdominal aorta. The ascending aorta was clinically unaffected. Van

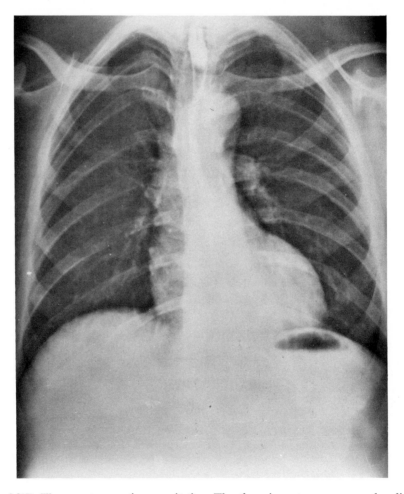

Fig. 3-30B. There was no aortic regurgitation. The thoracic aorta seems normal radiologically down to a point just above the diaphragm, where it became abruptly larger. (From McKusick, V. A.: Ann. Intern. Med. **49**:556, 1958.)

Buchem[571] described rupture of the abdominal aorta with cystic medial necrosis in a 20-year-old man who, because of striking skeletal changes, probably had the true Marfan syndrome, although the rest of the family was unaffected and no subluxation of the lenses was discovered. Langeron and colleagues[306] described 2 cases of abdominal aneurysm in the Marfan syndrome. Hardin,[229] in a case of full-blown Marfan syndrome in a 21-year-old man, described a fusiform abdominal aneurysm extending from the level of the renal arteries to the bifurcation of the aorta. It had ruptured into the inferior vena cava. At autopsy, although the abdominal aorta showed the histologic changes characteristic of the Marfan syndrome, "the thoracic aorta, pulmonary artery, and remaining arteries showed intact elastic fibers." In another patient with the Marfan syndrome, a 43-year-old male, Hardin[230] successfully resected an abdominal aneurysm. See also the cases of ruptured abdominal aortic aneurysm reported by Irwin and

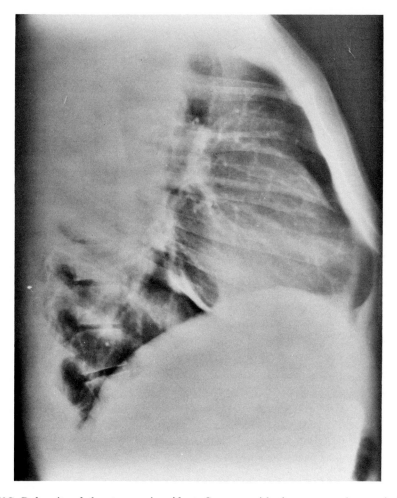

Fig. 3-30C. Deformity of the sternum is evident. Compare with the pectus carinatum in homocystinuria (Fig. 4-1). (From McKusick, V. A.: Ann. Intern. Med. 49:556, 1958.)

Continued.

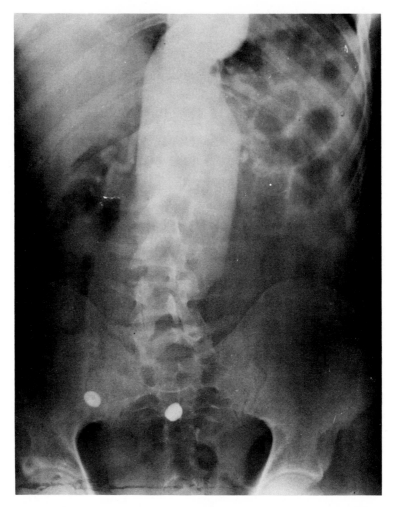

Fig. 3-30D. The enlargement of the aorta was shown by aortography to be cylindric and to extend the full length of the abdomen. The aneurysm was easily felt and seen on abdominal examination. (From McKusick, V. A.: Ann. Intern. Med. **49**:556, 1958.)

associates[261] and by Heitzman and Bryant.[240] Davis and colleagues[117] performed a total replacement of the abdominal aorta in a patient subsequently proved to have the Marfan syndrome. Recently in a 26-year-old male patient (D. W., 1471381), dissection occurred in the aorta below the renal arteries and extended into both iliacs. A graft was successfully installed. The thoracic aorta appeared to be unaffected. Dissection exclusively in the aorta beyond a mild coarctation at the usual site has been described.[570] In one reported case,[23] dissecting aneurysm was limited to the portion of the aorta between the mouth of the left subclavian artery and the level of the diaphragm; there seemed to be no other abnormality of the aorta.

Several cases (for example, see reference 382) have had cystic medial necrosis, dissection, and internal tears in the abdominal as well as the ascending aorta.

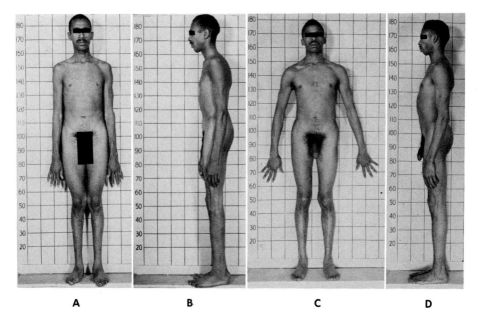

A   B   C   D

Fig. 3-31A to D. Brothers with the Marfan syndrome without ocular manifestations. **A** and **B**, J. M. (544088) had genu valgum, severe pes planus, and dolichostenomelia but no ectopia lentis. In 1950 an episode of chest pain accompanied by pericardial friction rub was interpreted as pericarditis and treated for presumed tuberculous etiology. Signs of aortic regurgitation developed thereafter. In 1953, there occurred at least one other episode of chest pain with pericardial friction rub. The effects of aortic regurgitation became progressively more severe and were the cause of death in April, 1955, at the age of 30 years. Autopsy revealed superannuated dissecting aneurysm of the ascending aorta and dilatation of the aorta above the aortic ring. The aorta had apparently "leaked" into the pericardial sac almost five years before death. (Known to us is a second case [S. T., 691351] in which the patient was still living following leakage about eighteen months before. The diagnosis of Erdheim's disease was established at operation for aneurysm of the ascending aorta. Sando and Helm[477] reported survival of a patient for four and one-half years after acute dissection accompanied by a pericardial friction rub.) **C** and **D**, W. M. (702409), 27 years of age, was discovered to have aortic regurgitation when examined in connection with his brother's illness. He had dolichostenomelia and spinal curvature. Although the left ventricle is large, no dilatation of the aorta is demonstrable. He is asymptomatic.

Continued.

Thrombosis of the abdominal aorta with production of the Leriche syndrome is described,[124] but such is more characteristic of homocystinuria (Chapter 4).

By examining a large number of patients with ectopia lentis and by studying the relatives in established cases of the Marfan syndrome, we discovered 6 patients who appeared to be in the early stages of aortic dilatation with aortic regurgitation.[335] In none was there then evident dilatation of the ascending aorta (Figs. 3-31C and D, 3-32A and B, and 3-33B). One of the 6 (Fig. 3-33B) died of aortic aneurysm about three years after first detection of aortic regurgitation. The others remained without particular cardiac symptoms, for periods as long as six years.

Recent years have witnessed a crescendo of interest in the subject of aneurysm of the sinuses of Valsalva.[35,120,164,484,613] Steinberg and Geller[530] have demon-

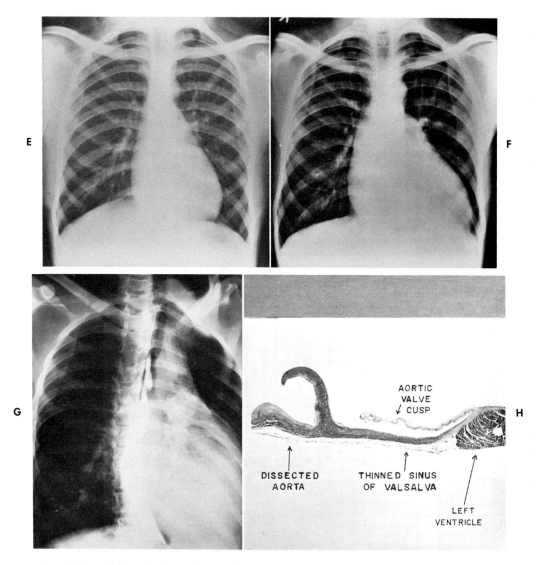

Fig. 3-31E to H. E to **G,** Series of x-ray films of J. M. **E,** Taken in 1950 about one month after the initial episode of leakage into the pericardial sac. **F** and **G,** The appearance in the last year of life. Enlargement of the aorta is not impressive in **F,** but the main pulmonary artery is prominent. In the right anterior oblique film, **G,** the barium-filled esophagus is displaced by a structure that necropsy demonstrated to be an aneurysm of the sinus of Valsalva. In the left anterior oblique (not shown here), again the aorta does not appear particularly dilated. **H,** Microscopic section (×4) of aortic valve area in J. M. (see **A**). The old dissection, the thinning of the sinus of Valsalva, and the minor fibrous thickening of the aortic valve are demonstrated.

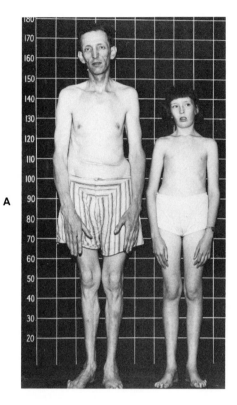

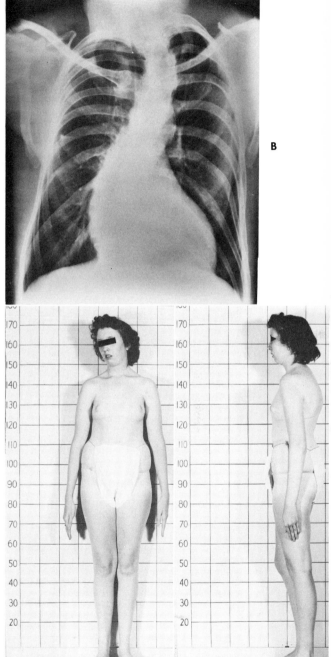

Fig. 3-32. A, Both the man (E. F., 194515) and his daughter (M. V. F., 565451) have bilateral subluxation of the lenses, spinal curvature, and dolichostenomelia (long, thin extremities). The man has had femoral and inguinal hernias repaired. The girl is only 9 years old. In 1950 the man had no cardiac murmurs. In 1953 he was found to have well-marked aortic regurgitation. Photograph, June, 1953. At this time the patient also had a crescendo holosystolic murmur of partially musical quality at the apex (see Fig. 317 in reference 336). **B,** The chest x-ray film of the man in **A** reveals no apparent dilatation of the ascending aorta. (The scoliosis obscures the picture.) Fluoroscopy likewise failed to establish dilatation of the aorta. **C,** Photograph of the daughter shown in **A,** August, 1958. She later gave birth to an infant with the Marfan syndrome and bilateral dislocation of the hips as reported by Heldrich and Wright.[241] (**A** and **B** from McKusick, V. A.: Circulation **11**:321, 1955.)

strated such aneurysms, by means of angiocardiography, in patients with the Marfan syndrome, and we have had similar experiences (Fig. 3-34*A* to *C*). Actually the "aortic sinus aneurysms" that occur in the Marfan syndrome behave clinically in quite a different manner than do those aneurysms to which this term is perhaps more legitimately applied. Rupture into the right side of the circulation has only rarely been observed; the aneurysm is not, with occasional exception, limited to one aortic sinus. The possibility of the Marfan syndrome should not be abandoned, however, in cases of rupture of an aortic sinus into the right side of the heart. In one reported case,[407] in a 36-year-old male, the following statement suggesting the Marfan syndrome was made: "Until his attack he was perfectly fit and served in the army during the Second World War in a low category on account of defective eyesight and flat feet." Rupture of dissecting aneurysm of the aorta into the right atrium[130] or the right ventricle[242]

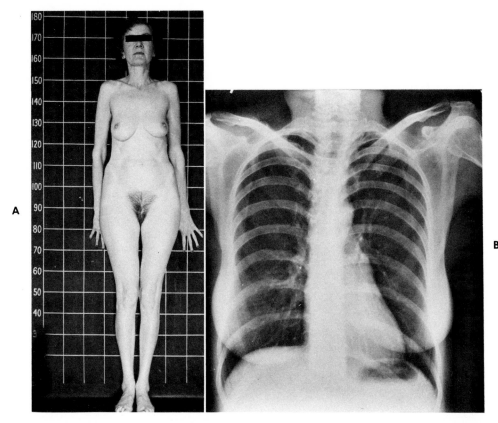

Fig. 3-33. A, M. B. (697662), 46 years old. Ectopia lentis, moderate dolichostenomelia, and spinal curvature. **B,** Although at the time of these studies (February, 1955) the patient was asymptomatic and the cardiovascular silhouette normal, an aortic diastolic murmur was present. The patient died in December, 1957. Diagnosis: aortic aneurysm. (Systolic clicks were recorded at the apex in 1955. The multiple clicks were described by the stethoscopist as a systolic crunch. Because of the mild chest deformity and the general loose-jointedness, the clicks are thought to have been produced by movement of joints of the thoracic cage. See Fig. 146 in reference 336.)

has been described in cases of the Marfan syndrome. Aortic sinus aneurysm leads to diagnostic radiologic signs in the plain films, including broadening of the waist of the heart, encroachment on the retrosternal space, prominence of the "pulmonary arc segment" due to its displacement by the aneurysm, and displacement of the left atrium, suggesting enlargement of the atrium.[484]

Dissecting aneurysm may occur as the first recognized aortic complication or may be superimposed on diffuse dilatation of the ascending aorta.[348] It is likely that dissecting aneurysm rarely occurs "out of the blue" in the Marfan syndrome. Some dilatation of the aorta, often expressed by aortic regurgitation, probably has already developed in the great majority of cases. This point is an important one in connection with prophylactic therapy with propranolol (p. 196).

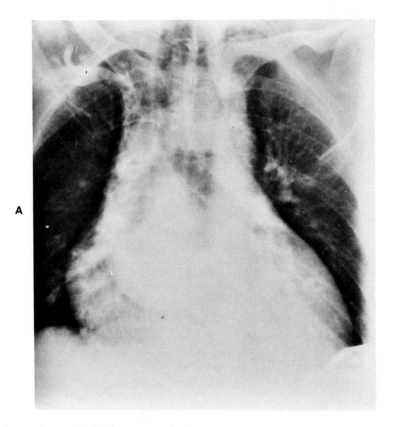

Fig. 3-34A and B. S. C. (575946), a veterinarian, had ectopia lentis and skeletal proportions of the Marfan syndrome. He died at the age of 37 years during an attempt at surgical repair of the ascending aorta. With the episode of dissection in October, 1955, a musical systolic murmur developed over the ascending aorta. This sign, a valuable diagnostic clue in such cases, probably owes its origin to vibration in intimal lip or fibrous bands in the ascending aorta. Angiocardiogram showed striking dilatation of the base of the aorta within the shadow of the heart, surprisingly little enlargement of the later portion of the ascending aorta, failure of opacification of the innominate artery, the lumen of which was tamponaded by a medial dissection, and finally, pseudocoarctation of the type so typical of the Marfan syndrome. (From McKusick, V. A.: Ann. Intern. Med. **49**:556, 1958.)

Continued.

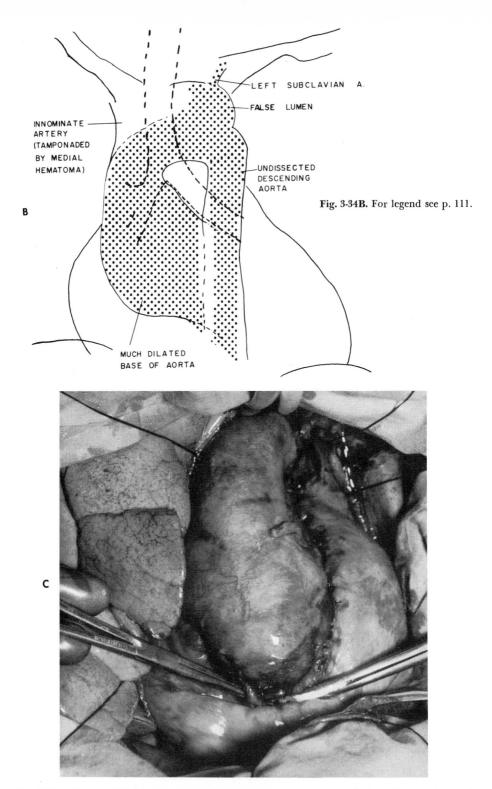

INNOMINATE
ARTERY
(TAMPONADED
BY MEDIAL
HEMATOMA)

LEFT   SUBCLAVIAN   A.

FALSE   LUMEN

UNDISSECTED
DESCENDING
AORTA

Fig. 3-34B. For legend see p. 111.

B

MUCH DILATED
BASE OF AORTA

C

Fig. 3-34C. The gourdlike appearance of the ascending aorta as exposed through a surgical incision in the right interior thorax. A clamp lies under the right coronary artery. Unusually high
displacement of this vessel made operation difficult, as did also the high extension of the aortic
commissures. The patient died during surgery. The mother of this patient died of the cardiac
complications of the Marfan syndrome at the age of 40 years. An older sister of the patient has
the Marfan syndrome. (From McKusick, V. A.: Ann. Intern. Med. **49:**556, 1958.)

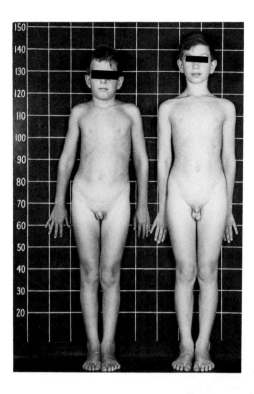

Fig. 3-34D. The proband's sons, one affected (left) and one unaffected, are seen here. R. C. (783343), the affected boy, 8¾ years old, has grossly visible dislocation of the lenses, myopia, and mild thoracic kyphosis. The normal brother is 12 years old; another brother, 4 years of age, is also normal. (From McKusick, V. A.: Ann. Intern. Med. **49**:556, 1958.)

There is evidence that dissection may occur in the first decade of life; Wong and associates[612] described fatal rupture of a dissecting aneurysm of the ascending aorta into the pericardial sac in a girl who was 4 years 9 months old. The patient shown in Fig. 3-35 was 61 years of age, however, when he died of probable dissecting aneurysm.

On aortography a radiolucent line can sometimes be demonstrated within the apparent aortic lumen and parallel to it. This line represents the intima and the inner part of the media, which separate the true from the false channel.[505] An incorrect angiographic diagnosis of dissection of the aorta may be made, however, on the basis of adventitial or venous opacification, which gives an impression of a double lumen, or false channel.[280]

The patient may survive for a number of years after first dissection of the aorta and even after a "leak" into the pericardium. Because of the aortic regurgitation, which results either from the dissection itself[224,450] or from the associated dilatation of the aortic ring, confusion with rheumatic[313] or syphilitic[199] heart disease is frequent. In a recently autopsied case at this hospital, leaking of the original dissecting aneurysm into the pericardial sac led to the misdiagnosis of tuberculous pericarditis. The patient survived five years after the first pericardial episode. One reported 8-year-old child survived massive hemopericardium and subsequently had successful resection of the dissected aorta.[134] Matsui and Ito[362] described a huge hydropericardium in a man who subsequently died of dissecting aneurysm. Although they admitted that the pericarditis could have been due to

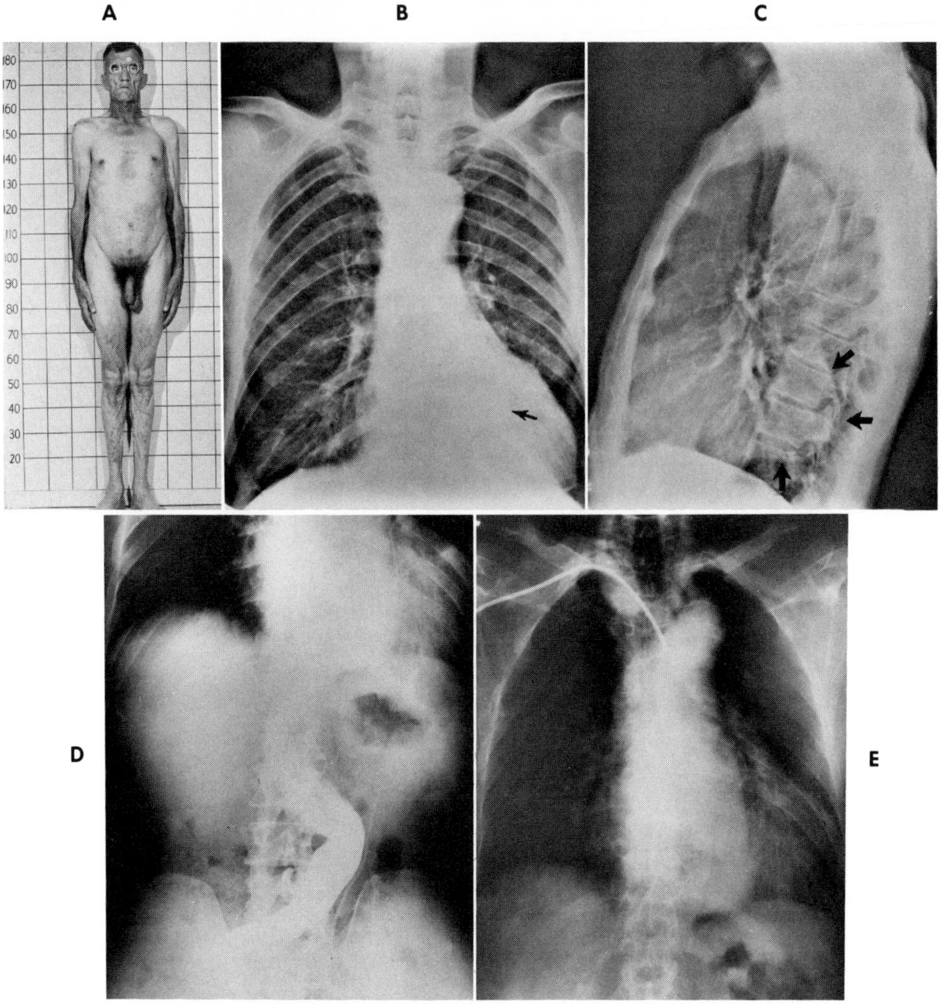

Fig. 3-35. Tortuous aorta in the Marfan syndrome. H. B. (621760), white male born in 1900, had ectopia lentis from birth and was educated until age 16 at the Iowa School for the Blind. Thereafter, following fitting for spectacles, he was able to attend regular school and was gainfully employed all his life as an electrical engineer. Both parents died in their eighties. No other certain instance of the Marfan syndrome is known in the family. The right eye was enucleated in 1951; several operations for glaucoma were performed on the left eye, and the lens was removed in 1952. In 1955 he had subtotal gastrectomy for peptic ulcer. Fourteen days after operation he experienced sudden and severe chest pain while sitting on the toilet. In retrospect this seems to have been either pulmonary embolism or aortic dissection, probably the former. Hearing was diminished, beginning about 1940.

When first seen by me in 1959, the patient was tall, with mild pectus excavatum, **A.** He had a loud murmur of aortic regurgitation and blood pressure of 136/40 mm. Hg. Chest x-ray films, **B** and **C**, showed left ventricular enlargement, prominent aortic knob, and apparent aneurysm of the descending thoracic aorta (arrow). Retrograde aortogram via the femoral artery showed, **D,** a markedly tortuous abdominal aorta without aneurysm. Since the catheter could not be passed farther up the aorta, aortography was performed via the brachial artery, with demonstration, **E,** that the apparent aneurysm was a buckled segment of the descending aorta. A suggestive double shadow in the area of the aorta above the diaphragm raised the question of dissection.

The patient died elsewhere in 1961. "Coronary thrombosis," occurring 4 days before death, was listed as the cause of death.

some unrelated cause, they favored obstruction of the pericardial vein by aneurysm of the root of the aorta as the mechanism.

Dissection occurs with increased frequency during pregnancy.[400,486,497] In chronic dissecting aneurysm of the aorta, there may be little enlargement of the aorta evident on x-ray examination (Figs. 3-26B and C and 3-31E to H). In our experience, when full family investigations are made, the Marfan syndrome is found to be a leading "cause" of dissecting aneurysm in persons under the age of 40 years. Gore[196] reported that 3 of 22 patients had arachnodactyly. This, however, was not a detailed clinicogenetic study. At least 17% of the reported cases of dissecting aneurysm in patients under the age of 40 years were recognized instances of the Marfan syndrome.[247] The true proportion is probably higher. For example, Spenser[523] described dissecting aneurysm during pregnancy in a "tall, thin" woman 32 years of age. Griffith and colleagues[210] reported on a dissecting aneurysm in a 34-year-old woman and in her 14-year-old daughter, both of whom were said to have been "delicate physically."

The occurrence of aortic regurgitation* with dissecting aneurysm is well recognized in the English-speaking medical world since the publication of Resnik and Keefer[450] in 1925. Hamman and Apperly's[224] explanation that the aortic

---

*I prefer the term "regurgitation" to "incompetence" or "insufficiency." A stenotic valve is also incompetent or insufficient in one of its functions—opening fully for forward flow.[238] "Regurgitation" connotes the precise functional defect.

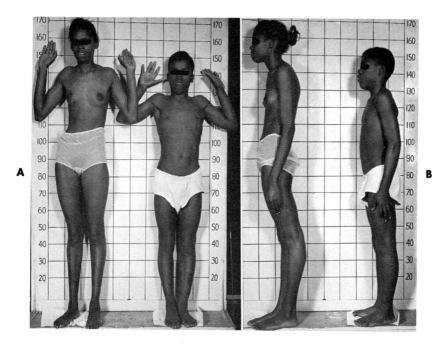

Fig. 3-36A and B. Fourteen-year-old S. S. (366788), II-6 of the pedigree (see **C**), and her normal 12-year-old brother, II-7. Note the kyphoscoliosis, genu recurvatum, excessively long legs, and strabismus. Ectopia lentis is present.

Continued.

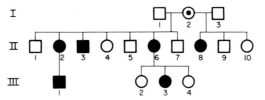

Fig. 3-36C. This pedigree illustrates how submerged the manifestations of Marfan's syndrome can be. Individual I-2 had had at least 3 affected offspring by one husband and one affected offspring by a second husband. Both husbands are unequivocally normal from the skeletal, ocular, and vascular points of view. The mother is 5 feet 8 inches tall, moderately long of limb, poorly muscled, and severely myopic (−6D), but has no ectopia lentis by careful ophthalmoscopic examination. (For the last I am indebted to Dr. J. E. Mishler of Atlantic City, N. J.) These manifestations are consistent with *forme fruste* of the Marfan syndrome but would not be recognizable as such without the knowledge of this pedigree. (Status of pedigree in 1959, six years after photographs in **A** and **B** were taken.)

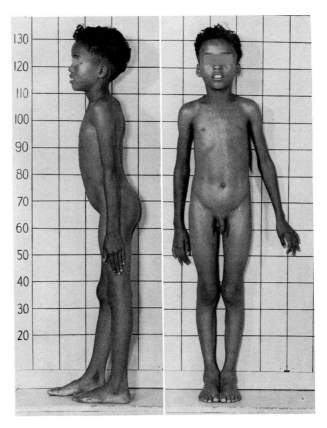

Fig. 3-36D. Two views of S. S. (719604), individual III-1 of the pedigree in **C.** Born March 1, 1948. Photograph, Aug. 6, 1956. When first examined at home in 1953, the patient was judged to be normal. It is now clear that slight bilateral lens dislocation is present. A faint aortic diastolic murmur was heard in 1958. The chest is asymmetrically deformed to a minor degree. Arachnodactyly and loose-jointedness are not impressive.

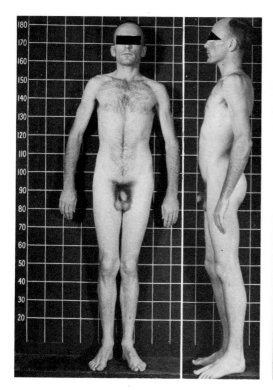

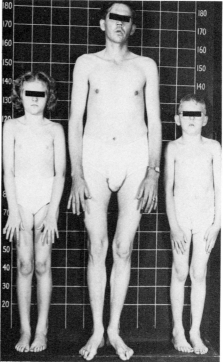

Fig. 3-37   Fig. 3-38

Fig. 3-37. C. H. (687485), 28 years old. Ectopia lentis. Lenses correcting for aphakia worn from age of 5 years. Brother, father, 2 paternal aunts, and 2 cousins are living and have the Marfan syndrome. Paternal grandmother and great grandmother likewise had it. Father blind in both eyes and aunt blind in one eye from secondary glaucoma. Patient in Army for forty-five months. Note deformity of knees. This patient and many of the others in this group of photographs make it clear that on superficial inspection the habitus may not seem impressively or abnormally dolichostenomelic.

Fig. 3-38. Father, E. C., and 2 children, Anna (593933), 9 years of age, and Robert (441759), 7 years of age, all with ectopia lentis and skeletal proportions that, albeit not striking, are consistent with the Marfan syndrome. The father's brother had had a "leaky heart" for several years and died suddenly at the age of 35 years.

regurgitation results from deformation of the aortic ring by the intramural hematoma is the generally accepted one. Obviously another mechanism for the association is preexisting dilatation of the aortic ring, on the basis of the same defect of connective tissue that led to the dissecting aneurysm.

In patients with the Marfan syndrome the sudden development of a murmur, especially a musical buzzing murmur over the ascending aorta, may be a valuable clue to the presence of dissection.[92,336] The murmur, which may be either systolic or, less commonly, diastolic (Fig. 3-26D), appears to be produced by vibrations excited in some of the anomalous structures—lips, fibrous cords, narrowed branches of the aortic arch—created by the dissection (Fig. 3-26E). The early diastolic murmur created at the aortic valve may be musical in quality[293] and, as in the case of many musical murmurs, may be very loud. Bean[32] had such a case in his series of precordial noises audible at a distance from the chest. Baer and associates[20] stated that one of their patients had a loud "systolic murmur" audible 2 inches from the chest. A diastolic murmur loudest at the *right* sternal border is more frequent in the Marfan syndrome than in aortic regurgitation of rheumatic causation.[238]

Another mechanism of aortic regurgitation in the Marfan syndrome is myxomatous transformation of the aortic valve itself.[443] It appears that aortic regurgitation due simply to aortic cuspid changes, without dilatation of the aortic

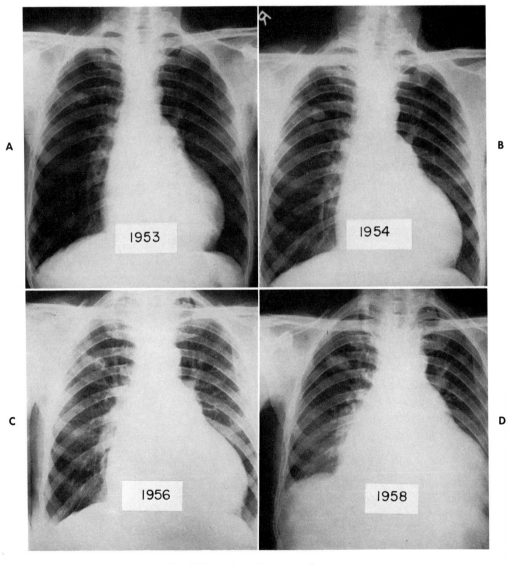

Fig. 3-39. For legend see opposite page.

ring, is rare in the Marfan syndrome. "Floppy aortic valve," functionally and histologically identical to the change in the mitral valve, has been described[443]; the affected patients were of asthenic habitus but had no unequivocal signs of the Marfan syndrome. It remains a question whether pure valvular aortic regurgitation often or ever occurs in the Marfan syndrome. If it does occur, it must be uncommon. The generalization is valid that aortic regurgitation in a patient with the Marfan syndrome indicates aortic dilatation and makes propranolol therapy worthy of consideration (p. 196).

In general, the clinical picture of dissecting aneurysm in the Marfan syn-

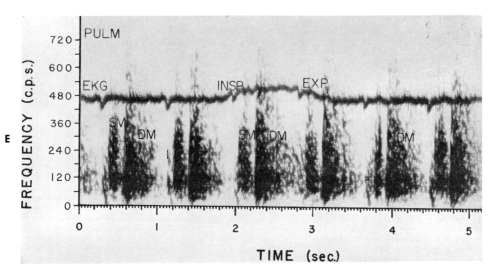

Fig. 3-39. Eight-year survival after onset of cardiac symptoms in the Marfan syndrome. A. D. (341643), a Negro male born in 1907, was well until 1950, when there was onset of chest pain and dyspnea. Late in 1951 chest pain and attacks of paroxysmal nocturnal dyspnea became especially frequent. The chest pain had the pattern typical of angina pectoris. At first it was relieved by nitroglycerin; later this drug seemed to have little effect. Throughout the eight years of observation the murmur and other signs of aortic regurgitation were present. Also, at the apex what was interpreted as an Austin Flint murmur was described. During the last three years of life a bizarre "crackling" systolic murmur was described at the apex. It was also described as "crunching" and compared to "footsteps in gravel." It disappeared on deep inspiration. Numerous serologic tests for syphilis and two treponemal immobilization tests were negative. Progressive widening of the QRS complexes, to a maximum of 0.13 second, occurred in the period of observation. Atrial fibrillation developed in the last two weeks of life. The patient died in 1958. The man was described as "tall," "thin," "asthenic," and "long-armed." His height was twice measured as 70½ inches. Visual acuity was essentially normal. Although no slit-lamp examination was performed, numerous standard ophthalmoscopic examinations showed no abnormality. There was no hernia or spinal deformity. The patient had had no children; his family was not available for study.

A to D, X-ray films: **A,** 1953; **B,** 1954; **C,** 1956; **D,** Three days before death in 1958. Dilatation of the aorta is conspicuous in its absence. The pulmonary artery segment is prominent throughout. **E,** Spectral phonocardiogram in pulmonary area, January, 1957. The findings are typical of severe aortic regurgitation, with no features pathognomonic for the Marfan syndrome.

Autopsy revealed findings similar to those shown in Fig. 3-28C except that the marked dilatation was limited more to the area of the sinuses of Valsalva. The histologic changes included loss of elastic fibers, spaces occupied by metachromatically staining material, whorls of disorganized smooth muscle fibers, and much dilated vasa vasorum.

drome is little different from that in persons without this syndrome, except that in the Marfan syndrome aortic regurgitation is more likely to be present (as a result of preexisting dilatation in the first part of the aorta), the average age is about twenty years younger than that for other dissecting aneurysms, and hypertension is usually absent. As in any dissecting aneurysm, the patient may demonstrate inequality of the radial pulses.[413]

I have not observed calcification of the ascending aorta in the Marfan syndrome. This fact may be helpful in differentiating the aortic involvement of the Marfan syndrome from that of syphilis, in which calcification is frequent.[332]

McKeown[334] described a 21-year-old white man with arachnodactyly but "no other stigmata of Marfan's syndrome." The patient died from myocardial infarction resulting from dissection limited to the right coronary artery. Dissection of the coronary arteries in patients with the Marfan syndrome is an adequately established although rare complication.[283,334,480]

Involvement of the aortic cusps has already been described. The aortic valve is sometimes bicuspid (Fig. 3-41); whether this is the case in the Marfan syn-

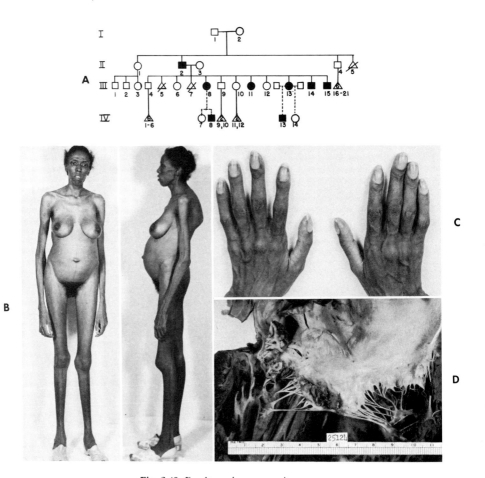

Fig. 3-40. For legend see opposite page.

drome more often than one would expect with this relatively frequent abnormality is not certain.

The mitral cusps and chordae tendineae may be redundant, with resulting mitral regurgitation. Subacute bacterial endocarditis may become engrafted on the valvular abnormality.[70,102,126a,241,335,405,577,614] (See Fig. 3-40 for a case of bacterial endocarditis with the Marfan syndrome.) Bacterial endocarditis in this syndrome is probably limited to the mitral valve in most cases. Murmurs of obscure origin are frequently encountered. Some may be on the basis of redundant chordae tendineae with incompetence of atrioventricular valves. These murmurs may be partially musical. In one patient (S. C., 575946) with a musical

---

Fig. 3-40. **A,** Pedigree of the family of patient M. E. R. (III-11). Individual II-2 may have been the original mutant. However, illegitimacy is so much more frequent than mutation that one can never be certain. **B,** Patient M. E. R. **C,** The combination of arachnodactyly and clubbing of the fingers relates to Marfan's disease and subacute bacterial endocarditis from which the patient M. E. R. suffered. **D,** The mitral valve, showing bacterial vegetation.

M. E. R. (J.H.H. 176836), a Negro woman born in 1929, is a member of a family that has been known to The Johns Hopkins Hospital for about twenty-five years and in which at least 9 cases of Marfan's syndrome (including this patient) have occurred. (The patient is individual III-11 in the pedigree presented in **A.**) The father of the patient, a well-documented instance of this syndrome, died of dissecting aneurysm of the aorta at the age of 43 years. Of 4 sibs of the patient with this disease, three have signs consistent with interatrial septal defect.

The patient demonstrated bilateral ectopia lentis, severe myopia, pronounced dolichostenomelia, very poor muscular development, severe kyphoscoliosis, pes planus, and, by x-ray films, pulmonary emphysema with bleb formation. She recalled nothing suggestive of acute rheumatic fever. Most of her life she had been subject to exertional dyspnea.

The patient became pregnant early in November, 1953. After about four months there was increase in her lifelong exertional dyspnea and the appearance of ankle edema and orthopnea, which required two pillows. In early April, 1954, there was onset of evening fever, night sweats, and aching of joints, especially knees and ankles. Tender red spots appeared on the palms and soles.

Physical examination revealed, as new findings, petechiae, embolic nodes of the palms, splinter hemorrhages of the nail beds, and clubbed fingers. A loud, harsh systolic murmur was audible over the entire precordium, and the second pulmonic sound was accentuated.

Six blood cultures demonstrated a *Streptococcus viridans*, which was late in growing out and atypical in morphology due probably to streptomycin and penicillin that had been administered before admission to the Osler Medical Clinic. The patient's white blood cell count was 10,000 to 12,000 and hematocrit 26%. Treatment with penicillin in large doses was instituted with seemingly successful results.

On the patient's twentieth day in the hospital premature labor began as a result of septic infarction of the placenta, and an infant weighing 1,700 grams was born. The infant, which demonstrated pronounced dolichostenomelia, lived only a very few minutes. Autopsy in the case of the infant revealed no cardiovascular lesion, and the cause of death is not completely clear. There was an abnormality of pulmonary lobation such as is frequently seen in the Marfan syndrome. (See Fig. 3-21*I.*)

The patient died of uncontrollable heart failure about two weeks after delivery. **D** shows the mitral valve with bacterial vegetation. No evidence of rheumatism was discovered. The tunica media of the aorta and the pulmonary artery showed extensive chromotropic degeneration.

Chest x-ray film in this patient (not illustrated) showed increased bronchovascular markings and evidences of bleb formation. At autopsy all lobes of the lungs, especially the upper ones, were cystic. Some of the cysts were as much as several centimeters in diameter. They were lined by columnar epithelium and contained strands of smooth muscle in the walls. (See Fig. 3-49.)

(From McKusick, V. A.: Circulation 11:321, 1955.)

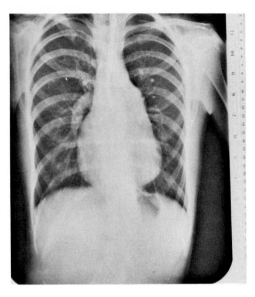

Fig. 3-41. X-ray film in case of Marfan syndrome in which atrial septal defect was incorrectly thought to be present.

M. E. C. (J.H.H. A98174), born in 1940, was first referred to Dr. Helen B. Taussig in November, 1952, for investigation of a congenital heart defect with paroxysmal tachycardia. The father was 76 inches tall and asthenic and had a spinal curvature and ectopia lentis but no evidence of cardiovascular abnormality. A single male sib was unaffected.

In this case a heart murmur had been described before the age of 2 years. Except that she never gained weight well and could not keep up with the other children at play, the patient was relatively well until April, 1952, when she had a first attack of paroxysmal tachycardia lasting several hours. Two more attacks occurred, one in May and a second in September, 1952.

The patient was a tall, slender white girl of better-than-average intellect. She was 64 inches tall and weighed 79 pounds. She wore glasses for ectopia lentis, which had been discovered at the age of 5 years. The palate was high. The chest was long, with convex scoliosis of the thoracic spine toward the right. The heart was not enlarged. However, a loud systolic murmur accompanied by a thrill was heard in the second and third intercostal spaces to the left of the sternum. The patient stood with rather marked pronation of the feet at the heels and moderate abduction. There was minimal genu valgum.

On fluoroscopy the right atrium was seen to be enlarged and the main pulmonary artery was prominent and active. There was moderate hilar dance. The left atrium and the ventricles appeared to be normal in size. During the recording of the electrocardiogram short paroxysms of atrial tachycardia occurred. There was a higher degree of right axis deviation than would have been anticipated as normal for this age. Leads II and III showed changes in the ST-T complex, interpreted as "right ventricular strain pattern." The QRS complexes were notched in most leads. X-ray films revealed no structural abnormality of the vertebrae.

It was my previous impression that this patient had atrial septal defect (ASD). It was commented that surgical repair is probably worthwhile in such a patient, provided there is no evidence of involvement of other parts of the cardiovascular system or severe skeletal involvement.

Subsequent events and the findings of autopsy proved the diagnosis of ASD to be incorrect. Late in 1955 a spinal operation for correction of deformity was performed. Thereafter, an infection with chronically draining sinuses necessitated readmission to the hospital. Following a debridement operation the patient died during a sudden bout of arrhythmia. The findings in the heart included bicuspid aortic valve and multicuspid mitral valve. The left coronary artery had two accessory ostia at the sinus of Valsalva. The mitral valve had five cusps, and the line of closure was thickened and nodular. Histologically this area showed "basophilic degeneration." The interatrial septum was perfectly intact. There was pulmonary emphysema.

Follow-up: The father of this patient died at 48 years of age of acute dissecting aneurysm of the aorta, with rupture into the pericardium. At autopsy the mitral valve ring was found to be calcified. The leaflets and chordae tendineae were thickened. (I am indebted to Dr. John Franklin of Norfolk, Va., for information on this patient.)

(From McKusick, V. A.: Circulation **11:**321, 1955.)

mitral systolic murmur, autopsy revealed a tear at the insertion of the posterior mitral cusp, amounting to a partial avulsion of the cusp.

A striking early systolic click heard not only at the aortic area but also at the apex is a frequent sign of dilatation of the ascending aorta in the Marfan syndrome. It is thought to represent a snapping of the aortic wall early in systolic ejection.[336] Extracardiac clicks and other extraneous sounds are frequent, and some may be attributable to a combination of thoracic deformity, the loose-jointedness of the bony thorax, and the cardiac enlargement. However, intracardiac origin of such systolic clicks, particularly those associated with a late systolic murmur, is more often the case.

It is now clear that involvement of the mitral and possibly the tricuspid valve with regurgitation may be the predominant cardiovascular lesion in the Marfan syndrome and may lead to early death.[495,507] Figs. 3-6A and 3-41 illustrate such cases. Redundancy of the chordae tendineae may be responsible, at least in part, for the valvular dysfunction. Tricuspid, or even quinquecuspid, mitral valves have been present in some cases. See Fig. 3-21C for reference to mitral anomaly. Grondin and co-workers,[211] as well as others, have described a peculiar and probably pathognomonic appearance of the mitral valve on angiocardiography and at autopsy. "The mitral leaflets were divided into several large serrations which bulged into the left atrium."[211] There are interchordal protrusions, essentially herniations, between the extensions of the chordae tendineae onto the valve leaf. Viewed from the atrial side, the valve in the simulated closed position looks like the anus surrounded by large hemorrhoids.[9a] Striking mitral regurgitation has been observed in infants with other severe manifestations of the Marfan syndrome.[248a]

It is now clear[169,253,312] that a late systolic murmur is often produced by mitral regurgitation of a particular type. Retroversion of a redundant posterior mitral cusp, with leak from the left ventricle to the atrium in late systole, has been demonstrated by cineangiocardiography[489] (e.g., Fig. 3-42). The murmur is of a type that was earlier interpreted as being of extracardiac origin.[336] It often is of rather musical quality and in these instances may be quite loud, being audible over most of the back as well as at the precordium centering around the apex. The musical quality may be present only intermittently and may be accentuated by exertion or excitement. Multiple systolic clicks in mid and late systole are frequent accompaniments of the late systolic murmur. These clicks may initiate the murmur. It is likely that they are also generated at the redundant posterior mitral leaflet.

Barlow and colleagues[24] found that 2 of 90 patients with late systolic murmurs and nonejection mid-late systolic clicks had the Marfan syndrome. Five others had a familial basis independent of the Marfan syndrome, a well-documented entity. Hunt and Sloman[255] and Shell and associates[500] described families with many affected persons in several generations, and there are rather numerous other families reported. Under observation, one patient reported by Hunt and Sloman[255] progressed to severe mitral regurgitation with pansystolic murmur. The 56-year-old brother and 55-year-old sister reported by Crocker[108] probably had the floppy mitral valve syndrome—not the Marfan syndrome.

Sometimes the mid-late systolic click/late systolic murmur is associated with a characteristic electrocardiographic pattern (depressed ST segments and in-

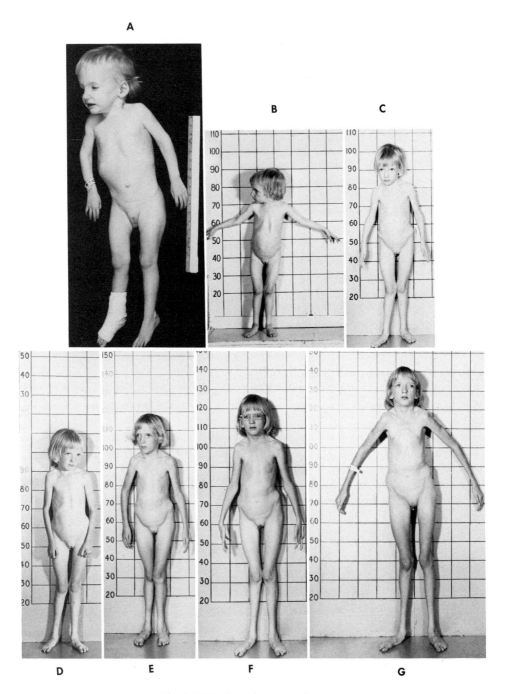

Fig. 3-42. For legend see opposite page.

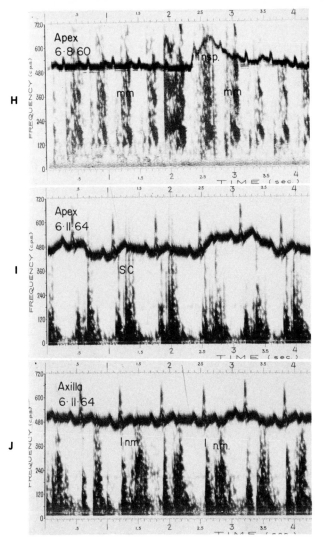

Fig. 3-42. Mitral regurgitation in Marfan syndrome (B. H., 941257). **A** to **F**, The appearance at ages, respectively, 14 months, 2 years, 3 years, 4 years, 5 years, and 6 years. Chest deformity— first pectus excavatum and later predominantly pectus carinatum—is shown. Dolichostenomelia and loose-jointedness are striking. Bilateral ectopia lentis is present. **G**, Appearance at age 8½ years (September, 1967), within a month of her death. **H** to **J**, Auscultatory findings as demonstrated by spectral phonocardiograms. At the age of 14 months, the patient showed a loud musical late systolic murmur which was initiated by a click and which extended across the second heart sound, **H**. Later the findings were predominantly multiple clicks in the latter two thirds of systole, **I**, and in other areas a noisy late systolic murmur extending over the second sound, **J**. Selective left ventricular cineangiocardiography, **K**, at age 5 years demonstrated prolapsed posterior mitral leaflet and mitral regurgitation. The catheter was introduced in retrograde fashion via the femoral artery. In the right anterior oblique view, **K**, the sinuses of Valsalva are seen to be markedly dilated. (**LA**, Left atrium; **LV**, left ventricle; **NC** and **LC**, non-coronary and left coronary sinuses of Valsalva.) (No auscultatory evidence of aortic regurgitation has developed.) Toward the end of systole the posterior leaflet of the mitral valve bulged markedly into the left atrium (indicated by arrows), and there was mitral regurgitation. The systolic clicks coincided temporally with maximum prolapse of the valve. In **L** is shown a diagram of the normal heart as viewed in the right anterior oblique position. (**K** and **L** from Criley, J. M., Lewis, K. B., Humphries, J. O., and Ross, R. S.: Brit. Heart J. **28:**488, 1966.)

Continued.

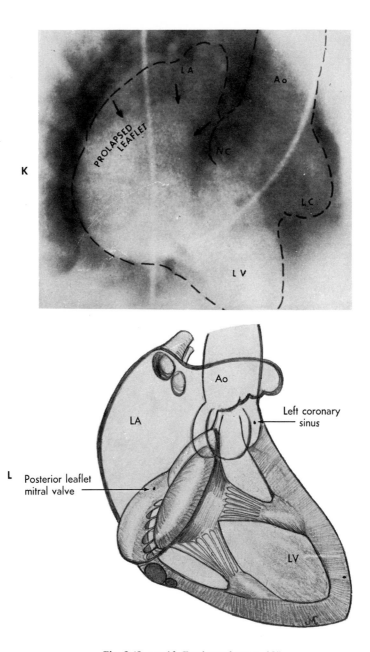

Fig. 3-42, cont'd. For legend see p. 125.

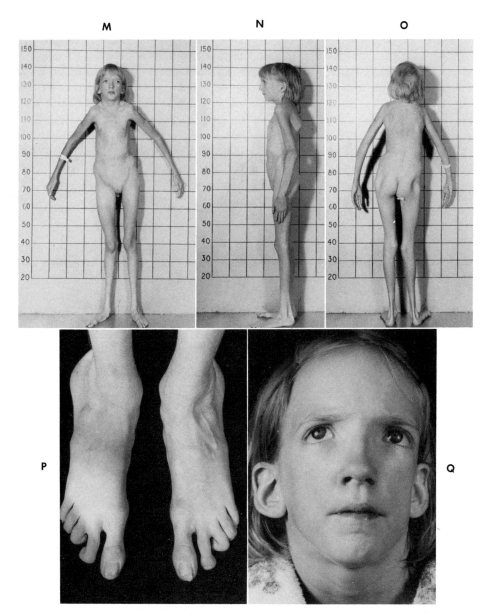

Fig. 3-42, cont'd. M to **Q,** Appearance at age 8½ years. **M** to **O,** Demonstrated here are excessive height, pectus carinatum, scoliosis, narrow flatfeet, sparsity of subcutaneous fat. **P,** The feet are very long, narrow, and everted, with a prominent heel and contracted toes III, IV, and V. **Q,** Characteristic Marfan facies. Note megalocornea and small, somewhat eccentric pupils.

Between ages 7 and 8 years the patient developed signs of aortic regurgitation and suffered episodes of severe chest pain, interpreted as indicating acute dissection of the aorta. Despite therapy with reserpine, rupture of the aorta occurred less than one month after these views were photographed.

verted T waves in leads II, III, and aV$_F$, interpreted as indicating posteroinferior myocardial ischemia).[68] Bowers[67] found this auscultatory-electrocardiographic syndrome in all of 13 patients with the Marfan syndrome who had mitral regurgitation from primary change in the mitral valve rather than secondary to aortic regurgitation.

This valvular defect, or the clinical syndrome it produces, is variously called the billowing mitral valve,[52] the floppy mitral valve syndrome,[443] the click syndrome,[145] the Barlow syndrome, the syndrome of apical systolic click, late systolic murmur and abnormal T waves,[145] and late systolic dysfunction of the mitral valve.[145] The syndrome can have many causes. As noted above, the Marfan syndrome is one, and inheritance as an isolated anomaly of the mitral valve is a second cause. We have seen it also in patients with osteogenesis imperfecta (p. 412). Criley and co-workers[107] observed it as a result of steering-wheel injury. Rheumatic fever is not a cause, it seems. Idiopathic mucoid degeneration, which may also involve the aortic valve,[265] is often the basis. The Ehlers-Danlos syndrome is yet another heritable disorder of connective tissue in which I have observed the "floppy mitral valve" syndrome (p. 334).

Other organic causes of a late systolic murmur[490] include hypertrophic subaortic stenosis, coarctation of the aorta, and the postmyocardial infarction state. Mitral regurgitation is of major functional significance in some cases.[375,437,443, 491,495,507] In Miller and Pearson's patient[375] the distribution of the systolic murmur simulated that of aortic stenosis, and at autopsy a jet lesion of the left atrial wall underlying the aortic ring was found. Further study by Keech and colleagues[284] tends to corroborate the diagnosis of the Marfan syndrome in at least some of the patients with "floppy valve syndrome" reported by Read and colleagues.[443] Myxomatous transformation of the mitral valve was the anatomic basis for the mitral regurgitation. Avulsion of a leaflet from the mitral annulus and also ruptured chordae tendineae have been observed in rare instances.[422,511] In two large series of cases of ruptured mitral chordae tendineae,[476,493] the Marfan syndrome was not recognized as a "cause." Most such patients are long considered to have rheumatic heart disease. It is undoubtedly relevant that the pathophysiologic effects of mitral valve involvement in the Marfan syndrome have been fully appreciated only in the era of left heart catheterization and contrast radiocardiography, as well as of prosthetic replacement of the mitral valve.

Calcification of the mitral annulus has been demonstrated in a number of instances.[50,58,189,214,375,553] We have observed one instance of calcified annulus fibrosus mitralis associated with "floppy" mitral valve and severe mitral regurgitation that was incorrectly interpreted as rheumatic (P. R., 559979). Although ocular stigmata of the Marfan syndrome were absent and the skeletal features only suggestive, the patient's son has the full-blown disorder.

I had previously thought that occasionally the pathophysiologic effects of interatrial septal defect can dominate the clinical picture. However, the only patient in my experience who might corroborate this impression (Fig. 3-41) proved on autopsy to have an intact atrial septum. Because of the gracile habitus that patients with atrial septal defect frequently display, the Marfan syndrome is frequently suspected. Such patients indeed have arachnodactyly; however, most do not have ectopia lentis or the characteristic family history to allow one to conclude that the true Marfan syndrome is present. (See Fig. 3-59D.) Bowden and

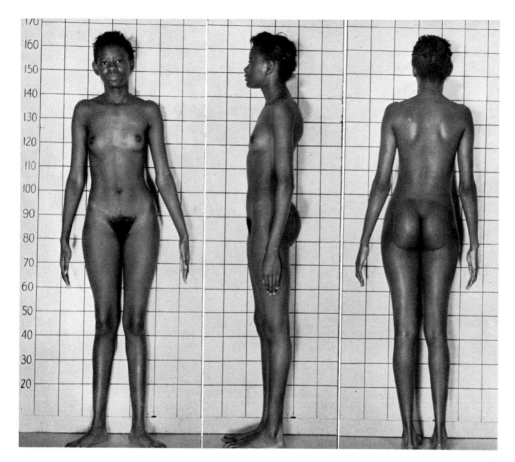

Fig. 3-43. G. H. (815634), 15 years of age, has bilateral subluxation of the lenses, spinal curvature, and the habitus typical of the Marfan syndrome. Clinical signs of interventricular septal defect are corroborated by the data of cardiac catheterization (courtesy Dr. Donald Nelson and Dr. Peter Luchsinger, District of Columbia General Hospital, Washington). In my personal experience this is the only case of interventricular septal defect in a patient with Marfan syndrome. (From McKusick, V. A.: Bull. N. Y. Acad. Med. 35:143, 1959.)

co-workers[63] reported a child who died at 6 months with profound mitral regurgitation and a large ostium secundum type of atrial septal defect. The clinical appearance and the histologic changes in the mitral valve, pulmonary artery, and ascending aorta supported the diagnosis of Marfan syndrome. Kumar and Berenson[300] also described ostium secundum defect.

In 1955 I wrote as follows: "Notwithstanding careless statements of previous reviews, no autopsy-confirmed or even clinically convincing case of interventricular septal defect has been reported." Since that time, however, at least one case of autopsy-proved interventricular septal defect with the Marfan syndrome* has

---

*In this case[558] the diagnosis of the Marfan syndrome is in some question, since there was no ectopia lentis and no positive family history. The patient had both patent ductus arteriosus and interventricular septal defect. The habitus suggesting the true Marfan syndrome may have been merely that rather often seen with these lesions.

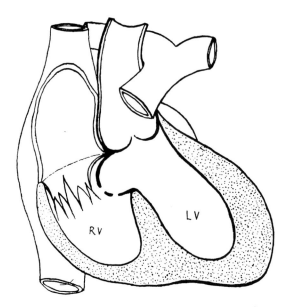

Fig. 3-44. Ruptured aneurysm of interventricular septum in the Marfan syndrome. Distortion of the septal leaflet of the tricuspid valve overlying the aneurysm is indicated. (From Ross, J. K., and Gerbode, F.: J. Thorac. Cardiov. Surg. **39:**746, 1960.)

been reported,[558] and I have had an opportunity to study the patient in one such case, a 15-year-old girl with typical Marfan syndrome, including ectopia lentis and clinically typical interventricular septal defect confirmed by cardiac catheterization (Fig. 3-43).* Broglio[76] reported a presumed case, and the grandfather of O'Doherty's proband[404] had the habitus of the Marfan syndrome and died at 37 years of age, with interventricular septal defect confirmed at autopsy. Ross and Gerbode[464] described a 15-year-old white girl with typical ocular and skeletal features of the Marfan syndrome. An unusual type of interventricular septal defect was repaired by open heart surgery. An aneurysm of the membranous septum bulged into the right ventricular outflow tract and displayed a fenestration (Fig. 3-44). It is attractive to suppose that the weakness of the membranous septum was part of the generalized disorder of connective tissue and that stress-fatigue was responsible for the fenestration. The murmur heard at an early age may have been produced by partial obstruction of right ventricular outflow, and the fenestration of the aneurysm may have occurred sometime after birth rather than being congenital. (Aneurysm of the membranous septum has been recognized in patients without stigmata of connective tissue disease.[25,85])

In Cockayne's case[100] the diagnosis of interventricular septal defect was only suspected clinically. There is a report[318] of possible tetralogy of Fallot with Marfan's syndrome. Two cases of tetralogy of Fallot with stigmata suggestive of the Marfan syndrome (see Fig. 3-45 for one of these) have come to my atten-

---

*I am indebted to Dr. Donald Nelson and Dr. Peter Luchsinger of the District of Columbia General Hospital, Washington, D. C., for calling this patient to my attention and providing catheterization data.

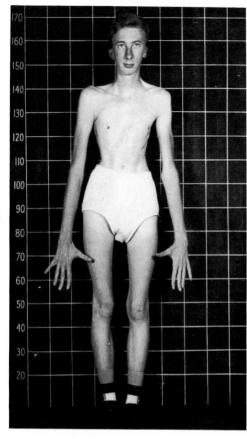

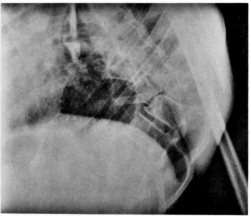

Fig. 3-45. A case (J.H.H. 525256) of tetralogy of Fallot with stigmata suggesting Marfan's syndrome. The absence of ectopia lentis and of other affected persons in the family makes the diagnosis of the Marfan syndrome dubious. There are malformed pinnae and long fingers, **A,** and hemivertebra, **B;** but these are nonspecific manifestations of the Marfan syndrome. Note also the facial asymmetry. (In yet another patient with tetralogy of Fallot [J.H.H. 482041], cleft palate, pes planus, talipes equinovarus, and long fingers are present, but in general the diagnosis of the Marfan syndrome is uncertain because of lack, as in the above patient, of ectopia lentis and positive family history.) (From McKusick, V. A.: Circulation 11:321, 1955.)

tion,[335] but the absence of involvement of other members of the family and the failure to find ectopia lentis in the patients make the diagnosis of the Marfan syndrome uncertain. I am inclined to think that these are not cases of the Marfan syndrome.

Van Buchem[571] concluded that mild pulmonary stenosis was present in one of his patients. However, the systolic gradient across the valve was only 35 mm. Hg. It is possible that there was only relative pulmonary stenosis from dilatation of the pulmonary artery (which was present).

The pulmonary valve was absent in a case of presumed Marfan syndrome.[93] The family history was negative and ectopia lentis was not found, but arachnodactyly was impressive, myopia was severe, and the aorta showed cystic medial necrosis. An aneurysm of the pulmonary artery was present.

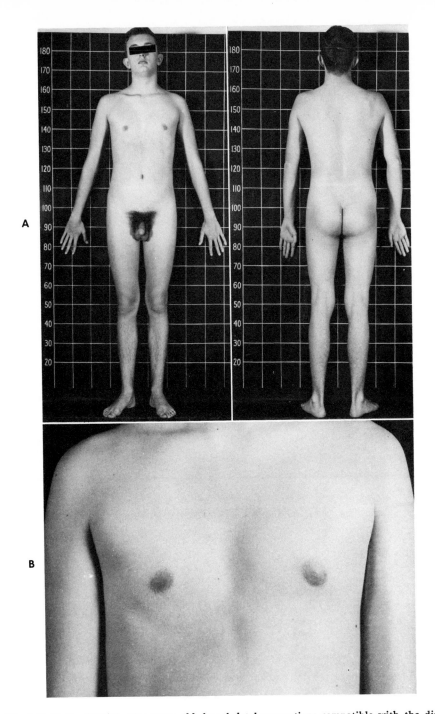

Fig. 3-46. D. D. (758872), 16½ years old, has skeletal proportions compatible with the diagnosis of the Marfan syndrome, **A,** slight bilateral ectopia lentis, very small posteroanterior dimension of the thorax, and asymmetric deformity of the anterior chest; the straight back is evident in the posterior view, **B.** Only mild pectus excavatum is present; however, its effects are greatly exaggerated by the small posteroanterior dimension, i.e., pronounced flat-chestedness. As in all cases of pectus excavatum, the thoracic spine is seen unusually clearly and little cardiac shadow is seen on the right of the midline, **C.** Both the spine and the sternum appear to impinge on the thoracic cavity, **D.** Multiple clicks in systole, **E,** were present in this, as in other cases of the Marfan syndrome.

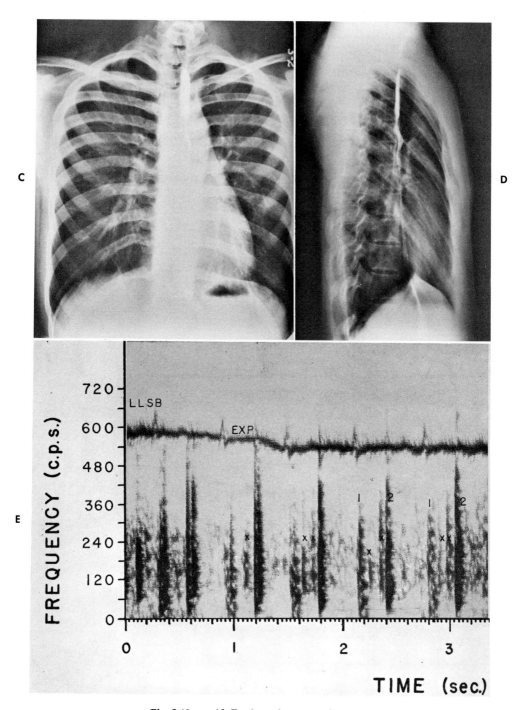

Fig. 3-46, cont'd. For legend see opposite page.

Much has been written about cardiac disability in pectus excavatum.[154,160, 379,546] Furthermore, since originally proposed by Flesch[168] in 1873, excessive longitudinal growth of the ribs has been thought to be the mechanism in many cases. As stated above, this appears to be the pathogenesis of the pectus excavatum in the Marfan syndrome. The hereditary nature of pectus excavatum has been appreciated.[420,474,519,638] Patients with pectus excavatum are often described as being unusually tall and thin, with spinal curvatures. Despite all these considerations, it has not been properly appreciated that the pectus excavatum may be but one manifestation of a generalized disorder of connective tissue, in which primary involvement of the cardiovascular system may occur. In Fig. 3-47 we have presented the case of a 24-year-old man with severe pectus excavatum, who died of rupture of the aorta shortly after surgical repair of the chest deformity.[49] Autopsy revealed aortic changes typical of the Marfan syndrome. An aortic diastolic murmur had been present before operation. In the surgical literature, there are 2 cases that may have been instances of the Marfan syndrome. One patient[313] was 6 years old and was described as having "systolic and diastolic murmurs and cardiac incompetence." The other,[439] 23 years old and 74 inches tall, had congestive heart failure and atrial fibrillation and was specifically de-

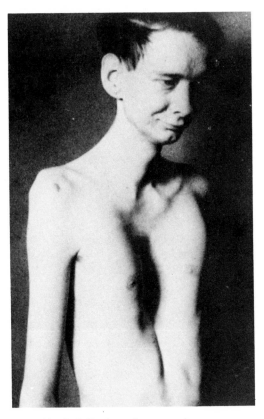

Fig. 3-47. For legend see opposite page.

scribed by his physician as thin, gangling, loose-jointed, and round-shouldered. In another instance, a case reported by Sweet,[547] the patient has been discovered to have typical Marfan's syndrome.[599]

Wachtel and associates[581] suggest that cardiac disability in pectus excavatum can result from four factors: (1) Due to twisting and distortion of the great veins, venous return may be impeded. (2) Restriction of diastolic expansion may further limit delivery of more blood on demand. (3) Impingement on the atria leads to supraventricular arrhythmias. (4) Respiratory reserve is decreased from impairment of the intercostal component of respiration. The heart may appear to be larger than, in fact, it is, because of (1) displacement of the heart into the left hemithorax, with mild clockwise rotation, and (2) pancaking of the heart, with increase in the transverse dimension. Electrocardiographic variations, such as rSr' or rSR' pattern in V_1, are secondary to the influence of the chest deformity on cardiac position and rotation.

Fig. 3-47. Severe pectus excavatum in the Marfan syndrome. K. B., a 24-year-old white man, was admitted to the Medical College of Virginia Hospital after a year of increasing dyspnea. Twenty-four days before admission he had suddenly become markedly dyspneic and had severe palpitation and substernal pain. About two weeks before admission he had a second episode of pain and palpitation. Following the first attack his dyspnea progressed more rapidly than before and he also became orthopneic.

Physical examination revealed a slender, underdeveloped, undernourished man who was dyspneic even at rest. There was pronounced pectus excavatum. The heart was markedly displaced to the left, with the point of maximum impulse in the midaxillary line and the seventh and eighth intercostal spaces. The left anterior chest wall heaved with each heartbeat. There was a loud continuous machinery-like murmur over the base of the heart, with a systolic thrill. Blood pressure was 90/40 in the right arm and 110/32 in the left.

On Nov. 5, 1949, surgical repair of the pectus excavatum was performed.[49] The patient withstood the operation well and remained in a satisfactory condition until 48 hours later, when he suddenly went into circulatory collapse and died in less than 2 hours after developing pronounced distention of the cervical veins.

At autopsy the body measured 72 inches in length. The arms and legs were very slender and long, with poor muscular development. The left leg was shorter than the right and showed partial clubfoot. Bilaterally the first and second toes were unusually long but the fourth toes were shorter than normal. There were flexion deformities of the fingers, deformed teeth with malocclusion, bifid uvula, and lumbar kyphosis.

The heart weighed 550 grams. The increase in weight and size was the result of left ventricular hypertrophy and dilatation. The pericardial sac contained 880 ml. of blood. The ascending aorta and first portion of the arch were markedly dilated, and, in addition, there was a dissecting aneurysm of the wall extending from an intimal tear about 3 cm. above the aortic ring to the point where there was slight coarctation of the aorta between the left subclavian and left common carotid ostia. Just distal to the left subclavian a second dissection began and extended throughout the rest of the aorta to involve the first portion of both iliac arteries. A small rent on the anterolateral surface of the ascending aorta represented the spot where perforation into the pericardial sac had occurred.

Histologically both dissections were endothelialized and showed some atheroma formation. In addition, the tunica media showed pronounced changes of the type described in other cases of aortic abnormality in this series.

Siegenthaler[504] reports an equally severe instance of pectus excavatum in the Marfan syndrome.

(From McKusick, V. A.: Circulation **11**:321, 1955.)

Prolongation of the P-R interval of the electrocardiogram occurs commonly in the Marfan syndrome[20,89,367] but is usually absent except in the presence of aortic regurgitation. It is interesting to speculate that aneurysmal dilatation of the aortic ring may compromise atrioventricular conduction by pressure on the conducting tissue. Bundle-branch block also occurs.[89,357,545] One patient (J. S., 543026), 18 years of age, with unequivocal ocular and skeletal signs of the Marfan syndrome has right bundle-branch block as the only cardiovascular abnormality demonstrable by extensive studies, including cardiac catheterization. A brother of this patient, who probably suffers from a *forme fruste,* demonstrates inverted P waves, bespeaking an ectopic pacemaker. The father, who was 78 inches tall, had aortic regurgitation and died suddenly at the age of 28 years; he had either ectopic pacemaker or prolongation of the P-R interval with superimposition of P waves on T waves. Bowers[64,65] reviewed the electrocardiographic findings in a group of cases. Moretti and colleagues[381] observed complete heart block and Stokes-Adams attacks in a 44-year-old man with the Marfan syndrome. The Wolff-Parkinson-White syndrome has also been observed.[244] The conduction abnormalities are of particular interest in connection with pathologic changes in the vascular supply to the sinus and atrioventricular nodes, described by James and associates[263,264] (p. 182). Chronic atrial flutter has been described,[473] and many patients have atrial fibrillation,[125] especially when significant mitral valve dysfunction is present.

There is one report[318] of dilatation of the left external carotid artery. No histologic study was made. Dilatation of the ascending aorta was also present in that patient. Hardin[230] described a 73-year-old woman with the Marfan syndrome, from whom an aneurysm of the extracranial portion of the internal carotid artery was successfully resected. We have observed pronounced dilatation of the left common carotid in a 13-year-old boy (B. F., 724330), with skeletal changes characteristic of the Marfan syndrome and with ectopia lentis but no clinical evidence of change in the aorta. Dissection may be limited to the innominate and common carotid arteries.[16] Dissection may extend out branches of the aorta for an appreciable distance.[317] Dissection limited to the coronary arteries has been described in the Marfan syndrome.[283,334,480] In one case (S. C., 575946), the splenic artery was friable at autopsy and was found to be the site of cystic medial necrosis. Cucolo and Kavazes[111] described cystic medial necrosis of the splenic artery with rupture of the spleen. Varicose veins probably occur more frequently and in more severe form in the Marfan syndrome than ordinarily would be expected.[606]

Mild coarctation of the aortic isthmus is common (Fig. 3-28). It is rarely of great functional significance.[140,571] Keech and co-workers[284] observed complete coarctation of the aorta in a 61-year-old Negro female with ectopia lentis and skeletal features of the Marfan syndrome. Seemingly the coarctation has not been resected in any case of the Marfan syndrome. Dissecting aneurysm occurs with increased frequency in coarctation,[235] and although the hypertension is doubtlessly a contributing factor, the possibility that a connective tissue abnormality may be responsible for both the coarctation and the dissection must be considered. One patient in my series (L. Y., J.H.H. 392843) had hypertension and a small left radial pulse but no significant discrepancy in arm and leg pressures.

Rib notching occurs with enlargement of any one of the elements of the neurovascular bundle on the undersurface of the ribs—artery, vein, or nerve. Enlargement of the artery in coarctation, of the vein in obstruction of the superior vena cava, or of the nerve in neurofibromatosis can lead to notching of the inferior margin of the rib. Rib notching has been described in the Marfan syndrome[308] but is probably part of the skeletal dysplasia and not related to one of the above mechanisms. This conclusion is based primarily on the fact that notching occurs on both the superior and the inferior margins. It might incorrectly suggest the presence of coarctation. Aortic regurgitation is probably rarely a cause of rib notching.

The changes at the aortic isthmus in the Marfan syndrome (Fig. 3-28C) have many of the features of what the angiocardiographers, who are largely responsible for discovering the disorder, call "pseudocoarctation." Even the "figure-of-three" sign may be present on conventional radiography of the chest. One would be suspicious of the presence of the Marfan syndrome in a patient such as the one described by Steinberg[526] in whom pseudocoarctation was associated with dilated sinuses of Valsalva.

The combination of aortic regurgitation with coarctation may confuse the diagnosis of coarctation. The pulses in the legs may seem normal unless the absence of the collapsing quality is noted.

Whitfield and associates[600] described a case of simple hypoplasia of the aorta with the Marfan syndrome. They suggested that the increased resistance resulting from the reduced aortic diameter might have been responsible, at least in part, for the cardiac hypertrophy observed in their case. Since hypoplasia of the aorta as a primary entity is a nebulous entity at best, this interpretation is suspect.

Hypertension, presumably without coarctation, was present at the age of 12 years in one reported case.[217] In another patient,[57] hypertension had been present from at least the age of 24 years, and the Smithwick operation was performed at the age of 27 years. Hypertension has been present at least from the age of 26 years in 2 of our cases (L. Y., 392843; C. S., 596716). Presumably the presence of hypertension[356] places the patient in double jeopardy from rupture of the aorta. (A Japanese patient described as an example of the Marfan syndrome with hypertension due to renal arterial stenosis[502] may have had homocystinuria instead.)

Thrombosis in arteries or veins should always suggest homocystinuria (Chapter 4) rather than the Marfan syndrome. However, bilateral renal vein thrombosis leading to the nephrotic syndrome was observed in a Mexican-Indian patient who clearly had the Marfan syndrome, with dissection in the aorta from the left subclavian artery to the bifurcation.[5]

In one reported case,[487] bacterial endaortitis was thought to be present.

Other cardiovascular abnormalities have been described, but in most of these cases a diagnosis of the Marfan syndrome is insecure. For example, Burry[81] described a 37-year-old mentally defective woman with negative family history and no ectopia lentis who did, however, have a moderate degree of myopia and presumably had characteristic skeletal proportions. Supravalvular aortic stenosis was present. Bingle[50] described a 32-year-old woman with patent ductus arteriosus, cystic medial necrosis of the aorta, dilatation of the aortic ring, and dissection of the ascending aorta with rupture into the pericardial sac. Grossly, there was

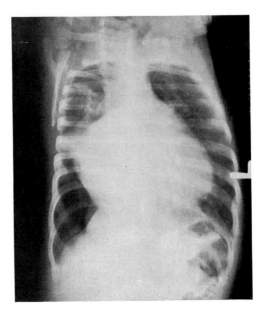

Fig. 3-48. For legend see opposite page.

an area of calcification and of scarring in the wall of the left atrium, and histologically, there was fragmentation and sparsity of elastic fibers. Family history was not provided. Although the patient was $68\frac{1}{2}$ inches tall, body proportions were not described. There were "no changes in eyes."

Some cardiac manifestations of the Marfan syndrome may be of the same origin as those of the "straight back" syndrome, described in 1960 by Rawlings[440] as a form of "pseudo heart disease." Patients with the Marfan syndrome often lack the normal kyphotic curve of the upper and mid thoracic spine and have a small anteroposterior, sternovertebral dimension (e.g., Fig. 3-46D). As a result the heart may appear to be enlarged, especially in its mid-left portion, and a basilar systolic murmur can be produced, probably through compression or torsion of the great vessels. Among the patients in the original report,[440] some had been refused insurance or employment, and there were some cases of iatrogenic invalidism. Errors in diagnosis of the opposite kind can be made; patients with the Marfan syndrome have been labeled as having "straight back" syndrome, pure and simple. Although caution must be exercised in making the straight-back syndrome the primary diagnosis,[562] the concept is a useful one.[441]

Other manifestations. Special attention is directed to certain manifestations which are of the nature of conventional congenital malformations in the cardiovascular system—coarctation of the aorta,[140,153,156,166,335,570,571] patent ductus arteriosus,[*9,568] anomaly of valvular cuspation, absent pulmonary valve,[93] interatrial defect,[14,306,426] and possibly pulmonary stenosis[571]; in the skeletal system—spina

---

*Patent ductus arteriosus must be very rare in the Marfan syndrome.[23] Apert[14] is frequently quoted as having described such a case; his patient in fact had "trou de Botal" (patent foramen ovale), not "ductus de Botal." Patent ductus arteriosus was present in one of the patients of Tune and Thal.[567]

Fig. 3-48. X-ray film of the chest in infant B. J. P. A pulmonary anomaly is evident, as well as pronounced cardiomegaly.

B. J. P. (H.L.H. A93754) was born Nov. 9, 1951. She weighed 6 pounds 11 ounces and was thought to be healthy. The mother had had no pregnancies in the nineteen years between this one and a pregnancy in 1933. The mother first learned of the child's heart murmur when the child was 4 months old. The child was never able to sit up or roll over by herself. When first seen at the age of 6 months, the following findings were recorded: the left side of the face was smaller than the right; respirations were rapid (about 50/min.); there was a pigeon-breast deformity of the thorax; the pulse was regular at a rate of 150/min.; femoral pulses were full; the heart was enlarged beyond the left midclavicular line; a systolic thrill was palpable over the entire precordium but was maximal in the left midprecordium; a harsh systolic murmur had the same location; the liver edge was 1.5 cm. below the right costal margin; there was no clubbing or cyanosis.

Fluoroscopy revealed great cardiac enlargement to both left and right, with globular shape. The right ventricle was definitely enlarged in the oblique views. The right lower lung field had a distinctly abnormal appearance. It lacked the usual lung markings and was unusually radiolucent. There was a question of atelectatic lung (? right middle lobe) at the right heart border. By electrocardiogram the P waves were broad and notched. The P-R interval was 0.16 second, which is long, considering the patient's age and heart rate of 150/min. Very large R waves in the leads from the left of the precordium suggested left ventricular hypertrophy. The hematocrit was 29.5%, with hypochromic, microcytic cell indices.

Late in May, 1952, the patient developed physical and x-ray signs of consolidation in the right upper lobe and became febrile. These signs were altered little by the administration of several different antibacterial agents. The heart was extremely overactive and shook the whole bed. Occasionally the murmur assumed a to-and-fro quality, especially at the lower left sternal border. The liver enlarged in size. Subsequently, signs of consolidation of the entire right lung appeared. On July 31, 1952, it was noted that both lenses were displaced mediad and that dilatation of the pupil with phenylephrine was only partially successful. Ophthalmologic consultants observed that the patient was extremely myopic, with small lenses. In the last weeks of life there was an episode of hematuria, perhaps related to sulfadiazine therapy. Death occurred on July 10, 1952, when the patient was only 8 months old.

Autopsy (23761) revealed that the right lung was partially atelectatic. The left lung was normal. The pulmonary artery was larger in circumference than the aorta. The foramen ovale was imperfectly closed. All chambers of the heart showed hypertrophy of their walls, and dilatation. The hypertrophy of the right atrium was particularly marked. Microscopically there were no lesions of the myocardium. However, the wall of the pulmonary artery and, to a lesser extent, that of the aorta showed typical changes of the Marfan syndrome. The media contained vacuoles filled with the metachromatically staining material, and there was derangement and relative sparsity of elastic fibers. The wall of the pulmonary artery was thicker than that of the aorta. At the time of the gross examinations the bronchial tree was injected with radiopaque material and radiograms were made. To the surprise of the prosector, no abnormality was identified.

Comment. Obviously the most informative feature of this case is the advanced change in the pulmonary artery, which undoubtedly resulted in pulmonary regurgitation and was a leading factor in the infant's death at the age of only 8 months. Ectopia lentis, myopia, microphakia, arachnodactyly, and retardation of ability to sit or roll over complete the picture of the Marfan syndrome.

This kinship illustrates one of the difficulties of genetic research in man. The illegitimacy of this infant and the presence of a legitimate wife of the father of the proposita made the utmost tact and resourcefulness necessary for collecting even these few data. The father of the infant is about 74 inches tall, has long hands and feet, and wears spectacles. Examination was not possible and no further pedigree information was obtained.

(From McKusick, V. A.: Circulation 11:321, 1955.)

bifida occulta, hemivertebra, and cleft palate[465,606]; in the eye—microphakia, hypoplasia, or aplasia of the dilator pupillae muscle, coloboma lentis, and coloboma iridis.[293] Encephalocele occurred in the forehead area in one patient (J. D., 184805). Internal hydrocephalus is also reported.[418,438] These are not among the more common manifestations; yet they occur sufficiently often in the Marfan syndrome to be considered more than coincidental associations. Their occurrence is difficult to reconcile with a unitary theory of a connective tissue defect unless one assumes that the presence of said defect during embryogenesis provides an abnormal environment in which these anomalies, congenital malformations in the usual sense, occur with increased incidence. In accordance with this last and not improbable proposition, these particular manifestations can be considered *secondary*.

Whether deafness is a specific manifestation of the Marfan syndrome and, if so, what its mechanism is,[320] cannot be stated at present. It is said to occur in 6% of cases.[436] Everberg[155] concluded that deafness is an integral feature and that it is of nerve (perceptive) type.

Pulmonary malformations are described in autopsy reports and various pulmonary complications in clinical reports[204,282,335,409,426,438,475,556] (Fig. 3-48). Repeated spontaneous pneumothorax has been described.[4,207,217,268,282,311] I have observed a number of dramatic examples of this complication of the Marfan syndrome (e.g., M. C., 1421753; D. W., 1471381). Spontaneous pneumothorax sometimes occurs as a familial disorder in the absence of evident Marfan syndrome[46,71] and also occurs in association with the Ehlers-Danlos syndrome (p. 329). Brock[75] favored the presence of hereditary lung cysts as the anatomic substrate. Statistically, spontaneous pneumothorax occurs most often in tall, slim young men. [172,607] The association between tall, asthenic habitus and pneumothorax is probably not the result of the presence of mild cases of the Marfan syndrome in the series studied.

Occasionally, congenital cystic disease of the lung occurs, probably as an integral part of the Marfan syndrome.[319a] In patient M. R. (J.H.H. 176836; see Fig. 3-49), very extensive disease of this type was discovered at autopsy. The stillborn child of this patient showed abnormal lobation of the lungs but no congenital cystic disease. Without an exhaustive review of the literature, it was possible to find 3 cases of cystic disease of the lung in which stigmata suggestive of the Marfan syndrome were described.

Case 1. A 26-year-old male medical student (Case 9 in reference 409) had had three attacks of spontaneous pneumothorax. He died following an attack of severe chest pain. Dissecting aneurysm of the aorta with rupture into the pericardium was discovered. Histologically there was cystic medial necrosis. Both lungs showed diffuse cystic changes regarded as congenital.

Case 2. A 26-year-old housewife (Case 13 in reference 409) with striking dolichostenomelia had had increasing dyspnea and, at the end of her second pregnancy, frank congestive failure. X-ray examination showed dilatation of the outflow tract of the right ventricle; electrocardiograms showed right axis deviation and the so-called P-pulmonale. Postmortem examination disclosed diffuse cystic changes in both lungs and widely patent foramen ovale.

Case 3. A 12-year-old child[467] was found at autopsy to have multiple simple cysts throughout both lungs, patent ductus arteriosus, aneurysm of the pulmonary artery, and anomalous coronary artery.

The case of Lillian[316] showed lung cysts, but the diagnosis of the Marfan syndrome is not completely certain.

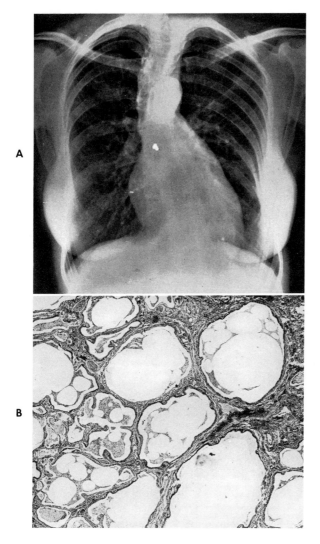

Fig. 3-49. A, X-ray film of the chest in M. R. (176836), from whom other illustrative materials are demonstrated in Figs. 3-21 and 3-40. Scoliosis, cardiac enlargement, increased pulmonary markings, and questionable bleb formation in the lungs are demonstrated. **B,** Same patient. At autopsy the lungs weighed 1,350 grams. There was exudation of copious edema from the cut surfaces. Bilaterally the upper lobes were involved by large, bleblike cavities filled with large amounts of greenish fluid. To a lesser extent, the middle lobe and both lower lobes were cystic. Histologically the cysts were large and conglomerate and lined with columnar epithelium. Some of the cysts were several centimeters in diameter. In the walls of many, thin strands of smooth muscle were identified. This photomicrograph was made at a magnification of ×25, reduced ⅓. The pulmonary cysts are clearly demonstrated.

Congenital cystic lung disease is probably a secondary component of this syndrome; that is, the presence of the connective tissue defect during embryogenesis conditions its development but is not as directly responsible for it as for some of the other manifestations. The Marfan syndrome can join Hand-Schüller-Christian disease[520,563] and tuberous sclerosis[42,43] in the group of systemic abnormalities associated with a type of cystic disease of the lung.

Neimann and associates[392] described a severely affected infant who died at 10 weeks of age of severe pulmonary emphysema. Bolande and Tucker[57] discussed the pathogenesis of emphysema in patients with the Marfan syndrome.[566] Six patients in one group of 7 cases had evidence of pulmonary dysaeration: 2 showed compression of the left main bronchus by a giant left atrium, with atelectasis of the lung and compensatory emphysema of the right lung, 2 showed chronic pulmonary emphysema, 3 had apical bullae bilaterally, and 1 developed pneumothorax. Bolande and Tucker suggested that emphysema, sometimes cystic, in young patients with the Marfan syndrome and without evidence of pulmonary infection, fibrosis, bronchitis, or bronchiolitis, is a result of the generalized disorder of connective tissue. No histologic changes leading to emphysema were found. Increased deposition of elastic fibers in the alveolar septa was interpreted as a response to mechanical stress and is seen in other comparable situations in non-Marfan patients. Flaccidity of the walls of the respiratory and terminal bronchioles may, they suggested, predispose to collapse during expiration and result in air trapping and emphysema. Pulmonary function was studied by Fuleihan and colleagues[178] and by Chisolm and colleagues.[94] The latter workers,[94] finding pulmonary function normal, concluded that "elasticity-determining tissues of the lung are not primarily affected by the Marfan lesion."

On rare occasions cardiopulmonary failure in the Marfan syndrome can be secondary to, or importantly contributed to, by severe kyphoscoliosis. The pathogenesis is the same as in cardiorespiratory failure from kyphoscoliosis of other cause.[44,227]

Hematologic abnormalities are unusual in the Marfan syndrome. Estes and colleagues[149] described a family with apparently typical and full-blown Marfan syndrome in 7 members. Five of the 7 had easy bruising, an increase in circulating immature granulocytes, an increase in leukocyte alkaline phosphatase, giant platelets, and functional platelet abnormalities.

The voice in patients with the Marfan syndrome sometimes is rather high pitched, with a timbre sufficiently characteristic that one author[69] thought he could recognize affected persons over the telephone.

Congenital cystic kidneys were described[59] in one case of arachnodactyly, but the evidence presented is inadequate for the reviewer to be certain that the genuine Marfan syndrome was present.

Fatal rupture of the stomach occurred in a 15-year-old boy with the Marfan syndrome after gross overeating.[576] This appears to be a unique observation. Cook[104] described two sisters who died in their early twenties of spontaneous perforation of the colon. They were thought to have no stigmata of the Marfan syndrome, but the father and a brother, a nephew, four aunts, and some cousins were apparently affected, some in full-blown form. Perforation of the colon is a recognized complication of the Ehlers-Danlos syndrome (p. 324).

There are other manifestations that occur less frequently, often in no more than single reported cases, than those termed "secondary" before. It is more likely that these anomalies occur only coincidentally with the bona fide features of the Marfan syndrome. When the case in question is a sporadic one, it may be valid to assume that the mutagenic factor might have caused more than one mutation simultaneously. Furthermore, in a given family, if the anomaly in question occurs in only one of the persons affected by the Marfan syndrome, or, better yet, if the anomaly also occurs in one or more members of the family unaffected by the Marfan syndrome, the manifestation in question should not be considered part of the Marfan syndrome.

Contrary to previous emphasis,[118,320,418,485] mental retardation is not, in my opinion, a component of this syndrome. Usually the patients are at least as bright as their siblings. Sometimes their innate intelligence is not fully realized because

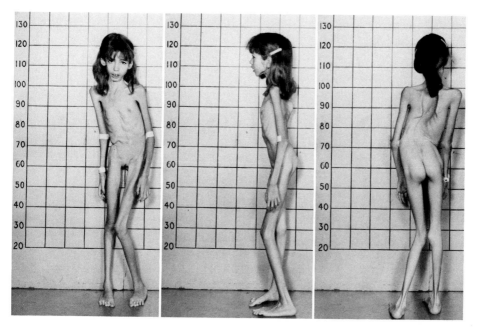

Fig. 3-50. Probable Marfan syndrome with muscular underdevelopment and hypotonia as leading features.

S. J. (1096410) was born in 1959 of a 26-year-old mother and a 27-year-old father. Of 2 sibs, one, a year older, had a small defect in the membranous ventricular septum, and the other, younger, had had a ventricular septal defect closed surgically. The father appeared to have a small patent ductus arteriosus. None had stigmata of the Marfan syndrome.

S. J. was born after a 10-month pregnancy during which the mother noted reduced fetal movements. Bilateral dislocated hips, striking muscular hypotonia, and torticollis were present at birth. The dislocated hips were repaired at 6 months and the torticollis at age 3 years. From birth she fed poorly but had normal subcutaneous and muscle bulk despite the severe *hypotonicity.* Neostigmine (Prostigmine) was given for about three years, beginning at 9 months, with apparent benefit at first but none later. The general clinical features are evident in the photographs made at the age of 10 years. The eyes were normal. The heart showed systolic clicks and a late systolic murmur consistent with floppy mitral valve. Muscle biopsy showed no specific change. Intelligence was normal. Respiratory difficulties secondary to the severe spinal deformity and the muscular hypotonia have been major problems.

of the limitation of opportunities imposed by severe visual impairment and other physical handicaps. One patient in our series (F. D.), who died at the age of 14 years, wrote a book of verse, which was published, and composed short dramas for enacting by her playmates. In severe sporadic cases in infants and children, there may be mental retardation, but this has, in my opinion, a separate basis, possibly an independent mutation. Another basis for confusion is the fact that a picture including arachnodactyly and suggesting the Marfan syndrome occurs with acquired developmental abnormalities such as those due to rubella and other maternal illness, maternal exposure to x ray, and Rh incompatibility. These patients are likely to show mental retardation. The occurrence of mental retardation as a conspicuous feature of homocystinuria (p. 225), which in several other respects simulates the Marfan syndrome, may be another reason that mental retardation has been thought to be a feature of the Marfan syndrome.

Haber[218] points out that a rare but characteristic *skin lesion* may be associated with the Marfan syndrome. It is called Miescher's elastoma, or elastoma intrapapillare perforans verruciforme. The lesions occur particularly on the neck and grossly appear as small nodules or papules. Histologically they are cysts oc-

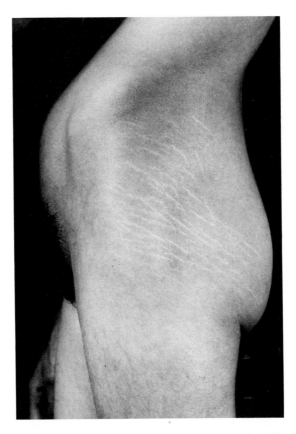

Fig. 3-51. Striae distensae. C. M. G. (J.H.H. 1257318), a girl born in 1951, has severe skeletal, ocular, and cardiac features of the Marfan syndrome. The patient was 16 years old at the time of this photograph, which demonstrates striae of the lateral buttock area.

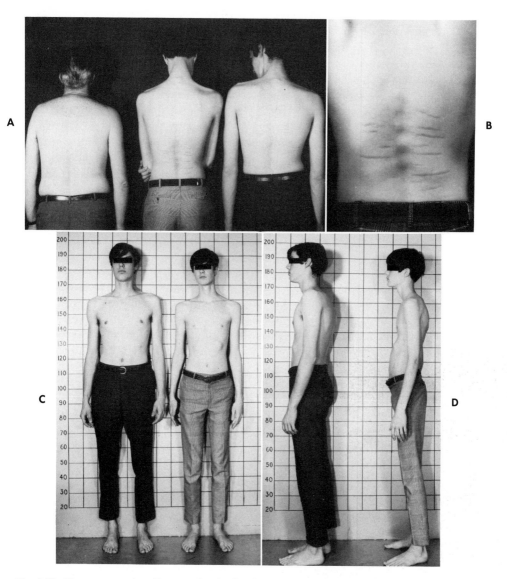

Fig. 3-52. Transverse striae distensae in the lumbar area in father and 2 sons. I. G. (J.H.H. 1198688), the younger of the sons, was referred by a gastroenterologist who had been consulted for "bellyache" and who suspected the Marfan syndrome. I. G. was then 15 years old and his brother 18 years old. They were 75 and 76 inches tall, respectively, and both had developed transverse purplish striae over the lower back at the age of about 15 years. The father developed identical striae in adolescence, but they faded as he grew older. The father was not unusually tall; the mother was 71 inches tall and came from an unusually tall family. Neither parent gave a family history of eye or cardiovascular complications. The 15-year-old proband showed moderate laxity of all joints, particularly the fingers, which he had dislocated on several occasions while playing football. He also had mild depression of the lower sternum, with flaring of the rib margins. Over the lower back were eight or ten broad, purplish transverse striae.

A, From left to right: father, 15-year-old son, 18-year-old son. Although clear enough on examination, the striae in the father are pale and barely visible in the photograph. **B,** Striae in 15-year-old son. (Infrared photograph.) **C** and **D,** Habitus in 2 sons. Note excessive height and, in the younger brother, poor posture, suggesting joint laxity.

cupied by whorls of material that have the tinctorial characteristics of elastic fibers and that seem to have erupted into the epidermis from the upper corium. In 1952 Storck[541] of Zurich described a patient with typical Marfan syndrome and skin lesions he classified as Kyrle's hyperkeratosis follicularis et perifollicularis in cutem penetrans. However, Miescher reported to Haber[218] that the skin lesions were histologically more characteristic of Miescher's elastoma. In 1958 Anning[10] of Leeds, England, described a young man in whom the diagnosis of Miescher's elastoma was made at the age of 18 years and who died at the age of 20 years of "dissecting aneurysm" of the aorta. It seems most likely that Anning's case[8] was an "ecchymotic" or "arterial" type of the Ehlers-Danlos syndrome (p. 311) and that the vascular accident was rupture of the aorta rather than conventional dissection of the aorta.

Striae of the skin in the pectoral and anterior deltoid areas,[276,324,380,482] radially oriented around the breasts and over the thighs, are frequently found in Marfan patients. They are observable in the teens and cannot be attributed to weight loss. (See Figs. 3-19B, 3-24D, and 3-51.) Elastoma perforans also occurs in the Ehlers-Danlos syndrome,[364] osteogenesis imperfecta, and pseudoxanthoma elasticum. It was also described in a child who at the age of 4 years suffered a subarachnoid hemorrhage from a berry aneurysm of the circle of Willis.[96] In a Marfan patient with nephrotic syndrome,[5] subcutaneous edema greatly exaggerated the striae. Striae distensae like those of the Marfan syndrome (except for the location) were seen in a father and two sons (Fig. 3-52). Although they were referred to me as possible examples of the Marfan syndrome, the findings did not seem to justify that diagnosis.

The dental and other oral findings of the Marfan syndrome have been discussed.[19,279,390] Normal standards of palatal measurements are available[445,496] for comparison with those in the Marfan syndrome.

Two patients (younger brother in Fig. 3-24; patient shown in Fig. 3-69) in my series have juvenile diabetes mellitus, which probably bears no relation to the Marfan syndrome. Diabetes insipidus has also been described in a single case of the Marfan syndrome[221] and also probably is unrelated to the connective tissue disorder.

Prognosis

One man almost certainly affected with the Marfan syndrome (Fig. 3-53) was killed accidentally at the age of 82 years. One of our oldest patients died at 61 years of age (Fig. 3-35). He had severe aortic regurgitation. Bowers[69] described 2 patients with the Marfan syndrome still living at 61 and 66 years of age. Among 16 dead affected members of a large family, Bowers[69] found the average age at death to be 43 years in the males and 46 years in the females. One individual survived to 73 years; another died at 9 years. We have a patient who is 71 years old. The youngest case of the Marfan syndrome I have seen is the stillborn infant shown in Fig. 3-21I. The Marfan syndrome was recognized at birth in the offspring of the daughter shown in Fig. 3-32.[241] The average age at death among 72 deceased patients in my personal series of the Marfan syndrome was 32 years.[387a] Cardiac problems led to fifty-two of the fifty-six deaths of known cause, with aortic dilatation and its complications accounting for about 80% of these.

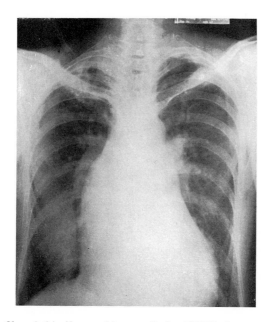

Fig. 3-53. The x-ray film of this 49-year-old man (B. L., 195805) shows prominence of the pulmonary artery and inconspicuous dilatation of the ascending aorta. These features, together with the murmur of aortic regurgitation and the associated Austin Flint murmur, led to the diagnosis of rheumatic heart disease with combined aortic and mitral lesions. This was the case in spite of the fact that the patient was 75½ inches tall, had spinal and thoracic deformities (a suggestion of which is indicated by the figure), and had had ectopic lenses removed ten and thirteen years previously. The patient had pneumonia twice in youth and had an operation for varicose veins at the age of 25 years. Scholastic performance was outstanding, with graduation from college at the age of 18 years. A bout of iritis prompted removal of the right lens in 1937. In 1940 the left lens was removed because of dislocation into the anterior chamber. Detachment of the retina on the left was discovered at that time. There was heterochromia iridis, with normal brown pigmentation on the right and greenish coloration on the left. The patient was accepted for service in the Army and, while there (1947), had his first bout of severe chest pain with extension to the arms, neck, and epigastrium. A second episode of probable aortic dissection occurred later in 1947 and a third in 1948. The episode in 1948 was characterized by severe low back pain radiating into the lower abdomen and genitalia. The diagnosis of rheumatic heart disease was based on the prominence of the pulmonary artery segment (due actually to displacement by the dilated aorta), a diastolic murmur at the apex (which was probably either radiation of the murmur of aortic regurgitation or an Austin Flint murmur or both), and displacement of the esophagus by what was interpreted as the left atrium (possibly indeed the left atrium enlarged from chronic left ventricular failure or possibly the aortic aneurysm, Fig. 3-31G). The patient died at home in 1950. The father, 6 feet 3 inches tall, was killed by a bus at the age of 82 years. He probably had the Marfan syndrome in mild form. He sired several affected children. His wife appears to have been unaffected. Of 11 sibs of the proband, 2, always puny, died at 8 and 10 years, of unknown causes; two had the same habitus as the proband; a fifth has definite Marfan syndrome. This man, now 49 years old, is 70½ inches tall, weighs 178 pounds, and wears an 11½C shoe. He was discharged from the Army when he lost the sight in one eye. Detachment of the retina was discovered at the age of 40 years. He has severe myopia and flat feet, is stoop-shouldered, is said to have a heart murmur, and has had left inguinal herniorrhaphy. (From McKusick, V. A.: Circulation 11:321, 1955.)

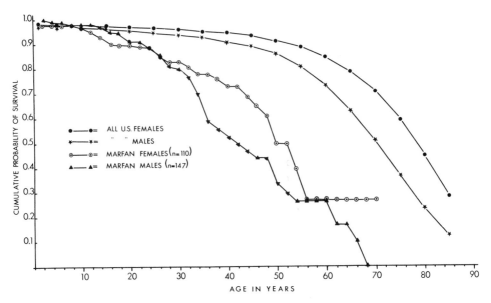

Fig. 3-54. Survivorship in the Marfan syndrome analyzed by the life table method. (From Murdoch, J. L., Walker, B. A., Halpern, B. L., Kuzma, J. W., and McKusick, V. A.: New Eng. J. Med. **286:**804, 1972.)

Fig. 3-54 shows survivorship curves* based on my personal experience with 257 cases of the Marfan syndrome diagnosed by stringent criteria. The more favorable prognosis in females is of interest. When sporadic and familial cases were considered separately, survivorship was found to be better in the familial cases. This is probably not surprising. Milder cases are found in families by their kinship to full-blown cases. The very fact that a given case was familial is an indication that the proband or someone else in the family was sufficiently mildly affected to have children.

Prevalence and inheritance

The sexes are equally affected.[327,436] The syndrome has been reported in Negroes,[179,335] Chinese,[91,231] Japanese,[395,513] Koreans (T. J., 132 2047), Hindus,[48] and Jews.[286,327] It has furthermore been reported in natives of virtually every European country. Its incidence in the American Negro is probably essentially the same as in the white population. It has occurred in American Indians.[185] Thus there is no evidence of particular ethnic incidence of the Marfan syndrome —and, of course, contrary to what is true of recessive disorders, one does not ex-

---

*As pointed out by Sartwell,[477a,477b] the life-table method of evaluating survivorship when the duration of observation varied widely was introduced into medicine in the early years of this century. Its application to the epidemiology and study of the natural history of disease was recognized and taught over a period of many years by Raymond Pearl and by W. H. Frost of the Johns Hopkins University School of Hygiene and Public Health. An early application to the determination of prognosis in chronic disease was made by Merrill and Shulman,[308a] also of Johns Hopkins, in 1955, systemic lupus erythematosus being the disorder studied. Among the heritable disorders of connective tissue, homocystinuria (p. 240) and pseudoxanthoma elasticum (p. 492) have also been analyzed by this approach.

pect ethnic nonhomogeneity in a detrimental Mendelian dominant such as the Marfan syndrome.

The Marfan syndrome is an uncommon, but by no means rare, disorder. Its incidence is certainly far greater than indicated in the general conception of the medical public. The connective tissue defect of the Marfan syndrome is a leading cause of dissecting aneurysm of the aorta in the younger decades. There is reason to believe that there is an appreciable number of very mild cases *(forme fruste)*, in which the connective tissue defect has little or no effect on health or longevity.

Preposterously high estimates of the number of sporadic cases (those derived presumably from *de novo* mutation), as opposed to inherited cases, have been made. My own experience would indicate that no more than 15% of all cases are new ones. Higher estimates, up to 70% by some writers, are the result of incomplete family studies. How often this mutation occurs in a total population is hard to determine. Attempts at estimation of gene frequency or of mutation rate are beset by difficulties, such as diagnostic doubts in mild cases, the impossibility of ascertaining mild cases unless severe cases are present in the family, variability in the age of onset of the aortic manifestations, and the mimicry of phenocopies. These difficulties attend the study of other incomplete dominant traits, such as dystrophia myotonica. On the basis of as complete ascertainment as possible and using Haldane's method,[220,329] which assumes that mutation replaces those genes lost because of reduced effective fertility of affected persons, Lynas[328] estimated the mutation rate to be 5 per million genes per generation in the population of northern Ireland:

$$\mu = \tfrac{1}{2}(1 - f)\, x = \tfrac{1}{2}(1 - \tfrac{1}{2})\, \frac{36}{1,370,921}$$

x = proportion of persons with the Marfan syndrome in the population
f = the effective fertility of affected persons, when unity is the average fertility

When the mutation rate was estimated from the incidence of sporadic cases, a similar estimate was obtained. A minimal figure for prevalence of the Marfan syndrome was 1.459 per 100,000 of the population and for gene frequency, one-half this value, 0.729 per 100,000 genes.

The Marfan syndrome is one of the conditions in which "paternal age effect" on mutation has been demonstrated. The average age of fathers of sporadic, "new mutation" cases is about seven years in excess of the mean age of fathers generally. Just as one is impressed with maternal age in cases of mongolism, paternal age is often impressive in nonfamilial cases of this point mutation. For example, in 4 sporadic cases seen by me in the last few years, the ages of the fathers were 73, 69, 63, and 43 years old at birth of the patients; the mothers were 40 and 42 years old in two instances each. Murdoch, Walker, and I[388] examined parental age and birth order in 23 apparently sporadic cases of the Marfan syndrome (Table 3-3).

The method of partial correlations, particularly useful in weighing the relative importance of maternal and paternal age effect, was also used. These values are given below, together with the comparable values for 102 sporadic cases of achondroplasia (in which Murdoch and colleagues[387] have confirmed the paternal age effect):

1. Partial correlation for father's age versus incidence when mother's age

Table 3-3. Parental age and birth order in 23 sporadic cases of the Marfan syndrome

	Father's age		Mother's age		Birth order	
	Mean	S.D.	Mean	S.D.	Mean	S.D.
Sporadic cases of						
Marfan syndrome	36.61	9.06	29.30	5.36	3.17	2.48
General population	29.85	6.95	26.54	6.07	2.64	1.73

and birth order are held constant $(r_{fi.mb}) = +0.32$ (for achondroplasia, +0.27)

2. Partial correlation for mother's age versus incidence when father's age and birth order are held constant $(r_{mi.fb}) = -0.09$ (for achondroplasia, −0.01)

3. Partial correlation for birth order versus incidence when both parents' ages are held constant $(r_{bi.fm}) = +0.05$ (for achondroplasia, +0.09)

These partial correlations indicate that mother's age and birth order are per se of little significance to the mutation rate. The older the father is, the older the mother is likely to be and the higher the birth order, but the father's age is the primary and predominant factor in determining mutation rate.

The pattern of inheritance is that of a simple Mendelian autosomal dominant (Figs. 3-27, 3-36, 3-40, 3-55, and 3-56). Parental consanguinity has not been an impressive feature, but exceptions are described.[62] In a few instances a recessive mode of inheritance seemed to be indicated by the presence of multiple affected members of one sibship with ostensibly normal parents. In only one of the pedigrees of this type that have come to my attention has it been practicable to do thorough investigations of parents and patients (Fig. 3-36). In the one kinship in which this was possible, I was forced to conclude that the mother was probably affected by a *forme fruste*. This woman had had at least 3 affected children by one man and 1 affected child by a second. The occurrence in one male and three females excluded the possibility of a sex-linked recessive trait. There was therefore no question that each of the victims inherited the disease rather than developed it through *de novo* mutation and that the mother carries the gene. On examination, she was found to be 5 feet 8 inches tall, to be moderately long of limb without typical arachnodactyly, and to be myopic but free of ectopia lentis on careful ocular examination. This pedigree demonstrates how it is possible for the student of the full clinical and genetic picture to recognize cases that would be missed otherwise. (There are risks, of course, of counting cases as affected that are, in fact, not affected.) Recessive inheritance of a disorder characterized by ectopia lentis, vascular abnormalities, and skeletal features somewhat similar to those of the Marfan syndrome should suggest homocystinuria (Chapter 4). In Hungary, for example, Varga[573] found 6 families in which both parents were normal and 9 out of 27 sibs were affected with what was interpreted as the Marfan syndrome. The families lived in villages with a highly inbred population. Tests for homocystinuria and more details on the clinical picture would be of interest.

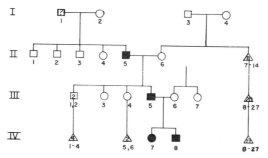

Fig. 3-55. By way of summary of the aortic complications of the Marfan syndrome, I present the story and pedigree of a family that was unusually heavily affected. Individual I-1 died suddenly in 1897 at the age of 47 years, presumably of apoplexy. This may have been dissecting aneurysm. A son of this man (II-5) died at the age of 27 years after a very brief illness of undiagnosed nature. He was 6 feet tall, was always very thin, and had been sent to Texas at one time, for suspected tuberculosis. He became ill at noon one day and was dead at 5 A.M. the following day. He was said to have had no pain but developed hematuria in the last afternoon of the day he became ill.

Most of the remainder of the story of this family is told in the words of individual III-6, an intelligent observer and cooperative informant. Her husband (III-5) died in 1945 at the age of 32 years. "His heart condition was diagnosed as endocarditis by a heart specialist. He was apparently in good health up to two months prior to his death. He was 6 feet 2½ inches tall and in the last two years of his life he weighed more than ever before—175 pounds—and appeared to be in excellent health, except for his failing eyesight. He was working exceptionally hard due to the wartime manpower shortage. He was appointed to a job that necessitated a great deal of coast-to-coast flying at high altitudes. It was on one of these trips that he was taken ill. He returned home, was put to bed and given medicine, to which he responded beautifully. He insisted on going on another trip and lived one month after his return. He was hospitalized, but his case was pronounced hopeless. He had a hernia operation two years before his death. A routine checkup before the anesthesia showed no heart condition then."

The daughter of this man (IV-7) "was born May 17, 1937. She was always frail. She and her brother had whooping cough when they were 6 and 5 years old. Her heart started enlarging at that time. She was extremely nearsighted and wore glasses from the age of 3 years. She had a severe spinal curvature that we first noticed when she was 10 years of age. The family doctor did not advise a brace or cast, as she was so frail and her heart was getting increasingly worse. During her last illness, which lasted six weeks, the doctor said that her heart was just as it would have been in a person in his forties who had had rheumatic fever in his youth, that her heart was just worn out. She died at the age of 12½ years and was 5 feet 2 inches tall in spite of a very bad curvature. She had a brilliant mind and was at the top of classes in spite of her many handicaps. Both of the children were thin to the point of looking emaciated."

The brother of this girl (IV-8) "was born Nov. 27, 1938. He and Catherine looked like twins and were as nearly like their father as was possible. He was well as a baby and up to the time that he had whooping cough at the age of 5 years. After that long siege of coughing the doctor discovered that he had a heart murmur. His heart enlarged so that his chest protruded. He complained of chest pain occasionally. He died suddenly in August, 1946. His sister said after he died that he had complained of severe chest pains a couple of days before but he didn't tell anyone else. He developed hernia when he was about 2 years old, but it never seemed to bother him. He had a bad case of influenza the winter before he died and had a bad cough that lingered all winter and we felt hastened his death."

At age 7 years, this last patient was 53 inches tall and weighed 51 pounds. He showed arachnodactyly, hypotonia, hammertoes, thin and translucent skin, ectopia lentis, cardiomegaly, dilatation of the aorta, aortic systolic and diastolic murmurs, left axis deviation (by electrocardiogram), deformity (not described in detail) of the hip joints and skull (by x-ray examination). The lenses in this case were displaced downward and outward.

(From McKusick, V. A.: Circulation **11**:321, 1955.)

Lynas[328] observed one pedigree (A2) of 3 affected children from apparently normal parents. Two of the 3 were, however, not definite cases. In another pedigree (A-9) each of 2 unaffected brothers produced 1 affected child. Again, however, only "slight signs" were present in one of these.

Capotorti and co-workers[86] described an Italian kindred in which 16 mem-

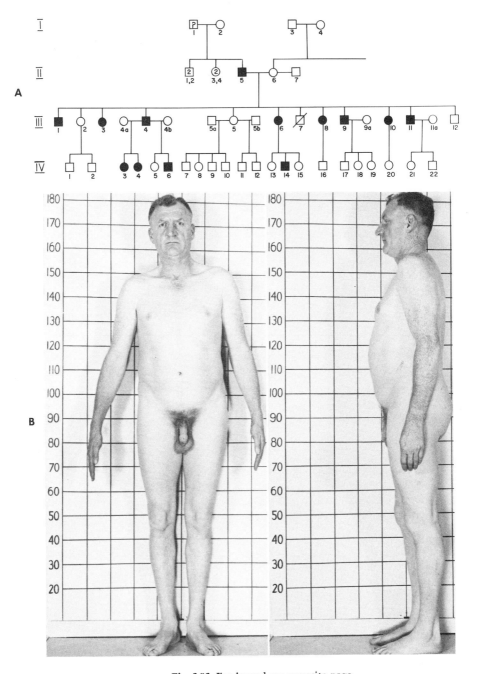

Fig. 3-56. For legend see opposite page.

bers of three generations showed the Marfan syndrome. The family contained the first known instance of marriage of 2 affected persons, who were first cousins. Of their 9 children, 4 were affected, 1 was normal, 3 died in infancy, and 1 was stillborn. Two of the 4 living affected children showed more severe manifestations than any of the other patients in the pedigree. Some members of this sibship may have been homozyzous for the Marfan gene.

Skipping of generations has never been observed in any thoroughly studied pedigree.[236]

Steinberg and colleagues[531] have reported on 2-year-old identical twins with the Marfan syndrome and "unperforated aortic sinus aneurysm." Becker[36] described identical twins, both affected, in a family with multiple cases of the Marfan syndrome. Kamen[279] also described identical twins, both affected. Papaioannou and associates[412] reported triplets, of whom two may have the Marfan syndrome.

Fig. 3-56A. The Marfan syndrome in three and probably four and more generations. **I-1,** Died at 39 years of age after brief illness. **II-5,** John Peter S., died at age 50 years, of dissecting aneurysm of aorta; had bad eyes. **III-1,** John A. S., born Sept. 29, 1913; has ectopia lentis and severe myopia; strabismus. **III-2,** Elizabeth S. M., born 1915; unaffected; requires hearing aid. **III-3,** Hilda S. S., born 1918; ectopia lentis, severe myopia, chest deformity, and dolichostenomelia. **III-4,** Joseph William S., born 1921; ectopia lentis, left myopia, and dolichostenomelia (see **B**). **III-5,** Frances S. Z. O., born May 9, 1922; small left posterior pole cataract; one of her 6 children deaf; probably unaffected. **III-6,** Naomi S. M., born Jan. 27, 1924; ectopia lentis, severe myopia, and "tonguetie," with indistinct speech. **III-7,** Died at one year of "summer complaint." **III-8,** Mildred S. D., born July 10, 1928; ectopia lentis and severe myopia. **III-9,** Frank Martin S., born April 9, 1931; ectopia lentis, severe myopia, dolichostenomelia, severe pneumonia twice as child, slight sternal depression and left chest deformity, and hernia. **III-10,** Nancy Patricia S. M., born 1932; ectopia lentis and myopia. **III-11,** Walter Raymond S., born Feb. 5, 1934; ectopia lentis, myopia, dolichostenomelia, history of severe pneumonia, and chest deformity. **III-12,** Jerome S., born 1935; unaffected apparently, but had operation for severe strabismus in 1949. **IV-3,** Katherine S.; affected. **IV-4,** Mary Dorothy Diane S., born Dec. 19, 1943; bilateral immature cataract and ectopia lentis; affected. **IV-6,** Probably affected. **IV-14,** Harry Douglas M., Jr., born 1945; trouble, like mother, in talking, chicken breast and myopia. **IV-15,** Sophronia M., born 1947; apparently unaffected; trouble talking distinctly. (In a family of 12 children—see generation III—the chance of 8 or more children being affected is almost one in four.) (From McKusick, V. A.: Ann. Intern. Med. 49:556, 1958.)

Fig. 3-56B. Individual III-4 (810977) in A, 41 years of age. The skeletal proportions are certainly not strikingly dolichostenomelic. Bilateral ectopia lentis is present. At age 41 years, the patient was having angina pectoris but had no murmur of aortic regurgitation. At the age of 47 years he was admitted to another hospital for suspected myocardial infarction. No murmur of aortic regurgitation was heard. At the age of 52 years he was admitted to yet another hospital for suspected aortic dissection. At this time aortic regurgitation was present and the mediastinum was widened. It was unfortunate that propranolol therapy (p. 196) was not instituted during this period. At the age of 53 years, after returning home from bowling, he had the abrupt onset of severe pain in the back, followed by pain in the left leg and chest. On admission to The Johns Hopkins Hospital he was found to have a cold, pulseless left leg, with total anesthesia of Poupart's ligament and a loud diastolic murmur. The pulses returned in the left leg shortly after admission. After 6 days' preparation, replacement of the ascending aorta and aortic valve was attempted, but the patient did not survive operation. The anterior descending and left circumflex coronary arteries had seperate origins from the left coronary sinus. (See Fig. 3-41 for a similar finding, which probably does not have an increased frequency in the Marfan syndrome, however.) Autopsy was not permitted.

Bowers[69] has traced the disease through six generations of a single family with a total of about 33 affected persons.

Lynas and Merrett[330] could find no evidence of genetic linkage between the Marfan trait and the following traits: sex, color vision, phenylthiocarbamide tasting, and ABO, Rhesus, Lewis a and b, Lutheran, Kell, P, and MNS blood groups.

Partial submersion of the manifestations of this syndrome, depending apparently on the rest of the genetic milieu in which the mutant gene is operating, has been observed.[335] For instance, when the mutation occurs in unusually

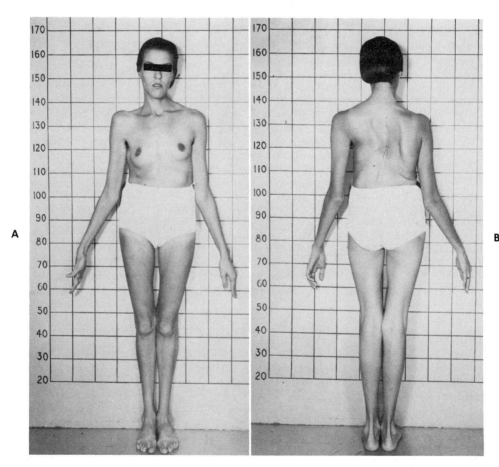

Fig. 3-57. Modification of phenotype by rest of genome. C. McD. (1352509), born in 1945, has bilateral upward displacement of the lenses and severe scoliosis, with major thoracic convexity to the right, for which spinal fusion was performed at the age of 10 years. All joints are moderately hyperextensible. The father and mother were 37 and 35 years old, respectively, at her birth. Her abnormality is thought to be the result of a fresh mutation. That this patient is only 64 inches tall is in part because of the short stature of her parents. The father is only 61 inches tall. **A,** Front view; **B,** posterior view. Note the right genu valgum and the scar of the spinal fusion. In a similar case we have seen recently (I. C., 1435250), the 63-inch-tall patient had very short parents (61 and 62 inches tall). The evidence for the Marfan syndrome was bilateral upward displacement of the lenses, "floppy mitral valve," narrow palate, pectus excavatum, and generalized loose-jointedness.

pyknic stock, the victim's habitus may be much less impressively unusual (Figs. 3-28 and 3-57).* No protection against ocular or aortic abnormality seems to be afforded thereby, however. Lynas[328] seems also to have observed the modifying effects of other genes. In one pedigree a woman with the Marfan syndrome married twice. By the first husband, a "non-Marfan" but tall man with tuberculosis, there were two children: one died in infancy and one had a severe complete form of the Marfan syndrome. By the second husband, "a small square-built man," one child was normal and a second had only mild skeletal and cardiac manifestations.

The fact that in some families pronounced aortic and skeletal abnormalities occur without demonstrable abnormality of the lens seems to be further evidence of the operation of the genetic milieu on expression of the syndrome. Considerable variability within families is also observed. For example, even sibs may vary in severity of affection, and some components of the syndrome, for example, the ocular ones, may be missing in one sib and present in another (Fig. 3-24). The variability is undoubtedly due both to exogenous (environmental, or nongenetic) factors and to differences in the remainder of the genotype of the individual—the genetic milieu in which the mutant gene operates. The "normal" allele with which the mutant allele is paired may be of diverse types; these normal alleles are called isoalleles. This source of variability may account in part for the fact that dominant conditions are usually more variable than recessive ones. In addition, many modifier genes may be present at other loci. Observations of the Marfan syndrome in monozygotic twins[36,531] who show closely similar type and degree of affection demonstrate the role of genetic modifiers. Variability in the Marfan syndrome is reminiscent of observations on single gene syndromes in mice, by Dunn and Charles[131] and others: depending on the genetic background on which the particular mutant gene is placed, some features of the syndrome may disappear or be strikingly modified in severity.

Differential diagnosis

Given stigmata suggestive of the Marfan syndrome, one can be most confident of the diagnosis if ectopia lentis is present in the patient or if other members of the family are unequivocally affected.[353]

For example, how can one be certain of the diagnosis of the Marfan syndrome in the case reported as such by Sinha and Goldberg,[510] when the patient "did not have tall features or long fingers," there was no ectopia lentis, "the family history was noncontributory," and the histologic changes possibly typical of the aorta in the Marfan syndrome (p. 181) were not described? Rather numerous uncertain cases are being reported.[50,59,81,188,328,448] I have been quoted as saying that "a diagnosis of the Marfan syndrome should not be made in the absence of ectopia lentis or, alternatively, a positive family history."[133] I would prefer that the

---

*By assigning, to affected and unaffected individuals, a score for upper segment–lower segment ratio based on the number of standard deviations by which each individual deviates from the mean for his race, age, and sex (Fig. 3-11), it will probably be possible to test this clinical impression. From initial observations it appears that when the scores for patients with the Marfan syndrome are lower (that is, deviate more on the negative side of the mean) then the average score for his normal first-degree relatives is in the low normal range. When the normal relatives have high normal scores, the Marfan patients do not have as markedly low US/LS values.

quote be worded that the diagnosis of the Marfan syndrome can usually not be made with complete confidence when ectopia lentis or a positive family history are not found. We do have some patients in whom we diagnose the Marfan syndrome with some certainty when the skeletal and cardiovascular features are typical, even though the case is sporadic and the eyes are normal.

The possibility of the Marfan syndrome is encountered in many situations, as in aortic regurgitation, otherwise unexplained, in an individual of asthenic and possibly dolichostenomelic habitus. Measurements alone are indicative but not completely conclusive. Measurements must be evaluated in the light of a rough evaluation of the average habitus of the family of which the possibly affected individual is a member. In the first decade of life, comparison of upper and lower segment measurements and of arm span with height is of greater sig-

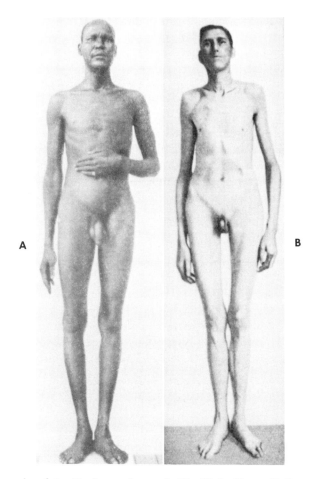

Fig. 3-58. Phenocopies of the Marfan syndrome. **A,** The Dinka Negro. **B,** Eunuch. Brief clinical description given by Bauer and the skeletal proportions suggest the Klinefelter syndrome. (**A** from Martin, R.: Lehrbuch der Anthropologie, ed. 2, Jena, 1928, Gustav Fisher; **B** from Bauer, J.: Innere Sekretion, ihre Physiologie, Pathologie und Klinik, Berlin, 1927, Julius Springer.)

nificance because of the relatively short extremities during this period.[543] (For normal values for these measurements during this period see references 144 and 602 or, better, Fig. 3-11.) The lack of complete specificity of such measurements is indicated by the occurrence of excessively long extremities on an anthropologic basis in the Dinka Negro[355] and on a pathologic basis in the eunuch,[29,192,373] in the Klinefelter syndrome (Fig. 3-58), and in patients with sickle cell anemia (Fig. 3-59A). In Wilkins' textbook[602] he pictures in the nude a Negro female patient who had had prepubertal castration for strangulated dermoid cysts. The skeletal proportions are strikingly suggestive of the Marfan syndrome. The rule of thumb for identification of arachnodactyly—longest digit at least 50% longer than the longest metacarpal—has proved to have both positive and negative error. In the Negro in particular, the Marfan syndrome is often suggested by skeletal proportions (Fig. 3-11). Sheldon[499] refers to this habitus as Nilotic dysplasia, since, according to him, inhabitants of the upper Nile area and their descendants display it most often. Members of the Watusi tribe of Uganda are very tall.

The habitus of successful basketball players suggests that of the Marfan syn-

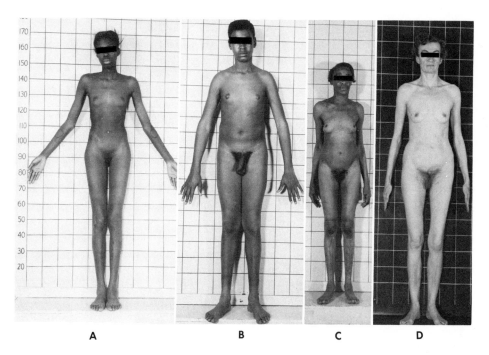

A   **B**   **C**   **D**

Fig. 3-59. A, Sickle cell anemia. D. M. (659463), 14½ years old, has no ectopia lentis or family history suggesting the Marfan syndrome but does have well-documented sickle cell anemia. **B,** Adolescence. E. K. (766137) was referred because of gynecomastia. There is no ectopia lentis or family history suggesting the Marfan syndrome. **C,** Syphilitic aortitis and ectopia lentis. S. J. (802999), 58 years old, has atrophy of the irides, bilateral ectopia lentis, optic atrophy, choroiditis, and secondary glaucoma. Aortic regurgitation is accompanied by blood pressure of 170/60 mm. Hg and enlargement of the left ventricle and left atrium. The family history is not indicative of the Marfan syndrome. **D,** Dolichostenomelia in atrial septal defect. M. L. (713241), 50 years of age, had a secundum type of ASD repaired surgically. There is no ectopia lentis or family history to suggest Marfan syndrome.

drome. Although I have made no systematic study of athletes in this group, one Negro all-state basketball star, previously a member of a champion university team, is 79½ inches tall and has myopia, high narrow palate, deformed chest, genu recurvatum, and the typically flat feet; at 24 years of age he shows profound heart failure and aortic regurgitation with characteristically dilated base of the aorta by aortography. Mitral regurgitation is also present.

Delayed puberty may be accompanied by Marfan-like body proportions. In one individual (E. K., Fig. 3-59B) adolescent gynecomastia was also present. As noted earlier, the gracile habitus of many patients with atrial septal defect often leads to a mistaken diagnosis of the Marfan syndrome (Fig. 3-59D). The high incidence of chest deformity in patients with congenital malformations of the heart[363] may further increase the confusion with the Marfan syndrome.

A picture mimicking in some respects that of the Marfan syndrome can result from Rh incompatibility and from intrauterine rubella infection. Ectopia lentis does not occur in these cases. However, deafness, ocular and cardiac defects, hypotonia, and even arachnodactyly may occur. The presence of some manifestations, such as anophthalmos, which is never encountered in the Marfan syndrome, is a point in favor of one of these other possibilities. Cases simulating Marfan's syndrome have occurred apparently as a result of febrile illness of unspecified type during early pregnancy[181] and as a result of x-ray therapy.[534]

Institutions for mental defectives often list an unbelievably high percentage of patients with arachnodactyly. This should not be taken to indicate the Marfan syndrome, in the majority of instances at any rate, since other evidence indicates that mental retardation is not an integral component of this syndrome and since it is clear that arachnodactyly is a nonspecific manifestation with many possible causes. The patient described by Benda,[40] for example, does not appear to have had the true Marfan syndrome. I would question the correctness of the diagnosis of the Marfan syndrome in the proband of family A5 of Lynas.[328] The patient, a female, was the only one of five children affected. She was a mental defective and "inclined just to sit and drool." The hands and fingers were very long and slender and showed marked clubbing due to bronchiectasis. The feet were abnormally small, however. Very severe kyphoscoliosis was present. The palate was broad and domed, not high and arched, and there were no eye or cardiac signs. "However, the clinicians are satisfied that she should be included as a case of arachnodactyly." Although by definition arachnodactyly was present, it is very doubtful that this is a case of the true Marfan disease.* (Fig. 3-60 demonstrates another patient with familial mental retardation and arachnodactyly. This case is also not the true Marfan syndrome, although the nature of the disorder is unknown.)

Several of the individual components of the Marfan syndrome occur alone or as part of other heritable syndromes and on a genetic basis distinct from the Marfan syndrome. Pectus excavatum,[420,474,519] scoliosis,[182,470] myopia,[129,248] and hernia,[153,594] are cases in point. Scoliosis is an important feature of von Recklinghausen's neurofibromatosis, which is inherited as a dominant.[109] Erdheim's cystic medial necrosis is almost certainly not a homogeneous entity from the etiologic

---

*This statement, written in 1959, has been proved true by the demonstration that this patient has homocystinuria.[184]

standpoint (p. 189). Marfan's disease is but one cause, there being other genetic (e.g., Ehlers-Danlos syndrome) and possibly acquired causes.

Several genetic varieties of ectopia lentis have been described.[38] One variety of isolated ectopia lentis is inherited as a simple Mendelian recessive.[175,569] I have observed[341a] 8 children of a first-cousin marriage, of whom 4 had ectopia lentis and 4 had sexual ateliotic dwarfism, or isolated growth hormone deficiency (a condition usually inherited as a recessive[454]). Coincidence of the two anomalies

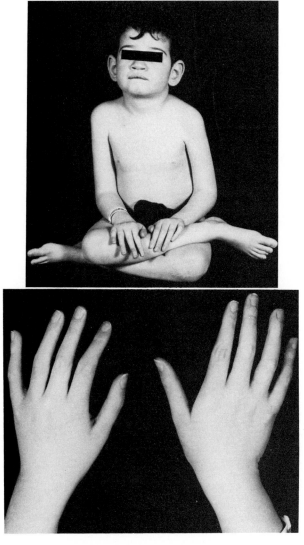

Fig. 3-60. Arachnodactyly with mental retardation. T. C. (1060982) was 6½ years old at the time of this study. Three sibs were unaffected; a brother, age 17 months, was apparently affected in an identical manner. The proband showed marked generalized hypotonia with hyperactive deep tendon reflexes and extensor plantar responses. Pneumoencephalogram suggested cerebellar atrophy. Precise classification of the disorder was impossible.

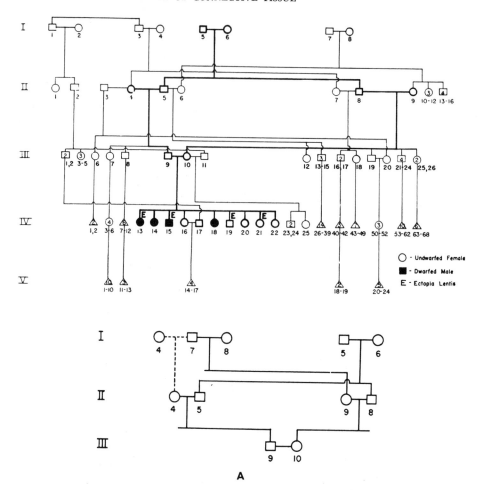

Fig. 3-61. These are illustrations of a sibship,[341a] children of a consanguineous marriage, in which 4 of 8 members had ectopia lentis and 4 had primordial, or ateliotic, dwarfism. In 2 individuals there was coincidence of the two pathologic traits. The pedigree is consistent with the view that the two traits were independently inherited as autosomal recessives. In the past, observations on the inheritance of primordial dwarfism have been consonant with this theory of inheritance, and it has been thought that ectopia lentis, as an isolated trait, is at times inherited as an autosomal recessive. This shows that the ectopia lentis of the Marfan syndrome is not the only genetic variety of this ocular anomaly. "The phenotype is not necessarily an indication of the genotype." **A,** The pedigree. The parents of the affected sibship were either first cousins or intermediate double first cousins. **B,** Left to right, individuals IV-15, IV-13, and IV-18 of the pedigree. The first two also have ectopia lentis with complicating glaucoma. Not photographed is individual IV-14 who, next to IV-15, is the shortest member of the family. The ages of these individuals are 31, 35, and 24 years, respectively, and their heights 39, 40, and 43¾ inches. **C,** These subjects, of approximately the same age, are 72 and 39 inches tall, respectively. Other than the proportionate dwarfism, the only abnormality revealed by radiographic study of the entire skeleton in individuals IV-15, IV-13, and IV-18 was delayed fusion of the epiphyses at the iliac crests in IV-15, who is 31 years old. When my colleagues and I[454] encountered recessively inherited isolated growth hormone deficiency, we suspected that these 4 midgets had that disorder. Although we could not persuade them to submit to growth hormone assays, we have studied a distant male relative (D. M., 1389271), age 61 years, who had 2 children and isolated deficiency of growth hormone by assay. He has no ectopia lentis. (From McKusick, V. A.: Amer. J. Hum. Genet. 7:187, 1955.)

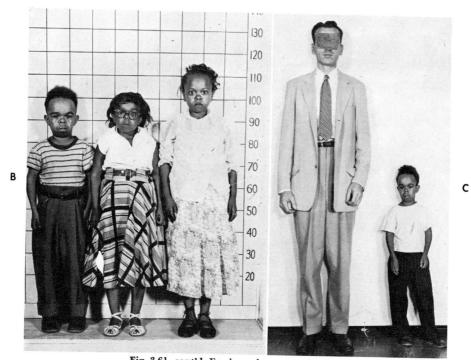

B   C

Fig. 3-61, cont'd. For legend see opposite page

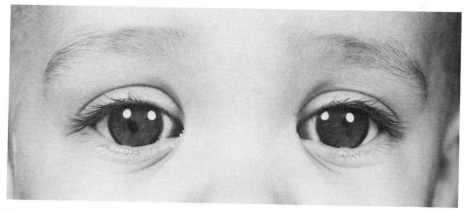

Fig. 3-62. Ectopia lentis et pupillae. Here are shown the temporally displaced irregular pupils in both eyes of B. M. (J.H.H. 1314449), a boy born in 1968, whose brother, the only sib, born in 1965, is identically affected. In both boys the lenses were subluxated nasally and inferiorly, and there was iridodonesis. Their physical and mental development was normal. Both parents are normal; they are not consanguineous. This disorder appears to be an autosomal recessive.[175]

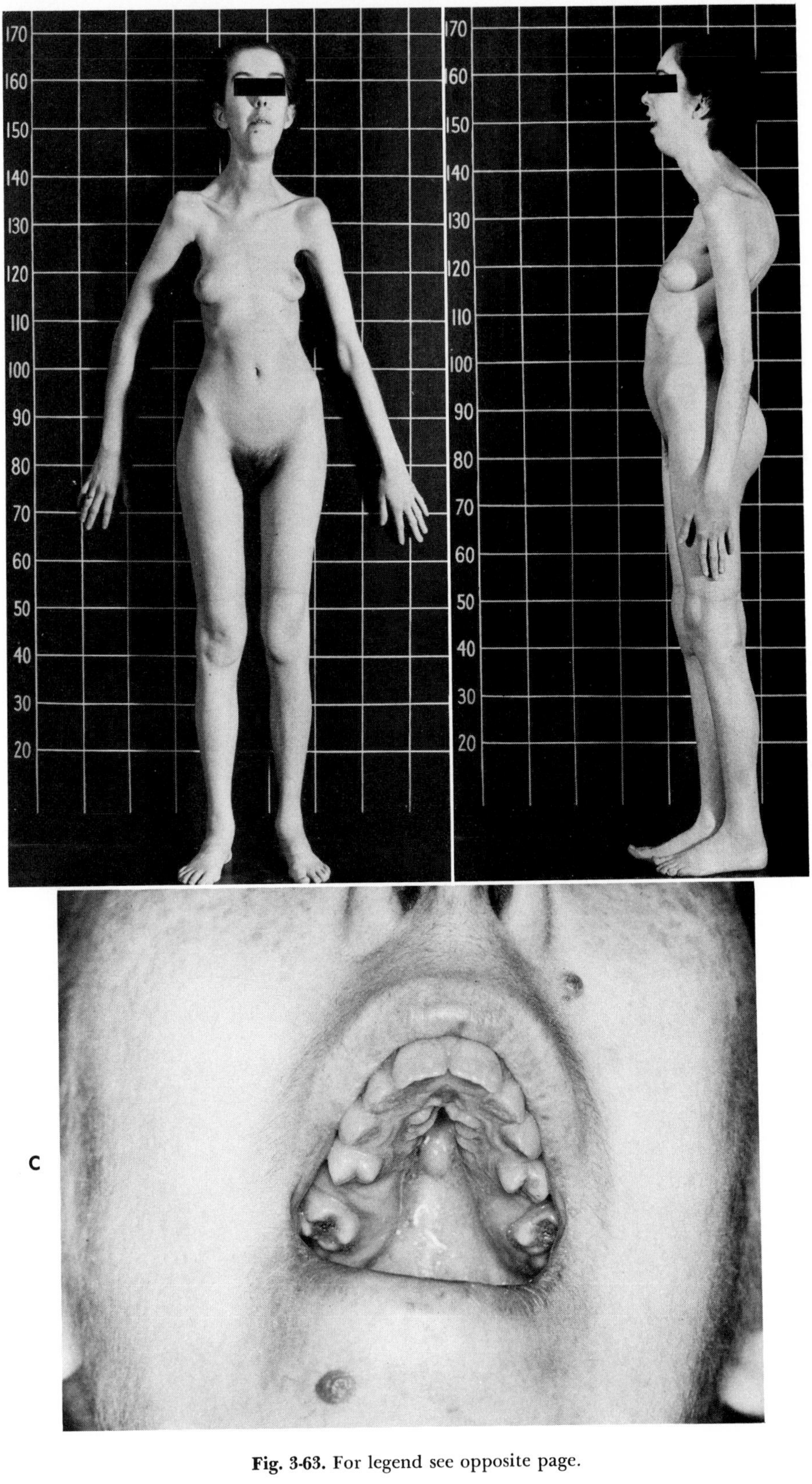

Fig. 3-63. For legend see opposite page.

occurred in 2 of the individuals. Another variety of ectopia lentis is that which is part of the Weill-Marchesani syndrome (Chapter 5), an autosomal recessive. Ectopia lentis et pupillae (Fig. 3-63) is also an autosomal recessive.[175] Ectopia lentis sometimes occurs with aniridia,[84] which is usually inherited as a dominant.

Muscular dystrophy was confused for the Marfan syndrome in the patient shown in Fig. 3-64*A* and *B*. Unusually pronounced spinal deformity and long fingers were apparent. The patient presented with bacterial endocarditis and aortic regurgitation—additional features suggesting the Marfan syndrome. Autopsy revealed no histologic evidence for this diagnosis but did show changes consistent with a rheumatic basis for the bacterial endocarditis. A brother, subsequently studied (Fig. 3-64*C* and *D*), shows unequivocal evidence of muscular dystrophy. In children, the pronounced muscular hypotonia may result in a picture suggesting Oppenheim amyotonia congenita or Werdnig-Hoffmann muscular atrophy.[206] Arachnodactyly with amyoplasia congenita has been described.[290] In brief, then, it is possible to make errors of diagnosis, in either direction, between the primary muscular disorders and the Marfan syndrome.

Slowly progressive congenital myopathy such as nemaline myopathy is often confused with the Marfan syndrome. The patient shown in Fig. 3-63 and her mother were recorded by Ford[171] as examples of congenital universal muscular hypoplasia of Krabbe. At one stage they were referred to me as possible instances of the Marfan syndrome. They were subsequently demonstrated[249] to be examples of nemaline myopathy. I strongly suspect that the two brothers reported by Cipolloni and colleagues[98] and thought to have the Marfan syndrome, complicated by chronic atrial flutter, had a myopathy and myocardiopathy. The eyes were normal in both boys, 17 and 19 years of age. The elder had severe bilateral foot drop, "pinched adenoidal facies, and a receding mandible." The younger had weakness of the back muscles and dorsiflexors of the feet, highly arched palate, crowded teeth, and nasal speech. Patients with myotonic dystrophy, especially that of early onset, often show dolichomorphism, arachnodactyly, high palate, and hyperextensible joints suggesting the Marfan syndrome.[434]

Another condition that has been mistaken for the Marfan syndrome is that of mucosal neuromas with pheochromocytoma and amyloid-producing medullary carcinoma of the thyroid.[112] See, for example, the patient reported as having the Marfan syndrome by Mielke and associates[372] and the patient shown in Fig.

Fig. 3-63. Nemaline myopathy in a patient suspected of having the Marfan syndrome. J. D. (J.H.H. 349573) was 31 years old at the time of these photographs. The mother was identically affected. The daughter breathed poorly, cried weakly, and sucked feebly in the neonatal period. She did not hold up her head until age 1 year and did not walk until 3 years of age. Amyotonia congenita was diagnosed. Joint hyperextensibility was present to such an extent that as a 10-year-old she could, for example, easily place her feet behind her head. After autopsy in the mother showed histologic changes typical of nemaline myopathy, biopsy performed in J. D. showed similar changes: rodlike bodies intermixed with myofibrillar fragments. J. D. died at the age of 42 years, 6 days after general anesthesia with thiamylal (Surital) and succinylcholine for dental extractions. Respiratory distress with previous anesthesia raised a question of unusual susceptibility in this disorder.[399] **A** and **B**, Front and side views; **C**, narrow and high-arched palate.

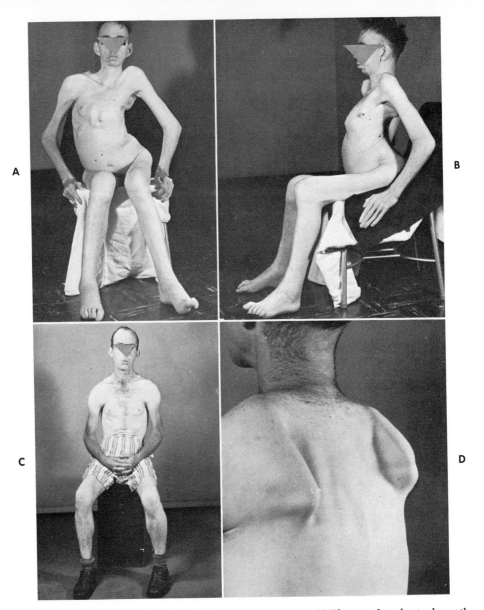

Fig. 3-64. A and **B,** W. M. (Mary Imogene Bassett Hospital 54659) was thought to have the Marfan syndrome because of aortic regurgitation, severe spinal deformity, and arachnodactyly. Clinical evidence for bacterial endocarditis was present. At autopsy the heart lesions appeared to be rheumatic with superimposed valvular infection. (I am indebted to Dr. James Bordley, III, for knowledge of this patient and permission to include him here.) Numerous pigmented nevi were present in this patient. **C** and **D,** D. M., brother of W. M. The finding of muscular dystrophy in this brother makes it likely that W. M. (in **A** and **B**) likewise had muscular dystrophy. The disease trait appears to be recessive in this family. In D. M. note the wasting of the upper arms, especially the left, the asymmetry of the face in whistling, and the winging of the scapulae. There is no arachnodactyly. Spinal deformity as severe as that in W. M. is sometimes seen with muscular dystrophy.[532] The proper classification of the muscular dystrophy in these brothers is uncertain. The parents are living and well. No other cases are known in the family. The brother in **C** and **D** has 6 children who show no sign of disease. Muscular dystrophy, which had its first manifestation at the age of 18 years in the form of weakness in raising the arms over the head, has been only slowly progressive in D. M. At age 50 years (1971) he is still able to maintain his garden and climb stairs. The disorder is most compatible with facioscapulohumeral muscular dystrophy (a dominant), but the apparent recessive inheritance suggests that this is in fact limb-girdle muscular dystrophy (an autosomal recessive) or one of the benign forms of X-linked muscular dystrophy.[37,341,536] (I am indebted to Dr. Charles Ellicott for studying this patient.)

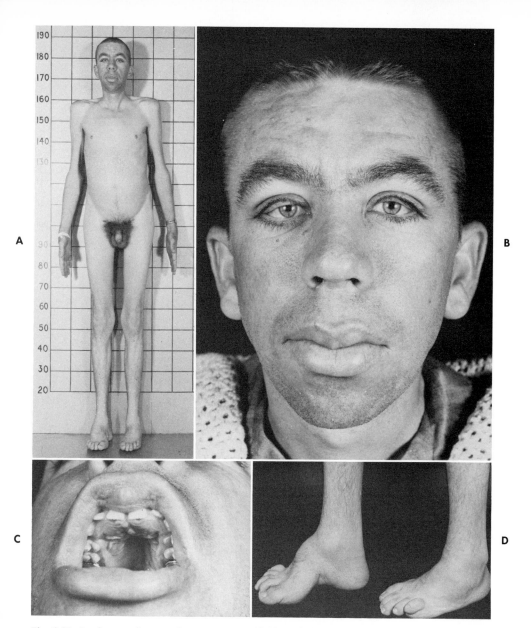

Fig. 3-65. Syndrome of mucosal neuromas, amyloid-producing medullary carcinoma of thyroid, pheochromocytoma, and Marfanoid habitus. K. S. (J.H.H. 110977), born in 1939, was noted during childhood to have an appearance different from that of other members of the family. He had intermittently troublesome diarrhea from age 10 years. At age 18 a medullary thyroid carcinoma was removed. At age 22 he was found to have a duodenal ulcer that was causing melena. At age 24 he was referred to me as a possible instance of the Marfan syndrome. He had been having increasing muscle weakness in the preceding months.

Examination showed a man 75 inches tall, **A**, with long, thin limbs, large, thick lips, and everted eyelids, **B**. The conjunctiva showed scattered small areas of yellowish thickening, and the corneal nerves were seen by slit-lamp microscopy to be thickened.

The gums were hypertrophied, the teeth widely spaced, and the palate narrow and high, **C**. Striking pes cavus was present, especially in the right, **D**. Megacolon was demonstrated by barium studies and intestinal malabsorption by other studies. Conjunctival biopsy was interpreted as consistent with neurofibroma. Chemical confirmation of pheochromocytoma could never be obtained.

The patient continued to have nausea, diarrhea, and weight loss and died in August, 1964. Autopsy showed metastatic tumors (presumably thyroid in origin) in the cervical lymph nodes, bone marrow, lungs, liver, spleen, and both adrenals. In addition, a small pheochromocytoma was present in each adrenal medulla.

3-65, who was referred to me with that diagnosis.[483] The basal cell nevus syndrome[72,518] is yet another condition that has been reported as the Marfan syndrome in individual instances.

Males with the XYY karyotype are unusually tall but lack other features of the Marfan syndrome.[106] One of the early cases of the XYY syndrome[258] was found in a boy who had the Marfan syndrome, which was also present in two

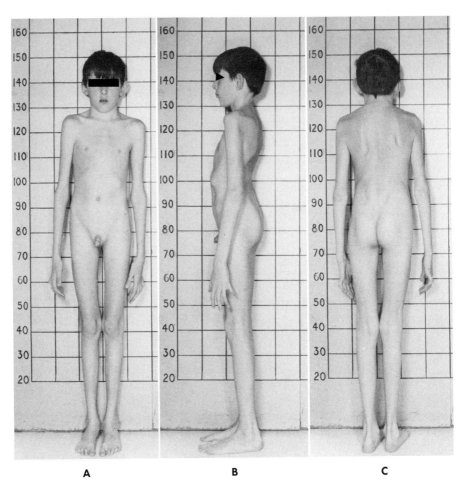

A   B   C

Fig. 3-66. Camptodactyly as a leading feature of the Marfan syndrome. The proband (J. T., J.H.H. 1418127), born in 1961, was first evaluated at the age of 9 years for finger contractures and scoliosis. His facial appearance and skeletal features were strongly suggestive of the Marfan syndrome. No ectopia lentis, heart murmur, or hernia was detected. He had mild pectus carinatum and sparsity of subcutaneous fat. At age 10 years, pneumonia necessitated hospitalization. His height was far above the 97th percentile for his age. The boy's father was 76½ inches tall and showed camptodactyly as well as limitation in raising the arms. The paternal grandfather had camptodactyly, had had extraction of the lenses (supposedly for cataract), and was blind from the age of 35 years. The paternal great-grandmother and a paternal uncle also had camptodactyly, and a paternal aunt had pectus excavatum. A, B, and C, J. T. at age 10 years. Note excessive height, mild pectus carinatum, bulging left costal margin, scoliosis, and camptodactyly. **D,** Arachnodactyly and camptodactyly in J. T. **E** and **F,** Camptodactyly in father of J. T. **G,** Maximal elevation of arms in J. T. and his father.

sisters who had normal karyotypes and in the father, who died presumably of aortic rupture.

A Marfanoid habitus has also been described in persons with the megaduodenum-megacystis syndrome.[398] This disorder, as the designation indicates, is characterized by dilated duodenum and/or urinary bladder and appears to be an autosomal dominant. Aganglionosis is probably not the basis; indeed, the basic defect is unknown. Newton[398] described affected brothers who were "tall and thin, with long, tapered fingers, in contrast with their living relatives, who tend to be short and hypersthenic."

The disorder in the sibship reported by Clunie and Mason[99] as the Marfan syndrome with unusual bowel manifestations was probably one of the several recognized forms of the Ehlers-Danlos syndrome. Marked ligamentous laxity and arachnodactyly were described. Although the affected individuals were tall (70 to 75 inches), the body proportions, as indicated by the photographs and by the published US/LS values, did not suggest the Marfan syndrome. Serious eye complications consisted of myopia and retinal detachment without ectopia lentis. Three brothers had recurrent inguinal and femoral hernias. Multiple diverticula of the urinary bladder and of the intestine were demonstrated, and 3 of 4 affected sibs had one or more episodes of bowel perforation that were thought to have occurred at the diverticula. The patients were 4 out of 10 offspring of parents who were normal but related as first cousins. The parental consanguinity and the

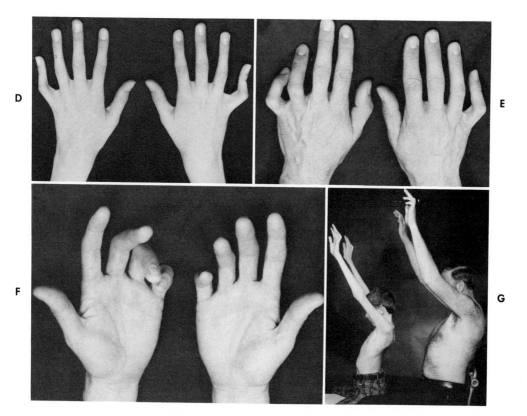

Fig. 3-66, cont'd. For legend see opposite page

serious eye complications, together with the joint laxity and recurrent hernias, suggest that this disorder was the recessively inherited "ocular" form of the Ehlers-Danlos syndrome (p. 341), not the Marfan syndrome.

The patients reported by Golden and Lakin[188] as having a *forme fruste* of the Marfan syndrome had either the pterygium syndrome or Noonan's syndrome, probably the former. Two brothers were affected. The clinical features were suggestive of those in the patients with pterygium syndrome, apparently inherited as a recessive, reported by Norum and colleagues.[402] The father had severe pectus excavatum and heart failure.

As was noted on p. 79 camptodactyly is sometimes a leading feature of the Marfan syndrome. A considerable number of families have been reported, indicating that camptodactyly can occur as an isolated autosomal dominant trait.[593,615] The fifth finger is always most severely involved, and often only it is affected. Fingers II to V may be affected in that order of increasing severity. It would be easy for the family pictured in Fig. 3-66 to be diagnosed as having simple hereditary camptodactyly. It is of note that camptodactyly was associated with familial subluxation of the knees in one family[389] and with taurinuria[397] and aminoaciduria[416] in one family each. However, I know of no previously reported family in which camptodactyly was inherited in successive generations as a cardinal feature of the Marfan syndrome. In another case (Y. S., J.H.H. 1412734), camptodactyly V is associated with other features of the Marfan syndrome. The mother also has severe camptodactyly V but no signs of the Marfan syndrome, and camptodactyly is reportedly present also in her father, some of his sibs, and her paternal grandmother, but these persons have not been examined.

The relationship, if any, of the Marfan syndrome to "status dysraphicus" is obscure.[425] The latter condition is too ill-defined to make an analysis of relationship possible. We (Fig. 3-16*A*) and others have observed bent fifth fingers (so-called camptodactyly or clinodactyly[243]) and heterochromia iridis,[118] both manifestations that are said to be characteristic of status dysraphicus. Apparently identical clinodactyly is sometimes inherited as an isolated anomaly.[243]

The following 2 cases illustrate yet other problems in the differential diagnosis of the Marfan syndrome. Both patients were initially considered to have this disorder.

Case 4. Bicuspid aortic valve with aortic regurgitation in tall, 15-year-old boy with "straight back."

T. A. (J.H.H. 987616), white male born in 1946, was first noted to have a murmur at age 7 years. The only symptom was excessive fatigability on overexertion.

Examination (1961) showed a tall, thin boy (Fig. 3-67) with unusually small anteroposterior chest dimension and "straight back" (absence of normal thoracic kyphosis). A decrescendo diastolic murmur beginning with the second sound was best heard at the left sternal border. Blood pressure was 110/70 mm. Hg.

Electrocardiogram showed peaked T waves in leads V_5 and V_6, consistent with left ventricular diastolic overload. Chest x-ray examination showed questionable left ventricular prominence.

A complete right and left cardiac catheterization study including cineangiocardiography (performed by Dr. J. Michael Criley) showed aortic regurgitation and no dilatation of the aortic sinuses but clear indications of a bicuspid aortic valve. The left coronary cusp was normal; the right and noncoronary cusps appeared to be one.

Case 5. Coronary arteriovenous fistula[616] in a dolichostenomelic male, producing a diastolic murmur mistaken for that of aortic regurgitation.

S. C. (J.H.H. 707722), a Negro male born in 1933, was seen in the Steering Clinic in 1960

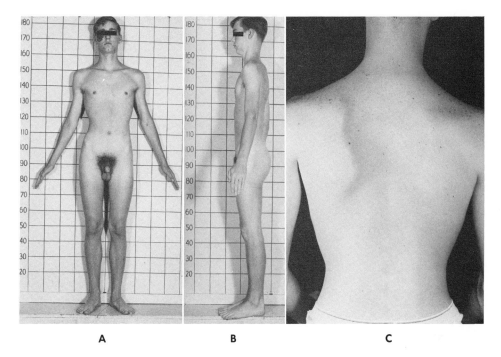

A   B   C

Fig. 3-67. Aortic regurgitation due to bicuspid aortic valve in 15-year-old with Marfanoid
habitus and "straight back." **A** and **B,** Note height and relatively small anteroposterior
dimension of chest. **C,** Note lack of normal thoracic kyphosis.

complaining of an upper respiratory infection. He was found to have a diastolic murmur at the
lower left sternal border, and dolichostenomelia (Fig. 3-68A and B) with highly arched palate
was noted. When I saw him in consultation, I thought that the Marfan syndrome was almost
certainly the diagnosis. It was noted that he had mild pectus excavatum. The murmur was
loudest and holodiastolic at the xiphoid area (Fig. 3-68C). It was high pitched, with a
"whirring" quality.

Aortography was performed to corroborate the impression of aortic sinus dilatation as the
basis of aortic regurgitation. To our surprise a coronary arteriovenous fistula was demonstrated (Fig. 3-68D and E). The aorta was entirely normal. The right coronary artery was
large and extremely tortuous, branching to form a large arteriovenous malformation on the
anteroinferior surface of the right ventricle. Dye remained pooled in the area throughout the
run.

In retrospect the location and other characteristics of the murmur were consistent with the
angiographic finding. Furthermore, a hemangioma on the thenar eminence of the right hand
acquired a new significance (Fig. 3-68F). Electrocardiogram has always shown a slight elevation
of the ST segment in leads V_5 and V_6.

Since the patient was asymptomatic, it was decided to postpone surgical therapy. When seen
in 1972, the patient was found to have no murmur whatever. Thrombosis of the fistula may
have occurred.

Parish[414] suggested that arachnodactyly with mandibulofacial dysostosis, particularly receding lower jaw, is a syndrome separate from Marfan's and properly
called Achard's syndrome. In the patient described, a 40-year-old woman, joint
laxity was confined to the hands and feet.[415] Although such a syndrome may
exist as a distinct entity, I have not recognized an example.

Epstein and associates[146] and Beals and Hecht[31] have observed a generalized
connective tissue disorder partially overlapping both the Marfan syndrome and

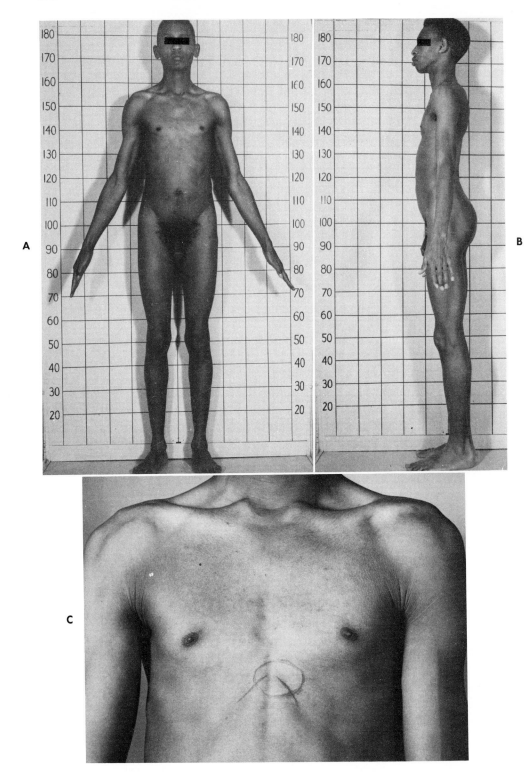

Fig. 3-68. For legend see opposite page.

osteogenesis imperfecta in its clinical manifestations: severe kyphoscoliosis, generalized osteopenia without fractures, slender long bones, arachnodactyly, congenital contracture of fingers and some other joints, underdeveloped musculature, and abnormally shaped ears. Inheritance is autosomal dominant. Beals and Hecht[31] refer to the condition as contractural arachnodactyly. They even suggest that Marfan's patient[351] had this disorder and not *the* Marfan syndrome! Beyer and co-workers[47] described a mother and 4 children with what appears to have been the same disorder. Several instances[208,290,447] of combined Marfan syndrome and arthrogryposis multiplex congenita have been reported. Some of these may be examples of contractural arachnodactyly.

In Fig. 3-70 are presented a pair of sibs who have a Marfan-like syndrome. They have arachnodactyly, loose-jointedness, chest deformity, and ocular abnormalities, but they are not exceptionally tall, and the ocular abnormalities are blue sclerae, high-grade myopia, and keratoconus; deafness is associated. It appears to be a distinct syndrome that may be inherited as a dominant, inasmuch as the father and paternal grandmother show some of the same features.

We have observed 2 patients (L. E., 677290; S. J., 802999) with ectopia lentis and syphilis. Is it possible that syphilis can cause or predispose to ectopia lentis? The association of syphilitic aortitis with ectopia lentis might occasion diagnostic confusion. Aside from the diagnostic implications, the theoretic ones are great, since, as previously indicated, the clinical behavior of the aortic involvement in syphilis has certain parallels to that in the Marfan syndrome. The rarity of dissecting aneurysm in syphilitic aortitis is a conspicuous difference, however.

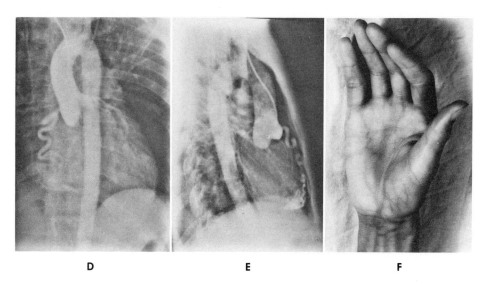

D   E   F

Fig. 3-68. Coronary arteriovenous fistula, producing a diastolic murmur in a man with skeletal features consistent with the Marfan syndrome. See Case 5 in text (p. 168). **A** and **B,** Note height of about 74 inches and reduced anteroposterior dimension of the thorax. **C,** Site of maximal audibility of diastolic murmur and indication of direction of radiation. **D** and **E,** Coronary arteriograms showing changes described in text. **F,** Infrared photograph of right hand showing, in addition to a local bulge in the thenar eminence, dilated vessels over the thenar eminence and palm.

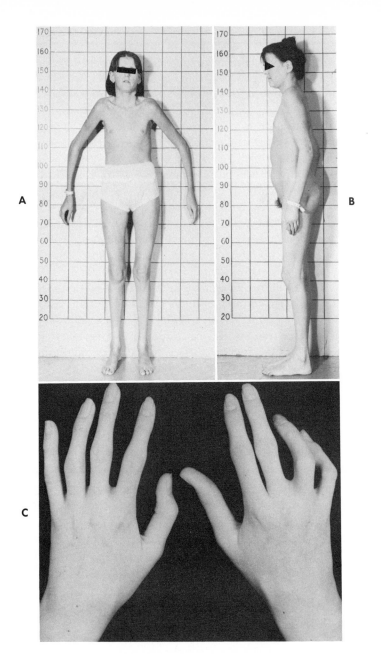

Fig. 3-69. Marfan syndrome with contractures and diabetes mellitus. J. M. (J.H.H. 944404), 12 years old at the time of these photographs, was investigated as having probable homocystinuria because of joint contractures and mild mental retardation (I.Q. = 75) in association with ectopia lentis. Stiff joints had been present from birth, and she received physical therapy for same during her first three years. Most joints are stiff to some degree. As noted in the pictures, there is camptodactyly, **C,** and incomplete extension of both elbows and the left knee, **A** and **B.** Systolic clicks suggesting a pericardial rub were heard on cardiac auscultation, and the aortic knob was prominent on x-ray examination. No other person in her family is known to have the Marfan syndrome. Her father was 39 years old at her birth.

This patient developed diabetes at the age of 12 years. Two sisters and several relatives of the father have juvenile diabetes.

The dark color of the patient's hair and the lack of dental crowding (the patient has absent superior lateral incisors) are points against a diagnosis of homocystinuria.

As noted on p. 87, a high frequency of syphilis was found among patients with traumatic ectopia lentis.[266] Trauma was not a recognized factor in the 2 cases previously mentioned.

It has been emphasized before that profound aortic regurgitation may be present in patients with the Marfan syndrome for many years before dilatation of the ascending aorta becomes evident by x-ray examination. Some patients with severe aortic regurgitation (Figs. 3-26, 3-27A and B, and 3-39) never show dilatation of the aorta. The differential diagnosis of the aortic lesion can therefore be confusing. Syphilis, rheumatism, or bacterial endocarditis is often suspected first. When one of these disorders appears unlikely from collateral evidence and when, as is so often possible in all sorts of disorders, a history of trauma is elicited, traumatic rupture of a normal aortic cusp is postulated (Fig. 3-28 and reference 34). Furthermore, a deceptive prominence of the pulmonic conus and main pulmonary artery may result from displacement of these structures by the dilated intrapericardial portion of the ascending aorta. Or the pulmonary artery may be dilated because of intrinsic involvement of its media. As in any severe, prolonged aortic regurgitation with chronic left ventricular failure, the left atrium is likely to become dilated. The prominence of the pulmonary artery and left atrium, the prolongation of the P-R interval (p. 136), and the Austin Flint murmur of aortic regurgitation conspire to lead to the incorrect diagnosis of rheumatic heart disease with combined aortic and mitral lesions.

All those conditions that produce aortic regurgitation, especially with aortic dilatation, come in for consideration in the differential diagnosis of the Marfan syndrome, including syphilitic aortitis, ankylosing spondylitis, and von Meyerborg's systemic chondromalacia (relapsing polychondritis).[419]

Fig. 3-70. Marfanoid syndrome in sister and brother, with some features in two preceding generations. **A,** N. M. E. (J.H.H. 549964), aged 20 years at the time of these photographs, had striking arachnodactyly and loose-jointedness from birth. Keratoconus and myopia also dated from an early age. Hearing impairment, first recognized when she was 7 years old, progressed to the point that she began wearing hearing aids in the teens. The right eye was enucleated (reason?) when she was 24. She is an excellent scholar and despite severe sensory impairments, completed a graduate course in library science. She is the eldest of 3 sibs; the youngest, T. M., is similarly affected. She is not excessively tall (67 inches). The US/LS ratio was 31:36. **B,** Keratoconus is demonstrated. Both corneas were thin centrally, with ruptures in Descemet's membrane posteriorly. The sclerae were blue. **C,** Fifth-finger camptodactyly, arachnodactyly, and loose-jointedness of the thumb are demonstrated. **D,** Hyperextensibility of the elbows, wrists, and fingers are demonstrated. **E,** The patient had bilateral hallux valgus, and the toes are thin and crooked.

T. M. (J.H.H. 1003942), brother of N. M. E., was 11 years old at the time of these photographs. He wore spectacles from an early age. Hearing impairment first noted at age 7 years, was considered to be predominantly of the nerve type. Examination showed average height, **F** and **G,** mild pectus excavatum, **H,** blue sclerae and severe myopia and astigmatism, **I,** arachnodactyly, **J,** with hyperextensibility of the fingers and wrists, and mild genu recurvatum. He had no keratoconus and, like his sister, no subluxation of the lenses. At the age of 18 years he was 72½ inches tall. **K,** Toes are long, with contracture of several of them.

The father of these sibs was 73½ inches tall and had arachnodactyly, loose-jointedness of the fingers, and mild genu recurvatum. Hearing was normal, but he had worn spectacles since the age of 16 years for progressive myopia. The paternal grandmother had worn spectacles for myopia since childhood and showed blue sclerae. Although she was only 63½ inches tall, she had pronounced arachnodactyly and hyperextensibility of the fingers. Her mother was said to have had long fingers and toes.

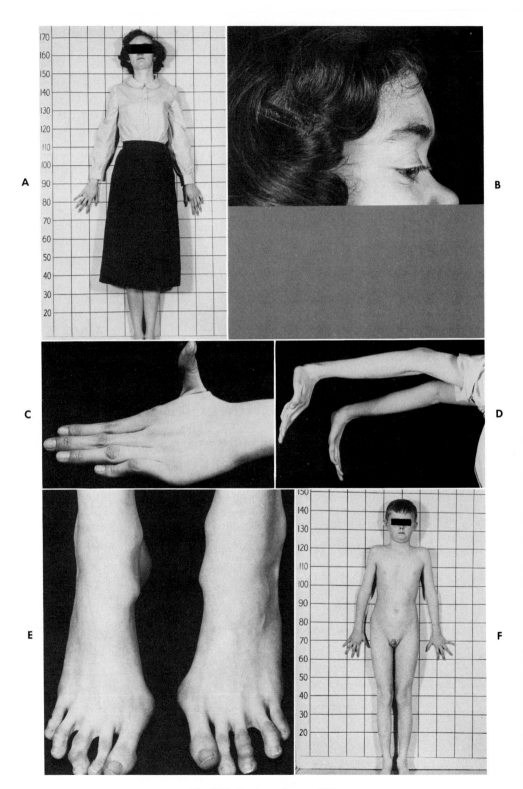

Fig. 3-70. For legend see p. 173.

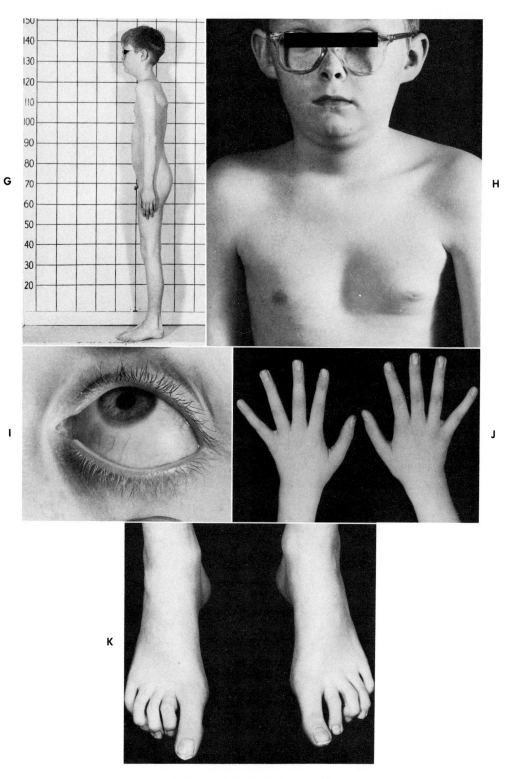

Fig. 3-70, cont'd. For legend see p. 173.

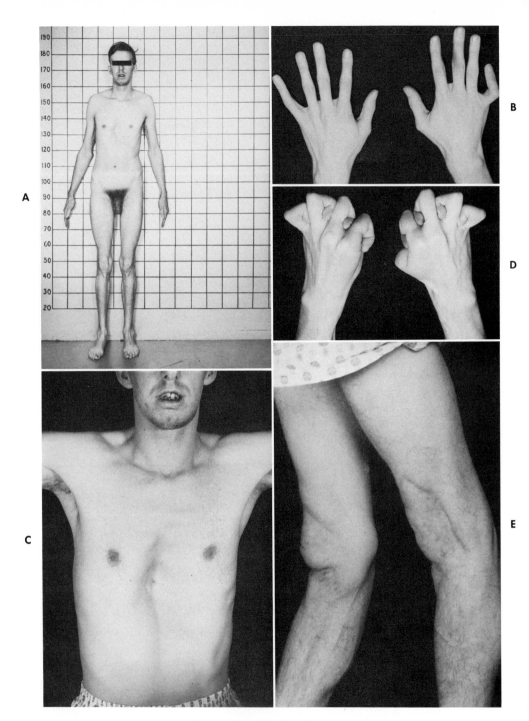

Fig. 3-71. Marfanoid hypermobility syndrome.[585] This 27-year-old man was the youngest of 8 children and the only sib with the features demonstrated here. The father and mother were likewise healthy. They were not consanguineous and were 40 and 41 years old, respectively, at the time of his birth. Extreme articular laxity, with ability to dislocate the sternoclavicular joints, had been present all his life. He was myopic. His U/L value was 0.92, **A.** Pronounced pectus excavatum, **C,** mild lower thoracic scoliosis, and arachnodactyly with camptodactyly V, **B,** were present. Steinberg's thumb sign was positive. He showed extreme loose-jointedness in the fingers, **D,** genu recurvatum, **E,** and hyperextensibility of the skin with numerous horizontal striae distensae over the lower back. A loud mid-systolic click was audible over the entire precordium. Ophthalmic examination showed mesodermal anomalies of the angle of the anterior chamber.[580]

Frieden and co-workers[177] described a puzzling case of ruptured aortic cusp that produced a musical aortic diastolic murmur in a 42-year-old man who had retinal detachment in the left eye secondary to trauma at 5 years of age and in the right eye at 40 years of age; hyperextensible joints; moderate kyphoscoliosis and pectus carinatum; severe flatfoot; and cystic medial necrosis of the aorta. He was only 65 inches tall. Both children had joint laxity and blue sclerae. No cutaneous changes of the Ehlers-Danlos syndrome were present. This patient may fall in the same category as those with "floppy aortic valve" reported by Read and colleagues.[443]

An evolution of aortic dilatation and rupture similar to that in Erdheim's cystic medial necrosis occurs in patients with the idiopathic medial aortopathy and arteriopathy reported by Marquis and co-workers.[354] Some of the patients had fever, elevated sedimentation rates, arthropathy, scleritis, etc., suggesting to these workers that autoimmunity may be involved in the pathogenesis.

Fatal rupture of the aorta or its large branches is a recognized complication of the Ehlers-Danlos syndrome, especially in the "ecchymotic," "arterial," or Sachs form (Chapter 6). Voigt and Hansen[578] described aortic rupture in 3 persons 13, 18, and 29 years of age. The youngest was probably, as they suggested, an instance of the Ehlers-Danlos syndrome, since the patient developed suggillations (ecchymoses) from minor blunt trauma. Up to 1967 about 130 cases of spontaneous aortic rupture had been reported in persons under the age of 18 years.[133,256]

Just as cystic medial necrosis of the aorta probably occurs as an inherited isolated defect (p. 189), the floppy mitral valve syndrome, with auscultatory and electrocardiographic signs indistinguishable from those of the mitral involvement in the Marfan syndrome, occurs as an isolated familial trait.[255,500] Sometimes the patients display loose-jointedness. In Fig. 3-72 is shown the case of a girl with the floppy mitral valve and associated loose-jointedness.

The Marfanoid hypermobility syndrome combines features of the Marfan and Ehlers-Danlos syndromes.[585] The patient illustrated in Fig. 3-71 is thought to have this distinct Marfan-like syndrome.

Walker and co-workers[585] described a 27-year-old man (Fig. 3-71) with a Marfanoid habitus but no evidence of involvement of the aorta or displacement of the lenses. Very marked hypermobility of joints and hyperextensibility of the skin, suggesting the Ehlers-Danlos syndrome, were present. They plausibly suggested that this is a distinct heritable disorder of connective tissue, designated by them as the *Marfanoid hypermobility syndrome*. Separation from the Ehlers-Danlos syndrome seems justified; in that disorder the subjects are not unusually tall, and in the patient of Walker and associates,[585] other features of the Ehlers-Danlos syndrome such as fragility of the skin, susceptibility to bruising, molluscoid pseudotumors, and subcutaneous spheroids were lacking.

Walker and associates[585] suggested that the Marfanoid hypermobility syndrome was present in at least 4 other reported patients.[106a,190,191,463a,479] Goodman and colleagues[191] had considered their patient to have both the Marfan syndrome and the Ehlers-Danlos syndrome. Serious cardiac abnormality with mitral regurgitation and cardiac failure beginning at 16 years of age was present in this case.[190] (It is noteworthy that the patient of Walker and associates[585] had a conspicuous systolic click (Fig. 3-71) compatible with "floppy mitral valve.")

The fibroblasts in a 10-day-old surgical wound showed ultrastructural abnormalities of the cytoplasm—poorly developed endoplasmic reticulum.[479] By light microscopy the nuclei were shown to be less basophilic than normal.

The genetics of the Marfanoid hypermobility syndrome is unclear. Only in one of the reported families were relatives thought to be affected,[191] some having, in the interpretation of the authors, the Marfan syndrome, some (such as the proband's mother) the Ehlers-Danlos syndrome, and some both.

The following case, earlier thought to be one of the Marfan syndrome, is almost certainly another distinct entity. The dramatic thinness of the sclerae and corneas, leading to rupture with minor trauma, is a main distinguishing feature.

Case 6. M. M. (J.H.H. 1387300), a white male, was born in 1950 to a 36-year-old father and a 31-year-old mother who were not consanguineous. A brother and 2 sisters were normal, and no similar affection was known in the family.

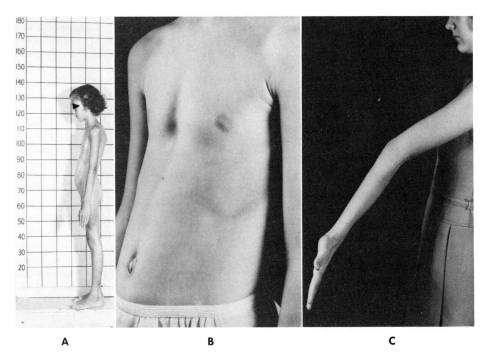

A   B   C

Fig. 3-72. "Floppy" mitral valve syndrome with pectus excavatum and loose-jointedness. J. W. (734856), a girl born in 1949, was first referred to me in 1956 because of an intermittent, very loud, musical systolic murmur. I thought it was probably of extracardiac origin secondary to a flulike illness which she had had shortly before the murmur was first noted and which I presumed to have been accompanied by pericarditis. I thought that the musical murmur was generated in the pericardium by a rubbing mechanism and that the systolic click which preceded it was the result of pericardial adhesion. The phonocardiograms (reference 336, p. 205, Fig. 178) showed changes similar to those in Fig. 3-42. The patient has maintained a slightly elevated ST segment and inverted T wave in leads 2, 3, and aV$_F$ of the electrocardiogram. She has mild pectus excavatum, **B,** and rather pronounced hyperextensibility at the elbows, **C,** but none at the knees. Although intracardiac radiographic studies have not been performed, it seems clear on the basis of present knowledge that this patient has the floppy mitral valve syndrome.

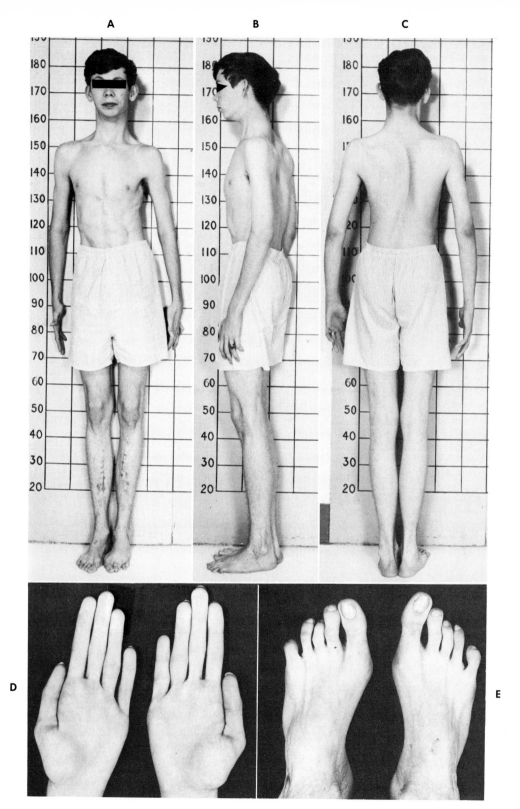

Fig. 3-73. Marfan-like syndrome with thin cornea and sclera. See text for **A, B,** and **C.** Note height and scoliosis. **D,** Hands showing arachnodactyly. **E,** Feet.

The sclerae were always very blue. At the age of about 7 years he suffered rupture of the right cornea from a minor blow. Rupture of the left cornea occurred while the patient was playing basketball at about age 13 years. In August, 1970, a left lamellar corneal graft was performed. Both corneas at that time were very thin, with leukoma. The lenses were cataractous and subluxated. A left penetrating corneal graft was implanted and the left lens was removed in June, 1971.

Loose-jointedness was always striking. Repeated dislocations occurred in the knees and elbows. A bloody effusion in the left knee required repeated tapping, with withdrawal of about 250 ml. of fluid in all. At 9 years of age triple arthrodesis was performed for flatfoot, by means of bone grafts from the tibias. Scoliosis appeared between August, 1964, and September, 1965, and was progressive despite the use of a Milwaukee brace. A 75% curve was reached by 1971, requiring consideration of spinal surgery.

Right inguinal hernia and undescended testis were repaired at about 12 years of age.

Two bouts of paroxysmal tachycardia had occurred: one following an eye operation at age 13 years and one following mild exertions of "shooting baskets" in 1971.

Examination (1971) showed a tall boy with US/LS measurements of 85/100 cm. (Fig. 3-73). (Despite his scoliosis, he was taller than both parents and both sibs.) The anterior chest was asymmetrically deformed and the spine scoliotic. The joints of the fingers were strikingly hyperextensible and the knees and elbows moderately so. Scars over the tibias marked the origin of bone grafts.

A mid-systolic click followed by a late systolic murmur was heard over the mid precordium and apex.

The patient had moderate reduction in hearing bilaterally. A junior in college, he is of normal intelligence.

Urinary test for homocystine was negative. Fluoroscopy showed unusually prominent pulsations of the aorta and questionably increased prominence of the left ventricle. Electrocardiograms showed a short P-R interval and an rSR′ pattern in lead V_1, with normal QRS duration and tall R wave (25 mm.) in lead V_5.

Comment. It is difficult to accept a view that the disorder in this patient is the Marfan syndrome. The thin sclerae and corneas and the joint laxity are more striking than is usual in the Marfan syndrome. It is more likely that the disorder is akin to that reported by Cordella and Vinciguerra[104a] (labeled Ehlers-Danlos syndrome with ectopia lentis by those authors), Arkin,[14a] Badtke,[19a] Hyams and colleagues,[259c] Stein and colleagues,[525a] Tucker,[566a] and Bertelsen.[46a] The disorders has features overlapping those of the Marfan syndrome, the Ehlers-Danlos syndrome, and osteogenesis imperfecta, but it is, in my opinion, a distinctive and specific heritable disorder of connective tissue. *Fragilitas oculi* would seem an appropriate tentative designation based on the most striking feature (see p. 341). In addition to dolichostenomelia, loose-jointedness, and spinal and thoracic deformity, "floppy mitral valve" occurs.

In all the reported cases autosomal recessive inheritance was consistent with the findings. Badtke,[19a] Bertelson,[46a] and Tucker[566a] all reported pairs of affected sibs with consanguineous unaffected parents. Hyams and co-workers[259c] and Stein and co-workers[525a] reported the disorder in separate Tunisian Jewish families. The disorder in M. M. bears some similarity to that in the sibs pictured in Fig. 3-70. Some signs of the disorder on one side of the family suggested dominant inheritance, however.

Pathology

Roark,[461] in 1959, estimated that at least seventy-one autopsies had been reported in the literature. Autopsy was performed in 18 of the 74 probands in my first series; necropsy information was available in at least 10 other affected members of these families. The gross changes in the aorta, as demonstrated in Figs. 26E and 28C, are the most dramatic. There are numerous reports of dissecting aneurysm in cases of the Marfan syndrome.[8,82,89,151,200,246,317,318,353,435,446,524,553,556,601]

With the exception of the changes in the tunica media of the great vessels and in the heart valves, no specific histologic abnormalities have been detected in this syndrome. In the tunica media of the aorta, the most advanced changes are seen in cases of diffuse dilatation of the ascending aorta in which the process has gone on over several years' time and the patient has succumbed to the effects of aortic regurgitation. In such cases, there are frequently early changes in the pulmonary artery. The early changes in the aorta are best demonstrated in those patients dying of dissecting aneurysm.

The advanced changes consist of fragmentation and sparsity of elastic fibers, irregular whorls of seemingly hypertrophied and perhaps hyperplastic smooth muscle, increase in collagenous tissue, pronounced increase in the vascularity of the tunica media, with wide dilatation of the vasa vasorum in both the tunica adventitia and the tunica media, and cystic spaces occupied by metachromatically staining material. The net result is an aorta which is thicker (but weaker) than normal. Moore[379] found a "florid inflammatory reaction in the adventitia" of the dissected aorta of a 24-year-old woman who died in the early puerperium. He pictured collagen fragments with surrounding cellular reaction. Rare reports of the same finding could be found.[403,501]

The early changes are those described by Erdheim[147] as cystic medial necrosis. There is mild to moderate degeneration of elastic fiber elements, with more or less striking cystic areas filled with metachromatically staining material. Wagenvoort and colleagues[583] concluded that the histologic changes in the Marfan syndrome and in cystic medial necrosis are indistinguishable.

Although cystic medial necrosis with dilatation may be observed in the pulmonary artery[568] and large branches of the aorta, and although abdominal aneurysm without thoracic involvement of note has occurred in a few patients,[358] overwhelmingly the main localization is to the ascending aorta. The predominant involvement of the ascending aorta is not inconsistent with a generalized defect of some element of connective tissue, since it is the ascending portion of the aorta that bears the main brunt of hemodynamic stress. Reynolds and associates[452] concluded that, with physiologic pulse pressures, it is only the ascending aorta that shows dilatation (i.e., increase in diameter) with each ventricular ejection. Other observers, while disagreeing with Reynolds' claim that virtually no expansile pulsation occurs beyond the arch, corroborate the finding that much greater expansion occurs in the ascending aorta (15% to 20% increase over diastolic diameter in the ascending aorta and 5% in the distal aorta). Engineers, textile scientists, and others concerned with testing the "strength of materials" are familiar with the fact that cyclic application of a stressing force results in structural disintegration much sooner than does steady application of the same force.

Another factor in the predominant localization in the ascending aorta may be implicit in Laplace's law (wall tension = pressure × radius). Since both pressure and radius find their largest values in the ascending aorta, the tension on the wall of that portion is greater than anywhere else in the vascular tree. In the case of aneurysm there is, by the same token, a vicious cycle or self-perpetuating action—the greater the radius, the greater the wall tension, the greater the radius, and so on.

The importance of hemodynamic stress to the genesis of cystic medial necrosis of the aorta is underscored by descriptions[344] of patients who develop this change in association with aortic stenosis and regurgitation of relatively mild nature.

The predominant localization of the pathologic changes of Marfan's syndrome, of other varieties of Erdheim's cystic medial necrosis (p. 189), and of syphilis, in the ascending aorta, probably has its basis in the physical and hemodynamic considerations outlined above. The pulmonary artery has the same defect of its tunica media but rarely gives trouble of clinical significance, probably because both blood pressure and pulse pressure are lower in the pulmonary artery than in the aorta. (In syphilis, other theories for preferential thoracic localization of the spirochete have been invoked, such as difference in the distribution of the vasa vasorum and a slightly cooler environment of the thoracic aorta. Proponents of the latter theory point to the difficulties in inducing syphilis in rabbits during hot weather and the preferential localization of spirochetes in parts of rabbit skin that have been shaved.)

In the pathogenesis of dissection, the abruptness of ventricular ejection may be important. Prokop and co-workers[433,433a] found that in a model with a standard intimal tear, steady flow at pressures of up to 400 mm. Hg results in no dissection, but pulsatile flow at a pressure as low as 50 mm. Hg does produce dissection. Thus the rate of development of intraluminal pressure would appear to be a key factor in tearing stress to the aorta.

Minor changes in the heart valves, in the form of marginal thickening or fibromyxomatous excrescenses, have been described grossly in many of the autopsied cases,[475,516,560] including Salle's case,[475] the first autopsied. Histologically, one case[568] was found to show "numerous lacunae in the collagenous substance of the mitral valve that were filled with a homogeneous basophilic material." This lesion resembles closely that which occurs in the tunica media of the aorta. In Fig. 3-31H is a representation of the changes in the aortic valve in one of our cases. The pronounced sacculation and stretching of the aortic cusps is probably per se evidence of weakness of the connective tissue stroma of the valve. In the process of the stretching, breaks, with fenestration of the cusp, may occur.[570] Corresponding to the redundant and subluxating posterior leaflet of the mitral valve demonstrated by cineangiocardiographic studies and correlated with a late systolic murmur (p. 123), this cusp was described at autopsy as "ballooned out like a billowing sail," by Tung and Liebow.[568] In a 34-year-old Marfan patient with aneurysm of the ascending aorta, Edynak and Rawson[138] found ruptured aneurysm of the mitral valve. "Diaphanous" appropriately describes the gross appearance of the valves at operation or autopsy in many cases.[443] Olcott,[405] Tobin and co-workers,[556] and Read and associates,[443] among others,[16,41] also described myxomatous transformation of the heart valves, especially the mitral. There are now numerous experiences (p. 121) indicating that the myxomatous valve transformation of the Marfan syndrome can be the basis for bacterial endocarditis.

Calcification and even ossification of the mitral annulus were detected radiologically and/or pathologically by several workers,[50,375,553] and we have observed one such case (P. R., 559979).

James and co-workers[264] studied the cardiac conduction system in two patients with the Marfan syndrome dying at 20 and 19 years of age. Significant narrowing of the nutrient arteries to the sinus node and atrioventricular node was demonstrated, as well as evidence of old and recent injury to these structures. The vessels showed medial degeneration and hyperplasia and intimal proliferation. In both patients the terminal illness was characterized by arrhythmias and conduction disturbances. Similar pathologic changes were present in the small arteries of the ventricular myocardium and lungs.

In one case (S. C., 575946) the splenic artery was grossly friable and showed advanced cystic medial necrosis on histologic examination. The splenic, iliac, innominate, both subclavian, both common carotid, both renal, and mesenteric arteries showed characteristic cystic medial necrosis in one well-studied case.[461] The intracranial arteries, inferior vena cava, and common iliac veins were normal. Austin and Schaefer[16] described a case in which both common carotids were extensively involved by cystic necrosis with subsequent dissection. Biopsy of the femoral artery during surgical repair of the heart or aorta under cardiopulmonary bypass has shown cystic medial necrosis in cases of the Marfan syndrome.[443] Edwards[137a] has informed me of a case of the Marfan syndrome in which the severely affected infant died immediately after birth and showed dissecting hematoma of the umbilical artery. The infant (AFIP 1147254) was 65 cm. long and had marked arachnodactyly. The heart showed enlarged valve rings, nodular thickening of the free margins of the aortic and mitral valves, and, histologically, fragmented elastic lamellae in the aorta.

The pathologic studies of the eyes[301] have not been very helpful from the fundamental standpoint. Hypoplasia of the dilator muscle of the iris provides explanation for the miosis and poor response to mydriatics.[478]

In the histopathologic study of an eye removed at autopsy from a 27-month-old infant, Theobald[552] found incomplete separation between the iris and trabecula. The dilator pupillae and the circular muscle of the ciliary body were not developed. Reeh and Lehman[446] reported similar findings in an older patient. The chamber angle contained numerous iris processes and strands extending from the anterior portion of the trabecula to the iris, similar to pectinate ligaments seen in lower animals. Prominent blood vessels were seen to cross through some of the larger processes. The dilator pupillae muscle was thinner than in the normal eye. In studies of the eye from 4 patients with the Marfan syndrome, Wachtel[582] found enlargement of the globe and microphakia, both factors that contribute to the myopia.

I question the diagnosis of the Marfan syndrome in the 11-month-old child in whom the hearing organ was studied histologically by Kelemen.[285] Fabré and colleagues[157] claimed that by electron microscopy the skin showed the collagen bundles to be abnormally gracile and fragmented, to be disoriented, and to be separated by abundant, presumably excessive ground substance. Furthermore, the elastic fibers had a moth-eaten appearance.

Joint capsules, ligaments, tendons, and periosteum have shown no abnormality, but studies in these areas are distressingly few. Roark[461] could find no definite abnormality in the anterior spinous ligament or intervertebral discs.

Read and associates[444] found enlargement of the anterior pituitary with nodular hyperplasia of acidophilic cells and suggested a role of the pituitary in the Marfan syndrome. Others[45,438,556] have described similar autopsy findings. None of the rather numerous autopsies performed in cases of the Marfan syndrome in this hospital has shown abnormality, however.

The basic defect

Bacchus[17] reported low levels of serum seromucoid in patients with the Marfan syndrome. However, comparing 40 persons having undoubtedly been affected with this disorder with an equal number of normal subjects matched for age, sex, and race, Leeming and McKusick[309] could demonstrate no abnormality of serum seromucoid. Lehmann[310] could demonstrate no abnormality of serum mucoproteins or urinary amino acids in the numerous affected members of a family.

Prockop and Sjoerdsma[432] found that whereas normal subjects excrete in the urine 16 to 34 mg. of peptide-bound hydroxyproline per day, 3 patients with the Marfan syndrome excreted 38 to 90 mg. Low hydroxyproline diet, isocaloric low protein diet, and state of hydration had no effect on hydroxyproline excretion, and no diurnal variations were found. Since hydroxyproline is an amino acid unique to collagen, the findings in the Marfan syndrome were greeted as of fundamental importance, suggesting that the primary defect involves collagen. Although such may indeed be the case, the work with hydroxyproline perhaps cannot be taken as proof, since (1) many conditions of increased growth are accompanied by elevated urinary hydroxyproline[267,271] and (2) adult Marfan patients may have normal urinary excretion of this amino acid.[512] (Jones and colleagues[270] did find elevation of urinary hydroxyproline in 5 adult patients, 23 to 38 years of age.) In the present view, the increased urinary excretion of hydroxyproline in patients with the Marfan syndrome under 20 years of age is merely a reflection of their increased growth.[367,517]

Segrest and Cunningham[492] suggested that urinary hydroxylysyl glycosides are a better indicator of collagen turnover than hydroxyproline peptides; less than 15% of the hydroxyproline of degraded collagen appears in the urine, according to the studies of the involuting uterus in the postpartum rat by Woessner.[609] The hydroxylysyl glycosides are little affected by diet. Very high excretion, indicating increased collagen turnover, was observed in a 19-year-old female patient with the Marfan syndrome. In the skin of a mother and son with Marfan syndrome, Macek and co-workers[333] found a 3:1 ratio of soluble to insoluble collagen, as compared with the normal 1:1 ratio. The ratio returned to a 1:1 ratio in later stages of culture, however. Laitinen and associates[304] reported increased soluble collagen in skin specimens obtained by punch biopsy, the value being two to three times normal.

In what element of connective tissue is the defect of the Marfan syndrome located? The histologic appearance of the aorta suggests that the primary defect may be in the elastic fiber. The pathogenic chain of events might be as follows[197]: The elastic fibers, constitutionally inadequate, undergo degeneration, particularly at the site of maximum hemodynamic stress, the ascending aorta. The smooth muscle elements, which normally have origin and insertion on the elastic lamellae, collapse together into disorganized whorls and undergo hyperplasia and hypertrophy. Reparative processes leave the tunica media scarred. Secondary to the frantic hypertrophy of smooth muscle fibers and the scarring process, dilatation of the vasa vasorum occurs. (In 1933 Wolff[611] suggested that Erdheim's cystic medial necrosis might be a generalized weakness of elastic fibers. He demonstrated abnormalities in larger peripheral arteries and in the main pulmonary artery.) Pinkus and colleagues[424] concluded that since elastic fibers of skin, although markedly stretched in striae distensae, do regenerate, the primary defect of the Marfan syndrome is not likely to reside in elastic tissue. The failure to find abnormality of elastic tissue in the trachea, skin spinal ligaments, and intervertebral disc[461] argues against the theory implicating elastic tissue.

What the suspensory ligament of the lens has in common with the tunica media of the aorta is obscure. If this common factor were known, the basic defect of the Marfan syndrome might be understood. Most information suggests that the suspensory ligament is collagenous in nature.[370] However, it cannot be like most collagen (Table 2-1, p. 34), because it is digested by chymotrypsin, as demonstrated by the surgical technique developed by Dr. Joaquin Barraquer of Spain and introduced into the United States by Dr. Derrick T. Vail. Furthermore, the zonular fibers are not digested by collagenase.[427]

The histologic changes in the aorta in the Marfan syndrome are not inconsistent with the possibility that the primary defect involves collagen. There is more collagen than elastic tissue in the aorta,[370] and by interconnecting the elastic lamellae, the collagen fibers may be important to the structural integrity of the skeleton of the aortic media.

It is possible to reconcile with a generalized connective tissue defect many of the other manifestations: the lax joint capsules, the weak ligaments, especially those with large elastic fiber representation such as the ligamenta flava of the spine, the malformed elastic cartilages of the pinnae, and the deformity of the foot, where elastic fibers are abundant in the ligaments.[544] But how is one to explain the most striking feature of this syndrome, dolichostenomelia, and the other dolichomorphic features? One receives the impression that the factor which is missing during morphogenesis and growth of bone in victims of this syndrome is a binding force that places a rein on longitudinal growth. Whether it is elastic fiber as such or some element with the properties of the elastic fiber matters not at the moment. Is some such element missing from the ground material of the cartilaginous precursors of bone? Or is the location of the defect in the periosteum? Longitudinal growth of the large bones of the extremities occurs at the epiphyseal-diaphyseal junctions. The periosteum, attached as it is to the epiphyseal cartilage, may exercise control over longitudinal growth.[587] Experiments of Ollier in 1867[406] and of others[303] more recently, although not without flaw, suggest such to be the case: If a cuff of periosteum is removed from the circumference of a growing long bone, that bone will grow longer than its undisturbed counterpart. An inborn weakness of the periosteum might have a similar effect. The bony abnormality does not appear to be one of simple overgrowth, since the excess is limited to longitudinal growth. The bones are abnormally small in cross section. Osteogenesis may be proceeding at a normal rate in the periosteum, which slides along the diaphysis, adding bone to the circumference; the diaphysis may not attain normal transverse dimensions because the periosteal bone is spread over a greater total area.* Periosteal stripping of the diaphysis has been used to increase length of the femur and tibia.[90b] Enhanced

---

*Lacroix[303] writes (p. 59) as follows: "A fibro-elastic membrane, the periosteum grows, while yielding to a traction imposed upon it, by stretching over its entire extent. Where only one zone of growth exists, as in the case of the long bones of the hand and foot, the periosteal sheath is attracted in only one direction; it is pulled in two opposite directions on the two sides of a 'neutral' zone in bones with two zones of growth. Since the diaphysis elongates only at the level of the growth cartilage, the periosteum during development slides along the bone surface at a rate and in a direction specific to each level." Later (p. 67), he writes: "Since the periosteum slides along the diaphysis which it encloses, the youngest trabeculae, those in formation at the moment of examination, are not deposited at exactly the same level as those which the same zone of periosteum elaborated in the preceding days." The obliquity of the canals of the nutrient arteries has its origin in this phenomenon.

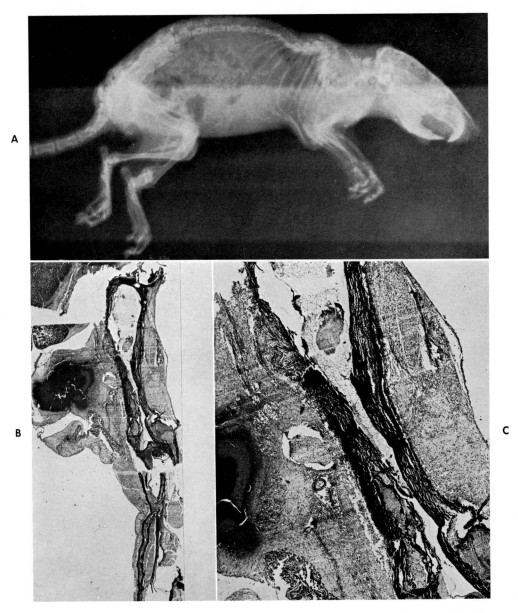

Fig. 3-74. Experiments conducted by Dr. James R. Brayshaw,[74] as student at The Johns Hopkins University School of Medicine. **A,** Deformity and pathologic fracture of spine and other bones in rat fed seeds of *Lathyrus odoratus*. **B,** Dissecting aneurysm of the aorta with rupture in rat fed seeds of *L. odoratus.* Shown is the dissection of the tunica media and the large mediastinal hematoma. Elastic tissue stain. The elastic lamellae are black. (×10; reduced ⅕.) **C,** Same at higher magnification. On the left below, the wall of the aorta is grossly scarred through almost its entire thickness. (×30; reduced ⅕.)

growth of the operated bone has been attributed to effects on blood supply. It is a frequent observation that when a fracture occurs in the shaft of the femur the bone grows more than its unfractured counterpart.

The report[17] that the affected members of one family showed abnormally low levels of serum mucoproteins was received with great interest. If confirmed, not only would the observation have diagnostic usefulness, but it also might assist in pinpointing the basic defect. Note that as stated on p. 45, the elastic fiber is, in one view, composed in part of "elastomucin." Unfortunately, Dr. James T. Leeming and I have been unable to demonstrate any abnormality of serum mucoprotein in 46 Marfan patients, as compared with controls matched for age, sex, and race.[309]

The production in rats of a somewhat analogous, but *acquired,* syndrome has been of great interest, for obvious reasons. Kyphoscoliosis, hernia, and aneurysm of the aorta (dissecting, diffuse, or saccular) can be produced in rats (Fig. 3-74) fed a toxic agent contained in the seed of *Lathyrus odoratus.*[74,429,430] The toxic material has been crystallized[132] and identified[481] as β (γL-glutamyl) amino-propionitrile:

$$HOOC-\underset{\underset{NH_2}{|}}{CH}-CH_2-CH_2-\overset{\overset{O}{||}}{C}-NH-CH_2-CH_2-C\equiv N$$

The aminopropionitrile will also cause skeletal changes and dissecting aneurysm of the aorta.[588] Gelatin and casein appear to afford partial protection against the effects of these toxins.[115] Whether the primary difficulty is in the elastic fibers or in the intermediate material is not clear.[18,97] Possibly significant with reference to the predominant male sex incidence of dissecting aneurysm in man is the finding[584] that aortic rupture occurs much more frequently in male rats fed sweet pea seeds than in female rats. Furthermore, the simultaneous administration of androgen considerably enhanced the incidence and severity of aortic medionecrosis[584] in sweet pea–fed rats. The demonstration of increased mucopolysaccharide[97] is of interest in light of the metachromatically staining material seen in human cases of Erdheim's cystic necrosis, including that caused by the Marfan syndrome (p. 181). Although the basic defect in this acquired syndrome is probably not the same as that in the Marfan syndrome, studies of this sort should be helpful in elucidating some of the many mysteries that surround dissecting aneurysm in particular[297] and disorders of connective tissue in general. Clinically, Bean and Ponseti[35] have been impressed with a relatively high incidence of kyphoscoliosis in the group of cases of dissecting aneurysm of the aorta.

If the defective connective tissue element in the Marfan syndrome is indeed collagen, the elucidation of the molecular defect in lathyrism, which simulates the Marfan syndrome rather closely, is of obvious pertinence. The aminonitriles, the toxic component of *Lathyrus odoratus* seeds, interfere with collagen cross-linking mechanisms.[212]

Arguing from the similarity of the lesions in the Marfan syndrome and in lathyrism, where the defect can be shown to concern an enzyme important in cross-linking of elastin and collagen, Nenci and Beltrami[396] suggested that the Marfan syndrome is "caused" by a genetic "defect of the amino-oxidase which activates the oxidative deamination of lysine." However, because of the dominant mode of inheritance, if the gene defective in the Marfan syndrome is one that determines protein structure as opposed to one with regulatory function, an enzymopathy seems unlikely. It is generally found that enzymopathies behave as recessives. The dominant pattern of inheritance makes change in a nonenzymic protein much more likely (p. 22).

Another possible model, or phenocopy, for the aortic lesion in the Marfan syndrome may be copper deficiency in swine.[105,319,503,592] Rupture of the aorta occurs at the age of 3 or 4 months in these animals. A defect in the elastica of the tunica media has been demonstrated mechanically, histologically, and biochemically. Linker and associates[319] demonstrated a threefold increase in the mucopolysaccharide content of the aorta. The basic defect in Menkes syndrome, an X-linked recessive, has been found by Danks and his colleagues[113a] to be copper deficiency resulting from a block of intestinal absorption. As in the animals with induced copper deficiency, patients with this disorder (see p. 710 for details) show changes in collagen and elastin that are well accounted for by the copper dependency of lysine oxidase, the enzyme that catalyzes the oxidative deamination of lysine to form allysine from which cross-links of collagen and elastin are formed (p. 40).

Yet another model of heritable connective tissue disorders with aortic aneurysm may be provided by the mouse with one or another mutant gene of the "mottled" series (Grahn and co-workers[202a,202b]). The alleles at the "mottled" locus on the X chromosome include: blotchy, *Blo;* brindled, *Mo*[br]; dappled, *Mo*[dp]; to tortoise, *To.* These alleles vary in their lethal effects, in their pathologic manifestations, and in their expression of mosaic coat color. (The mosaic coat color in the "mottled" series, together with certain other X-linked coat color variants in the mouse, was the basis of Dr. Mary Lyon's hypothesis as the inactive X chromosome [p. 10].) The most striking abnormalities of connective tissues occur in *To.* Of hemizygous males with this gene (*To*/Y), 81% had aortic aneurysm; of heterozygous females (*To*/+), 25% had aortic aneurysm, and another 17% had an S-curve (elongated and tortuous) aorta. Of *Blo*/Y and *Blo*/+ mice, 98% and 32%, respectively, had aortic aneurysm. On the other hand, no aortic aneurysm occurred in *Mo*[br]/Y or *Blo*/*Mo*[br] mice, and there was a low frequency (4%) in *Mo*[dp]/+. Histologic changes (Fry and colleagues[177a]) consist of irregularity and disruption of elastic laminae and metachromatic accumulations in the interlaminar areas. Deformity of the limb, thorax, and spine occur in these mice (Grahn and co-workers[202b]).

Matalon and Dorfman[360,361] described metachromatic granules in fibroblasts cultured from patients with the Marfan syndrome. Whereas dermatan sulfate is increased in fibroblasts in the mucopolysaccharidoses, hyaluronic acid is increased in the Marfan syndrome. Cartwright and associates[88] confirmed the metachromasia of Marfan fibroblasts. Danes[113] also confirmed the finding of metachromasia in some but not all cases of the Marfan syndrome. She found that all cases had normal total mucopolysaccharide but an elevated proportion of hyaluronic acid. The hyaluronic acid from fibrobasts that showed metachromasia was abnormally viscous.

Tjio and co-workers[555] described the presence of a chromosome with giant satellites in each of 2 patients designated as having familial Marfan's disease.

They stated that although "the present data do not prove the given abnormalities to be the underlying cause of Marfan's syndrome, a relationship is definitely suggested." Because of doubts about the diagnosis of the Marfan syndrome in the 2 patients, the failure to find giant satellites in a third undoubted case of the Marfan syndrome, and the observation of giant satellites in persons either without phenotypic abnormality or with features other than those of the Marfan syndrome, it seemed unlikely that a causal relationship existed.[337] Furthermore, Ford,[170] Böök (cited by Ford), and Handmaker[226] could find no abnormality of the chromosomes in a considerable number of Marfan patients. In 4 such patients Källén and Levan[278] found that chromosomes 21 and 22 were relatively shorter than those of normal persons. Of the 3 male patients one had an abnormally long Y chromosome and one an abnormally short Y chromosome. The findings in chromosomes 21 and 22, which apparently have not been sought by other workers, were interpreted by Källén and Levan[278] as a phenotypic expression at the level of the chromosomes, rather than as a causal feature. The XYY sex chromosome constitution found by Hustinx and van Olphen[258] was apparently only coincidental.

Relation to Erdheim's cystic medial necrosis[472, 578]

Erdheim's disease is probably not a single entity from the etiologic standpoint. There are probably a number of possible "causes"—some genetic (such as the Marfan syndrome) and some acquired in nature. With the control of syphilis and rheumatic fever, cystic medial necrosis will assume increasing importance as a cause of aortic regurgitation. It must be kept in mind, particularly when there is no history of syphilis, rheumatism, or bacterial endocarditis, and it must *not* be excluded from consideration on the grounds that there is no radiologic evidence of aortic dilatation. Unfortunately, the diagnosis of idiopathic Erdheim's disease (Erdheim's disease without the Marfan syndrome) will for the present need to be a diagnosis of exclusion.

Some pathologists, such as Dr. A. R. Rich and Dr. Ella Oppenheimer,[453] believe that the aorta in the Marfan syndrome has histologic features—specifically, large whorled bundles of disorganized smooth muscle and greatly dilated vasa vasorum—that are not seen in ordinary Erdheim's disease. The changes that are considered specific for the Marfan syndrome are most likely to occur in the first part of the aorta, the part that first undergoes dilatation. Farther on in the aorta, the changes are indistinguishable from those of idiopathic medial necrosis. It is uncertain whether this histologic picture indicates a fundamental difference. It seems to me to be possible for merely the prolonged evolution or some other feature of the Marfan syndrome to permit or to dictate the occurrence of this particular change.

Erdheim's disease is very familiar as a cause of dissecting aneurysm. That it can also cause diffuse or fusiform dilatation of the aorta is indicated by the surgically proved cases referred to above and by reports in the literature.[116,235, 466,610,617,619,623] In some of these cases, insufficient clinical information is provided to permit exclusion of the Marfan syndrome. The experience with the Marfan syndrome should prove very useful in the cases of idiopathic Erdheim's disease. In both disorders, dissecting aneurysm or fusiform dilatation, or a combination, can occur. In both, the ascending aorta is most severely affected.

In both, the process seems to pursue an unrelenting progression to death from rupture of the aorta or from the effects of aortic regurgitation.

Erdheim's medial necrosis may be the cause of death in the first months of life[392,660] or not until the ninth decade. There is now convincing evidence[515] that the metabolic turnover rate in the elastic skeleton of the aorta is so low* as to raise serious suspicions of complete metabolic inertia. The elastic structures of the aorta can be looked on as intended to outlive the rest of the organism. In certain unfortunate individuals, however, the elastica "gives out" prematurely. The result is Erdheim's cystic medial necrosis. Genetic inferiority is probably most frequently the basis. It has been described in brothers,[202,579] in father and son,[167] and in mother and daughter,[210] but the clinical information provided was sometimes too scant to permit exclusion of the Marfan syndrome. Hanley and Jones[228] reported dissecting aneurysm in 2 sisters and the son of one of them; no other stigmata of the Marfan syndrome or other connective tissue disorders were present. The following is a description of cystic medial necrosis in a father and son, neither of whom had clear signs of the Marfan syndrome:

Case 7. R. D. (J.H.H. 1308499), a male of Jewish extraction born in 1922, died in 1970 after operation for prosthetic replacement of the ascending aorta.

A heart murmur was discovered while he was in high school. He lived an active life, however, being successful in business and playing squash and tennis regularly. In September, 1968, he began to feel sluggish, with a sensation of congestion in his chest. He had several episodes of exertional dyspnea and nocturnal orthopnea. In October, 1968, electrocardiograms showed left ventricular hypertrophy and left axis deviation; chest x-ray examination showed marked cardiomegaly and calcification of the aortic valve. Aortogram showed aneurysmal dilatation of the ascending aorta. On November 1, 1968, the aortic valve was replaced with a Starr-Edwards prosthesis. The excised aortic valve was bicuspid, scarred, and calcified. The ascending aorta was dilated, and there was no evidence of dissection.

In February, 1970, dyspnea recurred. In May, 1970, recurrence of aortic regurgitation was demonstrated by catheterization studies. On September 5, 1970, cardiopulmonary bypass, with reinsertion of a Starr-Edwards valve and replacement of the ascending aorta with a prosthesis, was performed. The patient did not survive the operation. The ascending aorta had a transverse internal rent on the posterior wall of the aorta 1½ inches above the annulus of the valve, with complete dissection at the level of the innominate artery.

No seemingly relevant abnormality was known in the family, other than those in the son (Case 8). A daughter has scoliosis.

The patient was not considered to have the clinical features, either skeletal or ocular, of the Marfan syndrome. Right inguinal herniorrhaphy had been performed at 33 years of age. He had worn glasses for myopia of moderate degree.

At autopsy (J.H.H. 37429) the length of the body was 170 cm., with US/LS ratio of 0.73. The prosector thought that the palate was highly arched and that arachnodactyly was present. Fresh medial dissection involved the entire aorta and extended into the left innominate, left carotid and subclavian, celiac, and right iliac and femoral arteries, with occlusion of the bronchial and renal arteries. Microscopically, the changes of Erdheim's cystic medial necrosis were demonstrated. The eye showed no ectopia lentis or other histologic changes of the Marfan syndrome.

Comment. The association of a calcific, bicuspid, and at least mildly stenotic aortic valve brings to mind patients in whom the association of aortic valvular disease and cystic medial necrosis of the ascending aorta has been reported.[344]

Case 8. R. D. (S.H. 55371), born in 1948, the son of R. D. (Case 7, above), died of ruptured aorta at the age of 19 years.

Bilateral inguinal herniorrhaphies were performed in early childhood. He had mild con-

---

*Labella[302] suggests there may be a component of elastic fiber that is metabolically fairly active.

genital athetosis as well as mental retardation. At the age of 17 years he was found to be overweight and hypertensive. He was first recognized to have aortic regurgitation in January, 1967, during a physical examination for the draft. Further studies in March, 1967, showed left ventricular hypertrophy and enlargement of the ascending aorta but no skeletal or ocular features suggesting the Marfan syndrome.

He died in his sleep in July, 1967.

Autopsy showed a body length of 180 cm., with US/LS ratio of 0.65. The aortic valve was bicuspid and the left ventricle markedly dilated and hypertrophied. The ascending aorta showed fusiform dilatation, with a longitudinal rent of the tunica intima and external rupture into the pericardial sac. Microscopically, changes of Erdheim's cystic medial necrosis were visualized.

Comment. The question is whether the disorder in father and son is (1) the Marfan syndrome with submersion of the ocular and skeletal features or (2) a distinct disorder. The question will not be answered, it would seem, until biochemical or other methods for demonstrating the basic defect are available. I[342a] have speculated that, comparable to the association between bicuspid aortic valve and coarctation of the aorta, there may be an association between congenital bicuspid aortic valve and an innate weakness of the aorta leading to cystic medial necrosis.

Management of the patient with the Marfan syndrome

Therapeutic procedures in patients with the Marfan syndrome fall into four main categories: (1) inhibition of growth by hormonal induction of puberty; (2) use of anabolic steroids; (3) use of beta-blockade to reduce stress on the aorta; and (4) surgical procedures for the ocular, skeletal, and cardiovascular complications.

Particularly in girls with the Marfan syndrome, excessive height may reach grotesque proportions. Induction of precocious puberty by hormonal means seems indicated. Therapy should begin before 9 or 10 years of age if much is to be accomplished.[205] I suspect that severe progressive scoliosis can be avoided in part at least by this therapy. (Although my experience is limited to girls, hormonal induction of puberty might be considered in boys also, especially if scoliosis is developing.) Therapy has consisted of daily estrogen (Premarin), 10 mg./day, and medroxyprogesterone acetate (Provera), 10 mg/day, for one week out of each four. "Natural" bleeding occurs on this program. I have not seen excessive bleeding, such as may occur as a "breakthrough," if only estrogen is given. Menstruation in a young girl has not presented a psychosocial problem— even though the treatment has been initiated as early as 4 years of age (see following Case 9). Estinyl estradiol may be preferable to Premarin because of longer half-life and better defined chemical nature.[594a] Also, progesterone for 4 days out of each month is probably adequate.

The hormonal induction of puberty in the Marfan syndrome is illustrated by the following 2 cases:

Case 9. P. A. (J.H.H. 1233743), a white girl born December 16, 1964, has had extraordinarily rapid growth, making artificial induction of puberty a worthwhile procedure. She was treated with an anabolic steroid from the age of 16 months to the age of 34 months, with dramatic improvement in general strength and well-being but with an acceleration of bone age. Therapy with estrogen (Premarin) and progesterone (Provera) was initiated at the age of 4½ years. At the chronologic age of 6 years, her bone age was about 13 years and dental age about 7½ years. Her height was also about that of a 13-year-old.

She has always shown deep-set eyes with overhanging brow, large anterior ocular segment (megalocornea), small pupils, iridodonesis, upward displacement of the lenses, dolichocephaly with prominent sagittal ridge, pectus excavatum, pes planus with "curled-under" toes, striae distensae of the anterior thighs, apical systolic click, and late systolic murmur (Fig. 3-75). She is of superior intelligence.

Angiocardiographic studies at the age of 25 months showed no dilatation of the aortic sinuses. Mitral regurgitation was demonstrated.

The parents are normal, and no other instance of the Marfan syndrome is known in the family. The father was 56 years old at the time of the child's birth.

Case 10. M. T. (J.H.H. 1081724), born in 1954, was noted to have ectopia lentis at about age 30 months, and a diagnosis of Marfan syndrome was made. She appears to be a sporadic case. The father and mother were 31 and 30 years old, respectively, at her birth. When first

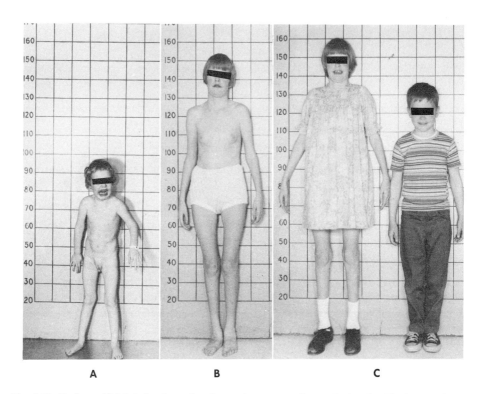

A   **B**   **C**

Fig. 3-75. Early artificial induction of puberty for arrest of growth in the Marfan syndrome. P. A. (J.H.H. 1233743) was born of a 40-year-old woman and her 56-year-old husband, both healthy. At 10 months of age arachnodactyly and muscular underdevelopment were noted, as well as a systolic murmur, shown by cardiac catheterization at age 25 months to be produced by retrolapse of the mitral valve ("floppy mitral valve"). Examination at 26 months showed a height of 100 cm., marked dolichostenomelia with asthenia, pes planus, facies characteristic of the Marfan syndrome, and megalocornea and bilateral ectopia lentis. An anabolic steroid, methandrostenolone, was administered from age 26½ months to age 46 months, with improvement in her muscular development and robustness. Growth acceleration was marked, however (see **D**), and virilization in the form of clitoral enlargement led to discontinuation. At the age of 4½ years the patient was placed on daily estrogen, with progesterone given daily during each fourth week. Regular menses began six weeks after initiation of therapy. At 6⅓ years of age the patient was 61¼ inches tall, with a bone age of 13½ years. At 6¹¹⁄₁₂ years of age she was 62¾ inches tall, with a bone age of about 14½ years.

Social adjustment has been excellent—in no small part because of intelligent and sympathetic management by the parents—and general health has been good. The child has grown from an asthenic, generally unhappy child into a happy, well-adjusted, robust young lady. **A,** age 26 months; **B,** age 71 months; **C,** age 77 months, with her brother, two years *older;* **D,** growth curves. Accelerated growth occurred during treatment with the anabolic steroid; a "leveling off" of growth has occurred during treatment with female hormones.

seen at this hospital at the age of 8 years 11 months, she was 63 inches tall (Fig. 3-76). Other features, particularly asymmetric hips, are shown in the photographs. Since her height was far above the 97th percentile (Fig. 3-76 *D*), therapy with estrogen (Premarin) was initiated. Estrogens were discontinued at age 12 years 9 months. On examination at age 13 years 8 months, her height was 71½ inches. She showed signs of floppy mitral valve (systolic click and late systolic murmur). The bone age was 18 years.

Anabolic steroids have been used in cases of the Marfan syndrome as a measure of general "strengthening." From observations in an adult patient,

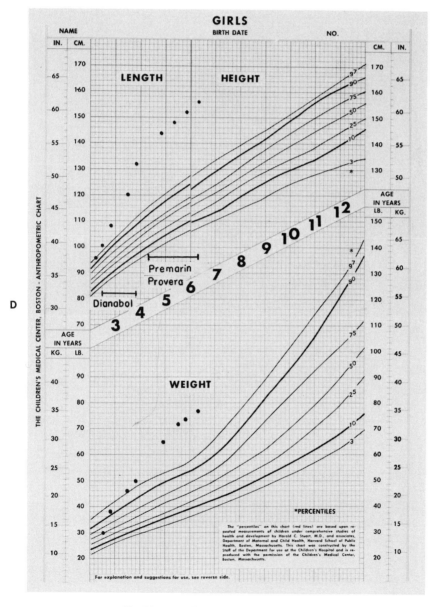

Fig. 3-75, cont'd. For legend see opposite page.

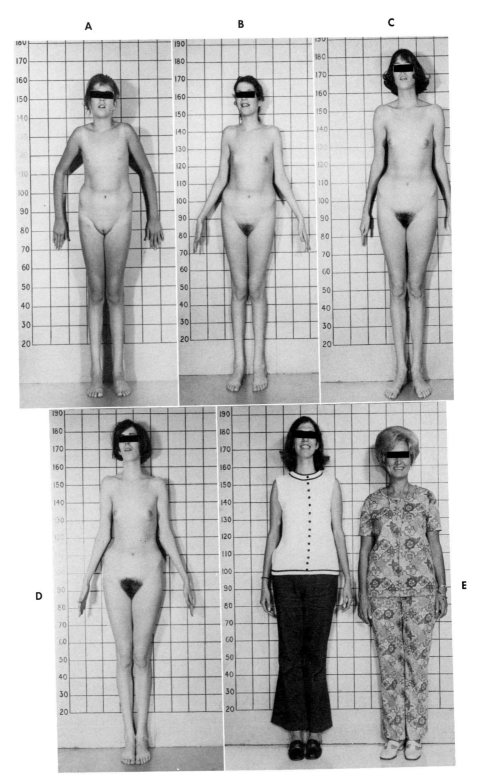

Fig. 3-76. Control of excessive height in the Marfan syndrome (Case 2). **A**, Age $8\frac{11}{12}$ years; **B**, age $9\frac{7}{12}$ years; **C**, age $12\frac{2}{12}$ years; **D**, age $13\frac{8}{12}$ years; **E**, age $15\frac{11}{12}$ years; **F**, growth chart.

Jones and co-workers[272] suggested that aortic deterioration was stayed by use of methandrostenolone (Dianabol). Decrease in urinary excretion of hydroxyproline may be an objective gauge of beneficial effects. I have observed gratifying general improvement in a 2½-year-old child who, before treatment, was strikingly asthenic. Further acceleration of growth is an undesirable effect in chil-

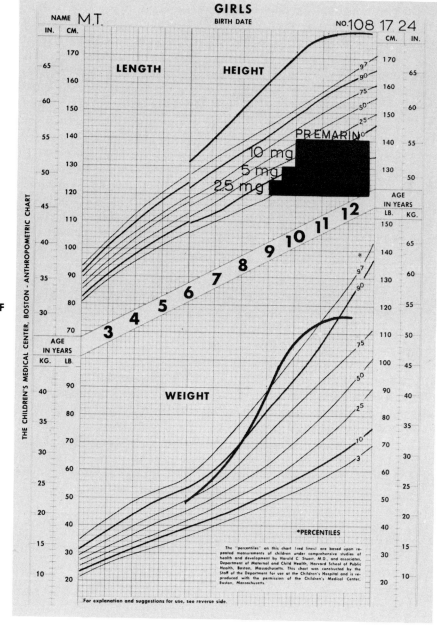

Fig. 3-76, cont'd. For legend see opposite page.

dren. Masculinization can be a limiting consideration in female patients. Oxandrolone (Anavar) has less masculinizing effect It is doubtful that anabolic steroids are often indicated, except in very asthenic female infants in whom hormonal closure of the epiphyses will be practiced later, according to the schedule described in Case 9, p. 191.

In turkeys with a high natural frequency of dissecting aneurysm* of the aorta,[347] the incidence thereof can be reduced dramatically by addition of a small amount of reserpine to the feed.[455,456] The amount of reserpine given is thought to be insufficient to reduce blood pressure but does affect the impulse, i.e., the rate of pressure rise. Palmer and Wheat[411] and Wheat and colleagues[598] have presented evidence that either reserpine or trimethaphan (Arfonad) is useful in the treatment of dissecting aneurysms even in nonhypertensive persons. McFarland et al.[333a] concluded there is a place for the medical treatment of dissecting aortic aneurysms with agents including propranolol. My colleagues and I[222] are accumulating experience that seems to indicate that propranolol (Inderal) can stay the progression of aortic dilatation in the Marfan syndrome.

Propranolol is a beta-adrenergic blocking agent that has been shown to decrease myocardial contractility[233,234] and to reduce the abruptness of ventricular ejection. Its effects can be gauged in the patient by the preejection period (PEP), which can be measured by "noninvasive" methods and shows prolongation with therapy. The PEP has two parts: (1) the time for electrical activation of the left ventricle, that is, the interval between the onset of the QRS of the electrocardiogram and the beginning of the pressure rise in the left ventricle, and (2) the time from the beginning of the rise in pressure to the opining of the aortic valve. The contractile, or inotropic, state of the left ventricle is reflected in the second portion, so-called dP/dT. The normal PEP measures about 100 msec.; propranolol therapy in doses of 120 to 160 mg./day increases PEP by about 10 msec.

The importance of pulse wave characteristics to extension and rupture of dissecting aneurysms was shown by the work of Prokop and associates.[433a] In a model of the aorta consisting of an outer layer of Tygon tubing and an inner layer of rubber cement, when an intimal tear was produced, nonpulsatile flow at pressure up to 400 mm. Hg produced no dissection, whereas pulsatile flow produced rapid dissection. Similar results were obtained using dog aortas. They could show that the extent of dissection was related to dP/dT_{max}.

In the management of patients with the Marfan syndrome, PEP is determined from simultaneous recordings of the electrocardiogram (lead II), phonocardiogram, and carotid pulse tracing, as recommended by Weissler and co-workers.[591] The Q-S_2 interval measures the entire electromechanical systole. The left ventricular ejection time (ET), the interval from aortic valve opening to aortic valve closure, is approximated by the interval between the onset of the carotid pulse and the dicrotic notch. PEP, the interval from the onset of the QRS complex to the opening of the aortic valve, is obtained by subtracting the ejection time from the Q-S_2 interval.

---

*Although aortic lesions can be produced in the turkey, as in other species, by feeding beta-aminopropionitrile,[506] endemic aortic rupture is probably not related to a specific dietary factor.

The pulse rate is another useful gauge of the effectiveness of therapy. We have aimed to keep the pulse rate below 70 at all times.

Because of difference in its mode of action, propranolol has theoretic advantages over reserpine. The latter agent depletes catecholamines from sympathetic nerve endings and cannot prevent an increase in ventricular contractility by circulating catcholamines. Propranolol, on the other hand, blocks beta receptors, thereby preventing the effects of both sympathetic nervous system discharge and circulating catecholamines.

Propranolol is remarkably free of complications. Since congestive heart failure can be precipitated by propranolol, significant myocardial dysfunction is a relative contraindication to its use. Exacerbation of asthma is sometimes produced, and Raynaud's phenomenon may occur. Mental depression has been associated with use of propranolol but is probably a more frequent complication of reserpine therapy.

The patients with Marfan syndrome who are candidates for propranolol therapy are those who demonstrate early signs of dilatation of the aorta, the murmur of aortic regurgitation being the usual first sign. As indicated earlier (p. 111), dissection and rupture of the aorta probably occur rarely, if ever, without preexisting dilatation of the aorta.

At this writing, my experience with propranolol therapy consists of 6 Marfan patients and 1 with idiopathic cystic medial necrosis. The longest period of treatment is two years. Progression in aortic dilatation appears to have been stayed; however, it is too early to evaluate the therapy conclusively.

One patient was switched to reserpine because of asthma. Rather severe Raynaud's phenomenon has developed in a second, but therapy has been continued because of the pronounced dilatation of the aorta.[222]

Symbas and colleagues[548] have provided an extensive review of surgical experience in the aortic abnormality of the Marfan syndrome. The aorta has been replaced with a prosthesis, of Teflon, for example,[54,134] the aortic valve has been bicuspidized[54,201,368,386] or replaced with a Starr-Edwards or other prosthesis,[286] the mitral valve has been replaced by a prosthesis,[58,125,223,292,462,494] and various combinations of these procedures have been performed.[90a,273,274,371,374,394] Sirak and Ressallat[511] replaced the mitral valve with a prosthesis in 2 adult females, 30 and 49 years of age, and Gerbode and co-workers[183] performed the operation in a 27-year-old man. In all three the valve was competent in the period soon after operation but again became regurgitant some months later. Aortic aneurysm has been resected in an 8-year-old child,[134] and dissecting aneurysm has been treated surgically in a 6-year-old child.[286] The mitral valve was replaced with a prosthesis in a 3-year-old child.[494]

De Bakey and colleagues[119,122] classify dissecting aneurysm into three types. The surgical management appropriate to each differs.

Type I dissecting aneurysms arise from an initimal tear in the ascending aorta, and dissection extends beyond the arch throughout a varying length of the entire aorta. The recommended surgery requires temporary cardiopulmonary bypass and consists of repair of the intimal tear with obliteration on the false lumen. Associated aortic regurgitation is usually corrected by resuspension of the aortic valve commissural attachment during repair of the intimal rent.

Type II dissecting aneurysms likewise begin at an intimal tear in the ascending aorta, but dissection is limited to the ascending aorta. Recommended operation in this group, into which most of the Marfan cases fall, consists of resection and graft replacement of the ascending aorta during cardiopulmonary bypass. Aortic annular involvement is usually more severe than in Type I, and concomitant aortic valve replacement with a prosthesis is often required.

Type III dissecting aneurysms arise from an initimal rent at or just distal to the origin of the left subclavian artery and extends distally for a varying distance but may be limited to the descending thoracic aorta. Recommended surgery makes use of temporary left atrial to femoral artery bypass with a pump and consists of resection and graft replacement of the portion of aorta containing the rent and as much as possible of the dissection, with obliteration of any remaining distal false lumen.

The surgery of coronary sinus abnormalities was also discussed by De Bakey and colleagues.[120] Of 25 patients with "three sinus" aneurysms, 8 were judged to have the Marfan syndrome. Their ages varied from 14 to 45 years. Seven were male. In all 25 cases, excision of the aneurysm was performed, and in a majority a Dacron graft and an aortic valve prosthesis were inserted.

One patient with the Marfan syndrome was represented among the 196 cases of scoliosis treated with casts and fusion by Moe and Gustilo.[377] Harrington instrumentation[550] has also been used[232] in the treatment of the Marfan syndrome.

Hammertoes have required corrective surgery in several patients (e.g., the daughter in Fig. 3-32).

Healing after surgical procedures is normal. Herniorrhaphy, orthopedic procedures, and correction of pectus excavatum are examples of surgery. (One patient with the Marfan syndrome sustained a lienorenal shunt procedure for unrelated hepatic cirrhosis.[568])

Correction of pectus excavatum should probably be postponed until after puberty, since an imperfect result may follow if opportunity for excessive longitudinal growth of ribs is still present after operation.

Ophthalmologic practice in regard to ectopia lentis has favored lens extraction only if glaucoma develops or satisfactory visual acuity cannot be achieved.[267a] There is probably an increased risk that detachment of the retina will occur in Marfan patients in connection with surgery for ectopia lentis, but it occurs also without surgery. Vitreous loss, often followed by blindness, has an unusually high frequency. However, the results of surgery are better than in cases of traumatic ectopia lentis.[266] The aspiration technique of Maumenee and Ryan[362] promises to give improved results when lens extraction is necessary because of glaucoma or serious visual impairment.

Other considerations

A point of medicolegal importance is the relationship of trauma to the development of various manifestations of the Marfan syndrome. The development of hernia, detachment of the retina,[69,342,485] dissecting aneurysm,[61,82,127,423,565] and total dislocation of the lenses may be intimately related to trauma as a precipitating factor. In Choyce's case[95] dislocation of the lenses into the anterior chamber occurred when the patient leaned forward to pick something up from the floor. Wilson[606] suggested that the strain of sexual intercourse may contribute to deterioration of the aorta. In one of his patients, death occurred 5 days after marriage; in another, symptoms of left ventricular failure began after intercourse. On the other hand, a murmur of aortic regurgitation is known to have been present for sixteen years in an unmarried affected sister. It has been said that in the Marfan syndrome a sedentary spinster may outlive an athletic husband. Contradicting this statement are the survivorship data, which are summarized in Fig. 3-54 and which indicate a poorer prognosis for females, at least between the ages of 10 and 30 years.

In connection with the relation of the Marfan syndrome to other diseases or special physiologic states, rheumatic fever, syphilis, hypertension, and pregnancy might be mentioned. The suggestion of Futcher and Southworth[179] that rheumatic fever may occur with increased incidence in these patients has not been confirmed by further observations. Syphilis and hypertension, if combined with the Marfan disease, might have particularly dire effects on the aorta.

There is now convincing evidence of a strikingly increased incidence of dissecting aneurysm of the aorta in pregnancy.[247,350,400,486,497] Conceivably, this is related to the hormone "relaxin" and to the general relaxation of ligaments and other joint structures during pregnancy.[1,2,237,421,428,449,619] Against this hypothesis is the fact that my colleagues and I[254,342] have been unable to induce aortic dissection in animals treated with large doses of "relaxin," with or without challenge with vasopressor agents. Rupture of the splenic artery, another rather frequently reported[498,557] accident of pregnancy, may be on a similar basis. The reduction of tensile strength of the skin during pregnancy is further evidence of a generalized change in connective tissue.

We observed 3 patients in whom pathologic changes occurred in the aorta in association with pregnancy. There was no evidence of the Marfan syndrome in any of them. (In addition, dissection may have occurred during pregnancy in the patient illustrated in Fig. 3-26A.)

Case 11. A. P. (621953), Negro female, at the age of 36 years had a difficult labor with her sixth child. During a period of hard straining in labor she suddenly "felt something snap" inside her body at the level of the lower back, and an excruciating pain spread over most of the trunk. The baby was delivered by cesarean section. A laparotomy five months later showed abdominal aneurysm, for which no treatment was attempted. She was aware of a pulsating mass in the abdomen. Palpitation, dyspnea, and profuse sweats developed. She was examined at The Johns Hopkins Hospital six years later. There was a pulsating abdominal mass, auscultatory signs of aortic regurgitation, and marked cardiomegaly. Serologic test for syphilis was negative. The patient died elsewhere; no autopsy was performed.

Case 12. C. T., a 41-year-old mother of seven, was found six weeks before her death to have a blood pressure of 180/100 mm. Hg. She was six months or more pregnant. She refused hospitalization at that time. On the morning of the day of death the patient had the onset of substernal pain and profuse perspiration. The blood pressure was 225/120 mm. Hg. On the way to the University Hospital the patient was suddenly seized with severe chest pain, collapsed in the car, and became very "blue." She was dead on arrival at the hospital. A postmortem cesarean section delivered a full-term live male child that weighed 5,089 grams. Autopsy of the mother revealed dissecting aneurysm of the aorta with rupture. (The case reported by Spenser[523] is rather similar, in that postmortem cesarean delivery was done in a woman dead of dissecting aneurysm.)

Case 13. D. W. (706005), a 33-year-old woman, sustained rupture of a coronary sinus into the right side of the heart, in the early puerperium.

Lindeboom and Bouwer,[317] Husebye and colleagues,[257] Novell and associates,[403] Moore,[379] Rivlin,[459] Massumi and co-workers,[358] Borglin and Bach,[60]

Grondin and colleagues,[211] and Baker and colleagues[23] reported on dissecting aneurysm in pregnant or recently pregnant women with the Marfan syndrome, and Spenser's case[523] may be another example. It is said[459] that dissection rarely occurs during labor, and that for this reason cesarean section is not justified. Dissection of the coronary arteries, with occlusion and sudden death, has also occurred in the puerperium,[126] and coronary dissection has been reported in the Marfan syndrome.[283,334,480] Avoidance of pregnancy seems indicated, especially by more severely affected women.[128,459,463]

The main features of the Marfan syndrome, its psychologic impact, and the trials and vicissitudes of cardiovascular investigations and aortic surgery are engaging by described in the diary of Yehuda Kesten,[286] a journalist in Tel Aviv, born in 1926.

> By my seventeenth birthday I stood six feet two inches in my stocking feet and weighed 136. My bones were flat, my shoulders broad, and my muscles hard and flexible. I had a broad chest in front and narrow in profile, while my hips were slightly wider than my waist. When I was being fitted for my first custom-made suit, the tailor pointed out that my right hip was slightly higher than my left. I tried to correct it by physical exercises.
>
> I too have a large skull. While serving in the Navy, the Quartermaster always had difficulty in finding a cap to fit me. But my ears are of normal size and I do not think I look older than I am.*

Between ages 22 and 30 years he had four operations for bilateral inguinal hernias that developed while in military service. In March, 1964, he suffered a bout of prolonged severe pain in the front and back of the chest and was found to have aortic regurgitation and aortic aneurysm. Demonstration of ectopia lentis confirmed the diagnosis of the Marfan syndrome, made on the service of Professor André DeVries at the Beilinson Hospital in Tel Aviv.

Kesten was referred to Dr. Michael DeBakey in Houston for surgery. Replacement of the ascending aorta was performed in late May, 1964, and, when the aortic regurgitation did not diminish adequately, the aortic valve was replaced by a Starr-Edwards prosthesis about thirteen months later. The book's dust jacket describes it as "the story of a double triumph: Dr. DeBakey's over the 'incurable' Marfan syndrome, and Yehuda Kesten's over his fear."

In June, 1972, when I had the privilege of examining Mr. Kesten, he was active and generally well, although he demonstrated moderate cardiomegaly, atrial fibrillation, and persistent aortic regurgitation and had been maintained on anticoagulant and digitoxin. In November, 1971, acute glaucoma from entrapment of the lens in the pupil necessitated removal of the right lens.

SUMMARY

The cardinal manifestations of the Marfan syndrome are skeletal, ocular, and aortic. Dolichostenomelia (long, thin extremities) and redundant ligaments and joint capsules characterize the skeletal changes. Ectopia lentis is the hallmark of the disorder in the eye. In the aorta, predominantly the ascending aorta, diffuse dilatation and/or dissection occur.

The only histopathologic changes described to date are those in the aorta,

---

*From Kesten, Y.: Diary of a heart patient, New York, 1968, McGraw-Hill Book Co., pp. 11, 30.

where degeneration of the elastic lamellae appears to be primary in the pathogenetic chain. Whether the basic defect resides in the elastic fiber or, as seems somewhat more likely, in collagen is unknown.

The pedigrees are consistent with inheritance of this trait as a simple Mendelian dominant with a relatively high grade of penetrance.

Although certainly there are some persons having true cases of the Marfan syndrome without ectopia lentis and without other, less equivocally affected members in the family, the lack of both of these features leaves the diagnosis in question in many instances.

REFERENCES

1. Abramson, D., Hurwitt, E., and Lesnick, G.: Relaxin in human serum as test of pregnancy, Surg. Gynec. Obstet. **65**:335, 1937.
2. Abramson, D., Roberts, S. M., and Wilson, P. D.: Relaxation of pelvic joints in pregnancy, Surg. Gynec. Obstet. **58**:595, 1934.
3. Achard, C.: Arachnodactylie, Bull. Mém. Soc. Méd. Hôp. Paris **19**:834, 1902.
4. Adams, R. A., and Porter, W. B.: Marfan's syndrome; report of a case, Southern Med. J. **42**:844, 1949.
5. Alarcon-Segovia, D., Fierro, F. J., Villalobos, J. de J., and Dies, F.: Bilateral renal vein thrombosis and nephrotic syndrome in a patient with the Marfan syndrome, Dis. Chest **54**:153, 1968.
6. Albanese, A.: Sulla dolichostenomelia, Arch. Ortop. **47**:539, 1931.
7. Allen, R. A., Straatsma, B. R., Apt, L., and Hall, M.: Ocular manifestations of the Marfan syndrome, Trans. Amer. Acad. Ophthal. Otolaryng. **71**:18, 1967.
8. Anderson, A., Spencer, H., and Staffurth, J. S.: Dissecting aneurysm and medial degeneration of the aorta in Marfan's syndrome, St. Thomas's Rep. **7**:146, 1951.
9. Anderson, M., and Pratt-Thomas, H. R.: Marfan's syndrome, Amer. Heart J. **46**:911, 1953.
9a. Anderson, R. E., Grondin, C., and Amplatz, K.: The mitral valve in Marfan's syndrome, Radiology **91**:910, 1968.
10. Anning, S. T.: Elastoma intrapapillare perforans verruciforme (Miescher), Proc. Roy. Soc. Med. (Sect. Derm.) **51**:932, 1958.
11. Anon.: Marfan's biography, Brit. J. Med. **2**:175, 1942.
12. Anon.: A. B. Marfan, Presse Méd. **50**:301, 1942.
13. Anon.: A. B. Marfan. Union Méd. Canada **73**:1706, 1944.
14. Apert, E.: Les formes frustes du syndrome dolichosténomélique de Marfan, Nourrisson **26**:1, 1938.
14a. Arkin, W.: Blue scleras with keratoglobus, Amer. J. Ophthal. **58**:678, 1964.
15. Atta, A. G., and Hoch, J.: Marfan's syndrome and dissecting aneurysm of the aorta, Arch. Intern. Med. **108**:781, 1961.
16. Austin, M. G., and Schaefer, R. F.: Marfan's syndrome, with unusual blood vessel manifestations; primary medionecrosis dissection of right innominate, right carotid, and left carotid arteries, Arch. Path. **64**:205, 1957.
17. Bacchus, H.: A quantitative abnormality in serum mucoproteins in the Marfan syndrome, Amer. J. Med. **25**:744, 1958.
18. Bachhuber, T. E., and Lalich, J. J.: Effect of sweet pea meal on the rat aorta, Arch. Path. **59**:247, 1955.
19. Baden, E., and Spirgi, M.: Oral manifestations of Marfan's syndrome, Oral Surg. **19**:757, 1965.
19a. Badtke, G.: Ueber einen eigenartigen Fall von Keratokonus und blauen Skleren bei Geschwistern, Klin. Mbl. Augenheilk. **106**:585, 1941.
20. Baer, R. W., Taussig, H. B., and Oppenheimer, E. H.: Congenital aneurysmal dilatation of the aorta associated with arachnodactyly, Bull. Hopkins Hosp. **72**:309, 1943.
21. Bahnson, H. T., and Nelson, A. R.: Cystic medial necrosis as a cause of localized aortic aneurysms amenable to surgical treatment, Ann. Surg. **144**:519, 1956.
22. Bahnson, H. T., and Spencer, F. C.: Excision of aneurysm of ascending aorta with prosthetic replacement during cardiopulmonary bypass, Ann. Surg. **151**:879, 1960.

23. Baker, C. B., Wilson, T. K., and Woods, J. M.: Marfan's syndrome; a successful aortic homograft for a dissecting aneurysm of the thoracic aorta, Canad. J. Surg. **1**:371, 1958.

24. Barlow, J. B., Bosman, C. K., Pocock, W. A., and Marchand, P.: Late systolic murmurs and non-ejection ("mid-late") systolic clicks; an analysis of 90 patients, Brit. Heart J. **30**:203, 1968.

25. Baron, M. G., Wolf, B. S., Grishman, A., and van Mierrop, L. H. S.: Aneurysm of the membranous septum, Amer. J. Roentgen. **91**:1303, 1964.

26. Barraquer, J., and Rutllán, J.: Alpha-chymotrypsin in cataract surgery, Postgrad. Med. **35**:57, 1964.

27. Barrett, J. S., Helwig, J., Jr., Kay, C. F., and Johnson, J.: Cineangiographic evaluation of aortic insufficiency; unsuspected idiopathic aneurysmal dilatation of the aortic root as a possible indication of the Marfan syndrome, Ann. Intern. Med. **61**:1071, 1964.

28. Barron, A. A.: Arachnodactyly (Marfan's syndrome), N. Carolina Med. J. **3**:353, 1942.

29. Bauer, J.: Innere Sekretion, ihre Physiologie, Pathologie und Klinik, Berlin and Vienna, 1927, Julius Springer, p. 361.

30. Bawa, Y. S.: Gupta, P. D., and Goel, B. G.: Complete heart block in Marfan's syndrome, Brit. Heart J. **26**:148, 1964.

31. Beals, R. K., and Hecht, F.: Contractural arachnodactyly, a heritable disorder of connective tissue, J. Bone Joint Surg. **53-A**:987, 1971.

32. Bean, W. B.: Precordial noises heard at a distance from the chest. In Monographs in medicine, Baltimore, 1952, The Williams & Wilkins Co., p. 22.

33. Bean, W. B., and Fleming, J. G.: Arachnodactyly; report of a case complicating pregnancy at term, Ohio Med. J. **36**:155, 1940.

34. Bean, W. B., and Mohaupt, F. X.: Rupture of the aortic valve, J.A.M.A. **150**:92, 1952.

35. Bean, W. B., and Ponseti, I. V.: Dissecting aneurysm produced by diet, Circulation **12**:185, 1955.

36. Becker (Naumberg): Linsenektopie in der I., (II.), und III. Generation, Klin, Mbl. Augenheilk. **94**:547, 1935.

37. Becker, P. E.: Dystrophia musculorum progressiva; eine genetische und klinische Untersuchung der Muskeldystrophien, Stuttgart, 1953, Georg Thieme Verlag.

38. Bell, J.: Anomalies and diseases of the eye, the treasury of human inheritance, Cambridge, 1932, Cambridge University Press, vol. 2, part V, p. 477.

39. Benavides, P.: Sindrome de Marfan, Principia Cardiologica **3**:193, 1956.

40. Benda, C. E.: Developmental disorders of mentation and cerebral palsies, New York, 1952, Grune & Stratton, Inc., p. 159.

41. Berenson, G. S., and Greer, J. C.: Heart disease in the Hurler and Marfan syndromes, Arch. Intern. Med. **111**:58, 1963.

42. Berg, G., and Vejlens, G.: Cystic disease of the lung in tuberous sclerosis, Acta Paediat. **36**:16, 1939.

43. Berg, G., and Zachrisson, C. G.: Cystic lungs of rare origin—tuberous sclerosis, Acta Radiol. **22**:425, 1941.

44. Bergofsky, E. H., Turino, G. M., and Fishman, A. P.: Cardiorespiratory failure in kyphoscoliosis, Medicine **38**:263, 1959.

45. Bergstrand, C. G.: Arachnodactylia; pathological anatomy in connection with a case, Acta Paediat **30**:345, 1943.

46. Berlin, R.: Familial occurrence of pneumothorax simplex, Acta Med. Scand. **137**:268, 1950.

46a. Bertelsen, T. I.: Dysgenesis mesodermalis corneae et sclerae. Rupture of both corneae in a patient with blue sclerae, Acta Ophthal. **46**:486, 1968.

47. Beyer, P., Klein, M. L., and Iszepy, E.: Maladie de Marfan avec raideurs articulaires importants atteignants les quatre enfants de la même fratrie et leur mère, Arch. Franc. Pediat. **22**:210, 1965.

48. Bhat, P. K.: Bilateral ectopia lentis with arachnodactyly; Marfan's syndrome with report of case and review of literature, Antiseptic **43**:651, 1946.

49. Bigger, I. A.: The treatment of pectus excavatum, or funnel chest, Amer. Surg. **18**:1071, 1952.

50. Bingle, J.: Marfan's syndrome, Brit. Med. J. **1**:629, 1957.

51. Binion, J. T.: Marfan's syndrome, Amer. Pract. Dig. Treat. **5**:135, 1954.

52. Bittar, N., and Sosa, J. A.: The billowing mitral valve leaflet; report on fourteen patients, Circulation **38**:763, 1968.
53. Black, H. H., and Landay, L. H.: Marfan's syndrome; report of five cases in one family, Amer. J. Dis. Child. **89**:414, 1955.
54. Blanchard, R. J. W., Felder, D. A., Culligan, J. A., and MacLean, L. D.: Cardiovascular surgery in Marfan's syndrome, Ann. Surg. **158**:990, 1963.
55. Boerger, F.: Ueber zwei Fälle von Arachnodaktylie, Zschr. Kinderheilk. **12**:161, 1914; Mschr. Kinderheilk. **13**:335, 1914.
56. Bolande, R. P.: The nature of the connective tissue abiotrophy in the Marfan syndrome, Lab. Invest. **12**:1087, 1963.
57. Bolande, R. P., and Tucker, A. S.: Pulmonary emphysema and other cardio-respiratory lesions as part of the Marfan abiotrophy, Pediatrics **33**:356, 1964.
58. Boone, J. A., and Clowes, G. H., Jr.: Calcified annulus fibrosus with mitral insufficiency in the Marfan syndrome—with prosthetic replacement of the mitral valve, Southern Med. J. **62**:682, 1969.
59. Booth, C. C., Louchbridge, L. W., and Turner, M. D.: Arachnodactyly with congenital lesions of the urinary tract, Brit. Med. J. **2**:80, 1957.
60. Borglin, N. E., and Bach, G.: Marfan's syndrome and pregnancy, Acta Obstet. Gynec. Scand. **40**:271, 1961.
61. Bornstein, F. P.: Dissecting aneurysm of the thoracic aorta due to tramua, Texas J. Med. **50**:720, 1954.
62. Bortree, L. W.: Discussion of Strayhorn and Wells.[545]
63. Bowden, D. H., Favara, B. E., and Donahoe, J. L.: Marfan's syndrome; accelerated course in childhood associated with lesions of mitral valve and pulmonary artery, Amer. Heart J. **69**:96, 1965.
64. Bowers, D.: The electrocardiogram in Marfan's syndrome, Amer. J. Cardiol. **7**:661, 1961.
65. Bowers, D.: An electrocardiographic pattern associated with mitral valve deformity in Marfan's syndrome, Circulation **23**:30, 1961.
66. Bowers, D.: Marfan's syndrome: the S family re-visited, Canad. Med. Ass. J. **89**:337, 1963.
67. Bowers, D.: Pathogenesis of primary abnormalities of the mitral valve in Marfan's syndrome, Brit. Heart J. **31**:679, 1969.
68. Bowers, D.: Primary abnormalities of the mitral valve in Marfan's syndrome; electrocardiographic findings, Brit. Heart J. **31**:676, 1969.
69. Bowers, D. (Kelowna, British Columbia): Unpublished observations.
70. Bowers, D., and Lim, D. W.: Subacute bacterial endocarditis and Marfan's syndrome, Canad. Med. Ass. J. **86**:455, 1962.
71. Boyd, D. H. A.: Familial spontaneous pneumothorax, Scot. Med. J. **2**:220, 1957.
72. Boyer, B. E., and Martin, M. M.: Marfan's syndrome; report of a case manifesting a giant bone cyst of the mandible and multiple (110) basal cell carcinomata, Plast. Reconstr. Surg. **22**:257, 1958.
73. Bramwell, C., and King, J. T.: The principles and practice of cardiology, London, 1942, Oxford University Press, p. 29.
74. Brayshaw, J. R., and McKusick, V. A.: Unpublished observations.
75. Brock, R. C.: Recurrent and chronic spontaneous pneumothorax, Thorax **3**:88, 1948.
76. Broglio, G.: Difetto del setto interventricolare in sindrome de Marfan, Boll. Soc. Ital. Cardiol. **6**:17, 1961.
77. Bronson, E., and Sutherland, G. A.: Ruptured aortic aneurysms in childhood, Brit. J. Child. Dis. **15**:241, 1918.
78. Burian, H. M.: A case of Marfan's syndrome with bilateral glaucoma; with description of a new type of operation for developmental glaucoma (trabeculotomy ab externo), Amer. J. Ophthal. **50**:1187, 1960.
79. Burian, H. M.: Chamber angle studies in developmental glaucoma; Marfan syndrome and high myopia, J. Missouri Med. Ass. **55**:1088, 1958.
80. Burian, H. M., von Noorden, G. K., and Ponseti, I. V.: Chamber angle anomalies in systemic connective tissue disorders, Arch. Ophthal. **64**:671, 1960.
81. Burry, A. F.: Supra-aortic stenosis associated with Marfan's syndrome, Brit. Heart J. **20**:143, 1958.
82. Cabot Case No. 43011: Marfan's syndrome with old and recent dissecting aneurysm, fibrin-

ous pericarditis with effusion, Hufnagel operation two months before death, thrombosis of valve, New Eng. J. Med. **256**:30, 1957.

83. Calhoun, F. P.: Causes of heterochromia iridis, with special reference to paralysis of the cervical sympathetics, Amer. J. Ophthal. **2**:255, 1919.

84. Callahan, A.: Aniridia with ectopia lentis and secondary glaucoma, Amer. J. Ophthal. **32**: 28, 1949.

85. Campbell, R. W., Steinmetz, E. F., and Helmen, C. H.: Congenital aneurysm of the membranous portion of the ventricular septum; a cause for holosystolic murmurs, Circulation **30**:223, 1964.

86. Capotorti, L., Gaddini de Benedetti, R., and Rizzo, P.: Contribution to the study of the heredity of Marfan's syndrome. Description of a family tree of 4 generations with marriage between consanguineous patients, Acta Genet. Med. (Roma) **8**:455, 1959.

87. Cartellieri, L., and Kleinsorge, H.: Neurologische Störungen beim Marfan-Syndrom, Nervenartz **24**:376, 1953.

88. Cartwright, E., Danks, D. M., and Jack, I.: Metachromatic fibroblasts in pseudoxanthoma elasticum and Marfan's syndrome, Lancet **1**:533, 1969.

89. Case Records of the Massachusetts General Hospital, New Eng. J. Med. **243**:346, 1950.

90. Castellanos, A., Jr., Ugarriza, R., de Cardenas, A., and Cano, L. A.: Sindrome de Marfan: reporte de seis casos en una misma familia, Arch. Hosp. Univ. (Habana) **9**:353, 1957.

90a. Caves, P. K., and Paneth, M.: Replacement of the mitral valve, aortic valve, and ascending aorta with coronary transplantation in a child with the Marfan syndrome, Thorax **27**:58, 1972.

90b. Chan, K. P., and Hodgson, A. R.: Physiologic leg lengthening, Clin. Orthop. **68**:55, 1970.

91. Chang, C. E.: Marfan's syndrome; review of literature and report of one case, Chin. Med. J. **68**:433, 1951.

92. Chapman, D. W., Beazley, H. L., Peterson, P. K., and Cooley, D. A.: Annulo-aortic ectasia with cystic medial necrosis; diagnosis and surgical treatment, Amer. J. Cardiol. **16**:679, 1965.

93. Childers, R. W., and McCrea, P. C.: Absence of the pulmonary valve; a case occurring in the Marfan syndrome, Circulation **29**:598, 1964.

94. Chisholm, J. C., Cherniack, N. S., and Carton, R. W.: Results of pulmonary function testing in 5 persons with the Marfan syndrome, J. Lab. Clin. Med. **71**:25, 1968.

95. Choyce, D. P.: Anterior dislocation of the lens in Marfan's syndrome, Brit. J. Ophthal. **41**:446, 1957.

96. Christianson, H. B.: Elastosis perforans serpiginosa: association with congenital anomalies; report of 2 cases, Southern Med. J. **59**:15, 1966.

97. Churchill, D. W., Gelfant, S. Lalach, J. J., and Angevine, D. M.: Alterations in the polysaccharides and elastic fibers in the aortas of rats fed toxic lathyrus factor, Lab. Invest. **4**:1, 1955.

98. Cipolloni, P. B., Jr., Shane, S. R., and Marshall, R. J.: Chronic atrial flutter in brothers with the Marfan syndrome, Circulation **31**:572, 1965.

99. Clunie, G. J. A., and Mason, J. M.: Visceral diverticulosis and the Marfan syndrome, Brit. J. Surg. **50**:51, 1962.

100. Cockayne, E. A.: Arachnodactyly with congenital heart disease (patent interventricular septum), Proc. Roy. Soc. Med. **29**:120, 1935.

101. Coffey, J. H. Barker, D. E., and Friedlander, J. H.: Dissecting aneurysm with Marfan's syndrome, Texas J. Med. **51**:79, 1955.

102. Cohen, D. N., and Kaye, D.: Staphylococcal endocarditis in narcotic addict with Marfan's syndrome, New York J. Med. **67**:2362, 1967.

103. Consul, B. N., Kutshrestha, O. R., and Kasliwal, R. M.: Marfan's syndrome, J. Indian Med. Ass. **35**:218, 1960.

104. Cook, J. M.: Spontaneous perforation of the colon; report of two cases in a family exhibiting Marfan stigmata, Ohio Med. J. **64**:73, 1968.

104a. Cordella, M., and Vinciguerra, E.: Le manifestazioni oculari nella sindrome d'Ehlers-Danlos, Minerva Oftal. **8**:103, 1966.

105. Coulson, W. F., and Carnes, W. H.: Cardiovascular studies on copper-deficient swine. II. Mechanical properties of the aorta, Lab. Invest. **11**:1316, 1962.

106. Court Brown, W. M.: Males with an XYY sex chromosome complement, J. Med. Genet. **5:**341, 1968.

106a. Coventry, M. B.: Some skeletal changes in the Ehlers-Danlos syndrome, J. Bone Joint Surg. **43-A:**855, 1961.

107. Criley, J. M., Lewis, K. B., Humphries, J. O., and Ross, R. S.: Prolapse of the mitral valve; clinical and cine-angiographic findings, Brit. Heart J. **28:**488, 1966.

108. Crocker, D. W.: Marfan's syndrome confined to the mitral valve region; two cases in siblings, Amer. Heart J. **76:**538, 1968.

109. Crowe, F. W., Schull, W. J., and Neel, J. V.: A clinical, pathological and genetic study of multiple neurofibromatosis, Springfield, Ill., 1956, Charles C Thomas, Publisher.

110. Crump, J. Mikelberg, R. M., and Recknagel, E. M. S.: Arachnodactyly (Marfan's syndrome), J. Amer. Med. Wom. Ass. **13:**62, 1958.

111. Cucolo, G. F., and Kavazes, J. P.: Marfan's syndrome with rupture of the spleen and cystic medionecrosis of the splenic artery, New York J. Med. **67:**2863, 1967.

112. Cunliffe, W. J., Hudgson, P., Fulthorpe, J. J., Black, M. M., Hall, R., Johnston, I. D. A., and Shuster, S.: A calcitonin-secreting medullary thyroid carcinoma associated with mucosal neuromas, Marfanoid features, myopathy, and pigmentation, Amer. J. Med. **48:**120, 1970.

113. Danes, B. S. (New York): Personal communication, 1971.

113a. Danks, D. M., Stevens, B. J., Campbell, P. E., Gillespie, J. M., Walker-Smith, J., Blomfield, J., and Turner, B.: Menkes' kinky-hair syndrome, Lancet **1:**110, 1972.

114. Das Gupta, B. K., and Basu, R. K.: Bilateral dislocation of the lens under voluntary control in Marfan syndrome with cardiovascular anomaly, Brit. J. Ophthal. **39:**566, 1955.

115. Dasler, W.: Partial protection against odoratism (sweet pea lathyrism) by diets high in gelatin or casein, Proc. Soc. Exp. Biol. Med. **85:**485, 1954.

116. Davies, D. H.: Idiopathic cystic medial necrosis of aorta, Brit. Heart J. **3:**166, 1941.

117. Davis, J. H. Benson, J. W., and Miller, R. C.: Thoracoabdominal aneurysm involving celiac, superior mesenteric, and renal arteries; report of a case successfully treated by resection and nylon-graft replacement, Arch. Surg. **75:**871, 1957.

118. Dax, E. C.: Arachnodactyly, J. Ment. Sci. **87:**434, 1941.

119. De Bakey, M. E., Beall, A. C.. Jr., Cooley, D. A., Crawford, E. S., Morris, G. C., Garrett, H. E., and Howell, J. F.: Dissecting aneurysms of the aorta, Surg. Clin. N. Amer. **46:**1045, 1966.

120. De Bakey, M. E., Diethrich, E. B., and Liddicoat, J. E.: Abnormalities of the sinuses of Valsalva; experience with 35 patients, J. Thorac. Cardiov. Surg. **54:**312, 1967.

121. De Bakey, M. E., Henley, W. S., Cooley, D. A., Morris, G. C., Jr., Crawford, E. S., and Beall, A. C., Jr.: Surgical management of dissecting aneurysm involving the ascending aorta, J. Cardiov. Surg. **5:**200, 1964.

122. De Bakey, M. E., Henly, W. S., Cooley, D. A., Morris, G. C., Jr., Crawford, E. S., and Beall, A. C., Jr.: Surgical management of dissecting aneurysms of the aorta, J. Thorac. Cardiov. Surg. **49:**130, 1965.

123. Deckers, P. F. L. H. M.: Het Syndroom van Marfan: Een Literatuurstudie, klinisch en biochemisch Onderzoek, Thesis, Rijksuniversiteit te Groningen, 1967.

124. Dexter, M. W., Lawton, A. H., and Warren, L. O.: Marfan's syndrome with aortic thrombosis, Arch. Intern. Med. **99:**485, 1957.

125. Dietzman, R. H., Peter, E. T., Wang, Y., and Lillethei, R. C.: Mitral insufficiency in Marfan's syndrome; a case report of surgical correction, Dis. Chest **51:**650, 1967.

126. DiMaio, V. J. M., and DiMaio, D. J.: Postpartum dissecting coronary aneurysm, New York J. Med. **71:**767, 1971.

126a. Di Matteo, J., Vacheron, A., Sacaut, D., Delvaux, J. C., and Audoin, J.: Anévrysmes multiples de la valve mitrale. Endocardite bactérienne et syndrome de Marfan, Coeur Med. Intern. **10:**519, 1971.

127. Dimond, E. G., Larsen, W. E., Johnson, W. B., and Kittle, C. F.: Post-traumatic aortic insufficiency occurring in Marfan's syndrome, with attempted repair with a plastic valve, New Eng. J. Med. **256:**8, 1957.

128. Donaldson, L. B., and Ramon DeAlvarez, R.: The Marfan syndrome and pregnancy, Amer. J. Obstet. Gynec. **92:**629, 1965.

129. Duke-Elder, W. S.: Textbook of ophthalmology, St. Louis, 1949, The C. V. Mosby Co., vol. 4, p. 4265.

130. Dulake, M., and Ashfield, R.: Dissecting aneurysm of the aorta with rupture into the right atrium, Brit. Heart J. 26:862, 1964.

131. Dunn, L. C., and Charles, D. R.: Studies on spotting patterns. I. Analysis of quantitative variations in the pied spotting of the house mouse, Genetics 22:14, 1937.

132. Dupuy, H. P., and Lee, J. G.: The isolation of a material capable of producing experimental lathyrism, J. Amer. Pharm. Ass. (Scient. Ed.) 43:61, 1954.

133. Du Rietz, B., and Lundström, N. R.: Ruptured aneurysm of the aorta in a 12-year-old girl, Acta Paediat. Scand. 56:541, 1967.

134. Durnin, R. E., Lindesmith, G., and Meyer, B.: Aorta surgery in a child with Marfan's syndrome, Amer. J. Dis. Child. 110:547, 1965.

135. Düx, A., Hilger, H. H., Schaede, A., and Thurn, P.: Zum Marfan-Syndrom, Z. Kreislaufforsch. 50:492, 1961.

136. Dwyer, E. M., Jr., and Troncale, F.: Spontaneous pneumothorax and pulmonary disease in the Marfan syndrome; report of two cases and review of the literature, Ann. Intern. Med. 62:1285, 1965.

137. Editorial: Marfan's syndrome, New Eng. J. Med. 256:39, 1957.

137a. Edwards, R. H. (Washington, D. C.): Personal communication, 1971.

138. Edynak, G. M., and Rawson, A. J.: Ruptured aneurysm of the mitral valve in a Marfanlike syndrome, Amer. J. Cardiol. 11:674, 1963.

139. Eisen, S., and Elliott, L. P.: The roentgenology of cystic medial necrosis of the ascending aorta, Radiol. Clin. N. Amer. 6:437, 1968.

140. Eldridge, R.: Coarctation in the Marfan syndrome, Arch. Intern. Med. 113:342, 1964.

141. Eldridge, R.: The metacarpal index, a useful aid in the diagnosis of the Marfan syndrome, Arch. Intern. Med. 113:248, 1964.

142. Ellis, R. W. B.: Four cases of fragilitas ossium and blue sclerotics, Proc. Roy. Soc. Med. 24 (part 2): 1054, 1931.

143. Ellis, R. W. B.: Arachnodactyly and ectopia lentis in father and daughter, Arch. Dis. Child. 15:267, 1940.

144. Engelbach, E.: Endocrine medicine, Springfield, Ill., 1932, Charles C Thomas, Publisher.

145. Engle, M. A.: The syndrome of apical systolic click, late systolic murmur, and abnormal T waves, Circulation 39:1, 1969.

146. Epstein, C. J., Graham, C. B., Hodgkin, W. E., Hecht, F., and Motulsky, A. G.: Hereditary dysplasia of bone with kyphoscoliosis, contractures, and abnormally shaped ears, J. Pediat. 73:379, 1968.

147. Erdheim, J.: Medionecrosis aortae idiopathica cystica, Virchow Arch. Path. Anat. 276:187, 1930.

148. Erdohazi, M., Cowie, V., and Lo, S. S.: Case of haemophilia with Marfan's syndrome, Brit. Med. J. 1:102, 1964.

149. Estes, J. W., Carey, R. J., and Desai, R. G.: Marfan's syndrome; hematological abnormalities in a family, Arch. Intern. Med. 116:889, 1965.

150. Esteve, R.: Idiopathic scoliosis in identical twins, J. Bone Joint Surg. 40-B:97, 1958.

151. Etter, L. E., and Glover, L. P.: Arachnodactyly complicated by dislocated lens and death from rupture of dissecting aneurysm of the aorta, J.A.M.A. 123:88, 1943.

152. Euzière, J., Pagès, P., Lafon, R., Mirouze, J., and Salvaing, J.: Myopathie scapulo-humérale d'Erb et dolichosténomélie; cas., Arch. Francedilla. Pédiat. 6:651, 1949.

153. Evans, P. A.: A hereditary tendency to hernia, Lancet 2:293, 1942.

154. Evans, W.: The heart in sternal depression, Brit. Heart J. 8:162, 1946.

155. Everberg, G.: Marfan's syndrome associated with hearing defect. Report of a case in one of a pair of twins, Acta Paediat. 48:70, 1959.

156. Fabré, J., Veyrat, R., and Jeanneret, O.: Syndrome de Marfan avec anevrysme et coarctation de l'aorte; étude anatomo-clinique, Schweiz. Med. Wschr. 87:49, 1957.

157. Fabré, M. T., Duret, J. C., Broustet, A., and Bouissou, H.: Ultrastructure du derme dans le syndrome de Marfan, Presse Med. 76:419, 1968.

158. Fahey, J. J.: Muscular and skeletal changes in arachnodactyly, Arch. Surg. 39:741, 1939.

159. Fairbank, T.: Atlas of general affections of the skeleton, Baltimore, 1951, The Williams & Wilkins Co., p. 175.

160. Faivre, G., Frenkiel, Pernot, C., and Hueber: Le coeur des dépressions sternales congénitales, Arch. Mal. Coeur **47**:322, 1954.

161. Falls, H. F.: A gene producing various defects of the anterior segment of the eye, with a pedigree of a family, Amer. J. Ophthal. **32**:41, 1949.

162. Fay, J. E., Horlick, L., Merrimban, J. E., and Nanson, E. M.: A case of Marfan's syndrome with an aneurysm at the ascending aorta, with physiologic, operative and postmortem studies, Canad. Med. Ass. J. **78**:862, 1958.

163. Feingold, M.: The "thumb sign" in children, Clin. Pediat. **7**:423, 1968.

164. Feldman, L., Friedlander, J., Dillon, R., and Wallyn, R.: Aneurysm of right sinus of Valsalva, with rupture into the right atrium and into the right ventricle, Amer. Heart J. **51**: 314, 1956.

165. Ferguson, M. J., and Clemente, A. R.: Rupture and dissection of the aorta in Marfan's syndrome, Amer. J. Cardiol. **4**:543, 1959.

166. Fischl, A. A., and Ruthberg, J.: Clinical implications of Marfan's syndrome, J.A.M.A. **146**: 704, 1951.

167. Fleming, J., and Helwig, F. C.: Medionecrosis aortae idiopathica cystica with spontaneous rupture, J. Missouri Med. Ass. **38**:86, 1941.

168. Flesch, M.: Ueber eine seltene Missbildung des Thorax, Virchow Arch. Path. Anat. **57**:289, 1873.

169. Fontana, M. E., Pence, H. L., Leighton, R. F., and Wooley, C. F.: The varying clinical spectrum of the systolic click–late systolic murmur syndrome: a postural auscultatory phenomenon, Circulation **41**:807, 1970.

170. Ford, C. E.: Human cytogentics: its present place and future possibilities, Amer. J. Hum. Genet. **12**:104, 1960.

171. Ford, F. R.: Diseases of the nervous system in infancy, childhood, and adolescence, ed. 4, Springfield, Ill., 1961, Charles C Thomas, Publisher, pp. 1259-1260.

172. Forgacs, P.: Stature in simple pneumothorax, Guy's Hosp. Rep. **118**:199, 1969.

173. Forsius, H., and Raitta, C.: Congenital spherophakia as a cause of severe myopia, Acta Ophthal. **42**:812, 1964.

174. Frable, W. J.: Mucinous degeneration of the cardiac valves—the "floppy valve" syndrome, J. Thorac. Cardiov. Surg. **58**:62, 1969.

175. Francheschetti, A.: Ectopia lentis et pupillae congenita als rezessives Erbleiden und ihre Manifestierung durch Konsanguinitäat, Klin. Mbl. Augenheilk **78**:351, 1927.

176. Frei, C.: Ueber das Aneurysma dissecans aortae, Inaugural Dissertation, Zürich, 1962, J. J. Meier.

177. Frieden, J., Hurwitt, E. S., and Leader, E.: Ruptured aortic cusp associated with an heritable disorder of connective tissue, Amer. J. Med. **33**:615, 1962.

177a. Fry, R. J. M., Slaughter, B., Grahn, D., Wassermann, F., Manelis, F., Hamilton, K. F., and Staffeldt E.: Inherited connective tissue defect in tortoise mice, Argonne National Laboratory Biological and Medical Research Division Annual Report, 1967, ANL-7049, pp. 114-117.

178. Fuleihan, F. J., Suh, S. K., and Shepard, R. H.: Some aspects of pulmonary function in the Marfan syndrome, Bull. Hopkins Hosp. **113**:320, 1963.

179. Futcher, P. H., and Southworth, H.: Arachnodactyly and its medical complications, Arch. Intern. Med. **61**:693, 1938.

180. Gailloud, C., DuFour, R., Barsewisch, B., and Meyer-Schevickerath, G.: Juvenile retinal detachment, Bibl. Ophthal. **79**:150, 1969.

181. Ganther, R.: Ein Beitrag zur Arachnodaktylie, Z. Kinderheilk. **43**:724, 1927.

182. Garland, H. G.: Hereditary scoliosis, Brit. Med. J. **1**:328, 1934.

183. Gerbode, F., Kerth, W. J., Hill, J. D., Sanchez, P. A., and Puryear, G. H.: Surgical treatment of nonrheumatic mitral insufficiency, J. Cardiov. Surg. **10**:103, 1969.

184. Gibson, J. B., Carson, N. A. J., and Neill, D. W.: Pathologic findings in homocystinuria, J. Clin. Path. **17**:427, 1964.

185. Gilston, R. J.: Marfan's syndrome, Med. Ann. D. C. **24**:127, 1955.

186. Goetz, R. H.: Dissecting aneurysm of the abdominal aorta in Marfan's syndrome; surgical treatment, Proc. Virchow Med. Soc. N. Y. **23**:102, 1964.

187. Goldberg, M. F., and Ryan, S. J.: Intercalary staphyloma in Marfan's syndrome, Amer. J. Ophthal. **67**:329, 1969.

188. Golden, R. L., and Lakin, H.: The *forme fruste* in Marfan's syndrome, New Eng. J. Med. **260**:797, 1959.

189. Goodman, H. B., and Dorney, E. R.: Marfan's syndrome with massive calcification of the mitral annulus at age twenty-six, Amer. J. Cardiol. **24**:426, 1969.

190. Goodman, R. M., Baba, N., and Wooley, C. F.: Observations on the heart in a case of combined Ehlers-Danlos and Marfan syndromes, Amer. J. Cardiol. **24**:734, 1969.

191. Goodman, R. M., Wooley, C. F., and Frazier, R. L.: Ehlers-Danlos syndrome occurring together with the Marfan syndrome; report of a case with other family members affected, New Eng. J. Med. **273**:514, 1965.

192. Gordan, G. S., and Lisser, H., editors: Endocrinology in clinical practice, Chicago, 1953, Year Book Medical Publishers, Inc.

193. Gordon, A. M.: Abraham Lincoln—a medical appraisal, J. Kentucky Med. Ass. **60**:249, 1962.

194. Gordon, A. M.: A case of Marfan syndrome, Parke-Davis Magazine, 1963.

195. Gordon, H., Davies, D., and Berman, M.: Camptodactyly, cleft palate, and clubfoot; syndrome shown the autosomal-dominant pattern of inheritance, J. Med. Genet. **6**:266, 1969.

196. Gore, I.: Dissecting aneurysm of the aorta in persons under forty years of age, Arch. Path. **55**:1, 1953.

197. Gore, I.: The pathogenesis of dissecting aneurysm of the aorta, Arch. Path. **53**:142, 1952.

198. Gore, I., and Seiwert, V. J.: Dissecting aneurysm of the aorta: pathologic aspects, an analysis of eighty-five fatal cases, Arch. Path. **53**:121, 1952.

199. Gouley, B. A., and Anderson, E.: Chronic dissecting aneurysm of aorta simulating syphilitic cardiovascular disease; notes on associated aortic murmurs, Ann. Intern. Med. **14**:978, 1940.

200. Goyette, E. M., and Palmer, P. W.: Cardiovascular lesions in arachnodactyly, Circulation **7**:373, 1953.

201. Goyette, E. M., Storer, J., and Grierson, A. L.: Thoracic aortic aneurysm in Marfan's syndrome; a case report, Ohio Med. J. **64**:804, 1968.

202. Graham, J. G., and Milne, J. A.: Dissecting aneurysm of the aorta: review of 29 cases, Glasgow Med. J. **33**:320, 1952.

202a. Grahn, D., Fry, R. J. M., and Hamilton, K. F.: Genetic and pathologic analysis of the sex-linked allelic series, mottled, in the mouse (abstract), Genetics **61**:S22, 1969.

202b. Grahn, D., Verley, F. A., Fry, R. J. M., Slaughter, B., Staffeldt, E., and Hamilton, K. F.: Inherited connective tissue defect in tortoise mice, Argonne National Laboratory Biological and Medical Research Division Annual Report, 1966, ANL-7278, pp. 145-146.

203. Gray, H.: Arachnodactyly (spider fingers), Arch. Intern. Med. **75**:215, 1945.

204. Green, H., and Emerson, P. W.: Arachnodactylia, Arch. Pediat. **60**:299, 1943.

205. Greenblatt, R. B., McDonough, P. G., and Mahesh, V. B.: Estrogen therapy in inhibition of growth, J. Clin. Endocr. **26**:1185, 1966.

206. Greenfield, J. G., Cornman, T., and Shy, G. M.: The prognostic value of the muscle biopsy in the "floppy infant," Brain **81**:461, 1958.

207. Grenet, P., Badoual, J., Gallet, J. P., and Alibert, L.: Pneumothorax et maladie de Marfan, Arch. Franc. Pediat. **26**:227, 1969.

208. Grenier, B., Laugier, J., Soutoul, J., and Desbuquois, G.: Maladie de Marfan et arthrogrypose; à propos d'un cas chez un nouveau-né, Sem. Hôp. Paris **45**:702, 1969.

209. Griffin, J. F., and Koman, G. M.: Severe aortic insufficiency in Marfan's syndrome, Ann. Intern. Med. **48**:174, 1958.

210. Griffith, G. J., Hayhurst, A. P., and Whitehead, R.: Dissecting aneurysm of aorta in mother and child, Brit. Heart J. **13**:364, 1951.

211. Grondin, C. M., Steinberg, C. L., and Edwards, J. E.: Dissecting aneurysm complicating Marfan's syndrome (arachnodactyly) in a mother and son, Amer. Heart J. **77**:301, 1969.

212. Gross, J.: An intermolecular defect of collagen in experimental lathyrism, Biochim. Biophys. Acta **71**:250, 1963.

213. Grossman, H., Fleming, R. J., Engle, M. A., Levin, A. H., and Ehlers, K. H.: Angiocardiography in the apical systolic click syndrome; left ventricular abnormality, mitral insufficiency, late systole murmur, and inversion of T waves, Radiology **91**:898, 1968.

214. Grossman, M., Knott, A. P., Jr., and Jacoby, W. J., Jr.: Calcified annulus fibrosus with mitral insufficiency in the Marfan syndrome, Arch. Intern. Med. **121**:561, 1968.

215. Groves, L. K., Effler, D. B., Hawk, W. A., and Gulati, K.: Aortic insufficiency secondary to aneurysmal changes in the ascending aorta: surgical management, J. Thorac. Cardiov. Surg. **48:**362, 1964.

216. Gueron, M., Hirsh, M., Shahin, W., and Levy, M. J.: The surgical treatment of dissecting aortic aneurysm due to idiopathic cystic medial necrosis in a six-year-old child, Dis. Chest **56:**152, 1969.

217. Gupta, S. K., and Sharma, V. N.: Chronic pneumothorax in Marfan's syndrome, Brit. J. Tuberc. **51:**346, 1957.

218. Haber, H.: Miescher's elastoma (elastoma intrapapillare perforans verruciforme), Brit. J. Derm. **71:**85, 1959.

219. Haik, G. M., Kalil, H. H., Ferry, J. F., and Childers, M. D.: Subluxations and luxations of the lens; with a special note on the Barraquer operation and on Marfan's and Marchesani's syndromes, Southern Med. J. **54:**642, 1961.

220. Haldane, J. B. S.: The rate of spontaneous mutation of a human gene, J. Genet. **31:**317, 1935.

221. Halle, M. A., and Collipp, P. J.: Marfan's syndrome associated with diabetes insipidus, New York J. Med. **71:**773, 1971.

222. Halpern, B. L., Char, F., Murdoch, J. L., and Horton, V. A.: A prospectus on the prevention of aortic rupture in the Marfan syndrome with data on survivorship without treatment, Johns Hopkins Med. J. **129:**123, 1971.

223. Hamilton, C. A.: Mechanical hemolytic anemia improved by corticosteroids; patient with mitral insufficiency at the prosthetic valve in a case of Marfan's syndrome, Nebraska Med. J. **54:**161, 1969.

224. Hamman, L., and Apperly, F. L.: Spontaneous rupture of the aorta with aortic insufficiency, Int. Clin. **4:**251, 1933.

225. Hamwi, G. J.: Marfan's syndrome (arachnodactyly), Amer. J. Med. **11:**261, 1951.

226. Handmaker, S. D.: The satellited chromosomes of man with reference to the Marfan syndrome, Amer. J. Hum. Genet. **15:**11, 1963.

227. Hanley, T., Platts, M. M., Clifton, M., and Morris, T. L.: Heart failure of the hunchback, Quart. J. Med. **28:**115, 1958.

228. Hanley, W. B., and Jones, N. B.: Familial dissecting aortic aneurysms; a report of three cases within two generations, Brit. Heart J. **29:**852-858, 1967.

229. Hardin, C. A.: Ruptured abdominal aneurysm occurring in Marfan's syndrome; attempted repair with the use of a nylon prosthesis, New Eng. J. Med. **260:**821, 1959.

230. Hardin, C. A.: Successful resection of carotid and abdominal aneurysm in two retarded patients with Marfan's syndrome, New Eng. J. Med. **267:**141, 1962.

231. Haridas, G.: Arachnodactylia in a Chinese infant, Arch. Dis. Child. **16:**257, 1941.

232. Harrington, P. R. (Houston): Personal communication, 1971.

233. Harris, W. S., Schoenfeld, C. D., Brooks, R. H., and Weissler, A. M.: Effects of beta adrenergic blockade on the hemodynamic responses to epinephrine in man, Amer. J. Cardiol. **17:**484, 1966.

234. Harris, W. S., Schoenfeld, C. D., and Weissler, A. M.: Effects of adrenergic receptor activation and blockade on the systolic preejection period, heart rate, and arterial pressure in man, J. Clin. Invest. **46:**1704, 1967.

235. Harrison, F. F.: Coarctation of the aorta of the adult type, associated with cystic degeneration of the media of the first portion of the arch, Arch. Path. **27:**742, 1939.

236. Harrison, J., and Klainer, M. J.: Arachnodactyly; its occurrence in several members of one family, New Eng. J. Med. **220:**621, 1939.

237. Hartman, C. G., and Straus, W. L.: Relation of pelvic ligaments in pregnant monkeys, Amer. J. Obstet. Gynec. **37:**498, 1939.

238. Harvey, W. P., Corrado, M. A., and Perloff, J. K.: "Right-sided" murmurs of aortic insufficiency, Amer. J. Med. Sci. **245:**533, 1963.

239. Headley, R. N., Carpenter, H. M., and Sawyer, C. G.: Unusual features of Marfan's syndrome, Amer. J. Cardiol. **11:**259, 1963.

240. Heitzman, E. J., and Bryant, R. B.: The Marfan syndrome, gigantism and ruptured abdominal aneurysm, New York J. Med. **64:**436, 1964.

241. Heldrich, F. J., Jr., and Wright, C. E.: Marfan's syndrome; diagnosis in the neonate, Amer. J. Dis. Child. **114:**419, 1967.

242. Henderson, J. W.: Marfan's syndrome: report of a case with congenital aneurysm of the coronary sinus and perforation into the right ventricle, J. Indiana Med. Ass. **54**:325, 1961.

243. Hersh, A. H., DeMarinis, F., and Stecher, R. M.: On the inheritance and development of clinodactyly, Amer. J. Hum. Genet. **5**:257, 1953.

244. Hiejima, K., Tsuchiya, S., Sakamoto, Y., and Shiina, S.: Two cases of Marfan's syndrome associated respectively with subacute bacterial endocarditis and the Wolff-Parkinson-White syndrome, Jap. Heart J. **9**:208, 1968.

245. Hindle, N. W., and Crawford, J. S.: Dislocation of the lens in Marfan's syndrome; its effect and treatment. Canad. J. Ophthal. **4**:128, 1969.

246. Hirst, A. E., Jr., and Bailey, H. L.: Arachnodactyly with associated healing dissecting aneurysm, Calif. Med. **84**:355, 1956.

247. Hirst, A. E., Jr., Johns, V. J., Jr., and Kime, S. W., Jr.: Dissecting aneurysm of the aorta; a review of 505 cases, Medicine **37**:217, 1958.

248. Hofmann, W. P., and Carey, E. T.: Congenital myopic astigmatism in identical twins, Amer. J. Ophthal. **25**:1495, 1942.

248a. Hohn, A. R., and Webb, H. M.: Cardiac studies of infant twins with Marfan's syndrome, Amer. J. Dis. Child. **122**:526, 1971.

249. Hopkins, I. J., Lindsey, J. R., and Ford, F. R.: Nemaline myopathy; a long-term clinico-pathologic study of affected mother and daughter, Brain **89**:299, 1966.

250. Hudson, J. R.: Marfan's syndrome with retinal detachment, Brit. J. Ophthal. **35**:244, 1951,

251. Hufnagel, C. A., and Conrad, P. W.: Dissecting aneurysms of ascending aorta: direct approach repair, Surgery **51**:84, 1962.

252. Hufnagel, C. A., Harvey, W. P. Rabil, P. J., and McDermott, T. E.: Surgical correction of aortic insufficiency, Surgery **35**:673, 1954.

253. Humphries, J. O'N., and McKusick, V. A.: The differentiation of organic and "innocent" systolic murmurs, Progr. Cardiovasc. Dis. **5**:152, 1962.

254. Humphries, J. O'N., and Pusch, A. L.: Effect of the hormone relaxin on the aorta of the guinea pig and rat, Clin. Res. **6**:233, 1958.

255. Hunt, D., and Sloman, G.: Prolapse of the posterior leaflet of the mitral valve occurring in eleven members of a family, Amer. Heart J. **78**:149, 1969.

256. Huntington, R. W., and Hirst, A. E.: Dissecting aneurysm of the aorta in a 16-year-old girl, Amer. J. Clin. Path. **48**:44, 1967.

257. Husebye, K. O., Wolff, H. J., and Friedman, L. L.: Aortic dissection in pregnancy; a case of Marfan's syndrome, Amer. Heart J. **55**:662, 1958.

258. Hustinx, T. W. J., and van Olphen, A. H. F.: An XYY chromosome pattern in a boy with Marfan's syndrome, Genetica **34**:262, 1963.

259. Huston, W. H.: The Marfan syndrome; a report of an atypical case, Henry Ford Hosp. Med. Bull. **5**:90, 1957.

259a. Hyams, S. W., Kar, H., and Neumann, E.: Blue sclerae and keratoglobus; ocular signs of a systemic connective tissue disorder, Brit. J. Ophthal. **53**:53, 1969.

260. I.A.A.: Bernard Jean Antoine Marfan, M.D., Amer. J. Dis. Child. **64**:354, 1942.

261. Irwin, J. W., Hancock, D. M., and Sharp, J. R.: Ruptured abdominal aortic aneurysm in Marfan's syndrome, Brit. Med. J. **1**:1293, 1964.

262. Jain, S. R., and Sepaha, G. C.: Marfan's syndrome; Report of 4 cases, with brief review of literature, Indian J. Med. Sci. **14**:418, 1960.

263. James, T. N.: An etiologic concept concerning the obscure myocardiopathies, Progr. Cardiovasc. Dis. **7**:43, 1964.

264. James, T. N., Frame, B., and Schatz, I. J.: Pathology of cardiac conduction system in Marfan's syndrome, Arch. Intern. Med. **114**:339, 1964.

265. Jamshidi, A., and Klein-Robbenhaar, J.: Myxomatous transformation of the aortic and mitral valve with subaortic "sail-like" membrane, Amer. J. Med. **49**:114, 1970.

266. Jarrett, W. H., II: Dislocation of the lens; a study of 166 hospitalized cases, Arch. Ophthal. **78**:289, 1967.

267. Jasin, H. E., and colleagues: Relationship between urinary hydroxyproline and growth, J. Clin. Invest. **41**:1928, 1962.

267a. Jensen, A. D., and Cross, H. E.: Surgical treatment of dislocated lenses in the Marfan syndrome and homocystinuria, Trans. Amer. Acad. Ophthal. Otolaryng. **76**:1972.

268. Jequier, M.: Observations sur le syndrome de Marfan, Helv. Med. Acta **10**:233, 1943.

269. Jervey, J. W., Jr.: Lens dislocation in Marfan's syndrome; a case report, Amer. J. Ophthal. 57:484, 1964.

270. Jones, C. R., Bergman, M. W., Kittner, P. J., and Pigman, W. W.: Urinary hydroxyproline excretion in Marfan's syndrome as compared with age-matched controls, Proc. Soc. Exp. Biol. Med. 116:931, 1964.

271. Jones, C. R., Bergman, M. W., Kittner, P. J., and Pigman, W. W.: Urinary hydroxyproline excretion in normal children and adolescents, Proc. Soc. Exp. Biol. Med. 115:85, 1964.

272. Jones, C. R., Van Itallie, T. B., Stevenson, S. S., and Pigman, W. W.: Decrease in hydroxyproline excretion in a patient with Marfan's syndrome after methandrostenolone therapy, J.A.M.A. 207:2085, 1969.

273. Jortner, R., Shahin, W., Eshkol, D., and Levy, M. J.: Cardiovascular manifestations and surgery for Marfan's syndrome, Dis. Chest 56:24, 1969.

274. Jortner, R., Shahin, W., Eshkol, D., and Levy, M. J.: Surgery for Marfan's syndrome, Israel J. Med. Sci. 5:871, 1969.

275. Joseph, M. C., and Meadow, S. R.: The metacarpal index of infants, Arch. Dis. Child. 44:515, 1969.

276. Kachele, G. E.: The embryogenesis of ectopia lentis, Arch. Ophthal. 64:135, 1960.

277. Kahrs, T.: Three cases of arachnodactylia, Acta Med. Scand. 121:240, 1945.

278. Källén, B., and Levan, A.: Abnormal length of chromosomes 21 and 22 in four patients with Marfan's syndrome, Cytogenetics 1:5, 1962.

279. Kamen, S.: Oral manifestations of Marfan's syndrome in twins, Oral Surg. 21:19, 1966.

280. Kanick, V., Hemley, S. D., and Kittredge, R. D.: Some problems in the angiographic diagnosis of dissecting ansuryems of the thoracic aorta, Amer. J. Roentgen. 91:1283, 1964.

281. Kaplan, B. M., Schlichter, J. G., Graham, G., and Miller, G.: Idiopathic congenital dilatation of the pulmonary artery, J. Lab. Clin. Med. 41:697, 1953.

282. Katz, H. L.: Thoracic manifestations in Marfan's syndrome, Quart. Bull. Sea View Hosp. 13:95, 1952.

283. Kaufman, G., and Engelbrecht, W. J.: Hemorrhagic intramedial dissection of coronary artery with cystic medial necrosis, Amer. J. Cardiol. 24:409, 1969.

284. Keech, M. K., Wendt, V. E., and Read, R. C.: Family studies of the Marfan syndrome, J. Chronic Dis. 19:57, 1966.

285. Kelemen, G.: Marfan's syndrome and hearing organ, Acta Otolaryng. 59:23, 1965.

286. Kesten, Y.: Diary of a heart patient, New York, 1968, McGraw-Hill Book Co.

287. Killen, D. A., Gobbel, W. G., Jr., and France, R.: Spontaneous aortico–left ventricular fistula associated with myxomatous transformation, Ann. Thorac. Surg. 8:570, 1969.

288. Killip, T., III (New York City): Personal communication.

289. Killip, T., III, and Holmquist, N. D.: Aortic surgery in Marfan's syndrome; hemodynamic and histologic response, Ann. Intern. Med. 54:431, 1961.

290. Kingsley-Pillers, E. M.: Arachnodactyly with amyoplasia congenita, Proc. Roy. Soc. Med. 39:696, 1946.

291. Kirk, J. A., Ansell, B. M., and Bywaters, E. G.: The hypermobility syndrome; musculoskeletal complaints associated with generalized joint hypermobility, Ann. Rheum. Dis. 26:419, 1967.

292. Kiser, J. C., Martin, F. E., and Kiser, R. C.: Mitral insufficiency in Marfan's syndrome—surgical correction (letter), J.A.M.A. 213:1039, 1970.

293. Knight, A. M., Jr.: The Marfan syndrome, J. Med. Ass. Georgia 46:413, 1957.

294. Knight, A. M., Clark, S. W., and Terry, D. B.: Case presentation: Marfan syndrome, dissecting aneurysm, intermittent occlusion of both coronary arteries, J. Med. Ass. Georgia 49:222, 1960.

295. Knott, V. B., and Johnson, R.: Height and shape of the palate in girls: a longitudinal study, Arch. Oral Biol. 15:849, 1970.

296. Kohn, J. L., and Strauss, L.: Marfan's syndrome (arachnodactyly); observation of a patient from birth until death at 18 years, Pediatrics 25:872, 1960.

297. Kountz, W. B., and Hempelmann, L. H.: Chromatrophic degeneration and rupture of the aorta following thyroidectomy in cases of hypertension, Amer. Heart J. 20:599, 1940.

298. Kravitz, D.: Marfan's syndrome, Amer. J. Ophthal. 39:576, 1955.

299. Krupers, F. M., and Schutz, I. J.: Prognosis in dissecting aneurysm, Circulation 27:658, 1963.

300. Kumar, V., and Berenson, G. S.: The Marfan syndrome: report of an interesting case with unusual anatomic findings, J. Louisiana Med. Soc. 118:511, 1966.
301. Kvorak-Theobald, G.: Histologic study of an eye from a child with arachnodactyly, Arch. Ophthal. 24:1046, 1940.
302. Labella, F. S.: Elastin, a metabolically active lipoprotein, Nature 180:1360, 1958.
303. Lacroix, P.: The organization of bone; translated by Stewart Gilder, Philadelphia, 1951, The Blakiston Co.
304. Laitinen, O., Uitto, J., Iivanainen, M., Hannuksela, M., and Kivirikko, K. I.: Collagen metabolism of the skin in Marfan's syndrome, Clin. Chim. Acta 21:321, 1968.
305. Lampen, H.: Das Marfan-Syndrom als kardiologisches Problem, Deutsch. Med. Wschr. 87: 2250, 1962.
306. Langeron, T., Girard, P., Liefooghe, J., and Masson, C.: Maladie de Marfan et anéurysme abdominal, Bull. Soc. Méd. Hôp. Paris 70:374, 1954.
307. Lavoie, R. G., and Boulanger, J.: Le syndrome de Marfan, Laval Méd. 25:453, 1958.
308. Leak, D.: Rib notching in Marfan's syndrome, Amer. Heart J. 71:387, 1966.
309. Leeming, J. T., and McKusick, V. A.: Serum seromucoid levels in the Marfan syndrome, Bull. Hopkins Hosp. 110:38, 1962.
310. Lehmann, O.: A family with Marfan's syndrome traced through an affected newborn, including analysis of the mucoproteins in serum and urinary excretion of amino acids, Acta Paediat. 49:540, 1960.
311. Lemenager, J., Renault, P., Neel, J. P., and Fentry, J. P.: Les accidents respiratories de la maladie de Marfan (A propos d'une observation de pneumothorax par rupture de bulle emphysémateuse), J. Franc. Med. Chir. Thorac. 22:438, 1968.
312. Lenchman, R. D., Francheschi, A. D., and Zamalloa, O.: Late systolic murmur and clicks associated with abnormal mitral valve ring, Amer. J. Cardiol. 23:679, 1969.
313. Lester, C. W.: The surgical treatment of funnel chest, Ann. Surg. 123:1003, 1946.
314. Levine, E., Stein, M., Gordon, G., and Mitchell, N.: Chronic dissecting aneurysm of the aorta resembling chronic rheumatic heart disease, New Eng. J. Med. 244:902, 1951.
315. Liboro, A., Torralba, T. P., Perez, A. P., Basa, G., and St. Ana, D.: The Marfan syndrome, J. Philipp. Med. Ass. 36:513, 1960.
316. Lillian, M.: Multiple pulmonary artery aneurysms; endocarditis of ductus arteriosus and congenital pulmonary cysts, Amer. J. Med. 7:280, 1949.
317. Lindeboom, G. A., and Bouwer, W. F.: Dissecting aneurysm (and renal cortical necrosis) associated with arachnodactyly (Marfan's disease), Cardiologia 15:12, 1949.
318. Lindeboom, G. A., and Westerveld-Brandon, E. R.: Dilatation of the aorta in arachnodactyly, Cardiologia 17:217, 1950.
319. Linker, A., Coulson, W. F., and Carnes, W. H.: Cardiovascular studies on copper-deficient swine. VI. The mucopolysaccharide composition of aorta and cartilage, J. Biol. Chem. 239:1690, 1964.
319a. Lipton, R. A., Greenwald, R. A., and Seriff, N. S.: Pneumothorax and bilateral honey-combed lung in Marfan syndrome. Report of a case and review of the pulmonary abnormalities in this disorder, Amer. Rev. Resp. Dis. 104:924, 1971.
320. Lloyd, R. I.: Arachnodactyly, Arch. Ophthal. 13:744, 1935.
321. Lloyd, R. I.: Clinical course of the ocular complications of Marfan's syndrome, Arch. Ophthal. 40:558, 1948.
322. Lloyd, R. I.: A second group of cases of arachnodactyly, Arch. Ophthal. 17:69, 1937.
323. Loughridge, L. W.: Renal abnormalities in the Marfan syndrome, Quart. J. Med. 28:531, 1959.
324. Loveman, A. B., Gordon, A. M., and Fliegelman, M. T.: Marfan's syndrome; some cutaneous aspects, Arch. Derm. (Chicago) 87:428, 1963.
325. Low, A.: Measurements of infants at birth, Ann. Eugen. 15:210, 1950.
326. Lowe, R. C.: Polycythemia vera (erythremia). Arachnodactyly with congenital defect of vertebral column, and familial muscular dystrophy in Negroes; case reports, Tri-State Med. J. 13:2679, 1941.
327. Lutman, F. C., and Neel, J. V.: Inheritance of arachnodactyly, ectopia lentis and other congenital anomalies (Marfan's syndrome) in the E. family, Arch. Ophthal. 41:276, 1949.
328. Lynas, M. A.: Marfan's syndrome in northern Ireland; an account of thirteen families, Ann. Hum. Genet. 22:289, 1958.

329. Lynas, M. A.: Unpublished observations referred to in reference 535.

330. Lynas, M. A., and Merrett, J. D.: Data on linkage in man; Marfan's syndrome in northern Ireland, Ann. Hum. Genet. **22**:310, 1958.

331. MacCallum, W. G.: Dissecting aneurysm, Bull. Hopkins Hosp. **20**:9, 1909.

332. McCann, J. S., and Porter, D. C.: Calcification of the aorta as an aid to the diagnosis of syphilis, Brit. Med. J. **1**:826, 1956.

333. Macek, M., Hurych, J., Chvapil, M., and Kadlecová, V.: Study of fibroblasts in Marfan's syndrome, Humangenetik **3**:87, 1966.

333a. McFarland, J., Willerson, J. T., Dinsmore, R. E., Austen, W. G., Buckley, M. J., Sanders, C. A., and De Sanctis, R. W.: Medical treatment of dissecting aortic aneurysms, New Eng. J. Med. **286**:115, 1972.

334. McKeown, F.: Dissecting aneurysm of the coronary artery in arachnodactyly, Brit. Heart J. **22**:434, 1960.

335. McKusick, V. A.: The cardiovascular aspects of Marfan's syndrome, Circulation **11**:321, 1955.

336. McKusick, V. A.: Cardiovascular sound in health and disease, Baltimore, 1958, The Williams & Wilkins Co.

337. McKusick, V. A.: Chromosomes in Marfan's disease (letter), Lancet **1**:1194, 1960.

338. McKusick, V. A.: The functional vocabulary of valvular heart disease (editorial), Clin. Res. Proc. **5**:239, 1957.

339. McKusick, V. A.: The genetic aspects of cardiovascular diseases, Ann. Intern. Med. **49**:556, 1958.

340. McKusick, V. A.: Hereditary disorders of connective tissue, Bull. N. Y. Acad. Med. **35**:143, 1959.

341. McKusick, V. A.: Mendelian inheritance in man; catalogs of autosomal dominant, autosomal recessive, and X-linked phenotypes, ed. 3, Baltimore, 1971, The Johns Hopkins Press.

341a. McKusick, V. A : Primordial dwarfism and ectopia lentis, Amer. J. Hum. Genet. **7**:187, 1955.

342. McKusick, V. A.: Unpublished observations.

342a. McKusick, V. A.: Association of congenital bicuspid aortic valve and Erdheim's cystic medial necrosis (letter), Lancet **1**:1026, 1972.

343. McKusick, V. A., Hahn, D. P., Bradshaw, J. R., and Humphries, J. O'N.: Some hemodynamic effects of the Hufnagel operation for aortic regurgitation; studies in models and a patient, Bull. Hopkins Hosp. **95**:322, 1954.

344. McKusick, V. A., Logue, R. B., and Bahnson, H. T.: Association of aortic valvular disease and cystic medial necrosis of the ascending aorta, Circulation **46**:188, 1957.

345. McKusick, V. A., Murray, G. E., Peeler, R. G., and Webb, G. N.: Musical murmurs, Bull. Hopkins Hosp. **97**:136, 1955.

346. MacLeod, M., and Williams, W. A.: The cardiovascular lesions in Marfan's syndrome, Arch. Path. **61**:143, 1956.

347. McSherry, B. J., Ferguson, A. E., and Ballantyne, J.: Dissecting aneurysm in turkeys, J. Amer. Vet. Med. Ass. **124**:279, 1954.

348. Maier, C., Rubli, J. M., Schaub, F., and Hedinger, C.: Kardiale Störungen beim Marfanschen Syndrom, Cardiologia **24**:106, 1954.

349. Mamou, H., and Hérault, P.: Maladie de Marfan et maladie de Scheuermann, Sem. Hôp. Paris **27**:3071, 1951.

350. Mandel, W., Evans, E. W., and Walford, R. L.: Dissecting aortic aneurysm during pregnancy, New Eng. J. Med. **251**:1059, 1954.

351. Marfan, A. B.: Un cas de déformation congénitale des quatre membres plus prononcée aux extrémités charactérisée par l'allongement des os avec un certain degré d'amincissement, Bull. Mém. Soc. Méd. Hôp. Paris **13**:220, 1896.

352. Marfan, A. B.: Sur la ponction du péricarde et en particulier sur la ponction par voie épigastrique sous-xiphoidienne, Arch. Mal. Coeur **29**:153, 1936.

353. Marks, J., and Gerson, K. L.: Importance of autopsies—an illustrative case, J.A.M.A. **168**:1450, 1958.

354. Marquis, Y., Richardson, J. B., Ritchie, A. C., and Wigle, E. D.: Idiopathic medial aortopathy and arteriopathy, Amer. J. Med. **44**:939, 1968.

355. Martin, R.: Lehrbuch der Anthropologie, Jena, 1928, Gustav Fischer.

356. Martin, V. A. F., and Cowan, E. C.: Bilateral secondary glaucoma and systemic hypertension in Marfan's syndrome, Brit. J. Ophthal. **44**:123, 1960.

357. Marvel, R. J., and Genovese, P. D.: Cardiovascular disease in Marfan's syndrome, Amer. Heart J. **42**:814, 1951.

358. Massumi, R. A., Lowe, E. W., and Misanik, L. F.: Multiple aortic ansurysms (thoracic and abdominal) in twins with Marfan's syndrome; fatal rupture during pregnancy, J. Thorac. Cardiovasc. Surg. **53**:223, 1967.

359. Master, A. M., and Stone, J.: The heart in funnel-shaped and flat chests, Amer. J. Med. Sci. **217**:392, 1949.

360. Matalon, R., and Dorfman, A.: The accumulation of hyaluronic acid in cultured fibroblasts of the Marfan syndrome, Biochem. Biophys. Res. Commun. **32**:150, 1968.

361. Matalon, R., and Dorfman, A.: Acid mucopolysaccharides in cultured human fibroblasts, Lancet **2**:838, 1969.

362. Matsui, E., and Ito, T.: Marfan's syndrome complicated by huge hydropericardium, Jap. Heart J. **8**:98, 1967.

362a. Maumenee, A. E., and Ryan, S. J.: Aspiration technique in the management of the dislocated lens, Amer. J. Ophthal. **68:808, 1969.**

363. Maxwell, G. M.: Chest deformity in children with congenital heart disease, Amer. Heart J. **54**:368, 1957.

364. Meara, R. A.: Ehlers-Danlos syndrome and ?elastoma verruciforme perforans (Miescher), Trans. St. Johns Hosp. Derm. Soc. (London) **40**:72, 1958.

365. Medawar, P. B.: The future of man, New York, 1960, Basic Books, Inc., p. 72.

366. Mehregan, A. H.: Elastosis perforans serpiginosa—a review of the literature and report of 11 cases, Arch. Derm. **97**:381, 1968.

367. Meilman, E., Urivetsky, M. M., and Rapoport, C. M.: Urinary hydroxyproline peptides, J. Clin. Invest. **42**:40, 1963.

368. Merendino, K. A., Winterscheid, L. C., and Dillard, D. H.: Cystic medial necrosis with and without Marfan's syndrome; surgical experience with 20 patients and a note about the modified bicuspidization operation, Surg. Clin. N. Amer. **47**:1403, 1967.

368a. Merrill, M., and Shulman, L. E.: Determination of prognosis in chronic disease illustrated by systemic lupus erythematosus, J. Chronic. Dis. **1**:12, 1955.

369. Méry, H., and Babonneix, L.: Un cas de déformation congénitale des quatre membres: hyperchondroplasie, Bull. Mém. Soc. Méd. Hôp. Paris **19**:671, 1902.

370. Meyer, K. (New York City): Personal communication.

371. Michaud, P., Gonin, A., Termet, H., Goudard, J., Gaillard, P., Chassignolle, J., Gravier, J., and Vignat, J.: Maladie de Marfan; remplacement prothétique simultané de l'aorte ascendante et des valvules aortiques pour fissuration d'anévrysme et insuffisance aortique majeure, Lyon Chir. **63**:161, 1967.

372. Mielke, J. E., Becker, K. L., and Gross, J. B.: Diverticulitis of the colon in a young man with Marfan's syndrome associated with carcinoma of the thyroid gland and neurofibromas of the tongue and lips, Gastroenterology **48**:379, 1965.

373. Millant, R.: Les eunques à travers les ages, Paris, 1908, Vigot Frères.

374. Miller, D. R., and Pugh, D. M.: Repair of ascending aortic aneurysm and aortic regurgitation complicated by acute cardiac compression by pectus excavatum in Marfan's syndrome, J. Thorac. Cardiovasc. Surg. **59**:673, 1970.

375. Miller, R., Jr., and Pearson, R. J., Jr.: Mitral insufficiency simulating aortic stenosis; report of an unusual manifestation of Marfan's syndrome, New Eng. J. Med. **260**:1210, 1959.

376. Mitchell, G. E., Lourie, H., and Berne, A. S.: The various causes of scalloped vertebrae with notes on their pathogenesis, Radiology **89**:67, 1967.

377. Moe, J. H., and Gustilo, R. B.: Treatment of scoliosis; results in 196 patients treated by cast correction and fusion, J. Bone Joint Surg. **46-A**:293, 1964.

378. Monz, W.: The Marfan syndrome; clinical and necropsy findings in the A. family, Med. J. Aust. **1**:571, 1965.

379. Moore, H. C.: Marfan syndrome, dissecting aneurysm of the aorta, and pregnancy, J. Clin. Path. **18**:277, 1965.

380. Moretti, G., LeCoulant, P., Staeffen, J., Catanzano, G., and Broustet, A.: La peau dans le syndrome de Marfan, Presse Méd. **72**:2985, 1964.

381. Moretti, G. F., Staeffen, J., Bertrand, E., and Broustet, A.: Bloc auriculo-ventriculaire complet dans le syndrome de Marfan, Presse Med. 72:605, 1964.

382. Moses, M. F.: Aortic aneurysm associated with arachnodactyly, Brit. Med. J. 2:81, 1951.

383. Moss, H. L.: Contact lenses for a rare case of Marfan's syndrome, Amer. J. Optom. 43: 531, 1966.

384. Mouquin, M., and colleagues: Les dissections aortiques du syndrome du Marfan, Arch. Mal. Coeur 54:141, 1961.

385. Muinos, A., and Sellyei, L.: Juvenile retinal detachment at the Barraquer clinic, Mod. Prob. Ophthal. 8:284, 1969.

386. Muller, W. H., Damman, J. F., and Warren, W. D.: Surgical correction of the cardiovascular deformities in Marfan's syndrome, Ann. Surg. 152:506, 1960.

387. Murdoch, J. L., Walker, B. A., Hall, J. G., Abbey, H., Smith, K. K., and McKusick, V. A.: Achondroplasia—a genetic and statistical survey, Ann. Hum. Genet. 33:227, 1970.

387a. Murdoch, J. L., Walker, B. A., Halpern, B. L., Kuzma, J. W., and McKusick, V. A.: Life expectancy and causes of death in the Marfan syndrome, New Eng. J. Med. 286:804, 1972.

388. Murdoch, J. L., Walker B. A., and McKusick, V. A.: Parental age effects on the occurrence of new mutations for the Marfan syndrome, Ann. Hum. Genet. 35:331, 1972.

389. Murphy, D. P.: Familial finger contracture and associated familial knee-joint subluxation, J.A.M.A. 86:395, 1926.

390. Nally, F. F.: The Marfan syndrome; report of two cases, Oral Surg. 22:715, 1966.

391. Neilson, G. H., and Sullivan, J. J.: Dissecting aneurysm of the aorta associated with Marfan's syndrome, Med. J. Aust. 1:925, 1956.

392. Neimann, N., Rauber, G., Marchal, C., Vidailhet, M., and Fall, M.: Maladie de Marfan chez un nouveau-né avec atteintes polyviscérales, Ann. Pediat. 15:619, 1968.

393. Nelson, J. D.: The Marfan syndrome, with special reference to congenital enlargement of the spinal canal, Brit. J. Radiol. 31:561, 1958.

394. Nelson, R. M., and Vaughn, C. C.: Double valve replacement in Marfan's syndrome, J. Thorac. Cardiov. Surg. 57:732, 1969.

395. Nemoto, H., and Yanai, N.: Marfan's syndrome, a family report, Jap. J. Hum. Genet. 5:199, 1961.

396. Nenci, I., and Beltrami, C. A.: Marfan's syndrome, a hereditary enzymopenia (letter), Lancet 2:1302, 1968.

397. Nevin, N. C., Hurwitz, L. J., and Neill, D. W.: Familial camptodactyly with taurinuria, J. Med. Genet. 3:265, 1966.

398. Newton, W. T.: Radical enterectomy for hereditary megaduodenum, Arch. Surg. 96:549, 1968.

399. Nickel, J. R., and McKusick, V. A.: Nemaline myopathy; second autopsied case in a previously reported family. In Bergsma, D., editor: Clinical delineation of birth defects. VII. Muscle. Baltimore, 1971, The Williams & Wilkins Co.

400. Nodes, J. D. S., and Henes, F.: Total rupture of an aneurysm of the splenic artery immediately after labor, Trans. Obstet. Soc. London 42:305, 1900.

401. Norcross, J. R.: Arachnodactylia—a report of three cases, J. Bone Joint Surg. 20:757, 1938.

402. Norum, R. A., James, V. L., and Mabry, C. C.: Pterygium syndrome in three children in a recessive pedigree pattern. In Bergsma, D., editor: The clinical delineation of birth defects. II. Malformation syndromes, New York, 1969, National Foundation.

403. Novell, H. A., Asher, L. A., Jr., and Lev. M.: Marfan's syndrome associated with pregnancy, Amer. J. Obstet. Gynec. 75:802, 1958.

404. O'Doherty, N. J.: Neonatal Marfan's syndrome, with malformation of the urinary tract, Proc. Roy. Soc. Med. 59:483, 1966.

405. Olcott, C. T.: Arachnodactyly (Marfan's syndrome) with severe anemia, Amer. J. Dis. Child. 60:660, 1940.

406. Ollier, L. X. E. L.: Traité expérimental et clinique de la régénération des os et production artificielle du tissu osseux, Paris, 1867, Masson & Cie.

407. Oram, S., and East, T.: Rupture of aneurysm of aortic sinus (of Valsalva) into the right side of the heart, Brit. Heart J. 17:541, 1955.

408. Ormond, A. W.: The etiology of arachnodactyly, Guy Hosp. Rep. 80:68, 1930.

409. Oswald, N., and Parkinson, T.: Honeycomb lungs, Quart. J. Med. 18:1, 1949.

410. Pahwa, J. M., and Gupta, D. P.: Marfan's syndrome, Brit. J. Ophthal. 46:105, 1962.

411. Palmer, R. F., and Wheat, M. W., Jr.: Treatment of dissecting aneurysms of the aorta, Ann. Thorac. Surg. **4**:38, 1967.

412. Papaioannou, A. C., Agustsson, M. H., and Gasul, B. M.: Early manifestations of the cardiovascular disorders in the Marfan syndrome, Pediatrics **27**:255, 1961.

413. Pappas, E. G., Mason, D., and Denton, C.: Marfan's syndrome: a report of three patients with aneurysms of the aorta, Amer. J. Med. **23**:426, 1957.

414. Parish, J. G.: Heritable disorders of connective tissue, Proc. Roy. Soc. Med. **53**:515, 1960.

415. Parish, J. G.: Skeletal hand charts in inherited connective tissue disease, J. Med. Genet. **4**:227, 1967.

416. Parish, J. G., Horn, D. B., and Thompson, M.: Familial streblodactyly with aminoaciduria, Brit. Med. J. **2**:1247, 1963.

417. Parker, A. S., Jr., and Hare, H. F.: Arachnodactyly, Radiology **45**:220, 1945.

418. Pasachoff, H. D., Madonick, M. J., and Drayer, C.: Arachnodactyly in four siblings with pneumoencephalographic observations of two, Amer. J. Dis. Child. **67**:201, 1944.

419. Pearson, C. M., Kroening, R., Verity, M. A., and Getzen, J. H.: Aortic insufficiency and aortic aneurysm in relapsing polychondritis, Trans. Ass. Amer. Physicians **80**:71, 1967.

420. Peiper, A.: Ueber die Erblichkeit der Trichterbrust, Klin. Wschr. **1**:1647, 1922.

421. Perl, E., and Catchpole, H. R.: Changes induced in the connective tissue of the pubic symphysis of the guinea pig with estrogen and relaxin, Arch. Path. **50**:233, 1950.

422. Perrin, A., Gravier, J., Verney, R. N., et al: L'insuffisance mitrale au cours du syndrome de Marfan, Actualités Cardiol. Angeiol. Int. **15**:229, 1966. Cited by Caulfield, J. B., Page, D. L., Kastor, J. A., and Sanders, C. A.: Connective tissue abnormalities in spontaneous rupture of chordae tendineae, Arch. Path. **91**:537, 1971.

423. Pierce, R. E.: Traumatic dissecting aneurysms of the thoracic aorta, U. S. Armed Forces Med. J. **5**:1588, 1954.

424. Pinkus, H., Keech, M. K., and Mehregan, A. H.: Histopathology of striae distensae, with special reference to striae and wound healing in the Marfan syndrome, J. Invest. Derm. **46**:283, 1966.

425. Pino, R. H., Cooper, E. L., and Van Wien, S.: Arachnodactyly and status dysraphicus; a review, Ann. Intern. Med. **10**:1130, 1937.

426. Piper, R. K., and Irvine-Jones, E.: Arachnodactylia and its association with congenital heart disease; report of a case and review of the literature, Amer. J. Dis. Child. **31**:832, 1926.

427. Pirie, A.: The vitreous body. In Davson, H., editor: The eye, New York, 1962, Academic Press, Inc.

428. Pommerenke, W. T.: Experimental ligamentous relaxation in guinea pig pelvis, Amer. J. Obstet. Gynec. **27**:708, 1934.

429. Ponseti, I. V., and Baird, W. A.: Scoliosis and dissecting aneurysm of the aorta in rats fed with lathyrus odoratus seeds, Amer. J. Path. **28**:1059, 1952.

430. Ponseti, I. V., and Shepard, R. S.: Lesions of the skeleton and of other mesodermal tissues in rats fed sweet-pea (Lathyrus odoratus) seeds, J. Bone Joint Surg. **36-A**:1031, 1954.

431. Poynton, F. J., and Maurice, W. B.: Arachnodactyly with organic heart disease, Trans. Clin. Soc. London **75**:21, 1923.

432. Prockop, D. J., and Sjoerdsma, A.: Significance of urinary hydroxyproline in man, J. Clin. Invest. **40**:843, 1961.

433. Prokop, E. K., Palmer, R. F., and Wheat, M. W., Jr.: Hydrodynamic forces on dissecting aneurysms (abstract), Circulation **38** (supp. 6):158, 1968.

433a. Prokop, E. K., Palmer, R. F., and Wheat, M. W., Jr.: Hydrodynamic forces on dissecting aneurysms; in vitro studies in a Tygon model and in dog aortas, Circ. Res. **27**:121, 1970.

434. Pruzanski, W.: Congenital malformations in myotonic dystrophy, Acta Neurol. Scand. **41**:34, 1965.

435. Pygott, F.: Arachnodactyly (Marfan's syndrome) with a report of two cases, Brit. J. Radiol. **28**:26, 1955.

436. Rados, A.: Marfan's syndrome, Arch. Ophthal. **27**:477, 1942.

437. Raghib, G., Jeu, K. L., Anderson, R. C., and Edwards, J. E.: Marfan's syndrome with mitral insufficiency, Amer. J. Cardiol. **16**:127, 1965.

438. Rambar, A. C., and Denenholz, E. J.: Arachnodactyly, J. Pediat. **15**:844, 1939.

439. Ravitch, M.: Pectus excavatum and heart failure, Surgery 30:178, 1951.

440. Rawlings, M. S.: The "straight back" syndrome, a cause of pseudo heart disease, Amer. J. Cardiol. 5:333, 1960.

441. Rawlings, M. S., and Travel, M. E.: Straight back syndrome? (letter), Ann. Intern Med. 74:300, 1971.

442. Read, R. C., and Thal, A. P.: Surgical experience with symtomatic myxomatous valvular transformation (the floppy valve syndrome), Surgery 59:173, 1966.

443. Read, R. C., Thal, A. P., and Wendt, V. E: Symptomatic valvula myxomatous transformation (the floppy valve syndrome): a possible *forme fruste* of Marfan's disease, Circulation 32:897, 1965.

444. Read, R. C., White, H. J., and Palacios, E.: Floppy valve syndrome; a possible expression of pituitary and mucopolysaccharide dysfunction, Surg. Clin. N. Amer. 47:1427, 1967.

445. Redman, R. S., Shapiro, B. L., and Gorlin, R. J.: Measurement of normal and reportedly malformed palatal vaults. II. Normal juvenile measurements, J. Dent. Res. 45:266, 1966.

446. Reeh, M. J., and Lehman, W. L.: Marfan's syndrome (arachnodactyly) with ectopia lentis, Trans. Amer. Acad. Ophthal. 58:212, 1954.

447. Reeve, R., Silver, H. K., and Ferrier, P: Marfan's syndrome (arachnodactyly) with arthrogryposis (amyoplasia congenita), Amer. J. Dis. Child. 99:101, 1960.

448. Reeves, J. E., and Irwin, H. R.: Marfan's syndrome; report of a probable case, Calif. Med. 86:183, 1957.

449. Reis, R. A., Baer, J. L., Arens, R. A., and Stewart, E.: Traumatic separation of symphysis pubis during spontaneous labor with clinical and x-ray study of normal symphysis pubis during pregnancy and puerperium, Surg. Gynec. Obstet. 55:336, 1932.

450. Resnik, W. H., and Keefer, C. S.: Dissecting aneurysm with signs of aortic insufficiency, J.A.M.A. 85:422, 1925.

451. Reynolds, G.: The heart in arachnodactyly, Guy Hosp. Rep. 99:178, 1950.

452. Reynolds, S. R. M., Light, F. W., Sr., Ardran, G. M., and Prichard, M. M. L.: Qualitative nature of pulsatile flow in umbilical blood vessels with observations on flow in the aorta, Bull Hopkins Hosp. 91:83, 1952.

453. Rich, A. R., and Oppenheimer, E. (Baltimore): Personal communication.

454. Rimoin, D. L., Merimee, T. J., and McKusick, V. A.: Growth-hormone deficiency in man: an isloated, recessively inherited defect, Science 152:1635, 1966.

455. Ringer, R. K.: Aortic rupture, plasma cholesterol, and arteriosclerosis following serpasil administration to turkeys, Second Conference on Use of Reserpine in Poultry Production, University of Minneapolis, May 6, 1960. Summit, N. J., Ciba, pp. 32-39.

456. Ringer, R. K.: Influence of reserpine on early growth, blood pressure, and dissecting aneurysms in turkeys. Conference on the Use of Serpasil in Animal and Poultry Production Rutgers University, May 7, 1959. Summit, N. J., Ciba, pp. 21-28.

457. Riquelme, A., and Green, L. J.: Palatal width, height, and length in human twins, Amer. J. Orthodont. 40:71, 1970.

458. Risser, J. C.: Clinical evaluation of scoliosis, J.A.M.A. 164:134, 1957.

459. Rivlin, M. E.: Marfan's syndrome and pregnancy, J. Obstet. Gynaec. Brit. Comm. 74:143, 1967.

460. Rizzuti, A. B.: Complications in the surgical management of the displaced lens, Int. Ophthal. Clin. 5:3, 1965.

461. Roark, J. W.: Marfan's syndrome; report of one case with autopsy, special histological study and review of the literature, Arch. Intern. Med. 103:123, 1959.

462. Roberts, W. C., and Morrow, A. G.: Late postoperative pathological findings after cardiac valve replacement, Circulation 35 (supp. 1):48, 1967.

463. Robins, S.: Cyesis and Marfan's syndrome, Virginia Med. Monthly 93:140, 1966.

463a. Roederer, C.: Syndrome d'Ehlers-Danlos, atypique, coincidant avec une dolichosténomélie, Arch. Franç. Pediat. 8:193, 1951.

463b. Ross, D. N., Frazier, T. G., and Gonzalez-Lavin, L.: Surgery of Marfan's syndrome and related conditions of the aortic root (annulo-aortic ectasia), Thorax 27:52, 1972.

464. Ross, J. K., and Gerbode, F.: The Marfan syndrome associated with an unusual interventricular septal defect, J. Thorac. Surg. 39:746, 1960.

465. Ross, L. J.: Archnodactyly: review of recent literature and report of case with cleft palate, Amer. J. Dis. Child. 78:417, 1949.

466. Rottino. A.: Medical degeneration in a non-ruptured aorta appearing syphilitic macroscopically, Arch. Path. **27**:320, 1939.

467. Rubin, E. H.: Diseases of the chest, Philadelphia, 1947, W. B. Saunders Co.

468. Rubin, P.: Dynamic classification of bone dysplasias, Chicago, 1964, Year Book Medical Publishers.

469. Russell, F.: An inquiry into the health of Mr. Lincoln, Delaware Med. J. **36**:103, 1964.

470. Rutherford, W. J.: Hereditary scoliosis, Brit. Med. J. **2**:87, 1934.

471. Ryback, R.: Inhibited maturation of collagen in lathyrism as a model for the Marfan syndrome and its implications, Gerontologia **11**:120, 1965.

472. Rywlin, A.: Medionecrosis idiopathica cystica unter Bilde des diffusen Aortenaneurysmas. Beziehungen zur Marfanschen Syndrom, Frankfurt Z. Path. **63**:187, 1952.

473. Sahadevan, M. G., Raman, P. T., and Hoon, R. S.: Chronic atrial flutter in a case of Marfan's syndrome, Amer. J. Med. **47**:965, 1969.

474. Sainsbury, H. S. K.: Congenital funnel chest, Lancet **2**:615, 1947.

475. Salle, V.: Ueber einen Fall von angeborener abnormen Grosse der Extremitaten mit einen an Akronemegalia erinnerden Symptomenkomplex, Jahrb. Kinderheilk. **75**:540, 1912.

476. Sanders, C. A., Austin, W. G., Harthorne, J. W., Dinsmore, R. E., and Scannell, J. G.: Diagnosis and surgical treatment of mitral regurgitation secondary to ruptured chordae tendineae, New Eng. J. Med. **276**:943, 1967.

477. Sando, D. E., and Helm, S.: Acquired coarctation in new channel of healed dissecting aneurysm, Ann. Intern. Med. **37**:793, 1952.

477a. Sartwell, P. E.: The time factor in studies of the outcome of chronic disease (editorial), Amer. Rev. Tuberc. **63**:608, 1951.

477b. Sartwell, P. E., Baltimore, personal communication, May 25, 1972.

478. Sautter, H.: Aplasie des Dilatator pupillae beim Marfanschen Symptomenkomplex, Klin. Mbl. Augenheilk. **114**:449, 1949.

479. Scarpelli, D. G., and Goodman, R. M.: Observations on the fine structure of the fibroblast from a case of Ehlers-Danlos syndrome with the Marfan syndrome, J. Invest. Derm. **50**:214, 1968.

480. Schatz, I. J., Yaworsky, R. G., and Fine, G.: Myocardial infarction and unusual myocardial degeneration in Marfan's syndrome, with dissection of the right coronary artery and aorta, Amer. J. Cardiol. **12**:553. 1963.

481. Schilling, E. D., and Strong, F. M.: Isolation, structure and synthesis of a lathyrus factor from L. odoratus, J. Amer. Chem. Soc. **76**:2848, 1954.

482. Schilling, V.: Striae distensae als hypophysäres Symptom bei basophilem Vorderlappenadenom (Cushingschem Syndrom) und bei Arachnodaktylie (Marfanschem Symptomenkomplex) mit Hypophysentumor, Med. Welt. **10**:183, 1936.

483. Schimke, R. N., Hartmann, W. H., Prout, T. E., and Rimoin, D. L.: Syndrome of bilateral pheochromocytoma, medullary thyroid carcinoma, and multiple neuromas, New Eng. J. Med. **279**:1, 1968.

484. Schneider, H. J., and Spitz, H. B.: Unruptured aortic sinus aneurysm, plain film diagnosis, Dis. Chest **53**:340, 1968.

485. Schneider, W. F.: Arachnodactyly; unusual complication following skull injury, J. Pediat. **27**:583, 1945.

486. Schnitker, M. A., and Bayer, C. A.: Dissecting aneurysm of the aorta in young individuals, particularly in association with pregnancy, with report of case, Ann. Intern. Med. **20**:486, 1944.

487. Schorr, S., Braun, K., and Wildman, J.: Congenital aneurysmal dilatation of the ascending aorta associated with arachnodactylia; angiocardiographic study, Amer. Heart J. **42**:610, 1951.

488. Schwartz, H.: Abraham Lincoln and the Marfan syndrome, J.A.M.A. **187**:473, 1964.

488a. Schwartz, H.: Abraham Lincoln and aortic insufficiency. The declining health of the president, Calif. Med. **116**:82, 1972.

489. Segal, B., Kasparian, H., and Likoff, W.: Mitral regurgitation in a patient with the Marfan syndrome, Dis. Chest **41**:457, 1962.

490. Segal, B. L., and Likoff, W.: Late systolic murmur of mitral regurgitation, Amer. Heart J. **67**:757, 1964.

491. Segal, B. L., Tabesh, E., Imbriglia, J. E., and Likoff, W.: The Marfan syndrome; necropsy

findings in three patients, with a review of the cardiovascular complications, Angiology **13**:444, 1962.

492. Segrest, J. P., and Cunningham, L. W.: Variations in human urinary O-hydroxylysyl glycoside levels and their relationship to collagen metabolism, J. Clin. Invest. **49**:1497, 1970.

493. Selzer, A., Kelly, J. J., Jr., Vannitamby, M., Walker, P., Gerbode, F., and Kerth, W. J.: The syndrome of mitral insufficiency due to isolated rupture of the chordae tendineae, Amer. J. Med. **43**:822, 1967.

494. Shahin, W., Eskhol, D., and Levy, M. J.: Valve replacement for mitral insufficiency in an infant with Marfan's syndrome, J. Pediat. Surg. **4**:350, 1969.

495. Shankar, K. R., Hultgren, M. K., and Lauer, R. M.: Lethal tricuspid and mitral regurgitation in Marfan's syndrome, Amer. J. Cardiol. **20**:122, 1967.

496. Shapiro, B. L., Redman, R. S., and Gorlin, R. J.: Measurements of normal and reportedly malformed palatal vaults. I. Normal adult measurements, J. Dent. Res. **42**:1039, 1963.

497. Sheehan, H. L.: The pathology of obstetric shock, J. Obstet. Gynaec. Brit. Comm. **16**:218, 1939.

498. Sheehan, H. L., and Falkiner, N. M.: Splenic aneurysm and splenic enlargement in pregnancy, Brit. Med. J. **2**:1105, 1948.

499. Sheldon, W. H., Atlas of men; a guide for somatotyping the adult male at all ages, New York, 1954, Gramercy Publishing Co., p. 338.

500. Shell, W. E., Walton, J. A., Clifford, M. E., and Willis, P. W., III: The familial occurrence of the syndrome of mid-late systolic click and late systolic murmur, Circulation **39**:327, 1969.

501. Shennan, T.: Dissecting aneurysms, London, 1934, His Majesty's Stationery Office.

502. Shibota, Y., Suto, K., Hiragami, H., Marfan's syndrome accompanied by renovascular hypertension, Tohoku J. Exp. Med. **98**:13, 1969.

503. Shields, G. S., Coulson, W. F., Kimball, D. A. Carnes, W. H., Cartwright, G. E., and Wintrobe, M. M.: Studies on copper metabolism XXXII. Cardiovascular lesions in copper-deficient swine, Amer J. Path. **41**:603, 1962.

504. Siegenthaler, W.: Die kardio-vaskulären Veränderungen beim Marfan-Syndrom (Arachnodatylie), Cardiologia **28**:135, 1956.

505. Simon, A. L., Hipona, F. A., and Stansel, H. C.: Dissecting aortic aneurysm in Marfan's syndrome, J.A.M.A. **193**:156, 1965.

506. Simpson, C. F, Pritchard, W R., Harms, R. H., and Sautter, J. H.: Skeletal and cardiovascular lesions in turkeys induced by feeding beta-aminopropionitrile, Exp. Molec. Path. **1**:305, 1962.

507. Simpson, J. W., Nora, J. J., and McNamara, D. G.: Marfan's syndrome and mitral valve disease—acute surgical emergencies, Amer. Heart J. **77**:96, 1969.

508. Sinclair, R. J. G.: The Marfan syndrome, Bull. Rheum. Dis. **8**:153, 1958.

509. Sinclair, R. J. G., Kitchin, A. H., and Turner, R W D: The Marfan syndrome, Quart J. Med. **29**:19, 1960.

510. Sinha, K. P., and Goldberg, H.: Marfan's syndrome; a case with complete dissection of the aorta, Amer. Heart J. **36**:890, 1958.

511. Sirak, H. D., and Ressallat, M. M.: Surgical correction of mitral insufficiency in Marfan's syndrome; late follow-up results in two cases, J. Thorac. Cardiovasc. Surg. **55**:493, 1968.

512. Sjoerdsma, A. (Bethesda): Personal communication.

513. Sjoerdsma, A., Davidson, J. D., Udenfriend, S., and Mitoma, C.: Increased excretion of hydroxyproline in Marfan's syndrome, Lancet **2**:994, 1958.

514. Skyring, A.: Personal communication.

515. Slack, H. G. B.: Metabolism of elastin in the adult rat, Nature **174**:512, 1955.

516. Sloper, J. C., and Storey, G.: Aneurysms of the ascending aorta due to medial degeneration associated with arachnodactyly (Marfan's disease), J. Clin. Path. **6**:299, 1953.

517. Smiley, J. D., and Ziff, M.: Urinary hydroxyproline excretion and growth, Physiol. Rev. **44**:30, 1964.

518. Smith, N. H.: Multiple dentigerous cysts associated with arachnodactyly and other skeletal defects; report of a case, Oral Surg. **25**:99, 1968.

519. Snyder, L. H., and Curtis, G. M.: An inherited "hollow chest," koilosternia, a new character dependent upon a dominant autosomal gene, J. Hered. **25**:445, 1934.

520. Sosman, M. C.: Xanthomatosis, J.A.M.A. **98**:110, 1932.

521. Soulié, P., and colleagues: Les manifestations cardiovasculaires de la maladie de Marfan (à propos de 8 observations personnelles). Arch. Mal. Coeur **54**:121, 1961.

522. Spencer, F. C., and Blake, H.: A report of the successful surgical treatment of aortic regurgitation from a dissecting aortic aneurysm in a patient with the Marfan syndrome, J. Thorac. Cardiovasc. Surg. **44**:238, 1962.

523. Spenser, J. T.: Post-mortem caesarian delivery after rupture of dissecting aortic aneurysm, Lancet **2**:565, 1952.

524. Spickard, W. B.: Arachnodactyly, description of the clinical characteristics with report of autopsied case, Stanford Med. Bull. **6**:422, 1948.

525. Starke, H.: Zur Pathogenese des Marfan-Syndroms, Von Gräfe's Arch. Ophthal. **151**:384, 1951.

525a. Stin, R., Lazar, M., and Adam, A.: Brittle cornea; a familial trait associated with blue sclera, Amer. J. Ophthal. **66**:67, 1968.

526. Stinberg, I.: Aneurysm of the aortic sinuses with pseudo-coarctation of the aorta, Brit. Heart J. **18**:85, 1956.

527. Steinberg, I.: Dilatation of the aortic sinuses in the Marfan syndrome, Amer. J. Roentgen. **83**:320, 1960.

528. Steinberg, I.: A simple screening test for the Marfan syndrome, Amer. J. Roentgen. **97**: 118, 1966.

529. Steinberg, I., and Finby, N.: Clinical manifestations of the unperforated aortic sinus aneurysm, Circulation **14**:115, 1956.

530. Steinberg, I., and Geller, W.: Aneurysmal dilatation of aortic sinuses in arachnodactyly: diagnosis during life in three cases, Ann. Intern. Med. **43**:120, 1955.

531. Steinberg, I., Mangiardi, J. L., and Noble, W. J.: Aneurysmal dilatation of the aortic sinuses in Marfan's syndrome; angiocardiographic and cardiac catheterization studies in idential twins, Circulation **16**:368, 1957.

532. Stephens, F. E.: Inheritance of diseases primary in the muscles, Amer. J. Med. **15**:558, 1953.

533. Stephenson, W. V.: Anterior megalophthalmos and arachnodactyly, Amer. J. Ophthal. **28**: 315, 1954.

534. Stettner, E.: Wachstum und Wachstumsstorungen, Mschr. Kinderheilk. **80**:387, 1937.

535. Stevenson, A. C.: Comparisons of mutation rates at single loci in man. In Effects of radiation on human heredity, Geneva, 1957, World Health Organization, p. 125.

536. Stevenson, A. C.: Personal communication.

537. Stewart, R. M.: A case of arachnodactyly, Arch. Dis. Child. **14**:64, 1939.

538. Stoddard, S. E.: The inheritance of "hollow chest", Cobbler's chest due to heredity—not an occupational deformity, J. Hered. **30**:139, 1939.

539. Stolz, H. R., and Stolz, L. M.: Somatic development of adolescent boys; a study of the growth of boys during the second decade of life, New York, 1951, The Macmillan Co.

540. Stonesifer, G. L., Jr.: Emergency correction of ascending aortic dissecting aneurysms, Surgery **56**:594, 1964.

541. Storck, H.: Ein Fall von Arachnodaktylie (Dystrophia mesodermalis congenita), Typus Marfan, Dermatologica **104**:321, 1952.

542. Straatsma, B. R., Christensen, R. E., and Pettit, T. H.: Lens subluxation and surgical aphakia treated wtih photocoagulation of the iris, Docum. Ophthal. **26**:664, 1969.

543. Stratz, C. H.: Der Körper des Kindes, Stuttgart, 1902, Ferdinand Enke.

544. Straub, H.: Die elastischen Fasern in den Bändern des menschlichen Fusses, Acta Anat. **11**:268, 1950.

545. Strayhorn, D., and Wells, E. B.: Arachnodactylia with aneurysmal dilatation of the aorta, Trans. Amer. Clin. Climat. Ass. **59**:205, 1947.

545a. Sutinen, S., and Piiroinen, O.: Marfan syndrome, pregnancy, and fatal dissection of aorta, Acta Obstet. Gynec. Scand. **50**:295, 1971.

546. Sutton, G. E. F.: Cardiac anomalies associated with funnel chest, Bristol Med. Clin. J. **64**:45, 1947.

547. Sweet, R. H.: Pectus excavatum; report of two cases successfully operated upon, Ann. Surg. **119**:922, 1944.

548. Symbas, P. N., Baldwin, B. J., Silverman, M. E., and Galambos, J. T.: Marfan's syndrome with aneurysm of ascending aorta and aortic regurgitation, surgical treatment and new histochemical observations, Amer. J. Cardiol. **25**:483, 1970.

549. Talbot, N. B., Sobel, E. H., McArthur, J. W., and Crawford, J. D.: Functional endocrinology, Cambridge, Mass., 1952, Harvard University Press.

550. Tambornino, J. M., Armbrust, E. N., and Moe, J. H.: Harrington instrumentation in correction of scoliosis, J. Bone Joint Surg. 46-A:313, 1964.

551. Tatoń, J.: Zagadnienie zespou Marfana w świetle wasnych spostrzezeń (Problem of Marfan's syndrome in the light of personal observations), Pol. Arch. Med. Wewnet. 30:1111, 1960.

552. Theobald, G.: Histologic eye findings in arachnodactyly, Amer. J. Ophthal. 24:1132, 1941.

553. Thomas, J., Brothers, G. B., Anderson, R. S., and Cuff, J. R.: Marfan syndrome; a report of three cases with aneurysm of the aorta, Amer. J. Med. 12:613, 1952.

554. Thursfield, H.: Arachnodactyly, St. Bartholomew's Hosp. Rep. 53:35, 1917-1918.

555. Tjio, J. H., Puck, T. T., and Robinson, A.: The human chromosomal satellites in normal persons and in two patients with Marfan's syndrome, Proc. Nat. Acad. Sci. USA 46:532, 1960.

556. Tobin, J. R., Jr., Bay, E. B., and Humphries, E. M.: Marfan's syndrome in the adult dissecting aneurysm of the aorta associated with arachnodactyly, Arch. Intern. Med. 80:475, 1947.

557. Toes, N. A.: Ruptured splenic artery aneurysm during parturition, Brit. Med. J. 1:495, 1956.

558. Tolbert, L. E., Jr., and Birchall, R. B.: Marfan's syndrome with interventricular septal defect found at autopsy, Oschner Clin. Rep. 2:48, 1956.

559. Tourniaire, A., Deyerieux, F., and Bastien, P.: Dilatation du segment initial de l'aorte: gigantisms de l'appareil valvulaire aortique, Arch. Mal. Coeur 44:153, 1951.

560. Traisman, H. S., and Johnson, F. R.: Arachnodactyly associated with aneurysm of the aorta, Amer. J. Dis. Child. 87:156, 1954.

561. Traub, E.: Epiphyseal necrosis in pituitary gigantism, Arch. Dis. Child. 14:203, 1939.

562. Travel, M. E.: Straight back—a "nonsyndrome"? Ann. Intern. Med. 73:335, 1970.

563. Troxler, E. R., and Niemetz, D.: Generalized xanthomatosis with pulmonary, skeletal and cerebral manifestations; report of a case, Ann. Intern. Med. 25:960, 1946.

564. Troy, J. M.: Marfan's disease complicated by hemothorax, J. Indiana Med. Ass. 48:488, 1955.

565. Trüb, C. L. P.: Aortenwanderkrankung (Medianecrosis aortae idiopathica), Aortenzerreissung und Arbeitsunfall, Mschr. Unfallheilk. 54:321, 1951.

566. Tucker, A. S., and Bolande, R. P.: Pulmonary dysaeration in Marfan's syndrome, Ann. Radiol. 7:450, 1964.

566a. Tucker, D. P.: Blue sclerotics syndrome simulating buphthalmos, Amer. J. Ophthal. 47:345, 1959.

567. Tune, N., and Thal, A. P.: Some unusual features of the Marfan syndrome; report of 4 cases, Circulation 24:1154, 1961.

568. Tung, H. L., and Liebow, A. A.: Marfan's syndrome; observations at necropsy, with special reference to medio-necrosis of the great vessels, Lab. Invest. 1:382, 1952.

569. Usher, C. H.: A pedigree of congenital dislocation of the lenses, Biometrika 16:273, 1924.

570. Uyeyama, H., Kondo, B., and Kamins, M.: Arachnodactylia and cardiovascular disease. Amer. Heart J. 34:580, 1947.

571. Van Buchem, F. S. P.: Cardiovascular disease in arachnodactyly, Acta Med. Scand. 161:197, 1958.

572. Van der Hyde, M. N., and Zwaveling, A.: Resection of an abdominal aneurysm in a patient with Marfan's syndrome, J. Cardiov. Surg. 2:359, 1961.

573. Varga, B.: The type of inheritance in Marfan's syndrome, Orv. Hetil. 103:438, 1962.

574. Vejdonsky, V.: Marfan's syndrome, Lek. Listy. 1:539, 1946.

575. Vesely, D. G., Bray, C. B., and Bryant, V. M.: Arachnodactyly; a case report, J. Med. Ass. Alabama 24:276, 1955.

576. Vigváry, L., Fazekas, A., and Ertner, I.: Fatal stomach rupture in a young patient with Marfan's syndrome (in Hungarian), Orv. Hetil. 111:2719, 1970.

577. Viva-Salas, E., and Sanson, R. E.: Sindrome d Marfan, sin cardiopatia congenita y con endocarditis lenta conformada por la autopsia, Arch. Inst. Cardiol. México 18:217, 1948.

578. Voigt, J., and Hansen, J. P.: Spontaneous rupture of the aorta in young people; its rela-

tion to so-called medionecrosis cystica and Marfan's syndrome, Acta Path. Microbiol. Scand. **212** (supp.):143, 1970.

579. Von Meyenburg, H.: Ueber spontane Aortenrupture bei zwei Brudern, Schweiz, Med. Wschr. **20**:976, 1939.

580. Von Noorden, G. K., and Schultz, R. O.: A gonioscopic study of the chamber angle in Marfan's syndrome, Arch. Ophthal. **64**:929, 1960.

581. Wachtel, F. M., Ravitch, M. M., and Grisham, A.: The relation of pectus excavatum to heart disease, Amer. Heart J. **52**:121, 1956.

582. Wachtel, J. G.: The ocular pathology of Marfan's syndrome, including a clinicopathological correlation and an explanation of ectopia lentis, Arch. Ophthal. **76**:512, 1966.

583. Wagenwoort, C. A., Neufeld, H. N., and Edwards, J. E.: Cardiovascular system in Marfan's syndrome and in idiopathic dilatation of the ascending aorta, Amer. J. Cardiol. **9**:496, 1962.

584. Wajda, I., Lehr, D., and Krukowski, M.: Sex difference in aortic rupture induced by Lathyrus odoratus in immature rats, Fed. Proc. **16**:343, 1957.

585. Walker, B. A., Beigthon, P. H., and Murdoch, J. L.: The Marfanoid hypermobility syndrome, Ann. Intern. Med. **71**:349, 1969.

586. Walker, B. A., and Murdoch, J. L.: The wrist sign; a useful physical finding in the Marfan syndrome, Arch. Intern. Med. **126**:276, 1970.

587. Warwick, W. T., and Wiles, P.: The growth of periosteum in long bones, Brit. J. Surg. **22**:169, 1934.

588. Wawzonek, S., Ponseti, I. V., Shepard, R. S., and Wiedenmann, L. G.: Epiphyseal plate lesions, degenerative arthritis, and dissecting aneurysm of the aorta produced by aminonitriles, Science **121**:63, 1955.

589. Weber, F. P.: Familial asthenia ("paralytic") type of thorax with congenital ectopia of lenses, a condition allied to arachnodactyly, Lancet **2**:1472, 1933.

590. Webster, B., Rich, C., Densen, P. M., Moore, J. E., Nicol, C. S., and Padget, P.: Studies in cardiovascular syphilis. III. The natural history of syphilitic aortic insufficiency, Amer. Heart J. **46**:117, 1953.

591. Weissler, A. M., Harris, W. S., and Schoenfeld, C. D.: Bedside technics for the evaluation of ventricular function in man, Amer. J. Cardiol. **23**:577, 1969.

592. Weissman, N., Shields, G. S., and Carnes, W. H.: Cardiovascular studies on copper-deficient swine, J. Biol. Chem. **238**:3115, 1963.

593. Welch, J. P., and Temtamy, S. A.: Hereditary contractures of the fingers (camptodactyly), J. Med. Genet. **3**:104, 1966.

594. West, L. S.: Two pedigrees showing inherited predisposition to hernia, J. Hered. **27**:449, 1939.

594a. Wettenhall, N. B. (Melbourne): Personal communication, 1972.

595. Weve, H.: Ueber Arachnodaktylie (Dystrophia mesodermalis congenita, typus Marfanis), Arch. Augenheilk. **104**: 1, 1931.

596. Weyers, H.: Zur Kenntnis der Arachnodaktylie und ihrer Beziehungen zu anderen mesodermalen Konstitutionsanomalien, Z. Kinderheilk. **67**:308, 1949.

597. Wheat, M. W., Jr., and Bartley, T. D.: Aneurysms of the aortic root, Dis. Chest **47**:430, 1965.

598. Wheat, M. W., Jr., Palmer, R. F, Bartley, T. D, and Seelman, R C: Treatment of dissecting aneurysms of the aorta without surgery, J. Thorac. Cardiovasc. Surg. **50**:364, 1965.

599. White, P. D.: Personal communication.

600. Whitfield, A. G. W., Arnott, W. M., and Stafford, J. S.: "Myocarditis" and aortic hypoplasia in arachnodactylia, Lancet **1**:1387, 1951.

601. Whittaker, S. R. F., and Sheehan, J. D.: Dissecting aortic aneurysm in Marfan's syndrome, Lancet **2**:791, 1954.

602. Wilkins, L.: The diagnosis and treatment of endocrine disorders in childhood an adolescence, Springfield, Ill., 1950, Charles C Thomas, Publisher.

603. Wilkinson, K. D.: Aneurysmal dilatation of the pulmonary artery, Brit. Heart J. **2**:255, 1940.

604. Williams, E.: Rare cases, with practical remarks, Trans. Amer. Ophthal. Soc. **2**:291, 1873-1879.

605. Wilner, H. I., and Finby, N.: Skeletal manifestations in the Marfan syndrome, J.A.M.A. **187**:490, 1964.

606. Wilson, R.: Marfan's syndrome: description of a family, Amer. J. Med. **23:**434, 1957.

607. Withers, J. N., Fishback, M. E., Kiehl, P. V., and Hannon, J. L.: Spontaneous pneumothorax; suggested etiology and comparison of treatment methods, Amer. J. Surg. **108:**772, 1964.

608. Witkin, M.: Arachnodactyly in a Bantu child, S. Afr. Med. J. **32:**45, 1958.

609. Woessner, J. F., Jr.: Catabolism of collagen and noncollagen protein in the rat uterus during postpartum involution, Biochem. J. **83:**304, 1962.

610. Wolff, K.: Unbekannte Erkrankung der Säuglingsaorta mit Schwund des elatischen Gewebes, Virchow Arch. Path. Anat. **285:**369, 1932.

611. Wolff, K.: Ueber die Ursachen der sogenannten spontanen Aortenzerreissungen, Virchow Arch. Path. Anat. **289:**1, 1933.

612. Wong, F. L., Friedman, S., and Yakovac, W.: Cardiac complications of Marfan's syndrome in a child; report of a case with rapidly progressive course terminating with rupture of dissecting aneurysm, Amer. J. Dis. Child. **107:**404, 1964.

613. Wright, J. S.: Ruptured aneurysm of the sinus of Valsalva, Quart. J. Med. **39:**493, 1970.

614. Wunsch, M. C., Steinmetz, E. F., and Fisch, C.: Marfan's syndrome and subacute bacterial endocarditis, Amer. J. Cardiol. **15:**102, 1965.

615. Yates, J. W., Treger, A., and Littman, A.: Camptodactyly; a kindred study, J.A.M.A. **206:**1565, 1968.

616. Yenel, F.: Coronary arteriovenous communication; report of a case and review of the literature, New Eng. J. Med. **265:**577, 1961.

617. Yettra, M., and Laski, S. L.: Aneurysmal dilatation of the aorta associated with cystic medial necrosis, Amer. Heart J. **33:**516, 1947.

618. Young, D.: Familial dissecting aneurysm complicating Marfan's syndrome, Amer. Heart J. **78:**577, 1969.

619. Young, J.: Relaxation of pelvic joints in pregnancy: pelvic arthropathy of pregnancy, J. Obstet. Gynaec. Brit. Comm. **47:**493, 1940.

620. Young, M. L.: Arachnodactyly, Arch. Dis. Child. **4:**190, 1929.

621. Zabriskie, J., and Reisman, M.: Marchesani syndrome, J. Pediat. **52:**158, 1958.

622. Zaidi, Z. H.: Bilateral ectopia lentis in Marfan's syndrome; review of features with report of two cases, Canad. Med. Ass. J. **82:**265, 1960.

623. Zanchi, M.: Medionecrosis idiopathica cystica dell'aorta ed aneurisma fusiforme puro giovanile in soggetto Basedowiano, Folio Hered. Path. (Milano) **7:**287, 1958.

4 · Homocystinuria

Historical note

The discovery and elucidation of an inborn error of metabolism reflected by the presence of homocystine in the urine and associated with systemic abnormalities of connective tissue were events of the last decade. In the course of a survey of institutionalized, mentally retarded persons in Northern Ireland, using urine chromatography, Carson and Neill[18] detected several instances of homocystinuria and noted the occurrence of ectopia lentis.[16] Simultaneously and independently, Gerritsen and co-workers[36,37] in Madison, Wisconsin, found the same metabolic defect in an infant with "cerebral palsy."

The occurrence of thromboembolic complications soon became evident, and the confusion with the Marfan syndrome, because of skeletal abnormalities and ectopia lentis, was pointed out on the basis of restudy of cases previously reported as instances of the Marfan syndrome.[39] That mental retardation is not an invariable feature of homocystinuria was demonstrated by Schimke and colleagues[100] when patients with ectopia lentis were screened for homocystinuria.

Mudd and co-workers,[82] from their previous studies of methionine metabolism, suspected that the defect might be in the enzymatic condensation of homocysteine and serine to form cystathionine. Their suspicions were confirmed by demonstration of deficiency of cystathionine synthetase activity in liver. Uhlendorf and Mudd[120] made the important observation that the enzymatic diagnosis of homocystinuria can be made using fibroblasts cultured from biopsies of skin. Spaeth and Barber[110] demonstrated that some patients with homocystinuria respond to vitamin B_6, clearing the urine of homocystine. The difference in responsiveness to vitamin B_6 corroborated other suspicions of heterogeneity in homocystinuria.

Clinical manifestations

More than phenylketonuria and many other inborn errors of metabolism, homocystinuria is a clinician's delight because of the abundance and variety of its manifestations. This survey of the clinical features is based in part on the descriptions of cases in the literature and in part on a personal series of 83 cases in 47 sibships and 45 kindreds.[77]

Changes in the central nervous system, skeletal system, eye, cardiovascular system, and skin are reflected in clinical manifestations.

Central nervous system. In addition to the obvious direct consequences of vascular thrombosis, central nervous system manifestations include mental retardation, seizures, and psychiatric disturbances.

Mental retardation of some degree occurs in a majority of patients with homocystinuria, but about 30% in our first series[100] had at least average intelligence. In the full series of 83 cases, 41 cases, close to half, have average intelligence or higher.[77] One subject in this series holds a doctoral degree and is a university instructor, and several others have university degrees. Mental retardation of profound degree would seem to be rather rare, if one judges by the study of Spaeth and Barber[110] in the United States, which showed a frequency of about 0.02% of institutionalized defectives. Of course, the thrombotic complications of homocystinuria lead to early death in some patients, thus reducing the frequency of institutionalized cases.

To what extent intracranial thrombosis and the underlying metabolic defect are individually responsible for mental retardation and for seizures is not clear. Both factors probably play a role in varying relative proportion.

Intracranial venous and arterial thromboses create a variety of clinical pictures in young children with homocystinuria. This metabolic error must be kept in mind in connection with acute hemiplegia of infancy and childhood.[11] Intracranial venous thrombosis can lead to a characteristic picture of headache, neck stiffness, and bloody cerebrospinal fluid.[4] Poliomyelitis may be mistakenly diagnosed in cases of acute paraplegia, as meningitis, meningoencephalitis, "brain fever," etc., may be mistakenly diagnosed in cases of intracranial venous thrombosis.[27] The young children frequently are thrown into that meaningless diagnostic hodgepodge "cerebral palsy." The original patient of Waisman and colleagues[20,38] had marked spasticity and died at 1 year of age; autopsy showed cystic degeneration of the brain.[20] One case of "temporal lobe agenesis" reported by Robinson[96] appears from the description to have represented homocystinuria; both the patient, who died at 20 years of age, and his brother were thought to have the Marfan syndrome.

Thrombosis of the carotid arteries has been known to occur in a number of instances[40]; for example, in an 18-year-old boy of our Kindred 1 and in a 12-year-old girl of our Kindred 14. In both, the evidence is clear that cerebral arteriograms accelerated the thrombotic process, and was the *coup de grace* that led to death soon after. In the 18-year-old, both internal carotid arteries were completely occluded, but the stenosis and occlusion had occurred episodically because there was fresh thrombus, canalizing thrombus, and organized thrombus of several vintages, showing new internal elastic lamellae. Intracranial thrombosis leading to death occurred in an 8-year-old boy of Irish extraction whose case was the subject of a clinicopathologic conference at the Massachusetts General Hospital in 1933. Homocystinuria was established retrospectively by Shih and Efron[104] by demonstration of the disorder in living members of the kindred. The histopathologic findings were reviewed by McCully,[73] who used them as the point of departure for his studies of the role of homocysteine in ordinary arteriosclerosis.[74]

Our first proved case of homocystinuria (J. H. M. of Kindred 1) was con-

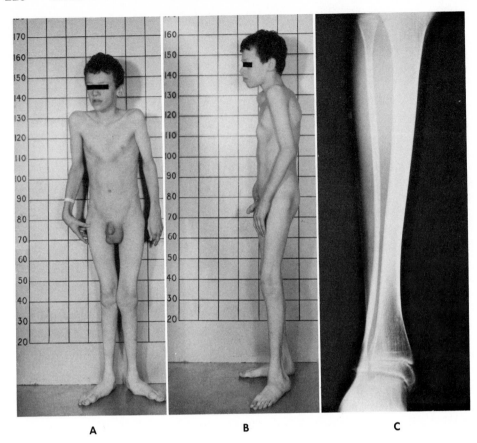

A   B   C

Fig. 4-1. Homocystinuria in S. H. (J.H.H. 1168161, Kindred 16) at the age of 12 years. **A** and **B,** Note pectus carinatum, left genu valgum, and "rocker-bottom" feet. Compare with Figs. 3-5 and 3-15. **C,** Roentgenogram of right leg showing slender fibula and tibia that are mildly bowed.

sidered to have schizophrenia for several years,[111] and others of the patients display schizoid behavior which has stimulated the interest of psychiatrists[55] because of findings from other sources suggesting abnormality of methionine metabolism in persons with behavioral disturbances. A striking family history of schizophrenia was noted by Carson and associates.[17] A systematic psychiatric investigation of homocystinurics and their relatives is yet to be done.

Skeletal features (Fig. 4-1). Osteoporosis, tendency to fracture, scoliosis, deformity of the anterior chest, kyphoscoliosis, excessive length of the round bones of the limbs resulting in tall stature, enlarged ossification centers, a "buried spicule" type of physeal-metaphyseal change, and a modest degree of limitation of joint mobility are all included in homocystinuria. The hands of homocystinurics tend to have a "tight feel" of restricted joint mobility in the fingers, in contrast to the loose-jointed hand of the Marfan syndrome. Contracture of the fingers[17] has been observed.

Excessive height and low US/LS value are usual findings in homocystinuria and are points of similarity with the Marfan syndrome. Platyspondyly and

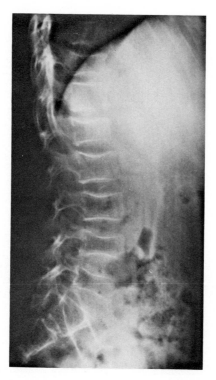

Fig. 4-2. Osteoporosis of the lumbar spine in G. M. (J.H.H. 950038, Kindred 28). 11-year-old girl. This patient had staphyloma. Another point of interest is the fact that her kindred is the one in which the Crigler-Najjar syndrome was first described, and a number of other rare recessive disorders have been identified in this inbred Old American kindred of the peninsula counties of southern Maryland: nonkeratosulfate-excreting Morquio syndrome (p. 599), Seckel's bird-headed dwarfism, metachromatic leukodystrophy, another unidentified cerebral degenerative disorder, and others.

particularly scoliosis reduce the height to some extent, and exaggerate the reduction in US/LS value.

The roentgenographic features of 26 of our patients, varying in age from 6 to 45 years, were subjected to particular analysis.[16]

In 25 of 26 patients the vertebral bodies were porotic, and in 19 the porosis* was associated with concavity of the vertebral end-plates (Figs. 4-2, 4-17M, and 4-21A). Scoliosis was noted in 17 patients and kyphosis in 5. Two patients had spondylolisthesis. It is likely that degeneration of the intervertebral discs is a feature in some cases. Chronic back pain was a major problem in some.

In most patients the long bones of the limbs were also porotic, and in many they were unusually long and thin (Fig. 4-1C). That fractures occur with relatively minor trauma is a not unexpected finding. Nine of 23 patients showed

---

*Osteoporosis of homocystinuria is listed in Table 4-2 as a feature distinguishing it from the Marfan syndrome. It is clearly a striking feature of homocystinuria. However, some physically active patients with the Marfan syndrome have mild osteoporosis of the lumbar vertebrae.

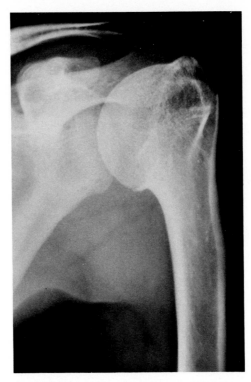

Fig. 4-3. Varus deformity of proximal humerus in 18-year-old man (D. R., J.H.H. 123012, Kindred 33).

varus deformity of the proximal humerus, (Fig. 4-3) which is an unusual finding in normal persons and which, in homocystinuria, may be related to round-shoulderedness. Flaring of the distal femur and large distal femoral epiphyses are exaggerated by the general thinness of the thighs and legs. Large, knobby knees are commonly noted.

Some of the most distinctive changes occur in the wrists (Fig. 4-4), particularly in children. In all of 12 children studied, the distal radial and ulnar physes contained focal calcifications, sometimes punctate but more often in the form of narrow spicules. Moreover, striking longitudinal linear radiodensities were present in the distal radius and ulna of most of the patients, both adults and children. These densities presumably represent physeal spicules that become buried in the metaphyseal bone with growth. All these patients were studied before therapy, dietary or other, had been given. The striking changes in 6 children resembled those which occur in patients with phenylketonuria whose dietary phenylalanine may have been excessively restricted.[113] Physeal changes in homocystinuria have been commented on also by Gaudier and co-workers[32] and by Holt and Allen,[51] among others.

The carpal bones were selectively enlarged and malformed in 8 patients: the capitate and hamate bones in 3, the capitate and triquetral bones in 1, the capitate bone alone in 3, and the triquetral bone alone in 1. (Like the knees, the

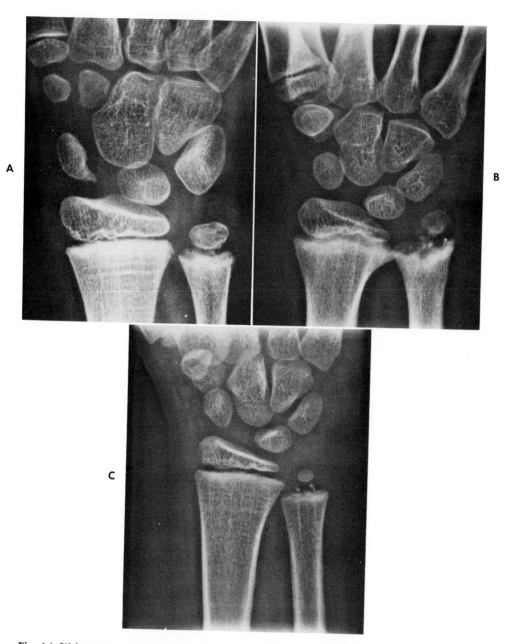

Fig. 4-4. Wrist roentgenograms in 3 untreated patients with homocystinuria. **A,** A. W. (J.H.H. 1155861, Kindred 10), a 6-year-old boy, has enlarged hamate and capitate bones, calcific spicules in both the radial and the ulnar physes, and buried spicules of the radial metaphysis. The ulnar physis is slightly widened, with cupping of the end of the metaphysis. **B,** T. B. (J.H.H. 1160985, Kindred 7), an 8-year-old girl, has widening of the physes, especially the ulnar, and multiple calcified dots in the ulnar physis. The ulnar metaphysis is cupped, and both metaphyses, especially the radial, contain streaklike buried spicules. **C,** R. H. (J.H.H. 994522, Kindred 11), a 9-year-old boy, has retarded ossification of all bones, particularly of the lunate bone. The ulnar physis is widened and contains conspicuous spicules and dots. Particularly striking buried spicules are evident in the radial and ulnar metaphyses.

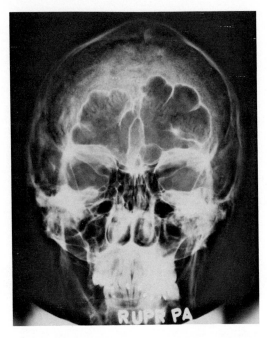

Fig. 4-5. Small head and very large paranasal sinuses in 26-year-old woman (J.H.M., 1037641, Kindred 1). Same patient as shown in Fig. 4-17N.

wrists tend to be enlarged clinically.) In 6 children, development of the lunate bones was retarded.

Among 15 prepubertal patients, skeletal maturation exceeded chronologic age by more than two standard deviations in 4 patients, was retarded in 1, and was normal in 10.

In 8 of 18 patients measured, the metacarpal index exceeded 8.5, a figure accepted by some as a criterion of arachnodactyly. The thumb sign (opposed across the palm, the thumb extends well beyond the ulnar border of the hand), usually found in the Marfan syndrome,[112] is not demonstrable in cases of homocystinuria,[28] probably because even if arachnodactyly is present, reduced joint mobility restricts opposition of the thumb. Joint laxity as seen in the Marfan syndrome is usually not found in homocystinuria. A "tight feel" of the hand suggesting restricted joint mobility is the rule.

In 6 of 24 cases the skull was abnormally small with abnormally thick calvaria, and in 4 cases, unusually large paranasal sinuses (Figs. 4-5 and 4-17N) were demonstrated. These 6 patients were mentally retarded, as were also at least 6 of the 18 patients whose skull films were judged normal.

Anterior chest deformity—pectus carinatum or pectus excavatum, or an asymmetric deformity that cannot be classed as either or has features of both—is present by adulthood in a majority of patients (Fig. 4-6).

Some patients have malformed, rocker-bottom feet somewhat like those of patients with the Marfan syndrome. Many of the patients "toe out" and walk with a "Charlie Chaplin gait."

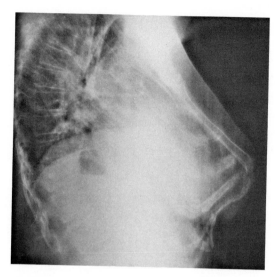

Fig. 4-6. Severe pectus carinatum, with osteoporosis and mild kyphosis, in **P. Tu.** (Kindred 18), a 39-year-old woman.

Comparable roentgenographic findings have been reported by Smith,[106] Mac-Carthy and Carey,[70] and others. The findings are summarized below.

The eye. Ocular features include myopia, ectopia lentis, glaucoma with or without pupillary entrapment of the dislocated lens, buphthalmos, staphyloma, retinal detachment, and optic atrophy.

Ectopia lentis is the ocular hallmark of homocystinuria. A curious difference from that of the Marfan syndrome is this: the lens tends to be dislocated *upward* in the Marfan syndrome but *downward* in homocystinuria (Fig. 4-7). There is another difference: ectopia lentis is probably *congenital,* as a rule, in the Marfan syndrome. Bowers[7] tells of a family with many members affected by the Marfan syndrome in which ectopia lentis is rather routinely sought in newborn or young babies by gentle shaking of the infant to demonstrate iridodonesis. To say that the ectopia lentis is congenital in the Marfan syndrome is not to deny, of course, that further dislocation, even into the anterior chamber, can occur in later life. On the other hand, ectopia lentis is an "acquired" and progressive abnormality in homocystinuria. Competent ophthalmologic examinations done because of suspected Marfan syndrome have failed to show ectopia lentis at the age of 6, for example, but have shown dislocation by 10 years of age in the same patient. The earliest detection of ectopia lentis in patients of this series was at 3 years of age. Ectopia lentis was not recognized until 24 years of age in one patient with the mild form of homocystinuria (p. 245), and not until 28 years in a published case.[20a] The view that ectopia lentis is "acquired" in homocystinuria and congenital in the Marfan syndrome might seem contradicted by some data on age of detection of ectopia lentis.[53a] I suspect, however, that age of detection is not valid evidence on the question.

As pointed out by Komrower,[61] myopia (discussed later) may precede detection of ectopia lentis by several years. Homocystinuria is a possibility to be

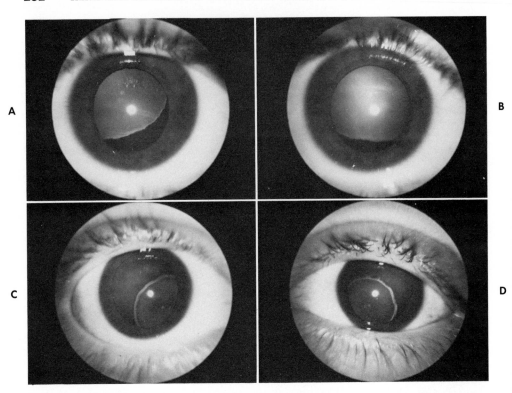

Fig. 4-7. A comparison of the ectopia lentis in the Marfan syndrome and in homocystinuria. **A** and **B**, A. G. (J.H.H. 1249930), 15 years old, has typical skeletal features of the Marfan syndrome and no homocystinuria. The lenses are displaced upward. **C** and **D**, V. S. (J.H.H. 1246970, Kindred 37), 14 years old, has homocystine in the urine and typical skeletal features of homocystinuria. Her lenses are displaced downward.

considered in children with myopia, especially, of course, if skeletal and other features are consistent.

Slightly less than 80% of our 157 patients with the Marfan syndrome have ectopia lentis. The great majority of patients with homocystinuria have demonstrable ectopia lentis by 10 years of age. However, we know now that some patients appreciably older than 10 years do not have ectopia lentis. In all these patients, other manifestations are likewise milder or absent. In this series 2 patients, sisters, lack ectopia lentis at the ages of 12 and 17 years; these sisters will be commented on further in connection with the mild form of homocystinuria.

Henkind and Ashton[49] showed histologically that the zonular fibers in homocystinuric eyes had "recoiled to the surface of the ciliary body, where they lay matted and retracted into a feltwork" that fused with a greatly thickened ciliary epithelium. Electron microscopy showed a disorganized, granular appearance of the fibers.

Like most Marfan patients, most homocystinuric patients are myopic. I have presumed that this is a function of an excessively long globe, but spherophakia from lack of the normal tension on the lens by the suspensory ligament may be a factor. The two factors are additive.

Glaucoma is a frequent ocular complication of homocystinuria. It is never present without ectopia lentis. It often develops acutely from pupillary entrapment of the dislocated lens, but it can develop in the absence of entrapment. The abnormally spherical lens seems to act like the ball of a ball valve in these cases. Martin and Carson[72] observed block of the pupil in 11 eyes of 14 patients with homocystinuria. Johnston[54] also commented on this feature. (Glaucoma is, of course, a complication of the ectopia lentis of the Marfan syndrome and of the Weill-Marchesani syndrome.) In younger children buphthalmos, a generalized bulging of the globe, can result. Buphthalmos and staphyloma, a localized bulging of the globe, are probably particularly likely to occur in homocystinuria and occur at lower pressures than in the normal eye because of the weakened state of the scleral collagen.

Detachment of the retina is a complication of lens surgery in homocystinuria, but it occurs spontaneously in a significant proportion of cases. I doubt that the long myopic globe is the main causative factor. A loosening of the mooring of the retina is probably another effect of the metabolic defect on the connective tissues.

Optic atrophy has been observed on the basis of glaucoma and also on the basis of arterial occlusion. Wilson and Ruiz[126] described bilateral central artery thrombosis in a 6-year-old Negro child.

Presley and co-workers[91-93] have reported confusing findings in regard to the ocular features of homocystinuria. In the first report,[91] 10 cases of presumed homocystinuria were identified in an eye clinic. Six patients had ectopia lentis. From the description provided, no more than 4 would appear to have a clinical picture consistent with that found in the present series. Some of their patients had the Weill-Marchesani syndrome (brachymorphism with spherophakia and ectopia lentis). One had aniridia, presumably of the standard hereditary type, since one parent also had aniridia. In the second paper,[92] urine screening in a school for the blind was reported; 54 of 375 students were found to have homocystinuria; only 4 of the 54 had ectopia lentis, one of these (L. B.) apparently being the same as one of the subjects in the eye clinic screening. One of the homocystinuric patients had ocular albinism with nystagmus (presumably the X-linked disorder), and a second had generalized albinism. In the third paper,[93] 65 cases of homocystinuria were reported, as well as 5 others with generalized aminoaciduria. Seven had albinism and 2 had the Weill-Marchesani syndrome. Enzymatic studies and detailed clinical investigations would be of interest in this group of subjects.

Cardiovascular system. Thrombosis has occurred, I suspect, at some time and in some homocystinuric patient in essentially every artery and vein of the body. Thrombophlebitis with pulmonary embolism, coronary artery occlusion, renal arterial stenosis with hypertension, and intracranial thromboses, venous and arterial, are the frequent forms of thrombosis of major clinical import.

Intracranial vascular thrombosis was discussed above.

Fatal coronary occlusion occurred in several teen-agers in our series. Carey and associates[12] described fatal coronary occlusion in an 11-year-old. Incapacitating angina pectoris occurred in another teen-ager of my series. Angina pectoris disappeared when the patient was placed on a low methionine diet. The histologic changes have consisted of great intimal thickening and, in addition, a thinning of the tunica media with increase in a ground substance of unidentified nature.

The aorta in autopsied cases has shown streaked intimal thickening. Thrombosis of the terminal aorta occurred in a 28-year-old man, and a girl 6½ years old had exploratory thoracotomy for coarctation of the aorta. The occlusion in the latter case was described as proximal to the left subclavian artery and not amenable to surgical repair. Although it is possible that two rare abnormalities, one a congenital malformation and the other an inborn error of metabolism, were present in this patient, homocystinuria alone might be responsible for the aortic occlusion. All the other clinical features of homocystinuria are severe in this patient; now at 21 years of age the blood pressure is found to be normal on most examinations.

Dilatation of the aorta has not been found in most patients with homocystinuria. In older patients with mild dilatation, long-standing hypertension provided an adequate explanation. Histologically, disorganization of the elastic weave in the aortic tunica media was described by Schimke and co-workers,[101] and the occurrence of thoracic and abdominal aneurysms in the 89-year-old patient with possible homocystinuria described in Family E should be noted.

Dunn and associates[27] described aortic regurgitation in one patient who also had unilateral Legg-Perthes disease. In one patient, 20 years old, with severe coronary artery disease that was fatal soon after, I heard a curious, semimusical early diastolic murmur that may have originated, not at the aortic valve (which was normal at autopsy), but in the pericardium or, more likely, in a stenotic coronary artery.[19] (See Family 1, p. 260.)

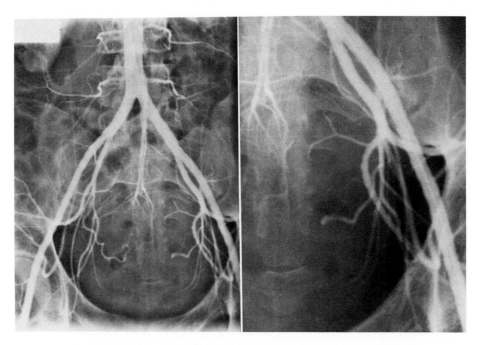

Fig. 4-8. Corrugation of the tunica intima of the iliac arteries and their branches in J. Mat. (Kindred 17), 11 years of age.

One patient with normal findings of catheterization (Case 4) had idiopathic dilatation of the pulmonary artery.

Heart failure has most often been due to cor pulmonale[12] from thromboembolism of the pulmonary arterial tree, aided and abetted by ischemic heart disease. Atrial fibrillation occurs as a feature of ischemic heart disease.

Acute gangrene of the leg, requiring amputation, was described in an 18-year-old boy by Finkelstein and colleagues.[29] We have observed, by means of x-ray films, calcification of the femoral artery in 2 patients and of the abdominal aorta in one young patient with homocystinuria, an unusual finding for their ages. Aortograms performed in a 13-year-old girl (before the dangers of the procedure were realized) showed corrugation of the wall of the iliac arteries (Fig. 4-8), which is thought to be due to striations of the type observed in the aorta. Thrombosis of the inferior vena cava and of the portal and mesenteric veins occurred in this series (Fig. 4-9). One 8-year-old boy in this series was pulseless in all four limbs and had occlusion of the inferior vena cava; yet he is still alive at 13 years of age. Thrombophlebitis, particularly in the legs, is

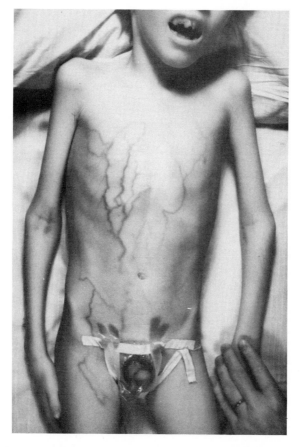

Fig. 4-9. Collateral venous pattern indicative of thrombosis of inferior vena cava in R. Hd. (Case 19).

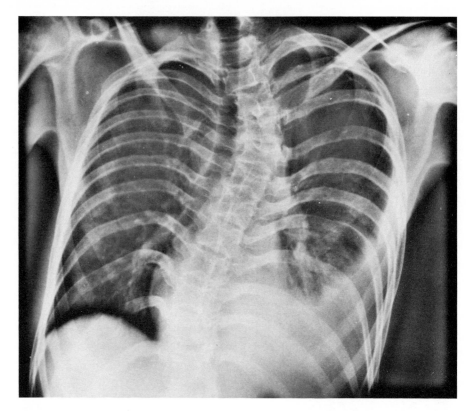

Fig. 4-10. Scoliosis and left pleural reaction from pulmonary embolism in D. R. (J.H.H. 1230124, Kindred 33), 18 years of age.

a frequent occurrence, even in the first decade of life, and pulmonary embolism often ensues (Fig. 4-10). "Varicose ulcers" of the leg are a frequent problem. It is likely that arteriolar thrombosis contributes to the development of these ulcers and to their refractoriness to treatment.

It has repeatedly been observed in this series and in published cases that vascular thrombosis is likely to follow surgical procedures.[12] Possibly the well-known postsurgical rise in platelet count may be a factor.

Contrast studies and other procedures that involve manipulation of arteries and veins probably lead to thrombosis; the evidence is most convincing for cerebral arteriography. The efficacy of long-term anticoagulant therapy has not been evaluated. It is noteworthy that prothrombin concentration is reduced, presumably because of liver disease, in many patients (*v. infra*).

Gastrointestinal bleeding has occurred in some homocystinurics, and roentgenographic studies (e.g., J. H. M., Kindred 1, and V. S., Kindred 37) have shown small wedge-shaped ulcerations of the gastric mucosa consistent with focal infarctions. Massive and fatal intestinal infarction from mesenteric artery occlusion occurred in one patient in this series.

The skin. Cutaneous features include malar flushing, wide pores of the facial skin, cutis marmorata, Price and co-workers' curious longitudinal crease of the fingers,[94] thin and focally even papyraceous skin, light-colored hair, and, of course, the ulcers of the ankles, dilated veins, and other changes secondary to vascular thrombosis.

I have the impression that malar flush is a more impressive feature of homocystinuria in the United Kingdom than in the United States, and I suggest, not entirely facetiously, that central heating in the United States and the lack thereof in the United Kingdom are responsible for the difference. Chilblains are something we rarely see in the United States, and British cardiologists were always more impressed with malar flush in mitral stenosis than were their colleagues on the other side of the Atlantic.

In homocystinuria the skin of the face is often coarse and wide-pored (Fig. 4-17L). Skin elsewhere, both on the trunk and the limbs, often shows cutis marmorata (livedo reticularis).[17] The skin is often generally thin, with venous pattern showing through clearly, and in some areas it may be papyraceous,[27] resembling that of patients after prolonged therapy with penicillamine. (The structural similarity of penicillamine and homocysteine and the documented effects of penicillamine on connective tissue[47,86] make the analogy more than merely descriptive.) Fine telangiectases are often noted around scars.[94]

The hair is often coarse and almost always of light color in homocystinuria. The latter feature is impressive in comparison with the hair of unaffected sibs, especially in patients of Mediterranean extraction. The darkening of the hair with restricted methionine intake and with vitamin B_6 therapy clinches the validity of light hair as a feature of homocystinuria. I call your attention to the dramatic picture published by Barber and Spaeth.[3] Premature graying of the hair even in teen-agers is also a feature of homocystinuria and also responds to low methionine diet and vitamin B_6.

Eczema seems to be unusually frequent in homocystinuric patients.

Miscellaneous features. A high, narrow palate like that in the Marfan syndrome is present in many homocystinuric patients. The teeth are often crowded and irregularly aligned. Early eruption of teeth has been noted in a number of cases. Mandibular prognathism occurs as an expression of the generalized overgrowth.

Hernia occurs with increased frequency,[37] and a large omphalocele was present in one of our cases.

Fatty changes have been observed in the liver at autopsy and hepatomegaly and disturbance of liver function *in vitam*. We have been impressed with the frequency of low prothrombin in homocystinurics. In 6 patients tested by Carson and associates,[17] serum isocitric dehydrogenase was elevated, presumably due to hepatic dysfunction.

One patient in this series showed changes consistent with medullary cystic disease of the kidney on intravenous pyelograms. Several patients have had urinary tract infections, possibly representing an increased frequency.[12] Vascular thrombosis in the kidney may predispose to infection. Unlike cystinuria and cystinosis, homocystinuria does not have renal calculi and tissue deposits as features. This is both because of the greater solubility of homocystine in body fluids and because of the lower concentrations of homocystine.

Many of the patients have had asthma. Although multiple pulmonary embolism is a likely explanation for some of what has been labeled asthma, the

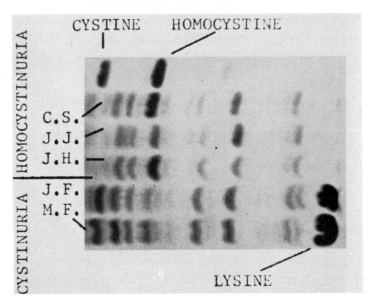

Fig. 4-11. High-voltage paper electrophoresis of urine from 3 patients with homocystinuria and 2 with cystinuria. For comparison, a mixture of cystine and homocystine is shown in the top run. The large amount of lysine in the cystinurics is another feature distinguishing homocystinuria from cystinuria.

frequency of true bronchial asthma may be increased in these patients. Pneumothorax has been observed in asthmatic homocystinuric patients (e.g., M. S., Kindred 14), perhaps contributed to by the connective tissue changes of this disorder.

Diagnosis

The specific diagnosis is made by demonstration of homocystine in the urine. The cyanide nitroprusside test used in the diagnosis of cystinuria is positive also in homocystinuria and is used for screening purposes.

The test is based on the fact that cystine and homocystine are reduced in the presence of sodium cyanide to cysteine or homocysteine, which in turn reacts with nitroprusside to give a violet color. It is important to realize that rather numerous other compounds, including creatinine and penicillamine, also give a positive reaction. The use of ammonium hydroxide removes the interference of creatinine. That creatinine is not a significant interference is indicated, however, by the fact that we used the test without alkali in our initial screening program,[100] which uncovered 20 affected kindreds. Presently the cyanide nitroprusside test is performed as follows: 5 drops of concentrated ammonium hydroxide are added to 5 ml. of urine. Then 2 ml. of freshly prepared 5% NaCN are added, mixed well, and allowed to react for 10 minutes at room temperature. Then 5 drops of 5% sodium nitroprusside are added, with further mixing. The presence of cystine or homocystine is indicated by a deep purple color that fades gradually.

The differentiation of cystine and homocystine can be performed by methods mentioned below; a recently described silver nitroprusside test[110] permits differentiation on the original screening. The silver nitroprusside test is performed as follows: 6 or 7 ml. of urine are saturated with solid sodium chloride. To this, 0.25 ml. of 1% sodium nitroprusside and 0.25 ml. of 0.7% sodium cyanide are added. Homocystine gives an immediate pink or purple color; cystine undergoes a slow reaction to give delayed development of color. The specificity of the test depends on the fact that only homocystine is reduced to the reactive thiol form (homocysteine) by the silver nitrate. Cyanide added in the final step binds the excess silver ion, thus allowing reaction between homocysteine and nitroprusside to give the colored product. Spaeth and Barber,[110] who introduced the silver nitroprusside test, found it to be sensitive to concentrations of 2 mg./100 ml. or more of homocystine.*

Cystine and homocystine give a spot at the same location on paper chromatography. They can be distinguished, however, by high-voltage paper electrophoresis or by specific assay by means of the Stein-Moore type of column chromatographic automatic amino acid analyzer. High levels of homocystine can also be demonstrated in the blood by the same techniques, but the blood must be promptly deproteinized, because otherwise homocystine binds to protein. By the same methods of amino acid analysis, high levels of methionine can be demonstrated in blood and urine. The literature contains few reports of well-substantiated cystathionine synthetase deficiency with normal levels of methionine in blood and urine.[81] For this reason a Guthrie type of test for methionine has been used in the neonatal screening for homocystinuria.[43] Bessman and colleagues[6] described a rapid method for assay of homocystine in biologic fluids.

Homocystinuria is probably present from birth and constant thereafter. However, under some circumstances, such as large urine volume and perhaps low protein intake, the qualitative cyanide nitroprusside test may be negative. Enzymatic diagnosis of homocystinuria can be made by assay of the activity of cystathionine synthetase in liver tissue. As will be noted, liver biopsy can, however, be circumvented by study of skin fibroblast cultures.

Prognosis

Patients dying at ages 1,[38] 2,[125] 3,[101] 7,[125] 8,[125] 9,[101] 9½,[17] 11,[100] 13,[100] 14,[100] 15,[100] 18,[101] 20,[101] and 28,[17,101] years have been reported. On the other hand, one patient in my series is living at age 52 years, and a patient with probable homocystinuria died at the age of 89 years (Family E, p. 249). Cline and colleagues[20a] described homocystinuria in a 74-year-old woman who had had 4 children (Fig. 4-12). At 28 years, after delivery of a child, she had sudden onset of glaucoma in one eye due to dislocation of the lens. Although the lens was removed, the eye became phthisic and was enucleated. At 32 years of age the same sequence of events occurred in the other eye, again following delivery: acute glaucoma from dislocated lens, surgical removal of the lens, development of phthisis, and enucleation.

Pathology

The most distinctive lesions are those of the arteries.[73] Usually many arteries show evidence of partial luminal obstruction, apparently due to episodic thrombosis followed by fibroelastic organization. The tunica media of these vessels shows drastic changes. The artery is dilated, with thinning out of muscular elements that became separated by a ground substance whose nature has not been determined.

The elastic weave of the aortic media, that is, the array of elastic lamellae,

---

*I am indebted to Dr. R. R. Howell, Houston, and Dr. G. H. Thomas, Baltimore, for information on diagnostic tests.

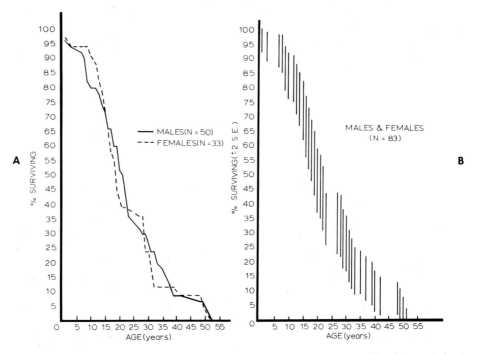

Fig. 4-12. Survivorship in 83 cases of homocystinuria (in 45 kindreds), a life-table analysis. **A,** Males and females demonstrate no significant or consistent difference in survivorship. **B,** Males and females are combined. The vertical lines indicate two standard errors on either side of the mean.

is abnormal in some cases. Aneurysmal dilatation of the aorta is not a conspicuous feature, however, and dissecting aneurysm has not been observed. Peculiar transverse intimal striations were noted in the descending aorta in one case,[17] and areas of disruption of elastic fibers in the media underlay the intimal striations. Thrombosis of the abdominal aorta occurred in a 28-year-old man (Case 8). Fibroelastic thickening of the endocardium of the left atrium has been found in most cases.

The ocular histopathology was studied by at least two groups.[49,94a]

The brain shows focal necrosis and gliosis.[17] Degenerative changes were described in the zonular fibers of the lens by light and electron microscopy.[123] Chou and Waisman[20] described severe spongy degeneration of the brain, together with micropolygyria and hypoplasia of the corpus callosum in a child who died at 1 year of age. Although the changes in some ways resembled those of van Bogaert–Bertrand spongy degeneration,[132] it was thought that they were probably different.

The first case of Gerritsen and Waisman[37] showed multiple pulmonary emboli, the patient having died at 1 year of age. Two 9-year-old patients of Brenton and associates[8] died of pulmonary embolus after eye surgery. Thrombosis of the portal vein was the cause of death in one patient of our series (Case 8).

Fatty liver has been found in several cases and is correlated with hepatomegaly observed clinically. A twofold increase in the neutral lipids of liver was measured by Carson and colleagues.[17]

Basic defect and pathogenesis

Deficient activity of the enzyme cystathionine synthetase (or synthase; both terms are used in the literature) has been demonstrated in the liver[82] and brain[80] of affected persons. Affected persons have less than 5% of normal activity. (The enzyme is normally absent from erythrocytes, leukocytes, platelets, skin, and intestinal mucosa.) Although threonine deaminase[42] and serine deaminase[103] activities are demonstrated by cystathionine synthetase of the rat, threonine deaminase activity was found[83] to be normal in a homocystinuric patient. Cystathionine synthetase is normally demonstrable by direct assay mainly in two tissues, liver and brain. (Kidney, pancreas, small intestinal mucosa, and fat also show cystathionine synthetase activity.) Enzymatic diagnosis of homocystinuria previously necessitated liver biopsy. Uhlendorf and Mudd[120] found, however, that cultured fibroblasts derived from skin biopsy material display cystathionine synthetase activity in normal persons and absence of this activity (or very low levels) in affected persons. (Heterozygotes can be identified by an intermediate level of enzyme activity on liver biopsy material, but the skin culture material shows too much overlap with the two homozygous groups. Goldstein et al.[41a] found that in phytohemagglutinin-stimulated lymphocytes heterozygotes could be identified by an intermediate level of enzyme activity.) The explanation for the discrepancy between intact and cultured skin may be one of the following: (1) a cell type that is present in only small numbers in the intact skin but preferentially proliferates in culture may have high cystathionine synthetase activity or (2) fibroblasts that normally do not have cystathionine synthetase activity undergo modulation or dedifferentiation.

Reasoning from the elevation of homocystine and methionine in the blood and the position of cystathionine synthetase in the metabolic chain leading from methionine to cystine (Fig. 4-13), one is forced to conclude that homocystinuria is not due to a renal tubular defect, as exists in cystinuria, but is a variety of overflow aminoaciduria consequent to a specific Garrodian inborn error of metabolism. (Actually there is no renal threshold for homocystine.)

The conversion of methionine to cystine has been shown to proceed as outlined in abbreviated form in Fig. 4-13. (See reference 78.) Homocystinurics fail to demonstrate the normal increase in urinary inorganic sulfate when a methionine load is administered.[65] With cystine loading, however, urinary inorganic sulfate rises in a normal manner. Peptide-bound methionine is increased in the urine to levels actually exceeding that of homocystine.[65] The accumulation of homocystine is probably partially counteracted by transmethylation of homocysteine back to methionine, since Brenton and co-workers[8] found that the activities of betaine-homocysteine transmethylase and of thetin methyl transferase are normal in homocystinuric liver.

As in most inborn errors of metabolism, two main alternatives exist as to origin of pathologic changes: (1) deficiency of substances distal to the block may result in pathologic manifestations or (2) substances accumulating proximal to the block may have toxic effects. The two possibilities are, of course, not mutually exclusive.

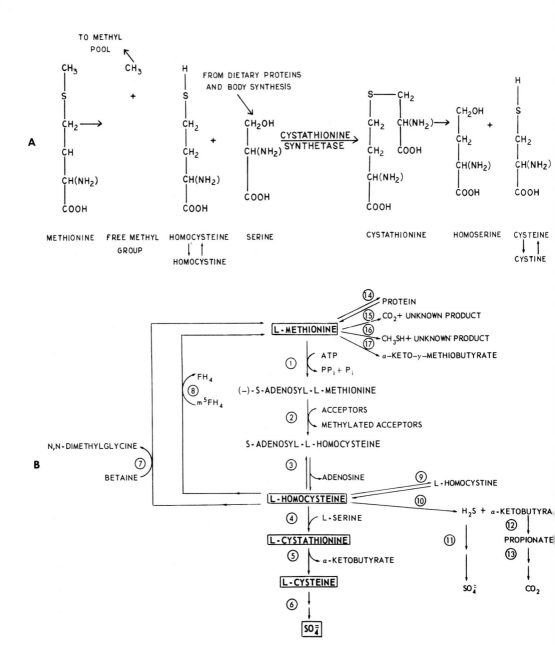

Fig. 413. **A,** Abbreviated schema of the metabolic pathway from methionine to cystine. Cystathionine synthetase activity in liver is very low in patients with homocystinuria. **B,** Detailed diagram of known pathways of mammalian metabolism of methionine and homocysteine. Abbreviations: ATP, adenosine triphosphate; PP_i, inorganic pyrophosphate; P_i, inorganic phosphate; FH_4, tetrahydrofolic acid; m^5FH_4, N^5-methyltetrahydrofolic acid. (**B** courtesy Dr. J. D. Finkelstein, Washington, D. C.)

Only limited information is available on pathologic effects of increased concentrations of homocystine[60] or other metabolites of methionine.

Cystathionine is normally found in brain tissue, in relatively abundant amounts,[52,116] and is absent from the brain of the homocystinuric.[8,37] In fact its concentration is normally higher in the brain than in other tissues and higher in the brain of man than of other species.[116] Cystathionine synthetase is normally present in the brain but was absent in one case of homocystinuria studied by Mudd.[80] Whether the deficiency of cystathionine is itself responsible for the mental retardation and psychic changes in homocystinuria is unknown. It is also useless to speculate about the reason for the variation in degree of mental retardation, from none to very severe. Whereas most of the homocystinurics studied have essentially no cystathionine synthetase activity in the liver, a 24-year-old patient with homocystine in the urine, who had normal mentality and had no other clinical features of homocystinuria, showed about 12% residual activity.[30] The interpretation of this puzzling case, in a patient who had a relative with typical features, remains in doubt.

Preliminary studies of homocystinurics using S^{35}-labeled methionine suggest that little if any radioactivity appears in cystine.[8] Absence of cystathionine synthetase might make the affected person dependent on absorbable dietary cystine for protein synthesis. Unfortunately, the disulfide cystine is relatively insoluble and therefore not well absorbed. During periods of rapid growth, dietary cystine might be insufficient for anabolic requirements. It has been suggested[16] that affected infants receiving cow's milk in the first weeks of life may be less adequately nourished than those breast-fed, since cow's milk is a much poorer source of cystine.[108]

Are the changes in connective tissue elements of the eye, skeleton, and arteries due to a relative deficiency of cysteine and cystine? Since collagen is notably deficient in sulfur-containing amino acids,[17] a deficiency in an amino acid-building block for collagen is not likely to be responsible for the connective tissue changes. (Deasy[25] found homocystine or homocysteine in steerhide corium and kangaroo rat tendon.) It is possible that the metabolism of acid mucopolysaccharides suffers from a deficiency of sulfate donor and that as a secondary result collagen synthesis, in which mucopolysaccharide plays a role (p. 49), suffers. Since glutathione contains cystine, it is also possible that glutathione-dependent reactions are retarded. Interference with collagen cross-linking by homocysteine is yet another possibility.

Ectopia lentis might be a consequence of cystine deficiency. Normally, rapid increases in beta crystallin of the lens, which has a high cystine content,[90] occurs in early embryonic growth.[98] Furthermore, the lens becomes isolated early in embryonic life and is dependent on its own enzymes for synthesis of necessary protein constituents. Dardenne and Kirsten[24] found that the lens has the capacity to convert methionine to cystine by the pathway shown in Fig. 4-13. They stated that "the autonomy of the metabolism of the sulfur-containing amino acids is a consequence of the ontogenetically very early separation of the lens. In the human embryo of 12 mm. length, the lens is already completely separated from surrounding tissue."*

---

*From Dardenne, V., and Kirsten, G.: Exp. Eye Res. 1:415, 1962.

Another possible connection between cysteine deficiency and ectopia lentis is suggested by the lens's high content,[20,59,90] especially in its cortex, of glutathione, a tripeptide containing cysteine as one of its three constituent amino acids. It is of interest, although the precise significance is not known, that ectopia lentis occurs with an enzymatic defect later in the pathway for metabolism of sulfur amino acids—sulfite oxidase deficiency.[84] The deficient enzyme normally catalyzes conversion of sulfite to sulfate.

It is of possible significance to the pathogenesis of ectopia lentis in homocystinuria that in hyperlysinemia the patients may have ectopia lentis as well as "muscular and ligamentous asthenia," i.e., joint laxity.[107,128,128a] Woody[128a] suggested that incorporation of lysine into protein is defective in hyperlysinemia. Lysine of collagen is involved in its intermolecular and intramolecular cross-linkage (p. 41).

The above suggestions on the relationship between cystine deficiency and connective tissue changes are largely speculative. Current thinking about the pathogenesis of the connective tissue manifestations, such as ectopia lentis and osteoporosis, centers more on the effects on collagen of an excess of sulfhydryl-containing compounds. Harris and Sjoerdsma[48] demonstrated a decrease in cross-linking of collagen in skin from patients with homocystinuria. Specifically they found an excess of alpha, or monomer, collagen relative to the amount of beta, or dimer, collagen. Homocysteine bears a structural resemblance to penicillamine, which has been found to affect cross-linking in collagen;[47,86] clinical abnormalities presumably related to changes in skin collagen and referred to as thiolism have been observed in patients under prolonged therapy with penicillamine for Wilson's disease[97] or cystinosis. A particularly dramatic case of connective tissue disorder produced by penicillamine is that reported by Mjølnerød et al.[78a] A young woman who had been treated with 2 grams of D-penicillamine daily during pregnancy gave birth to an infant with lax skin, hyperflexibility, venous fragility and varicosities, and impaired wound healing.

Clinically there is no evidence of abnormality of insulin or posterior pituitary hormone—proteins with high cystine content. The coarse hair of the homocystinuric may reflect an abnormality of keratin, which also has a high cystine content. However, the main feature of the hair in homocystinurics, its light color, is probably an effect of high levels of amino acids, e.g., methionine, on tyrosinase activity. A comparable mechanism appears to be responsible for the light pigmentation in phenylketonuria.

Many of the clinical and anatomic changes are the result of arterial stenosis or occlusion. McDonald and colleagues[75] claimed that platelet adhesiveness is increased in homocystinuria. Using a different method, we demonstrated no abnormality of platelet adhesiveness in patients in our series. Cline et al.,[20a] however, confirmed increased platelet adhesiveness and found that the platelets from 3 patients with homocystinuria aggregated more rapidly and formed larger aggregates in response to thrombin, epinephrine, and collagen suspension than did platelets of normal subjects. By electron microscopy, Gröbe and von Bassewitz[42a] found vacuolation of the cytoplasm of platelets in 6 patients with homocystinuria. This they interpreted as evidence of a role of platelets in the thromboses.

The drastic changes in vessel walls may be a partial explanation for the thrombotic changes. Microscopic cracks in the tunica intima might, for example, create foci[131] for aggregation of platelets, initiating thrombosis. The clinical course in several patients suggests that hypertension accelerates the thrombotic process, probably through increased dilatation of the defective vessels.

McCully and Ragsdale[74] pointed out that arteriosclerosis-like changes occur in both homocystinuria and in the homocystinuric disorder due to deficiency of N^5-methyltetrahydrofolate homocysteine methyl transferase.[85] They postulated that homocysteine affects the structure of proteoglycans of the vessel wall. *In vitro* support for the hypothesis was obtained by the study of cultured fibroblasts from skin. A role of methionine derivatives of wider significance, in arteriosclerosis in general, was suggested by these workers.[73,73a]

Ratnoff[95] found that homocystine accelerated clotting *in vitro* and suggested that activation of the Hageman factor (factor XII) is responsible. The fact that homocystine promotes kinin formation, as assayed by the rat uterus method, supports the suggestion. Vasoactive substances in the kinin system may be responsible for the malar flush in homocystinuria.

Heterogeneity

Genetic heterogeneity, which is becoming recognized as a feature of most hereditary disorders, is, of course, illustrated by the separation of homocystinuria from the Marfan syndrome. Further, heterogeneity undoubtedly exists within the homocystinuria category. In addition to (1) the rare defect in vitamin B_{12} metabolism that leads to homocystine in the urine and (2) deficiency of sulfite oxidase, which leads to clinical features somewhat like those in classic homocystinuria, including ectopia lentis, there appear to be at least two varieties of homocystinuria. The existence of two forms is suggested by the response to vitamin B_6 in pharmacologic dosage in some patients and not in others (p. 254) and by the presence of profound mental retardation in some patients and superior intelligence in others. As stated later, most patients of normal intelligence respond to vitamin B_6; response is not predictable in the retarded patients.

It seems inescapable that a mild form of homocystinuria exists and represents an entity distinct from that first described by Carson and Neill[18] and from that found in some of the severely affected patients in this series.

I have had an opportunity to observe several families with an unusually mild variety of homocystinuria. Of these, I shall detail four and a possible fifth.

Family A.* One family was ascertained through a 26-year-old doctoral candidate (born 1941), the oldest of 8 sibs, when he developed acute glaucoma from pupillary block in the right eye (Fig. 4-14*A*). Ectopia lentis had first been found at the age of 24 years, a diagnosis of Marfan syndrome was made at that time. He was a graduate of a well-known preparatory school and of one of our most prestigious universities. He was studying for his doctorate in psychology at the time of ascertainment. He had had asthma in childhood beginning at age 18 months and continuing until the late teens; it was precipitated by situational factors. Chest deformity (Fig. 4-14*B*) had rather abrupt onset at the age of 11 or 12 years and was attributed to asthma. There have been no fractures or vascular episodes. This man is now a university instructor; he is married and has one child, apparently healthy.

Of his sibs, the 2 youngest girls have homocystine in the urine. They were born in 1953 and 1958. Neither has ectopia lentis but both have severe myopia. The only peculiarity found was mild generalized osteoporosis and gracile bones of the limbs with mild bowing in the younger of the 2 sibs. Full-scale IQ was estimated at 130 in both.

---

*The first four families are among the 45 kindreds on whom the analyses presented on p. 252 are based. They are indicated here by letters rather than numbers to avoid confusion with the first 20 of the 45 families, which are detailed on pp. 256 to 275.

Fig. 4-14. Mild homocystinuria in T. K. (J.H.H. 1273175; Kindred 39), 26 years old. **A,** Note height and lack of conspicuous skeletal deformity of the type shown in Fig. 4-1. **B,** Note crowded teeth and chest deformity.

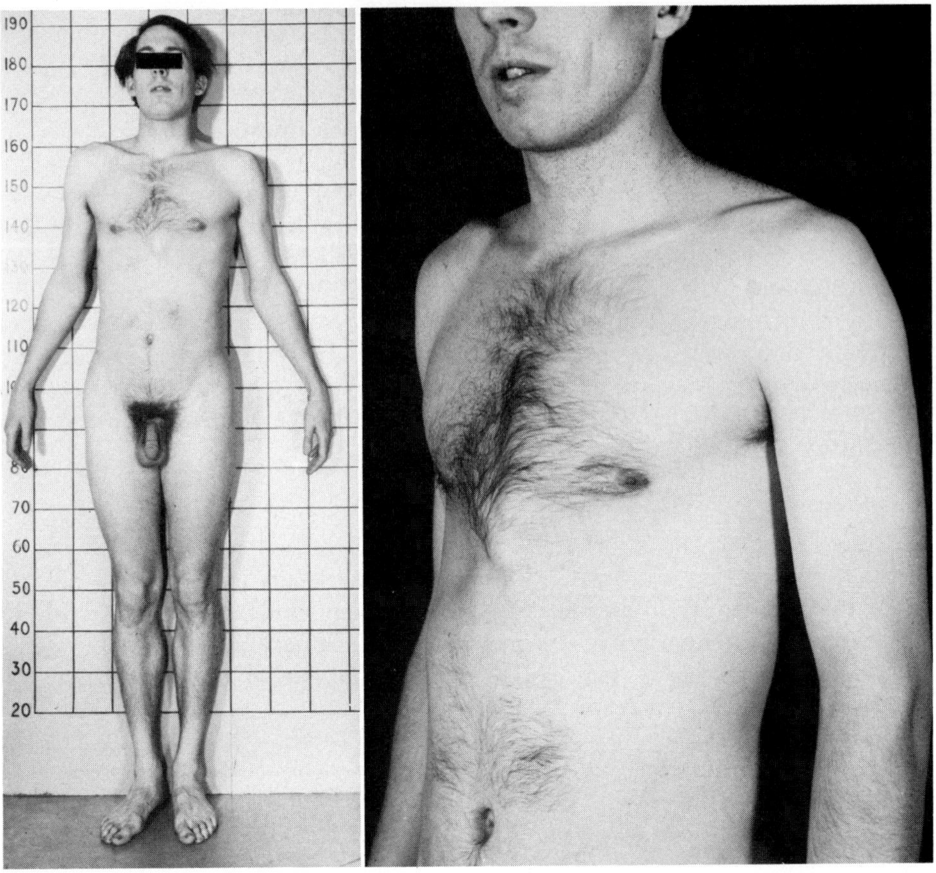

The administration of vitamin B_6 effected a clearing of homocystine from the urine in all 3 sibs.

Family B. A second family contained only a single affected person, a girl born in 1959. Although ectopia lentis was discovered at the age of 3 years, she has had no evident impairment of intellect (IQ = 110), no seizure disturbance, no osteoporosis, and no vascular complications. Low methionine diet and later vitamin B_6 therapy cleared the urine of homocystine and led to darkening of the hair.

Family C. A third family likewise has a single affected person (Fig. 4-15), a man now 52 years old (Kindred 15). Visual difficulties began at about 20 years of age, and subluxation of the lenses was first detected at 25 years. He served as a captain in an airborne division in France during World War II. He earned a B.S. degree in chemistry before the war and a B.S. degree in chemical technology after the war. After an automobile accident in 1944, swelling of the legs developed; thrombosis of the inferior vena cava was diagnosed. In 1954 venous stripping was performed in both legs for varicose veins. In recent years the patient has had several episodes of thrombophlebitis in the legs; he has chronic edema and intermittent ulceration. His face is notably plethoric, with "high coloration." He is employed as a food technologist. He has 2 sons and 4 daughters, all healthy (Fig. 4-16, Kindred 15).

Family D. The fourth kindred with mild homocystinuria is one I saw in Sydney, Australia, with Dr. Brian Turner, who has investigated the family and kindly allows me to include

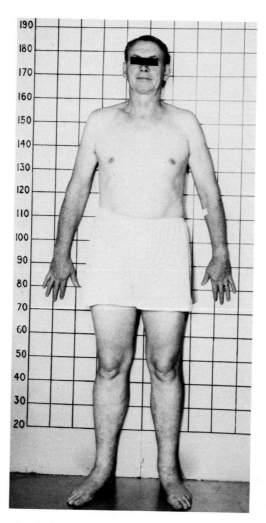

Fig. 4-15. Mild homocystinuria in I. M. (J.H.H. 1159640; Kindred 15), at the age of 48 years. Note height and lack of conspicuous skeletal deformity, and chronic edema of the legs and ankles. The face is unusually red.

a brief description here. The proband was a severely retarded 9-year-old boy. He was born, the second of male twins, weighing 3.07 kg. In the first day of life he developed congestive cardiac failure, and he had mild twitching in the first week. Definite seizures began at 7 months, and the electroencephalogram was abnormal; at the age of 3½ years he was admitted to an institution for the severely and permanently retarded. He first came to attention at the age of 9 years when a urinary tract infection was being investigated. The nitroprusside test was positive. Further studies confirmed the presence of homocystine in the urine and elevated plasma methionine. A large bladder calculus of mixed composition was found. Examination at 9 years of age showed no ectopia lentis, although high-grade myopia was present.

In the proband's sibship the oldest is a 13-year-old boy who is clinically and biochemically normal. The second child is an 11-year-old female who has mild pectus excavatum, a highly arched palate, US/LS value of 0.83, no ocular abnormality, and high normal intelligence. Homocystine is demonstrable in the urine, and a plasma methionine level of 0.053 micromole/ml. was measured. Hematologic findings were normal, and no methylmalonic acid was demon-

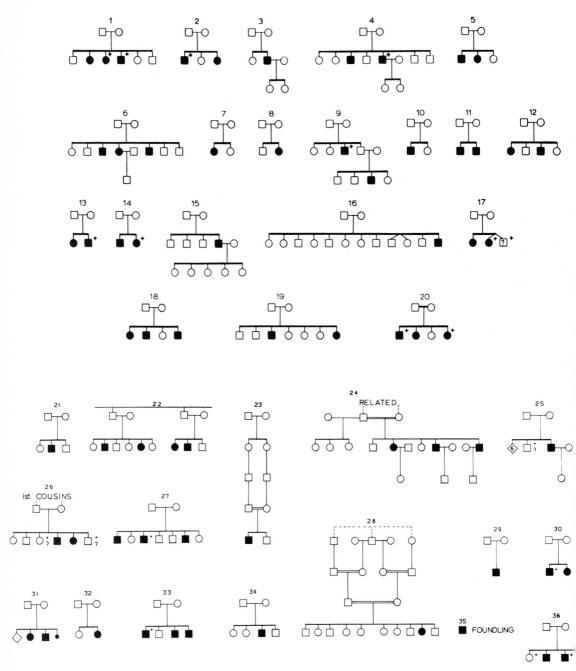

Fig. 4-16. Fragment pedigrees of forty-five personally studied kindreds with one or more homo-cystinuric. The parents were first cousins in Families 20 and 26 and were related as indicated in Families 23, 24, and 28. The slant line in Pedigree 44 indicates a person who may be a mani-festing heterozygote (M. A. G. in reference 30).

strated in the urine. The third child is the first-born co-twin of the proband; the twins have been shown to be dizygotic by blood grouping. He has high normal intelligence, mild pectus excavatum, and a US/LS value of 0.89. He has occasional petit mal seizures. The biochemical findings are identical to those in his severely retarded twin and his 11-year-old sister. Pyridoxine, 499 mg./day, cleared the urine of homocystine in all 3 homocystinuric sibs, caused cessation of petit mal episodes in the nonretarded twin, and resulted in authenticated improvement in concentration and scholastic performance in both him and his 11-year-old sister.

I interpret this kindred as having, like the first kindred, mild homocystinuria, brought to attention because of a severely retarded member of the family. I suggest that the retardation is due to the combination of the traumatic birth of the second twin and homocystinuria; that is, intracranial thromboses may have exaggerated the brain damage that would have occurred even in the absence of homocystinuria.

Family E. Not included in the 45 kindreds is one ascertained through a woman then 86 years old. In 1936, at 57 years of age, she had two operations for retinal detachment performed at the Mayo Clinic. At that time she also showed dislocated lenses in both eyes. When next seen at the Medical Center in Iowa City in 1957 (at the age of 78 years), she showed bilateral elevation of intraocular pressure, partial subluxation of the right lens, and dislocation of the left lens inferiorly into the vitreous. The left eye was sightless as a result of retinal detachment. It was because of the ectopia lentis that she was included in the nationwide urine screening survey that we initiated in 1964. Two screening tests were positive, and high-voltage paper electrophoresis confirmed the presence of homocystine. At that time the patient was in a home for the elderly in Iowa. Before further studies could be undertaken, she died at the age of 89 years. She was known to have both thoracic and abdominal aortic aneurysms. Her terminal illness was characterized by uremia; dissection of the aorta was suspected, but no autopsy was performed.

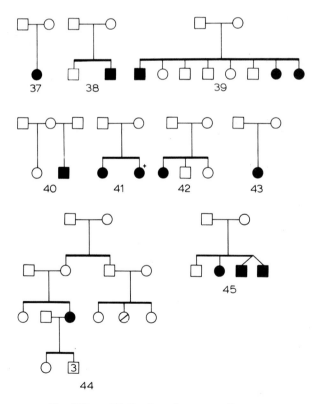

Fig. 4-16, cont'd. For legend see opposite page.

In her later years the patient had multiple attacks of phlebitis, complained of ankle pain but had no ulcers, and wore elastic stockings. A cerebrovascular accident occurred at 72 years of age. She had no other illnesses, although she was said to have had spastic colitis for many years.

The patient was about 66 inches tall. No spinal curvature or chest deformity was recorded in the medical records or recalled by her daughter, who is the main informant. She had 3 children. One, a boy was, dead at birth because of eclamptic convulsions in the mother; the second, also a boy, died of meningitis at 12 years of age; the third is the daughter, who provided most of the information. Through the daughter, the patient had 4 grandchildren and 12 great-grandchildren.

Proof of homocystinuria would be possible by demonstrating depressed levels of cystathionine synthetase in biopsy material from the proband's daughter, who must be heterozygous, if the mother was a homozygote.

Seashore et al.[102a] suggested that there may be two types of vitamin B_6 responders: those in whom cystathionine synthetase activity is increased by vitamin B_6 and those in whom increased metabolism of homocysteine must have some other mechanism.

Prevalence and inheritance

I previously had thought that homocystinuria might have a frequency of about 1 in 30,000 births, and that it might compete with galactosemia for second position in frequency, next to phenylketonuria, among specifically identified inborn errors of metabolism that lead to mental retardation. Newborn screening programs, however, have shown an extraordinarily low frequency of homocystinuria—2 in about 400,000 newborns.[43] The test used measures methionine by a Guthrie type of bacterial assay. Part of the screening was done in the Commonwealth of Massachusetts, which has a large segment of its population drawn from the area where the original cases of homocystinuria were identified, i.e., Ireland.

Possibly cases of homocystinuria are being missed in the newborn screening. Levy[66] found one infant who had normal methionine levels at 4 days and elevated methionine at 4 weeks of age, whereas 2 others had elevated methionine levels at both times. The first infant was "a vitamin-B_6 responder" and also responded unusually well to a low methionine diet. The other two were nonresponders to vitamin B_6. It is entirely possible that low methionine intake, deficient vitamin B_{12} or folic acid, low betaine or choline intake, high vitamin B_6 intake, or some combination thereof, might result in false negative tests for homocystinuria in the newborn period.

If homocystinurics have a fitness of 0, that is, if none reproduces, and heterozygotes have a fitness of 1.0 (the population average), then the mutation rate (μ) is equal to the frequency of homozygotes. One in 200,000 would be a lower mutation rate than has been calculated for most other traits in man. Estimating that the fitness of homocystinurics is 10% that of the general population, then the estimate of the mutation rate becomes even lower. These considerations suggest that 1 in 200,000 is too low an estimate of the frequency of homocystinuria.

An educated guest on the frequency of homocystinuria is provided by the mutation rate formula, assuming fitness of 0.1 and average fitness (1.0) of heterozygotes:

$$\mu = q^2(1 - f)$$

$$\hat{q}^2 = \frac{2 \times 10^{-5}}{0.9} = \frac{1}{45,000}$$

The value for mutation rate (1 in 50,000) is approximately average.[123]

Special factors, such as founder effect and random genetic drift, based on small population size at some stage in its history, could account for an increase in the frequency in particular groups. There is no evidence for or against a heterozygote advantage. In view of the seemingly low frequency of homocystinuria, a general advantage of heterozygotes in unlikely. An advantage under certain environmental circumstances, past or present, could, of course, also account for a relatively high frequency in some groups. The only group in which an increased frequency has been suspected is that of the Irish. Carson[14] stated that 20 cases of homocystinuria are known in Northern Ireland, which has a population of about 1.5 million, or 1 in 75,000, not a particularly high value. In Iceland, with a population of 200,000, 2 apparently unrelated cases of homocystinuria were diagnosed by Halldorsson,[45] but this was not necessarily a total ascertainment because the cases were recognized by clinical features, not in a screening program.

Among institutionalized mental defectives in this country, Spaeth and Barber[110] found that homocystinuria had a frequency of about 0.02% (1 in 5000).

In an apparently comparable population of mental defectives in Northern Ireland, Carson and associates[16] found a frequency of 0.3% (15 in 5000).

Among about 700 families with ectopia lentis, my colleagues and I[102] found that 35 had one or more member with homocystinuria. Thus about 5% of nontraumatic ectopia lentis is "caused" by homocystinuria.

The ethnic distribution of cases is wide. A number of Irish kindreds are included in our series, and the frequency of the homocystinuria gene may be somewhat higher in Americans of Irish extraction than in other Americans. The frequency is not likely, however, to be more than a few times higher—certainly there is no concentration of the gene in the Irish comparable to that of the Tay-Sachs gene in Ashkenazim. The remarkable feature is the wide representation of ethnic extractions in this series and in the literature: Swedish,[46] German, Dutch, Jewish, Polish, French,[32] southern Italian, and Lithuanian.[82] O'Brien (discussion of reference 33) commented on rather numerous cases among Spanish-Americans living in Denver. We had no Oriental cases but have screened few Oriental families; homocystinuria has been observed in Japanese.[115,130] Several Negro families have been reported (No. 26 of this series).[44,93,117,126] Homocystinuria has been observed in India.[122]

Like all other Garrodian inborn errors of metabolism, homocystinuria is inherited as a recessive, in this case an autosomal recessive. The evidence consists of the facts that both males and females are affected, brothers and sisters with normal parents are observed, parental consanguinity has an increased frequency, and both parents of affected persons, although clinically normal, show about half the normal level of hepatic cystathionine synthetase activity.[30]

Although the above evidence, particularly the enzymatic findings in parents, is adequately convincing of recessive inheritance, it is of interest to perform segregation analysis as a check on randomness or completeness of ascertainment,

Table 4-1. A segregation analysis by a priori method that assumes random ascertainment of affected sibships[147]

Sibship size	Number of sibs	Number of sibs affected	No sibs affected	
			Expected	**Variance**
1	5	5	5.0000	0.00000
2	13	18	14.8572	1.59185
3	7	12	9.0790	1.84100
4	10	22	14.6280	4.20050
5	1	3	1.6389	0.50178
6	3	7	4.9167	2.32770
7	4	10	8.0784	3.88096
8	2	4	4.4450	2.34480
9	—	—	—	—
10	1	1	2.6490	1.59170
11	—	—	—	—
12	1	1	3.5630	2.44600
	47	83	68.8552	20.72629

S.D. = 4.55261

$$\text{Deviation of observed from expected} = \frac{83 - 68.8552}{4.55261} = 3.107 \text{ S.D.}$$

or distortion of segregation. In other words, a deviation from the expected proportion of affected offspring would require explanation.

As can be seen from Table 4-1, the number of affected, on the assumption of either complete ascertainment or random ascertainment of affected *sibships,* exceeds that expected by more than three standard deviations. Although inaccurate diagnosis in presumed affected sibs of living cases is possible, it is more likely that the probability of ascertainment in this study was related to the number of sibs affected. When the correction appropriate for random ascertainment of affected *individuals* is used—subtracting one affected for each sibship (N) from both the affected group (R) and the total group of sibs (I)—the proportion of affected sibs approaches the expected 25% closely.

$$\hat{q} = \frac{R - N}{T - N} = \frac{84 - 48}{184 - 48} = 0.26471$$

$$\text{S.D.} = \sqrt{\frac{(83 - 47) \times (181 - 83)}{[(83 - 47) + (181 - 83)]^3}} = 0.03829$$

$$\text{Deviation of observed from expected} = \frac{0.25 - 0.2687}{0.03829} = 0.4872 \text{ S.D.}$$

Incomplete single ascertainment, that is, random ascertainment of affected individuals, means that whereas the chance of ascertaining any particularly affected person is low, a given sibship has a probability of entering the series, which is directly proportional to the number of sibs affected. For example, a 3-sib family with all 3 sibs affected has three times' greater probability of being included in the sample than a 3-sib family with only 1 sib affected. In retrospect it is plausible that this situation would have obtained in this series since such a large proportion of the families were ascertained through eye clinics.

Until recently, no reliable method for identifying the heterozygote, short of enzyme assays of liver biopsy material, has been devised. The enzyme activity of fibroblasts grown from heterozygotes shows too much overlap with that of fibroblasts from normal homozygotes to be depended on.[120] Goldstein and his collaborators[41a] found that in phytohemagglutinin-stimulated blood lymphocytes, heterozygotes can be identified by an intermediate level of enzyme activity.

Nine of the 83 affected persons in this series (7 males, 2 females) in 8 kindreds have had a total of 17 children. None of the 17 children is homocystinuric, as predicted by the recessive hypothesis; they represent, however, a series of obligatory heterozygotes for study of possible manifestations. In estimating the fitness of a given genotype, selection of the appropriate comparison group is usually a problem. It is clear, however, that the average reproductive fitness of the homocystinuric homozygote is severely reduced; fitness is probably between 0.05 and 0.1, the normal value being 1.0. The reduced reproductive fitness is apparently due mainly to reduced survivorship (Fig. 4-12).

Because of the mental defects and the malformations that occur in the children of phenylketonuric women,[53] the status of the offspring of homocystinuric women in this series was examined closely. No relevant abnormality was detected in the son of the homocystinuric woman in Kindred 6, studied in a hospital. This same patient, since the preparation of the pedigrees shown in Fig. 4-16, was delivered of a markedly hydrocephalic infant, stillborn as a result of a decompression procedure done to permit delivery. Although no autopsy was done, the infant was said to have been normally formed except for the hydrocephalus.

One patient with normal mentality and no other clinical signs of homocystinuria, the cousin of a "typical" case, had a lesser degree of homocystinuria and enzyme activity about 12% of normal.[30] The genetic basis of this difference is unclear.

The vitamin B_6-responsive and B_6-nonresponsive forms of homocystinuria may be the result of allelic mutations. However, cystathionine synthetase of rat liver has two structurally different subunits, presumably under the control of different genetic loci.[56a] The same is probably true for man. Thus there may be nonallelic varieties of homocystinuria.

Management

Specific therapy for the metabolic defect of homocystinuria has been largely low methionine diet and supplementation with pyridoxine (vitamin B_6).

The rationale of a low methionine diet is the same as for a low phenylalanine diet in phenylketonuria: the accumulated metabolites proximal to the site of enzyme block (Fig. 4-13) are toxic and can be reduced by restriction of input to the relevant metabolic pathway.[17,46,100] Since cystine becomes an essential amino acid in the homocystinuric patient, supplementation of the low methionine diet with cystine seems logical. Komrower and associates[63] and Schimke and colleagues,[102] among others, provided details on the composition and preparation of the low methionine diet. Perry and associates[89] have also used a methyl donor, choline, in connection with the low methionine diet. The rationale is that choline assists the remethylation of homocysteine to methionine. Others[97] have used betaine on the basis of a similar rationale. Perry[88] has strong evidence for the beneficial effects of the low methionine diet; a homocystinuric sib of a severely affected child has had diototherapy from birth and has developed normally without signs of the metabolic defect. The child was 6 years old in 1971.

It has also been shown that the homocystinuric can synthesize cystathionine from homoserine and cysteine because of the bidirectional nature of the enzyme reaction, shown as unidirectional in Fig. 4-13. Reasoning that deficiency of cystathionine may be an important factor in the mental retardation (p. 243), Wong and co-workers[127] have suggested treatment with homoserine and cystine.

Treatment with folic acid, which is involved in the salvage pathway by which homocystine is remethylated to methionine, has also been recommended.[12] With folic acid administration, homocystine in the urine is reduced and methionine increased.

The simplest and in some patients the most effective therapy for homocystinuria is vitamin B_6 in pharmacologic dosage (50 to 300 mg./day). Homocystinuria is a vitamin-dependent inborn error of metabolism, one of a group that also includes methylmalonic aciduria, cystathioninuria, pyridoxine-responsive anemia, and xanthurenic aciduria.[96a] Like some of the others, homocystinuria exists in both vitamin B_6–responsive forms and in nonresponsive forms.[15,21,34,51,56,119] Most clinically mildly affected cases of homocystinuria have the vitamin B_6–responsive type. It is difficult to predict responsiveness in more severely affected patients, but in very severely affected patients, vitamin-B_6 responsiveness is rare. The genetic distinctness between the vitamin B_6–responsive types and the nonresponsive types is indicated by the fact that concordance always obtains within families.[14]

Morrow[79a] has data indicating that "response" to vitamin B_6 may be blunted or abolished by folate depletion. One should be sure that folate is adequate before conclusion is made about vitamin B_6 response. Homocystinuria patients who received diphenylhydantoin (Dilantin) for seizures may become depleted of folic acid[41b] and require repletion before therapy with vitamin B_6 is effective (see Patient 15, p. 268).

Pyridoxine (vitamin B_6) is a cofactor for cystathionine synthetase. In vitamin-B_6 responders the mutation is thought so to affect the enzyme molecule that collaboration with the cofactor is defective. Only very slight increases in enzyme activity can be demonstrated after treatment—as a result, perhaps, of stabilization and delayed degradation of the enzyme. Yet Mudd and colleagues[80a,81] believe that even so slight a change may be adequate to produce clearing of the urine of homocystine. (Gaull and associates[34,35] were of the opposite view—that some other mechanism must be operative in the clearing of homocystine.) It is hoped (with some justification) that the development of complications may be prevented—for example, ectopia lentis in the teen-age vitamin B_6–responsive homocystinuric sisters of the patient shown in Fig. 4-14. One of the objective signs of effects of vitamin B_6 is darkening of the hair. Pictures have been published of a band of dark hair in an affected girl who was on vitamin B_6 intermittently.[3]

Since enhanced platelet aggregation may be the leading factor in thrombosis in homocystinuria, anticoagulants are unlikely to be of much benefit. Long-term heparin therapy is probably contraindicated because of its osteoporotic effect in a situation where osteoporosis already exists. A rational approach to therapy would appear to be use of agents such as phenylbutazone, sulfinpyrazone, dipyridamole, and chloroquine, which inhibit platelet aggregation and/or release of platelet constituents when the agent is given in doses without major side effects.[85d] Acetylsalicylic acid also has platelet suppressive effects,[27a] but its irritative effects on the gastrointestinal tract limit its usefulness in homocystinuria. Homocystinuric patients who are unresponsive to vitamin B_6 should, it would seem, be maintained on a diet reduced in methionine with supplemental cystine and with maintenance doses of one of the above platelet-suppressing agents. A controlled study of these agents in vitamin B_6–unresponsive homocystinurics is indicated. Their use in patients undergoing surgery might be particularly worthwhile. The pill should probably be avoided by women with homocystinuria because of its thrombogenic hazards.

Other considerations

Differentiation from the Marfan syndrome is summarized in Table 4-2. Patients with homocystinuria have been reported as instances of the Marfan syndrome.[68,69] All the patients described in detail below were considered at one time to have the Marfan syndrome. Family A, reported by Lynas[69] as showing the Marfan syndrome, has been found to have homocystinuria. One can speculate about the diagnosis in other reported cases, for example, the patient with presumed Marfan syndrome and thrombotic occlusion of the aorta described by Dexter and associates.[26] The parents were related but unaffected. Follow-up in 1964 showed* that the patient died in 1962 at the age of 42 years of acute myocardial infarction and hypertension; autopsy was not performed.

Phenylketonuria in the mother results in congenital defects in the children. We have been unable to convince ourselves of any unusual incidence of congenital defects among the children of homocystinuric women; however, see Case 12, p. 268, for description of hydrocephalus in the offspring of such a woman.

Other "causes" of homocystinuria. In addition to deficiency of cystathionine synthetase, homocystinuria has been observed with three other rare genetic disorders: (1) deficiency of $N^{5,10}$-methylenetetrahydrofolate reductase,[85b] (2) a defect in vitamin B_{12} metabolism, and (3) a selective defect in intestinal absorption of vitamin B_{12}.

Freeman et al.[30a] studied a 15-year-old, mildly retarded Negro female with a two-year history of progressive withdrawal, hallucinations, delusions, and catatonia unresponsive to psychotherapy. Homocystinuria without elevation of plasma methionine was found. Psychotic symptoms gradually disappeared with administration of pyridoxine and folic acid. A sister had homocystinuria but no symptoms. Cystathionine synthetase and the enzymes methylating homocysteine were normal in liver and fibroblasts. A decrease was shown in methylenetetrahydrofolate reductase, the enzyme synthesizing N^5-methyltetrahydrofolate. Shih et al.[104a] found the same enzyme deficiency in a 16-year-old boy with proximal muscle weakness, waddling gait, and episodes of flinging movements

---

*Follow-up information courtesy Dr. Lyman O. Warren, Bay Pines, Fla.

of the upper limbs. Although the same enzyme was implicated in the patients of Freeman and Shih,[85b] the phenotypic differences and the fact that only Shih's patient showed reduction in homocystinuria with administration of flavin adenine dinucleotide suggests that the disorders may be determined by different but allelic mutations.

Mudd et al.[85,85a,85c] described the biochemical findings in an infant boy, E. M., who died at $7\frac{1}{2}$ weeks of age. This oft reported case[66a,70b,73,85,85a,85c] showed homocystinemia, cystathioninemia and cystathioninuria, decrease in blood methionine, and methylmalonicaciduria. Deficient activity was found in the two enzymes dependent on B_{12} derivatives as enzymes: (1) methyltetrahydrofolate methyltransferase, which catalyzes the formation of methionine from 5-methyltetrahydrofolate and homocysteine, and (2) methylmalonyl-CoA isomerase, which catalyzes the isomerization of methylmalonyl-CoA to succinyl-CoA. These are the two reactions known to require vitamin B_{12}. Thus the homocystinuria and methylmalonicaciduria are explained. Since vitamin B_{12} was present in normal concentrations in the liver, Mudd and his colleagues concluded that the gene-determined defect probably concerned the conversion of vitamin B_{12} to coenzymatically active derivatives. The tissue concentration of 5'-deoxyadenosylcobalamin was much reduced. The child died before definitive therapy with vitamin B_{12} and B_{12} coenzymes could be tried. Goodman et al.[40a] reported two brothers with a milder form of the same disorder. The older brother, a 14-year-old Mexican-American, was first admitted to hospital in an acute psychotic episode. He had an IQ of about 50 (Wechsler Intelligence Scale for Children), a somewhat Marfanoid habitus, and mild abnormalities on neurologic examination. Ectopia lentis and chest deformity were lacking. The parents were first cousins once removed.

Familial selective malabsorption of vitamin B_{12},[70a] something called Imerslund syndrome, may be accompanied by homocystinuria.[49b] The mechanism is the same as in the disorder with a defect in vitamin B_{12} metabolism. Proteinuria is another feature of the Imerslund disease.

In all three of these disorders lack of elevation of serum methionine can distinguish them from cystathionine synthetase deficiency. Low methionine diet might be disastrous in these cases.

Furthermore, all three of these other "causes" of homocystinuria indicate that remethylation of homocysteine by N^5-methyltetrahydrofolate methyltransferase is a physiologically important reaction.

ILLUSTRATIVE CASES

To illustrate the clinical features and natural history of homocystinuria, an account of 38 cases in 20 families is provided below. These were the first 20 families ascertained up until 1965 in this department, mainly through a urine screening program of cases of presumed Marfan syndrome and/or nontraumatic ectopia lentis seen at this hospital and at many eye clinics in this country.

Family 1

Case 1. D. Ho. (B.C.H. 328838), an 18-year-old white male, was in good health until 10 days before death. (Ectopia lentis had been noted, and mild mental retardation was evident from his school record.) Following physical exertion he noted the onset of weakness and numb-

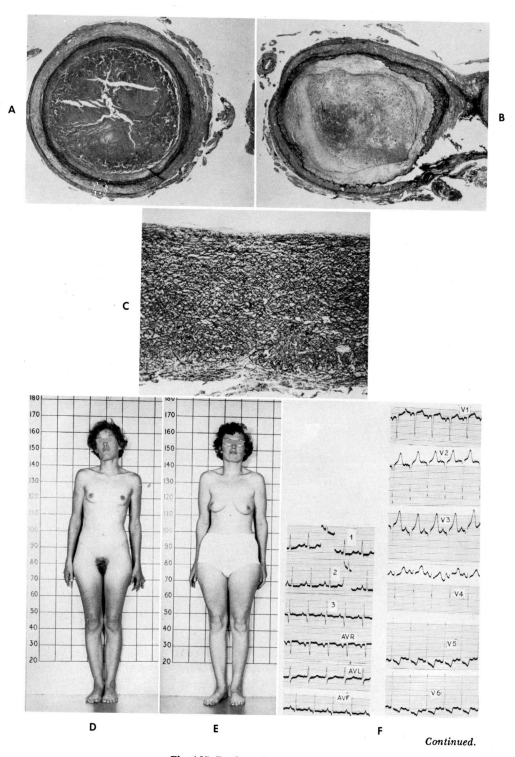

Fig. 4-17. For legend see p. 258.

Continued.

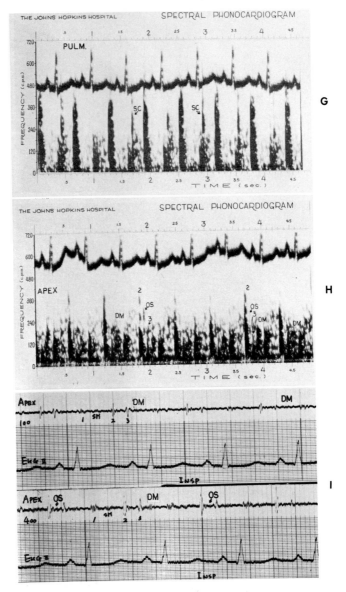

Fig. 4-17. Data on 3 homocystinuric sibs (Family 1, p. 256). **A,** Thrombosed right internal carotid artery in D. Ho., Case 1. Note thinning of tunica media with dilatation of artery. **B,** Thrombosed left internal carotid artery in same patient. Thrombosis has occurred episodically with formation of new internal elastic lamellae. **C,** An abnormal elastic weave of the aortic media was demonstrated by both longitudinal and transverse section. **D,** Body habitus in E. Ho., Case 2, age 20 years. **E,** Body habitus in J. Ho., Case 3, age 22 years. **F,** Electrocardiogram in E. Ho., Case 2, age 20 years, indicating old posterior myocardial infarction. **G** to **I,** Spectral phonocardiograms demonstrate a conspicuous systolic ejection click in the pulmonary area, **G,** and a mitral opening snap, third heart sound, and mid-diastolic murmur at the apex. **H.** The findings at the apex are confirmed by the oscillographic phonocardiogram shown in **I. J** and **K,** Coronary artery in E. Ho., Case 2. The tunica media is markedly thickened. The branch is spared. The dark-staining muscle fibers of the tunica media are separated by a ground substance. **L,** Face showing coarse wide-pored skin in J. Ho., Case 3. **M,** Spine showing osteoporosis in J. Ho., Case 3. **N,** Skull showing osteoporosis and large sinuses in J. Ho., Case 3.

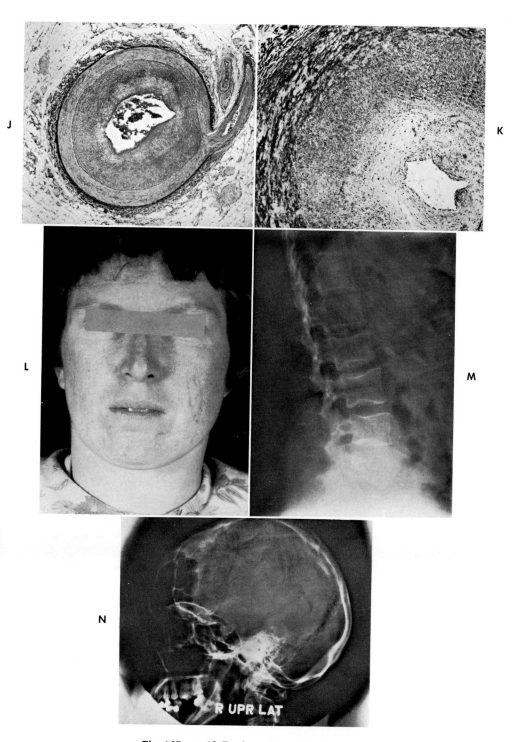

Fig. 4-17, cont'd. For legend see opposite page.

ness of the right arm and leg. Examination at that time showed the blood pressure to be 180/120 mm. Hg; no abnormal neurologic signs were detected. One week later he was admitted to the hospital for investigation of hypertension.

Physical examination showed a healthy-appearing, normally developed, and well-nourished young man. The blood pressure was 180/110 mm. Hg in both arms. Bilateral subluxation of the lenses was detected. A grade II systolic murmur was heard at the left sternal border and was not transmitted into the neck. Wide variability in intensity and some variability in quality of this murmur were noted. Pulsation was thought to be diminished in the left common carotid artery and both femoral arteries, and a loud bruit was audible over the bifurcation of the abdominal aorta and both femoral triangles. No pulses were palpable in the feet. The only abnormal neurologic finding was weakness of the right trapezius muscle.

On the day after admission to the hospital, the patient noted the sudden onset of weakness of the right arm and hand. This progressed to involve the right side of the face, and Babinski's sign was noted on the right. Retrograde aortogram demonstrated no abnormality of the major branches of the aortic arch. The right hemiparesis increased, and the patient became unresponsive to all except painful stimuli. Ophthalmodynamometry showed marked depression of arterial pressure in the left eye. A left common carotid arteriogram showed obstruction of the internal carotid artery immediately above the bifurcation. At this time cyanotic discoloration and a lack of pulsations in the right upper extremity were noted.

Surgical exploration of the left common carotid artery was performed on the fourth hospital day. A thrombus was removed from the left internal carotid for a distance of about 3 cm. beyond the bifurcation, but adequate backflow was not achieved. The patient died about 24 hours after operation.

Autopsy. Both internal carotid arteries were completely occluded proximal to the circle of Willis. On the left the thrombosis was old and organized, and on the right there was evidence of both old and recent thrombosis. Both femoral arteries and the right brachial and the right coronary artery ostia were partly occluded. The aorta showed only scattered atheromata, and no aneurysm was found in any vessel. Histologically, all large vessels showed peculiar disorganization of the medial elastic fibers but no medial necrosis. There was marked endocardial elastosis of the left atrium. The right kidney weighed 150 grams and the left kidney, 230 grams. Hypertrophy of the left ventricle suggested rather long-standing hypertension.

Comment. The hypertension is adequately accounted for by the smallness of the right kidney.

Case 2. E. Ho. (J.H.H. 1037640), the 20-year-old sister of D. Ho. (Case 1), was examined after her brother's death. She was a nervous, emotionally unstable girl. She described breathlessness and "jabby" sensations around the left breast about the time of menstruation and said she felt tired all the time. She had suffered three fractures. Her academic record in school was poor, but she completed high school at 19 years 9 months of age. Bilateral lens extraction was performed at the age of 17 years. Her blood pressure was 120/70 mm. Hg. She was 65½ inches tall, with upper segment–lower segment ratio of 1.01. Except for bilateral surgical aphakia and tachycardia, no abnormality was detected on physical examination. On a later examination, the patient complained of an ache below the left breast which occurred intermittently with either rest or exercise. The heart rate was 100/min. Third and fourth heart sound gallops were easily heard at the apex. A short musical early diastolic murmur was audible in the third left interspace close to the sternum.

An electrocardiogram showed changes interpreted as left ventricular hypertrophy and an old posterior myocardial infarction.

Six months after the first examination the patient suddenly developed chest pain and was dead on arrival at the hospital.

Autopsy (Medical Examiner). All major coronary arteries showed moderately severe atherosclerosis. Old scarring was present in the anterior part of the interventricular septum and the anterior wall of the left ventricle. Close histologic study of the coronary arteries showed the same type of change as was seen in Case 1.

Comment. If the patient had the same type of change in the left atrial endocardium as did her brother, the mitral opening snap may be no surprise. The origin of the presumed early diastolic murmur in Erb's area is not clear.

Case 3. J. Ho. (J.H.H. 1037641), the only surviving affected sib of Cases 1 and 2, was born in

1940. In 1961 she had hematemesis for which investigations uncovered no satisfactory explanation. She had always stuttered somewhat, but this became more pronounced after her hematemesis. Because of backache, intravenous pyelography was performed in 1956 and 1958, with demonstration of a bifid collecting system on the left. She also complained of ache in the left arm, unrelated to exertion. Weakness in the left leg and pain in both legs were likewise noted.

Examination in 1962 showed height of 64 inches with upper segment–lower segment ratio of 0.94. The lenses had been removed. All deep tendon reflexes were hyperactive, especially in the left leg, where ankle clonus and Babinski's sign were demonstrated.

Because of increasing nervousness and peculiar behavior, psychiatric care was required, with apparent improvement. Pain in the region of the left breast has been a frequent complaint. A fracture of the left wrist occurred with adequate trauma and healed satisfactorily. On another occasion, fracture of the coccyx resulted from slipping on the ice. Bilateral partial detachment of the retina was detected in 1964.

Her left leg becomes cyanotic if she crosses her legs for any length of time, and it becomes stiff if she is nervous or walks a long distance. Occasionally she has numbness without tingling, beginning in the fingers of the left hand and slowly progressing to involve her face. The episodes last about 10 minutes. Difficulty in picking up small objects with the left hand has been noted.

Blood pressure, normal during the early part of the period of observation, was about 155/100 mm. Hg in both arms on recent examinations. Furthermore, pulses are weak in the left carotid, radial, femoral, dorsalis pedis, and posterior tibial arteries. A faint early or mid-diastolic murmur is audible at the apex. The left leg is weak and she walks with a limp. The toenails are smaller on the left foot than on the right, and the left thumbnail is somewhat smaller than the right one. Hypalgesia of the entire left side is inconsistently present.

Laboratory evaluation showed normal hematologic studies, fasting and postprandial glucose, serum cholesterol, total serum lipids, serum electrolytes, liver function studies, urinalysis, protein-bound iodine, serum proteins, and electrocardiogram. The electroencephalogram (EEG) was abnormal, demonstrating diffuse disorganization without localization or laterlization. There were no seizure potentials. Intermittent photic stimulation did not cause activation. Hyperventilation gave rise to only a minimal increase in slowing but no abnormal discharges. The EEG pattern was essentially unchanged 2 hours after a methionine load.

Coagulation studies were performed both before and 90 minutes after an oral methionine load. They showed clotting times of 11.13 and 9.12 minutes (glass) and were essentially unchanged in silicone. Prothrombin time was 25 and 23 seconds and bleeding time was 2½ and 4½ minutes, before and after methionine. Platelets were 250,000 and 183,000/cu. mm., and partial thromboplastin time was 75 and 85 seconds. Fibrinogen was 210 mg./100 ml. and did not change. Euglobulin clot lysis time was normal both before and after methionine. None of these values or changes therein were significant. Platelet adhesiveness was considered to be within normal limits. Platelet survival was also normal.*

Chest x-ray results were normal except for some scoliosis of the thoracic spine. Skeletal x-ray films demonstrated generalized osteoporosis with early "cod-fish" changes in the lumbar vertebrae. There was rarefaction of the skull bones, and the frontal and ethmoidal sinuses were unusually large.

1972: The patient has been married since 1966 but has remained childless through the use of an intrauterine contraceptive device. Oral contraceptives have been avoided because of probable aggravating effects on the thrombotic tendency. The patient responded incompletely to low methionine diet, which she found difficult to follow, and is a vitamin B_6 nonresponder. She is incapacitated by psychiatric disturbances, including many hypochondriacal complaints, and stutters badly.

Family 2

Cases 4 and 5. J. Har. (Case 4), a white female born in November, 1953, first came to specific medical attention in 1959 because of a heart murmur. Chest x-ray films in 1960 showed

---

*Determination, courtesy Dr. N. Raphael Shulman, National Institutes of Health, Bethesda, Md.

dilatation of the pulmonary artery (Fig. 4-18F and G). At that time the diagnosis of the Marfan syndrome was suggested because of striking skeletal features (Fig. 4-18A). Right heart catheterization, performed without complication in 1964, showed normal pressures and no evidence of intracardiac shunt.

The patient has worn glasses for high-grade myopia since 1960. Repeated eye examinations in 1965 after the diagnosis of homocystinuria was established showed minimal but definite dislocation of the lenses.

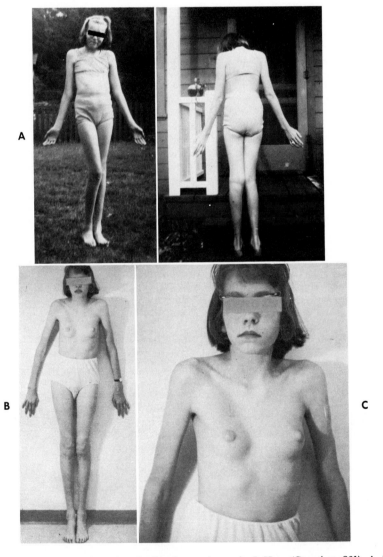

Fig. 4-18. Homocystinuria simulating the Marfan syndrome in J. Har. (Case 4, p. 261). **A,** Marfan-like skeletal features at 9¾ years of age. **B,** Same at 11½ years. Height 68½ inches. **C,** Pectus excavatum. **D,** Hands showing contracture of the fifth fingers, which become irregularly white on forced extension. **E,** Long narrow feet. **F** and **G,** X-ray films at 7 years of age. Dilatation of the pulmonary artery and reduced anteroposterior dimension are demonstrated.

Spinal curvature has developed in recent years. Loose-jointedness has never been conspicuous. The fifth fingers of both hands cannot be fully extended.

The parents have observed her "high coloration" and a tendency to become unusually flushed with exertion in hot weather. The hair and complexion are appreciably lighter than those of both parents and the surviving unaffected sib. Orthodontal correction of malaligned front teeth was necessary in recent years. Despite numerous traumata, she has sustained no fracture. Menarche occurred at 11 years of age.

The patient is definitely retarded in her learning ability. Coordination of brain and body seems poor. She has never learned, for example, to use scissors. She learns by rote reasonably well, and through patient instruction she has learned to read and spell well. In school, "social studies" and arithmetic are more difficult for her.

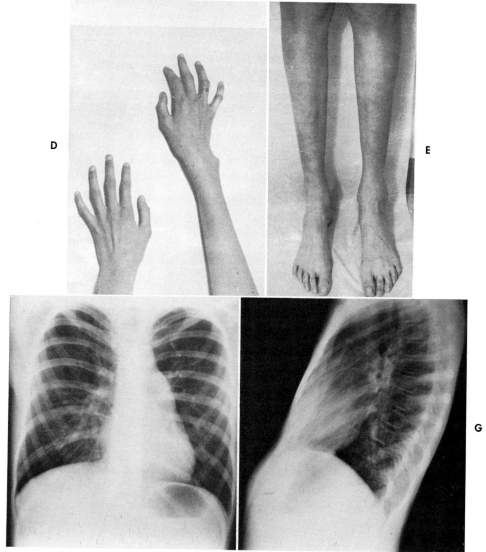

Fig. 4-18, cont'd. For legend see opposite page.

Examination in 1965 showed mild upper malar flush. At 11 years 6 months of age she was 69½ inches tall with a US/LS ratio of 0.72. The palate was abnormally high. The hands and feet were cold, but the pulses were normal. The hands had a "tight feel"—probable reduced joint mobility; both fifth fingers were mildly incurved and could not be fully extended. Pectus excavatum was striking, and considerable scoliosis was present.

The parents are not related, and the ancestry of both originated in the British Isles. The mother had had three pregnancies: (1) A male, born in 1950, died in 1953. He had "cerebral palsy" and never learned to walk, although he could sit. At birth a large omphalocele requiring surgical repair was present. Autopsy showed "fatty metamorphosis of the liver." It is suspected that he had homocystinuria (Case 5 of this series) and that intracranial thromboses were responsible for the cerebral palsy. (2) A female, born in 1952, is normal in every respect. (3) The proband was born in 1953.

1972: J. Har. is now 73 inches tall. She has been found to be a vitamin B_6 responder. She had decrease in her nervousness and other apparent subjective improvement with administration of pyridoxine. She completed high school in June, 1972, and takes special training in nursery school teaching beginning in the fall of 1972.

Family 3

Case 6. C. S., a white male farmer born in 1921, was reasonably well, except for ectopia lentis, until early 1965. The left lens was extracted in 1945, with complications leading to residual corneal opacification. Right inguinal herniorrhaphy was performed in 1947. The right lens was extracted in 1952. About 1959 he suffered from right-sided "sciatica." Manipulations by a chiropractor afforded relief. About 1963 he was refused insurance because of albuminuria and hypertension.

In January, 1965, the patient developed weakness and palpitations without pain and was thought to have had a heart attack. The electrocardiogram showed atrial fibrillation, probable old myocardial infarction, and unifocal ventricular premature contractions.

Examination in 1965 showed intense violaceous flushing of the face and most of the body. The trunk and proximal portions of the extremities showed livedo reticularis, and with brief dependency the feet became purple. The nose, lips, buccal mucosa, and hands showed deep purple cyanosis.

The height was 73½ inches, with a US/LS value of 0.98. The chest showed a combination of pectus excavatum and carinatum, and mild scoliosis was present. A grade III/VI systolic ejection murmur was heard over the precordium. Blood pressure was 220/110 mm. Hg (sitting)

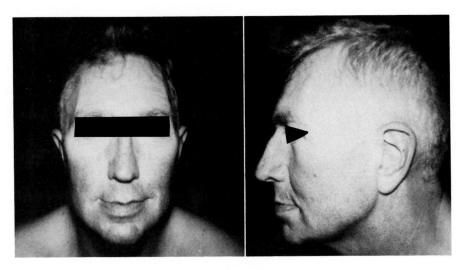

Fig. 4-19. Telangiectatic facial flush in C. S. (Case 6).

in the right arm and 190/100 in the left arm. The liver was enlarged, 2 to 3 fingerbreadths below the right costal margin. Intelligence seemed to be normal. Hemoglobin was 17.7 gm./100 ml.; hematocrit, 51 vol./100 ml.; red blood cell count, 4.9 million.

The parents were not known to be related. However, both came from the Dalarne region of Sweden. The proband was an only child.

1972: The patient is able only to care for his garden. He has gout and mild diabetes mellitus for which he takes a uricosuric agent and an oral hypoglycemic agent. He is also maintained on digitalis and warfarin sodium (Coumadin). He had phlebitis in his legs in February, 1968.

Family 4

Case 7. J. Je. (1153704), a white male truck driver born in 1925, had had hypertension since at least 18 years of age, when it was first discovered during a Selective Service examination. An ocular defect was also discovered at that time. The left lens was extracted in 1956. In 1957 acute glaucoma developed in the right eye and because of a delay in medical attention total loss of vision in that eye resulted. He was otherwise asymptomatic, however, until 1959, when he developed pneumonia necessitating hospitalization. Shortly thereafter, apparently related to the death of his brother, W. Je. (Case 8), J. Je. suffered a "nervous breakdown." He recovered without specific psychiatric therapy. During a hospitalization during the same period, an abnormal substance, presumably homocystine, was revealed in the urine by paper chromatography but was not identified. About 1963 he suffered a brief episode of blindness and weakness while driving. This cleared spontaneously and did not recur. He was told in 1959 that pulses were absent in the left leg, but no symptoms were attributable thereto. He had been aware of tachycardia for at least twenty years. He did heavy work as a furniture truck driver and denied claudication and impotence.

In February of 1965 he injured his remaining (left) eye on a car mirror, producing retinal detachment for which surgery was performed.

The parents were healthy and were not related. The ancestry was English and Irish. Of 7 sibs, the patient and brother W. Je. (Case 8) have homocystinuria. The other 5 sibs are apparently healthy.

Examination in 1965 showed a well-developed, alert, cooperative man of normal intelligence. The face showed malar flush with coarse, large-pored skin. The skeletal findings were in no way remarkable. The heart showed persistent tachycardia and grade II (out of six) systolic ejection murmur at the left sternal border. Blood pressure was 180/110 mm. Hg in both arms, standing and recumbent. A large varicocele was present on the left. Both femoral pulses were decreased, the left being almost absent. A loud bruit was heard over the right femoral triangle and a softer one on the left. The left foot was cooler than the right. The neurologic findings were within normal limits.

1972: The patient is able to work only part-time as a carpenter. He has angina pectoris after heavy meals and pains in the legs after walking and has been hypertensive for several years.

Case 8. W. Je., the brother of J. Je. (Case 7), had bilateral ectopia lentis and long-standing hypertension. He died at age 28 following surgery for infarction of the bowel. For several months he had been markedly nervous, with recurring attacks of abdominal pain and backache. At operation the arterial supply to the bowel seemed adequate, whereas extensive venous thrombosis was present. Autopsy showed thrombosis of the portal vein, thrombosis in the terminal aorta, occlusion of the left iliac artery, and multiple small infarctions of the myocardium and kidneys.

Family 5

Cases 9 and 10. L. Br., a white male born in 1941, and his sister, K. Br., born in 1943, were first examined in 1954 when they sought treatment for ectopia lentis. At that time the Marfan syndrome was diagnosed. The skeletal features were more suggestive in the brother than in the sister (Fig. 4-20A and B).

L. Br. developed weakness in the left leg in 1951 and a diagnosis of poliomyelitis was rendered. Function returned to normal in the following few years. In 1957 he sustained a fracture of the right tibia and fibula, which required open reduction with application of a plate.

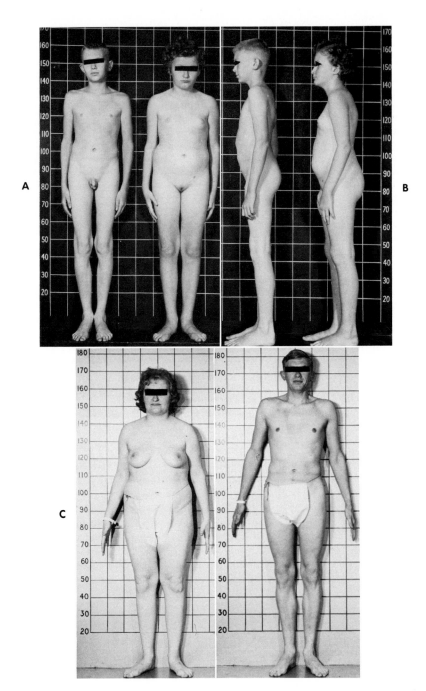

Fig. 4-20. Homocystinuria in brother and sister (Cases 9 and 10, p. 265). **A** and **B,** L. Br. (left), 13½ years old; K. Br. (right), age 10¾ years old. Long everted feet and mild scoliosis and pectus excavatum are demonstrated. **C,** K. Br., 22 years old (left), and L. Br., 25 years old (right).

A few weeks later admission to a hospital was required because of the development of acute respiratory symptoms. X-ray studies showed a "segmental type of pneumonia" with pleural effusion on the right. (Pulmonary embolism seems likely.)

Ectopia lentis was first noted at 6 years of age and glasses were worn from that age, but no surgery has been performed. Despite school absences necessitated by the neurologic episode in 1951 and the fracture and its complications in 1957, the patient graduated from a state teachers college in 1965 and plans to teach at the high school level. He was active in intramural athletics. He has always been of nervous inclination.

Examination in 1965 showed a height of 72 inches and a US/LS value of 0.84. The feet and hands were long. He wore a size 12D shoe. He had high color of the cheeks and coarse, wide-pored facial skin. Pectus excavatum was present. Deep tendon reflexes were hyperactive but symmetric. The intelligence quotient (IQ) was estimated to be between 105 and 110. Platelets were normal in number, morphology, and adhesiveness.

K. Br. was noted to have ectopia lentis at the age of 3 years. At 11 years, the right lens was removed. The lenses were described as somewhat globular and dislocated downward and nasally. She did poorly in school and at the age of 21 years had not yet succeeded in completing requirements for graduation from high school. Menarche occurred at 11 years of age.

Examination in 1965 showed a height of 65 inches with a US/LS value of 0.88. As indicated by the measurements and by the photographs (Fig. 4-20C), her body habitus was much less suggestive of the Marfan syndrome than the brother's. The patient "toed out" and the feet were flat and everted. An ejection pulmonary systolic murmur was present when the patient was recumbent. The intelligence quotient was estimated to be about 80.

The parents are not related. The father and mother are 68 and 66 inches tall, respectively. The father is of Dutch extraction, and the mother, German. A third child, a female born in 1947, is normal.

1972: Now 31 years of age, L. Br. works as a draftsman and is reasonably well. K. Br., 29 years of age, has hypertension and frequent headaches and is becoming obese, in part because of inactivity. Therapeutic abortion for an unwanted pregnancy and tubal ligation were tolerated without apparent ill effects in the way of thrombotic episodes. These sibs are vitamin B_6 responders. Data on K. Br. is presented by Mudd et al.[51]

Family 6

Case 11. D. Ap. (1153651), a white male born in 1940, had normal birth and development and finished two years of college, being forced to stop because of failing vision. In 1961 and 1963 lenses were extracted without complication. At 17 years of age he developed recurrent thrombophlebitis and varicosities in the left leg. Traumatic fracture of the right femur has been sustained. He has his own insurance business.

The parents, of English-Irish-German extraction, are well and are not known to be related. Of their 7 children, 3 (Cases 11, 12, and 13) have homocystinuria.

Examination showed normal blood pressure, prominent malar flush with coarse, wide-pored skin of the face, fine blond hair, and moderately high palate. The height was 71 inches and the US/LS value was about 1.0. The left leg showed stasis dermatitis and venous varicosities. The left foot was red-blue on dependency, with thick nails. All pulses were adequate and no arterial bruits were heard. Intelligence is apparently normal and he has a pleasing personality.

X-ray films showed calcification of the left femoral artery (and/or vein), over an extended segment, and generalized osteoporosis.

1972: This patient was on warfarin sodium (Coumadin) for over thirteen years following an episode of phlebitis at age 17. He discontinued the anticoagulant about 18 months ago and since then has been on vitamin B_6, to which he responds. Varicose veins that were operated on several years ago have recurred. He is successfully employed as an accountant.

Case 12. Mrs. J. A. McC. (1153679), a sister of D. Ap. (Case 11), born in 1942, quit school in grade 11 presumably because of visual difficulties. Upper canine teeth were removed because of crowding. She is married and has 1 child, 4 years old.

Examination in 1965 showed normal blood pressure, height 68 inches, US/LS about 1.0, thin blond hair, high color of the cheeks, bilateral dislocation of the lenses with iridodonesis, and highly arched palate. She is probably mildly retarded, and by x-ray examination she is shown to have generalized osteoporosis.

1972: In 1969 the son (J.H.H. 1328039), then 7 years of age, was found normal on examination and testing. In 1970 Mrs. McC. completed her second pregnancy, delivering a dead hydrocephalic fetus (see p. 255).

Case 13. C. Ap. (J.H.H. 1188576), a brother of the preceding 2 patients, was born April 24, 1945. He had ectopic lenses, which were removed in 1952-1953. In 1965 he was hospitalized for thrombophlebitis in the legs. While hospitalized he suffered onset of clonic movements in both legs, which spread to involve the arms and trunk and continued for several hours. The focal seizures were thought to be due to sagittal sinus thrombosis. Bruits were heard over both femoral arteries, louder on the right. In 1966 his height was 189 cm., span 194 cm.

1972: The patient works regularly. Because of a chronic ulceration at the ankles, vein stripping was performed in 1972. Also in 1972 grand mal seizures had their onset. These were well controlled by medication.

Family 7

Case 14. T. Bu., a female born July 15, 1957, sat at 6 months of age and walked at 14 months, although she was noted to be clumsy. She first wore glasses at 3 years 6 months of age, when her parents were told she had dislocated lenses. During the following three years progressive downward dislocation of the lenses took place. She was always a "slow learner" and was placed in a special school. In November, 1963, she developed acute glaucoma in the left eye. Surgery was not done. In February, 1964, acute glaucoma occurred in the right eye. After needling, the lens fell back into position.

Examination in 1965 showed a cooperative child with short attention span. The IQ was estimated to be below 70. Malar flush was striking and livedo reticularis mild. The eyes showed obvious iridodonesis, displaced lenses, and high-grade myopia. Lumbar lordosis was exaggerated, with protuberant abdomen and mild scoliosis. Genu valgum was noted. The hair is blonder than that of any other member of the family.

The parents are well and are not known to be related. Both are of Irish extraction. One sib of the proband, 5 years old, is normal.

December, 1970: T. Bu. attends a special ungraded school. She wears a size 10AAA shoe as compared with her father's 9½ and mother's 8½. Yet she is only slightly over 5 feet tall.

July, 1972: Severe scoliosis with curvature of 70 degrees in the lumbar area and 65 degrees in the thoracic area was corrected surgically in a two-stage procedure. Hypertension followed the first operation.

Family 8

Case 15. M. Ba., a female born in May, 1953, was ascertained through a urine screening of patients with ectopia lentis. Birth weight was 7 pounds 8 ounces, and except for vomiting in the neonatal period no abnormality was noted early in life. She was always irritable, and in hot weather her face became beet-red. She was noted to have myopic astigmatism from the age of about 4 years. Although she was seen by several competent ophthalmologists, ectopia lentis was not detected until 1964, suggesting that the dislocation may have been progressive. Several teeth were removed because of crowding.

Examination in 1965 showed crowded teeth, venous flush of the face when recumbent, dry skin, and thick nails. The lenses were dislocated downward bilaterally. She walked with exaggerated lumbar lordosis attributable to spondylolisthesis demonstrated by x-ray study. Her height was 54 inches with US/LS ratio of 0.76. IQ was estimated to be less than 70.

X-ray films showed generalized demineralization of the lumbar vertebrae, with some flattening of the vertebral bodies. Calcification was visualized in the lateral occipital ligaments. Spina bifida occulta and spondylolisthesis were present in the lumbar spine. The electroencephalogram was considered abnormal because of an unusual amount of slow activity and biooccipital slowing and sharp wave activity more on the left side.

The parents are not known to be related. Both are of Russian-Jewish extraction. Both are well. The mother and maternal grandfather have von Recklinghausen's neurofibromatosis. The mother is only 59 inches tall, and the father is 65 inches tall. A brother of the proband is unusually intelligent at 16 years of age.

1972: In 1966 the patient developed grand mal seizures controlled by diphenylhydantoin (Dilantin), 50 mg. three times daily. She has been plagued by recurrent bronchial asthma and atopic dermatitis. In 1967 a diet restricted in methionine and supplemented with cystine was instituted and resulted in decreased urinary homocystine. Since 1968 she has been on an unrestricted diet supplemented with 250 mg. of pyridoxine twice daily. In February, 1969, she was studied by Dr. Grant Morrow III for fatigue, weakness, and pallor. She was found to have macrocytic anemia with hemoglobin of 8.0 to 9.0 grams/100 ml., low plasma folate (less than 1.0 mμg. per milliliter), and normal plasma vitamin B$_{12}$ activity. Urinary methylmalonate was absent, and a Schilling test showed adequate vitamin B$_{12}$ absorption and excretion (24%). Oral folic acid, 40 mg. per day for 6 days and then 5 mg. per day, produced a reticulocyte response and correction of the anemia. Several trials of pyridoxine, folate, and vitamin B$_{12}$ demonstrated that full correction of the homocystinuria necessitated administration of both folate and vitamin B$_{12}$ in pharmacologic dosage.[79a]

Family 9

Case 16. S. Bo. (1152914), a white male born Aug. 1, 1954, was noted to have "flickering of the iris" when as a baby he would sit on his mother's lap. Furthermore he held his picture books close to his eyes. Because of ectopia lentis in this patient's paternal uncle, his parents were alert to the possibility of ectopia lentis. Glasses were worn from the age of 5 years. The diagnosis of Marfan syndrome was made soon thereafter.

The boy has been a "slow learner." He repeated the first grade and at age of 10 entered the fourth grade of a special class. He is hyperkinetic, strongly motivated to learn, enjoys reading, learns well by rote, and does well in spelling but poorly in "social studies," apparently because of difficulties in reasoning.

The parents are well. Both are of German extraction. Three sibs, 2 older brothers and a younger sister, are well.

Examination revealed bilateral ectopia lentis with iridodonesis, malaligned teeth undergoing orthodontic correction, a late systolic murmur introduced by a click, and mild pectus excavatum. Genu valgum and mild livedo reticularis and malar flush were noted. The IQ was estimated as less than 70.

1972: The patient has been remarkably well physically during the last six years and has been receiving special schooling to prepare him for work and life in the community.

Case 17. F. Bo., the paternal uncle of S. Bo. (Case 16), had bilateral ectopia lentis and had lens extraction. Always sickly and retarded in mental development, he died in 1927 at the age of 9 years, of scarlet fever. The diagnosis of homocystinuria is considered quite certain.

Family 10

Case 18. A. Wz. (1155861), born July 30, 1959, was first seen by me in March, 1961, when the diagnosis of Marfan syndrome had been made because of the finding of ectopia lentis, highly arched palate, and long hands and feet. Physical and intellectual development had been retarded. He did not yet walk or sit unaided. Prominent veins over the forehead and anterior upper chest were noted. Height was 33¾ inches and the head, which seemed relatively large, measured 20¼ inches. The hair was blond and the eyes blue. Muscular hypotonia was striking. On x-ray study the thoracolumbar spine was considered normal at 1 year 6 months of age.

The child began to walk at about 3 years of age. Mental retardation was evident throughout. Dislocation of the lenses may have progressed. In May, 1965, examination revealed an unusually tall boy, measuring 52½ inches, with long narrow feet and hands, narrow, highly arched palate, and crowded front teeth. Iridodonesis, dilated veins over the chest, pulmonary systolic ejection murmur when recumbent, and lumbar kyphosis in sitting were also noted. The hands, specifically the fingers, had a "tight feel."

The parents are not related and are apparently healthy. The mother has severe myopia. They are of old American stock—English, French, and Irish. A younger female sib of the proband is healthy. A maternal first cousin of the proband, 24 years old, is institutionalized for a psychiatric disorder, and a brother of this first cousin, 19 years, is mentally retarded, requiring attendance at a special school. A maternal second cousin of the proband, 22 years old, is also mentally retarded and attends a "farm school." A first cousin of the proband's mother, 43 years of age, is mentally retarded. On the paternal side, a cousin has had detached retina from an early age. In several of these relatives, screening tests show no homocystine in the urine.

Subsequent course: The patient died elsewhere early in 1968.

Family 11

Case 19. R. Hd. (994522), a white male born in 1956, crawled at 7 months, walked at 17 months, and talked at 2 years 6 months. He always seemed backward mentally. The mother noted dislocation of his left lens at 5 years of age. Both lenses were extracted in 1961. At 3 or 4 months of age he had left-sided seizures. At 7 years six teeth were extracted to relieve crowding. On several occasions the mother was told he had a heart murmur. He does very poorly in school.

Examination in 1965 showed a slender, blond-haired, obviously retarded boy. The skin was pale and unusually transparent but showed no flushing or livedo reticularis. The front teeth were prominent. Other findings included pigeon breast, systolic ejection pulmonary murmur, and genu valgum.

The parents, of English and Irish extraction, were healthy and were not related. This boy and D. Hd. (Case 20) were the only children.

Case 20. D. Hd. (1154438), the brother of R. Hd., born in 1957, developed pneumonia at 11 months of age and shortly thereafter began to have seizures and left-sided paresis. Seizures were reasonably well controlled with phenobarbital and by 19 months he was walking. At 4 years he developed severe seizures with a period of coma and right-sided paresis. About the same time, aseptic necrosis of the right femoral head, necessitating traction for fourteen months, was discovered. Bilateral lens extractions were performed at 5 years of age. By 6 years he was able to play actively with little evident incapacity. At 7 years he again had pneumonia with uneventful recovery. About four months later his right leg became blue and swollen. About three weeks later the same phenomenon occurred in the left leg. He also had prolapse of the rectum, and the physician told the mother he had a "clot in the bowels." The veins of the anterior abdominal wall became prominent. In March, 1965, he developed fever leading to coma. The right arm became blue and swollen.

Examination in April, 1965, showed an emaciated, obtunded boy who responded only to painful stimuli. The only satisfactory pulse was the left radial. Others were absent or only very weakly palpable. The front teeth were protruding, with malocclusion and high palate. The hair was blond and the skin transparent. Prominent venous collaterals on the anterior surface of the trunk filled from below, becoming particularly prominent when he cried. All four extremities were cold. Deep tendon reflexes were essentially unobtainable.

Both brothers showed generalized osteoporosis of moderately severe degree. The skull had a granular or finely reticular appearance.

1972: Now aged 16 and 15 years, the boys are about status quo. The older boy goes to a special school. The younger boy is confined to bed and wheelchair and goes to school only intermittently. Both are vitamin B_6 responders.

Family 12

Case 21. J. Gil., born in 1950, had breath-holding attacks as an infant. Physical and mental development was at all stages retarded. Bilateral ectopia lentis was detected at an early age.

Examination at age 15 years showed a boy who looked old for his age. The eyes were sunken. He was nervous and apprehensive and, obviously, severely retarded. The face and trunk developed a venous flush when he was supine. The skin of the face was coarse and large pored. The blood pressure was 160/80 mm. Hg and labile. Tachycardia and an ejection pulmonary systolic murmur in recumbency were present. The liver was not enlarged. Pectus carinatum was present. An unusually wide space separated the first and second toes. The foot showed a striking pes cavus deformity. (Fracture had been sustained in the right foot.) Varicose veins were present. The liver was not enlarged. There were no localizing neurologic signs.

Case 22. S. Gil., a sister of J. Gil. (Case 21), born in 1943, had breath-holding attacks in infancy. She also is severely retarded, although somewhat less so than her brother, and is nervous and apprehensive. Examination in 1965 showed crowded teeth, dilated venules over the legs, especially the ankles, a flaring of the lower ribs but no sternal deformity, and pulmonary ejection systolic murmur in the recumbent position. There were no localizing neurologic signs.

Marked osteoporosis of the spine, skull, and hands was demonstrated radiologically in both sibs. The electrocardiogram was normal in both.

Both parents, of Irish extraction, are well and are not known to be related. The sibship of the above patients contains 2 other children, both normal, a boy 19 years of age and a girl 14 years.

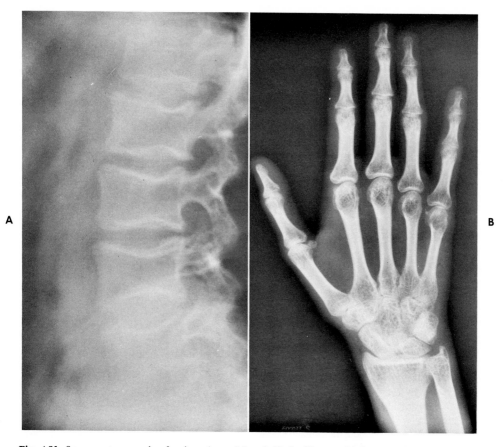

Fig. 4-21. Severe osteoporosis of spine, **A,** and hand, **B,** in 22-year-old homocystinuric (Case 22, p. 270).

Family 13

Case 23. J. Te. (764615), a white female office worker born July 28, 1920, has suffered all her life from eye abnormalities consisting of myopia, etopia lentis, and retinal detachment; she had a well-documented anteroseptal myocardial infarction at 31 years of age. During hospitalization for this, intermittent arterial spasm in the left foot was noted. At 42 years the patient was hospitalized for arterial occlusion in the right arm. Despite these handicaps she attended college for three years and has worked as a civilian employee for a defense agency of the government since May, 1942. Palpitations due to extrasystoles (present since 18 years of age) and intermittent angina pectoris have been the main nonocular symptoms.

Examination in 1965 showed an alert, intelligent, emotionally stable woman with excellent recall. Habitus is dumpy, with fat hips and a height of 66 inches. The skeletal features are not remarkable. The heart is moderately enlarged, with auscultatory and electrocardiographic signs of right bundle-branch block.

The patronymic was derived from a French ancestor who settled in New Haarlem in 1652. The mother came from a well-known family, of Irish origin, which settled in Maryland before 1700. The parents were not related. A brother (Case 24) is thought to have died of the complications of homocystinuria at 18 years of age. Another brother died at a few weeks of age, presumably of meningitis.

Subsequent course: The patient died July 14, 1969. Clinically acute myocardial infarction was considered. Autopsy showed extensive myocardial disease with a healed infarct and left ventricular hypertrophy, the heart weighing 650 grams. The right renal artery was found to be completely occluded by a recent thrombus, and the entire right kidney was infarcted.

Case 24. C. Te., the brother of J. Te. (Case 23), had "bad eyes" and was 76 inches tall. At 18 years he was seized with severe chest pain while doing farm chores and died one week later after recurrence of the pain. He had graduated from high school a few months previously. Cause of death was certified as "coronary occlusion due to vascular spasm."

Family 14

Case 25. M. St., a white male born Sept. 10, 1947, is 73½ inches tall and in the tenth grade of school. He may be normally intelligent but "has had many emotional problems all his life." His school standing suggests retardation. He has bilateral ectopia lentis. The left lens was needled in 1961. Glaucoma on the right occurred in 1964 and a cataractous dislocated lens was extracted. At age 15, spontaneous pneumothorax occurred. He had suffered from bronchial asthma for several years. The left testis was removed after trauma.

The parents of this patient, of Jewish extraction, were not known to be related. Both are now dead, the father having died in an airplane accident and the mother of breast cancer. The only sib is Case 26.

Case 26. N. St., a white female, died in September, 1964, at age 11 years 9 months, while a patient in the Neurologic Institute at Columbia. She had had bilateral ectopia lentis, the right lens being dislocated up and out and the left lens nasally displaced. The left lens was needled in 1960; a cataractous right lens was extracted in 1962. At the time of the terminal admission in 1964, recurrent leg fractures, gigantism, and decreased strength in the left arm were noted. Since childhood, she had had difficulty in walking. A limp "favoring" the left leg was attributed to previous fractures. The child had complained of numbness in the left hand, for six to eight weeks, with difficulty in use of the left hand for one week. Left central facial weakness and weakness of the left arm and leg were present. In the last 12 days of life, she developed hypertension (blood pressure 210/130 mm. Hg) and evidence of thrombosis in the carotid arteries, lower aorta, common iliacs, and femoral and subclavian arteries. A brachial arteriogram for demonstration of the aortic arch and cranial vessels showed "essentially complete obstruction of the right internal carotid artery near its origin." Left carotid arteriogram showed the left internal carotid artery to be very small through its entire course. The electroencephalogram was strikingly abnormal.

Family 15

Case 27. I. MacD., a white male born in 1920, had a history of visual difficulties from the age of about 20 years. Subluxated lenses were detected in 1945. In 1964 the right lens was found to be dislocated infranasally and the left lens, nasally. The fundi were normal. The left lens was extracted in 1964. At that time blood pressure, electrocardiogram, and chest x-ray films were normal.

This man received a B.S. degree in chemistry before World War II and a B.S. degree in chemical technology after World War II. He now works as a food technologist. During the war he served as captain in an airborne division in France. In 1942 he fractured a tibia in a jump. Shortly after an automobile accident in 1944 he noticed swelling behind the knees, and possible inferior vena caval thrombosis was subsequently diagnosed. Venous stripping was performed bilaterally in 1954. The patient, who is 74 inches tall and wears a 12B shoe, is of Scottish-English-Irish descent. Three male sibs are well. He has 5 children, all well.

June, 1972: The patient is a vitamin B_6 responder and has probably had less trouble with phlebitis since taking the vitamin. The left lens was extracted in 1964. In November, 1971, he suffered detachment of the right retina. This was promptly treated surgically with good results.

Family 16

Case 28. S. Han., a white male born Aug. 14, 1954, was slow in physical and mental development from the beginning. He did not walk until age 4 years. An eye problem was not noted until age 7, when acute glaucoma developed. Asthmatic attacks occurred on several occasions. Beginning in 1963 he has had multiple "spells" consisting of stiffening of the left side without loss of consciousness. He appears to be intolerant to sun, developing facial swelling on exposure but no blisters or red urine.

Physical examination in 1965 showed a hyperactive boy with dull, expressionless face. The teeth were carious and crowded. Corneal edema suggested chronic glaucoma. Other features were pectus carinatum, genu valgum, height of 57 inches, long narrow toes, and everted feet with thick calluses on the inner aspect of both insteps.

The proband is the youngest of 12 children of a Jewish father and an Irish mother. The ages of the other children range from 32 to 12 years. Four of them are married and had children. None has homocystinuria, by screening test, and none has symptoms suggesting this disorder.

Subsequent course: The patient died January 9, 1971, of massive intracranial thrombosis. Autopsy was not performed.

Family 17

Case 29. J. Mat., a white female born March 14, 1943, was found to have ectopia lentis in 1949, at which time the left lens was extracted. The right lens was needled in 1955. In 1959 she was admitted to a hospital because of thrombophlebitis in the right leg. In May, 1960, thrombophlebitis in the left leg, probably secondary to trauma and accompanied by pulmonary embolus, again prompted hospitalization. In November, 1960, superficial thrombophlebitis occurred in the left leg. Her IQ was estimated to be 74. (She eventually completed the tenth grade.) Psychiatric consultation was sought because of a possible schizophrenia, but no evidence to support that diagnosis was found. In June, 1962, another pulmonary embolus occurred and inferior vena caval ligation was performed. In December, 1962, the patient was complaining of "pins and needles" in the feet. No pulses were felt in either leg below the popliteals. Arteriograms showed complete occlusion of the right superficial femoral artery, with a "rippled appearance of fibromuscular hyperplasia" in patent portions of the arterial tree. Multiple areas of narrowing and dilatation were present bilaterally, more on the right side than the left.

In 1965 at the age of 22 years the patient showed blood pressure of 160/110 mm. Hg (both arms); height, 69 inches; obesity; prognathism; faint malar flush; high palate; chronic ulcer of right heel; edema of both legs; livedo reticularis of arms, with cool hands.

Case 30. M. Mat., a female born Oct. 7, 1947, died Oct. 1, 1960, of massive venous thromboses and pulmonary emboli. She had had recurrent convulsions. Autopsy* showed height 70 inches and weight 189 pounds. The arms were long and tapering, with long thin tapering fingers. The legs were thick and stocky. Superficial veins formed a prominent network over the anterior thorax centrally and over the left hip anteriorly. Thrombi were palpable in the superficial saphenous veins. The inferior vena cava and both iliac and both femoral veins contained organizing thrombi. No changes in the vein wall were described. Old and recent pulmonary emboli and a large thrombus in the main pulmonary artery were also found. The heart showed "interstitial collagenosis," the muscle fibers being separated by wide collagenous areas. Parenchymal cells of the liver (which weighed 2,760 grams) showed large lipid vacuoles; fatty liver, type undetermined, was diagnosed.

Family 18

Case 31. P. Tu., a white female born March 25, 1921, has bilateral ectopia lentis and skeletal features suggesting the Marfan syndrome. Congestive heart failure and renal insufficiency have been problems in the last few years. Blood pressure is normal. She has had asthma since childhood. Adrenocortical steroid given for asthma probably aggravated congestive heart failure. She is 67 inches tall and weighs 125 pounds. Intelligence is apparently normal. The patient enjoys opera and good books. She completed high school. She is of high-strung and dominating temperament, in the view of her brothers.

The parents were of English stock and were not related. One unaffected sib was born Sept. 16, 1929. No sibs are dead.

Case 32. C. Tu., a white male born in June, 1934, has bilateral ectopia lentis and skeletal features suggesting the Marfan syndrome. He completed high school. He has a "ruddy complexion" and dry skin. He is considered the "black sheep" of the family and is an alcoholic and a sociopsychopath. He completed high school and is considered to have normal intelligence.

---

*Courtesy Dr. Joseph Spellman, Chief Medical Examiner, City of Philadelphia.

Case 33. W. Tu., a white male born April 14, 1922, has bilateral ectopia lentis and skeletal features suggesting the Marfan syndrome. He is 69 inches tall and weighs 160 pounds. Both lenses have been removed. The right eye is sightless as a result of detached retina. He has a "ruddy complexion" that has often been commented on by friends. Dry skin with abundant flaking has been present most of his life. He has had no fractures. He graduated from college and is a kitchen employee of a Veterans Administration hospital.

1972: P. Tu. showed, on intravenous pyelograms, changes consistent with medullary sponge kidney. According to her physician, the aorta was enlarged and chronic phlebitis in the legs with ulceration was a problem. She was discovered to be mildly diabetic; her father had diabetes mellitus. Diabetes may have been aggravated by prednisolone, which she took intermittently for many years for asthma. Despite physical handicaps, including severe impairment of vision, the patient has been able to care for herself in a small apartment.

C. Tu. worked formerly as a nightwatchman and more recently as a maintenance man. W. Tu. continues employment in a VA hospital.

Family 19

Case 34. D. How., a white male born Feb. 15, 1949, has bilateral ectopia lentis. At 16 years of age he is 75 inches tall and weighs 211 pounds. Because of mental retardation he attends a special school and is in the third grade. The patronymic is the same as that of Family 6. It has been impossible to establish a connection between Families 6 and 25; on the other hand, a connection has not been disproved, but if present, it must be remote.

1970: D. How. was then totally blind. At age 21 years he was 78 inches tall and wore a size 14B shoe. He was married and had a healthy daughter. He attended special classes until age 16. He was unable to hold a job thereafter.

Case 35. De. How., sister of Case 34, born Sept. 9, 1955, is 57 inches tall and weighs 100 pounds. She has ectopia lentis and is mentally retarded.

1970: De. How. was almost 6 feet tall at the age of almost 15 years. She attended regular classes in the eighth grade. When she was a small child, pains in the legs and difficulty walking led to a diagnosis of poliomyelitis, which was later revised to rheumatic fever. It is quite possible that this was either a vascular or a neurologic complication of homocystinuria.

Family 20

Case 36. J. S. (160377), born Aug. 24, 1920, is of Jewish extraction. The parents are first cousins. Ectopia lentis was first detected in 1928. Bilateral lens extraction was performed in 1939, prompted by acute secondary glaucoma in the right eye. Both lenses had been dislocated, first nasally and later downward. Severe myopia was also present. When seen in 1955 she displayed, on the right eye, exotropia, scarring of the cornea, and phthisis of the globe. The left eye was normal.

The patient was recognized to be slow in mental development from the beginning. In 1929 she was diagnosed as having encephalitis. The family impressed physicians as highly neurotic, and in addition to mental retardation there seemed to be a psychiatric problem.

In 1938 "slight athetosis" and a "systolic cardiac blow" were described. Asymmetry of the face, with flattening of the right labial folds, suggested seventh nerve abnormality.

In 1958 it was stated that a movement disturbance manifested mainly by tremor and diagnosed as Parkinsonism had been present since the "encephalitis" in 1929.

The patient was hospitalized from March until May, 1956, for total hysterectomy for fibromata. After surgery she developed phlebitis in the legs and subacute bacterial endocarditis, which was treated successfully with antibiotics. In 1958 she was described as having a "double murmur" in the mitral area.

The patient died July 15, 1967, of acute myocardial infarction. In May, 1967, she had been hospitalized in congestive cardiac failure. Aortic systolic and diastolic murmurs were described.

Case 37. P. S. (Sinai 55812, 13540), born in 1916, was admitted in 1930 for repair of right inguinal hernia and hydrocele. He was noted to have high-grade myopia with "cloudy lenses," and "extremely" long extremities leading to a diagnosis of gigantism. Because of malocclusion, the mouth was usually half open. The chest showed marked xiphisternal depression. Seventeen days after operation he developed tachycardia, fever, and severe headaches followed by Jacksonian seizures and showed a positive Babinski's sign bilaterally, with inequality of the pupils.

The spinal fluid was negative. He died 22 days after operation. The final diagnosis was encephalitis. Autopsy was not performed. Extensive intracranial thrombosis is likely.

Case 38. A. S. (Sinai 7320-3) was born Feb. 7, 1932, and died Nov. 10, 1947. Harelip was present at birth. She walked at 2 years 6 months of age but had poor coordination. All her education was done at home. She learned very little reading and could not write well. In 1947 a few weeks before death she showed positive Babinski's signs bilaterally, choreoathetosis, and a short pulmonary systolic murmur. In 1938 she had sustained fractures of the humerus and of the neck of the right femur. At that time she had an expressionless facies, was uncooperative, and uttered only a few indistinct words. Four weeks before the terminal admission, abdominal pain, vomiting, pallor, and polyuria developed. Jaundice also appeared. Multiple skeletal deformities, particularly scoliosis and pectus excavatum, were present. The blood urea nitrogen was found to be 280 mg./100 ml. Autopsy was not performed.

Intra-abdominal arterial and/or venous thromboses seem likely.

Table 4-2. Comparison of homocystinuria with the Marfan syndrome*

	Homocystinuria	Marfan syndrome
Inheritance	Recessive	Dominant
Skeletal abnormality	Osteoporosis, fractures, occasional arachnodactyly	Arachnodactyly and loose-jointedness more striking
Pectus excavatum or carinatum	Frequent	Frequent
Ectopia lentis	Develops progressively, with downward displacement	Usually congenital and displaced upward
Vascular disease	Dilatation with thrombosis in medium-sized arteries and veins	Dilatation and/or dissection of aorta
Skin	Malar flush, livedo reticularis	Striae distensae
Mental retardation	Frequent	Absent

*Also see reference 8a.

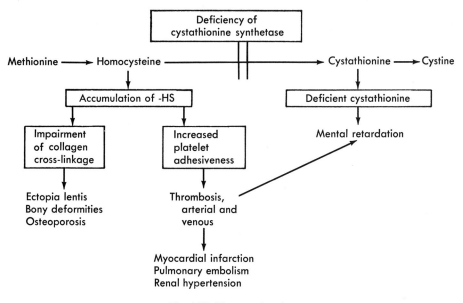

Fig. 4-22. Homocystinuria.

SUMMARY

Homocystinuria is an inborn error of metabolism simulating the Marfan syndrome in many respects. Ectopia lentis, disruption of the arterial tunica media, and skeletal changes are connective tissue disorders secondary to the metabolic defect. The precise mechanisms of the connective tissue changes are not fully understood. Fig. 4-22 is a "pedigree of causes" that attempts to relate all features of homocystinuria to the deficiency of cystathionine synthetase. Table 4-2 summarizes the differences between the Marfan syndrome and homocystinuria.

REFERENCES

1. Arnott, E. J., and Greaves, D. P.: Ocular involvement in homocystinuria, Brit. J. Ophthal. **48**:688, 1964.
2. Barber, G. W., and Spaeth, G. L.: Pyridoxine therapy in homocystinuria (letter), Lancet **1**:337, 1967.
3. Barber, G. W., and Spaeth, G. L.: The successful treatment of homocystinuria with pyridoxine, J. Pediat. **75**:463, 1969.
4. Barnett, H. J. M., and Hyland, H. H.: Noninfective intracranial venous thrombosis, Brain **76**:36, 1953.
5. Beals, R. K.: Homocystinuria: a report of two cases and review of the literature, J. Bone Joint Surg. **51A**:1564, 1969.
6. Bessman, S. P., Koppanyi, Z. H., and Wapnir, R. A.: A rapid method for homocystine assay in physiological fluids, Anal. Biochem. **18**:213, 1967.
7. Bowers, D. (Kelowna, British Columbia): Unpublished observations.
8. Brenton, D. P., Cusworth, D. C., and Gaull, C. E.: Homocystinuria; biochemical studies of tissues, Pediatrics **35**:50, 1965.
8a. Brenton, D. P., Dow, C. J., James, J. I. P., Hay, R. L., and Wynne-Davies, R.: Homocystinuria and Marfan's syndrome: a comparison, J. Bone Joint Surg. **54B**:277, 1972.
9. Brett, E. M.: Homocystinuria with epilepsy, Proc. Roy. Soc. Med. **59**:484, 1966.
10. Brune, C. G., and Himwich, H. E.: Effects of methionine loading on behavior of schizophrenic patients, J. Nerv. Ment. Dis. **134**:447, 1962.
11. Canter, S., and Gold, A. P.: Acute infantile hemiplegia, Pediat. Clin. N. Amer. **14**:851, 1967.
12. Carey, M. C., Donovan, D. E., Fitzgerald, O., and McAuley, F. D.: Homocystinuria. I. A clinical and pathological study of nine subjects in six families, Amer. J. Med. **45**:7, 1968.
13. Carey, M. C., Fennelly, J. J., and Fitzgerald, O.: Homocystinuria. II. Subnormal serum folate levels, increased folate clearance, and effects of folic acid therapy, Amer. J. Med. **45**:26, 1968.
14. Carson, N. A. J.: Homocystinuria, Proc. Roy. Soc. Med. **63**:41, 1970.
15. Carson, N. A. J., and Carre, I. J.: Treatment of homocystinuria with pyridoxine: a preliminary study, Arch. Dis. Child. **44**:387, 1969.
16. Carson, N. A. J., Cusworth, D. C., Dent, C. E., Field, C. M. B., Neill, D. W., and Westall, R. D.: Homocystinuria; a new inborn error of metabolism associated with mental deficiency, Arch. Dis. Child. **39**:425, 1963.
17. Carson, N. A. J., Dent, C. E., Field, C. M. B., and Gaull, C. E.: Homocystinuria; clinical and pathological review of ten cases, J. Pediat. **66**:565, 1965.
18. Carson, N. A. J., and Neill, D. W.: Metabolic abnormalities detected in a survey of mentally backward individuals in northern Ireland, Arch. Dis. Child. **37**:505, 1962.
18a. Carson, N. A. J., and Raine, D. N., editors: Inherited disorders of sulphur metabolism, S.S.I.E.M. symposium no. 8, Edinburgh, 1971, Churchill Livingstone.
19. Cheng, T. O.: Diastolic murmur caused by coronary artery stenosis, Ann. Intern. Med. **72**:543, 1970.
20. Chou, S.-M., and Waisman, H. A.: Spongy degeneration of the central nervous system; case of homocystinuria, Arch. Path. **79**:357, 1965.
20a. Cline, J. W., Goyer, R. A., Lipton, J., and Mason, R. G.: Adult homocystinuria with ectopia lentis, Southern Med. J. **64**:613, 1971.

20b. Cross, H. E., and Jensen, A. D.: Ocular manifestations in the Marfan syndrome and homocystinuria, Amer. J. Ophthal. 74: 1972.

21. Cusworth, D. C., and Dent, C. E.: Homocystinuria, Brit. Med. Bull. 25:42, 1969.

22. Daisley, K. W.: Synthesis of glutathione by normal and x-irradiated lens, Biochem. J. 60:x1, 1955.

23. Dancis, J., Hutzler, J., Cox, R. P., and Woody, N. C.: Familial hyperlysinemia with lysine-ketoglutarate reductase insufficiency, J. Clin. Invest. 48:1447, 1969.

24. Dardenne, V., and Kirsten, G.: Presence and metabolism of amino acids in young and old lenses, Exp. Eye Res. 1:415, 1962.

25. Deasy, C.: Evidence for the existence of homocystine (or homocysteine) in steerhide corium and in kangaroo tail tendon, J. Amer. Leather Chem. Ass. 59:691, 1964.

26. Dexter, M. W., Lawton, A. H., and Warren, L. O.: Marfan's syndrome with aortic thrombosis, Arch. Intern. Med. 99:485, 1957.

27. Dunn, H. G., Perry, T. L., and Dolman, C. L.: Homocystinuria; a recently discovered cause of mental defect and cerebrovascular thrombosis, Neurology 16:407, 1966.

27a. Evans, P., Packham, M. A., Nishizawa, E. E., Mustard, J. F., and Murphy, E. A.: The effect of acetylsalicylic acid on platelet function. J. Exp. Med. 128:877, 1968.

28. Feingold, M.: The "thumb sign" in children, Clin. Pediat. 7:423, 1969.

29. Finkelstein, J. D., Fenichel, G. M., and Reichmister, J.: Homocystinuria, Clin. Proc. Child. Hosp. (Wash.) 25:291, 1969.

30. Finkelstein, J. D., Mudd, S. H., Irreverre, F., and Laster, L.: Homocystinuria due to cystathionine synthetase deficiency; the mode of inheritance, Science 146:785, 1964.

30a. Freeman, J. M., Finkelstein, J. D., Mudd, S. H., and Uhlendorf, B. W.: Homocystinuria presenting as reversible "schizophrenia." A new defect in methionine metabolism with reduced methylene-tetrahydrofolate-reductase activity (abstract), Pediat. Res. 6:423, 1972.

31. Frimpter, G. W.: Homocystinuria: vitamin B_6—dependent or not? (editorial), Ann. Intern. Med. 71:209, 1969.

32. Gaudier, B., Remy, J., Nuyts, J.-P., Caron-Poitreau, C., Bombart, E., and Foissac-Gegoux, M.-C.: Étude radiologique des signes osseux de l'homocystinurie (à propos de six observations), Arch. Franc. Pédiat. 26:963, 1969.

33. Gaull, G. E.: The pathogenesis of homocystinuria; implications for treatment, Amer. J. Dis. Child. 113:103, 1967.

34. Gaull, G. E., Rassin, D. K., and Sturman, J. A.: Enzymatic and metabolic studies of homocystinuria; effects of pyridoxine, Neuropädiatrie 1:199, 1969.

35. Gaull, G. E., Rassin, D. K., and Sturman, J. A.: Pyridoxine dependency in homocystinuria [letter], Lancet 2:1302, 1968.

36. Gerritsen, T., Vaughn, J. G., and Waisman, H. A.: The identification of homocystine in the urine, Biochem. Biophys. Res. Commun. 9:493, 1962.

37. Gerritsen, T., and Waisman, H. A.: Homocystinuria; absence of cystathionine in the brain, Science 145:588, 1964.

38. Gerritsen, T., and Waisman, H. A.: Homocystinuria, an error in the metabolism of methionine, Pediatrics 33:413, 1964.

39. Gibson, J. B., Carson, N. A. J., and Neill, D. W.: Pathologic findings in homocystinuria, J. Clin. Path. 17:427, 1964.

40. Girard, P. F., Schott, B., Bady, B., and Boucher, M.: A case of familial homocystinuria with carotid alterations and dislocations of the crystalline lens [in French], Lyon Med. 218:1369, 1967.

40a. Goodman, S. I., Moe, P. G., Hammond, K. B., Mudd, S. H., and Uhlendorf, B. W.: Homocystinuria with methylmalonicaciduria. Two cases in a sibship, Biochem. Med. 4:500, 1970.

41. Glynn, M. F., Movat, H. Z., Murphy, E. A., and Mustard, J. F.: Study of platelet adhesiveness and aggregation, with latex particles, J. Lab. Clin. Med. 65:179, 1965.

41a. Goldstein, J. L., Campbell, B. K., and Gartler, S. M.: Cystathionine synthetase activity in human lymphocytes: induction by phytohemagglutinin, J. Clin. Invest. 51:1034, 1972.

41b. Gordon, N.: Anticonvulsant drugs and folic acid deficiency, Develop. Med. Child. Neurol. 10:497, 1968.

42. Greenberg, D. M., and Nagabhushanam, A.: Isolation and properties of a homogeneous preparation of cystathionine synthetase-serine and threonine dehydratase, 1964, Proceedings of the Sixth International Congress of Biochemistry, Moscow (abstract 461), p. 310.

42a. Gröbe, H., and von Bassewitz, D. B.: Thromboembolische Komplikationen und Thrombocytenanomalien bei Homocystinurie, Ztschr. Kinderheilk. 112:309, 1972.

43. Guthrie, R. (Buffalo): Personal communication, 1970.

44. Hall, W. K., Coryell, M. E., Hollowell, J. G., Jr., and Thevaos, T. G.: A metabolic study of homocystinuria (abstract), Fed. Proc. 24:470, 1965.

45. Halldorsson, S., (Reykjavik, Iceland): Personal communication, 1971.

46. Hambraeus, L., Wranne, L., and Lorentsson, R.: Biochemical and therapeutic studies in two cases of homocystinuria, Clin. Sci. 35:457, 1968.

47. Harkness, R. D.: In vitro and in vivo observations on the effect of penicillamine on collagen, Postgrad. Med. J. 44 (supp.):31, 1968.

48. Harris, E. D., Jr., and Sjoerdsma, A.: Collagen content solubility: cross-linking in human dermis, J. Lab. Clin. Med. 45:1020, 1966.

49. Henkind, P., and Ashton, N.: Ocular pathology in homocystinuria, Trans. Ophthal. Soc. U. K. 85:21, 1965.

49a. Hollowell, J. G., Jr., Coryell, M. E., Hall, W. K., Findley, J. K., and Thevaos, T. G.: Homocystinuria as affected by pyridoxine, folic acid, and vitamin B_{12}, Proc. Soc. Exp. Biol. Med. 129:327, 1968.

49b. Hollowell, J. G., Jr., Hall, W. K., Coryell, M. E., McPherson, J., Jr., and Hahn, D. A.: Homocystinuria and organic aciduria in a patient with vitamin-B_{12} deficiency, Lancet 2:1428, 1969.

50. Holt, J. F., and Allen, R. J.: Signes radiologiques des amino-aciduries primitives, Ann. Radiol. 10:317, 1967.

51. Hooft, C., Carton, D., and Samyn, W.: Pyridoxine treatment in homocystinuria [letter], Lancet 1:1384, 1967.

52. Hope, D. B.: Cystathionine accumulation in brains of pyridoxine-deficient rats, J. Neurochem. 11:327, 1964.

53. Huntley, C. C., and Stevenson, R. E.: Maternal phenylketonuria; course of two pregnancies, Obstet. Gynec. 34:694, 1969.

53a. Jensen, A. D., and Cross, H. E.: Surgical treatment of dislocated lenses in the Marfan syndrome and homocystinuria, Trans. Amer. Acad. Ophthal. Otolaryng. 76, 1972.

54. Johnston, S. S.: Pupil-block glaucoma in homocystinuria, Brit. J. Ophthal. 52:251, 1968.

55. Kaeser, A. C., Rodnight, R., and Ellis, B. A.: Psychiatric and biochemical aspects of a case of homocystinuria, J. Neurol. Neurosurg. Psychiat. 32:88, 1969.

56. Kang, E. S., Byers, R. K., and Gerald, P. S.: Homocystinuria; response to pyridoxine, Neurology 20:503, 1970.

56a. Kashiwamata, S., Kotake, Y., and Greenberg, D. M.: Studies of cystathionine synthetase of rat liver: dissociation into two components by sodium dodecyl sulfate disc electrophoresis, Biochim. Biophys. Acta 212:501, 1970.

57. Kelly, S., and Copeland, W.: Preliminary report; a hypothesis on the homocystinuric's response to pyridoxine, Metabolism 17:794, 1968.

58. Kennedy, C., Shih, V. E., and Rowland, L. P.: Homocystinuria; a report in 2 siblings, Pediatrics 36:736, 1965.

59. Kinsey, V. E., and Merriam, F. C.: Studies on the crystalline lens. II. Synthesis of glutathione in the normal and cataractous lens, Arch. Ophthal. 44:370, 1950.

60. Klavins, J. V.: Pathology of amino acid excess. I. Effects of administration of excessive amounts of sulphur containing amino acids: homocystinuria, Brit. J. Exp. Path. 44:507, 1963.

61. Komrower, G. M.: Dietary treatment of homocystinuria, Amer. J. Dis. Child. 113:98, 1967.

62. Komrower, G. M. (Manchester, England): Personal communication, 1970.

63. Komrower, G. M., Lambert, A. M., Cusworth, D. C., and Westall, R. G.: Dietary treatment of homocystinuria, Arch. Dis. Child. 41:666, 1966.

64. Komrower, G. M., and Wilson, V. K.: Homocystinuria, Proc. Roy. Soc. Med. 56:996, 1964.

65. Laster, L. (Bethesda, Md.): Personal communication, 1966.

65a. Laster, L., Mudd, S. H., Finkelstein, J. D., and Irreverre, F.: Homocystinuria due to cystathionine synthase deficiency: the metabolism of L-methionine, J. Clin. Invest. 44:1708, 1965.

66. Levy, H. L. (Boston, Mass.): Personal communication, 1971.

66a. Levy, H. L., Mudd, S. H., Schulman, J. D., Dreyfus, P. M., and Abeles, R. H.: A derangement in B_{12} metabolism associated with homocystinemia, cystathioninemia, hypomethioninemia, and methylmalonic aciduria, Amer. J. Med. **48**:390, 1970.

67. Lieberman, T. W., Podos, S. M., and Hartstein, J.: Acute glaucoma, ectopia lentis, and homocystinuria, Amer. J. Ophthal. **61**:252, 1966.

68. Loughridge, L. W.: Renal abnormalities in the Marfan syndrome, Quart. J. Med. **28**:531, 1959.

69. Lynas, M. A.: Marfan's syndrome in northern Ireland; an account of thirteen families, Ann. Hum. Genet. **22**:289, 1958.

70. MacCarthy, J. M., and Carey, M. C.: Bone changes in homocystinuria, Clin. Radiol. **19**:128, 1968.

70a. Mackenzie, I. L., Donaldson, R. M., Jr., Trier, J. S., and Nathan, V. I.: Ileal mucosa in familial selective vitamin B_{12} malabsorption, New Eng. J. Med. **286**:1021, 1972.

70b. Mahoney, M. J., Rosenberg, L. E., Mudd, S. H., and Uhlendorf, B. W.: Defective metabolism of vitamin B_{12} in fibroblasts from children with methylmalonicaciduria, Biochem. Biophys. Res. Commun. **44**:375, 1971.

71. Martenet, A. C., Witmer, R., and Speiser, P.: Ocular changes in homocystinuria, Ophthalmologica **154**:318, 1967.

72. Martin, V. A., and Carson, N. A.: Inborn metabolic disorders with associated ocular lesions in Northern Ireland, Trans. Ophthal. Soc. U. K. **87**:847, 1967.

73. McCully, K. S.: Vascular pathology of homocysteinemia; implications for the pathogenesis of arteriosclerosis, Amer. J. Path. **56**:111, 1969.

73a. McCully, K. S.: Homocysteinemia and arteriosclerosis, Amer. Heart J. **83**:571, 1972.

74. McCully, K. S., and Ragsdale, B. D.: Production of arteriosclerosis by homocysteinemia, Amer. J. Path. **61**:1, 1970.

75. McDonald, L., Bray, C., Field, C., Love, F., and Davies, B.: Homocystinuria, thrombosis and the blood platelets, Lancet **1**:745, 1964.

76. McKusick, V. A.: Human genetics, ed. 2, Englewood Cliffs, N. J., 1969, Prentice-Hall, Inc.

77. McKusick, V. A., Hall, J. G., and Char, F.: The clinical and genetic characteristics of homocystinuria. In Carson, N. A. J., and Raine, D. N., editors: Inherited disorders of sulphur metabolism, London, 1971, J & A Churchill, Ltd., p. 179.

78. Meister, A.: Methionine and cysteine. In Biochemistry of the amino acids, vol. 2, ed. 2, New York, 1965, Academic Press, Inc., pp. 757-818.

78a. Mjølnerød, O. K., Rasmussen, K., Dommerud, S. A., and Gjeruldsen, S. T.: Congenital connective-tissue defect probably due to D-penicillamine treatment in pregnancy, Lancet **1**:673, 1971.

79. Moreels, C. L., Jr., Fletcher, B. D., Weilbaecher, R., and Dorst, J. P.: The roentgenographic features of homocystinuria, Radiology **90**:1150, 1968.

79a. Morrow, G., III (Tucson, Ariz.): Personal communication, 1972.

80. Mudd, S. H. (Bethesda, Md.): Personal communication.

80a. Mudd, S. H.: Pyridoxine-responsive genetic disease, Fed. Proc. **30**:970, 1971.

81. Mudd, S. H., Edwards, W. A., Loeb, P. M., Borwn, M. S., and Laster, L.: Homocystinuria due to cystathionine synthase deficiency; the effect of pyridoxine, J. Clin. Invest. **49**:1762, 1970.

82. Mudd, S. H., Finkelstein, J. D., Irreverre, F., and Laster, L.: Homocystinuria; an enzymatic defect, Science **143**:1443, 1964.

83. Mudd, S. H., Finkelstein, J. D., Irreverre, F., and Laster, L.: Threonine dehydratase activity in humans lacking cystathionine synthase, Biochem. Biophys. Res. Commun. 1965.

84. Mudd, S. H., Irreverre, F., and Laster, L.: Sulfite oxidase deficiency in man: demonstration of the enzymatic defect, Science **156**:1599, 1967.

85. Mudd, S. H., Levy, H. L., and Abeles, R. H.: A derangement in B_{12} metabolism leading to homocystinemia, cystathioninemia, and methylmalonic aciduria, Biochem. Biophys. Res. Commun. **35**:121, 1969.

85a. Mudd, S. H., Levy, H. L., and Morrow, B. G.: Deranged B_{12} metabolism: effects on sulfur amino acid metabolism, Biochem. Med. **4**:193, 1970.

85b. Mudd, S. H., Uhlendorf, B. W., Freeman, J. M., Finkelstein, J. D., and Shih, V. E.:

Homocystinuria associated with decreased methylenetetrahydrofolate reductase activity, Biochem. Biophys. Res. Commun. **46**:905, 1972.

85c. Mudd, S. H., Uhlendorf, B. W., Hinde, K. R., and Levy, H. L.: Deranged B_{12} metabolism: studies of fibroblasts grown in tissue culture, Biochem. Med. **4**:215, 1970.

85d. Mustard, J. F.: Platelets and thrombosis in acute myocardial infarction, Hosp. Practice, p. 115, Jan., 1972.

86. Nimni, M. E., and Bavetta, L. A.: Collagen defect induced by penicillamine, Science **150**:905, 1965.

87. Park, L. D., Baldessarini, R. J., and Kety, S. S.: Methionin effects on chronic schizophrenics, Arch. Psychiat. **12**:346, 1965.

88. Perry, T. L., (Vancouver): Personal communication, 1971.

89. Perry, T. L., Hansen, S., Love, D. L., Crawford, L. E., and Tischler, B.: Treatment of homocystinuria with a low-methionine diet, supplemental cystine, and a methyl donor, Lancet **2**:474, 1968.

90. Pirie, A., and van Heyningen, R.: Biochemistry of the eye, Springfield, Ill., 1956, Charles C Thomas, Publisher, pp. 12-31, 19-22, 60-63.

91. Presley, G. D., and Sidbury, J. B.: Homocystinuria and ocular defects, Amer. J. Ophthal. **63**:1723, 1967.

92. Presley, G. D., Stinson, I. N., and Sidbury, J. B.: Homocystinuria at the North Carolina School for the Blind, Amer. J. Ophthal. **66**:884, 1968.

93. Presley, G. D., Stinson, I. N., and Sidbury, J. B., Jr.: Ocular defects associated with homocystinuria, Southern Med. J. **62**:944, 1969.

94. Price, J., Vickers, C. F., Brooker, B. K.: A case of homocystinuria with noteworthy dermatological features, J. Ment. Defic. Res. **12**:111, 1968.

94a. Ramsey, M. S., Yanoff, M., and Fine, B. S.: The ocular histopathology of homocystinuria. A light and electron microscope study, Amer. J. Ophthal. **74**:377, 1972.

95. Ratnoff, O. D.: Activation of Hageman factor by L-homocystine, Science **162**:1007, 1968.

96. Robinson, R. G.: The temporal lobe agenesis syndrome, Brain **87**:87, 1964.

96a. Rosenberg, L. E.: Inherited aminoacidopathies demonstrating vitamin dependency, New Eng. J. Med. **281**:145, 1969.

97. Sardharwalla, I. B., Jackson, S. H., and Sass-Kortsak, A.: Cited by Perry, 1968.

98. Sauer, F. C.: Development of beta crystallin in the pig and prenatal weight of the lens, Growth **3**:381, 1939.

99. Scheinberg, I. H.: Toxicity of penicillamine, Postgrad. Med. **44** (supp.):11, 1968.

100. Schimke, R. N., McKusick, V. A., Huang, T., and Pollack, A. D.: Homocystinuria, a study of 38 cases in 20 families, J.A.M.A. **193**:711, 1965.

101. Schimke, R. N., McKusick, V. A., and Pollack, A. D.: Homocystinuria simulating Marfan's syndrome, Trans. Ass. Amer. Phys. **78**:60, 1965.

102. Schimke, R. N., McKusick, V. A., and Weilbaecher, R. G.: Homocystinuria In Nyhan, W. L., editor: Amino acid metabolism and genetic variation, New York, 1967, McGraw-Hill Book Co.

102a. Seashore, M. R., Durant, J. L., and Rosenberg, L. E.: Studies of the mechanism of pyridoxine-responsive homocystinuria, Pediat. Res. **6**:187, 1972.

103. Selim, A. S. M., and Greenberg, D. M.: An enzyme that synthesizes cystathionine and deaminates L-serine, J. Biol. Chem. **234**:1474, 1959.

104. Shih, V. E., and Efron, M. L.: Pyridoxine-unresponsive homocystinuria; final diagnosis of M.G.H. Case 19471, 1933, New Eng. J. Med. **283**:1206, 1970.

104a. Shih, V. E., Salem, M. Z., Mudd, S. H., Uhlendorf, B. W., and Adams, R. D.: A new form of homocystinuria due to $N^{5,10}$-methylenetetrahydrofolate reductase deficiency (abstract), Pediat. Res. **6**:395, 1972.

105. Shipman, R. T., Townley, R. R. W., and Danks, D. M.: Homocystinuria, Addisonian pernicious anaemia, and partial deletion of a G chromosome, Lancet **2**:693, 1969.

106. Smith, S. W.: Roentgen findings in homocystinuria, Amer. J. Roentgen. **100**:147, 1967.

107. Smith, T. H., Holland, M. G., and Woody, N. C.: Ocular manifestation of familial hyperlysinemia, Trans. Amer. Acad. Ophthal. Otolaryng. **75**:355, 1971.

108. Soupart, P., Moore, S., and Bigwood, E. J.: Amino acid composition of human milk, J. Biol. Chem. **206**:699, 1954.

109. Spaeth, G. L., and Barber, G. W.: Homocystinuria: a new syndrome. Presented to Amer. Acad. Ophthal. Otolaryng., October, 1964.

110. Spaeth, G. L., and Barber, G. W.: Prevalence of homocystinuria among the mentally retarded; evaluation of a specific screening test, Pediatrics **40**:586, 1967.

111. Spiro, H. R., Schimke, R. N., and Welch, J. P.: Schizophrenia in a patient with a defect in methionine metabolism, J. Nerv. Ment. Dis. **141**:285, 1965.

112. Steinberg, I.: A simple screening test for the Marfan syndrome, Amer. J. Roentgen. **97**:118, 1966.

113. Sutherland, B. S., Umbarger, B., and Berry, H. K.: The treatment of phenylketonuria; a decade of results, Amer. J. Dis. Child. **111**:505, 1966.

114. Tada, K.: Discussion, Amer. J. Dis. Child. **113**:108, 1967.

115. Tada, K., Yoshida, T., Hirono, H., and Arakawa, T.: Homocystinuria; amino acid pattern of the liver, Tohoku J. Exp. Med. **92**:325, 1967.

116. Tallan, H. H., Moore, S., and Stein, W. H.: L-cystathionine in human brain, J. Biol. Chem. **230**:707, 1958.

117. Thomas, R. P., Hollowell, J. G., Peters, J. H., Coryell, M. E., and Lester, R. H.: Homocystinuria and ectopia lentis in Negro family, J.A.M.A. **198**:560, 1966.

118. Tristarn, G. R., and Smith, R. H.: The amino acid composition of some purified proteins, Advances Protein Chem. **18**:227, 1963.

119. Turner, B.: Pyridoxine treatment in homocystinuria (letter), Lancet **2**:1151, 1967.

120. Uhlendorf, B. W., and Mudd, S. H.: Cystathionine synthetase in tissue culture derived from human skin; enzyme defect in homocystinuria, Science **160**:1007, 1968.

121. Varga, F., and McKusick, V. A.: Homocystinuria and Marfan's syndrome, Orv. Hetil. **108**:969, 1967.

122. Verma, I. C., and Sinclair, S.: Homocystinuria; report of two cases in siblings, Indian J. Pediat. **37**:263, 1970.

123. Vogel, F., and Röhrborn, G., editors: Chemical mutagenesis in mammals and man, New York, 1970, Springer Publishing Co., Inc.

124. White, H. H., Rowland, L. P., Araki, S., Thompson, H. L., and Cowen, D.: Homocystinuria, Arch. Neurol. **13**:455, 1965.

125. White, H. H., Thompson, H. L., Rowland, L. P., Cowen, D., and Araki, S.: Homocystinuria, Trans. Amer. Neurol. Ass. **89**:24, 1964.

126. Wilson, R. S., and Ruiz, R. S.: Bilateral central retinal artery occlusion in homocystinuria; a case report, Arch. Ophthal. **82**:267, 1969.

127. Wong, P. W., Komrower, G. M., and Schwarz, V.: The biosynthesis of cystathionine in patients with homocystinuria, Pediat. Res. **2**:149, 1968.

128. Woody, N. C. (New Orleans): Personal communication, 1971.

128a. Woody, N. C.: Hyperlysinemia, Amer. J. Dis. Child. **108**:543, 1964.

129. Wright, L. D.: An inborn error of metabolism associated with deficiency of enzyme cystathionine synthetase leading to homocystinuria, New York J. Med. **65**:559, 1965.

130. Yoshida, T.: A simple thin-layer–chromatographic method for detection of urinary homocystine, Tohoku J. Exp. Med. **91**:31, 1967.

130a. Yoshida, T., Tada, K., Yokoyama, Y., and Arakawa, T.: Homocystinuria of vitamin B_6–dependent type, Tohoku J. Exp. Med. **96**:235, 1968.

131. Zucker, M. B., and Borrelli, J.: Platelet clumping produced by connective tissue suspensions and by collagen, Proc. Soc. Exp. Biol. Med. **109**:779, 1962.

132. Zu Rhein, G. M., Eichman, P. L., and Puletti, F.: Familial idiocy with spongy degeneration of central nervous system of van Bogaert–Bertrand type, Neurology **10**:998, 1960.

5 · The Weill-Marchesani syndrome

Like the Marfan syndrome and homocystinuria, this generalized and heritable disorder of connective tissue has ectopia lentis as a conspicuous feature. The skeletal features are the antithesis of those in the Marfan syndrome: the patients are short of stature, with particularly short hands and feet, and many have stiff joints, especially in the hands. Persons with the full Weill-Marchesani syndrome are homozygous, but heterozygotes are short of stature.

Historical note

In 1932[26] G. Weill of Strasbourg reported, among 8 cases of supposed Marfan syndrome, a 42-year-old woman with ectopia lentis, height of 142 cm., and "short, swollen fingers permitting only imperfect opening and closing" of the hands. In 1939[13,14] Oswald Marchesani, then in Münster, later in Hamburg, gave the first definitive description based on two families. In one the syndrome occurred in an 8-year-old male, both of whose parents were short and had short hands. In the other family 2 brothers and a sister were affected; both parents were short. The genetics, including the short stature of heterozygotes, was established by Kloepfer and Rosenthal[9,20] on the basis of a family in Louisiana (Fig. 5-1).

This disorder is often called simply the Marchesani syndrome. Others have called it the spherophakia-brachymorphia syndrome.[9] The abbreviated designation that will be used here is W-M.

Clinical manifestations

Skeletal features. Generalized short stature is present. Weill's original patient[26] was only 142 cm. tall. The head is brachycephalic and the face round. The fingers are short, with prominent knuckles and interphalangeal joint area. Many of the patients show limitation of joint mobility, especially in the hands,[15,26] where neither full extension nor full flexion of the fingers is possible. Seeleman[24] described the fingers and toes in a 3-year-old boy as being capable of only slight flexion. In 1971 I had an opportunity to see the proband of Kloepfer and Rosenthal's study.[9] Then 61 years old, he showed marked restriction of motion in all joints. He also showed evidence of carpal tunnel compression bilaterally (Fig. 5-1). Joint stiffness seems to be a variable feature of W-M.

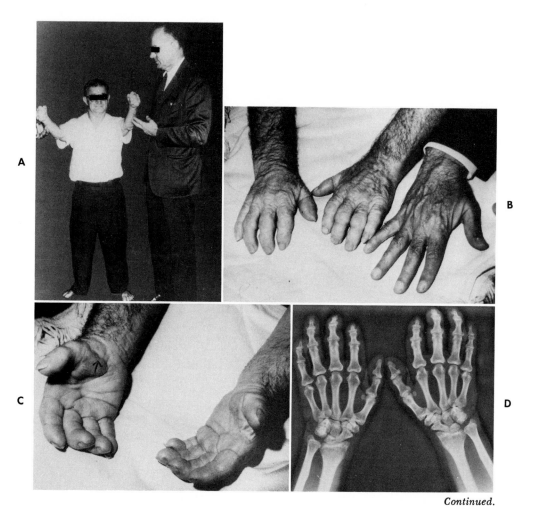

Continued.

Fig. 5-1. Weill-Marchesani syndrome in proband of family reported by Kloepfer and Rosenthal.[9] **A,** Short stature and limitation in closure of the fists are demonstrated. Motion was limited at the wrists and elbows. **B,** The short fingers with "knobby" joints are well demonstrated in comparison with the hand of a normal male. **C,** The fingers are held at almost maximal extension. Atrophy of the abductor pollicis brevis muscle, consistent with compression of the median nerve in the carpal tunnel ("carpal tunnel syndrome"), is present bilaterally (arrow). The palmar fascia is irregularly thickened, with puckering of overlying skin. **D,** X-ray films of the hands show hypertrophic osteoarthropathy. **E,** The short feet are compared with the foot of a normal male. **F,** X-ray film of the pelvis, showing irregularity of the ischial tuberosities and the left acetabulum. Soft tissue calcification overlies the greater trochanters. **G,** Lateral x-ray film of the lumbar spine, showing lipping of the vertebral bodies. (Courtesy Dr. H. W. Kloepfer and Dr. T. F. Thurmon, New Orleans.)

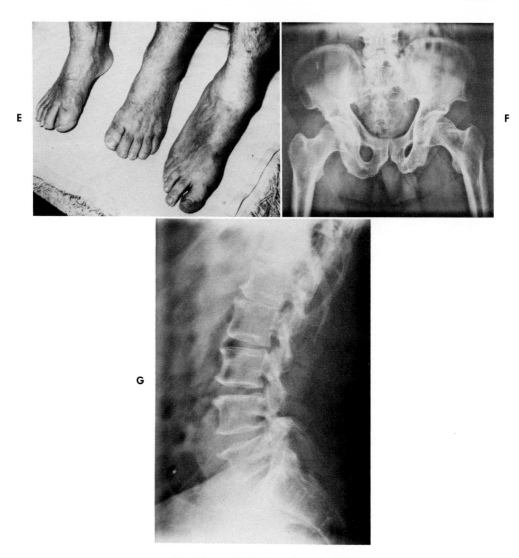

Fig. 5-1, cont'd. For legend see p. 283.

(See Figs. 5-3 and 5-4, in contrast to Figs. 5-1 and 5-2.) Reduced joint mobility, like short stature, is a feature exactly opposite to the usual finding in the Marfan syndrome.[20] Rennert[19] described "difficulty in extending his arms over his head" in a 9-year-old boy.

An unusual bony protuberance on the lateral aspect of the foot has been present in cases observed in the Amish (Fig. 5-2). It is an excrescence on the calcaneus.

The eye. The lens is small and almost spherical, and often is dislocated. Displacement of the lens tends to be downward; cataract is frequent. Myopia, present in all cases, usually measures between 10 and 20 diopters, and occasionally is higher.[12] Glaucoma is a frequent complication. The redundant zonular fibers

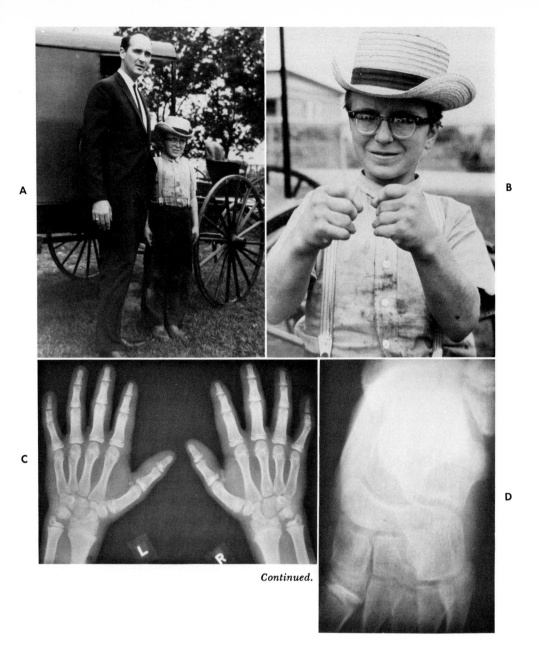

Continued.

Fig. 5-2. Weill-Marchesani syndrome in an Amish brother and sister. *Case 1.* L. E. (J.H.H. 1260976) was 15½ years old at the time of the pictures shown in **A** and **B**. He had worn spectacles for myopia from the age of 10 years. He had always been of short stature. Limitation of joint mobility was striking, especially in the hands, **B**. In addition to spherophakia and iridodonesis, he has intermittently had elevated intraocular pressure, with serious decline in vision. In addition to short fingers, the fifth fingers showed clinodactyly, **C**. An unusual bony protuberance was demonstrated on the os calcis, **D**, and was evident clinically on the side of the foot below the fibula. *Case 2.* A. E. (J.H.H. 1260975), almost four years younger than her brother, showed features identical to his. In September, 1967, she was found to have advanced optic atrophy secondary to glaucoma. The hands, **E** to **G**, showed the same short fingers, limitation in joint mobility, and clinodactyly as in the brother. Also as in the brother, the toes were short, and a ledge of bone projected laterally from each os calcis below the fibula, **H**. The parents are related as first cousins once removed. An affected second cousin has catheterization-confirmed pulmonic stenosis.

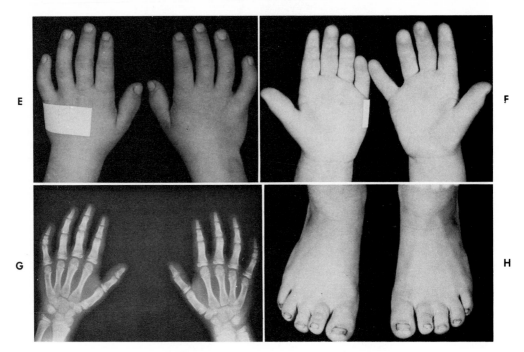

E

F

G

H

Fig. 5-2, cont'd. For legend see p. 285.

permit the lens to come forward into close contact with the pupil and thus to block the passage of aqueous from the posterior to the anterior chamber. The angle is forced shut and intraocular tension rises. Repeated self-limited attacks may occur, but ultimately, extensive synechiae develop, leading to closure of the angle and permanent glaucoma.[2] Chamber-angle anomalies such as those seen in other heritable disorders of connective tissue[1] have been described[5]—bridging pectinate strands, numerous iris processes, fraying of the iris root, and anomalous angle vessels—but they may be secondary to glaucoma. Chandler[2] and others[3]

Fig. 5-3. Brother and sister with the Weill-Marchesani syndrome; parents are short of stature. The boy shown here (O. O., J.H.H. 1320735), born in 1956, was 21 inches long at birth and weighed almost 9 pounds. He was found to be myopic when he started school. At the age of 12 years, aspiration of the anteriorly displaced lens and iridectomy were performed in the left eye. The father and mother were unrelated, were 28 and 31 years old, respectively, at his birth, and were 64 and 61 inches tall, with stubby fingers. Of 5 sibs, one, L. O. (J.H.H. 1319574), also had the Weill-Marchesani syndrome. At the age of 18 years she was 60 inches tall, with short hands. Bilateral operations for small dislocated lenses were performed. Examination of O. O. in 1969 at the age of 13, **A,** showed a height of 54 inches (below the third percentile for age). The hands, **B** and **C,** and feet were stubby. Only slightly limited extention of joints was noted. In the right eye the lens was microspheric and the anterior chamber was shallow. The left eye showed the signs of extracapsular cataract extraction and superior sector iridectomy. **A,** Father and son; **B** and **C,** hands of son; **D** and **E,** hands of father.

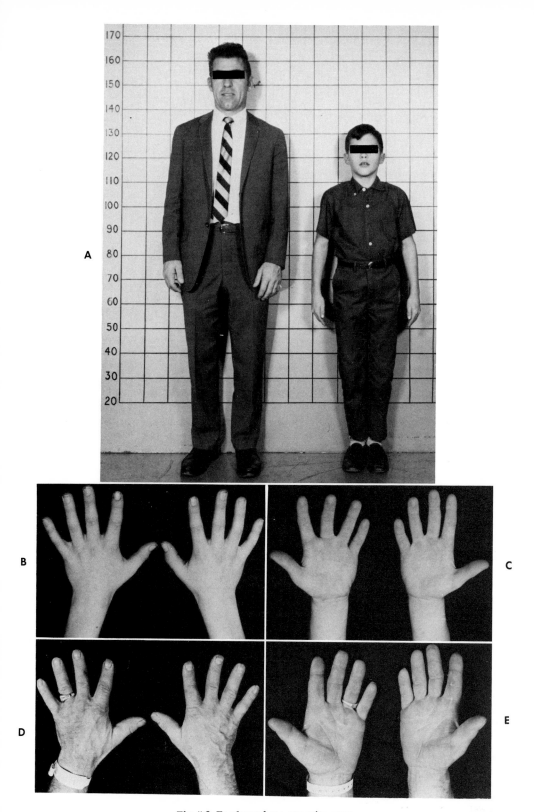

Fig. 5-3. For legend see opposite page.

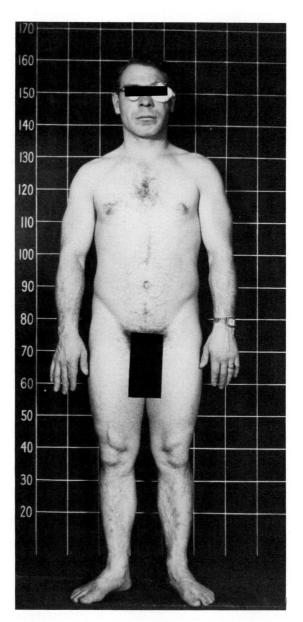

Fig. 5-4. W. B. (141009), born in 1925, and his brother, L. B., have the Weill-Marchesani syndrome. A sister, who has not been examined, also is bilaterally blind, but this abnormality, which dates from childhood, has been attributed to a febrile illness. Because of secondary glaucoma, subluxated spherophakic lenses were removed from both eyes in W. B. He suffered a retinal detachment in the left eye.

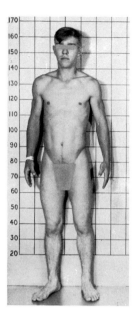

Fig. 5-5. Weill-Marchesani syndrome. R. L. U. (1122410) and 2 of his 4 sibs have high-grade myopia and ectopia lentis. No other ocular abnormality is known in the family. All 3 affected sibs are short of stature as compared with unaffected members of the family. The right eye in the proband showed central serous retinopathy resulting in a rather abrupt drop in vision. None of the 3 affected sibs has joint stiffness. The mother is about 62 inches tall. Her maiden name, an unusual one, was the same as her husband's name, but consanguinity was denied.

have noted that, paradoxically, intraocular pressure goes even higher when miotic treatment is given during attacks of glaucoma. By gonioscopy the angle can be observed to "close" with miosis and "open" again with pupillary dilatation.

Iridectomy is considered the treatment of choice for glaucoma in W-M.[2]

Other features. One of the Amish cases of W-M has congenital pulmonic stenosis, established by cardiac catheterization. It is doubtful that mental retardation is a feature. Pigmentary retinopathy, present in one case,[18] was probably unrelated to the W-M.

The sisters reported by Feinberg[6] clearly did not have W-M. The same sisters were described by Gorlin and colleagues[7] as a "new" syndrome. The features included craniofacial dysostosis, hypertrichosis, hypoplasia of the labia majora, dental and eye anomalies, and patent ductus arteriosus.

Prevalence and inheritance

Kloepfer and Rosenthal[9] concluded that only the homozygotes show the full-blown disorder, although the height of heterozygotes is roughly intermediate between that of unaffected persons and of homozygotes. Their findings suggest that about 92% of heterozygotes have abnormally short stature. Probert[17] described a family in which 4 sibs (3 females, 1 male) had the full syndrome, and one of their parents and many relatives had brachymorphism in a dominant pedigree pattern. Meyer and Holstein[15] described 4 affected sibs whose parents were first cousins; Diethelm[4] described 2 affected children with first-cousin parents. The high rate of consanguinity among the Amish and in other reported cases[5,9,25,27] also speaks for recessive inheritance.

Families have been reported in which persons in successive generations had presumed W-M syndrome.[10,21] I reinvestigated the family of Italian extraction reported by McGavic[10] and concluded that it represents an instance of "simple" autosomal dominant ectopia lentis in a generally short-statured family. No difference in stature was observed between those with and those without the ocular feature. I suspect that the family of Rousseau and Hermann[21] may have been similar.

Kloepfer and Rosenthal[9] concluded that a particularly good way to recognize the heterozygous state, or at least to quantitate the short, broad hands, is by measuring the angle formed between straight lines joining the distal axial triradius on the palm to the triradii at the base of the index and fifth fingers. The sum of this so-called a.t.d. angle* of the two hands averaged 80 degrees in normal males, 91 degrees in normal females, 103 degrees in heterozygotes, 125 degrees in male patients, and 151 degrees in female patients.

Three types of recessively inherited dwarfism have been found to be frequent among the Amish, an American religious isolate (actually, isolates). One is the Ellis–van Creveld syndrome[11]; a second is a "new" form of skeletal dysplasia, cartilage-hair hypoplasia[12]; and the third is W-M.[23] Because heterozygotes are much more frequent than homozygotes, the Lancaster County (Pennsylvania) community has rather numerous persons of short stature, apparently on the basis of heterozygosity for the W-M gene. Before the cases of W-M were recognized and before their genealogic relationship to the persons of intermediate short stature was identified, I considered the latter group to represent polygenic dwarfism.

The W-M syndrome has been described mainly in Caucasian Europeans. The large kindred studied by Kloepfer and Rosenthal[9] is of French extraction. Cases have been reported from Pakistan,[18] in a Bengali Muslin boy from India,[22] and from Israel[5] (ethnicity not stated). Two Japanese cases are on record.[8]

Basic defect and pathogenesis

Nothing is known.

SUMMARY

Weill-Marchesani syndrome is a generalized disorder of connective tissues characterized by spherophakia, ectopia lentis, brachymorphism, and joint stiffness. The full syndrome is inherited as an autosomal recessive; heterozygotes show brachymorphism.

---

*The "a" and "d" are points on the palm near the base of the second and fifth fingers, respectively. "t" refers to the axial triradius that is normally near the base of the palm.[3a] The a.t.d. angle is larger than normal when the hand is short as in the Weill-Marchesani syndrome, or the axial triradius is displaced distally as in mongolism (Down syndrome). (The letters "a.t.d." are not abbreviations; it might be preferable to write it "ATD angle," according to the practice of electrocardiographers who write of the "QRS complex.")

REFERENCES

1. Burian, H. M., Von Noorden, G. K., and Ponseti, I. V.: Chamber angle anomalies in systemic connective tissue disorders, Arch. Ophthal. **64:**671, 1960.
2. Chandler, P. A.: Choice of treatment in dislocation of the lens, Arch. Ophthal. **71:**765, 1964.
3. Cotlier, E. (Chicago, Ill.): Personal communication through Harold E. Cross, 1971.
3a. Cummins, H., and Midlo, C.: Finger prints, palms and soles. An introduction to dermatoglyphics, New York, 1961, Dover Publications, Inc.
4. Diethelm, W.: Über Ectopia lentis ohne Arachnodaktylie und ihre Beziehungen zur Ectopia lentis et pupillae, Ophthalmologica **114:**16, 1947.
5. Feiler-Ofry, V., Stein, R., and Godel, V.: Marchesani's syndrome and chamber-angle anomalies, Amer. J. Ophthal. **65:**862, 1968.
6. Feinberg, S. B.: Congenital mesodermal dysmorpho-dystrophy (brachymorphic type), Radiology **74:**218, 1960.
7. Gorlin, R. J., Chandhry, A. P., and Moss, M. L.: Craniofacial dysostosis, patent ductus arteriosus, hypertrichosis, hypoplasia of labia majora, dental and eye anomalies—a new syndrome? J. Pediat. **56:**778, 1960.
8. Hazato, N., Ko, T., Vesugi, M., Okada, R., and Kitamura, K.: Two cases of Marchesani syndrome (in Japanese), Jap. J. Intern. Med. **60:**45, 1971.
9. Kloepfer, H. W., and Rosenthal, J. W.: Possible genetic carriers in the spherophakia-brachymorphia syndrome, Amer. J. Hum. Genet. **7:**398, 1955.
10. McGavic, J. S.: Weill-Marchesani syndrome; brachymorphism and ectopia lentis, Amer. J. Ophthal. **62:**820, 1966.
11. McKusick, V. A., Egeland, J. A., and Eldridge, R.: Dwarfism in the Amish. I. The Ellis–van Creveld syndrome, Bull. Hopkins Hosp. **115:**306, 1964.
12. McKusick, V. A., Eldridge, R., Hostetler, J. A., Ruangwit, U., and Egeland, J. A.: Dwarfism in the Amish. II. Cartilage-hair hypoplasia, Bull. Hopkins Hosp. **116:**285, 1965.
13. Marchesani, O.: Brachydaktylie und angeborene Kugellinse als Systemerkrankung, Klin. Mbl. Augenheilk. **103:**392, 1939.
14. Marchesani, O.: Jubilee volume for Prof. Vogt, part II, Basle, 1939, Benno Schwage Co., p. 32.
15. Meyer, S. J., and Holstein, T.: Spherophakia with glaucoma and brachydactyly, Amer. J. Ophthal. **24:**247, 1941.
16. Obituary: Oswald Marchesani (1900-1952), Klin. Mbl. Augenheilk. **120:**653, 1952; Graefe Arch. Ophthal. **152:**551, 1951-52.
17. Probert, L. A.: Spherophakia with brachydactyly; comparison with Marfan's syndrome, Amer. J. Ophthal. **36:**1571, 1953.
18. Rahman, M., and Rahman, S.: Marchesani's syndrome, Brit. J. Ophthal. **47:**182, 1963.
19. Rennert, O. M.: The Marchesani syndrome; a brief review, Amer. J. Dis. Child. **117:**703, 1969.
20. Rosenthal, J. W., and Kloepfer, H. W.: The spherophakia-brachymorphia syndrome, Arch. Ophthal. **55:**28, 1956.
21. Rousseau and Hermann: Ectopie congénitale du cristallin avec brachymorphie (syndrome de Marchesani), Bull. Mém. Soc. Franç. Ophtal. **62:**369, 1949.
22. Saxena, K. M., Saxena, P. N., Gorg, K. C., and Dube, S. K.: Dwarfism with brachydactyly, spherophakia, and glaucoma; Marchesani syndrome in an Indian girl, Indian Pediat. **3:**231, 1966.
23. Scott, C. I.: Weill-Marchesani syndrome. In Clinical delineation of birth defects. II. Malformation syndromes, New York, 1969, National Foundation–March of Dimes, pp. 238-240.
24. Seeleman, K.: Brachydaktylie und angeborene Kugellinse, Z. Kinderheilk. **67:**1, 1949.
25. Stadlin, W., and Klein, D.: Ectopie congénitale du cristallin avec sphérophaquie et brachymorphie accompagnée des parésies du regard (syndrome de Marchesani), Ann. Ocul. **181:**692, 1948.
26. Weill, G.: Ectopie du cristillins et malformations générales, Ann. Ocul. **169:**21, 1932.
27. Zabriskie, J., and Reisman, M.: Marchesani syndrome, J. Pediat. **52:**159, 1958.

6 · The Ehlers-Danlos syndrome

Historical note

None of the hereditary disorders of connective tissue, except possibly osteogenesis imperfecta, has as ancient a history as does the Ehlers-Danlos syndrome. The first definitive case* of this syndrome seems to have been described in 1682[275] by Job van Meekeren, a surgeon of Amsterdam. In Fig. 6-1 is presented van Meekeren's illustration of the "extraordinary dilatability of the skin" in a 23-year-old Spaniard who could pull the right pectoral skin to the left ear, the skin under the chin up over the head like a beard, and the skin of the knee area out about one-half yard. On being released, the skin retracted promptly to fit snugly over the underlying structures. This phenomenon was limited to the skin of the right side of the body.

In retrospect, Smith and Worthington[249] suggested that Nicolò Paganini (1782-1840), the violinist "virtuoso in excelsis," had the Ehlers-Danlos syndrome. His slender physique, thoracic deformity, and joint laxity, which in the hypermobility of the fingers is thought to have contributed to his virtuosity, are well documented.

Late in the last century, various dermatologists published scattered references to this condition, which was usually observed as a curiosity in "India rubber men" of side shows. Gould and Pyle[111] published the photograph made in Budapest in 1888 of an exhibitionist named Felix Wehrle, "who besides having the power to stretch his skin could readily bend his fingers backward and forward."

---

*In *Airs, Waters and Places* Hippocrates,[163] in the fourth century B.C., described the Scythians as having markedly lax joints. "I will give you a strong proof of the humidity (laxity?) of their constitutions. You will find the greater part of the Scythians, and all the Nomades, with marks of the cautery on their shoulders, arms, wrists, breasts, hip-joints, and loins, and that for no other reason but the humidity and flabbiness of their constitution, for they can neither strain with their bows, nor launch the javelin from their shoulder owing to their humidity and atony: but when they are burnt, much of the humidity in their joints is dried up, and they become braced, better fed, and their joints get into a more suitable condition." Is it possible that the cigarette-paper scars of the Ehlers-Danlos syndrome were misinterpreted? Against this suggestion is the fact that burning the skin around joints became an established treatment for dislocation of joints, in the ancient world. Another statement is of much interest: ". . . they afterwards became lame and stiff at the hip-joint, such of them, at least, as are severely attacked with it." (From Adams, F.: The genuine works of Hippocrates, New York, 1891, William Wood & Co.)

Kopp,[147] who is widely quoted as first drawing attention to familial incidence by describing an affected father and son, was probably dealing with cutis laxa, not the Ehlers-Danlos syndrome.

With considerable justification Jansen[131] argues that Tschernogobow[269,270] is most deserving of credit for the first detailed clinical description of this syndrome. In 1891 he presented to the Moscow Dermatologic and Venereologic Society 2 cases of the syndrome. He described the fragility as well as the hyperelasticity of the skin, the failure of the skin to hold sutures, the hypermobility and luxation of joints, and the molluscoid pseudotumors of the knees, elbows, and other areas. Most important, he tied all these features together as manifestations of a fundamental and generalized inadequacy of connective tissue; "Erschlaffung des Bindegewebes" were his words.

One of Tschernogobow's patients[269] was a 17-year-old epileptic male who, in

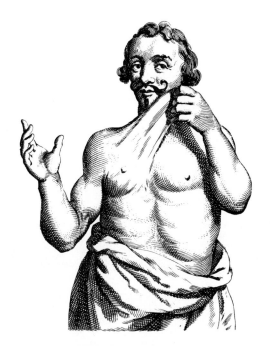

Fig. 6-1. Job van Meekeren's case of "extraordinary dilatability of the skin."

"In the year 1657, in the presence of the very distinguished John van Horne and Francis Sylvius, professors of medicine in the famous academy of Leyden, as well as of William Piso and Francis vander Schagen, practitioners of Amsterdam, we saw in our hospital a certain young Spaniard, 23 years of age, by the name of George Albes, who with his left hand grasped the skin over his humerus and right breast and stretched it till it was quite close to his mouth. With each hand he first pulled the skin of his chin downward like a beard to his chest, hence he lifted it upwards to the vertex of his head so as to cover each eye with it. As soon as he removed his hand the skin contracted to reassume its proper smoothness. In the same way he pulled the skin of his right knee upwards or downwards, to the length of half an ell; then it easily returned to its natural position. It was worthwhile noting that the skin which covered the forementioned parts on the left side could not be extended since it firmly adhered to them. It has, thus far, not been possible to learn the cause [of this anomaly?]."—Translated from original Latin by Dr. Owsei Temkin.

falling frequently on his face, had left there and elsewhere broad fissures running in all directions. The skin of the knees, elbows, and wrists was unusually spongy and loose, suggesting elephantiasis mollis or fibroma molluscum. Joint changes were especially pronounced on the left side, where dislocations of the elbow and hip, dating from childhood, were present. In the second patient,[270] a 50-year-old woman, "tumors" were present not only on the elbows and knees but also on the buttocks, presumably in the vicinity of the ischial tuberosities. When one of these "tumors" was removed, it was discovered that sutures did not hold well and dehiscence of the wound occurred in a couple of days.

Du Mesnil[80] in 1890, Williams[293] in 1892, working in Unna's laboratory in Hamburg, and Unna[274] himself in 1894 reported on histologic studies. In general, these authors were puzzled by the absence of specific changes and encountered difficulties in the interpretation of what they did find. The contribution in 1901 by Ehlers[85] of Denmark[68] consisted of pointing out the associated loose-jointedness and the subcutaneous hemorrhages that are prone to occur. Danlos[67] in 1908 rounded out the clinical description with inclusion of the tumors that may develop at subcutaneous sites.

In London, Sir Malcolm Morris demonstrated a case in 1900 and pictured the boy in the 1909 edition of his *Diseases of the Skin* (Fig. 6-2, *A*). Beighton[22] provided a picture of the same patient in his eighty-second year (Fig. 6-2, *B*).

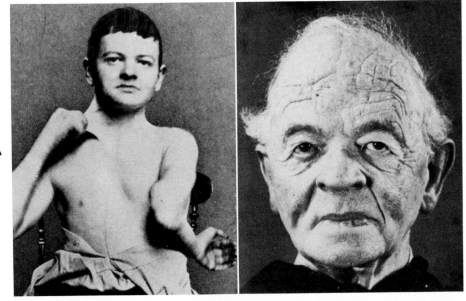

Fig. 6-2. "Lad with elastic skin and multiple cutaneous nodules," a case presented to the Old Dermatological Society of London in 1900 by Sir Malcolm Morris.[184] Beighton[22] suggests that this is the earliest recognizable case of E-D in the British medical literature. The picture of the boy, **A,** appeared in the 1909 edition of Morris' *Diseases of the Skin,*[185] where the disorder was described as "fibroma with elastic skin and congenital dislocations." The photograph in **B** is of the same "lad" in his eighty-second year. His activity was limited by degenerative arthritis of the spine, knees, elbows, and hands. (From Beighton, P.: The Ehlers-Danlos syndrome, London, 1970, William Heinemann Medical Books Ltd.)

The first case report from the United States was that of Tobias.[268] In 1936 Ronchese[226] of Rhode Island found 24 cases in the literature and added 3 of his own. In the first edition of *Heritable Disorders of Connective Tissue* (1956) I estimated that the world's literature contained less than 100 well-documented reports, but by the third edition (1966) the estimate had risen to over 300.

In 1949 autosomal dominant inheritance was demonstrated by Johnson and Falls[137] on the basis of an extensive kindred containing 32 affected persons. In 1954 Jansen[131] suggested that the defect concerns the collagen wickerwork, or basketry, which is excessively loose in this disorder.

Genetic heterogeneity of the Ehlers-Danlos syndrome was proposed in the second edition of *Heritable Disorders of Connective Tissue*. Barabas[14] suggested the existence of three forms of the disorder, and Beighton* recognized at least five clinically distinct forms, of which one is an X-linked recessive. Beighton's classification has been adopted here as a useful tentative grouping, and a sixth autosomal recessive form has been added to the classification. In this last variety of the Ehlers-Danlos syndrome a molecular defect of collagen was identified by Pinnell, Krane, and their colleagues[149a,209b] and confirmed by Lichtenstein et al.[160a] This is the first heritable disorder of collagen—other than alkaptonuria—to be elucidated at the molecular level.

Many terms have been used for this syndrome or, more often, for its individual features. In 1936 F. Parkes Weber[284] attempted to bring nosologic order out of the group of conditions with lax skin and loose joints, together or alone, and defended the use of the eponym "Ehlers-Danlos syndrome" as useful for the specific disorder discussed in this chapter (Tschernogobow's reports were not known to Weber). As in the case of the Marfan syndrome, the eponymic designation seems preferable, since it does not convey any connotations of the invariable occurrence of an individual manifestation or any ill-founded notion of the nature of the basic defect. "E-D" is the abbreviated label that will be used frequently in this presentation.†

Clinical manifestations[149,261]

The Ehlers-Danlos syndrome is characterized mainly by hyperextensible skin, hypermobile joints, fragile tissues, and a bleeding diathesis. Variability in the individual features and differences in inheritance patterns permit delineation of separate forms of the disorder, as detailed below.

The manifestations of the Ehlers-Danlos syndrome can conveniently be discussed under the following categories: cutaneous, musculoskeletal, ocular, and internal.

The skin.[34,49,144,218,226,229] Characteristically, the skin in E-D is velvety in appearance and feel. It may also resemble wet chamois in feel. In the infant, it may be impressively white. It is hyperextensible, yet not lax (Fig. 6-3*A*).

---

*Beighton has made important contributions to the nosography of E-D, culminating in a monograph[22] based on the reported cases, numbering about 300, and a unique personal experience with 130 cases. He dedicated his monograph to the "India Rubber Men for bending over backwards to help in my investigations, and to the Elastic Ladies, who were always prepared to stretch a point to assist my work."

†ED is used for "ectodermal dysplasia" by some (e.g., Gold and Scriver, Amer. J. Hum. Genet. 24:549, 1972).

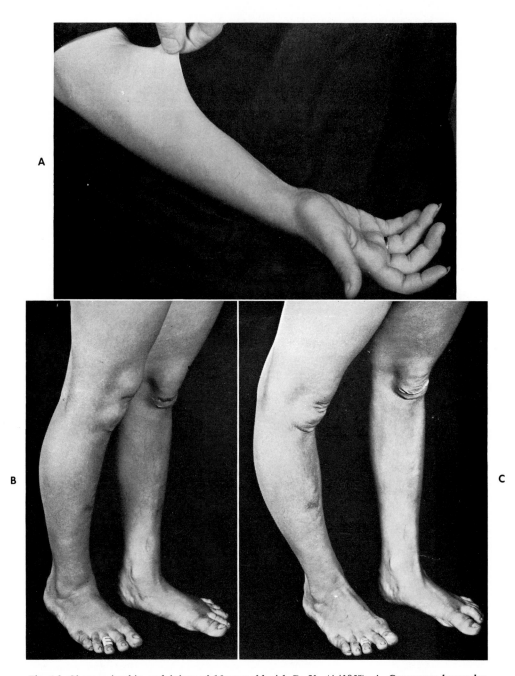

Fig. 6-3. Changes in skin and joints of 16-year-old girl, D. V. (A41965). **A,** Cutaneous hyperelasticity. **B,** Normal position of knees. Note papyraceous scars over the knees, and flat feet. **C,** Genu recurvatum, more on the right knee. **D,** Hyperextensibility of fifth finger. **E,** Hyperextensibility of thumb. Note, in the left hand, the hyperextension of the index finger and the abnormal separation of the knuckles. **F,** Hyperextensibility of fingers. **G,** Unusual mobility of hip and knee joints.

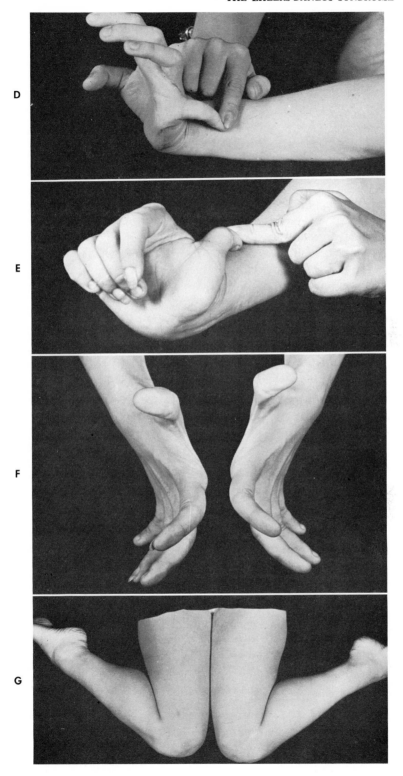

Fig. 6-3, cont'd. For legend see opposite page.

The term *cutis laxa* is inappropriate in the typical case in young persons. Except as noted below, the skin is truly hyperelastic, in the popular sense of the word.* Cutis laxa is a term properly reserved for a separate genetically determined entity.[70,220] (See Chapter 7.)

In addition, the skin is fragile, leading to the phenomenon called dermatorrhexis.[226] Minor trauma may produce gaping, fish-mouth wounds. One of my patients was for a time a professional boxer, a mutilating occupation for one with this disorder. Another, 16 years old at the time of study (Fig. 6-3), had had a total of 148 cutaneous stitches taken during her lifetime. The skin of the forehead, chin, knees, and shins is particularly vulnerable. Often stitches hold poorly in the skin,[137,227] and the patients and physicians resort to the use of adhesive tape. In the patient of Brown and Stock,[46] 282 stitches had been taken before count was stopped. Thomas and associates[264] described slow healing of a skin biopsy site and dehiscence of an ocular incision for removal of an ectopic lens. Packer and Blades[200] observed disruption of an appendectomy scar four times in thirty months. In one of my cases, a surgeon described the tissue at laparotomy as being like wet blotting paper. The tissues at autopsy are likely to be abnormally friable (*v. seq.*).

Very little bleeding occurs from the skin wounds. On the other hand, easy bruisability is the rule and, together with other hemorrhagic phenomena, frequently leads these patients to consult hematologists. The subsequent organization and calcification of the hematomas at times result in one type of pseudotumor.

So-called molluscoid pseudotumors,[204,212] which develop at pressure points—heels (Figs. 6-2*B*, 6-4*A*, 6-16, and 6-22†), knees, elbows, etc.—were the basis for the misconceived term of Hallopeau and Mace de Lépinay[67,119]: "juvenile pseudodiabetic xanthomatosis." Another type of tumor, small to be sure, seen

---

*There is so much confusion in the biologic literature with reference to the term *elasticity* that some care must be exercised. Burton writes as follows:

> Elasticity is properly defined as the property of materials which enables them to resist deformation by the development of a resisting force or "tension." All coefficients of elasticity are defined as the ratio of this resisting force (which at equilibrium is equal to the applied deforming force, or "load") to the measure of deformation produced. Thus, by the physical definition, material of "high elasticity" resists deformation, e.g., stretching, by a large force; so that it takes a large force to produce a given deformation. A material of "low elasticity" cannot resist deformation so well, and it takes only a small force to produce the same degree of deformation. Thus glass or steel has a much higher elasticity than does rubber.
>
> Most unfortunately, popular usage of the adjective "elastic" connotes the opposite. If a material like rubber is easily stretched, it is popularly said to be "elastic" and glass is "not so elastic" as rubber. (From Burton, A. C.: Physiol. Rev. 34:619, 1954.)

As used in this discussion of E-D, *elasticity* refers to physical properties like those of rubber, specifically stretchability, and restoration after deformation.

†In a young man who presumably did not have E-D, Shelley and Rawnsley[247] described painful feet due to small papular herniation of subcutaneous tissue into the skin on the medial aspects of the heel. Since the herniation occurred only with weight bearing, they used the designation piezogenic papules. A similar mechanism may be responsible for painful feet in E-D, other causes being related to the skeletal deformity (Figs. 6-5 and 6-16) or to the thin skin of the soles (Fig. 6-22).

in these cases is the so-called spherule, which is usually pea-sized or smaller and slips about under the skin an inch or more without causing the patient any discomfort. These small fat-containing cysts may become calcareous.[285] They are most frequently the basis for subcutaneous calcifications that may be demonstrable radiologically,[39,126] another basis being calcified hematomas as noted above. (Congenital lipomatosis has been described in association with Ehlers-Danlos syndrome by Tobias.[268] It is entirely possible, however, that the fatty tumors in his case were an integral part of the connective tissue disease.) At times actual ossification occurs.[142] The subcutaneous calcifications are characteristically ovoid in shape and 2 to 8 mm. in largest dimensions. They occur principally on the legs and, to a lesser extent, on the arms. Radiologically they display a diffuse inner calcification with a more dense surrounding shell. They are not laminated like phleboliths. These characteristics, together with the facts that they are not in muscle (as are calcified parasitic cysts) and are too widely distributed to be phleboliths, should permit the radiologist to make the diagnosis of E-D.[152]

Easily recognized changes develop in the skin overlying the knees, shins, and elbows; it becomes shiny, parchment-thin, and hyperpigmented (Figs. 6-3*B* and 6-4*B*). Resulting are the so-called "cigarette paper" or "papyraceous" scars. Telangiectases sometimes develop in the region of these atrophic scars. The skin changes may suggest those produced by exposure to x rays.

Bleeding may occur from the gums with brushing of the teeth, from tooth sockets after dental extractions, from the pharynx after tonsillectomy, and at the site of operations on the joints.[280] Petechiae in late pregnancy and prolonged postpartum hemorrhage have been described.[236] Gastrointestinal bleeding occurs in some patients.[129,236,277] Recurrent hemoptysis has been described.[221] Contrariwise, in one of my patients it is difficult to get blood for cell counts by finger puncture, and venipunctures are also difficult, seemingly because of very small and collapsed superficial veins. In another of my patients (Fig. 6-5), a strain of the tendons of the hamstring muscles at the knee resulted in the subcutaneous dissection of blood down to the ankle. E-D must be included in the differential diagnosis of familial hemophilia-like states. All tests of coagulation are usually normal[47,129,258,271] except that the Rumpel-Leede test may be positive.[93,122,200,203,232,236,273] In a family with E-D transmitted through four generations, a mother and daughter studied by Lisker and associates[162] showed deficiency of plasma thromboplastin component (Christmas factor, factor IX). A deficiency of Hageman factor was described by Fantl et al.[89] in a boy with E-D, but a brother without E-D also had the clotting defect. Kashiwagi and associates[141] and Green and colleagues[115] reported on studies of a patient with E-D and probable deficiency of platelet factor III, as well as morphologic alteration of platelet structure demonstrable by electron microscopy: the platelets tended to clump and showed osmiophilic blunting of processes with few or no dendrites. Estes[88] found abnormally large platelets, some of which also showed a functional abnormality, in patients with E-D as well as in patients with other heritable disorders of connective tissue. Goodman and co-workers[105] found defective platelet thromboplastic function and clot retraction, as well as a vascular defect. On the other hand, Day and Zarafonetis[69] and Wigzell and Ogston,[292] like others just referred to, found normal tests of coagulation in patients with the syndrome and con-

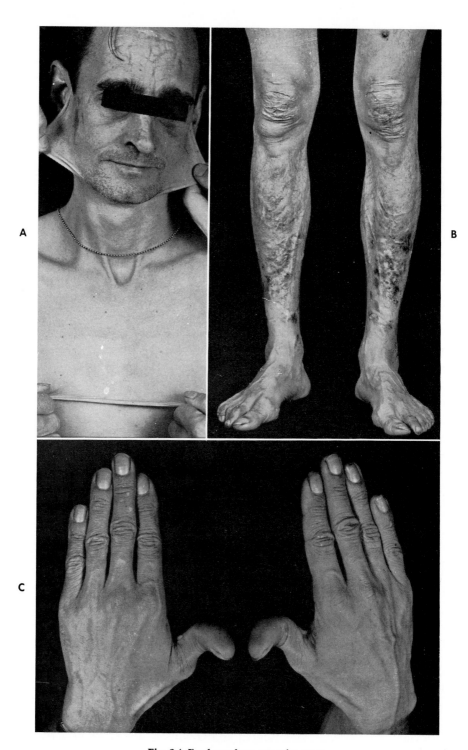

Fig. 6-4. For legend see opposite page.

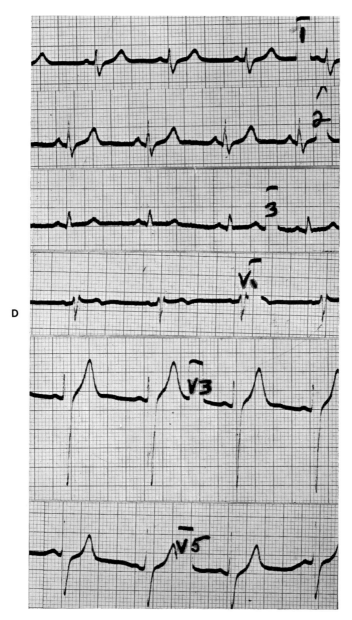

Fig. 6-4. Patient 35 years of age (a son has the E-D syndrome). **A,** Note scars of forehead and hyperextensibility of the skin. The patient was a professional boxer for a time. **B,** Note the spherical tumor in the skin of the anterior aspect of the left thigh. **C,** Ability to hyperextend the thumb occurs frequently as an isolated inherited characteristic.[100,290] **D,** Incomplete right bundle-branch block present since at least the age of 19 years and almost certainly all of life. No other cardiovascular or internal medical disorder was demonstrable.

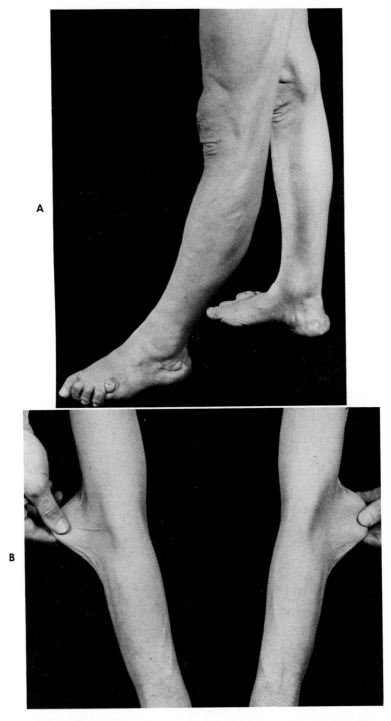

Fig. 6-5. K. W. (667280), 48-year-old man. **A,** Note deformity of feet, molluscoid tumors around heels (seen less distinctly in Fig. 6-3B). The soles appeared to be loose-fitting and resembled moccasins. There are cigarette-paper scars over the knees. **B,** Dewlaps of both elbows.

cluded that the subcutaneous bleeding is the result of some defect other than one of platelets or plasma clotting factors. They expressed the opinion that reported clotting defects in E-D are coincidental associations, and I am inclined to agree. Dr. Dudley P. Jackson has been unable to demonstrate a coagulation defect in several of my patients. Shapiro and colleagues[245] described a form of

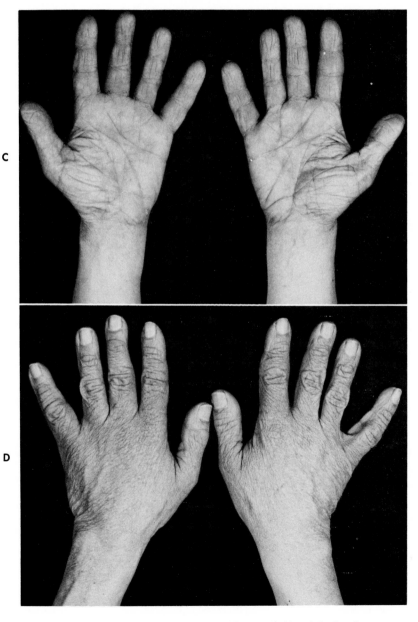

Fig. 6-5, cont'd. C and **D,** Lax and furrowed skin of the hands.

Continued.

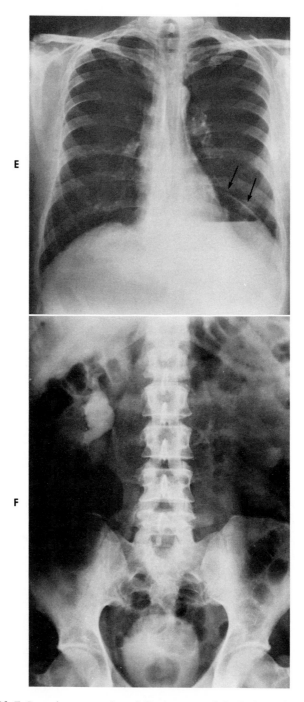

Fig. 6-5, cont'd. E, Posterior eventration of diaphragm on left. **F,** Anomaly of ureteropelvic junction, bilaterally. Nonfunctioning kidney on left.

dysprothrombinemia, with a variant prothrombin called Cardeza, in many members of three generations of a family with an autosomal dominant pedigree pattern. A maternal uncle of the proband (Case 2 of Day and Zarofonetis[69]) had typical skin and joint manifestations of E-D and also serious hemorrhagic problems; he died of intracranial hemorrhage at the age of 32 years. Although the proband of Shapiro and colleagues[245] had mild hyperextensibility of the finger joints, no member of the family other than the patient of Day and Zarofonetis[69] had stigmata of E-D. I suspect that the concurrence of E-D and prothrombin Cardeza in this family is coincidence, just as deficiencies that have been found in other plasma clotting factors in association with E-D are a matter of coincidence.

Blisterlike lesions may develop, suggesting epidermolysis bullosa (see Weber's interpretation of Burrows' case[48]).

The limitation of the cutaneous changes, particularly hyperelasticity, to one side of the body, as recounted by van Meekeren[275] in 1682, is almost completely incredible but is probably possible (*v. infra*). Beighton[22] observed a patient with striking cutaneous hyperextensibility on the right side and only mild changes on the left side of the body. Limitation of integumental hyperelasticity to the mucous membranes, specifically those of the mouth and tongue, has been described,[78] and many patients show evidences of changes (hyperelasticity and/or

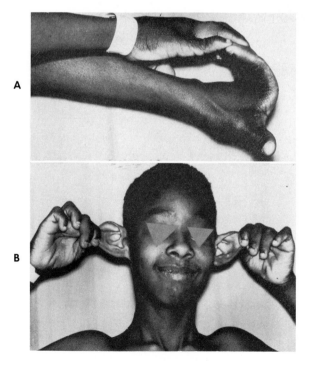

Fig. 6-6. Negro boy, 12 years old, with typical features of E-D syndrome, including hyperextensible joints, **A**, and stretchable ears, **B**. The skin was unusually stretchable, but fragility and bruisability were not present. (Courtesy Dr. Glenn R. Stoutt, Louisville, Ky.)

fragility) at these sites.[78,94,161,267,288] Affected women usually do not develop striae gravidarum.[137]

The skin of the hands and of the soles of the feet tends to be redundant (unlike most of the skin elsewhere, which fits snugly); with pressure it flattens out like a loose glove or moccasin (Fig. 6-5A, C, and D). A comparable change may develop in later years at the elbows, where the skin may hang lax like a dewlap (Fig. 6-5B). In general, late cases tend to show cutis laxa more than cutis hyperelastica, whereas, as emphasized above, cutis laxa is not an accurate designation in the typical case in young persons. Most patients with E-D have markedly wrinkled palms, that is, they have a large number of adventitious palmar creases. These creases are evident in Figs. 6-16B, 6-21B, and 6-23B. Goodman et al.[104a] referred to these as secondary skin creases, showed that they may de-

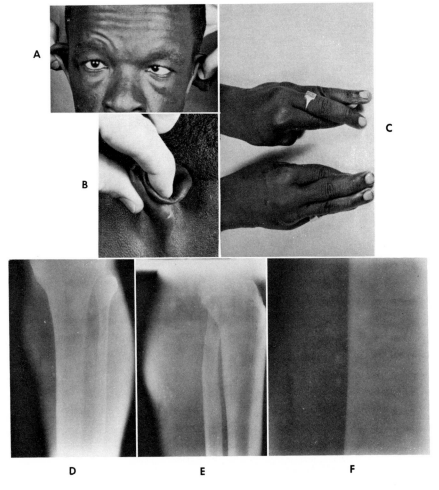

Fig. 6-7. E-D in Negro male, 28 years old. Strabismus and compressibility of the ears are demonstrated in **A** and **B**. The ease of folding the hand is shown in **C**. X-ray films demonstrated soft tissue calcifications, or spherules, **D, E,** and **F.**

velop as early as the age of 2½ years, and that they are well demonstrated by the standard dermatoglyphic techniques.

As indicated later, several distinct forms of E-D can be identified on clinical and/or genetic grounds. The skin and other manifestations show qualitative and quantitative differences. The skin changes in E-D type IV (the ecchymotic, arterial, or Sack's type) are distinctive (p. 339 and Figs. 6-10 and 6-21). Although fragility and bruisability are striking, the skin is generally thin and translucent, with clearly evident subcutaneous venous pattern. The skin is not excessively stretchable; indeed it is usually tight over the fingers and face and, with associated absence of subcutaneous fat, may suggest the Werner syndrome (p. 726). The ears are firm and not stretchable.

"Lop ears," ears that project farther than normally from the head and tend to face downward to some extent, occur commonly in E-D and occur also as an isolated heritable anomaly[165] (Fig. 6-25A). Normally the ear makes a 30-degree angle with the head.[167] The ears are, furthermore, unusually stretchable (Fig. 6-6B) and can be folded into a ball-like mass (Fig. 6-7B).

Gorlin and Pindborg[110] point out that many E-D patients display unusual ease in touching the tip of the nose with the tip of the tongue (Fig. 6-8B).

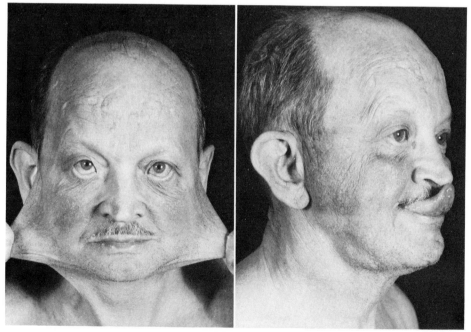

Continued.

Fig. 6-8. R. A. (911928), 60 years of age, has all the typical features of E-D syndrome. He subsequently died of metastatic squamous cell carcinoma of the nasopharynx. No other member of his family is known to be affected. **A,** Excessively stretchable skin and scars of the forehead are demonstrated. **B,** Gorlin's sign, unusual facility in touching the tip of the nose with the tip of the tongue, is demonstrated. **C,** Delicate epicanthal fold is demonstrated on the right. **D,** Typical skin changes are present over the legs.

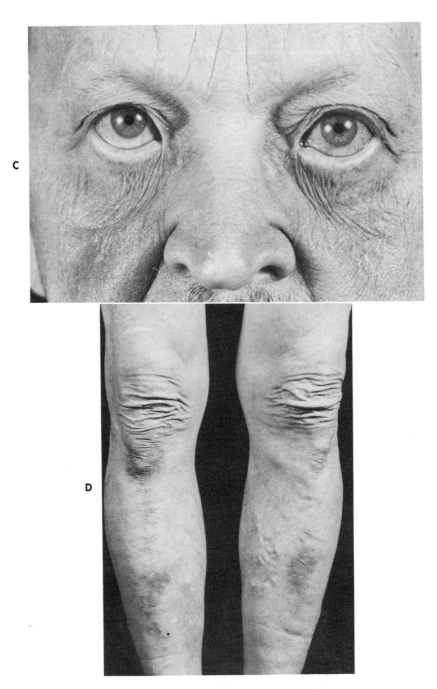

Fig. 6-8, cont'd. For legend see p. 307.

Duperrat[81] described a patient who was able to hold six golf balls in his mouth—a further demonstration of hyperextensibility of mucous membranes.

Acrocyanosis and chilblains have been described as a seemingly integral component, by French authors in particular,[91,99,187,215] but by others as well.[46,57,229,260,273] There seem to be few American reports of this complaint. In general, chilblains are much less common in this country than in Europe, possibly because of our more universal use of central heating. E-D is at least one basis for acrocyanosis that "runs in a family." It may be the presenting complaint in E-D. For example, Gilbert and associates[99] described a 22-year-old man who had had cyanosis of the hands, feet, and ears from birth and displayed the other characteristic features of E-D. In the patient's family there were several other cases of "cyanosed limbs and ulcerated chilblains" in association with E-D. Burrows[48] provided an excellent photograph of the hand of one of these patients, showing both joint hyperextensibility and cyanosis of the fingers. I have seen 2 patients (A. H., 796695; Mrs. R., P3479), both women, in whom acrocyanosis was a striking feature. They suffered severely from cold and displayed the Raynaud phenomenon. A woman with E-D reported by Newton and Carpenter[189] had severe Raynaud's symptoms and marked acro-osteolysis of the terminal phalanges.

Conceivably the abnormality with hyperelasticity, either of the supporting tissues about the arterioles or of the connective tissue in the vessel wall itself, interfers with blood flow. My observations of difficulties in obtaining blood by finger puncture or venipuncture, mentioned above, are significant in this connection.

Miescher's elastoma, which was described earlier (p. 146) as an occasional but surely rare finding in the Marfan syndrome, and which occurs more fre-

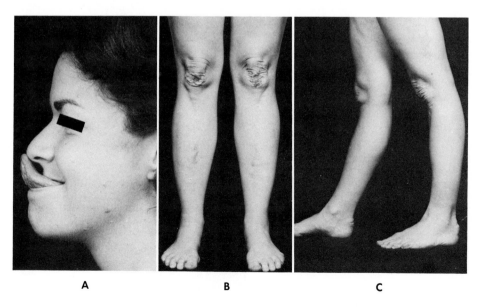

A   **B**   **C**

Fig. 6-9. E-D syndrome in V. B. (J.H.H. 1397865), 29 years old, apparently originating as a new mutation. **A,** Gorlin's sign; **B** and **C,** typical joint and skin changes.

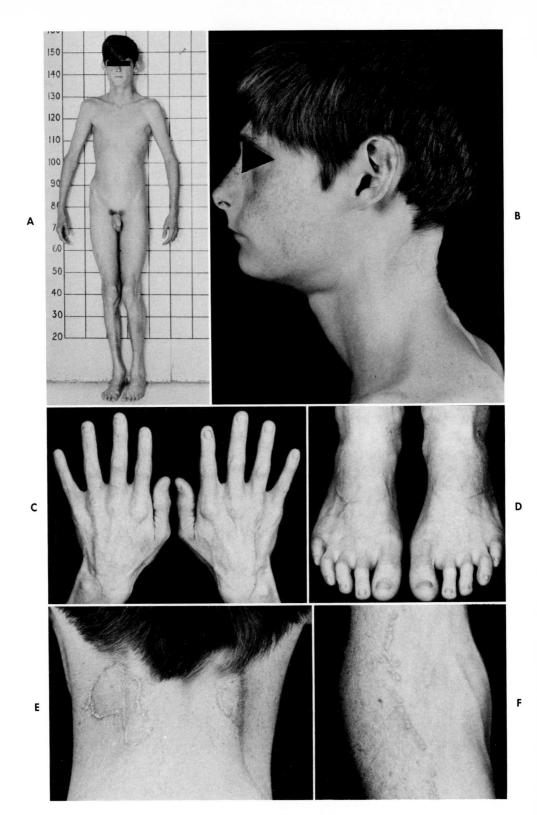

Fig. 6-10. For legend see opposite page.

quently in pseudoxanthoma elasticum (p. 483) and also in osteogenesis imperfecta, has been observed in E-D.[148,176,177,297] In a 65-year-old man with E-D, Castrow and Ritchie[56] described symmetric striae in a curved pattern situated symmetrically over the back. Folds of skin were present when the shoulders were extended, like those shown in Figs. 6-16C and 6-19B; when the shoulders were brought forward, thin striae were evident in the fold areas. I have seen elastosis perforans serpiginosa in only one patient, a 13-year-old boy with particularly extensive involvement of the arms and nape of neck (Fig. 6-10E and F). The patient had E-D type IV, the ecchymotic variety (p. 339); this form may be especially likely to occur in conjunction with elastosis perforans; the extreme deficiency of subcutaneous collagen may be responsible. I am told of a boy with elastosis perforans who had frequent ecchymoses and died at 18 years of age of a hemorrhage from the thyrocervical trunk.[96a]

Associated neurofibromatosis has been reported in at least three instances.[65,103,273] The association is probably coincidental. I have had one patient in whom squamous cell carcinoma developed in a prepatellar scar (Fig. 6-11A). It is difficult to defend any direct relationship between E-D and the carcinoma. It may be significant that Ross and Dooneief,[228] in reporting successful chest surgery in this patient, commented on unusual tumors in areas of friction such as the elbows and dorsa of the feet. Histologically these tumors showed acanthosis and hyperkeratosis. Examples of these warty lesions are shown in Fig. 6-11B.

The musculoskeletal system. Hyperextensibility of the joints is characteristic (Figs. 6-3D to F, 6-4C, and 6-12). This condition and the corresponding change in the skin make the victims of advanced forms of this disease the "India rubber men," "human pretzels," and contortionists of sideshows. The hyperextensibility tends to become less marked as the patient becomes older. For semiquantitation

---

Fig. 6-10. Extensive elastosis perforans in a 13-year-old boy with E-D syndrome, type IV. P. P. (J.H.H. 1426591), born Oct. 11, 1957, had required 300 stitches before 3 years of age and had had 500 stitches before the parents stopped counting. He had typical E-D scars of the forehead, chin, shins, and knees. The skin was generally thin and translucent, with a striking venous pattern, and was rather tight over the fingers and face, deficiency of corium being evident. The lesions of elastosis perforans extended in streaks down the lateral extensor surfaces of both arms to the midforearm and involved the neck in a figure-of-eight and annular pattern. Tinea had been an earlier diagnosis, based on the clinical appearance and on a mistaken interpretation of elastic fibers as mycelia in potssium hydroxide preparations.

The patient's ears were firm. He could touch the tip of his nose with the tip of his tongue. The fingers were hyperextensible but other joint laxity was unimpressive. He had recently "pulled a muscle" on the inner aspect of the upper right thigh in running, resulting in a large ecchymosis. He had no hernia, and had had no abdominal surgery or bowel symptoms. X-ray studies, including those of the small bowel, showed no diverticula. (Courtesy Dr. Harry M. Robinson, Jr.)

This patient's disorder appears to have originated as a new mutation. **A,** General appearance at the age of 13½ years. Note sparsity of subcutaneous fat, and thin, slimy, seemingly tight skin over the distal portion of the limbs. **B,** Lateral view of face and neck, showing tight, scarred skin over pinnae, pinched nose, sparsity of fat over face, and figure-of-eight elastoma lesion in nuchal area. **C** and **D,** Hands and feet showing tight, thin skin. **E,** Nape of neck showing bilateral lesions of elastosis perforans. **F,** Right antecubital area showing linearly arranged lesions of elastoma.

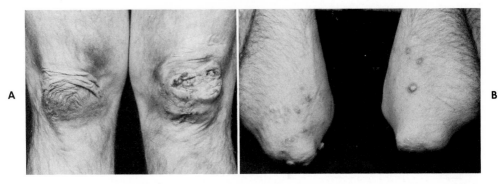

Fig. 6-11. Squamous cell carcinoma developing in a cigarette-paper scar. S. L. (J.H.H. 1421056), an attorney born in 1929, was diagnosed as having the Ehlers-Danlos syndrome at the age of 9 years. He had required over 300 sutures for skin lacerations, and often the sutures did not hold well. Loose-jointedness was moderate, and special shoes were required for foot drop deformity. Thoracoplasty was performed in 1952 for pulmonary tuberculosis. Moderate scoliosis appeared to be related in part to the tuberculosis and in part to the connective tissue disorder. No other member of the family was affected. In early 1970 he first noted an ulceration in the cigarette-paper scar over the left knee. This scar gradually enlarged and acquired heaped-up margins. It was surgically excised in June, 1971, by Dr. John E. Hoopes, and the area was successfully engrafted. Histology showed squamous cell carcinoma. The patient had used silver nitrate and other irritants on the ulcer daily for several months before surgical excision. This patient is the same as the one reported as having had successful thoracoplasty for pulmonary tuberculosis.[228] The early report commented on unusual tumor formation at pressure points such as the elbows and the dorsa of the feet. **A,** Knees showing bilateral cigarette-paper scars and, on the left, an ulceration with heaped-up margins. **B,** Unusual warty or pediculated lesions in vicinity of elbows.

of joint laxity, Beighton and Horan[28] made use of a scoring system adopted from that described by Carter and Wilkinson.[54] Patients were given a score of 0 to 5, one point being assigned for each of the following:

1. Passive dorsiflexion of the fifth finger beyond 90 degrees with the forearm flat on a table, as suggested by Ellis and Bundick[86] (Figs. 6-3*D* and 6-29)
2. Passive opposition of the thumb to the flexor aspect of the forearm (Fig. 6-3*E*)
3. Hyperextension of the elbow beyond 10 degrees (Fig. 6-14)
4. Hyperextension of the knees beyond 10 degrees (Fig. 6-3*C*)
5. Forward flexion of the trunk so that the palms of the hands rest easily on the floor

Wynne-Davies[294a] likewise modified the Carter-Wilkinson method[54] for evaluating joint mobility. Her all-or-none approach is diagrammed in Fig. 6-13.

Frequently the patients have joint effusions, especially in the knees, because of traumatization as a result of joint instability. Hemarthroses also occur.[188,209] Flatfoot occurs commonly (Fig. 6-3*B*), and clubfoot has been described[40,209] (Fig. 6-24, legend). The foot deformity is often a particularly troublesome feature (e.g., Figs. 6-5 and 6-20). The loose-jointedness, in the knees in particular, may result in a gait and stance suggesting tabes dorsalis[143] (Figs. 6-3*C* and 6-5*A*). Habitual dislocation of the hip,[54,67,193,203,287] patellae[52,53,79,193,241] (Fig. 6-15*E*), shoul-

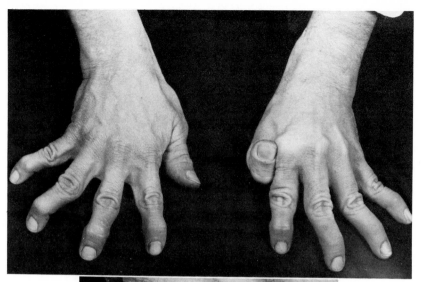

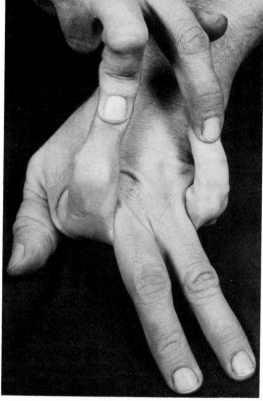

Fig. 6-12. C. G. (287731), 47 years old, with a long history of "congenital dislocation of right hip," treated with a spica at the age of 2 years and with several operations in his twenties. Bilateral inguinal hernias repaired. Hiatal hernia is apparently responsible for epigastric and substernal pressure, which occurs especially in the recumbent position and is relieved by belching. Dehiscence followed attempts at surgical repair of the hiatal hernia. Two operations on knee for presumed trauma of automobile accident. At the age of 27 years, "relaxation of right radiocarpal joint" necessitated application of a cast. Hyperelasticity of the skin, although present, was a subsidiary feature in this patient.

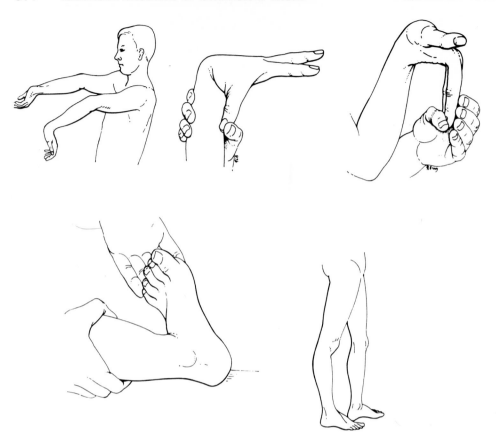

Fig. 6-13. Method for evaluating joint mobility.[21,294a] Excessive joint laxity is judged to be present when at least three of the five conditions obtain: (1) elbow extended beyond 180 degrees, (2) thumb touching the forearm on flexing the wrist, (3) the fingers parallel to the forearm on extending the wrist and metacarpophalangeal joints, (4) the foot dorsiflexed to 45 degrees or more, and (5) the knees extended beyond 180 degrees. (From Wynne-Davies, R.: J. Bone Joint Surg. 52B:704, 1970.)

der,[53,205] radii,[143] clavicle,[111] and other joints is a frequent feature. Chronic temporomandibular joint subluxation has been described.[103] Congenital dislocation of the hip was reported several times.[4,158,260] The recurrent dislocations of the patellae[241] are spontaneously reducible and usually represent no particular incapacitation to the patient. As in the Marfan syndrome, the sternal ends of the clavicle may be very loose.[143] There is likely to be genu recurvatum[287] (Fig. 6-3C). The patients are often able to pull their fingers out longitudinally for an appreciable distance, even to almost twice their length,[203] and allow them to snap back into place on release. The loose-jointed hand is evident in the handshake. Indeed, the limp feel has been compared to that of a fine foam-rubber sponge.[157] The hand can be folded up as shown in Fig. 6-16A. Some patients may show restricted motion in joints such as the elbows and hips.[169] Radioulnar synostosis[159] has been said[235] to occur. Posterior dislocation of the radial heads[59] may be a feature. Kyphoscoliosis is likely to develop[71,143,193,225,244,259,260,273,289] (Fig. 6-16).

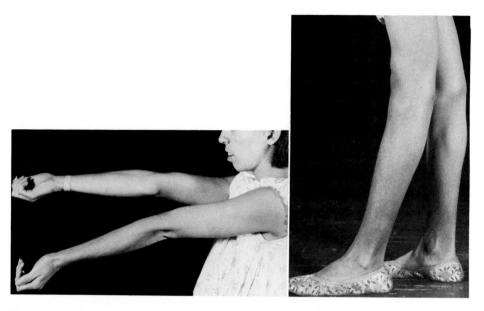

Fig. 6-14. M. W. (688052), 28-year-old female, presents another example of "simple" joint hypermobility. Loose-jointedness is most striking in the knees and elbows, as shown. Unusual stretchability, bruisability, fragility, and scarring of the skin were not present. The mother and at least one sib and one offspring are similarly affected.

Coventry[64] observed thoracolumbar kyphoscoliosis with anterior wedging of several vertebrae, long, giraffelike neck, downward curvature of the upper ribs, and a tendency to reversal of the normal spinal curves. It seems plausible that laxity in the joints of the shoulder girdle and downward dragging with gravity may result in sloping shoulders and a long neck. Spina bifida occulta is described,[145] as well as wedge-shaped deformity of vertebral bodies.[169] Dental deformities are frequent,[92,143,190] and Gothic palate may be present.[140] Muscular hypotonicity and underdevelopment seem to exist in these patients. In one of my cases, a 4-year-old child, amyotonia congenita of Oppenheim was the initial diagnosis. Smith[248] describes a similar experience. Hernias occur frequently.[285] In some, repair of an umbilical hernia at a young age is necessary.

Spondylolisthesis was a painful problem to 2 of my patients (R. W., 709823; L. S., 1117754) during their teens. The patient shown in Fig. 6-17 had spinal fusion at the age of 18 years and has felt well since that time. The second patient had spontaneous relief of symptoms. Scalloping, an exaggeration of the normally slight concavity of the dorsal aspect of the vertebral bodies, has been observed in E-D,[180] and also in the Marfan syndrome (p. 83).

Ectopic bone formation with formation of osseous bridges between the acetabula and the femoral trochanters has been described by Katz and Steiner.[142] The pathogenesis may have involved hemorrhage from increased joint mobility.

Short stature has been a feature of some cases.

Severe leg cramps, occurring at night and at other times, such as while watching television, have been a major problem over a period of many years in one

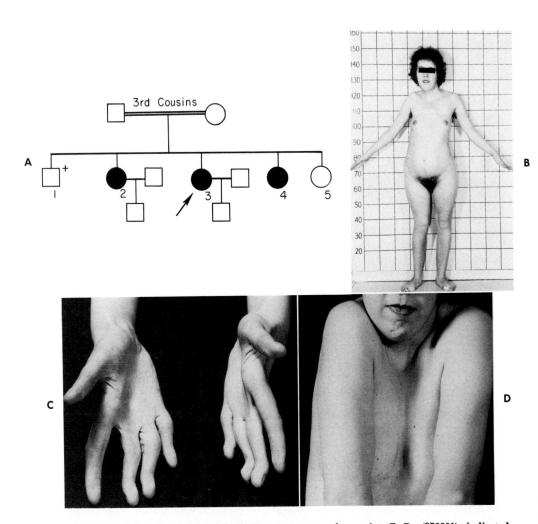

Fig. 6-15. Marked loose-jointedness inherited as an autosomal recessive. E. D. (970801), indicated by arrow in perigree, **A,** and 25 years old at the time of study, has marked hyperextensibility of many joints, especially those of the hands, feet, shoulders, and spine. Dislocations at both hips and both elbows have resulted in limitation of motion in these joints. The bridge of the nose is broad, and she has myopia, microphthalmia, and intermittent exotropia. She is 58 inches tall. The fingers are somewhat webbed. The skin is not excessively stretchable or fragile, but there is some increased bruisability. There are no cigarette-paper scars; no striae resulted from pregnancy. No chromosomal abnormality could be identified. A sister (2 in the pedigree) has had dislocation of the knees about twenty-five times, beginning at 6 years of age. She also has bilateral dislocation of the patella, and scoliosis. A young sister (II-4) also has habitual dislocation of the patellae. Neither parent shows any abnormality resembling those in the children, and the 2 offspring of affected sibs show no abnormality. In **B, C,** and **D** are demonstrated general features and the loose-jointedness. Acrocyanosis is suggested in **C.** **E** to **H** show the radiologic features of the proband. Both patellae, **E,** both hips, **F,** and the head of each radius, **G,** are dislocated. Scoliosis is marked, **H.** It is suggested that a form of severe loose-jointedness behaving as an autosomal recessive is present in this family. (Family studied by Dr. R. M. Goodman and Dr. Yves Duchastel.) Recent findings suggest that E. D. may have deficiency of procollagen protease (p. 341).

patient (Fig. 6-4). Beighton[22] found this feature in 43 of his patients, and Kirk and associates[146] noted it as a feature of simple joint hypermobility. Quinine and quinidine afford relief. The cramps may result indirectly from the loose-jointedness. Individuals with flat feet or disorders of the low back are prone to night cramps. Easy fatigability is a frequent complaint of E-D patients.

The eye. Changes have been described in the ocular adnexa, the cornea, the sclera, the suspensory mechanism of the lens, and the fundus.

The skin about the eyes often lies in redundant folds and can be pulled out to a considerable distance, like the skin elsewhere. Epicanthal folds are fre-

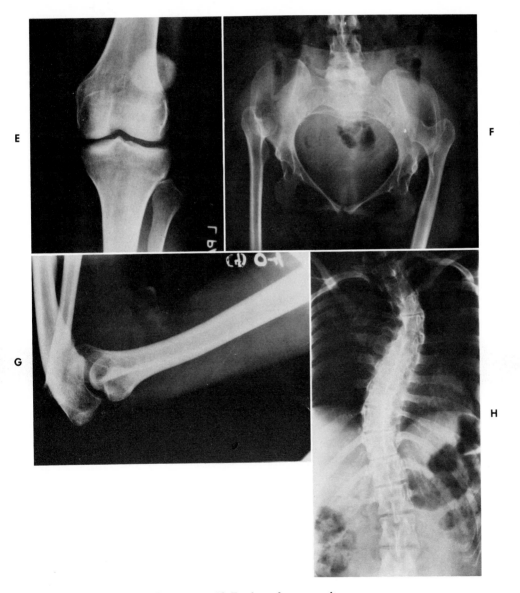

Fig. 6-15, cont'd. For legend see opposite page.

quent[7,34,97,137,191,213,238,246] (Fig. 6-18C). (Epicanthal folds occur, of course, in mongolism. They are also part of the facies characteristic of thalassemia; in other instances, they are inherited as a trait with no syndromal significance.) Epicanthus may disappear as the patient grows older; it is replaced by "widely spaced eyes," a frequent feature that appears to represent, not true hypertelorism, but a change in the tissues at each side of the nose, resulting in telecanthus. The eyes have

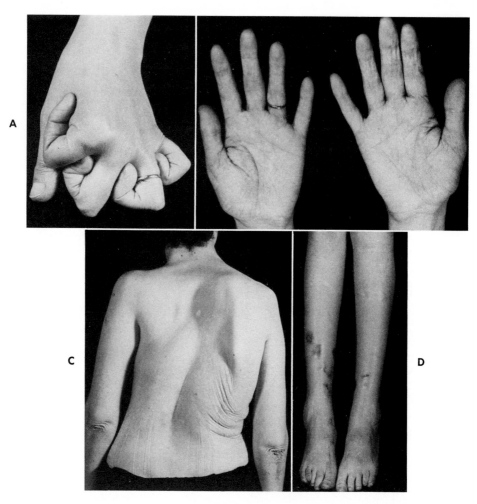

Fig. 6-16. Severe scoliosis and acrocyanosis in E-D syndrome. I. B. (983764), 37-year-old white female, has had loose-jointedness, **A,** stretchable and fragile skin, and acrocyanosis, **B,** all her life. She spent several months in an orthopedic hospital at 12 years of age for treatment of "clubfoot" and again at 15 years for treatment of scoliosis, **C.** In **D** are shown multiple breaks and excessive bruising in the skin over the legs. Ocular complications also were present. From the age of 6 years she wore spectacles for myopia. Microcornea, blue sclerae, and glaucoma were noted at 27 years of age and were described in brief by Durham.[52] Between 35 and 37 years of age complete detachment, first of the left and then of the right retina, occurred. A brother likewise sustained bilateral retinal detachment after minor trauma and is, like his sister, totally blind. Both parents and 6 sibs of the 2 are normal, as are also 4 children of the brother. At age 19 the brother developed left-sided hemiplegia following head injury.

a parrotlike or owllike appearance, as demonstrated in Figs. 6-2*B* and 6-19*E*. Méténier[178] has lent his name to a frequent phenomenon, namely, unusual ease in everting the upper lid. Strabismus has been encountered frequently.[17,61,63,131,246]

Blue sclerae have been described commonly.[42,82,174,265] Microcornea with associated glaucoma was described in one patient[82] in whom the small size of the cornea was thought to be responsible, at least indirectly, for an impediment to ocular drainage. Microcornea and myopia were present in Schaper's first patient.[238] Keratoconus is also described,[265] as are corneal thinning and megalocornea,[41] and corneal laceration from minor trauma.[69] Retinal detachment occurred, after minor trauma, in the brother of the patient pictured in Fig. 6-16. As noted on p. 340, there may be a specific variety of E-D appropriately called the ocular type because of a high frequency of ocular manifestations including microcornea, glaucoma, retinal detachment, and rupture of the globe from minor trauma. The cornea was abnormally large and thin in one reported case.[41]

Ectopia lentis occurred in at least one twice-reported patient.[264,265] Operative repair was complicated by wound dehiscence. Unilateral slight dislocation of the lens and mild iridodonesis was described by Cordella and Vinciguerra.[62] Minor indirect trauma caused luxation of the lens and rupture of the cornea in a 4-year-old child.[181]

In one patient, the author[40] described and illustrated changes in the fundus, consisting of retinitis proliferans, pigment spots that were interpreted as residua of microhemorrhages, and detachment of the retina of secondary type (no retinal

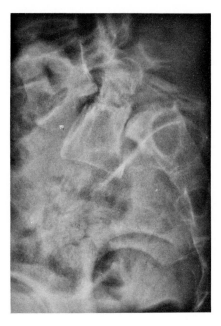

Fig. 6-17. Severe spondylolisthesis in L. S. (1117734), 17-year-old white girl with all the cardinal features of E-D syndrome. The fifth lumbar vertebra has almost slipped off the first sacral vertebra.

tear was detected). Retinal detachment occurred bilaterally in the patient shown in Fig. 6-16. Retinal detachment followed trauma to the eye in a patient described by Cordella and Vinciguerra.[62] Pemberton and colleagues[206] described a kindred in which several members had myopia and retinal detachment. One of the patients died at the age of 39 years after operation for dissected aorta.

Green and co-workers[116] found typical angioid streaks in 2 of 6 affected members of a kindred. To their knowledge, this was the first description of angioid

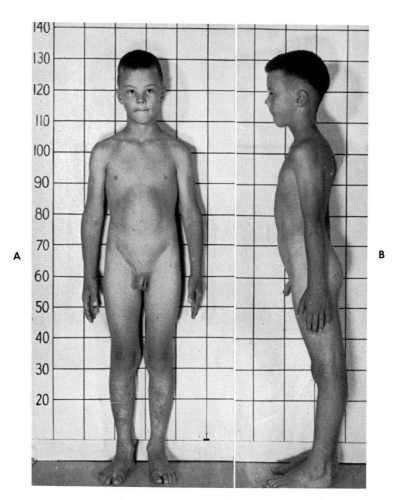

Fig. 6-18. R. R. (B53739), 8 years 9 months of age, shows characteristic pretibial scarring, mild genu recurvatum, flat feet, and looseness of the soles. The skin generally is abnormally stretchable and the joints hypermobile. Easy bruisability was the presenting complaint. An epicanthal fold, **C,** which is not present in unaffected members of his family, is a frequent finding in this syndrome, as is also mild retardation of growth. The characteristic scars are evident also on the forehead and right side of the face. Bilateral inguinal hernias and an umbilical hernia were repaired at 2 years of age. No other members of the family are definitely affected. The patient has 4 brothers and no sisters. One brother had pectus excavatum severe enough to warrant surgical repair, and a second brother has mild pectus excavatum. (From McKusick, V. A.: Bull. N. Y. Acad. Med. **35:**143, 1959.)

streaks in patients with E-D and no skin manifestations of pseudoxanthoma elasticum.

Internal ramifications. The internal manifestations of E-D can be discussed under the following categories: gastrointestinal, pulmonary, cardiovascular, neurologic, and obstetric.

One of my patients has eventration of the left leaf of the diaphragm (Fig. 6-5E). Differentation from a large posterior diaphragmatic hernia is uncertain. We have observed *hiatal hernia* in a second patient, of whom other illustrations are shown in Fig. 6-12. Zalis and Roberts[296] also observed eventration of the diaphragm and hiatal hernia. The stomach, located in the thorax, became strangulated. Beighton and associates[33] found eventration of the diaphragm on routine chest x-ray examination in 1 out of 40 patients. Brombart and associates[44] described a patient in whom hiatal hernia, diverticulum of the stomach, duodenal diverticulum, and colonic diverticulosis occurred in association with E-D. *Gastrointestinal diverticula* were present in Case 4 (see below) and are demonstrated in Fig. 6-19F to H. In a 64-year-old man with E-D, Green and colleagues[115] described diverticulosis of the sigmoid colon complicated by hemorrhage that was controlled only by subtotal colectomy. Mega-esophagus, mega-trachea, and megacolon were described in another case.[187] Bladder diverticulum is described,[257,296] as are also ptosis viscerum[3,198] and gastric atony.[229]

There are in the literature cases of abnormal friability of the intestine and uncontrollable internal hemorrhage in E-D. Jacobs,[129] in describing a case of

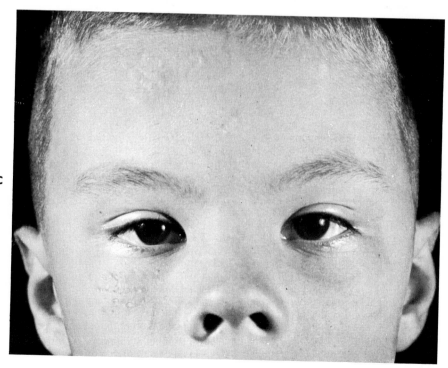

C

Fig. 6-18, cont'd. For legend see opposite page.

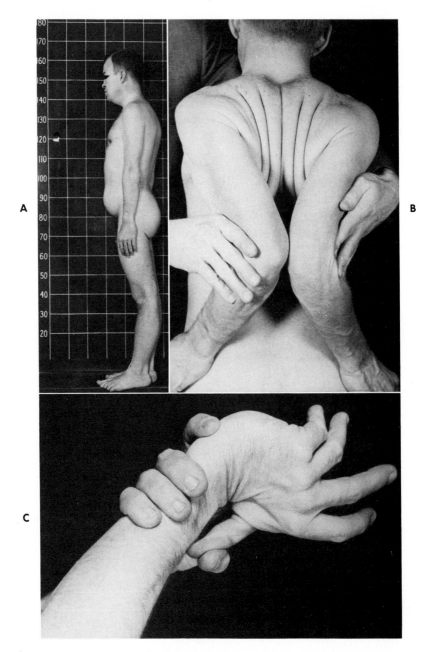

Fig. 6-19. Case 4. **A,** Lateral view. Note genu recurvatum and short stature. **B,** Hyperextensibility of the shoulders. **C,** Joint hypermobility. Note also the loose, coarse-grained appearance of the skin resembling that in the patient shown in Fig. 6-5.

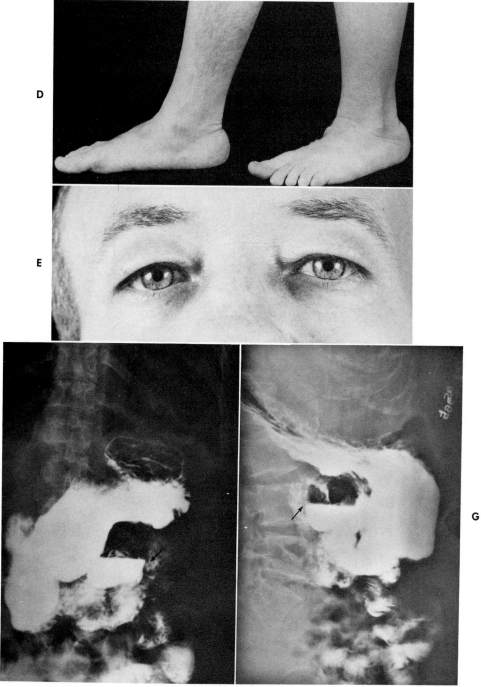

Fig. 6-19, cont'd. D, Flat feet; loose, redundant soles. **E,** Redundant skin of lids. **F,** Film from gastroduodenal series to show large duodenal diverticulum arising in region of ligament of Treitz and extending up behind the stomach. **G,** Same as **F,** lateral view.

Continued.

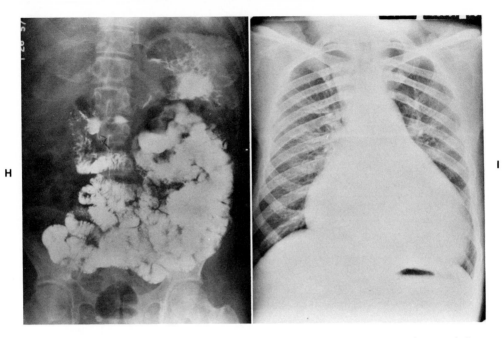

Fig. 6-19, cont'd. H, Gastrointestinal x-ray film showing diverticulum of second part of duodenum (arrow). **I,** Chest x-ray film to show general cardiomegaly.

E-D, stated that a brother, during appendectomy at the age of 37 years, was found to have very friable bowel covered with numerous hemorrhages. In the postoperative period wound disruption occurred and the patient died of uncontrolled gastrointestinal hemorrhage. *Spontaneous perforation of the bowel,* as discussed by Robertson and associates,[219] probably has multiple predisposing causes. The Ehlers-Danlos syndrome is sometimes one cause.

André and colleagues[6] described a young Frenchwoman who had a spontaneous intestinal perforation during childhood. Later hemorrhagic episodes of several types—rectal bleeding, hemoperitoneum from a ruptured ovarian cyst, and hemothorax—occurred. Aldridge[4] described successful surgical repair of spontaneous rupture of the sigmoid colon in a patient who died three years later from another perforation. In another patient spontaneous rupture of the jejunum was observed. Perforations occur in areas of the bowel without diverticula. Harlano[120] described perforation of the sigmoid colon in a 17-year-old boy whose father died of perforation of the sigmoid colon.

In addition to the case of Dr. Bouton, described later (p. 331), we have observed rupture of the bowel in 3 patients.[33] One woman (L. D. P., 1121524) had rupture of the sigmoid colon at the age of 24 years and again at 26 years. Each episode was preceded by rectal bleeding, suggesting that intramural bleeding may be a factor in rupture, along with friability of the bowel wall. The patient died at the age of 36 years after an operation for perforated sigmoid colon (Fig. 6-20). At autopsy multiple intestinal hematomas were found, as well as a large hepatic hematoma. The second patient (J.H.H. 1287186), at 17 years of age, had an attack of severe abdominal pain three weeks after a mild bout of

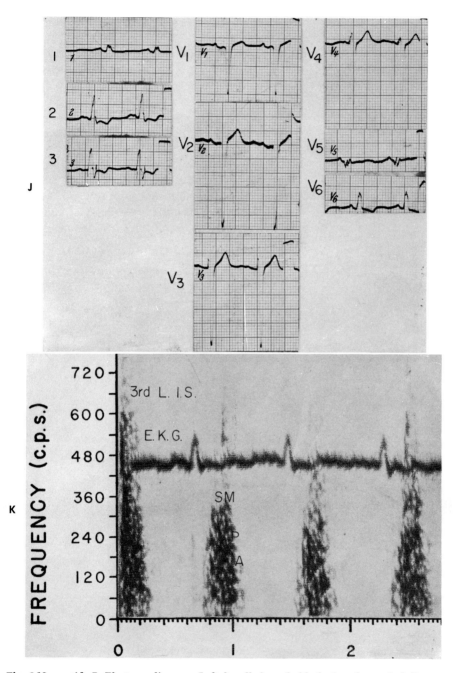

Fig. 6-19, cont'd. J, Electrocardiogram. Left bundle-branch block; broad, notched P waves. **K,** Spectral phonocardiogram, aortic area. The systolic murmur is consistent with aortic stenosis. There may be paradoxical splitting of S_2. The systolic murmur may extend to the pulmonary component (which is first) but not to the aortic. Recordings at the third left interspace and in the left mid-precordial areas showed a diastolic murmur of arterial type, probably indicative of aortic regurgitation.

gastroenteritis. Surgery was not performed, but a subsequent barium enema showed narrowing of the distal colon. When she was 19 years old, a second attack of severe abdominal pain developed while she was sitting quietly at home. Laparotomy revealed a massive intramural hematoma of the jejunum, necessitating resection of an 18-inch-long segment of bowel. At this operation the narrowed area in the colon was found to show mural fibrosis consistent with intramural hematoma at that site two years previously. The patient continues to have episodes of partial intestinal obstruction, apparently due to intramural bowel hemorrhage. She has learned to recognize the event when it develops, and conservative measures have usually sufficed in "tiding her over." This patient had had pyloric stenosis of apparently conventional type, operated on at the age of 7 weeks. Also, when she was 12 years old, splenic rupture occurred after a fall from a bicycle (Fig. 6-21). The third patient (Fig. 6-22) had well-established E-D, but intestinal perforation is less well substantiated. A. H. H. (J.H.H. 796695), a white woman, 48 years old, had the acute onset of abdominal pain and died 15 hours later on the way to the hospital by ambulance. Autopsy was not performed.

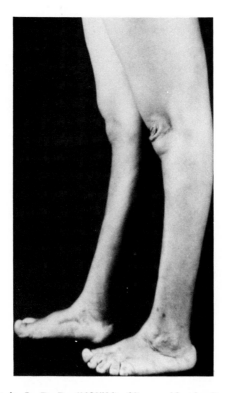

Fig. 6-20. Deformed foot in L. D. P. (1121524), 30-year-old schoolteacher. Several operations for "clubfoot" were performed in childhood. Other cardinal features of E-D were present. Dislocation of the shoulder and of the patella occurred on several occasions. Intracranial hemorrhage, presumably from berry aneurysm, occurred in this patient. The patient died at 36 years of age after an operation for perforated sigmoid colon.

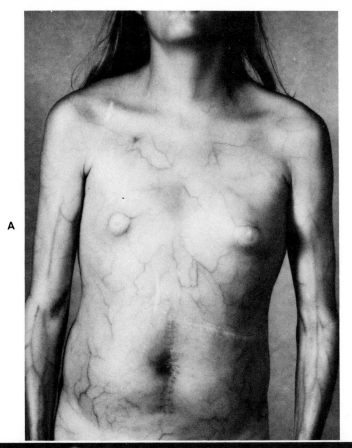

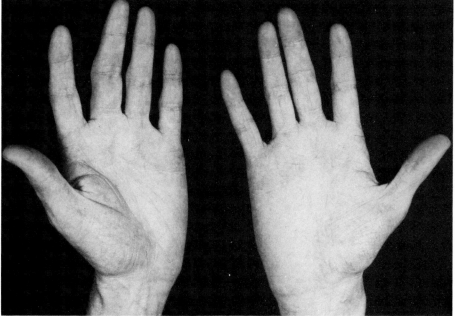

Fig. 6-21. "Arterial," "ecchymotic," or Sack's variety of E-D syndrome (J.H.H. 1287186). **A,** Thin, translucent skin with easily visible venous pattern is demonstrated. Surgery had been performed for pyloric stenosis in infancy, traumatic rupture of the spleen at the age of 12 years, and spontaneous intestinal rupture at 19 years (p. 326). **B,** Hands showing many creases and blotchy appearance. (See also Fig. 6-16*B*.)

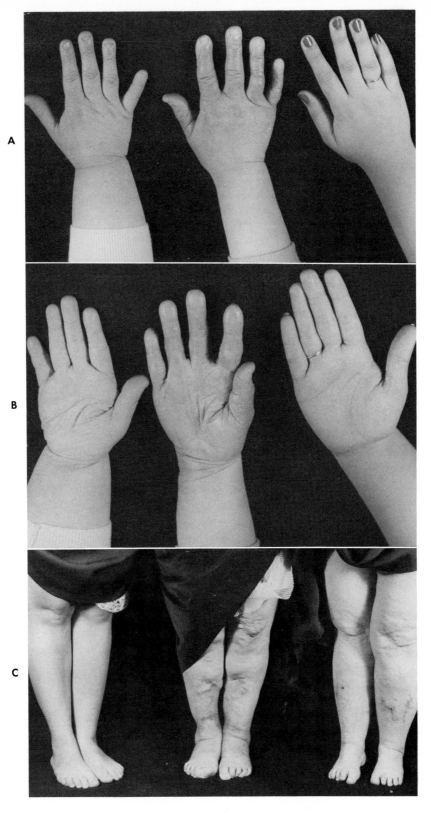

Fig. 6-22. For legend see opposite page.

Rectal bleeding is an occasional complication in E-D, and repeated rectal prolapse has been a problem in infancy or childhood but usually is not observed beyond the age of 4 or 5 years[33]

In one reported patient,[200] repeated episodes of mediastinal and subcutaneous emphysema occurred. Spontaneous pneumothorax occurred in one patient of mine and in one reported by Graf.[112] It is to be noted that in the first case of dissecting aneurysm described below, the lungs revealed subpleural blebs, and subcutaneous emphysema was present. Hemoptysis is a rare complication of E-D,[114,129,221] a manifestation of the bleeding diathesis. André and colleagues[6] observed a young woman who had many bleeding episodes from various sites and developed left- and right-sided hemothorax without recognized precipitating factors. Dilatation of the trachea and bronchi has been described[1,187] in patients with presumed E-D. This tracheobronchiomegaly is sometimes called the Mounier-Kuhn syndrome.[1]

Dissecting aneurysm of the aorta is now a well-established, although fortunately rare, complication of E-D.[22,206] Uncontrollable bleeding from large arteries also occurs and in some instances has been initiated by puncture of the artery for arteriography.[164] The histologic changes in the aorta in at least some of the cases are those of Erdheim's cystic medial necrosis and are indistinquishable from those in cases of the Marfan syndrome. Abstracts of illustrative cases follows:

Case 1. H. L. R.,* a 15-year-old Negro student, with a history of always having been sickly, was thrown forcibly to the ground by a schoolmate. He complained immediately of pain in the chest extending down the right arm and soon developed signs and symptoms of circulatory collapse. He was taken to the neighboring office of a physician, where he died within 10 minutes.

Autopsy revealed an adequately developed and nourished Negro male weighing 140 pounds and measuring 5 feet 6 inches in height. The skin showed many scars; some resembled burn scars. One on the right thigh was covered with thin epidermis and measured 15 by 3.8 cm. An ulcer with hemorrhagic base, 25 mm. in diameter, was located on the medial aspect of the left ankle. There was considerable subcutaneous emphysema below the right rib margin.

---

*For calling this case to my attention I am indebted to Robert K. Osborne, then a fourth-year student, Medical College of Virgina. For much information bearing on the case I am indebted to Dr. George W. Thoma, formerly Assistant Chief Medical Examiner, Commonwealth of Virgina.

Fig. 6-22. Wrinkled skin of hands in E-D syndrome in mother and daughter. **A** and **B,** Shown in the center of each photograph is the hand of a woman 44 years old with E-D (A. H. H., J.H.H. 796695). The hand of an unaffected daughter is on the right and that of an affected daughter is on the left. **C,** The legs of the same three persons are shown. The unaffected daughter is now on the left. The daughter with E-D syndrome is mentally retarded, possibly as a result of prematurity. She also has strabismus. The mother died of "acute peritonitis," probably secondary to spontaneous rupture of the bowel. She had always been loose-jointed and bruised easily. She suffered from Raynaud's phenomenon, varicose veins, and ankle edema. Hysterectomy had been performed at 31 years of age for descensus uteri, without complications. She was 61 inches tall, had a peculiar delicate fold of skin at the inner canthus of each eye (like that shown in Fig. 6-8), and had thin skin of the soles of the feet, which the patient blamed for her painful feet. Inflation of the arm cuff in determining blood pressure occasioned pain, a finding in other patients with E-D syndrome.

During the dissection, the connective tissues were found to be very friable. They tore easily, and even the skeletal muscles pulled apart with incredible ease. (The autopsy was performed only a few hours after death. The tissue was not autolyzed histologically. Dr. Thoma, the prosector, had never encountered such fragility of tissues and considered it highly significant.) Fourteen hundred milliliters of blood were found in the right hemithorax. The mediastinal structures were infiltrated with blood, which also had dissected along the fascial planes of the neck. The lungs showed multiple large emphysematous subpleural bullae and were easily torn. The heart weighed 300 grams. The gastrointestinal tract tore easily.

Histologic studies, including stains by the periodic acid–Schiff method and elastic tissue stains, were unrevealing of definite abnormality.

Further investigation of the boy's previous health and of his family revealed that he had always been sickly, did not play as actively as his contemporaries, and often complained of severe headache. He "cut" his skin easily and healed poorly. At the age of 11 years he had sprained his ankle; x-ray films of the injured part were not considered abnormal on review.

The father of the patient died at the age of 21 or 22 years, of asthma. The mother died at the age of 22 years after a 24-hour illness beginning with abdominal pain, nausea, and vomiting, and characterized by progressive circulatory failure. Autopsy was not performed, but the diagnosis given on the death certificate was "internal hemorrhage of unknown cause." There were no siblings of the propositus.

Case 2. J. M. M.,* a 24-year-old white man, was well until 6 A.M. on the morning of Dec. 31, 1946, when he awoke with a vague discomfort in the abdomen. In the course of 2 hours this discomfort developed into pain in the right flank and the lower quadrant of the abdomen. By the time he was admitted to the hospital, a few hours after onset, he was in profound shock. The administration of fluids intravenously raised the blood pressure from an indeterminably low level of 90/60 mm. Hg. The white count was 25,000 and 28,000 per cubic millimeter on two determinations. The hemoglobin concentration fell from 82% to 69% of normal during the afternoon. By 3 P.M. the patient was complaining of pain in the region of the right shoulder. Abdominal exploration was undertaken at 5 P.M. The abdomen contained blood-stained fluid. A large retroperitoneal hematoma involved the right kidney. There was dissection into the mesentery, which was torn in several places. The surgeon compared the tissues to wet blotting paper. Bleeding and clotting times, determined postoperatively, were 1 and 4 minutes, respectively. The patient died a 4:15 A.M. on Jan. 1, 1947.

Subsequent investigation revealed that the patient had always bled and bruised easily. He also had sustained a number of fractures. The possibility of minor trauma during the previous evening could not be excluded.

Autopsy revealed a body measuring only 62 inches in length. Despite this, arachnodactyly was thought to be very impressive. The prosector may have been unduly impressed because of the recognized association of arachnodactyly and dissecting aneurysm. During the opening of the chest at autopsy the ribs were thought to fracture with abnormal ease. The abdomen contained 500 ml. of bloody fluid. The aorta and the renal and iliac arteries were described as hypoplastic. A dissection of the right renal artery with infarction of the kidney was discovered. Histologically the media of the aorta was thin, with numerous areas of "myxomatous degeneration" and basophilically staining material. There was some fragmentation of the elastic fibers, which seemed to be normally abundant but morphologically abnormal. The renal artery showed marked fragmentation of elastic fibers.

Although the second patient was included as an instance of arachnodactyly in reports[108,109] of a series of cases of dissecting aneurysm, the short stature, the easy bruisability, and the friability of the tissues at operation and at autopsy suggest E-D. The case of MacFarlane at the Radcliffe Infirmary, Oxford (described by Mories[182,183]), has parallels to these 2 cases. A 15-year-old white boy, the elder of twins, developed a swelling in the right groin after falling from his bicycle.

---

*I am indebted to Dr. John F. Brownsberger of Takoma Park, Md., for much information on this patient.

Trueta attempted to stop the bleeding, which was obviously the cause of the inguinal swelling, by ligature. However, all the vessels were so extremely friable that hemostasis was impossible. At autopsy, all tissues, especially muscle and fascia, were very friable, and the abdominal aorta tore readily. Histologically there was said to be an increase in the elastica of the aorta, with degeneration and hyalinization of the collagenous elements.

Dr. S. Miles Bouton, Jr., of Lynchburg, Va., has informed me of yet another case:

Case 3. The boy died at the age of 14 years, of dissecting aneurysm of the aorta. At the age of 7 years spontaneous rupture of the outer two coats of the sigmoid colon, with intraabdominal bleeding, produced severe pain in the left lower abdomen and required surgical exploration. Two weeks after operation symptoms of partial obstruction of the large bowel appeared but were resolved with conservative measures. Six months later partial bowel obstruction necessitated surgical release of adhesions. Less than four weeks later, the child was sitting in school when he was seized with left upper quadrant pain radiating to the shoulder, which doubled him over. Operation revealed peritonitis secondary to perforation of the splenic flexure of the colon. About three years later, at the age of 10 years, perforation of the sigmoid colon and pelvic abscess again required operation.

It was noted repeatedly that lacerations of the knees, legs, and scalp occurred unusually readily. Healing of the skin occurred normally, however. The boy tended toward constipation.

Later, at the age of 11 years, the boy again suffered a perforation of the colon; the transverse and descending portions of the colon were removed. Four months later the monotonous accident was repeated: the ascending colon ruptured spontaneously; the remainder of the colon was resected and the ileum was anastomosed to the rectum. In the postoperative period there was intra-abdominal hemorrhage with shock, and drainage of a subdiaphragmatic hematoma was necessary.

Three years after the last surgical episode, at the age of 14 years, this apparently healthy boy, who did, however, receive skin lacerations at slight provocation, went to summer camp. One night, while in bed, he suffered the onset of severe pain in the back and abdomen. He died on the way to his home.

Autopsy revealed two transverse intimal tears, one in the descending portion of the arch and the other just proximal to the renal arteries. A large volume of blood occupied the left pleural cavity. The entire aorta and its branches appeared to be unusually delicate. Dissection extended from the reflection of the pericardial sac to the bifurcation of the aorta and into the right iliac artery.

Histologically the bowel removed at surgery revealed disarrangement, irregular development, and, in places, marked hypoplasia of the smooth muscle elements.

The next case of dissecting aneurysm is in a patient with E-D, particularly remarkable because of the familial incidence.

Case 4. T. F. (J.H.H. 1432502), born in May, 1918, is a white male stockbroker. As a child he was noted to be "double-jointed" and to have stretchable skin. He had been able to dislocate and reduce his knees at will, but had had no difficulty with skin lacerations, bruising, or cigarette-paper scarring. Bilateral inguinal hernias and umbilical hernia were repaired in adult life.

The patient was in general good health until June, 1969, when he had the acute onset of knifelike substernal pain. Initially myocardial infarction was diagnosed on the basis of rise in myocardial enzymes despite lack of concomitant electrocardiographic change. He was then well until May, 1971, when the pain recurred after mild exertion. Enlarged thoracic aorta was then discovered on chest x-ray examination, and the murmur of mitral regurgitation was first noted. In July, 1971, an aortogram showed chronic dissection beginning in the ascending aorta. At that time the diagnosis of Ehlers-Danlos syndrome with dissecting aneurysm of the aorta and "floppy" mitral valve was made. Surgery was considered inadvisable and propranolol therapy (p. 196) was substituted.

In January, 1972, the patient had an attack of severe pain in the back with drop in blood pressure and in hematocrit. An upper gastrointestinal series suggested the presence of a retroperitoneal mass. Urinary retention necessitated suprapubic prostatectomy (complicated by bleeding that required transfusion). The patient had suffered from low back pain intermittently for several years, and x-ray films in April, 1972, suggested degenerative disc disease in the lumbar spine, and back pain continued to plague him.

The patient has 2 children, of whom a daughter 13 years of age has stretchable skin and loose joints consistent with E-D. T. F.'s only sib, a sister, and his mother had the same skin and joint changes. The sister died at age 56 years immediately after operative repair of a chronic dissection of the aorta by Dr. Michael E. DeBakey. The mother died suddenly, possibly of rupture of the aorta, also at age 56 years.

Examination of T. F. (June, 1972) showed redundant skin of the upper eyelids, a positive Gorlin test (Fig. 6-23B), stretchable skin, loose-jointedness especially in the fingers (Fig. 6-23A), cardiomegaly, and a grade V/VI pansystolic murmur loudest at the cardiac apex but heard over a wide area. No diastolic murmur has been heard. A linear scar above the right knee was abnormally wide, with paper-thin skin.

In addition to these cases of dissecting aneurysm in E-D, a few instances of dilatation in the ascending aorta with aortic regurgitation simulating that of the Marfan syndrome have been described.[57a,271]

McFarland and Fuller[168] described 2 patients who died of spontaneous rupture of large arteries. One was a 12-year-old boy who suffered rupture of the right popliteal artery that apparently occurred spontaneously during sleep. Trauma at play during the previous day could not be excluded. The second was a 17-year-old boy who died of rupture of the right subclavian artery, which occurred during the course of strenuous cheering at a basketball tournament. Lynch and colleagues[164] described a boy who died after a tear of the lower thoracic aorta. Autopsy showed fistulas between the abdominal aorta and inferior vena cava and the left common iliac artery and vein. Rupture of major arteries, either spontaneously or on relatively minor trauma, has also been described by Rybka and O'Hara[233] and by Barabas.[14] Heilmann and Kolig[125a] described rupture of the renal artery in a 24-year-old man.

Rubinstein and Cohen[232] described a 47-year-old white female with typical E-D and multiple intracranial aneurysms. (A brother also had E-D. One of her children died at the age of 1 month of massive ectasia of the gastrointestinal tract through the abdominal wall. Another child, who had hyperelastic skin, died at the age of 2 years, of a congenital cardiac defect.) François and colleagues[91] observed a case with an intracranial arteriovenous aneurysm. Spontaneous cure occurred through thrombosis. Intracranial arteriovenous fistulas were described also by Schoolman and Kepes[240] and by Graf.[112] In the last instance multiple intracranial aneurysms were found at autopsy.[10] A brother had a spontaneously developing arteriovenous fistula. Bannerman and colleagues[11] reported a brother and sister with the "arterial" form of E-D and spontaneously developing carotid-cavernous fistula. A mother and daughter in a collateral branch of their family had died of subarachnoid hemorrhage. I have observed a 30-year-old woman with E-D subarachnoid hemorrhage, presumably from an intracranial aneurysm (Fig. 6-20). Cerebrovascular accidents that may have had the same basis were described in normotensive middle-aged women by several authors.[114,235,240]

Because of friability of tissues, including those of arterial walls, cerebral arteriograms, like other procedures requiring arterial puncture,[164,233] can be hazardous in E-D. One woman died from a tear in the ascending aorta sustained

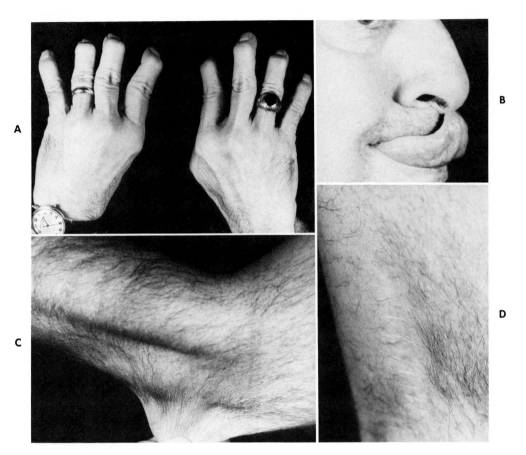

Fig. 6-23. Familial dissecting aneurysm with E-D in T. F. (J.H.H. 1432502). See text. **A,** Loose-jointedness in hands; **B,** Gorlin's sign; **C,** stretchable skin at elbow; **D,** papyraceous scar above right knee.

during investigation of her intracranial arteriovenous fistula.[240] Familial dissecting aneurysm in persons with stigmata of E-D is illustrated by Fig. 6-23.

Brodribb[43] successfully cured an aneurysm of the left vertebral artery in an Asiatic Indian, by means of proximal and distal ligation. The patient was thought to have the "arterial," or "ecchymotic," form of E-D (p. 339). The aneurysm was probably a false aneurysm, although the distinction from "true" aneurysm can be difficult. The same patient was described by Edwards and Taylor.[84] Dales and O'Neill[66] described a comparable false aneurysm that developed in the left axilla of a 15-year-old boy while he was lifting a mattress. Ballooning of the aneurysm occurred 12 days later. Because of arterial friability, suture of the torn artery was not possible; proximal ligature of the axillary artery was performed.

The 18-year-old patient of Garrick[96a] who had elastosis perforans and frequent ecchymoses, and died at 18 years of age from rupture of the thyrocervical trunk, probably had E-D type IV, the ecchymotic variety. Anning[7a] gave a dermatologic report of a patient who was found to have elastosis perforans at the age of 18 years and died of "dissecting aneurysm of the aorta" at 20 years. Whether this was the Marfan syndrome or E-D type IV, or another distinct entity, is unclear, but E-D type IV would seem the most likely possibility. There were said to be "multiple tears of the aorta, which was thin walled. Histologic examination of the aorta: degenerative elastic tissue." The description suggests the form of arterial rupture that occurs with E-D type IV rather than dissecting aneurysm, as seen in the Marfan syndrome.

In one patient, an 11-year-old girl, Bell's palsy followed a large subgaleal hematoma that was produced by a fall, with blow to the occiput.[258] One patient (Fig. 6-16) developed left-sided hemiplegia at 19 years of age, after a head injury which had occurred three weeks previously. Dodge and Shillito[75] described acquired encephalocele—essentially a cerebral hernia—which developed gradually in an infant who died at the age of 2 years 4 months.

Varicose veins are a frequent finding in E-D.[235]

In the *heart* two reported patients had interatrial septal defect[92,239]; another had tetralogy of Fallot.[282] One patient had partial persistent atrioventricular canal,[89] and another had aneurysm of a sinus of Valsalva and other abnormal cardiac findings on physical examination, without more definitive diagnosis of the defect.[271] One patient had a bicuspid right atrioventricular valve.[168] One patient in the series reported by Sestak[243] had atrial septal defect. A loud systolic murmur in the pulmonary area, audible also in the left interscapular area of the back, was described in one patient.[172] One of my patients has demonstrated for many years, probably all his life, the electrocardiographic pattern of incomplete right bundle-branch block without subjective or other objective cardiovascular manifestations (Fig. 6-4D). Sestak[243] also observed incomplete right bundle-branch block block in 2 patients, in one of whom atrial septal defect was present.

Signs of the "floppy mitral valve" syndrome (p. 128) are demonstrated by some patients, probably particularly by those with E-D type III, or benign hypermobile type (e.g., J. L., J.H.H. 1434401).

Madison and co-workers[171] described a 17-year-old Negro patient with features of E-D and intractable heart failure from mitral and tricuspid regurgitation. Autopsy findings seemed to exclude rheumatic heart disease and showed redundant chordae tendineae and valve cusps—changes compatible with the same defect as in other connective tissue structures. The chordae tendineae of the atrioventricular valves are indeed tendons, and the cusps themselves and fibrous skeleton of the heart are largely collagenous. Possibly the marvel is that serious cardiac difficulties occur so relatively uncommonly in these patients. Green and associates[115] found nodular thickening of the mitral valve in a 64-year-old man who in life had a grade 3 rough, high-pitched systolic murmur at the left sternal border. A small atrial septal defect was also present. Case 5 described below, represents a case of grave cardiac abnormality in association with E-D. The precise nature of the cardiac abnormality is not known.

Case 5. W. E. W. (765864), a white male born in 1917, was referred to Dr. Helen B. Taussig and Dr. Richard S. Ross, for study of his heart condition.

To the patient's knowledge, no condition similar to his existed in his family. The father died of cerebral hemorrhage at 54 years. The mother, who had diabetes, died in childbirth at 37 years of age. Six brothers, 20 to 44 years of age, were living and well, and 6 sisters were likewise well. Some of the siblings were half-brothers and half-sisters. The patient had no children.

He was the shortest member of his family. He had always had unusually soft, smooth, elastic skin, with abnormal hyperextensibility of all joints. Both the joints and the skin had tended to become less elastic as he grew older. At no time was there any bleeding tendency, fragility of the skin, or unusual scarring over exposed areas. The patient had had prolapse of the rectum on several occasions.

Shortly after birth a murmur was discovered, and it was described at each of many examinations as he was growing up. He was rejected for the armed services in World War II because of the murmur. In 1948 his physician described a harsh systolic murmur, loudest at the apex but audible over the entire heart, with no diastolic murmur. By x-ray examination a left ventricular enlargement was demonstrated. In 1955 the first signs of congestive heart failure appeared. Left bundle-branch block was discovered; how long it had been present is unknown.

Early in 1957 the patient had an onset of abdominal pain. Gastrointestinal x-ray films showed redundancy of the colon, a small diverticulum in the second portion of the duodenum, and a huge diverticulum at the ligament of Treitz.

Physical examination revealed an intelligent, moderately deaf, rather short man (Fig. 6-19*A*), who appeared to be about his stated age of 40 years. The head was short and round. The skin was smooth, velvety, and loose, with redundant skin of the upper lid. When stretched, the skin returned promptly to its normal position on release. All joints displayed hyperextensibility. There was pes planus, genu recurvatum, and ability to hold a pencil between the knuckles. The hands could be folded together transversely, with opposition of the thenar and hypothenar portions. Audiogram showed impairment of all tones bilaterally. (The patient was aware of impairment of hearing only in the left ear. This had begun after a purulent discharge at the age of 18 years.) The hard palate was unusually highly arched.

The heart was massively enlarged (Fig. 6-19*I*), with a localized point of maximum impulse in the seventh interspace, just outside the anterior axillary line. At the base a grade III harsh systolic murmur was transmitted into the neck. At the apex a higher-pitched systolic murmur was of approximately grade II intensity (on a base of six). A soft, decrescendo diastolic murmur was audible down the left sternal border. The liver edge was 2 fingerbreadths below the costal margin. Blood pressure was 100/70 mm. Hg.

The left testis was undescended.

Serum cholesterol was 217 mg./100 ml. X-ray films revealed great enlargement of the heart, involving all chambers. Right heart catheterization showed no evidence of shunt. Pressure in the right ventricle was 56/2/5 mm. Hg.

It was concluded that aortic stenosis and/or mitral regurgitation would best account for the physical findings.

In Fig. 6-19 are the photographs, electrocardiograms, phonocardiograms, and x-ray films of this patient. Although no special search for calcified subcutaneous spherules typical of E-D was made by x-ray examination, one such body, oval in shape, was visible on chest x-ray examination in the skin of the left upper arm.

The patient died suddenly at home about five months after these studies. Autopsy was not performed.

Lees and colleagues[156] described multiple severe pulmonary arterial stenoses in a child with cutaneous and skeletal features of E-D. Tortuosity of the aorta and its major intrathoracic branches, including the coronary arteries, was also present. The pulmonary arterial stenoses were like those which occur as a familial trait in association with supravalvar stenosis of the aorta[166] and like those produced by fetal rubella.[231]

Another of my patients has a bilateral congenital anomaly of the ureteropelvic junction (Fig. 6-5*F*), and Levine and Michael[158] described a similar anomaly. Lewitus,[160] Graf,[112] and Bannerman and colleagues[10] reported finding polycystic kidneys in E-D. Medullary sponge kidneys have been observed in patients with E-D.[158,186] Morris and co-workers[186] found E-D in 2 of 20 cases

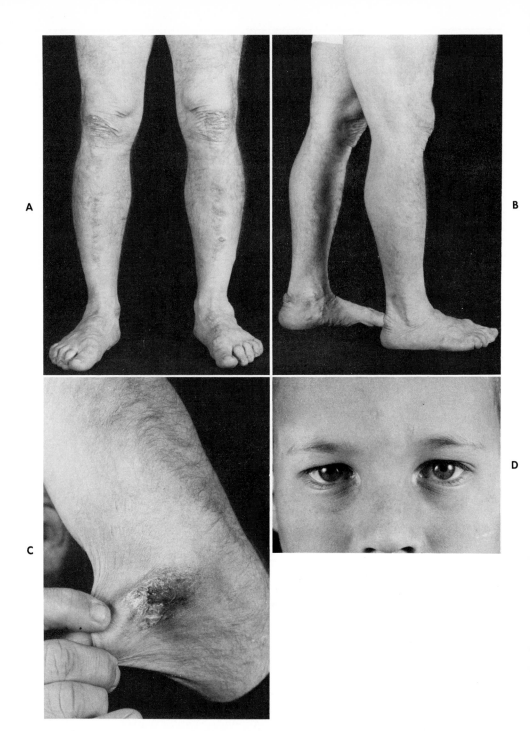

Fig. 6-24. E-D syndrome in father and son. The father (J. D., 122647) showed stretchable and fragile skin with cigarette-paper scars, but only mild loose-jointedness, **A** to **C.** The son (S. D., J.H.H. 971359) demonstrated a conformation of the eyes typical of E-D, **D,** and typical changes of moderate severity in the skin, **E,** and joints, **F.** The father apparently acquired the abnormality through new mutation. He had had repair of a right inguinal hernia. The son was born with left-sided clubfoot.

of medullary sponge kidney. They felt that this must be more than coincidence and suspected that medullary sponge kidney is a condition that can have different causes, among them the connective tissue defect of E-D. Imahori and colleagues[128] noted multiple cysts of the kidney in a patient with the "arterial" form of E-D, and multiple arterial aneurysms. Congenital cystic kidneys and intracranial aneurysms represent a well-known[37] but poorly understood association.

Bladder neck obstruction was noted in E-D by Eadie and Wilkins.[83]

In the case of the Marfan syndrome it was pointed out that there are a number of manifestations which are congenial malformations in the conventional sense and which occur often enough to be considered bona fide components of the syndrome. It was proposed that these are secondary manifestations, that the hereditary disorder of connective tissue creates an ontogenetic setting in which certain predictable congenital anomalies occur with increased frequency. In E-D, ureteropelvic anomaly, tetralogy of Fallot, and interatrial defect may fall into this category of secondary manifestations. However, since, to my knowledge, these malformations have been described in very few patients, it is equally reasonable to suspect that they may have occurred by coincidence. Diverticula of the bladder are probably frequent in E-D[296] but are usually turned up only incidentally by contrast studies because they rarely produce symptoms. This condition has been described in a 47-year-old man[83] and in a young infant in whom the diverticulum extended into a sliding left inguinal hernia and umbilical hernia.[75] Spina bifida occulta has been described,[131,178,191] but from the experience of Beighton,[22] it cannot be considered more than coincidence. The

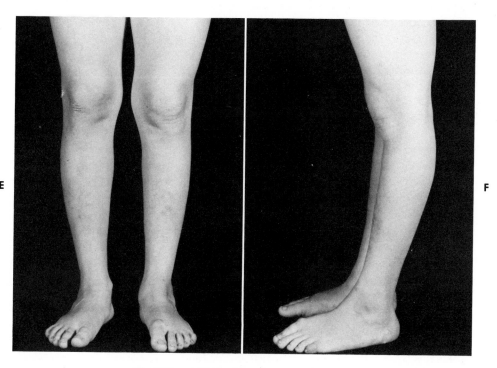

E   F

Fig. 6-24, cont'd. For legend see opposite page.

teeth may be irregularly formed,[155] irregularly positioned,[99,149,238] abnormally small,[154,172,212] or even absent. Crenation of the incisors has been noted,[161,172] but it is a frequent finding in normal persons. Easy fracturing of the teeth was thought by Barabas and Barabas[16] to be an expression of the generalized connective tissue defect.

Gingival fragility, with bleeding after use of a toothbrush[137] and excessive bleeding after dental extractions, sometimes requiring transfusion,[22,107,268] is well known in E-D. A soft toothbrush is recommended to these patients, and the dentist is urged to use special precautions such as avoidance of nerve blocks and extra care during scaling lest the fragile gum be split. Grant and Aldor[114] described tearing of the buccal mucosa, with severe hemorrhage, during dental extraction. Hyperextensibility of the tongue (Fig. 6-8B) and stretchability of the buccal mucosa have already been noted.

Chronic or recurrent temporomandibular joint dislocation[103] was commented on earlier. Thexton[262] performed bilateral condylectomy in a young woman who had recurrent dislocations of the jaw. She was found to be a notorious "Munchausen," or peripatetic medical confabulator, who had visited many London hospitals, displaying a variety of dislocated joints.

As a rule, mental retardation is not a feature of this syndrome. However, occasionally patients show it. In some cases the association may be only coincidental,[154,161] whereas in others it may be the result of prematurity.[72]

Severe essential hypertension occurred in one patient as a probable incidental finding.[142]

Pregnancy carries risks for both the mother and the baby with E-D. The mother with E-D may display an increase in bruisability during pregnancy,[236] may develop abdominal hernia, and varicosities not only of the leg veins but also of those in the vulva,[22] and may suffer exacerbation of joint manifestations. Rupture of great vessels probably is a risk of pregnancy in E-D, as is in the Marfan syndrome.

Excessive bleeding from episiotomy, spontaneous extension of episiotomy, perineal hematoma, and postpartum hemorrhage have been observed as expressions of the mother's friable tissues and bleeding diathesis. At cesarean section, sutures have been found not to hold in the uterus, and hysterectomy has been necessary.[240] Stoddard and Myers[253] performed an elective cesarean section at 39 weeks of gestation in a woman in whom a similar procedure had been carried out as an emergency during her previous pregnancy. The scar in the uterine wall had completely disrupted, leaving the baby's head covered only by perineum and the fetal membranes. Whereas uterine rupture has, it seems, not been observed in E-D, it is a risk, especially in patients who have had a previous cesarean section. Forceps must be used with caution. Beighton[22] referred in passing to an instance in which the baby was extracted by forceps along with the uterus, posterior wall of the bladder, and part of a ureter. In his large series Beighton[22] recorded experience with pregnancy in 29 affected women who produced 27 affected and 34 unaffected children. Complications included (1) distraction of the pubic symphysis during delivery, with prolonged postpartum discomfort, (2) postpartum uterine prolapse,[141] and (3) slow healing of perineal wounds. Tyson[273a] tells me of unpublished examples of uterine rupture, vaginal rupture, or avulsion of the bladder in patients with E-D.

Tyson[273a] points out to me that precocious and precipitous labor can be a complication of maternal E-D. In the presence of lax tissues the increasing weight of the products of conception act to force cervical effacement and dilatation leading to early delivery. Some of the prematurity noted by several observers and attributed to precocious rupture of fetal membranes (see below) may be due to maternal factors in those cases in which the mother is affected.

The remarkable freedom from striae gravidarum enjoyed by most women with E-D was noted earlier.

The fetus with E-D runs risks because of the friablity of the fetal membranes. The high incidence of prematurity in E-D was noted by Kanof[140] and by Mories.[183] Barabas[12] confirmed this and advanced the reasonable hypothesis that the E-D defect in the connective tissue of the fetal membranes (which are, of course, of fetal origin) predisposes to early rupture of the membranes and precocious delivery. (Spontaneous rupture of the membranes before onset of contractions was noted in the case of one E-D mother whose offspring was apparently unaffected.[250]) Difficulties in ligature of the umbilical cord may be encountered because of its friability. Congenital dislocation of the hips has been observed.[4,54] Thomas and associates[265] described dislocation of the shoulder in a baby delivered by breech presentation. Macfarlane[169] reported Erb's palsy, which may be more likely to occur because of the preternatural joint mobility. As stated earlier, the infant with E-D is often floppy, leading to the misdiagnosis of amyotonia congenita. Bleeding in male infants with E-D has led to the misdiagnosis of hemophilia.

Heterogeneity in the Ehlers-Danlos syndrome

A recurrent theme of medical genetics in recent years has been heterogeneity. Many disorders hitherto considered single entities have been found to be two or more fundamentally distinct ones. The Ehlers-Danlos syndrome is no exception.

The following classification of E-D is that of Beighton,[22] to which has been added a sixth form revealed in recent biochemical studies by Pinnell, Krane, and colleagues[149a,209b] and by Lichtenstein et al.[160a]

Ehlers-Danlos syndrome I, or gravis type. Skin hyperextensibility, fragility, and bruisability are striking, and joint hypermobility is generalized and severe. Friable tissues create difficulties at operation. Prematurity due to early rupture of the fetal membranes is frequent.

Ehlers-Danlos syndrome II, or mitis type. The cutaneous and joint manifestations are mild. Joint hypermobility may be limited to the hands and feet. Tissue friability and prematurity are not problems.

Ehlers-Danlos syndrome III, or benign hypermobile type. Joint hypermobility is generalized and marked; hyperextensibility and other cutaneous manifestations are usually only minimal. Although skeletal deformity is usually not present, complications of the joint hypermobility are frequent.

Ehlers-Danlos syndrome IV, or ecchymotic (arterial, or Sack's) type. Joint hypermobility is largely limited to the digits, and skin hyperextensibility is minimal or absent. However, the skin is characteristically thin and pale, with prominent venous network (Fig. 6-21). Bruisability, the cardinal feature of this form, is severe. Minor trauma leads to extensive ecchymoses. Bony prominences become covered with thin, darkly pigmented scars. Rupture of the bowel and rupture of great vessels occur predominately in this form of E-D. The ecchymotic type in the Beighton nosology is probably the same as the "arterial type" of Barabas.[14] The condition reported by Sack[234] as "status dysvascularis" is clearly the same[13]; indeed some[43] suggest that this condition be called Sack's disease, and others Sack-Barabas disease.

Ehlers-Danlos syndrome V, or X-linked form. Joint hypermobility is limited, but skin stretchability is striking. Fragility, cigarette-paper scarring, and bruising occur to a moderate degree.

Ehlers-Danlos syndrome VI, or hydroxylysine-deficient collagen (or ocular) type. This form is characterized genetically by autosomal recessive inheritance, biochemically by paucity of hydroxylysyl residues in collagen because of deficiency of lysyl hydroxylase (p. 345), and clinically by abnormality of the eyes out of proportion to the ocular abnormalities seen in the other forms. Thus far the diagnosis has been established biochemically in only two families,[149a,160a,209b] each with 2 affected sibs, but some reported cases outlined below may have the same disorder.

Pinnell et al.[209b] first found hydroxylysine-deficient collagen in 2 sisters, 9 and 12 years of age, with severe scoliosis, recurrent joint dislocation, and hyperextensible skin and joints. Pregnancy with the older child had been characterized by lack of fetal movements, frequent spotting, and rupture of fetal membranes at 3 months, forcing the mother to bed rest for the remainder of the pregnancy. The infant was floppy and fed poorly in early life. At age 12 years eye examination showed small corneas (10 mm.), with scattered infiltrates in the anterior part of the stroma and slightly blue sclerae. Her sister, age 9 years, had required removal of the left eye following trauma sustained in an automobile accident. The right cornea was small (10 mm.) and "deeply curved." The sclerae were slightly blue. (The second sib had a late systolic click and late systolic murmur consistent with floppy mitral valve.)

Lichtenstein et al.[160a] demonstrated hydroxylysine-deficient collagen in a patient long known to me. In that family a brother and sister (latter shown in Fig. 6-16) had typical cutaneous and articular features of E-D and both had lost their sight after ocular catastrophes.[22] The brother, born in 1915, sustained rupture of the right globe from a minor blow from a car-tire patch, at 22 years of age. Enucleation was necessary. At the age of 51 years the patient tripped and hit the left side of the head; the left globe ruptured, and although the scleral rent was sutured, he remained blind. The sister (Fig. 6-16), born in 1924, had, like her brother, severe myopia from an early age. Glaucoma, microcornea, and blue sclerae were described by Durham in 1953.[82] At the age of 36 years she sustained detachment of the left retina, followed a year later by detachment of the right retina. Attempts at repair, during which the surgeons commented on the fragility of the sclera and excessive bleeding, were unsuccessful, and the woman has remained totally blind. These sibs are 2 among 8 children, the others being unaffected, as are also their parents and the 4 children of the brother. Although the parents were not consanguineous, recessive inheritance is likely.

Reports in the literature strengthen the possibility of an "ocular variety" of E-D with autosomal recessive inheritance. Thomas and co-workers[266] described a 2-year-old girl who suffered corneal damage from a minor blow to the head.

She had blue sclerae, keratoconus, and undue scleral fragility. Her brother also had E-D and the parents were consanguineous, although free of signs of E-D. Bossu and Lambrechts[42] described a 19-year-old girl who had detached retina on the right and spontaneous vitreous hemorrhage on the left. Two of her 12 'sibs had E-D. The parents and other relatives were normal; there was no consanguinity. Cordella and Vinciguerra[62] described a 30-year-old man who in addition to typical signs of E-D had thin blue sclerae, right-sided retinal detachment, and displacement of the lens of the left eye. Eight sibs were normal and 2 others had been stillborn; the parents were first cousins. The postulated recessively inherited "ocular" form of E-D may have been present also in the 4 offspring of first-cousin parents reported by Cluney and Mason.[58a] They had marked joint laxity and arachnodactyly, recurrent inguinal and femoral hernias, high-grade myopia and retinal detachment leading to blindness, and multiple intestinal and bladder diverticula complicated by perforation of the bowel. The existence of a recessive ocular form of E-D is supported by the rarity of serious eye complications except in families such as those with only sibs affected, and those with consanguineous parents.

The "ocular" form of the Ehlers-Danlos syndrome shares many features with the disorder described on p. 433 and referred to as *fragilitas oculi*. Both have fragility of the sclera and cornea, with blue sclerae, rupture from minor trauma, and deformation of the cornea, either keratoconus or keratoglobus, and, often, megalocornea. Both have joint hyperextensibility and both seem to be autosomal recessive disorders. Fragilitas ossium was displayed by some patients with fragilitas oculi, and the physicians reporting these cases have considered them a "variant" of osteogenesis imperfecta, whereas the authors of the papers just reviewed considered the condition they were reporting a variant of the Ehlers-Danlos syndrome. It is not certain that they are separate and distinct, however.

A seventh distinguishable form of E-D may have the same molecular defect as in dermatosparaxis of cattle (p. 346)—persistence of procollagen as a result of deficiency of the protease that cleaves the registration peptide from procollagen (p. 39). Studying collagen from three of our patients in the laboratory of Dr. George Martin (Lichtenstein[160b]) has found evidence of persistence of procollagen. The clinical picture is identical in the three patients, although different from that in cattle that show skin fragility as the main feature. The patients show floppiness as infants, marked loose jointedness, and moderate stretchability and bruisability of the skin. Stature is abnormally short. The disorder is presumably an autosomal recessive. (See Fig. 6-28 for one of the patients.)

Goodman and colleagues[104,106] described a patient thought to have both the Ehlers-Danlos syndrome and the Marfan syndrome. The possibility that this patient had a connective tissue disorder distinct from both E-D and the Marfan syndrome and called the Marfanoid hypermobility syndrome[281] is discussed on p. 177.

Pathology

In none of the ten main disorders of connective tissue discussed in this book is the microscopic anatomy in such a disputed state as in E-D.[149]

Increase in elastic tissue of the corium has been described by many writers.[17,42,137,178,179,213,215,227,252,264,268] Some of them described morphologic ab-

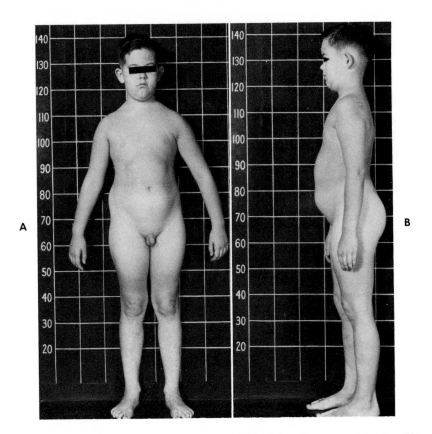

Fig. 6-25. Typical E-D in 10-year-old boy (J. I., A75064). There is a normal brother 1½ years of age. The mother and father are unaffected and no similar cases are identified in the family of either parent. There is striking fragility of the skin, as evidenced by many scars, e.g., of the knees, forehead, and shins. The wounds, of which dozens have occurred, are almost round, and subcutaneous areolar tissue herniates up through the break in the epidermis. The joints are strikingly hyperextensible. When not bearing weight, the pedal arches appear higher than normal, but with bearing weight the feet become strikingly flat. There is knobby redundancy of the skin of soles, especially around the heels. The fragility and hyperelasticity extend to the buccal and lingual mucosa (at one time stitches had to be taken in a cut in the tongue) and possibly to the pharyngeal and laryngeal areas, where redundancy of the mucosal lining appears to be responsible for a chronic cough, especially during the winter months. The ears are large and "floppy," with less prominent landmarks than is normally the case. There are bilateral epicanthal folds. The skin under the chin is loose and redundant. Bilateral cervical ribs are present; members of the father's family show this anomaly. Easy bruising has been a striking feature. The patient is less active than normal because of voluntary restriction and has become somewhat obese as a result. The regular use of bandages on the legs has helped avoid much trouble with cuts on the shins. Biopsy of skin and skeletal muscle in the left pectoral area revealed increase in the number of elastic fibers in the corium and in the perimyal areas. Some of the arteries showed what appeared to be anomalous elastic fibers. **A,** Front view. **B,** Lateral view. Note the scars of the face and knees, the knobby appearance of the soles, the flat feet, the peculiarly shaped pinnae, and the epicanthal folds. **C,** Loose collagen meshwork and unusually abundant elastic fibers (stained black) in the subcutaneous area overlying pectoral muscle (Verhoeff–van Giesen stain; ×200; reduced 3/7). **D,** Increased elastic fibers in small artery in pectoral muscle (Verhoeff–van Giesen stain; ×200; reduced 3/7).

normalities of the elastic fibers, as did Smith[248] and Pittinos,[210] who, however, did not consider the elastic fibers to be more numerous than normal. Williams[293] and Pautrier[204] found the elastic fibers *normal,* and Brown and Stock[46] believed them to be *decreased.* To some extent at least, the apparent excess of elastic fibers may be relative. In E-D type IV, the ecchymotic variety (p. 339), for instance, the marked deficiency in collagen inevitably leaves the elastic fibers as a predominant fibrous element of the corium. Elastosis perforans may be more likely to occur in E-D type IV than in the other forms.

Diminution and morphologic abnormalities of collagen fibers have been described.[197,248,268] Katz and Steiner[142] report histochemical studies that they interpret as indicating increase of mucopolysaccharide of corium.

Studying skin biopsies from 3 cases of E-D, Wechsler and Fisher[286] confirmed a relative decrease in collagen and increase in elastic tissue. Other histochemical stains, enzyme studies (with elastase and pepsin), and electron microscopic studies of collagen periodicity showed no differences from the normal. In E-D the tensile strength of the skin has been found to be about one fifth that of normal skin.[225] (See p. 352.)

Jansen[133] points out, with excellent illustrations, that "in normal skin, a system of robust, well directed, crossing and tightly interlacing collagen fibre bundles is present. The whorled disorderly structure in hyperelastic (E-D) skin is remarkable; the collagen bundles seem to have been insufficiently united." By electron microscopy collagen and elastin were morphologically normal. This corroborates the finding of Tunbridge and collaborators,[272] but Jansen was unable to agree that there was an absolute increase in the number of elastic fibers.

Collections of giant cells are sometimes found.[225] The subcutaneous nodules or spherules are apparently fat-containing cysts.[285] They frequently become calcified. It seems likely that they are related to minor traumata and to the general fragility of the connective tissue in which the fat deposits normally exist. Molluscoid pseudotumors that develop at pressure points are characterized by cyst formation.[131]

How much of the bleeding is due to a defect in the supporting tissues and how much to weakness of the vessel walls themselves is not clarified by histologic studies. Abnormal, dilated, weak-appearing vessels have been described by

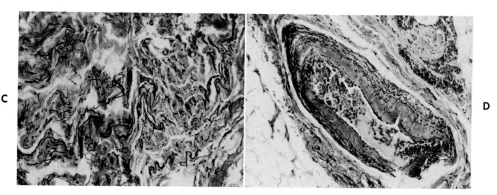

C   D

Fig. 6-25, cont'd. For legend see opposite page.

Tobias[268] and by others.[161] An abnormality (Fig. 6-25*D*) of the connective tissue of the wall of small arteries was demonstrated in one of my cases, and similar changes are seen in Fig. 21 of Jansen's report.[131]

Few histologic studies of tissues other than skin have been reported with the exception of an autopsy case described by Lienhart,[161] one by Nicod,[191] two by McFarland and Fuller[168] and, of course, the cases of dissecting aneurysm described above. In Lienhart's patient, a 22-year-old woman who died of pulmonary tuberculosis, no internal abnormality referable to the connective tissue defect was discovered. Nicod[191] studied bone and cartilage and could detect no abnormality.

Behar and Rachmilewitz[19] described arterial changes in a 32-year-old male with E-D. Since the patient died of chronic glomerulonephritis, the changes may have been exaggerated by the accompanying hypertension. The findings consisted of hypoplasia and aplasia of the internal elastic lamina; multiple dissections of the aorta, pulmonary artery, and atrial endocardium; and Erdheim's cystic medial necrosis of the aorta.

The basic defect(s)

Superficial consideration of the clinical manifestations of E-D might suggest an abnormality of elastic tissue as the fundamental defect—probably a superabundance of elastic fibers in the skin and joint capsules. However, the histologic studies by no means afford unequivocal substantiation of this theory. Brown and Stock[46] suggested, and others (notably, and most recently, Jansen[133]) maintain,[96] that the defect may reside in the collagen fibers, which, because of lack of normal tensile strength, permit the skin, joint capsules, ligaments, and so forth to be stretched beyond the normal limits (Fig. 6-26). The elastic fibers may function

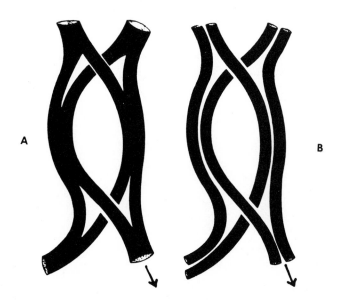

Fig. 6-26. Jansen's schematic representation of the postulated defect in collagen fasciculation in E-D syndrome. **A,** Normal. **B,** E-D syndrome. (From Jansen, L. H.: Dermatologica **110**:108, 1955.)

in connection with the process of restoration to normal configuration of these tissues. According to the "collagen theory," the histologic changes, both quantitative and qualitative, are interpretable as secondary effects of the abnormality of collagen. I am inclined to favor the view that the Ehlers-Danlos syndrome is another heritable disorder of collagen, biochemically, morphologically, clinically, and, of course, genetically distinct from the others which are under discussion in this book.

The fact that collagen is genetically defective as the primary fault has been unequivocally established in the case of type VI E-D. Here the collagen has deficiency of hydroxylysine and an excess of lysine.[209b] The enzyme lysyl hydroxylase (p. 39), which catalyzes hydroxylation of lysine after its incorporation into the peptide chain, is functionally deficient.[149a] Certain hydroxylysine residues of collagen are involved in cross-linkage (p. 41, Fig. 2-5). Cross-linkage is defective in hydroxylysine-deficient collagen. Other types of defects affecting cross-linking are being actively sought in other varieties of E-D.

The comparative inextensibility of nomal collagen may depend on some specific molecular or intermolecular structure which is altered in E-D, with resulting increase in extensibility. This alteration is assumed in the theory of Brown and Stock[46] and has been explicitly stated by Froelich[94] and by others. Jansen[133] has recently advanced a related theory, incriminating collagen but placing the defect at a higher level of organization of collagen—that E-D is a disorder of the organization of collagen fibrils into bundles and of the bundles into a strong network. He refers to the disease as one of a "defective wickerwork" of collagen. The evidence he assembles (see discussion of pathology) and the clinical aspects of the disease outlined here make Jansen's version of the "collagen theory" highly probable. The electron microscopic and thermographic normality of collagen[174,192] may support the view of Wechsler and Fisher[286] that there is no qualitative abnormality of collagen but, rather, inadequate collagen production. In fibroblasts from patients with E-D, Martin[173] could not, however, demonstrate deficient collagen synthesis.

It is possible that, in some patients and at some subcutaneous and articular locations, production of an excessive number of elastic fibers is stimulated by the repeated and excessive stretching. In tissue culture, Maximow[175] and Bloom[38] thought that the tugging of contractile myocardial cells was a factor in the formation of elastic fibers. Varadi and Hall[276] compared elastin isolated from the skin of 4 patients with E-D and elastin isolated from normal controls. No abnormality of quantity, amino acid composition, or desmosine cross-linking could be demonstrated. No difference in elastin content could be demonstrated between skin of thigh and knee, an argument against the possibility of stimulation of elastin synthesis at sites of flexion.

The changes that occur in the skin of the feet and hands and at the elbows of older patients fit in well with the view that the primary defect resides in the collagen fibers: the normal elastic tissue may, with the passage of time, "wear out" from excessive stress imposed on it, and the cutis laxa (as opposed to cutis hyperelastica) of late cases becomes evident.

In Hungary, Banga and Baló,[9] who discovered the elastolytic enzyme in pancreas, also demonstrated that normal serum contains an elastase inhibitor. In Tunbridge's department in Leeds, Hall and co-workers[118] found in 2 patients with

E-D a concentration of elastase inhibitor in the blood that was "between 50 and 100 times as great as that in pooled normal serum." Goltz and Hult[102] also found elevated serum elastase inhibitor. Carter and Walford[55] could, however, demonstrate no increase in elastase inhibitor in 7 patients.

Scarpelli and Goodman[237] found abnormalities of fibroblasts from healing wound tissue in a patient presumed to have combined E-D and the Marfan syndrome. (See p. 177 for a reinterpretation of this case.) By electron microscopy they observed a paucity of rough-surfaced endoplasmic reticulum with a resultant decrease in the number of collagen fibers in the extracellular compartment. They considered the findings "not inconsistent" with the decreased dermal collagen, deficient hydroxyproline content (a reflection of decreased collagen), and lowered thermal stability of collagen found by other workers.[174]

The weakness of vessel walls seems an adequate basis for the hemorrhagic diathesis in E-D, and the lack of any consistent abnormality of clotting factors suggests that the defect does not lie in that domain. Owren[199] has advanced the plausible suggestion that because of an abnormal structure or a quantitative deficiency, collagen in E-D is ineffective in attracting platelets and triggering liberation of adenosine diphosphate from them. The role of collagen in hemostasis is discussed in Chapter 2 (p. 34). Caen and associates[50a] have recently reported a case of bleeding diathesis and abnormal wound healing in which the patient's collagen had an abnormal electron microscopic appearance and failed to induce aggregation of normal platelets; the patient's platelets adhered to normal skin collagen.

If there is a defect in collagen in E-D, accounting for the fragility of the skin and other cutaneous features, it cannot be surprising that the bowel is friable in E-D. Recall that "surgical gut" is made from the submucosa and serosa of sheep and hogs and is almost pure collagen. Obviously collagen is very important to the integrity of the bowel.

Clinically abnormalities of the bones themselves are notable in their absence in E-D. It is therefore difficult to interpret the findings[138] that in E-D the collagen of bone is abnormally irregular, that tetracycline uptake is less than in controls, and that by microradiography there is decreased mineralization of trabeculae.

Potentially, the existence of an analogous hereditary disorder in an animal that can be studied experimentally offers promise of providing important new information on the nature of the basic defect. For this reason, descriptions of the Ehlers-Danlos syndrome in springer spaniels[283] and in mink[201] are of great interest. In these animals, Hegreberg and colleagues[123 to 125] found the same fragility of skin and peripheral arteries and the same hyperextensibility and laxity of skin and joints. In both species, inheritance was autosomal dominant, as are most forms of E-D in man.[123] The skin in affected dogs had tensile strength only one twenty-seventh that of the normal; in affected mink the tensile strength of skin was one thirteenth that of normal.[124,125] The histologic appearance was similar to that in the human disease.[124,125]

A disorder characterized by extremely fragile skin and called dermatosparaxis has been described in cattle.[7b,7c,119a,193a] Lapière and colleagues[152a] have demonstrated the basic defect to be a deficiency of the protease that cleaves procollagen to remove the extra segment which distinguished the procollagen molecule from the molecule that exists extracellularly. The disorder is inherited as an autosomal recessive. The same defect probably occurs in man (p. 341).

Prevalence and inheritance

Thus far, this syndrome has been described principally in Europeans and persons of European extraction. There is one report from India[57] of the disease in a 12-year-old Hindu girl. The disorder has been seen in Japan.[198] In addition to those reported here, a number of cases of E-D in Negroes have been reported.[47,69,171]

Schaper[238] stated in 1952 that only 93 cases of this syndrome had been reported. Although the number is now probably well in excess of 150, it is possible that fewer of these cases have been reported than of any of the other syndromes discussed in this series. This is, in part, the result of greater difficulties of recognizing the syndrome, since cutaneous and articular hyperelasticity is a graded trait. I hazard to say, however, that in actuality this is one of the most frequent of the heritable disorders of connective tissue. My photographer, in the course of the study of other patients with E-D, recalled that his brother-in-law could do contortionist tricks with his hands. On investigation this individual was found to have had congenital dislocation of the right hip, bilateral inguinal hernias, diaphragmatic hernia, and trouble with one knee and the right wrist (Fig. 6-12). Although these conditions had all been considered unrelated, the diagnosis of the Ehlers-Danlos syndrome is quite certain, and all these manifestations are clearly part of the syndrome. This patient illustrates how easy it is to overlook the generalized disorder.

In a majority of the kindreds I have studied, now numbering over thirty, multiple members are affected and, in most, affected persons were found in successive generations. Since mild manifestations tend to be overlooked by laymen and since only the propositus was examined in several instances, the above evidence can be taken only as a rough indication of autosomal dominant inheritance.

In 1949 Johnson and Falls[137] reviewed sixteen families reported in the literature as having more than 1 affected member.[145] In these families, a total of 80 affected individuals had been identified, of whom exactly half were male. Brown[45] found 19 affected members in a family numbering 47 individuals. Johnson and Falls[137] studied the pattern of inheritance in detail and concluded that the disorder is inherited as a dominant. Two sisters with an unusually severe form of the disease were children of cousins, each with a mild form of the disease; this suggested to the authors that the trait might have occurred in homozygous state in these girls. Consanguinity was thought to be a factor in the cases observed by Ronchese[227] and by Weber and Aitken.[285] For an extensive review of most of the then published pedigrees, see Jansen.[131,132] Since then extensively affected kindreds with an autosomal dominant pedigree pattern have been reported by several authors.[22,202]

Although the survey of the literature by Johnson and Falls[137] indicated a sex ratio of 1:1, in the kindred they studied personally there were 21 affected males and 11 affected females. Furthermore, Jansen,[132] on the basis of a more extensive survey, concluded that the incidence of this disorder is consistently higher in males.

Coe and Silver[60] and Ormsby and Tobin[197] presented illustrations of members of three generations displaying the E-D syndrome; Stuart,[254] Mories,[183] and Husebye[127] traced it through four generations; the largest pedigree is that of Johnson and Falls,[137] with six generations affected. Here there was again clear evidence of dominant inheritance. The disease has been described in one of twins who were probably fraternal.[77]

Penetrance in this disease is probably considerably lower than in the Marfan syndrome, for example. This, however, is merely the result of the greater difficulty of recognizing mild and graded abnormality of the joints and skin as opposed to less equivocal manifestations, e.g. ectopia lentis, in the Marfan syndrome.

As always, the possibility of the existence of more than one genotype in this disease must be kept prominently in mind. Some minor phenotypic differences—for example, the lack of skin fragility in cases such as that shown in Fig. 6-19—suggest this possibility but are not sufficiently clear-cut to make one certain. Somatic mutation is a possible explanation for unilateral involvement, as in the famous case of van Meekeren. However, there are no clearly described similarly unilateral cases reported in recent times. That of Du Bois[79] is too sketchily reported to permit analysis.

Although autosomal dominant inheritance obtains in the first four varieties of E-D discussed earlier (p. 339), a fifth X-linked form is well established as well as a sixth form with autosomal recessive inheritance and a proved abnormality of the mechanism by which lysine of collagen is hydroxylated. In the sixth form, deficiency of lysyl hydroxylase has been demonstrated. There may be allelic forms of the sixth form of E-D, because the phenotype is somewhat different in the two families in which deficiency of this enzyme had been demonstrated (p. 340).

The karyotype is normal in E-D.[211] An exception was the child, reported by Vissian and colleagues,[279] with E-D and the *cri-du-chat* syndrome (deletion of part of the short arm of a chromosome 5). Because of the potential for deletion mapping of the chromosomes, patients with the *cri-du-chat* syndrome and other deletion syndromes should be investigated for the presence of rare recessive disorders that may become evident in the hemizygous state in such patients. However, it is difficult to believe that the occurrence of E-D in this infant was more than coincidence, since no autosomal recessive form of E-D is clearly established.

Miscellaneous considerations

"Simple" hypermobility of joints, known also as congenital laxity of ligaments, may occur as an isolated finding,[53,64,143,222,256] with a genetic background distinct from that in E-D. See Figs. 6-14 and 6-27 for examples. (Some of the familial cases reported as instances of simple joint laxity may, in fact, be examples of E-D. For example, Key[143] described "hypermobility of joints as a sex-linked hereditary characteristic." The disorder was clearly E-D because photographs showed cigarette-paper scars over the knees, and the inheritance could not have been sex-linked in the strict genetic sense because father-to-son transmission was observed.) Loose-jointedness occurs also in the Marfan syndrome and with osteogenesis imperfecta, whereas reduced joint mobility is characteristic

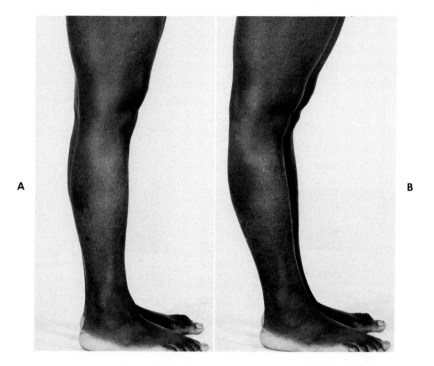

Fig. 6-27. H. L. W. (395947), affected with "simple" joint hypermobility. There is seemingly no similar disorder in family. Although the knees and feet are most markedly affected, with genu recurvatum and pes planus, all joints of the body are more mobile than the average. The pes planus is of the dynamic type; the arch of the foot appears fairly normal except during weight bearing. The joint instability at the knees resulted in recurrent hydrarthroses. The patient has worn knee braces with benefit. There are no associated cutaneous or internal manifestations to suggest E-D syndrome. Strabismus (intermittent exotropia) was treated by means of resection and advancement of the left medial rectus muscle. This case illustrates how difficult it is to be sure of the proper diagnostic classification in a patient with manifestations that may represent an incomplete form of the E-D syndrome, especially when there is no other full-blown example of the disorder in the family. **A,** Position at rest. **B,** Forced backward displacement of knees to demonstrate genu recurvatum. In addition to flat feet, a few scars were suggestively papyraceous.

of the Hurler syndrome. In the differential diagnosis of loose-jointedness, especially in children, cerebrocortical degeneration or malformation, mongolism, cretinism, rickets, and nonspecific cachexia must be kept in mind. Carter and Wilkinson[54] emphasized the importance of persistent joint laxity in the occurrence of congenital dislocation of the hip.

Hass and Hass[121] suggest that there is a distinct entity of loose-jointedness, or, as they term it, *arthrochalasis multiplex congenita,* which is a "constitutional dyscrasia of mesenchyme," has wide variability and severity, and may occur with or without skin changes. In this view E-D is apparently construed as merely those cases of arthrochalasis multiplex congenita in which skin involvement happens to be present. It seems more likely, however, that there are a number of genetic causes of loose-jointedness, and that although E-D may occur without much or any skin change, most cases do show changes in both the skin and joints. If any condition deserves the designation arthrochalasis multiplex congenita, it would seem to be that affecting the patients shown in Figs. 6-15 and 6-28. We have seen several such patients born with dislocation of the hips and severe laxity at other joints. The patients are short of stature and show epicanthal folds. The skin is soft and mildly stretchable but not excessively fragile. This disorder may be classified as a seventh distinguishable form of the Ehlers-Danlos syndrome, as outlined on p. 341. The defect, in some at least, may involve pro-collagen protease,[160b] which is normally responsible for clearing the registration peptide from collagen (p. 39).

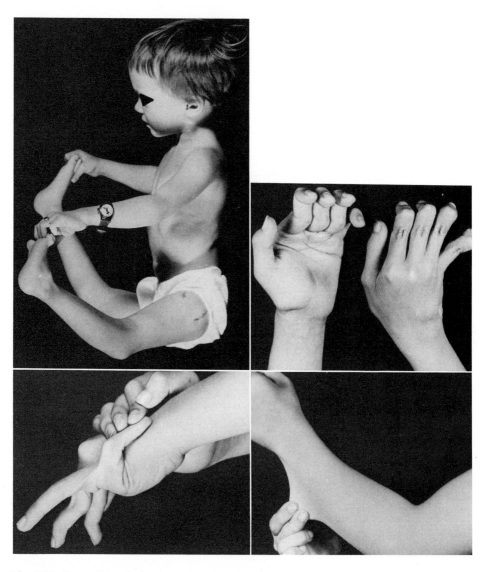

Fig. 6-28. Severe joint laxity in S. E. (J.H.H. 967533), born in 1954. Dislocated hips and hypermobile knee joints were noted at birth. Recent findings suggest that S. E. has deficiency of procollagen protease (p. 341).

The Larsen syndrome[153] comprises multiple congenital dislocations with osseous anomalies and unusual facies. The elbows, hips, and knees show dislocation, usually bilaterally. Anterior dislocation of the tibia on the femur is especially characteristic. The fingers are cylindrical, with short nails, the thumbs are spatulate, and the metacarpals short. The facies is characterized by prominent or bossed forehead, flat or depressed nasal bridge, and wide-set eyes. A juxtacalcaneal accessory ossification center and abnormality of vertebral seg-

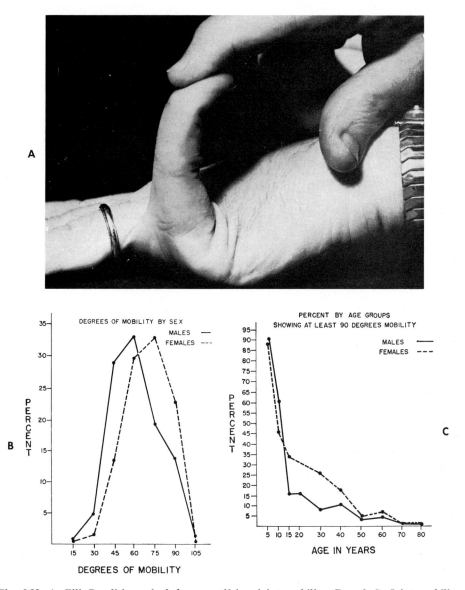

Fig. 6-29. **A,** Ellis-Bundick method for quantifying joint mobility. **B** and **C,** Joint mobility by age and sex, as determined by the Ellis-Bundick method in 500 subjects. **B,** Most young children under 5 years of age show at least 90-degree mobility. In the groups of intermediate age the incidence is appreciably greater in women. **C,** Female subjects show higher grades of mobility. (**B** and **C** from Ellis, F. A., and Bundick, W. R.: Arch. Derm. **74:**22, 1956.)

mentation, especially in the upper thoracic and cervical spine, are demonstrable radiographically. Cleft palate, congenital heart malformation, and hydrocephalus occur in some. Decreased rigidity of cartilage in the rib cage epiglottis, arytenoid, and perhaps trachea occasion respiratory difficulties in the young child. The disorder is probably an autosomal recessive in most cases, although the possibility of dominant inheritance in some instances has been raised.[153a]

Ellis and Bundick[86] have measured joint mobility in 500 subjects, about half male and half female, spanning eight decades of age. The gauge of mobility was extensibility of the fifth finger as shown in Fig. 6-29*A*. The subject placed his extended hand on a flat surface with the forearm parallel to the examining surface. The examiner then extended the fifth finger as far as comfortably possible and measured the angle made by the proximal phalanx with the flat surface with a protractor to the closest multiple of 15 degrees. The results are charted in Fig. 6-29*B* and *C*. Most children have a high degree of mobility. Between ages 15 and 50 years a high degree of mobility is considerably more frequent in female subjects than in males. Although no quantitative study of the subject has been made, there is a clinical impression that Negroes are more loose-jointed than whites.

Measures of joint elasticity and of other characteristics such as plasticity and viscosity will be valuable in the study of E-D. Promising progress in the quantitation of loose-jointedness and delineation of the components of joint stiffness has been made by Wright and Johns.[135,136,294]

Interesting physiologic studies of skin elasticity and tensile strength have been done in recent years.[74,76,113,134,145,195,225,289] Skin elasticity can be measured with the "pinchmeter" of Olmsted and associates,[194] with the elastometer of Schade, or by the simple although subjective method of Ellis and Bundick.[86] In this last technique, the skin of the dorsum of the wrist is elevated between the forefinger and thumb and relative elasticity estimated. Normal elasticity is indicated by 2+, reduced elasticity by 1+, and increased elasticity by 3+. Scleroderma on this scale is 0 and full-blown E-D, 4+. Rollhäuser[225] found least tensile strength in the skin of infants under 3 months (about 0.25 kg./sq. mm.); more in adults (about 1.6 kg./sq. mm.); and yet more in aged individuals (over 2 kg./sq. mm.). With aging, furthermore, skin became progressively less extensible. These observations may explain the tendency for the cutaneous fragility and extensibility in E-D to become less striking as the affected individual ages. Rollhäuser[225] studied the skin tensile strength of a 35-year-old man with E-D and found it to be very low (0.34 kg./sq. mm.). It is of interest that this worker found parallel changes in the tensile strength and extensibility of tendons, suggesting that the properties measured in the skin may be constitutional and generalized. Wenzel[289] found lesser tensile strength in female skin and made important observations indicating reduction in the strength of the skin in normal pregnancy and in Cushing's syndrome. In connection with the latter condition, it is noteworthy that the fragility of the skin and easy bruisability are rather similar in E-D and in Cushing's syndrome.[150] However, in all likelihood, the similarity is only superficial.

Blue sclerae are not uncommon in E-D,[42,82] and the presence of this feature cannot be taken as evidence of associated osteogenesis imperfecta. Biering and Iversen[36] have reported a more convincing case of association of the two connective tissue disorders. There was no familial history of manifestations of osteogenesis imperfecta, but in the father's line there was joint and skin hyperextensibility. The description[132,161,224] of associated dolichostenomelia (long, thin extremities, as in the Marfan syndrome) cannot be taken as evidence that E-D and the Marfan syndrome coincided in those patients, since no ectopia lentis was detected and no unequivocal cases of the Marfan disease in other members of the family were described. Some of these cases of presumably combined E-D and Marfan syndromes were probably instances of the Marfaroid hypermobility syndrome (p. 177).

Seemingly bona fide instances of coincident E-D and pseudoxanthoma elasticum have been described.[63,193,205] In Cottini's patient[63] there were angioid streaks, and lesions of the skin of the neck characteristic of pseudoxanthoma elasticum (Chapter 10); in addition there were cigarette-paper scars of the elbows and knees and hyperextensible skin and joints characteristic of E-D. The pseudoxanthoma elasticum, which appears to be a recessive trait, was not transmitted to a daughter who suffered from acrocyanosis or to a son who had hyperextensible skin and joints, hernia, and varices of the leg veins. The 22-year-old woman described by Pelbois and Rollier[205] consulted them because of the cosmetically undesirable lesions of pseudoxanthoma elasticum involving the skin of the neck and other areas of flexure. As well as angioid streaks of the fundus (characteristic of pseudoxanthoma), the patient had multiple cicatrices indicative of cutaneous fragility, striking cutaneous hyperelasticity, and articular hypermobility. The parents were first cousins, a fact significant in the appearance of the recessive trait of pseudoxanthoma. The parents were themselves unaffected by pseudoxanthoma, although a maternal aunt of the patient was affected. As for E-D, the patient's mother displayed features of this syndrome and had probably transmitted it as a dominant trait to her daughter. These cases are, then, examples of accidental coincidence of the two syndromes, one behaving as a dominant and one as a recessive trait.

In *cutis laxa,* which is discussed as a distinct entity in Chapter 7, the skin hangs in loose folds, and internal manifestations of a generalized connective tissue abnormality are present in some cases. The skin in pseudoxanthoma elasticum acquires the character of cutis laxa in the late stages in extreme cases (Fig. 10-15, pp. 494 and 495).

In one patient, 61 years old,[190] E-D coexisted with muscular atrophy of the Aran-Duchenne type (amyotrophic lateral sclerosis). I find it impossible to agree with the authors[190] that an etiologic connection between the two conditions existed. In one of my cases, Oppenheim's disease (amyotonia congenita)[117] was the original diagnosis when the patient was first seen at the age of 4 years. Abnormality of creatine metabolism was reported in one patient,[210] and in another[207] there was coincident parathyroid tumor with osteitis fibrosa cystica. After correction of the hyperparathyroidism surgically, it appeared that the joint laxity, particularly the scoliosis, and the fragility of the skin decreased.

The Bonnevie-Ullrich-Turner syndrome[151] often has hyperelasticity of joints and skin as a feature. Furthermore, the skin of the hands may be loose and wrinkled as an aftermath of the lymphedema that is frequently present in the first year or so after birth. (More characteristic features are dwarfism, webbing of the neck, cubitus valgus, gonadal dysgenesis, and female phenotype with male

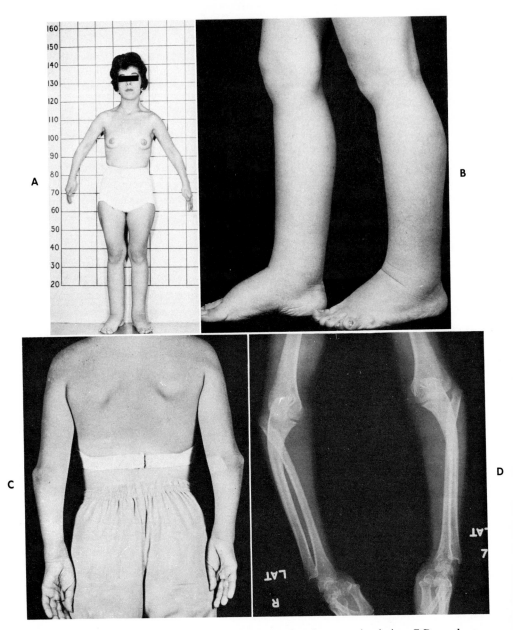

Fig. 6-30. Patient with the Noonan syndrome, showing features simulating E-D syndrome. **A,** Short stature, low-set ears, and leg edema. **B,** Lymphedema shown here and in **A** probably is aggravated only to a minor extent by the heart disease. Secondary sexual characteristics are normally developed. **C,** Bilateral posterior dislocation of radial heads.[59] **D,** X-ray film of same. **E,** Hands. Note the loose, coarse-grained appearance of the skin. **F,** Deformed, edematous feet. **G,** Chest x-ray film. Note cardiomegaly. **H,** Spectral phonocardiogram showing systolic and diastolic murmurs. The same auscultatory findings were present at the left lower sternal border and apex. **I,** Electrocardiogram.

sex chromatin pattern and usually XO sex chromosome constitution.) Rossi and colleagues[229,230] have emphasized the similar features. Rossi and Angst[229] write as follows: "The Ehlers-Danlos syndrome sufficiently closely resembles the pterygium syndrome that the former should be considered a forerunner of the latter." Although it is probably far-fetched to presume any fundamental relationship, the possibility of diagnostic confusion cannot be disputed.

In recent years a group of patients with what might be termed the pseudo-Turner syndrome have been recognized. These female patients have short stature, low-set ears, low posterior hairline, facial features reminiscent of the Turner syndrome, sometimes webbing of the neck, and short, square hands and feet with wrinkled skin of the palms and soles. Lymphedema of the feet may be present in early life or may appear in the teens. However, secondary sex char-

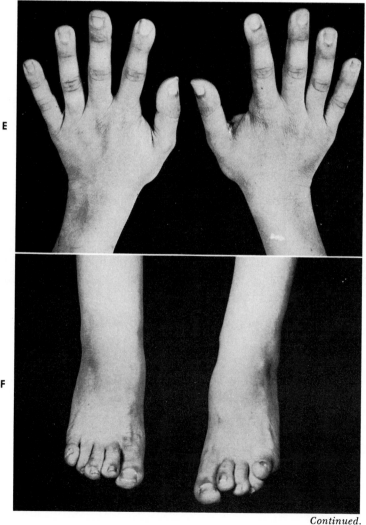

E

F

Continued.

Fig. 6-30, cont'd. For legend see opposite page.

acteristics are normally developed, menstruation is normal, and sex chromatin and chromosomes are those of the normal female. Congenital malformation of the heart, particularly pulmonary stenosis, is present in many. A similar syndrome occurs in males and is called the male Turner syndrome; in these cases the chromosomal findings have usually been those of a normal male. This pseudo-Turner syndrome occurring in either sex is also referred to as the Noonan syndrome or the Turner phenotype with normal karyotype. Evidence is accumulating that the disorder is Mendelian, possibly autosomal dominant.[8a,57a]

Several of the features of the disorder suggest the Ehlers-Danlos syndrome. The case of C. E. (Fig. 6-30*A* to *I*), which was presented earlier (1960) as E-D with cardiac malformation, is more likely an example of the pseudo-Turner or Noonan syndrome.

Case 6. C. E. (B32309; 745114), a white female born in 1939, was first seen in this hospital in 1956 for opinion on her heart condition and for plastic surgery.

Apparently no other members of her family have skin, joint, or cardiac changes similar to hers. The parents and brother and sister are of average stature. Various members of the father's family were short. For example, the paternal grandfather was only 5 feet tall.

The patient was "very flabby" at birth. X-ray films were taken in the first days of life, probably because of dislocation of the elbows (Fig. 6-30*C* and *D*) and possibly other joints. No mention of a murmur or other sign of cardiac abnormality was made to the parents until the patient was 15 months old. At that time she was still flabby and did not stand or walk. The flabbiness was no longer apparent after the age of 9 or 10 years. An endocrinopathy, probably hypopituitarism, was suspected, mainly because of the short stature. However, sexual maturation occurred normally.

The patient lived a sheltered life. Palpitation was the only symptom definitely attributable to the heart. Both systolic and diastolic murmurs are known to have been present from the age of 10 years. At that time she weighed only 43 pounds and was 45 inches tall.

G

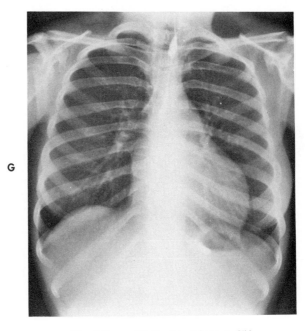

Fig. 6-30, cont'd. For legend see p. 354.

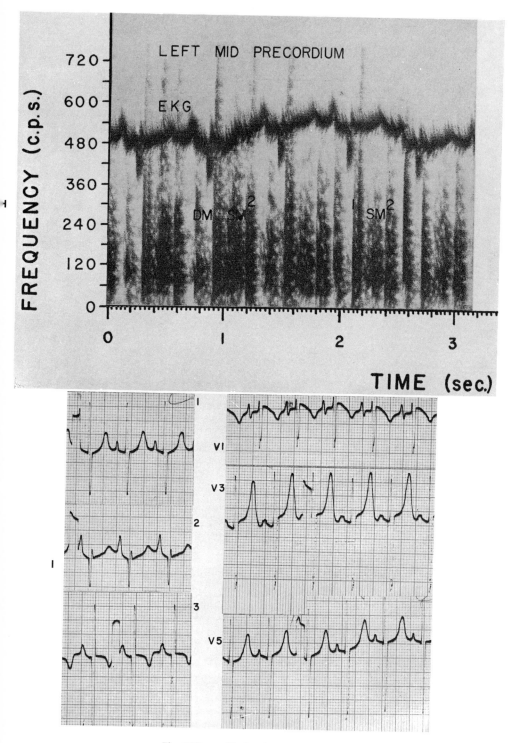

Fig. 6-30, cont'd. For legend see p. 354.

Physical examination in 1956 revealed an intelligent girl only 56 inches tall. There were generalized hypermobility of the joints and elasticity of the skin. The head of each radius was dislocated posteriorly. The patient could not extend the elbow beyond a point 18 degrees from full extension. Pronation of the wrists and forearms was moderately impaired.

The nose was hooked. Malocclusion, with narrowing of the anterior vertical arch of the hard palate, was present. The pinnae were also mildly deformed; they were low in position and rotated so that the lobule was located somewhat anteriorly to the external meatus and helix.

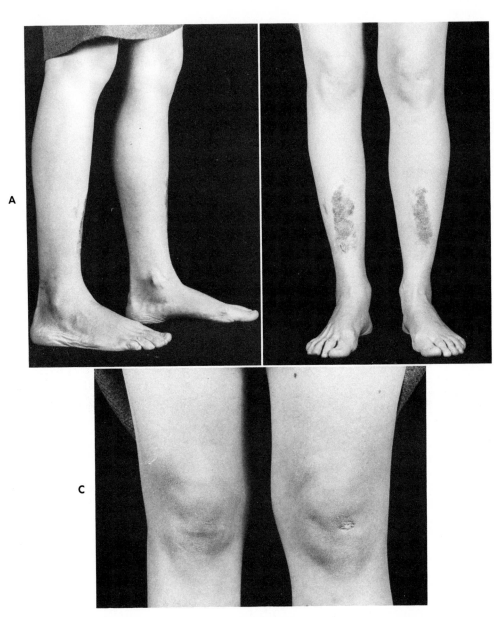

Fig. 6-31. Patient with absorptive periodontosis, showing wrinkling of the skin on the lateral aspects of the feet, **A,** skin lesions over the shins, **B,** and scars on the knees, **C.** The wrinkles on the feet and the scars on the knees are somewhat suggestive of E-D syndrome. Several relatives have the same combination of features.

The heart was enlarged to the left anterior axillary line. The auscultatory findings were dominated by bizarre murmurs, in systole and diastole, of a scratchy quality, suggesting pericardial friction rub (Fig. 6-30*H*). The murmurs were maximal at the apex and left mid-precordium.

Photographs, an electrocardiogram, a phonocardiogram, and x-ray films are presented in Fig. 6-30*A* to *I*. Angiocardiograms revealed dilatation of the entire right side of the heart.

Rhinoplasty and repair of both elbows by resection of the heads of the radii were performed with success. Healing after surgery was perfectly normal, and there were no late complications.

Edema in the right leg began about 1959, and in the left leg in 1960. At first the edema would subside overnight or after a weekend of rest and was helped by a diuretic. More recently it has become more marked, and episodes of cellulitis and/or lymphangiitis have occurred.

In 1968 the patient delivered vaginally a normal female infant weighing 6½ pounds. The child has shown no signs of the Noonan syndrome.

A condition unique in my experience, and apparently in the literature as well, is demonstrated by the wife of a colleague of mine and several of her relatives. Lesions on the shins suggest those of E-D, and slow-healing breaks in the skin at that site have occurred after blunt trauma. The skin is not generally fragile, and no unusual bruisability or stretchability of the skin has been noted. The joints are not hyperextensible. A second feature, apparently syndromally related to the lesions on the shins, is absorptive periodontosis, with early loss of the teeth. The dental and skin changes are present also in the proband's father, in several sibs of her father, and in a cousin. The lesions on the shins suggested necrobiosis diabeticorum on histologic study, but there is no diabetes in the family, and no abnormality of carbohydrate metabolism is demonstrable in the proband. The lesions on the shins are demonstrated in Fig. 6-31*B*. The small scars on the knees are somewhat like those of E-D, and the skin of the lateral aspect of the soles is wrinkled in the manner demonstrated by E-D patients.

Surgery in the Ehlers-Danlos syndrome has often been accompanied by wound dehiscence[129,200] (Fig. 6-12). The tissues may be strikingly friable and hold sutures poorly. Hemostasis may be a problem. With particular care, Ricketson[217] was able to repair a large flaplike wound of the right shin; the scars of the other shin were removed and likewise replaced by a split-thickness graft, with excellent results. Thoracoplasty was successfully performed in one patient with severe E-D[228] (Fig. 6-11).

Almost always the skin and joint changes in E-D are evident from an early age. However, Jacobs[129] described a patient in whom the manifestations seemed quite clearly to appear first at the age of 29 years. Although the patient had been a pugilist, no friability of the skin had been noted earlier. A brother was also affected. Golden and Garret[101] described a rather similar case, a patient with onset of easy bruising, cutaneous fragility, and poor wound healing after the age of 26 years. It seems possible that one or both of these reports relate to a condition other than E-D.

In the management of pregnancy in severe E-D, elective cesarean section has much to recommend it. Two patients so treated without complications are known to Tyson.[273a] The procedure is best performed through a lower midline abdominal incision avoiding, insofar as possible, the use of forceful tissue retraction. The uterus is entered through an incision of the lower uterine segment, with the usual repair following delivery of the infant and placenta. Closure of the abdominal wall should include the use of large retention sutures secured over plastic retention bridges, which remove tension from the suture line. After retention sutures are placed, subcuticular stitching can be performed with a non-absorbable suture. The retention sutures should be left in for 6 weeks or longer.

SUMMARY

The cardinal manifestations of the Ehlers-Danlos syndrome are loose-jointed-ness; hyperextensibility; fragility and bruisability of the skin, with "cigarette-paper" scarring; and generalized friability of tissues. Internal manfestations include rupture of great vessels; diaphragmatic and other hernias; gastrointestinal diverticula; friability of the bowel, leading to spontaneous rupture; and rupture of the lung with mediastinal emphysema and/or pneumothorax. When the fetus is affected, precocious rupture of the membranes may occur.

The basic defect is thought to concern the organization of collagen bundles into an intermeshing network.

By clinical and genetic means, several (perhaps as many as six) distinct forms of the Ehlers-Danlos syndrome can be identified. One form is inherited as an X-linked recessive and one probably distinct "ocular" form may be inherited as an autosomal recessive. The others, which constitute the majority of cases, show autosomal dominant inheritance.

REFERENCES

1. Aaby, G. V., and Blake, H. A.: Tracheobronchiomegaly, Ann. Thorac. Surg. **2**:64, 1966.
2. Adams, F.: The genuine works of Hippocrates, New York, 1891, William Wood & Co.: Airs, waters, and places, paragraphs 20 and 22, vol. 1, pp. 176-178.
3. Agostini, A.: Cited by Jansen.[181]
4. Aldridge, R. T.: Ehlers-Danlos syndrome causing intestinal perforation, Brit. J. Surg. **54**:22, 1967.
5. Almquist, E. E., Gordon, L. H., and Blue, A. I.: Congenital dislocation of the head of the radius, J. Bone Joint Surg. **51-A**:1118, 1969.
6. André, R., Duhamel, G., Verzog, D., and Lavallee, R.: Incidences hémorragiques et viscérales de la maladie d'Ehlers-Danlos, Bull. Soc. Méd. Hôp. Paris **116**:971, 1965.
7. Angst, H.: Das Ehlers-Danlos Syndrome, Dissertation, Zürich, 1951. Cited by Jansen.[181]
7a. Anning, S. T.: Elastoma intrapapillare perforans verruciforme (Miescher), Proc. Roy. Soc. Med. (Sect. Derm.) **51**:932, 1958.
7b. Ansay, M., Gillet, A., and Hanset, R.: La dermatosparaxie héréditaire des bovides; Biochemie descriptive de la peau, Ann. Méd. Vet. **112**:449, 1968.
7c. Ansay, M., Gillet, A., and Hanset, R.: La dermatosparaxie héréditaire des bovides; observations complimentaires sur le collagene et les mucopolysaccharides acides, Ann. Méd. Vet. **112**:465, 1968.
7d. Arlein, M. S.: Generalized acute cutaneous asthenia in a dog, J.A.M.A. **111**:52, 1947.
8. Avogaro, P., Lauro, S., and Castellani, A.: Ehlers-Danlos syndrome with some unusual skeletal abnormalities, Clin. Orthop. **65**:183, 1969.
8a. Baird, P. A., and DeJong, B. P.: Noonan's syndrome (XX and XY Turner phenotype) in three generations of a family, J. Pediat. **80**:110, 1972.
9. Banga, I., and Baló, J.: Elastin and elastase, Nature **171**:44, 1953.
10. Bannerman, R. M., Graf, C. J., and Upson, J. F.: Ehlers-Danlos syndrome, Brit. Med. J. **3**:558, 1967.
11. Bannerman, R. M., Ingall, G. B., and Graf, C. J.: The familial occurrence of intracranial aneurysms, Neurology **20**:283, 1970.

12. Barabas, A. P.: Ehlers-Danlos syndrome associated with prematurity and premature rupture of foetal membranes; possible increase in incidence, Brit. Med. J. 2:682, 1966.

13. Barabas, A. P.: Ehlers-Danlos syndrome with vertebral artery aneurysm, Proc. Roy. Soc. Med. **62**:735, 1969.

14. Barabas, A. P.: Heterogeneity of the Ehlers-Danlos syndrome; description of three clinical types and a hypothesis to explain the basic defect(s), Brit. Med. J. 2:612, 1967.

15. Barabas, G. M.: The Ehlers-Danlos syndrome; abnormalities of the enamel, dentine, cementum, and the dental pulp—an histological examination of 13 teeth from 6 patients, Brit. Dent. J. **126**:509, 1969.

16. Barabas, G. M., and Barabas, A. P.: The Ehlers-Danlos syndrome; a report of the oral and haematological findings in nine cases, Brit. Dent. J. **123**:473, 1967.

17. Barber, H. S., Fiddes, J., and Benians, T. H. C.: The syndrome of Ehlers-Danlos, Brit. J. Derm. **53**:97, 1941.

18. Barker, S. A., and Kennedy, J. F.: Human skin acidic mucopolysaccharides and clinical conditions, Life Sci. **8**:989, 1969.

19. Behar, A., and Rachmilewitz, E.: Ellis–van Creveld syndrome, Arch. Intern. Med. **113**: 606, 1964.

20. Beighton, P.: Cardiac abnormalities in the Ehlers-Danlos syndrome, Brit. Heart J. **31**: 227, 1969.

21. Beighton, P.: Ehlers-Danlos syndrome, Ann. Rheum. Dis. **29**:332, 1970.

22. Beighton, P.: The Ehlers-Danlos syndrome, London, 1970, William Heinemann Medical Books Ltd.

23. Beighton, P.: Lethal complications of the Ehlers-Danlos syndrome, Brit. Med. J. 3:656, 1968.

24. Beighton, P.: Obstetric aspects of the Ehlers-Danlos syndrome, J. Obstet. Gynaec. Brit. Comm. **76**:97, 1969.

25. Beighton, P.: Serious ophthalmological complications in the Ehlers-Danlos syndrome, Brit. J. Ophthal. **54**:263, 1970.

26. Beighton, P.: X-linked recessive inheritance in the Ehlers-Danlos syndrome, Brit. Med. J. **2**:9, 1968.

27. Beighton, P., and Bull, J. C.: Plastic surgery in the Ehlers-Danlos syndrome; case report, Plast. Reconstr. Surg. **45**:606, 1970.

28. Beighton, P., and Horan, F.: Orthopaedic aspects of the Ehlers-Danlos syndrome, J. Bone Joint Surg. **51-B**:444, 1969.

29. Beighton, P., and Horan, F. T.: Surgical aspects of the Ehlers-Danlos syndrome. A survey of 100 cases, Brit. J. Surg. **56**:255, 1960.

30. Beighton, P., Price, A., Lord, J., and Dickson, E.: Variants of the Ehlers-Danlos syndrome; clinical, biochemical, haematological, and chromosomal features of 100 patients, Ann. Rheum. Dis. **28**:228, 1969.

31. Beighton, P., and Thomas, M. L.: The radiology of the Ehlers-Danlos syndrome, Clin. Radiol. **20**:354, 1969.

32. Beighton, P. H.: Gastrointestinal bleeding in the Ehlers-Danlos syndrome, Brit. Med. J. **1**:315, 1968.

33. Beighton, P. H., Murdoch, J. L., and Votteler, T.: Gastrointestinal complications of the Ehlers-Danlos syndrome, Gut **10**:1004, 1969.

34. Benjamin, B., and Weiner, H.: Syndrome of cutaneous fragility and hyperelasticity and articular hyperlaxity, Amer. J. Dis. Child. **65**:247, 1943.

35. Bernard, J., Bassett, A., and Duperrat, B.: Syndrome de fragilité cutanée avec hémorragies multiples, Bull. Soc. Franc. Derm. Syph. **61**:486, 1954.

36. Biering, A., and Iversen, T.: Osteogenesis imperfecta associated with Ehlers-Danlos syndrome, Acta Paediat. **44**:279, 1955.

37. Bigelow, N. H.: The association of polycystic kidneys with intracranial aneurysms and other related disorders, Amer. J. Med. Sci. **225**:485, 1953.

38. Bloom, W.: Studies on fibers in tissue culture. II. The development of elastic fibers in cultures of embryonic heart and aorta, Arch. Exp. Zellforsch. **9**:6, 1929.

39. Bolam, R. M.: A case of Ehlers-Danlos syndrome, Brit. J. Derm. **50**:174, 1938.

40. Bonnet, P.: Les manifestations oculaires de la maladie d'Ehlers-Danlos, Bull. Soc. Franc. Ophtal. **1**:211, 1953.

41. Bopp, P., Hatam, K., and Bussat, P.: Cardiovascular aspects of the Ehlers-Danlos syndrome; report of a case with pulmonary artery bifidity and aortic arch anomaly, Circulation **32:** 602, 1965.

42. Bossu, A., and Lambrechts: Manifestations oculaires du syndrome d'Ehlers-Danlos, Ann. Ocul. **187:**227, 1954.

43. Brodribb, A. J.: Vertebral aneurysm in a case of Ehlers-Danlos syndrome, Brit. J. Surg. **57:**148, 1970.

44. Brombart, M., Coupatez, G., and Laurent, Y.: Contribution à l'étude de l'étiologie de la hernie hiatale et de la diverticulose du tube digestif; un cas de maladie d'Ehlers-Danlos associée à une hernie hiatale, un diverticule de l'estomac, un diverticule duodénal, une diverticulose colique et une anémie sidéropénique, Arch. Mal. Appar. Dig. **41:**413, 1952.

45. Brown, A.: Ehlers-Danlos syndrome; description of 3 cases, Glasgow Med. J. **27:**7, 1946.

46. Brown, A., and Stock, V. F.: Dermatorrhexis; report of a case, Amer. J. Dis. Child. **54:**956, 1937.

47. Bruno, M. S., and Narashimhan, P.: The Ehlers-Danlos syndrome: a report of four cases in two generations of a Negro family, New Eng. J. Med. **264:**274, 1961.

48. Burrows, A.: Epidermolysis bullosa with cutis hyperelastica, Proc. Roy. Soc. Med. **25:**1319, 1932.

49. Burrows, A., and Turnbull, H. M.: Cutis hyperelastica (Ehlers-Danlos syndrome), Brit. J. Derm. **50:**648, 1938.

50. Burton, A. C.: Relation of structure to function of the tissues of the wall of blood vessels, Physiol. Rev. **34:**619, 1954.

50a. Caen, J. P., Legrand, Y., and Sultan, Y.: Platelet collagen interactions, Thromb. Diath. Haemorrh., supp. 40, p. 181, 1970.

51. Carney, R. G., and Nomland, R.: Acquired loose skin (chalazodermia): report of a case, Arch. Derm. Syph. **56:**794, 1947.

52. Carter, C. O., and Sweetnam, R.: Familial joint laxity and recurrent dislocation of the patella, J. Bone Joint Surg. **40-B:**664, 1958.

53. Carter, C. O., and Sweetnam, R.: Recurrent dislocation of the patella and of the shoulder, J. Bone Joint Surg. **42-B:**721, 1960.

54. Carter, C. O., and Wilkinson, J.: Persistent joint laxity and congenital dislocation of the hip, J. Bone Joint Surg. **46-B:**40, 1964.

55. Carter, P. K., and Walford, R. L.: Serum elastase inhibitor levels in Ehlers-Danlos syndrome, Ann. Rheum. Dis. **22:**198, 1963.

56. Castrow, F. F., II, and Ritchie, E. B.: Nonatrophic striae symmetrica in Ehlers-Danlos syndrome, Arch. Derm. **98:**494, 1968.

57. Chakraborty, A. N., Banerjee, A. K., and Ghosh, S.: Ehlers-Danlos syndrome (cutis hyperelastica), J. Indian Med. Ass. **23:**344, 1954.

57a. Char, F., Rodriguez-Fernandez, H. L., Scott, C. I., Borgaonkar, D. S., Bell, B. P., and Rowe, R. D.: The Noonan syndrome—a clinical study of 45 cases. In Bergsma, D., editor: Clinical delineation of birth defects. XIII. The cardiovascular system, Baltimore, 1972, The Williams & Wilkins Co.

58. Christiaens, L., Marchant-Alphant, A., and Fovet, A.: Emphysème congénital et cutis laxa, Presse Méd. **62:**1799, 1954.

58a. Cluney, G. J. A., and Mason, J. M.: Visceral diverticulosis and the Marfan syndrome, Brit. J. Surg. **50:**51, 1962.

59. Cockshott, W. P., and Omololu, A.: Familial congenital posterior dislocation of both radial heads, J. Bone Joint Surg. **40-B:**483, 1958.

60. Coe, M., and Silver, S. H.: Ehlers-Danlos syndrome (cutis hyperelastica), Amer. J. Dis. Child. **59:**129, 1940.

61. Corcelle and Fourcade: Maladie de Ehlers-Danlos et strabisme, Bull. Soc. Franç. Ophtal. **10:**931, 1956.

62. Cordella, M., and Vinciguerra, E.: Le manifestazioni oculari nella sindrome d'Ehlers-Danlos, Minerva Oftal. **8:**103, 1966.

63. Cottini, G. B.: Association des syndromes de Groenblad-Strandberg et d'Ehlers-Danlos dans le même sujet, Acta Derm. (Stockholm) **29:**544, 1949.

64. Coventry, M. B.: Some skeletal changes in the Ehlers-Danlos syndrome, J. Bone Joint Surg. **43-A:**855, 1961.

65. Crowe, J. F., Neel, J. V., and Schull, W. J.: A clinical and genetic study of multiple neurofibromatosis, Springfield, Ill., 1956, Charles C Thomas, Publisher, p. 112.

66. Dales, H. C., and O'Neill, J. J.: Management of arterial complications in a case of the arterial type of Ehlers-Danlos syndrome, Brit. J. Surg. **57**:476, 1970.

67. Danlos, M.: Un cas de cutis laxa avec tumeurs par contusion chronique des coudes et des genoux (xanthome juvenile pseudo-diabetique de M. M. Hallopeau et Mace de Lépinay), Bull. Soc. Franc. Derm. Syph. **19**:70, 1908.

68. Darier, M. J.: Notice nécrologiques sur M. Ehlers (1868-1937), Bull. Acad. Med. **117**:626, 1937.

69. Day, H. J., and Zarafonetis, C. J. D.: Coagulation studies in four patients with Ehlers-Danlos syndrome, Amer. J. Med. Sci. **242**:565, 1961.

70. Debré, R., Marie J., and Seringe, P.: "Cutis laxa" avec dystrophie osseuse, Bull. Soc. Méd. Hôp. Paris **61**:1038, 1937.

71. Debré, R., and Semelaigne, G.: A propos de la maladie d'Ehlers chez le nourrisson, Bull. Soc. Méd. Hôp. Paris **57**:849, 1936.

72. Dewart, P.: Maladie d'Ehlers-Danlos, Arch. Derm. Syph. **21**:397, 1965.

73. Dick, J. C.: Observations of the elastic tissue of the skin with a note on the reticular layer at the junction of the dermis and epidermis, J. Anat. **81**:201, 1947.

74. Dick, J. C.: The tension and resistance to stretching of human skin and other membranes, with results from a series of normal and edematous cases, J. Physiol. **112**:102, 1951.

75. Dodge, J. A., and Shillito, J., Jr.: Ehlers-Danlos syndrome associated with acquired encephalocele, J. Pediat. **66**:1061, 1965.

76. Doerks, G.: Zur klinischen Prüfung der Hautdehnug, Arch. Kinderheilk. **136**:1, 1949.

77. Dorsch, H. H.: Ueber das Ehlers-Danlos-Syndrom, Veröffentlichung eines Falles bei einem Zwillingskind, Kinderaerztl. Prax. **21**:49, 1953.

78. Dreyfus, G., Weill, J., Martineau, J., and Mathivat, A.: Un cas de maladie d'Ehlers-Danlos, Bull. Soc. Méd. Hôp. Paris **52**:1463, 1936.

79. Du Bois: Cutis laxa (abstract), Zbl. Haut-u. Geschlkr. **35**:52, 1931.

80. Du Mesnil: Beitrag zur Anatomie und Aetiologie bestimmter Hautkrankheiten, Dissertation, Würzburg, 1880. Cited by Unna.274

81. Duperrat, B.: Le syndrome d'Ehlers-Danlos, Gaz. Med. France **72**:4037, 1965.

82. Durham, D. G.: Cutis hyperelastica (Ehlers-Danlos syndrome) with blue scleras, microcornea, and glaucoma, Arch. Ophthal. **49**:220, 1953.

83. Eadie, D. G., and Wilkins, J. L.: Bladder-neck obstruction and the Ehlers-Danlos syndrome, Brit. J. Urol. **39**:353, 1967.

84. Edwards, A., and Taylor, G. W.: Ehlers-Danlos syndrome with vertebral artery aneurysm, Proc. Roy. Soc. Med. **62**:734, 1969.

85. Ehlers, E.: Cutis laxa, Neigung zu Haemorrhagien in der Haut, Lockerung mehrerer Artikulationen, Derm. Zschr. **8**:173, 1901.

86. Ellis, F. A., and Bundick, W. R.: Cutaneous elasticity and hyperelasticity, Arch. Derm. **74**:22, 1956.

87. Ermert, W.: Das Ehlers-Danlos-Syndrom, Deutsch. Med. Wschr. **85**:1386, 1960.

88. Estes, J. W.: Platelet size and function in the heritable disorders of connective tissue, Ann. Intern. Med. **68**:1237, 1968.

89. Fantl, P., Morris, K. N., and Sawers, R. J.: Repair of cardiac defect in patient with Ehlers-Danlos syndrome and deficiency of Hageman factor, Brit. Med. J. **1**:1202, 1961.

90. Flemming, J. W.: The Ehlers-Danlos syndrome, J. Florida Med. Ass. **42**:290, 1955.

91. François, P., Woillez, M., Warrot, and Maillet, P.: Maladie d'Ehlers-Danlos avec anévrysme artério-veineux intra-crânien. Bull. Soc. Franc. Ophtal. **5**:392, 1955.

92. Freeman, J. T.: Ehlers-Danlos syndrome, Amer. J. Dis. Child. **79**:1049, 1950.

93. Frick, P. G., and Krafchuk, J. D.: Studies of hemostasis in the Ehlers-Danlos syndrome, J. Invest. Derm. **26**:453, 1956.

94. Fritchey, J. A., and Greenbaum, S. S.: Two cases of Ehlers-Danlos syndrome, Arch. Derm. **42**:742, 1940.

95. Froelich, H.: Fibrodysplasia elastica generalisata (cutis laxa) und Nervensystem, Nervenarzt **20**:366, 1949.

96. Gadrat, J., and Bazex, A.: Sur le syndrome d'Ehlers-Danlos, Ann. Derm. Syph. **78**:430, 1951.

96a. Garrick, J. L. (Montgomery, Ala.): Personal communication, 1972.

97. Geldmacher, M.: Ein Fall von Dystrophia adiposa generalisata mit Cutis laxa und hochgradiger Vulnerabilität der Haut, Inaugural Dissertation, Bonn, 1921. Cited by Jansen.[181]

98. Gellis, S. S., and Feingold, M.: Picture of the month, Ehlers-Danlos syndrome, Amer. J. Dis. Child. **118:**891, 1969.

99. Gilbert, A., Villaret, M., and Bosviel, G.: Sur un cas d'hyperélasticité congénitale des ligaments articulaires et de la peau, Bull. Soc. Méd. Hôp. Paris **59:**303, 1925.

100. Glass, H. B.: Personal communication.

101. Golden, R. L., and Garret, R.: Forme fruste of Ehlers-Danlos syndrome, New York J. Med. **64:**3017, 1964.

102. Goltz, R. W., and Hult, A. M.: Generalized elastolysis (cutis laxa) and Ehlers-Danlos syndrome (cutis hyperelastica); a comparative clinical and laboratory study, Southern Med. J. **58:**848, 1965.

103. Goodman, R. M., and Allison, M. L.: Chronic temporomandibular joint subluxation in Ehlers-Danlos syndrome; report of case, J. Oral Surg. **27:**659, 1969.

104. Goodman, R. M., Baba, N., and Wooley, C. F.: Observations on the heart in a case of combined Ehlers-Danlos and Marfan syndromes, Amer. J. Cardiol. **24:**734, 1969.

104a. Goodman, R. M., Katznelson, M. B. M., and Frydman, M.: Evolution of palmar skin creases in the Ehlers-Danlos syndrome, Clin. Genet. **3:**67, 1972.

105. Goodman, R. M., Levitsky, J. M., and Friedman, I. A.: The Ehlers-Danlos syndrome and neurofibromatosis in a kindred of mixed derivation, with special emphasis on hemostasis in the Ehlers-Danlos syndrome, Amer. J. Med. **32:**976, 1962.

106. Goodman, R. M., Wooley, C. F., and Frazier, R. L.: Ehlers-Danlos syndrome occurring together with the Marfan syndrome; report of a case with other family members affected, New Eng. J. Med. **273:**514, 1965.

107. Gordon, H.: Ehlers-Danlos syndrome, Proc. Roy. Soc. Med. **35:**263, 1942.

108. Gore, I.: Dissecting aneurysm of the aorta in persons under forty years of age, Arch. Path. **55:**1, 1953.

109. Gore, I., and Seiwert, V. S.: Dissecting aneurysm of the aorta; pathologic aspects; an analysis of 85 fatal cases, Arch. Path. **53:**121, 1952.

110. Gorlin, R. J., and Pindborg, J. J.: Syndromes of the head and neck, New York, 1964, McGraw-Hill Book Co., pp. 96-97.

111. Gould, G. M., and Pyle, W. L.: Anomalies and curiosities of medicine, Philadelphia, 1897, W. B. Saunders Co., p. 217.

112. Graf, C. J.: Spontaneous carotid-cavernous fistula; Ehlers-Danlos syndrome and related conditions, Arch. Neurol. **13:**662, 1965.

113. Grahame, R., and Beighton, P.: Physical properties of the skin in the Ehlers-Danlos syndrome, Ann. Rheum. Dis. **28:**246, 1969.

114. Grant, A. K., and Aldor, T. A.: Haemorrhage into the upper part of the gastrointestinal tract in three patients with heritable disorders of connective tissue, Aust. Ann. Med. **16:**75, 1967.

115. Green, G. J., Schuman, B. M., and Barron, J.: Ehlers-Danlos syndrome complicated by acute hemorrhagic sigmoid diverticulitis, with an unusual mitral valve abnormality, Amer. J. Med. **41:**622, 1966.

116. Green, W. R., Friedman-Kien, A., and Banfield, W. G.: Angioid streaks in Ehlers-Danlos syndrome, Arch. Ophthal. **76:**197, 1966.

117. Greenfield, J. G., Cornman, T., and Shy, G. M.: The prognostic value of the muscle biopsy in the "floppy child," Brain **81:**461, 1958.

117a. Gupta, K. K., and Lal, R.: Two cases of Ehlers-Danlos syndrome with cardiac abnormalities, Indian Heart J. **23:**296, 1971.

118. Hall, D. A., Keech, M. K., Reed, R., Saxl, H., Tunbridge, R. E., and Wood, M. J.: Collagen and elastin in connective tissue, J. Geront. **10:**388, 1955.

119. Hallopeau and de Lépinay, M.: Sur un cas de xanthoma tubéreaux et de tumeurs juvéniles offrant les charactères du xanthome diabétique, Bull. Soc. Franc. Derm. Syph. **17:**283, 1906.

119a. Hanset, R., and Ansay, M.: Dermatosparaxie (peau déchirée) chez le veau; un defaut général du tissu conjonctif, de nature héréditaire, Ann. Méd. Vet. **110:**451, 1967.

120. Harland, D.: Ehlers-Danlos syndrome, Proc. Roy. Soc. Med. **63:**286, 1970.

121. Hass, J., and Hass, R.: Arthrochalasis multiplex congenita, J. Bone Joint Surg. **40-A:**663, 1958.

122. Hathaway, W. E.: Bleeding disorders due to platelet dysfunction, Amer. J. Dis. Child. **121**:127, 1971.

123. Hegreberg, G. A., Padgett, G. A., Gorham, J. R., and Henson, J. B.: A connective tissue disease of dogs and mink resembling the Ehlers-Danlos syndrome of man. II. Mode of inheritance, J. Hered. **60**:249, 1969.

124. Hegreberg, G. A., Padgett, G. A., and Henson, J. B.: Connective tissue disease of dogs and mink resembling Ehlers-Danlos syndrome of man. III. Histopathologic changes of the skin, Arch. Path. **90**:159, 1970.

125. Hegreberg, G. A., Padgett, G. A., Ott, R. L., and Henson, J. B.: A heritable connective tissue disease of dogs and mink resembling Ehlers-Danlos syndrome of man. I. Skin tensile strength properties, J. Invest. Derm. **54**:377, 1970.

125a. Heilmann, K., and Kolig, G.: Nierenarterienruptur bei Ehlers-Danlos-Syndrome, Z. Kreislaufforsch. **60**:519, 1971.

125b. Heilmann, K., Nemetschek, T., and Völkl, A.: Das Ehlers-Danlos-Syndrom aus morphologischer und chemischer Sicht, Virchow. Arch. Path. Anat. **354**:268, 1971.

126. Holt, J. F.: The Ehlers-Danlos syndrome, Amer. J. Roentgen. **55**:420, 1946.

127. Husebye, K. C.: Tre familiäere tilfelle av Ehlers-Danlos syndrom, T. Norsk. Laegeforen. **72**:185, 1952.

128. Imahori, S., Bannerman, R. M., Graf, C. J., and Brennan, J. C.: Ehlers-Danlos syndrome with multiple arterial lesions, Amer. J. Med. **47**:967, 1969.

129. Jacobs, P. H.: Ehlers-Danlos syndrome; report of a case with onset at age 29, Arch. Derm. **76**:460, 1957.

130. Jaeger, H.: Syndrome d'Ehlers-Danlos (deux cas familiaux), Dermatologica **100**:330, 1950.

131. Jansen, L. H.: De Ziekte van Ehlers en Danlos, Uitgeverij Excelsor's-Gravenhage, 1954.

132. Jansen, L. H.: Le mode de transmission de la maladie d'Ehlers-Danlos, J. Genet. Hum. **4**:204, 1955.

133. Jansen, L. H.: The structure of the connective tissue, an explanation of the symptoms of the Ehlers-Danlos syndrome, Dermatologica **110**:108, 1955.

134. Jochims, J.: Elastometrie an Kindern bei wechselnder Hautdehnung, Arch. Kinkerheilk. **135**:228, 1948.

135. Johns, R. J., and Wright, V.: An analytical description of joint stiffness, Biorheology **2**:87, 1964.

136. Johns, R. J., and Wright, V.: Relative importance of various tissues in joint stiffness, J. Appl. Physiol. **17**:824, 1962.

137. Johnson, S. A. M., and Falls, H. F.: Ehlers-Danlos syndrome; a clinical and genetic study, Arch. Derm. Syph. **60**:82, 1949.

138. Julkunen, H., Rokkanen, P., and Jounela, A.: Bone changes in Ehlers-Danlos syndrome, Ann. Med. Intern. Fenn. **56**:55, 1967.

139. Kalz, F.: Cutis laxa als Symptom allgemeiner Stützgewebsschwäche, Arch. Derm. Syph. **171**:155, 1935.

140. Kanof, A.: Ehlers-Danlos syndrome; report of a case with suggestion of a possible causal mechanism, J. Dis. Child. **83**:197, 1952.

141. Kashiwagi, H., Riddle, J. M., and Abraham, J. P.: Functional and ultrastructural abnormalities of platelets in Ehlers-Danlos syndrome, Ann. Intern. Med. **63**:249, 1965.

142. Katz, I., and Steiner, K.: Ehlers-Danlos syndrome with ectopic bone formation, Radiology **65**:352, 1955.

143. Key, J. A.: Hypermobility of joints as a sex-linked hereditary characteristic, J.A.M.A. **88**:1710, 1927.

144. King-Louis, F. J.: Two cases of Ehlers-Danlos syndrome, Proc. Roy. Soc. Med. **39**:135, 1946.

145. Kirk, E., and Kvorning, S. A.: Quantitative measurements of the elastic properties of the skin and subcutaneous tissue in young adults and old individuals, J. Geront. **4**:273, 1949.

146. Kirk, J. A., Ansell, B. M., and Bywaters, E. G.: The hypermobility syndrome; musculoskeletal complaints associated with generalized joint hypermobility, Ann. Rheum. Dis. **26**:419, 1967.

147. Kopp: Demonstration zweier Fälle von "Cutis laxa," München Med. Wschr. **35**:259, 1888.

148. Korting, G. W.: Elastosis perforans serpiginosa als ektodermales rand Symptom bei Cutis laxa, Arch. Klin. Exp. Derm. **224**:437, 1966.

149. Korting, G. W., and Gottron, E.: Cutis laxa, Arch. Derm. Syph. **193**:14, 1951.

149a. Krane, S. M., Pinnell, S. R., and Erbe, R. W.: Decreased lysyl-protocollagen hydroxylase activity in fibroblasts from a family with a newly recognized disorder: hydroxylysine-deficient collagen, J. Clin. Invest. **51**:52a, 1972.

150. Laane, C. L.: Cushing's syndrome associated with obliterative arterial disease and multiple subcutaneous nodules (Ehlers-Danlos syndrome?), Acta Med. Scand. **148**:323, 1954.

151. Lamy, M., and Frézal, J.: Le syndrome de Bonnevie-Ullrich et ses rapports avec le syndrome de Turner, Analecta Genetica, vol. 6 (International Symposium, Turin, 1957).

152. Lapayowker, M. S.: Cutis hyperelastica; the Ehlers-Danlos syndrome, Amer. J. Roentgen. **84**:232, 1960.

152a. Lapière, C. (Liège, Belgium): Personal communication, 1972.

152b. Lapière, C. M., Lenaers, A., and Kohn, L. D.: Procollagen peptidase: an enzyme excising the coordination peptides of procollagen, Proc. Nat. Acad. Sci. **68**:3054, 1971.

153. Larsen, L. J., Schottstaedt, E. R., and Bost, F. C.: Multiple congenital dislocations associated with characteristic facial abnormality, J. Pediat. **37**:574, 1950.

153a. Latta, R. J., Graham, C. B., Aase, J., Scham, S. M., and Smith, D. W.: Larsen's syndrome: a skeletal dysplasia with multiple joint dislocations and unusual facies, J. Pediat. **78**:291, 1971.

154. Launay, C.: Syndrome d'Ehlers-Danlos chez un garçon de onze ans, associé à une arriération mentale, Bull. Soc. Méd. Hôp. Paris **56**:709, 1941.

155. Le Coulant, P.: Hyperelasticité cutanée et articulaire avec fragilité anormale de la peau et tumeurs molluscoides, chez un enfant de treize ans (syndrome d'Ehlers-Danlos), Gaz. Sci. Méd. Bordeaux **29**:1934.

156. Lees, M. H., Menashe, V. D., Sunderland, C. O., Morgan, C. L., and Dawson, P. J.: Ehlers-Danlos syndrome associated with multiple pulmonary artery stenoses and tortuous systemic arteries, J. Pediat. **75**:1031, 1969.

157. Leider, M.: Forme fruste of Ehlers-Danlos syndrome, Urol. Cut. Rev. **53**:222, 1949.

158. Levine, A. S., and Michael, A. F.: Ehlers-Danlos syndrome with renal tubular acidosis and medullary sponge kidneys; a report of a case and studies of renal acidification in other patients with the Ehlers-Danlos syndrome, J. Pediat. **71**:107, 1967.

159. Levy-Coblentz, G.: Radio-ulnar synostosis, Bull. Soc. Franc. Derm. Syph. **39**:1252, 1932.

160. Lewitus, Z.: Ehlers-Danlos syndrome; report of two cases with hypophyseal dysfunction, Arch. Derm. **73**:158, 1956.

160a. Lichtenstein, J., Nigra, T. P., Sussman, M. D., Martin, G. R., and McKusick, V. A.: Molecular defect in a form of the Ehlers-Danlos syndrome: hydroxylysine deficient collagen (abstract), Amer. Soc. Hum. Genet., Philadelphia, Oct., 1972.

160b. Lichtenstein, J. (Baltimore and Bethesda): Personal communication, 1972.

161. Lienhart, O.: La maladie d'Ehlers-Danlos; étude clinque, anatomo-pathologique et génetique, Thesis de Nancy, 1945 (No. 30).

162. Lisker, R., Noguerón, A., and Sánchez-Medal, L.: Plasma thromboplastin component deficiency in the Ehlers-Danlos syndrome, Ann. Intern. Med. **53**:388, 1960.

163. Littré, E.: Oeuvres complète d'Hippocrate, Paris, 1840, J. B. Bailliére, vol. 2.

164. Lynch, H. T., Larsen, A. L., and Wilson, R.: Ehlers-Danlos syndrome and "congenital" arteriovenous fistulae, a clinicopathologic study of a family, J.A.M.A. **194**:1011, 1965.

165. MacCollum, D. W.: The lop ear, J.A.M.A. **110**:1427, 1938.

166. McDonald, A. H., Gerlis, L. M., and Somerville, J.: Familial arteriopathy with associated pulmonary and systemic arterial stenosis, Brit. Heart J. **31**:375, 1969.

167. McEvitt, W. G.: The problem of the protruding ear, Plast. Reconstr. Surg. **2**:480, 1947.

168. McFarland, W., and Fuller, D. E.: Mortality in Ehlers-Danlos syndrome due to spontaneous rupture of large arteries, New Eng. J. Med. **271**:1309, 1964.

169. Macfarlane, I. L.: Ehlers-Danlos syndrome presenting certain unusual features, J. Bone Joint Surg. **41-B**:541, 1959.

170. McKusick, V. A.: Hereditary disorders of connective tissue, Bull. N. Y. Acad. Med. **35**:143, 1959.

171. Madison, W. J., Jr., Bradley, E. J., and Castillo, A. J.: Ehlers-Danlos syndrome with cardiac involvement, Amer. J. Cardiol. **11**:689, 1963.

172. Margarot, J., Deneze, P., and Coll de Carrera: Hyperlaxité cutanée et articulaire (syn-

drome de Danlos) existant chez trois membres d'une même famille, Bull. Soc. Franc. Derm. Syph. **40**:277, 1933.

173. Martin, G. R. (Bethesda): Personal communication, 1971.

174. Mason P., and Rigby B. J.: Ehlers-Danlos syndrome; physical and biochemical aspects, Arch. Path. **80**:363, 1965.

175. Maximow, A.: Development of argyrophile and collagenous fibers in tissue culture, Proc. Soc. Exp. Biol. Med. **25**:437, 1928.

176. Meara, R. H.: Ehlers-Danlos syndrome and elastoma verruciforme perforans (Miescher), Trans. St. John Hosp. Derm. Soc. **40**:72, 1958.

177. Mehregan, A. H.: Elastosis perforans serpiginosa; a review of the literature and report of 11 cases, Arch. Derm. **97**:381, 1968.

178. Méténier, P.: A propos d'un cas familial de maladie d'Ehlers-Danlos, Thése d'Alger, 1939, No. 55.

179. Miguet, A.: Le syndrome d'Ehlers-Danlos, Thése, Paris, 1933, Louis Arnette.

180. Mitchell, G. E., Lourie, H., and Berne, A. S.: The various causes of scalloped vertebrae, with notes on their pathogenesis, Radiology **89**:67, 1967.

181. Moestrup, B.: Tenuity of cornea with Ehlers-Danlos syndrome, Acta Ophthal. **47**:704, 1969.

182. Mories, A.: Ehlers-Danlos syndrome, with a report of a fatal case, Scot. Med. J. **5**:269, 1960.

183. Mories, A.: An investigation into the Ehlers-Danlos syndrome, Edinburgh Thesis, 1954.

184. Morris, M.: Case report; elastic skin and numerous cutaneous nodules, Brit. J. Derm. **12**:209, 1900.

185. Morris, M.: Diseases of the skin, ed. 4, New York, 1909, William Woods & Co., Plate XI.

186. Morris, R. C., Yamauchi, H., Palubinskas, A. J., and Howenstine, J.: Medullary sponge kidney, Amer. J. Med. **38**:883, 1965.

187. Mounier-Kuhn, P., and Meyer, L.: Méga-organes (oesophage, trachée, colon), syndromes de Mickulicz et d'Ehlers-Danlos chez une hérédo-syphilitique, Bull. Soc. Méd. Hôp. Lyon, Nov. 9, 1943.

188. Murray, J. E., and Tyars, M. E.: A case of Ehlers-Danlos syndrome, Brit. Med. J. **1**:974, 1940.

189. Newton, J. E., and Carpenter, M. E.: Ehlers-Danlos syndrome with acro-osteolysis, Brit. J. Radiol. **32**:739, 1959.

190. Nicaud, P., Lafitte, A., and Buhot, S.: Syndrome d'Ehlers-Danlos fruste associé à une atrophic musculaire du type Aran-Duchenne, Bull. Soc. Méd. Hôp. Paris, March 10, 1944.

191. Nicod, M.: Un cas de syndrome d'Ehlers-Danlos, Ann. Paediat. **167**:358, 1946.

192. Nordschow, C. D., and Marsolais, E. B.: Ehlers-Danlos syndrome; Some recent biophysical observations, Arch. Path. **88**:65, 1969.

193. Noto, P.: Cited by Pelbois and Rollier.[205]

193a. O'Hara, P. J., Read, W. K., Romane, W. M., and Bridges, C. H.: A collagenous tissue dysplasia of calves, Lab. Invest. **23**:307, 1970.

194. Olmsted, F., Page, I. H., and Corcoran, A. C.: A device for objective clinical measurement of cutaneous elasticity; a "pinchmeter," Amer. J. Med. Sci. **222**:73, 1951.

195. Ona, C. K., and Cowdry, E. V.: Aging of elastic tissue in human skin, J. Geront. **5**:203, 1950.

196. Orlandi, O. V., and Rodrigues, Y. T.: Ehlers-Danlos syndrome; capillary microscopy in cases, Pediatria (Rio) **17**:189, 1952.

197. Ormsby, O. S., and Tobin, W. W.: Cutis hyperelastica; case report, Arch. Derm. Syph. **38**:828, 1938.

198. Ota, M., and Yasuda, T.: Erster Fall von "Syndrome d'Ehlers-Danlos" in Japan, Zbl. Haut. Geschlechtskr. **66**:120, 1941.

199. Owren, P. A.: The nature of the defects in hemorrhagic disorders, Acta Haemat. **36**:141, 1966.

200. Packer, B. D., and Blades, J. F.: Dermatorrhexis; a case report; the so-called Ehlers-Danlos syndrome, Virginia Med. Monthly **81**:21, 1954.

201. Padgett, G. A., Gorham, J. R., and Henson, J. B.: Mink as a biomedical model, Lab. Anim. Care **18**:258, 1968.

202. Papp, J. P., and Paley, R. G.: Ehlers-Danlos syndrome; incidence in three generations of a kindred, Postgrad. Med. **40**:586, 1966.

203. Pascher, F.: Ehlers-Danlos syndrome, Arch. Derm. Syph. **67**:214, 1953.

204. Pautrier, M.: Note histologique sur un cas de cutis elastica, avec pseudotumeurs aux genoux et aux coudes, presenté par M. Danlos, Bull. Soc. Franc. Derm. Syph. **19**:72, 1908.

205. Pelbois, F., and Rollier, F.: Association d'un syndrome d'Ehlers-Danlos et d'un syndrome de Groenblad-Strandberg. Bull. Soc. Franc. Derm. Spyh. **59**:141, 1952.

206. Pemberton, J. W., Freeman, H. M., and Schepens, C. L.: Familial retinal detachment and the Ehlers-Danlos syndrome, Arch. Ophthal. **76**:817, 1966.

207. Perreau, P., Bangas, J., and Lecuit, P.: Osteitis fibro-kystique atypique et syndrome d'Ehlers-Danlos; lesion parathyroidienne, Bull. Soc. Méd. Hôp. Paris **57**:135, 1941.

208. Péyri: Un cas de syndrome d'Ehlers-Danlos, probablement d'origine syphilitique, Bull. Soc. Franc. Derm. Syph. **44**:1744, 1937.

209. Pierce, L. E., Tyrrell, M. E., and Day C. E.: Gastrectomy in Ehlers-Danlos syndrome, Arch. Surg. **96**:95, 1968.

209a. Pinnell, S. R.: Personal communication, 1971.

209b. Pinnell, S. R., Krane, S. M., Kenzora, J., and Glimcher, M. J.: A new heritable disorder of connective tissue with hydroxylysine-deficient collagen, New Eng. J. Med. **286**:1013, 1972.

210. Pittinos, G. E.: Ehlers-Danlos syndrome with disturbance of creatine metabolism, J. Pediat. **19**:85, 1941.

211. Pommerening, R. A., and Antonius, J. I.: Normal chromosomes in a family with Ehlers-Danlos syndrome, Arch. Derm. **94**:425, 1966.

212. Poumeau-Delille, G., and Soulié, P.: Un cas d'hyperlaxité cutanée et articulaire avec cicatrices atrophiques et pseudo-tumeurs molluscoides (syndrome d'Ehlers-Danlos), Bull. Soc. Méd. Hôp. Paris **50**:593, 1934.

213. Pray, L. G.: Cutis elastica (dermatorrhexis, Ehlers-Danlos syndrome), Amer. J. Dis. Child. **75**:702, 1948.

214. Rahn, E. K., Meadow, E., Falls, H. F., Knaggs, J. G., and Proux, D. J.: Leber's congenital amaurosis with an Ehlers-Danlos–like syndrome; study of an American family, Arch. Ophthal. **79**:135, 1968.

215. Raybaud, A., and Guidoni, P.: Hyperlaxité ligamentaire et cutanée; trouble du métabolisme calcique; maladie d'Ehlers-Danlos, Bull. Soc. Med. Hôp. Paris **54**:738, 1938.

216. Rees, T. D., Wood-Smith, D., and Converse J. M.: The Ehlers-Danlos syndrome, Plast. Reconstr. Surg. **32**:39, 1963.

217. Ricketson, G.: The behavior of skin grafts and donor sites in a case of Ehlers-Danlos syndrome, Plast. Reconstr. Surg. **20**:32, 1957.

218. Ringrose, E. J., Nowlan, F. B., and Perry, H.: Ehlers-Danlos syndrome; report of a case, Arch. Derm. Syph. **62**:443, 1950.

219. Robertson, J. A., Eddy, W. A., and Vossler, A. J.: Spontaneous perforation of the cecum without mechanical obstruction; review of literature and case report, Amer. J. Surg. **96**:446, 1958.

220. Robinson, H. M., Jr., and Ellis, F. A.: Cutis laxa, Arch. Derm. **77**:656, 1958.

221. Robitaille, G. A.: Ehlers-Danlos syndrome and recurrent hemoptysis, Ann. Intern. Med. **61**:716, 1964.

222. Rocher, H. L.: Une nouvelle dysmorphose articulaire congénitale: laxité articulaire congénitale multiple. In Livre jubilarie d'Henri Hartmann, Paris, 1932, Masson et Cie.

223. Rodermund, O. E.: Ehlers-Danlos syndrome, Z. Haut Geschlechtskr **44**:17, 1969.

224. Roederer, C.: Syndrome d'Ehlers-Danlos atypique coincidant avec une dolichosténomélie, Arch. Franc. Pédiat. **8**:192, 1951.

225. Rollhäuser, H.: Die Zugfestigkeit der menschlichen Haut, Gegenbaur Morph. Jahrb. **90**:249, 1950.

226. Ronchese, F.: Dermatorrhexis, with dermatochalasis and arthrochalasis (the so-called Ehlers-Danlos syndrome), Amer. J. Dis. Child. **51**:1403, 1936.

227. Ronchese, F.: Dermatorrhexis with dermatochalasis and arthrochalasis (the so-called Ehlers-Danlos syndrome); additional data on a case reported 12 years previously, Rhode Island Med. J. **32**:80, 1949.

228. Ross, M., and Dooneief, A. S.: Chest surgery in the presence of cutis hyperelastica (Ehlers-Danlos syndrome), New York J. Med. **57**:2256, 1957.

229. Rossi, E., and Angst, H.: Das Danlos-Ehlers Syndrome, Helv. Paediat. Acta **6**:245, 1951.

230. Rossi, E., and Caflisch, A.: Le syndrome du pterygium; satus Bonnevie-Ullrich, dystrophia

brevicolli congenita, syndrome de Turner et arthromyodysplasia congenita, Helv. Paediat. Acta **6**:119, 1951.

231. Rowe, R. D.: Maternal rubella and pulmonary artery stenoses; report of eleven cases, Pediatrics **32**:180, 1963.

232. Rubinstein, M., K., and Cohen, N. H.: Ehlers-Danlos syndrome associated with multiple intracranial aneurysms, Neurology **14**:125, 1964.

233. Rybka, F. J., and O'Hara, E. T.: Surgical significance of the Ehlers-Danlos syndrome, Amer. J. Surg. **113**:431, 1967.

234. Sack, G.: Status dysvascularis; ein Fall von besonderer Zerreisslichkeit der Blutgefässe, Deutsch. Arch. Klin. Med. **178**:663, 1936.

235. Saemundsson, J.: Ehlers-Danlos syndrome; a congenital mesenchymal disorder, Acta Med. Scand. **154** (supp. 312):399, 1956.

236. Samuel, M. A., Schwartz, M. L., and Meister, M. M.: The Ehlers-Danlos syndrome, U.S. Armed Forces Med. J. **4**:737, 1953.

236a. Sanders, C. A., Austen, W. G., Harthorne, J. W., Dinsmore, R. E., and Scannell, J. G.: Diagnosis and treatment of mitral regurgitation secondary to ruptured chordae tendineae, New Eng. J. Med. **276**:943, 1967.

237. Scarpelli, D. G., and Goodman, R. M.: Observations on the fine structure of the fibroblast from a case of Ehlers-Danlos syndrome with the Marfan syndrome, J. Invest. Derm. **50**:214, 1968.

238. Schaper, G.: Familiäres Vorkommen von Ehlers-Danlos Syndrome; ein Beitrag zur Klinik und Pathogenese, Zschr. Kinderheilk. **70**:504, 1952.

239. Scheinin, T. M., and Dahl, M.: Repair of atrial septal defect in a patient with the Ehlers-Danlos syndrome, Scand. J. Thorac. Cardiovasc. Surg. **1**:114, 1967.

240. Schoolman, A., and Kepes, J. J.: Bilateral spontaneous carotid-cavernous fistulae in Ehlers-Danlos syndrome; case report, J. Neurosurg. **26**:82, 1967.

241. Seaton, D. G.: Bilateral recurrent dislocation of the patellas in the Ehlers-Danlos syndrome, Med. J. Aust. **1**:737, 1969.

242. Segrest, J. P., and Cunningham, L. W.: Variations in human urinary O-hydroxylysyl glycosile levels and their relationship to collagen metabolism, J. Clin. Invest. **49**:1497, 1970.

243. Sestak, Z.: Ehlers-Danlos syndrome and cutis laxa; an account of families in the Oxford area, Ann. Hum. Genet. **25**:313, 1962.

244. Shapiro, S. K.: A case of Meekrin-Ehlers-Danlos syndrome with neurologic manifestations, J. Nerv. Ment. Dis. **115**:64, 1952.

245. Shapiro, S. S., Martinez, J., and Holburn, R. R.: Congenital dysprothrombinemia; an inherited structural disorder of human prothrombin, J. Clin. Invest. **48**:2251, 1969.

246. Shaw, A. B., and Hopkins, P.: A case of a boy, aged seven, showing (a) double-jointedness, (b) dermatolysis ("elastic skin") with great friability of the skin and excessive tendency to bruising, and (c) multiple subcutaneous tumours on the limbs (fibromata, neuronomata), Proc. Roy. Soc. Med. (Clin. Sect.) **6**:20, 1913.

247. Shelley, W. B., and Rawnsley, H. M.: Painful feet due to herniation of fat, J.A.M.A. **205**:308, 1968.

248. Smith, C. H.: Dermatorrhexis (Ehlers-Danlos syndrome), J. Pediat. **14**:632, 1939.

249. Smith, R. D., and Worthington, J. W.: Paganini; the riddle and connective tissue, J.A.M.A. **199**:820, 1967.

250. Smith, S. A., Powell, L. C., and Essin, E. M.: Ehlers-Danlos syndrome and pregnancy; report of a case, Obstet. Gynec. **32**:331, 1968.

251. Sodeman, W. A., and Burch, G. E.: Skin elasticity in scleroderma, Amer. Heart J. **17**:21, 1939.

252. Stillians, A. W., and Zakon, S. J.: Cutis laxa (cutis hyperplastica), Arch. Derm. Syph. **35**:342, 1937.

253. Stoddard, F. J., and Myers, R. E.: Connective tissue disorders in obstetrics and gynecology, Amer. J. Obstet. Gynec. **102**:240, 1968.

254. Stuart, A. M.: Three cases exhibiting the Ehlers-Danlos syndrome, Proc. Roy. Soc. Med. **30**:984, 1937.

255. Stucke, K.: Ueber das elastische Verhalten der Achillessehne im Belastungsversuch, Arch. Klin. Chir. **265**:579, 1950.

256. Sturkie, P. D.: Hypermobile joints in all descendants for two generations, J. Hered. **32**:232, 1941.

257. Sullivan, J. D.: The Danlos-Ehlers syndrome; report of case with transient paralysis of vocal cord, Arch. Neur. Psychiat. **47**:316, 1942.

258. Summer, G. K.: The Ehlers-Danlos syndrome; a review of the literature and report of a case with a subgaleal hematoma and Bell's palsy, J. Dis. Child. **91**:419, 1956.

259. Sutro, C. J.: Hypermobility of bones due to "overlengthened" capsular and ligamentous tissues; cause for recurrent intra-articular effusions, Surgery **21**:67, 1947.

260. Svane, S.: Ehlers-Danlos syndrome; a case with some skeletal changes, Acta Orthop. Scand. **37**:49, 1966.

261. Taylor, F. R.: The Meekrin-Ehlers-Danlos syndrome, Urol. Cut. Rev. **47**:378, 1943.

262. Thexton, A.: A case of Ehlers-Danlos syndrome presenting with recurrent dislocation of the temporomandibular joint, Brit. J. Oral Surg. **2**:190, 1965.

263. Thivolet, J., Perrot, H., Leung, T. K., and Claudy, A.: Dysplasie mésenchymateuse complexe: type artériel de l'Ehlers-Danlos syndrome de Sack-Barabas? Bull. Soc. Franç. Derm. Syph. **76**:817, 1969.

264. Thomas, C., Cordier, J., and Algan, B.: Une étiologie nouvelle du syndrome de luxation spontanée des cristallins: la maladie d'Ehlers-Danlos, Bull. Soc. Belg. Ophtal. **100**:375, 1952.

265. Thomas, C., Cordier, J., and Algan, B.: Les altérations oculaires de la maladie d'Ehlers-Danlos, Arch. Ophtal. (Paris) **14**:691, 1954.

266. Thomas, C., Neimann, N., Cordier, J., and Algan, B.: Les manifestations oculaires de la maladie d'Ehlers-Danlos, Bull. Soc. Ophtal. Franç. p. 211, 1953.

267. Thurmon, F. M.: Ehlers-Danlos syndrome, Arch. Derm. **40**:120, 1939.

268. Tobias, N.: Danlos syndrome associated with congenital lipomatosis, Arch. Derm. Syph. **30**:540, 1934; ibid. **40**:135, 1939.

269. Tschernogobow, A.: Cutis laxa (Presentation at first meeting of Moscow Dermatologic and Venereologic Society, Nov. 13, 1891), Mhft. Prakt. Derm. **14**:76, 1892.

270. Tschernogobow, A.: Ein Fall von Cutis laxa. Protokoly Moskowskawo wenerologitscheskawo i dermatologitscheskawo Obtschestwa, vol. 1. Quoted in Jahresb. Ges. Med. **27**:562, 1892.

271. Tucker, D. H., Miller, D. E., and Jacoby, W. J., Jr.: Ehlers-Danlos syndrome with sinus of Valsalva aneurysm and aortic insufficiency simulating rheumatic heart disease, Amer. J. Med. **35**:715, 1963.

272. Tunbridge, R. E., Tattersall, R. N., Hall, D. A., Astbury, W. T., and Reed, R.: The fibrous structure of normal and abnormal human skin, Clin. Sci. **11**:315, 1952.

273. Turkington, R. W., and Grude, H. E.: Ehlers-Danlos syndrome and multiple neurofibromatosis, Ann. Intern. Med. **61**:549, 1964.

273a. Tyson, J. E. A. (Baltimore): Personal communication, 1972.

274. Unna, P. G.: The histopathology of the diseases of the skin. Translated from the German by N. Walker with the assistance of the author, New York, 1896, The Macmillan Co., pp. 984-988.

275. van Meekeren, J. A.: De dilatabilitate extraordinaria cutis, chap. 32, Observations medico-chirugicae, Amsterdam, 1682.

276. Varadi, D. P., and Hall, D. A.: Cutaneous elastin in Ehlers-Danlos syndrome, Nature **208**:1224, 1965.

277. Verger, P., Channarond, N. I., Guillard, J. M., Sandler, B., and Beylot, N. I.: Syndrome d'Ehlers-Danlos compliqué d'hémorragies digestives chez l'enfant, Pediatrie **25**:215, 1970.

278. Villegas, R., and Albornoz, R.: Posibles mecanismos causales del sindrome de Ehlers-Danlos, Acta Med. Venezolana **4**:1956.

279. Vissian, L., Manasséro, J., Blaive, B., and Borja, A.: Un nouvel état morbide lié à une anomalie chromosomique: syndrome d'Ehlers-Danlos associé à une maladie du "cri du chat" chez un nouveau-né, Presse Med. **73**:2991, 1965.

280. Vissian, L., and Rovinski, J.: Syndrome d'Ehlers-Danlos chez quatre membres d'une même famille, Bull. Soc. Franc. Derm. Syph. **62**:62, 1955.

281. Walker, V. A., Beighton, P. H., and Murdoch, J. L.: The Marfanoid hypermobility syndrome, Ann. Intern. Med. **71**:349, 1969.

282. Wallach, E. A., and Burkhart, E. F.: Ehlers-Danlos syndrome associated with tetralogy of Fallot, Arch. Derm. Syph. **61**:750, 1950.

283. Ward, G. W.: Cutaneous asthenia (cutis hyperelastica) of dogs, Aust. Vet. J. **46**:115, 1970.
284. Weber, F. P.: The Ehlers-Danlos syndrome, Brit. J. Derm. Syph. **48**:609, 1936.
285. Weber, F. P., and Aitken, J. K.: Nature of the subcutaneous spherules in some cases of Ehlers-Danlos syndrome, Lancet **1**:198, 1938.
286. Wechsler, H. L., and Fisher, E. R.: Ehlers-Danlos syndrome; pathologic, histochemical, and electron microscopic observations, Arch. Path. **77**:613, 1964.
287. Weill, J., and Martineau, J.: A propos d'un cas de maladie d'Ehlers-Danlos; étude anatomoclinique et biologique, Bull. Soc. Franc. Derm. Syph. **44**:99, 1937.
288. Weiss, R. S.: Danlos' syndrome, Arch. Derm. **40**:137, 1939.
289. Wenzel, H. G.: Untersuchungen über die Dehnbarkeit und Zerreissbarkeit der Haut, Zbl. Allg. Path. **85**:117, 1949.
290. Whitney, L. F.: Inheritance of double-jointedness in thumb, J. Hered. **23**:425, 1932.
291. Wiener, K.: Gummihaut (cutis laxa) mit dominanter Vererbung, Arch. Derm. Syph. **148**:599, 1925.
292. Wigzell, F. W., and Ogston, D.: The bleeding tendency in Ehlers-Danlos syndrome, Ann. Phys. Med. **7**:55, 1963.
293. Williams, A. W.: Cutis laxa, Monatsschr. Prakt. Derm. **14**:490, 1892.
294. Wright, V., and Johns, R. J.: The quantitative measurement of joint stiffness (abstract), J. Clin. Invest. **38**:1056, 1959.
294a. Wynne-Davies, R.: Acetabular dysplasia and familial joint laxity: two etiological factors in congenital dislocation of the hip. A review of 589 patients and their families, J. Bone Joint Surg. **52B**:704, 1970.
295. Zaida, A. H.: Ehlers-Danlos syndrome with congenital herniae and pigeon breast, Brit. Med. J. **2**:175, 1959.
296. Zalis, E. G., and Roberts, D. C.: Ehlers-Danlos syndrome with a hypoplastic kidney, bladder diverticulum, and diaphragmatic hernia, Arch. Derm. **96**:540, 1967.
297. Zambal, Z.: Sind Hyperkeratosis follicularis in cutem penetrans und Elastoma intrapapillare perforans verruciforme identisch? Hautarzt **9**:304, 1958.

7 · Cutis laxa

Historical note

The nosography of cutis laxa (CL) is intimately entwined with that of the Ehlers-Danlos syndrome, with which CL has often been confused. The confusion has been in considerable part semantic; in both of the case reports that earned Ehlers and Danlos their eponymic distinction,[14,18] the Ehlers-Danlos syndrome was referred to as cutis laxa. The father and son whom Kopp[28] described in 1888 are often cited as the first example of hereditary transmission of the Ehlers-Danlos syndrome; their cases seem instead to have been instances of cutis laxa. In 1923 F. Parkes Weber[52a] pointed out the clinical differences between E-D and cutis laxa, and in 1936 Francesco Ronchese[42] attempted to clarify terminology. In recent years the term *cutis laxa* has only rarely been used for E-D, mainly because of increased familiarity with the distinctive clinical picture in the two disorders, especially the latter. Confusion also existed in the early literature between cutis laxa and the localized pendulous skin in patients with neurofibromatosis; e.g., 2 patients reported by Mott in 1854[36] and the patient reported by Alibert in 1855,[1] as pictured in the review of Robinson and Ellis.[41] Stokes's report in 1876[50] seems to have concerned neurofibromatosis also.

The internal changes in CL and other aspects of the disease have been elucidated particularly by Goltz and co-workers.[21,22]

Synonyms for *cutis laxa* include *dermatomegaly*,[42] *dermatochalasia* and *chalasoderma* (relaxed or loose skin),[20] and, when there are internal manifestations, *systemic elastolysis*.[33] The last term runs a risk of semantic confusion with Touraine's for pseudoxanthoma elasticum (PXE), *élastorrhexie systematisée*. The term *anetoderma* ("slack skin"), as usually used, refers to circumscribed cutis laxa.[41]

Clinical manifestations

As the main clinical characteristic of CL, the skin hangs in loose folds over all parts of the body, particularly in those areas where the skin is normally loose, e.g., on the face and around the eyes. The sagging jowls create a "bloodhound" facies. The changes in the face give a prematurely aged appearance, as is well demonstrated by Fig. 7-1. One author[4] referred to an adolescent girl with CL who was frequently mistaken for her grandmother. The picture of the 7½-year-old boy presented by Chadfield[11] could easily be that of a 40-year-old man. The 16-year-old girl shown in Fig. 7-5 looks considerably older than her mother. The patient[9] sometimes must suspend the skin around the eyes with cellophane tape in order to see. The severely affected infant has continual drooling due to laxity of the lower lip (Fig. 7-1D). The pendulous skin over the abdomen may cover the genitalia.

The skin is extensible in CL, but unlike that of E-D it does not spring back into place on release. It shows no fragility or bruisability. Some[2,16] have

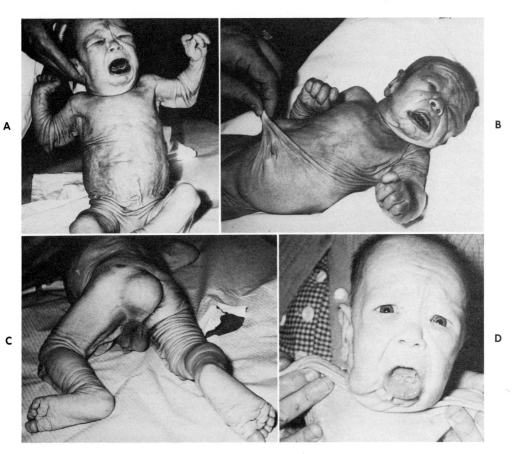

Fig. 7-1. Severe cutis laxa in a young child. Generalized involvement of the skin, which is redundant and pendulous, is shown in **A** and **B**. In addition, **C** demonstrates an obturator hernia. In **D,** taken at a later age than the other pictures, drooling because of laxity of the lower lip is demonstrated. This child was born of a 35-year-old mother and a 45-year-old father. No other family member was similarly affected. The skin was generally loose from birth. He always had a hoarse cry and grunting respiration. At 3 weeks of age, operation for pyloric stenosis was performed. Respiratory distress with bronchopneumonia led to hospitalization at 4 months of age. He had bilateral inguinal hernias and a large left obturator hernia. Chest x-ray examination showed emphysema and pneumonitis. Electrocardiogram indicated right ventricular hypertrophy. The patient died at home at the age of about 20 months. (Courtesy Dr. Florence Char.)

been impressed with apparent diminution in the cutis laxa as the affected child grows to "fill out the loose integument".[16]

In addition to pendulous skin and wrinkles, the facies is characterized by an unusually long upper lip, a tendency toward hook nose, and shortening of the columella, the distal fleshy part of the nasal septum. The nose tends to have a dorsal hump and hanging tip. Pointed out by Beighton and associates,[4] these features are clearly demonstrated in published photographs,[23,27] as well as in Fig. 7-5. The earlobes are unusually long, as well.

The joints are usually not involved in CL.[21,22] However, Sestak[47] observed joint hypermobility in a father and daughter with otherwise typical CL. Growth is normal in the affected children.

Internal manifestations relate particularly to the lungs, which are emphysematous in severe cases.[4,23,33a,44] This condition may lead to cor pulmonale, which has caused death as early as 18 months of age.[12,21,22] Some instances of heart failure in children with CL may be the result of obstruction at a higher level by a mechanism comparable to the one by which enlarged tonsils and adenoids cause heart failure.[30a,32] In one reported case of heart failure,[11] laryngoscopy at the age of 22 months showed "an excess of soft tissue around the aryepiglottic folds." Tracheostomy might be beneficial in such cases. The voice is often husky from birth because of redundancy of tissues of the larynx.

Umbilical, inguinal, and obturator (Fig. 7-1C) hernias, prolapse of the rectum, and diverticula of the bladder and gastrointestinal tract have been noted.[21,22] Prolapse of the uterus was described in an adult.[9] A 6-month-old child showed redundant tortuous ureters by intravenous pyelograms.[23]

One patient[11] had had Ramstedt operation for pyloric stenosis at the age of 6 weeks. Partial right bundle-branch block was observed in 2 reported patients.[21,22,47] Multiple pulmonary artery stenoses were described in a 4-year-old child[24] and are probably present in Case 2, below. Pulmonic stenosis was diagnosed clinically in another case.[27]

The disorder is present from birth in typical CL. Acquired cutis laxa is probably a distinct disorder and may be nongenetic in most cases, although familial occurrence was noted by Graf,[22a] who first reported adult onset. Although he examined only the proband, who showed onset between the ages of 40 and 50 years, and although the father was said to be unaffected, a paternal aunt and uncle and the paternal grandfather were said to have been affected. In acquired CL, changes in the skin are in all ways like those of the congenital form, but they begin in adulthood. Changes in the elastic tissue of the lung and great vessels occur in the acquired form also. Rossbach's patient,[43a] who acquired cutis laxa at 18 years of age, was a baker's apprentice. Exposure to heat was suggested as a causative factor. Bettman[5] described the relentless progression of cutaneous laxity that developed in a 49-year-old electrician. He died thirteen years later from rupture of the aorta. By that time his skin was so lax he resembled a 90-year-old man. In the acquired form of cutis laxa, or generalized elastolysis, the onset is often characterized by an erythematous rash. Case 3, below, represents this category. Marshall and colleagues[33] described 5 such cases, and Jablónska,[26] one. Wanderer and co-workers[52] described the case of a 14-year-old boy with CL beginning after persistent urticaria and accompanied by marked dilatation of the tracheobronchial tree. Tracheobronchiomegaly goes by the eponymic Mounier-Kuhn syndrome. It occurs also in the Ehlers-Danlos syndrome (p. 329).

Prevalence and inheritance

Familial cutis laxa is exceedingly rare. Probably the entire experience recorded in the world's medical literature does not exceed 25 families. Both autosomal dominant and autosomal recessive forms exist, and the recessive form is usually more malignant in terms of internal involvement.[3b]

"Dominant" families include those of Sestak[47] (father and daughter), Lewis[30] (mother and daughter), Schreiber and Tilley[44] (four generations*), Kopp[28] (father and son; the father had onset of cutis laxa at 16 years of age, whereas it was present at birth in the son), and Reidy[40b] (father and daughter). New dominant mutation was considered possible in Case 2, below, because the father and mother were 36 and 34 years old, respectively, at the time of her birth. Beighton[3b] described 2 kindreds with affected persons in successive generations, including in each kindred an affected father and son. However, these males were not examined. Their status was by lay report only.

"Recessive" families include those of Goltz and associates[21,22] (2 brothers) and of Sestak[47] (brother and sister—one was pictured by Cashman[10]—with parents who were first cousins once removed and with a common ancestor of the 2 parents reputedly affected). Beighton[3b] described 2 cases of cutis laxa with severe pulmonary complications, one the offspring of first-cousin parents and the other the product of father-daughter incest.

Pathology

The histopathology, both in the skin and in involved internal organs such as the lung and large arteries, is dominated by sparsity, fragmentation, and granular disruption of elastic fibers.[21,22] Furthermore, there is a striking accumulation of material with the staining properties of acid mucopolysaccharides.[20b] Collagen is apparently normal.

The basic defect

Undoubtedly the element of connective tissue primarily involved in CL is the elastic fiber, but knowledge of the basic defect goes little further. Deficiency of an elastase-inhibiting substance of blood was suggested by the findings of Goltz and colleagues[21,22] but was not confirmed by Beighton.[3a] An abnormality of copper (which is important to the metabolism of elastin—witness the consequences of copper deficiency, p. 42) has also been suggested, but this remains hypothetic.

Differential diagnosis

Older adults with E-D develop "dewlaps" at the elbows that might be termed cutis laxa, but of course they represent no source of serious confusion with the specific entity CL. Similarly, patients with PXE, especially women, may have

---

*Another family (No. 1) reported by Schreiber and Tilley[44] as cutis laxa transmitted through four generations is clearly the same family as that reported by Rosenthal and Kloepfer,[43] with the distinctive acromegaloid, cutis verticis gyrata, corneal leukoma syndrome.

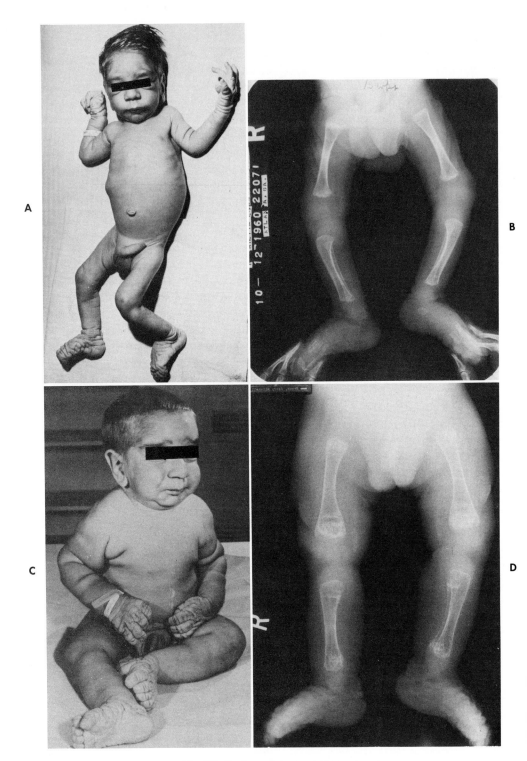

Fig. 7-2. For legend see opposite page.

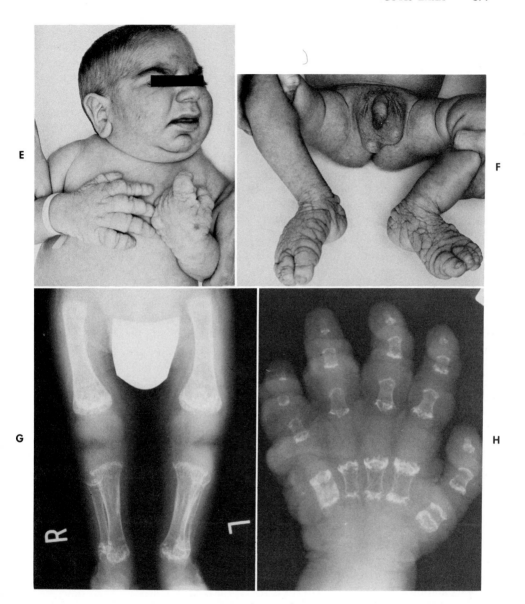

Fig. 7-2. Patterson's leprechaunoid syndrome. **A,** Appearance in infancy. The patient was in the 97th percentile for length. The nipples were prominent and the penis was unusually large. The cry was mature—deep and husky. Left inguinal hernia was present. **B,** X-ray film made at 15 weeks, showing absent ossification centers. Serum alkaline phosphatase levels were always low, but no phosphoethanolamine was demonstrable in the urine. **C,** Appearance at 3 years of age was cushingoid; the patient developed acne, striking hirsutism, "buffalo hump," intermittent hypertension, and glycosuria followed by frank diabetes mellitus. Bladder diverticula and probable bladder neck obstruction were demonstrated. Terminally he developed cryptococcal meningitis, which responded satisfactorily to therapy with amphotericin B, but he succumbed at 7½ years of age to gram-negative sepsis as a complication of an indwelling catheter. A main finding at autopsy was marked enlargement of the adrenal glands, which was most evident in the zona fasciculata. **D,** X-ray film made at 3 years of age. **E** and **F,** Appearance at 7 years of age. **G** and **H,** X-ray films made at 7 years of age. (Courtesy Dr. J. H. Patterson and The National Foundation–March of Dimes.)

strikingly pendulous, folded skin over the abdomen and, to a lesser extent, in the axillary folds, around the neck, and over the thighs. The pendulous fibroma molluscum (plexiform neuroma) of von Recklinghausen's neurofibromatosis[46] is a local form of cutis laxa, if you will; it is an expression of overgrowth like that sometimes seen in the fingers and other structures in that disorder.

The condition reported by Debré and co-workers[15] and by Fittke,[20] cutis laxa with dysostosis, is a distinct entity probably inherited as a recessive. Fittke's proband, a 10½-month-old girl, had loose, redundant skin from birth. Skeletal abnormalities included persistently wide fontanelles, slight oxycephaly, and dislocation of one hip with flattening of the other acetabulum. Although the parents were not known to be related, they lived in an area of Europe where most persons are related. The mother had "weak knee joints," and the proband's first cousin, 7 years 9 months of age, had cutis laxa, pigeon breast, static scoliosis, flat feet, and delay in closure of the fontanelles until she was 3 years old. Theopold and Wildhack[50a] restudied the family, demonstrating consanguinity of the parents of one of the affected cousins.

In 3 brothers whose parents were second cousins, Welch and associates[52b] described a disorder with many of the features of cutis laxa, particularly the facial appearance and sagging skin. In addition, all 3 demonstrated premature rupture of fetal membranes, hypermobility of joints, and death in infancy. Strikingly tortuous large arteries and aneurysms were present in 2 of the 3 brothers. Two other brothers, the father, and many members of the father's family, through the line not related to the probands' mother, had manifestations considered consistent with the benign hypermobile form of the Ehlers-Danlos syndrome (Chapter 6). The arterial abnormality in the 3 brothers suggested that described by Ertugrul,[18a] Beuren and associates,[5a] and Lees and colleagues,[29] but the cutaneous and other features seemed to distinguish the disorder. Homozygosity of the E-D gene, and interaction between the E-D gene inherited from the father and the homozygous state of another gene, were possibilities considered by Welch and co-workers.[52b]

Cutis laxa was also a striking feature of a child, reported by Barsy and colleagues,[3] who also showed mental retardation, dwarfism, degeneration of the elastic tissue of skin and of Bowman's membrane of the cornea, producing clouding, and generalized muscular hypotonicity with adventitious movements. The parents were of different ethnic origins. Two older sibs were normal.

The acromegaloid, cutis verticis gyrata, corneal leukoma syndrome described by Rosenthal and Kloepfer[43] need not be confused with CL. It is in autosomal dominant disorder that has apparently been described only in a Louisiana Negro family in which at least 13 persons in four generations were affected. The first patient reported by Schreiber and Tilley,[44] presumably being a member of the same kindred, seems to have had this disorder, and not CL. (Their third patient came from a family in which CL occurred in four generations, as noted earlier.)

In blepharochalasis, cutis laxa is limited to the eyelids. Autosomal dominant transmission was noted in an extensively affected French-Canadian family by Panneton.[38] Schulze[45] described blepharochalasis limited to the upper lid in 14 members of six generations of a German family. Blepharochalasis combined with "double lip" constitutes Ascher's syndrome,[19] a quite distinct disorder.

In leprechaunism,[17] the skin is abnormally loose and the patient has a pre-

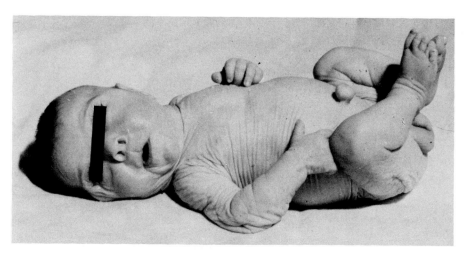

Fig. 7-3. Leprechaunism versus cutis laxa. The question is whether this child suffered from Donohue's leprechaunism, Patterson's leprechaunoid syndrome, or cutis laxa. See text. (Courtesy Dr. Louis Dallaire and The National Foundation–March of Dimes.)

cociously senile appearance somewhat like that of cutis laxa. The peculiar facies is gnomelike, giving the condition its name. On clinical grounds alone it is not likely to be confused with cutis laxa. A condition almost certainly distinct from leprechaunism was described by Patterson and Watkins,[40] with follow-up given by Patterson.[39] As is demonstrated by Fig. 7-2, cutis laxa was particularly striking over the hands and feet, and severe skeletal changes evolved as the patient became older.

The confusion between leprechaunism and cutis laxa may be illustrated by the patient of Dallaire[13] (Fig. 7-3). The patient was hospitalized at 8 months of age because of a respiratory infection. The skin was generally loose, and umbilical hernia was present. The penis was enlarged. Chest x-ray films showed bronchopneumonia and cardiac enlargement. The patient died soon after admission, and no autopsy was performed. As shown in Fig. 7-3, the facies, particularly the long upper lip, is suggestive of cutis laxa.

The condition described by O'Brien and colleagues[37] as "multiple congenital skin webbing with cutis laxa" may be a distinct entity. The proband, a boy, had a midline neck web with micrognathia and malocclusion, broad webs in both axillae, and a web across the perineum between the upper aspects of the thighs, causing retroposition of the penis and scrotum. Another broad web was present in the left popliteal fossa, as well as the left talipes equinus. Otherwise the skin of the entire body was like that seen in typical cutis laxa. A brother had rather typical cutis laxa without webs or other deformities.

Management

Plastic surgery[4,30] can make a dramatic improvement in the appearance of patients with cutis laxa, inevitably with important psychosocial benefits. In addition to face-lifting and blepharoplasty, excessive skin can be removed from the neck, arms, breasts, abdomen, etc., and Beighton and associates,[4] who first

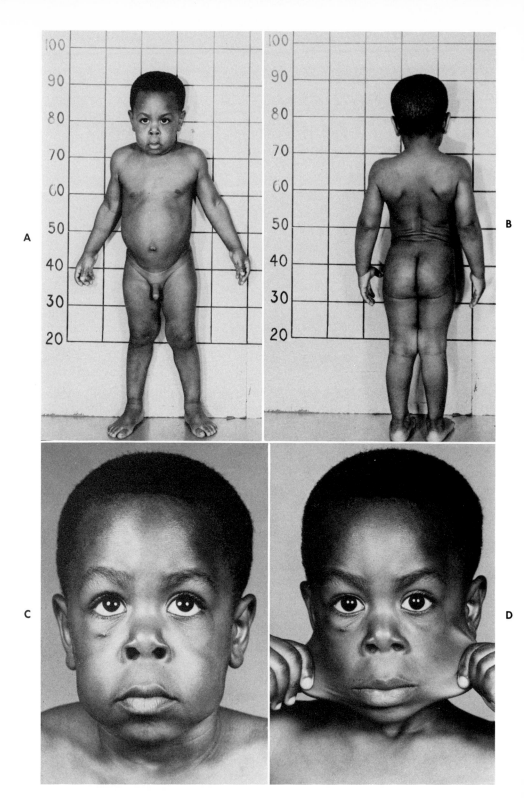

Fig. 7-4. Cutis laxa in S. H. (J.H.H. 1203951). **A** and **B,** Appearance at the age of 3 years. **C** and **D,** Facial appearance at the age of 4 years. **E,** Chest x-ray film showing emphysema and diminished vascularity.

emphasized the characteristic conformation of the nose, reconstructed that part also. Tissue fragility, excessive bleeding, and tenuous healing, which plague surgery in E-D, are usually not problems in CL. Operations are uncomplicated and postoperative scars are fine and normally strong.[40b] An exception to these statements is the case of acquired cutis laxa (Case 3, below) in which hematoma formation followed surgery. Sagging skin may recur after face-lifting operations,[30] but repeated operations can be performed.[21,22] Patients should be evaluated from the cardiovascular viewpoint before surgery, both because of possible risks in general anesthesia and because of poor prognosis generally if internal involvement, such as emphysema, is present.

No other therapeutic measures can be proposed. In children with heart failure the possibility of upper airway obstruction should be kept in mind and tracheostomy considered.

Illustrative cases

Case 1.* S. H. (J.H.H. 1203951), a Negro male born in 1966, was first admitted to the hospital at the age of 5 months because of episodes of wheezing and tachypnea. Peculiar facies with lax, sagging skin had been present from birth. During the first year of life he had repeated pulmonary infections.

Examination (1970) showed an adequately developed and nourished, alert and active child with a low-pitched voice (Fig. 7-4). Unusual sagging cheeks and skin of the chin gave him the appearance of a bloodhound. The skin of the trunk and limbs, especially that over the anterior chest, was also loose. A grade II/VI systolic murmur was audible over the entire precordium.

*This patient was reported by Maxwell and Esterly.[33a]

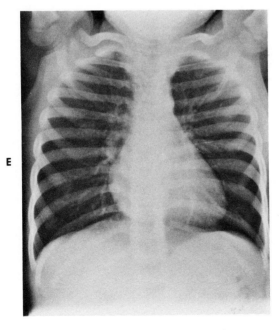

Fig. 7-4, cont'd. For legend see opposite page.

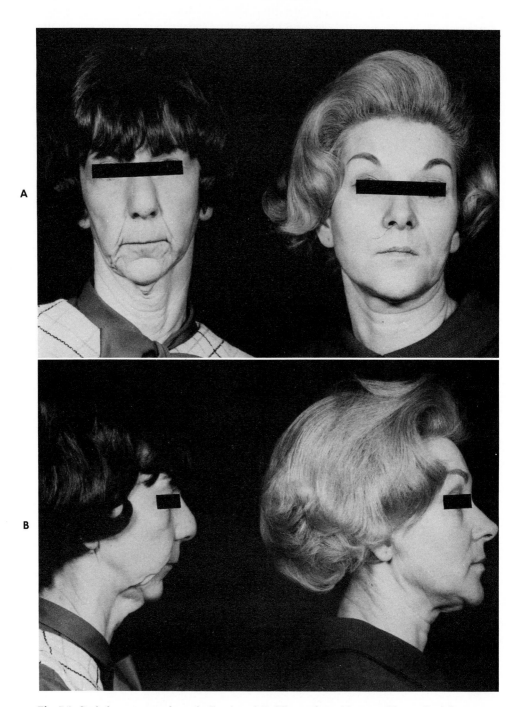

Fig. 7-5. Cutis laxa corrected surgically. **A** and **B,** The patient, 16 years old, on the left, appears older than her mother, on the right. **C** and **D,** Improvement of appearance after plastic surgery of the face and nose is demonstrated. (See also Beighton, P., Bull, J. C., and Edgerton, M. T.: Brit. J. Plast. Surg. 23:285, 1970.)

The chest x-ray film showed the heart to be at the upper limit of normal for size. The lung fields showed a probable decrease in vascularity. Peripheral pulmonary arterial stenoses have been suspected, but no special studies were done for confirmation. Skin biopsy showed no definite abnormality of elastic fibers.

Case 2. L. G. (J.H.H. 1313500), a white female born in 1952, was reported by Robinson and Ellis,[41] who made the diagnosis of cutis laxa when they saw her at the age of 3½ years (see photograph in reference 8a) and kindly arranged for her to be seen here in her teens for investigations and treatment. The results of plastic surgery were reported by Beighton and co-workers.[4] Somewhat increased skin wrinkling had been noted at birth. By the age of 6 months the laxity was marked; however, after a few years the laxity did not seem to increase. The skin was not unusually fragile or bruisable, and scarring was normal. Her general health was good and she had no serious illnesses. At no time has she had cardiac or pulmonary symptoms or complications suggesting diverticula of the bladder or gastrointestinal tract. She was normally intelligent and did well in school, although she was limited in social activities by embarrassment over her appearance.

Two older sibs and their children were normal. The parents, also normal, were both Italian but presumably not related. The father was 36 and the mother 34 years old at her birth.

Examination (1968) showed a shy 16-year-old girl with lax, redundant skin of the face and neck that made her look about three times as old as she really was. Indeed, she looked older than her mother (Fig. 7-5A and B). The skin was unremarkable except for the laxity and wrinkles. Her peculiar appearance was exaggerated by the conformation of her nose, which was hooked, with prominent bridge and short columella, and of her upper lip, which was unusually long. Her voice was deep. No other abnormality was detected.

Chest x-ray examinations, an electrocardiogram, pulmonary function tests, the karyotype, and dermatoglyphics were all normal.

A consultant psychiatrist applied the standard "Self-image questionnaire" and concluded that the patient was unusually well adjusted.

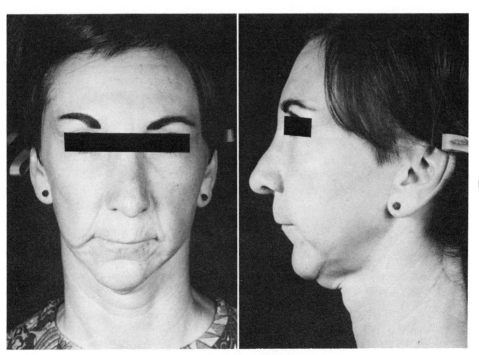

C   D

Fig. 7-5, cont'd. For legend see opposite page.

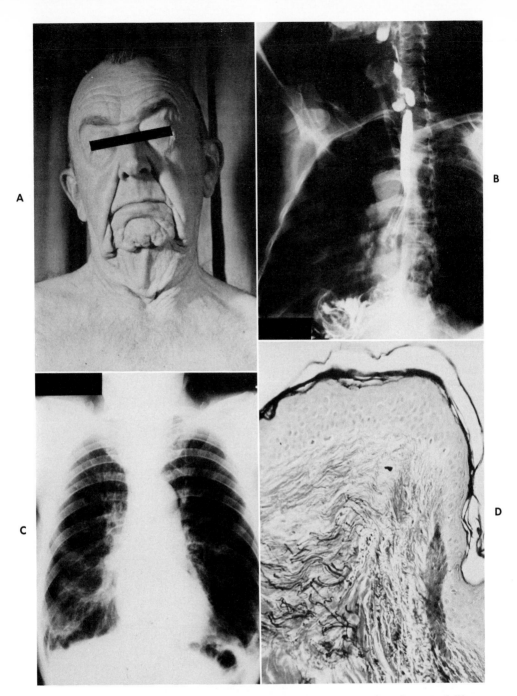

Fig. 7-6. Acquired cutis laxa with systemic elastolysis. **A,** Appearance at the age of 50 years before first plastic surgical repairs. **B,** Barium-swallow x-ray film showing bilobed Zenker's diverticulum of the upper esophagus and hiatus hernia. **C,** Chest roentgenogram, one month before death, showing advanced pulmonary emphysema, pneumonitis, and dilatation of the pulmonary artery and aorta. **D,** Section of skin showing virtual absence of elastic fibers in the superficial part of the corium and, in the mid and lower dermis, reduced numbers of elastic fibers, which are fragmented and granular. (Weigert's elastica stain; ×560.) **E,** Section showing medium-sized pulmonary artery. The elastic fibers of the internal elastica are severely disrupted. There is probable muscular hyperplasia. (Weigert's elastica stain; ×125.) **F,** Section of aortic tunica media, showing fragmented and granular elastic fibers. (Weigert's elastica stain; ×560.)

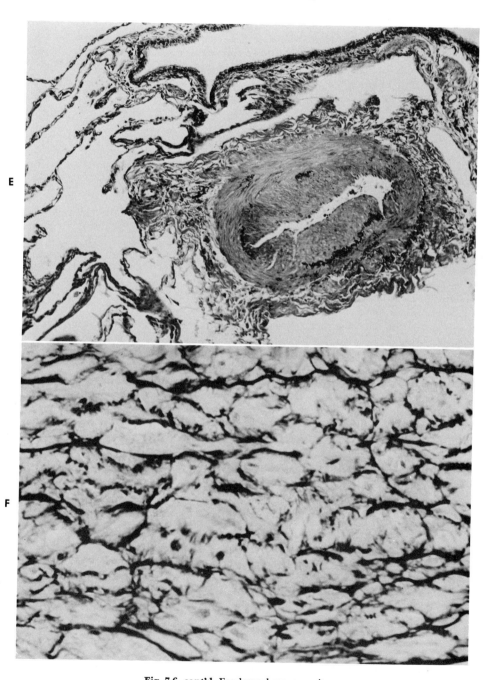

Fig. 7-6, cont'd. For legend see opposite page.

At a first operation, rhinoplasty was performed, removing the dorsal hump and hanging tip. Excess skin was removed from the upper arms at the same operation. At a second operation a formal face-lifting was performed. The patient was delighted with her improved appearance (Fig. 7-5C and D).

Case 3.* I. H. K., a 59-year-old engineer, noted the onset of progressive and generalized laxity of the skin at 40 years of age, after a particularly severe penicillin reaction that lasted for a month (Fig. 7-6A). A mass removed from the side of the neck when he was 50 years old proved to be a subcutaneous varix with organizing thrombus. Face-lifting and blepharoplasty were complicated by the development of a large hematoma. A later Z-plasty of the neck was also complicated by secondary bleeding with formation of a hematoma.

At the age of 53 years the patient underwent surgery for a bilobed Zenker's diverticulum of the esophagus (Fig. 7-6B). At that time recurrence of cutis laxa of the face, neck, axillae, and scrotum was noted. The buccal mucosa was thrown into folds. Continuing difficulty in swallowing was found to be due to a large hiatal hernia (Fig. 7-6B), which was repaired with vagotomy and pyloroplasty.

At the age of 56 years the patient developed severe generalized erythema multiforme of unknown cause. This lasted for about four weeks. Also at this time he continued to have upper abdominal distress; prolapse of gastric mucosa into the base of the duodenal bulb, with a probable ulcer at the apex of the bulb, was demonstrated by x-ray examination.

Bilateral inguinal hernias and orthopnea were also first noted at 56 years of age. X-ray films of the chest (Fig. 7-6C) showed moderately severe pulmonary emphysema. The hernias were repaired uneventfully when he was 59 years old. Thereafter he had increasing cardio-respiratory symptoms. X-ray examination showed increase in the size of the heart and aorta and in the signs of emphysema. He died suddenly at the age of 59 years.

Grossly, autopsy showed generalized cutis laxa, moderate hypertrophy of the right ventricle, moderate ectasia of the aorta with severe atherosclerosis, striking pulmonary emphysema, markedly dilated gallbladder (measuring 15 cm. × 7 cm), and numerous diverticula of the colon, especially in the descending part.

Histologically the skin (Fig. 7-6D) showed generalized loss of pegs and flattening of the papillae. Elastic fibers were exceedingly sparse in all layers of the corium and virtually absent in the upper layers. In deeper parts, the elastic fibers were fragmented and granular. Elastic fibers of the fibrous septae in the subcutaneous fat were markedly diminished and similarly fragmented and granular. In the lungs, diminution, fragmentation, and granularity of pleural elastic fibers, extensive pulmonary emphysema, and marked muscular hypertrophy of pulmonary arterioles, suggesting pulmonary hypertension, were demonstrated (Fig. 7-6E). Almost no elastic tissue could be demonstrated in the alveolar septae, and pronounced changes in the form of disruption and discontinuity were found in the internal elastica of the pulmonary arteries. The tunica media of the aorta showed areas where elastic fibers were replaced with metachromatic material. In other areas elastic fibers were fragmented and granular (Fig. 7-6F).

SUMMARY

Cutis laxa is a generalized disorder of connective tissue characterized mainly by striking laxity of all the skin but also by abnormalities of the lung and arteries. The fundamental defect resides in elastic fibers. At least two genetic forms, one autosomal dominant and the other autosomal recessive, appear to exist. Several other genetic disorders resemble cutis laxa in some ways. An acquired form of systemic elastolysis has many features like that of the genetically determined and usually congenital disorder, but it probably is a distinct etiopathogenetic, possibly nongenetic, entity.

---

*I am indebted to Dr. William B. Reed, of Burbank, California, for information on this patient and permission to include the case report here. This patient was reported by Reed and co-workers.[40a]

REFERENCES

1. Alibert, J. L.: Histoire d'un berger des environs de Gisors (dermatose hypermorphe), Monogr. Derm. **2**:719, 1855.
2. Bakker, B. J.: Cutis laxa universalis und Lungenemphysema, Hautarzt **10**:371, 1959.
3. Barsy, A. M., Moens, E., and Dierckx, L.: Dwarfism, oligophrenia, and degeneration of the elastic tissue in skin and cornea; a new syndrome, Helv. Paediat. Acta **23**:305, 1968.
3a. Beighton, P.: Personal communication, 1970.
3b. Beighton, P.: The dominant and recessive forms of cutis laxa, J. Med. Genet. **9**:216, 1972.
4. Beighton, P., Bull, J. C., and Edgerton, M. T.: Plastic surgery in cutis laxa, Brit. J. Plast. Surg. **23**:285, 1970.
5. Bettman, A. G.: Excessively relaxed skin and the pituitary gland, Plast. Reconstr. Surg. **15**:489, 1955.
5a. Beuren, A. J., Hort, W., Kalbfleisch, H., Muller, H., and Stoermer, J.: Dysplasia of the systemic and pulmonary arterial system with tortuosity and lengthening of the arteries; a new entity, diagnosed during life, and leading to coronary death in early childhood, Circulation **39**:109, 1969.
6. Bondi, R., Gori, F., and Treves, G.: Concomitanza e signifactao della cutis laxa e dell'enfisema polmonare alveolare infantile in una rara osservazione anatomopatologica, Arch. De Vecchi Anat. Pat. **51**:801, 1968.
7. Boreux, G.: Osteodysplastic geroderma of sex-linked heredity; a new clinical and genetic entity, J. Génét. Hum. **17**:137, 1969.
8. Butterworth, T., and Strean, P.: Clinical gerodermatology, Baltimore, 1962, The Williams & Wilkins Co.
9. Carney, R. G., and Nomland, R.: Acquired loose skin (chalazoderma); report of a case, Arch. Dermat. Syph. **56**:794, 1947.
10. Cashman, M. E.: Cutis laxa, Proc. Roy. Soc. Med. **50**:719, 1957.
11. Chadfield, H. W.: Cutis laxa, Brit. J. Derm. **81**:387, 1969.
12. Christiaens, L., Marchant-Alphant, A., and Fovet, A.: Emphyseme congénital et cutis laxa, Presse Méd. **62**:1799, 1954.
13. Dallaire, L.: Discussion (of leprechaunism). In Bergsma, D., editor: Clinical delineation of birth defects. IV. Skeletal dysplasias. New York, 1969, National Foundation, p. 121.
14. Danlos, M.: Uncas de cutis laxa avec tumeurs par contusion chronique des coudes et des genoux (xanthome juvenile pseudo-diabetique de M. M. Hallopeau et Mace de Lépinay), Bull. Soc. Franç. Derm. Syph. **19**:70, 1908.
15. Debré, R., Marie, J., and Seringe, P.: "Cutis laxa" avec dystrophies osseuses, Bull. Soc. Méd. Hôp. Paris **61**:1038, 1937.
16. Dingman, R. O., Grabb, W. C., and O'Neal, R. M.: Cutis laxa congenita—generalized elastosis, Plast. Reconstr. Surg. **44**:431, 1969.
17. Donohue, W. L., and Uchida, I.: Leprechaunism; a euphuism for a rare familial disorder, J. Pediat. **45**:505, 1954.
18. Ehlers, E.: Cutis laxa, Neigung zu Hämorrhagien in der Haut, Lockerung mehrerer Artikulationen, Derm. Wschr. **8**:173, 1901.
18a. Ertugrul, A.: Diffuse tortuosity and lengthening of the arteries, Circulation **36**:400, 1967.
19. Findlay, G. H.: Idiopathic enlargements of the lips; cheilosis granulomatosa, Ascher's syndrome, and double lip, Brit. J. Derm. **66**:129, 1954.
20. Fittke, H.: Uber eine ungewöhnliche Form "multipler Erbabartung" (Chalodermie und Dysostose), Z. Kinderheilk. **63**:510, 1942.
20a. Franceschetti, A.: Manifestation de blepharochasis chez le père, associé à des doubles lèvres apparaissant également chez sa filette agée d'un mois, J. Genet. Hum. **4**:181, 1955.
20b. Goltz, R. W. (Denver): Personal communication, 1971.
21. Goltz, R. W., and Hult, A. M.: Generalized elastolysis (cutis laxa) and Ehlers-Danlos syndrome (cutis hyperelactica); a comparative clinical and laboratory study, Southern Med. J. **58**:848, 1965.
22. Goltz, R. W., Hult, A. M., Goldfarb, M., and Gorlin, R. J.: Cutis laxa; a manifestation of generalized elastolysis, Arch. Derm. **92**:373, 1965.
22a. Graf (N.I.): Örtliche erbliche Erschlaffung der Haut, Wschr. Ges. Heilk. (Berlin), p. 225, 1836.

23. Hajjar, B. A., and Joyner, E. N., III: Congenital cutis laxa with advanced cardiopulmonary disease, J. Pediat. **73**:116, 1968.

24. Hayden, J. G., Talner, N. S., and Klaus, S. N.: Cutis laxa associated with pulmonary artery stenosis, J. Pediat. **72**:506, 1968.

25. Hult, A. M., Goltz, R. A., and Midtgaard, K.: The dermal elastic fibers in cutis hyperelastica (E.D.S.) and in cutis laxa (generalized elastosis), Acta Dermatovener. **44**:415, 1964.

26. Jablońska, S.: Inflammatorische Hautveränderungen, die eine erworhenen Cutis laxa vorausgehen, Hautarzt **17**:341, 1966.

27. Koblenzer, P. J., and LoPresti, P. J.: Dermatochalasia (dermatomegaly) and congenital pulmonic stenosis, Arch. Derm. **97**:602, 1968.

28. Kopp, W.: Demonstration zweier Fälle von "Cutis laxa," München, Med. Wschr. **35**:259, 1888.

29. Lees, M. H., Menashe, V. D., Sunderland, C. O., Morgan, C. L., and Dawaon, P. J.: Ehlers-Danlos syndrome associated with multiple pulmonary artery stenoses and tortuous systemic arteries, J. Pediat. **75**:1031, 1969.

30. Lewis, E.: Cutis laxa, Proc. Roy. Soc. Med. **41**:864, 1948.

30a. Luke, M. J., Mehrizi, A., Folger, G. M., and Rowe, R. D.: Chronic nasopharyngeal obstruction as a cause of cardiomegaly, cor pulmonale, and pulmonary edema, Pediatrics **37**:762, 1966.

31. McCarthy, C. F., Warin, R. P., and Read, A. E. A.: Loose skin (cutis laxa) associated with systemic abnormalities, Arch. Intern. Med. **115**:62, 1965.

32. Macartney, F. J., Panday, J., and Scott, O.: Cor pulmonale as a result of chronic nasopharyngeal obstruction due to hypertrophied tonsils and adenoids, Arch. Dis. Child. **44**:585, 1969.

33. Marshall, J., Hey, L. T., and Weber, H. W.: Postinflammatory elastolysis and cutis laxa, S. Afr. Med. J. **40**:1016, 1966.

33a. Maxwell, E., and Esterly, N. B.: Cutis laxa, Amer. J. Dis. Child. **117**:479, 1969.

34. Miller, E. J., Martin, G. R., Mecca, C. E., and Piez, K. A.: The biosynthesis of elastin cross-links; the effect of copper deficiency and a lathyrogen, J. Biol. Chem. **240**:3623, 1965.

35. Monnet, P., Gauthier, J., and Colomb, D.: Cutis laxa à forme généralisée, Pediatrie **17**:567, 1962.

36. Mott, V.: Remarks on a peculiar form of tumour of the skin denominated pachydermatocele, London Med. Chirurg. Trans. **37**:155, 1854.

37. O'Brien, B. M., Garson, O. M., Baikie, A. G., and Dooley, B. J.: Multiple congenital skin webbing with cutis laxa, Brit. J. Plast. Surg. **23**:329, 1970.

38. Panneton, P.: La blepharochalasis; à propos de 51 cas dans une même famille, Arch. Ophtal. (Paris) **53**:729, 1936.

39. Patterson, J. H.: Presentation of a patient with leprechaunism. In Bergsma, D., editor: Clinical delineation of birth defects. IV. Skeletal dysplasias. New York, 1969, National Foundation, p. 117.

40. Patterson, J. H., and Watkins, W. L.: Leprechaunism in a male infant, J. Pediat. **60**:730, 1962.

40a. Reed, W. B., Horowitz, R. E., and Beighton, P.: Acquired cutis laxa; primary generalized elastolysis, Arch. Derm. **103**:661, 1971.

40b. Reidy, J. P.: Cutis hyperelastica (Ehlers-Danlos) and cutis laxa, Brit. J. Plast. Surg. **16**:84, 1963.

40c. Reisner, S. H., Seelenfreund, M., and Ben-Bassat, M.: Cutis laxa associated with severe intrauterine growth retardation and congenital dislocation of the hip, Acta Paediat. Scand. **60**:357, 1971.

41. Robinson, H. M., and Ellis, F. A.: Cutis laxa, Arch. Derm. **77**:656, 1958.

42. Ronchese, F.: Dermatomegaly, Arch. Derm. **77**:666, 1958.

43. Rosenthal, J. W., and Kloepfer, H. W.: An acromegaloid, cutis verticis gyrata, corneal leukoma syndrome, Arch. Ophthal. **68**:722, 1962.

43a. Rossbach, M. J.: Ein merkwürdiger Fall von griesen hafter Veränderung der allgemeinen Körpdecke bei einem achtzehnjährigen Jüngling, Deutsch. Arch. Klin. Med. **36**:197, 1884.

44. Schreiber, M. M., and Tilley, J. C.: Cutis laxa, Arch. Derm. **84**:266, 1961.

45. Schulze, F.: Beitrag zur hereditären Blepharochalasis, Klin. Mbl. Augenheilk. **147**:863, 1965.

46. Sequeira, J. H.: A case of dermatolysis and molluscum fibrosum, with congenital morbus cordis and kyphosis, Brit. J. Derm. **28**:68, 1916.

47. Sestak, Z.: Ehlers-Danlos syndrome and cutis laxa; an account of families in the Oxford area, Ann. Hum. Genet. **25**:313, 1962.

48. Shelley, W. B., and Crissey, J. T.: Classics in clinical dermatology, Springfield, Ill., 1953, Charles C Thomas, Publisher.

49. Souques, A., and Charcot, J. B.: Géromorphisme cutané, Nouv. Iconogr. Salpêt. **4**:169, 1891.

50. Stokes, W.: On excision of a pachydermatocele from the scalp, Dublin J. Med. Sci. **61**:1, 1876.

50a. Theopold, W., and Wildhack, R.: Dermatochalasis im Rahmen multipler Abortungen, Mschr. Kinderheilk. **99**:213, 1951.

51. Tourtellotte, C. D., and Dziawiatkowski, D. D.: A disorder of enchondral ossification induced by dextran sulfate, J. Bone Joint Surg. **47-A**:1185, 1965.

51a. Von Kétly, L.: Ein Fall von eigenartiger Hautveränderung: "Chalazodermie" (Schlaffhaut), Arch. Derm. Syph. **56**:107, 1901.

52. Wanderer, A. A., Ellis, E. F., Goltz, R. W., et al.: Tracheobronchiomegaly and acquired cutis laxa in a child. Physiologic and immunologic studies, Pediatrics **44**:709, 1969.

52a. Weber, F. P.: Chalasodermia, or "loose skin," and its relationship to subcutaneous fibroids or calcareous nodules, Urol. Cutan. Rev. **27**:407, 1923.

52b. Welch, J. P., Aterman, K., Day, E., and Roy, D. L.: Familiar aggregation of a "new" connective tissue disorder; a nosologic problem. In Bergsma, D., editor: Clinical delineation of birth defects. XII. Skin, hair, and nails, Baltimore, 1971, The Williams & Wilkins Co.

53. Wile, H.: The elastic skin man, Medical News **43**:705, 1883.

54. Wiskemann, A.: Gerodermie, Arch. Klin. Exp. Derm. **213**:870, 1961.

8 · Osteogenesis imperfecta

Historical note

It has been suggested[152,294] that an early case of osteogenesis imperfecta was that of Ivar the Boneless, the mastermind behind the Scandinavian invasion of England in the last quarter of the ninth century. He is said to have had cartilage where bones should have been. He could not walk and was carried into battle on shields. Complete verification of the diagnosis is impossible because so much poetic glorification enshrouds any remaining records, and Ivar's skeleton is no longer available for study, having been dug up and burned by William the Conqueror. A study of Ivar's descendants turned up no cases of osteogenesis imperfecta or other bone disease.

A left femur thought to be that of a person with osteogenesis imperfecta was found in an Anglo-Saxon burial ground in England dating from the seventh century A.D.[357] The evidence is, at the best, tenuous. Better evidence was provided in the case of an Egyptian mummy dating from about 1000 B.C. and residing in the British Museum for more than sixty years.[139] The skull showed a mosaic of innumerable Wormian bones and tam-o'-shanter deformity on reconstruction. The teeth were amber-colored, with the roots disproportionately smaller than the crowns. The legs were bowed, and x-ray studies showed the "thick bone" type of change.[139] These manifestations are indicative of osteogenesis imperfecta congenita.

The recorded history of the development of knowledge of this disease is given in Table 8-1. Isolated cases were reported even before Ekman, from as early as 1678.[294]

The terms that have been applied to this syndrome are numerous and include, to mention a few, osteogenesis imperfecta (Vrolik[349]), mollities ossium (Ormerod[248]), fragilitas ossium (Gurlt[143]), and osteopsathyrosis idiopathica (Lobstein[213]). To complicate matters further, the disease is called *la maladie de Lobstein* in the French-speaking portion of the medical world. It is also known as Eddowes' syndrome (brittle bones and blue sclerae), van der Hoeve's syndrome (brittle bones, blue sclerae, and deafness), and Vrolik's disease (osteogenesis imperfecta congenita). Looster[214] suggested the terms osteogenesis imperfecta congenita (OIC) and osteogenesis imperfecta tarda (OIT).

390

Table 8-1. Landmarks in the history of osteogenesis imperfecta

1788	O. J. Ekman.[96] In medical doctorate thesis at Uppsala, described "osteomalacia congenita" in three generations. (See Seedorff[294] for an extensive translation of Ekman's Latin thesis.)
1831	Edmund Axmann,[15] Wertheim, Germany. Described the disease in himself and his brothers, Paul and Anton. Made reference to the occurrence of articular dislocations and blue sclerae. One of the brothers had been reported by Strack in 1807.[329]
1833	J. C. Lobstein (1777-1838), gynecologist and pathologist, Strasbourg. Wrote about adult form of the disease in his textbook of morbid anatomy.[213]
1849	Willem Vrolik (1801-1863). Dutch anatomist. Described disease in newborn infant.[349] See Fig. 8-1.
1859	Edward Latham Ormerod,[248] Brighton, England. Early description of case of 68-year-old woman only 39½ inches tall. Disease was passed to a son and a daughter. The skeleton, in the Royal College of Surgeons, London, is reproduced in Bell's monograph.[26] Use of term "mollities ossium."
1862-1865	Ernest Julius Gurlt[143] (1825-1899), Professor of Surgery, Berlin. Use of term "fragilitas ossium."
1889	H. Stilling,[325] Strasbourg. Histologic studies.
1896	John Spurway,[317] Tring, England. Described blue sclerae with fragility of bones.
1897	M. B. Schmidt,[286] Strasbourg. Proposed fundamental identity of the disease in adults and newborn infants.
1900	Alfred Eddowes,[95] London. Described blue sclerae. Suggested that OI is generalized hypoplasia of mesenchyme.
1903	Leslie Buchanan,[55] Glasgow. Demonstrated that blue sclerae are due to thinness of sclera. Fractures, deafness, or familial incidence not mentioned in his "A. M'C—, a girl aet. 9 years."
1906	E. Looser,[214] Heidelberg. Defended identity of disease in adult and newborn infant. Proposed terms osteogenesis imperfecta congenita (OIC) and osteogenesis imperfecta tarda (OIT).
1912	Charles A. Adair-Dighton,[1] Liverpool. Described deafness.
1918	J. van der Hoeve, Groningen, and A. de Kleyn, Utrecht.[341] Emphasized brittle bones, blue sclerae, and deafness as a syndrome.
1920	K. H. Bauer,[22,23] Breslau. Provided histologic support for view that OI is a "hypoplasia mesenchymialis." Described dental histology.
1919, 1922	E. Ruttin,[281,282] Vienna. Described otosclerotic nature of the deafness in OI.
1928	Julia Bell,[26] of the Galton Laboratory, London. Described dominant pattern of inheritance, especially of blue sclerae, on basis of large number of pedigrees.

The condition called periosteal dysplasia of Porak and Durante by French authors is probably the same as osteogenesis imperfecta congenita.

Clinical manifestations

The clinical aspects of osteogenesis imperfecta will be discussed under the following categories: skeletal, ocular, cutaneous, otologic, dental, and internal. The osseous manifestations greatly outweigh the others in significance.

Clinically two varieties of OI have been distinguished. In so-called osteogenesis imperfecta congenita, the disease is so severe that the relatively minor traumata to which the fetus is exposed in utero produce numerous fractures. The victum is often born dead or survives only a short time. The cranium is soft and membranous. Short, clumsy extremities suggest achondroplasia (Fig. 8-2). In the second variety, so-called osteogenesis imperfecta tarda (or tardiva), the manifestations are so mild that blue sclerae may be the only manifestation, and fractures may occur only late in life or not at all. Seedorff[294] further divides osteogenesis imperfecta tarda into levis and gravis types. In the latter, the first fractures are likely to occur when the patient is an infant. In the former, the fractures occur only considerably later.

On the basis mainly of radiologic changes, Fairbank[107] distinguishes a "thick bone type," a "slender bone type," and a form he calls osteogenesis imperfecta cystica (Fig. 8-10). This categorization, like the antenatal and postnatal distinction he makes, may have no basis so far as difference in the fundamental defect is concerned. During prepubertal years a patient may demonstrate an evolution from the "slender bone type" to the cystic type or the "thick bone type." The "thick" and "slender" bone types of OIC are illustrated by Figs. 8-3 and 8-5, respectively.

Experience with categories of genetic disease has repeatedly shown that what at first appears to be a single homogeneous entity is in fact several fundamentally distinct disorders. Examples are the cases of homocystinuria that have been

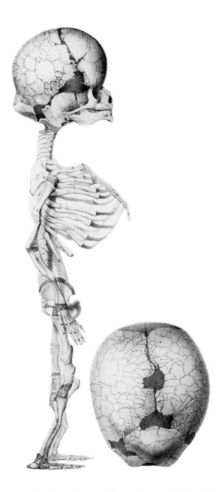

Fig. 8-1. Skeleton in osteogenesis imperfecta. Note the multiple Wormian bones of the caput membranaceum. (From Vrolik, W.: Tabulae ad illustrandam embryogenesim hominis et mammalium, tam naturalem quam abnormem, Amstelodami, 1849.)

classified as the Marfan syndrome in the past (Chapter 4) and the six distinct mucopolysaccharidoses (Chapter 11) that have at times been called Hurler's syndrome. A priori, therefore, heterogeneity in the category of osteogenesis imperfecta is almost a certainty. Later (p. 421), evidence will be reviewed that bears on the question of multiple distinct forms of osteogenesis imperfecta—the alternative being that the clinically somewhat different conditions are all the same entity, which has an exceedingly great range of clinical severity.

Musculoskeletal system.[40] As will be seen later, osteogenesis imperfecta is a hereditary defect of the bone matrix. Calcification of whatever bone matrix is formed probably proceeds normally. Osteogenesis imperfecta is then a form of hereditary osteoporosis, inasmuch as osteoporosis is defined as a deficiency in the formation (or an acceleration of the breakdown) of bone matrix. This is an important consideration in the understanding of some of the clinical manifestations of the disease and in its rational therapy. For example, in later life, partic-

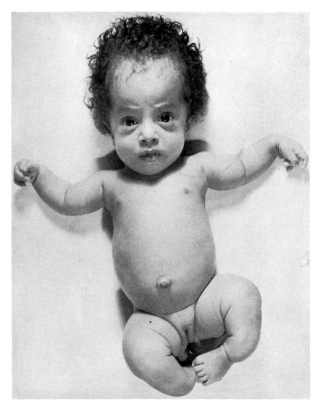

Fig. 8-2. P. D. (A42000), 3 months old, an instance of so-called osteogenesis imperfecta congenita. Micromelia is striking. The head appears disproportionately large. Numerous fractures were demonstrated immediately after birth. The patient was referred with the diagnosis of chondrodystrophia fetalis, however. The skull bones were described as "crumbly" on palpation. The parents and the parents' families were normal. By the age of 1 year there were evidences of well-advanced hydrocephalus. Death occurred at the age of 38 months.

ularly if few fractures have occurred, the disease may masquerade as postmenopausal osteoporosis; immobilization is as bad for OI as it is for other forms of osteoporosis.

Caput membranaceum and micromelia ("tiny extremities") are the characteristics of OIC (Figs. 8-1 to 8-5). The limbs are described as bowed on the chest and abdomen at birth. If the patient survives, the bowing is likely to persist. The disorder may at first be considered "simple" idiopathic congenital bowing of the legs,[7,59] if blue sclerae and Wormian bones are not noted. I know of such a case. Prenatal bowing shows cutaneous dimpling, apparently from pressure atrophy, at the summit of the curves. Dimpling had also been described with the prenatal bowing of hypophosphatasia[356] and might be expected in OIC. Prenatal bowing is associated with abnormalities of the pelvis, spine, and scapula (which is very small) in a usually fatal disorder[17,316] for which Maroteaux suggested[315] the designation *camptomelic dwarfism*. Other features are cleft palate, micrognathia, flat face, and hypertelorism. A misdiag-

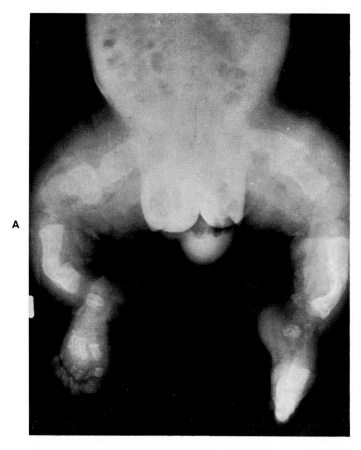

A

Fig. 8-3. "Congenital" osteogenesis imperfecta in K. K. (A95443), 2½ weeks of age. **A,** Multiple fractures, bowing of the extremities, and bilateral inguinal hernias are evident. **B** and **C,** Demonstration of multiple Wormian bones in the membranaceum. (**A** and **B** from McKusick, V. A.: Bull. N. Y. Acad. Med. **35:**143, 1959.)

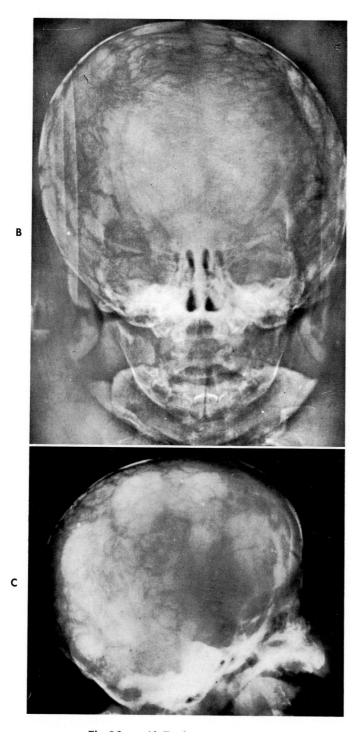

Fig. 8-3, cont'd. For legend see opposite page.

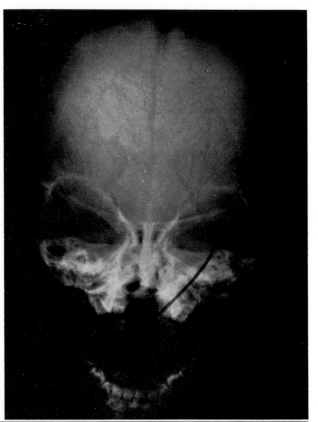

A

Fig. 8-4. W. B. (A79352), 2-month-old white male, radiographic views (**A** and **B**) of the skull in a case of osteogenesis imperfecta congenita, showing a mosaic of Wormian bones and the thin calvarium characteristic of so-called *caput membranaceum*.

B

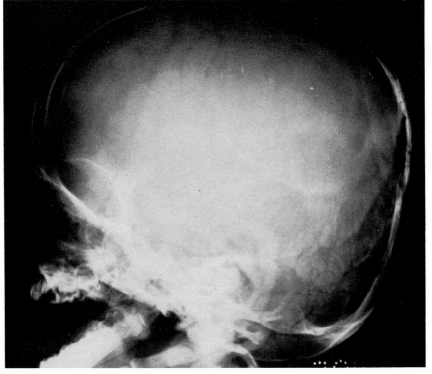

nosis of chondrodystrophia fetalis (achondroplasia) is often made. By x-ray examination (Fig. 8-3B and C and Fig. 8-4) the skull is likely to show a mosaic pattern as a result of the presence of numerous Wormian bones.[280] This mosaic phenomenon was very striking in the case described and illustrated by Vrolik in 1849.[349] (See Fig. 8-1.) (This was the first case to which the name osteogenesis imperfecta was given.) The mosaic pattern persists throughout life. The patient whose skull was studied anatomically by Ruth[280] was variously estimated to be 46 to 55 years old. The diagnosis of OIC has been made at times in utero by means of x-ray films[88,116,130,140,231,254,284] (Fig. 8-5). The bones may be of either the broad (Fig. 8-3) or slender (Fig. 8-5) type but more often are of the former.[110,145,198] In this form, OI is a lethal or sublethal trait. Death is usually the result of intracranial hemorrhage and other injury, since the calvarium offers little protection during delivery and later. Beading of the ribs by calluses is often misinterpreted as a rachitic rosary. Progressive hydrocephalus often occurs in OIC[115,284] (Figs. 8-2 and 8-5B). Hernia is frequent.[115]

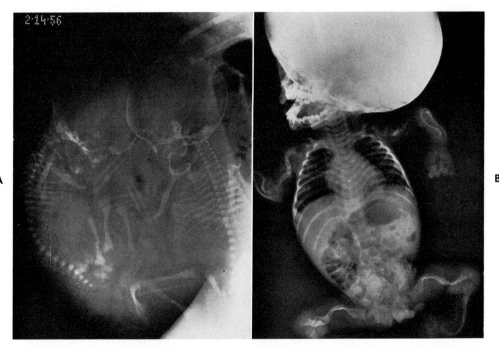

A

B

Fig. 8-5. Presumedly monozygotic twins with osteogenesis imperfecta congenita diagnosed in utero. The mother (M. B., B.C.H. 209850), father, and an only sibling show no stigmata of OI. The mother was admitted to the hospital on Feb. 13, 1956, because of irregular labor pains. The abdomen was very large and tense. **A,** X-ray film revealed twins in breech presentation, facing each other in boxing position. Both fetuses showed multiple fractures in various stages of healing. Delivery was spontaneous. The baby born second lived for thirty-three days. Autopsy revealed the characteristic changes of OI. There was a patent ductus arteriosus and mild hydrocephalus. The first-born twin lived for twenty-seven months. From the first the head was large and soft. Progressive enlargement occurred, so that the proportions indicated in **B** were attained. The sclerae were never impressively blue. Others[108,288,306,358] have described affected twins.

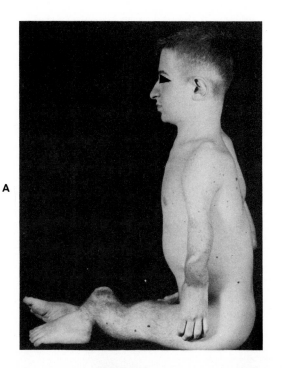

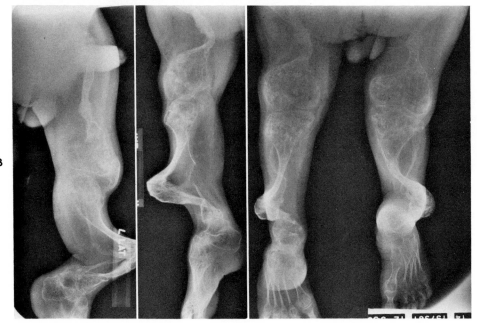

Fig. 8-6. Severely affected 14-year-old male (J. L., 757361). The family history reveals no similar manifestations. Two other children are normal. The father had cleft palate and harelip. The infant was born by vertex presentation. At birth the left thigh showed a swelling, which was later found to be a fracture of the femur with callus formation. The mother estimated that about 107 fractures had occurred, all with minimal trauma at the most. The sclerae are not blue, and there is no deafness. The teeth are small and widely spaced, with translucent enamel. The entire body is covered with nevi, but there were no palpable subcutaneous neurofibromata and no definite café-au-lait spots. The skeletal deformity is adequately described by the photographs and the x-ray films. Calcium, phosphorus, and acid phosphatase of serum were normal. The alkaline phosphatase was 13.7 Bodansky units. Multiple osteotomies, with stabilization by means of metal plates and medullary bars, were performed. **A,** General view. **B,** Anteroposterior view of both legs. **C,** Lateral view of both legs.

Because of the poorly ossified calvarium and also perhaps the proneness to bleeding, intracranial hemorrhage often occurs during delivery. (The association of OI and panhypopituitarism, described later, may have its basis in hemorrhage in, or other damage to, the hypothalamus and/or pituitary during delivery.) Because of the soft bones of the thoracic cage, "flail chest" is frequently the basis for severe, often lethal, respiratory embarrassment in the neonate.

In OIT, the triviality of the trauma that may cause fracture is well known: fracture of the forearm in whittling or throwing a chip, of the phalanges in writing, of the femora when another person sits on the patient's lap[319] or when the patient stretches out in bed. Apert[9] called these patients "les hommes de verre." In one family severely affected children were referred to, appropriately, as "china dolls." (R. Y., B.C.H. 143029.)

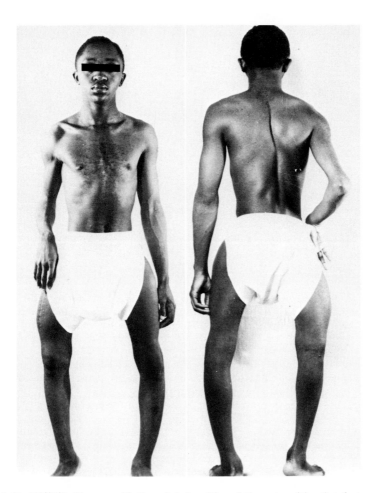

Fig. 8-7. J. B. (459707), 21 years old. Bowed deformities of the extremities, flat feet, and moderately bulging skull are evident. As a result of the bulging skull, the ears point forward and downward. Beginning at the age of 8 years the patient has had approximately thirteen fractures, with no decrease in incidence at puberty. The sclerae are deeply blue.

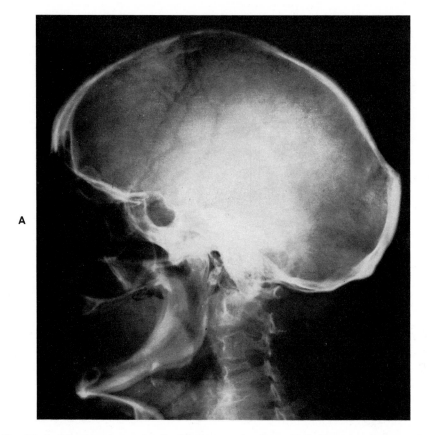

Fig. 8-8. A, "Overhanging occiput" with decrease in the vertical dimension is demonstrated by the skull of this 51-year-old patient (G. I., 587372). She is edentulous. Definite platybasia was judged to be present. The patient has deeply blue sclerae and has had a large number of fractures dating from birth and resulting in marked deformity. She is scarcely taller than a 3-year-old child (42 inches). Deafness of conduction type dates from the age of 13 years following pertussis, and there has been intermittent tinnitus. She has had weakness of the left quadriceps muscle group, with absence of the left knee kick and anesthesia about the left knee, resulting presumably from a compression fracture of the lumbar spine.

Follow-up: The patient demonstrated the occurrence of fractures before puberty and after the menopause. Between these she was able to get about on crutches and was gainfully employed. At 54 years of age she suffered fracture of the neck of the right femur, and at age 59, fracture of the neck of the left femur. She spent the last ten years of her life in a nursing home. Death due to pulmonary emboli occurred at age 69.

Autopsy by Dr. Michael R. Flick showed many bone deformities. The vertebral bodies were markedly flattened in hourglass fashion. Both femoral necks showed ununited fractures with pseudoarthrosis. **B,** Gross section of spine showing thin biconcave vertebral bodies. **C,** X-ray view of same. **D,** X-ray film of specimen of proximal femur showing ununited fracture of the femoral neck with pseudoarthrosis. (**B** to **D** from Milgram, J. W., Flick, M. R., and Engh, C. A.: Osteogenesis imperfecta. A histopathological case report. To be published.)

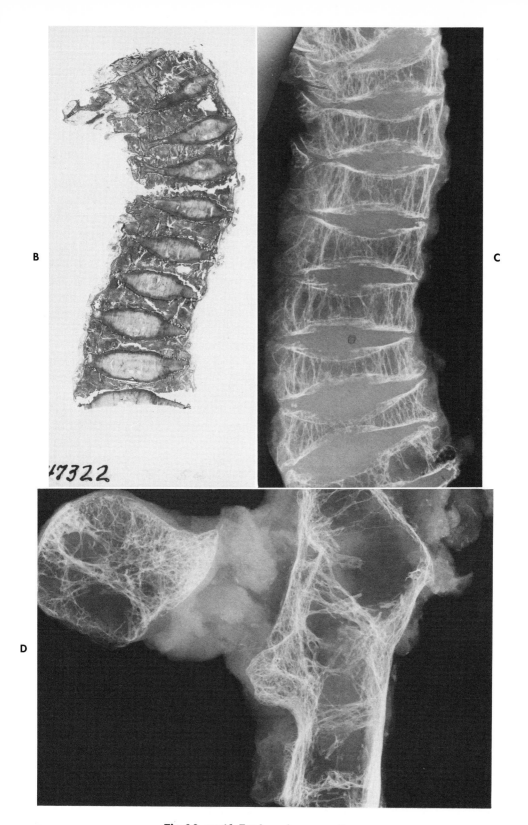

Fig. 8-8, cont'd. For legend see opposite page.

Sudden muscle pulls may fracture bones: the olecranon, for instance, has been pulled off by the triceps muscle in swimming[1] or even less strenuous exercise. Levin pictured an avulsion fracture of the olecranon (Fig. 5 in reference 210). Relatively little pain tends to accompany the fracture, due probably to the facts that there is minimal soft tissue trauma and that the patients become accustomed to the frequent fractures. Occasionally they learn to set their own fractures.[346] The fractures appear to heal with normal speed, but occasionally the callus is so large (Fig. 8-10*A*) as to suggest osteosarcoma.[1,18,107,193,290,294,328,346] (*Callus luxurians* is the term used by some authors.[99]) However, unlike Paget's disease, malignant degeneration is not recognized as a definite complication of this disease, although bone neoplasms have been described.[177,359] Metastases occurred in a case of Jewell and Lofstrom,[177] and Klenerman and associates[197] reported 2 children with OI who died of metastases from osteosarcoma arising in the femur. The dosage of diagnostic x-ray and the interval between radiation exposure and the malignant change were thought to be insufficient to indicate an etiologic relationship. Patients (e.g., J. B. in Fig. 8-7) are sometimes operated on for suspected osteosarcoma.[193] At times overgrowth of bone occurs without evident fracture, and exostosis-like abnormalities develop. (Wide hypertrophic scars occur at the sites of surgical operations such as laparotomy.[291] These may be fundamentally analogous to the hypertrophic callus formation.) Functionally awkward pseudoarthroses may develop. Pseudoarthrosis of the tibia or other bones may be the presenting manifestation[89,192] (S. E., H.L.H. A18674). (Neurofibromatosis[86] is another hereditary disorder in which pseudoarthrosis occurs.) The development of numerous Wormian bones in the occipital area of the skull[280] is a similar phenomenon seen particularly in the "congenital" form of the disease. In the series studied at this hospital, one cannot corroborate, in adults at least, the impression[20] that fracture of the neck of the femur is uncommon as compared with other types of osteoporosis. (See, for example, patient G. I., Fig. 8-8.) There is no sex difference in the severity of the fragilitas ossium.

In general, a decrease in the incidence of fractures is observed after puberty,[53] with, possibly, an increase in incidence after the menopause. The father of one of my patients (C. B., 351637) had numerous fractures up to the age of 16 years but thereafter was well enough that he served in the Navy for several years! Both sexes show the improvement at puberty. Both clinical experience in man[4] and experimental evidence from animals[125] indicate an important role of sex hormones in the normal formation of bone matrix. This hormonal influence may explain in large part the observation cited above; increased vigilance on the part of the patient may be in part responsible for the improvement after puberty.

By x-ray examination all bones have thin cortices, and the long bones usually have a slender shaft, with rather abrupt widening as the epiphysis is approached. There are instances, as Fairbank[106,107] has indicated, in which the shaft of the long bones is thick, and yet others in which a cystic appearance is presented on the x-ray film (Fig. 8-10*B*).

As in other types of osteoporosis, "codfish" or "hourglass" vertebrae develop as a result of the biconcave deformity produced by the pressure of the normally elastic nucleus pulposus on the abnormally soft bone of the vertebral body (Fig.

8-9). Furthermore, "schmorlsches Knötchen," actual herniations of the nucleus pulposus into the substance of the vertebral body, may occur. (Schmorl's nodes derive their eponym from Christian G. Schmorl, who also did a classic study of Paget's disease of bone. See Chapter 12.)

Characteristically the adults have short legs as compared with the upper part of the body. The shortness of the lower extremities is due in part to bowing and to fractures in the shafts of the long bones, but it is also due in considerable degree to interference with growth by multiple microfractures at the epiphyseal ends of the bones. This feature may lead to the misdiagnosis of achondroplastic dwarfism. One patient (Fig. 8-8), who died at age 69, was "scarcely taller than a 3-year-old child." Marked bowing of the legs often results in a scissors-gait. On x-ray examination the femora often have a shepherd's-crook appearance.

Anterior bowing of the tibiae, producing saber shins, is a frequent occurrence. Gross deformities, which resemble somewhat those of Marfan's syndrome, such as kyphoscoliosis, koilosternia (pectus excavatum), and pigeon breast, are not uncommon. Arachnodactyly also has been described by several writers.[98,190,263,294] It must be remembered that arachnodactyly is a symptom, not a disease; that its presence does not indicate the coexistence of Marfan's disease. Unequivocal, or at least less equivocal, manifestations of the latter disease, such as ectopia lentis and involvement of the aortic media, have, with rare exceptions,[25] not been reported with osteogenesis imperfecta.

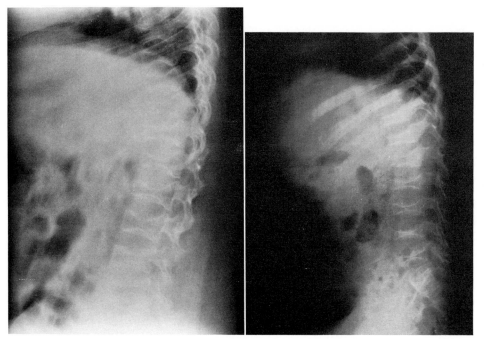

Fig. 8-9. Lateral views of the spine in 2 patients wtih codfish vertebrae. **A,** Patient J. L. L. (Children's Hospital School), 13 years of age. **B,** Patient H. R. (Children's Hospital School), 2 years of age. The marked change, called platyspondyly,[375] is shown.

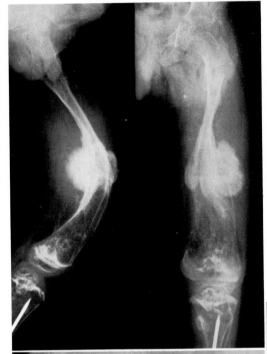

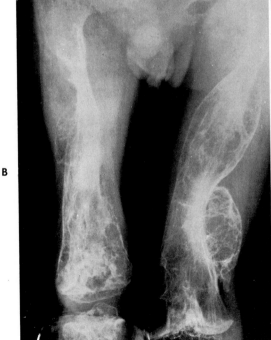

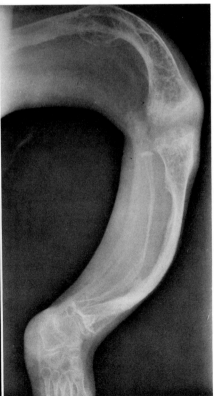

Fig. 8-10. A, Frontal and lateral views of femur showing hypertrophic callus. **B,** Pseudocystic changes. **C,** Marked curvature of a leg due to bowing both in the femur and in the tibia and fibula.

The back is usually round, and the thorax has a characteristic conic or bee-hive shape (see Fig. 8-5*B*). The face is usually triangular, due largely to the bulging calvarium and to faciocranial disproportion. The forehead is broad and domed and the temporal areas are overhanging. The "temporal bulge"[85] and the "overhanging occiput"[98] (Fig. 8-8) are characteristic. The victims have trouble getting hats large enough to fit. As a result of the bulging calvarium, the ears tend to be displaced outward and to point downward. On skull x-ray films the inferosuperior dimension is reduced. This, together with the "occipital overhang," the frontal bossing, and the platybasia that may be present in severe cases, re-sults in a mushroom appearance of the skull on lateral x-ray examination. Apert[9] referred to the skull as "crâne en rebord," and Nielsen[243] used the analogy "soldier's helmet," or "helmet head." "Tam-o'-shanter skull" is yet another fre-quently used simile.[139] In general, as with so many other hereditary disorders, victims of this disease tend to resemble each other closely, even though they are quite unrelated. The facies and skeletal proportions are so characteristic that one can usually recognize the victims from a photograph, a feature useful in pedigree investigations.[294]

Because of pelvic deformity, successful termination of pregnancy may be a serious problem.[180] Fracture of the rami of the pubis during delivery has been described.[88] Severe pelvic deformity with marked *intrusio acetabulorum* is dem-onstrated by Ramser et al.[257]

By x-ray examination the bones are demonstrated to be more radiolucent than normal. If x-ray films are taken at times when no fractures are present, the skeleton may, at the most, be described only as very "porotic."[186] In fact, the x-ray films may show no definite abnormality, and it may be concluded that the findings do not justify the diagnosis of OI. In severe cases the cortex is thin, and gross deformities, such as are shown in Fig. 8-10, are demonstrated. Bone age is proportionate to chronologic age. In adults with OI, Keats[186,187] noted diffuse thickening of the calvarium, with diffuse granular osteoporosis. Levin[209] pointed out excessively large frontal, sphenoid, and mastoid sinuses similar to those in homocystinuria (p. 230; Fig. 4-17*N*). Marked protrusio acetabuli—projection of the acetabulum and head of the femur into the pelvis—results from the soft state of the bones.[257]

The joints, typically, are excessively mobile[31,144,158,294] in this condition, just as in the Marfan syndrome and the Ehlers-Danlos syndrome. Both OI and E-D were thought to be present in one case.[34] It is said[294] that this characteristic is at times so striking that the subject can perform as a contortionist. The basis is in part the presence of weak, stretched tendons and joint capsules and in part the deformity and maladaptation of the bony surfaces of the joints. In one re-ported case,[41] the patient won prizes as a gymnast; his repertoire included the ability to put his feet into his trouser pockets. Pseudoarthrosis may have been present. Key[191] described the Achilles tendon in one patient as, grossly, the "diameter of a lead pencil (0.6 cm.) and translucent in appearance, there being a striking absence of the dense white fibrous tissue usually seen." From the standpoint of histology and of pathologic involvement in a number of diseases, the sclera bears many resemblances to tendon.[120]

Rupture of the inferior patellar tendon may follow exertion with more force-ful quadriceps activity than usual.[220,319] This accident occurred in at least 4 patients in our series (E. Z., H.L.H. 81588; K. Y., J.H.H. 594806; R. C., U.M.H. 40485; E. R., J.H.H. 602544). Habitual dislocation of joints[19,25,51,165,323,334] or of the patella,[118] pes planus, and pseudoclubfoot[294] are frequent occurrences. In at least 2 patients (H.L.H. 19845; A94292) bilateral clubfoot was thought to be present at birth. The reason for confusion is evident from Fig. 8-2. The father of one of our patients (J. B., 541962), himself a victim of OI, has suffered from recurrent dislocation of the shoulder. The articular laxity probably exposes the victim to falls, which are so likely to result in fracture.

Wyllie and Schlesinger[372] reported 2 cases in children whose mothers con-

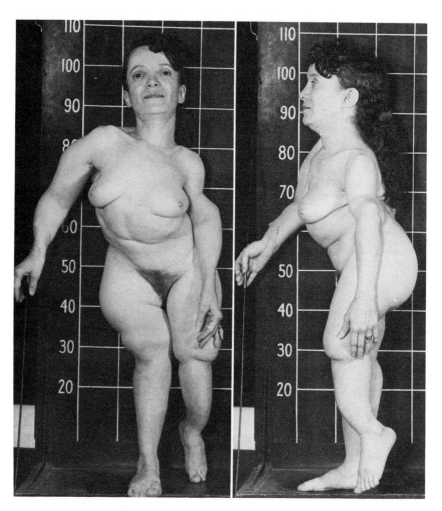

Fig. 8-11. Osteogenesis imperfecta in K. C. (673043), 35 years of age. Innumerable fractures have occurred, the first having been recognized at the age of 9 months. The sclerae are blue; hearing is intact. The patient is scarcely taller than a 4-year-old child. She has never walked and is carried about by a husky female friend. There are pseudoarthroses of the left humerus and left tibia. Of two pregnancies, one was terminated for therapeutic reasons and the other ended in spontaneous abortion. (From McKusick, V. A.: Bull. N. Y. Acad. Med. 35:143, 1959.)

sulted them because of the child's tardiness in walking. No fractures had occurred; at least, none had been recognized. The presenting complaint, not an unusual one for OI, was apparently due to difficulty in fixing the joints for walking. The diagnosis of OI was based on the occurrence of clear cases in the family and of supporting radiologic changes in the patients. In one of our patients (R. F., J.H.H. 194765) there was such loose-jointedness and tardiness in walking and sitting that flaccid diplegia was suspected for a time.

As in the Marfan syndrome, muscular hypotonia and underdevelopment have been emphasized by several writers.[12,13,82] As in the Marfan syndrome, these features are quite clearly secondary to the anomalies of the tendons and joints and to general debility with reduced muscular activity. The fibrous skeleton of the muscles may be defective, but there is no evidence that the muscle cell itself is at fault. At times, in children (N. T., A46910), enlargement and weakness of the limbs have suggested pseudohypertropic muscular dystrophy.

Scoliosis may develop as a result of laxity of ligaments, as well as of vertebral osteoporosis (Fig. 8-11). The spinal deformity is often extreme. Back pain is frequent in these patients.

Hernia occurs with high incidence in these patients (see pedigree 603 in reference 26), as with most other hereditary connective tissue disorders under discussion, except pseudoxanthoma elasticum. The infant with OIC shown in Fig. 8-3 clearly demonstrates the combination of multiple fractures and bilateral scrotal hernias. Cryptorchidism may occur in the males, in association with inguinal hernia (E. J. W., S.B.G. 6914).

The eye. Blue sclerae constitute the ocular hallmark of this syndrome. The color of the sclera is described at times as robin's egg blue and at times as slate blue. "Wedgwood blue" is another vivid description. Of the manifestations of this disease, the presence of blue sclerae is the most frequent. Occasionally blue sclerae are absent in unmistakable instances of the syndrome, which is not surprising, since a high degree of variability in severity (expressivity) of this manifestation is to be expected, and overlapping with the curve of normal distribution is likely to occur. Impressively blue sclerae are not infrequently encountered in persons free from all other stigmata of this syndrome.

Vaughan[343] noted an increase in the blueness of the sclerae in a case of OI, with episodes of stress such as fractures. This increase as well as the declining frequency of fractures at puberty (and possible increase after the menopause), may represent an interaction of hormonal effects with the hereditary disorder of connective tissue.

Often the part of the sclera immediately surrounding the cornea is whiter, resulting in the so-called "Saturn's ring." There is probably some increased risk of traumatic perforation of the sclera, a complication that occurred in Buchanan's historic case.[55]

Embryotoxon, a congenital opacity in the periphery of the cornea, sometimes called arcus juvenilis, is very frequent.[49,252,271,339,367] By slit-lamp examination, the cornea is demonstrated to be measurably thinner than normal.[224,367] Hypermetropia appears to be significantly frequent.[1,5,79,323,326] Chorioretinitis, probably inherited independently, was reported by Colden.[77]

Other clinical manifestations probably closely related to the same defect of scleral connective tissue are keratoconus[13,25,55,92] megalocornea,[92] and maculae corneae.[348] Keratoconus was present in one of our patients (E. Z., H.L.H. 81588). Behr's patient[25] and a patient of Remigio and Grinvalsky[262] had ectopia lentis. Premature arcus senilis is described.[348] However, this may have been merely the embryotoxon just mentioned. In 2 cases observed at this hospital[220] glaucoma has been present. In one, it was discovered soon after birth (R. F., 194765) and has been termed congenital; in the other (H. J., 428403), the right eye was rendered blind (phthisis bulbi), presumably by glaucoma, at the age of about 20 years, and the other eye later was affected by so-called chronic, wide-angle glaucoma. There are a few reports of associated glaucoma in the literature.[334,361]

The skin. The skin in this condition is characteristically thin and translucent. It may resemble prematurely the atrophic skin of the aged. Healing of skin wounds has been found, by study of surgical incisions in these patients, to result in wider scars than usual.[281] Subcutaneous hemorrhages* tend to occur after minor injuries,[66] and tests of capillary fragility may be positive.[294,303] Macular atrophy of the skin is described by Blegvad and Haxthausen.[39] This may be comparable to the spotty blueness of the sclera in some instances.[348]

Biebl and Streitmann[33] described elastosis perforans in a 16-year-old male with OI. Members of three generations of his family were affected with OI. Reed and Pidgeon,[259] and others,[195,196,228,261] also observed this skin change in OI. Elastosis perforans has been observed in the Marfan syndrome (p. 146), the Ehlers-Danlos syndrome (p. 309), and pseudoxanthoma elasticum (p. 483), as well as in mongolism.

The ear.[47,49] Deafness is the least constant of the major features of OI.[63] Although the histologic patterns may be distinct, the clinical[36,40,51,74,114,281,326,334,341] pattern of the deafness which accompanies this syndrome differs in no respect from that of otosclerosis. Stenvers[322] demonstrated that characteristic sclerosis of the petrous portion of the temporal bone can be detected radiologically even before the impairment of hearing has its onset; also, of course, these changes may be present but not so located as to cause deafness. Deafness may have its onset in the teens; often it begins during pregnancy.[113,294] In Nager's patient,[239] hearing loss had its onset at the age of 9 years. As with otosclerosis of other origin, two types, a common stapes-ankylosing variety and a rarer cochlear type, have been described alone or in combination. Therefore, the hearing loss may be either of the conduction type or of the nerve type.[119] Fenestration operation[176] has been performed in 2 patients, with good results, by Shambaugh,[297] and in one, with indifferent results, by Watkyn-Thomas.[352] Shea[299] performed stapedectomy in 6 patients, and Patterson and Stone[249] in 7 patients (8 ears); the results were good in both series. (Nager[240a] concludes, however, that long-term results are not satisfactory, recurrence being the rule.) Patterson and Stone concluded that the conductive hearing loss was secondary in part to fracture or absorption, or both, of the stapedial crura and in part to footplate fixation caused by an immature-appearing, soft, chalky, vascular bone that seemed to be quite different from the typical otosclerotic bone. These surgeons never found this bone as hard as in ordinary otosclerosis. As with other types of otosclerosis, middle ear infection aggravates the hearing loss. There has been described[322] an interesting blueness of the tympanic membrane, analogous to the blue sclerae as

---

*See discussion of hemorrhagic disease in OI, p. 414.

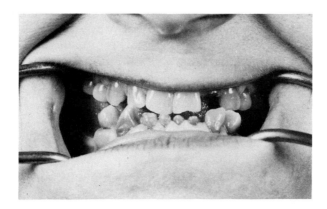

Fig. 8-12. Teeth in M. W., 32-year-old female with fragilitas ossium, blue sclerae, and mild deafness. One of her 2 children (D. W., 736452) has OI. However, 5 sibs, both parents, and all other relatives are apparently unaffected. The stunting and discoloration of the lower incisor teeth are well demonstrated.

far as indicating thinness of the structure is concerned. The patient may complain of almost constant tinnitus for long periods and of attacks of vertigo. Labyrinthine disease uncomplicated by deafness has been described.[119,348] Leicher and Haas[207] described patients who had no dizziness and only mild difficulty walking in the dark, but little or no response to vestibule-stimulating maneuvers.

The teeth. The teeth in OI often have an abnormal amber, yellowish brown, or translucent bluish gray coloration.[342] Both deciduous and permanent teeth may show this peculiarity. Witkop[368] states that the teeth which erupt first, e.g., the lower incisors, are the ones most affected (Fig. 8-12). On x-ray examination the teeth are likely to show no pulp canal. Often during drilling, the patient feels no pain, only vibration. One patient (S. W., 782036) stated that although his teeth had always been embarrassingly yellow, they were unusually hard to drilling. Inspection revealed a good state of repair. Although most of each tooth was yellowish, the tip of each incisor was slightly translucent and blue. The lamina dura, as in acquired types of osteoporosis, remains intact. The enamel is thought to be fundamentally normal,[24] and the abnormality is thought to reside in the dentine. Thus Roberts and Schour[267] were prompted to suggest the name *dentinogenesis imperfecta** for the dental aspect of this disease rather than the terms *hereditary opalescent dentine* or *hereditary hypoplasia of the dentine,* which had been used before. For the disorder of the teeth which resembles that in OI but has no extradental manifestations, Rao and Witkop[258] prefer the term "opalescent dentin" (called hereafter OD); the opalescent character of the OD tooth is particularly evident in transmitted light. The brownish or bluish coloration comes from blood (Fig. 8-12). In OD the teeth are uniformly affected. On the other hand, in OI some teeth may be spared, and in some patients all teeth are spared, something that

---

**Odontogenesis imperfecta* is a less specific term, inasmuch as the first portion refers to both enamel and dentine.

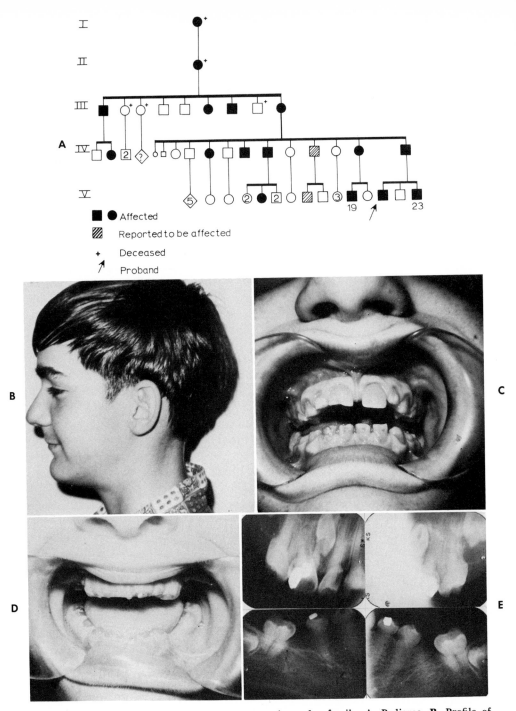

Fig. 8-13. Dentinogenesis imperfecta in five generations of a family. **A,** Pedigree. **B,** Profile of R. E., the proband, 14 years old (see arrow in **A**), showing decreased vertical occlusive dimension of face. The sclerae were normally white. Hearing was acute. There had been no fractures. As shown in **C,** both the permanent and the deciduous teeth showed discoloration and excessive attrition. The changes were not as extreme, however, as those in his cousin, C. G., 8 years old, who showed, **D,** complete loss of crowns and discoloration of remaining portions of the teeth. X-ray views of the teeth of R. E. showed, **E,** diminished or absent pulp chambers, with short roots and bulbous crowns, and submersion of the second upper bicuspids. (Courtesy Ronald J. Jorgenson, D.D.S., Baltimore.)

never occurs in OD. Wide variability in the extent of dental involvement is noted even in the same family with OI. Further, Witkop[369] finds a possibly pathognomonic histologic change in the teeth in OI, whether the teeth are clinically affected or not. This change consists of what he calls "trapped capillary loops." These loops are never seen in OD but are present in the OI tooth even when the tubules are regularly arranged.

The root canals and pulp chambers in OD and in the OI tooth tend to become obliterated (Fig. 8-13). The enamel, although not primarily affected, fractures or chips off because of the defective underpinning of dentin. Caries tends to be less frequent in these teeth. Because of the soft dentin the tooth is self-cleaning to some extent through the wearing off of the carious area. The teeth are soft and wear down, sometimes to the gum margin. Although qualitatively the same, the tooth involvement in OI is never as marked as in many cases of OD.

Witkop's experience with opalescent dentin extends to over 1000 personally examined examples of the disorder. The lesser variability in expression of OD than is seen in the dental involvement of OI is probably reflected by the fact that Witkop[369] found no instance of a skipped generation among 251 three-generation transmissions personally examined.

Opalescent dentin is called Capdepont teeth in the continental literature.[64] Witkop[370] found a frequency of about 1 in 8000 in Michigan, but in that state and elsewhere, nonrandomness in the distribution is striking. In one area of Michigan the frequency was about 1 in 500 persons, and in a biracial isolate of southern Maryland, 5.7% of 5128 persons were affected. The trait has never been observed in Africans (cases in American Negroes could be traced to European ancestors), and it must be very rare in Orientals, only one family, Japanese, having been observed in which there was no known European ancestry.[258]

Opalescent dentin occurring in the northern part of the United States can be traced mainly to a passenger on the *Mayflower* born in 1607. In the Middle Atlantic States, families trace their ancestry to an early Pennsylvania settler from southern Germany. Other families, including those in the biracial isolate mentioned, trace back to a sea captain from Liverpool who settled in southern Maryland in 1732. He was said to trace descent from, or at least relationship to, a butler of Henry II of England; Butler was the surname of the southern Maryland progenitor.

The most extensively investigated genealogies have been English, French, Irish, Dutch, German, Danish, Swedish, and Italian. The disorder occurs in fairly high frequency in Romania, leading Rao and Witkop[258] to suggest that these families and the kindreds of northwestern Europe may have had common ancestry in Roman times.

Internal manifestations. As for cardiovascular involvement, Sundberg[332] and Johansson[179] have described calcification of large peripheral arteries in victims of OIC. In one of our cases of OIC (557774; aut. 22803) in which there was neonatal death, necropsy revealed calcification of pulmonary and cerebral arteries. Arteries in the limbs were not studied histologically. Although Bauer[21] and Kaul[185] described changes in the connective tissue elements of the arterial wall, others have not been impressed with these changes. Lobeck,[212] Colden,[77] and Voorhoeve[348] described premature arteriosclerosis. Congenital heart disease was present in one patient. Hass[151] described heart disease in several members of a kinship. From the descriptions of one of the members of that pedigree, rheumatic heart disease seems to have been present in that individual. In general, the heart disease was probably unrelated to the OI. Severe aortic regurgitation of obscure etiology was present in one patient with OI seen at The Johns Hopkins Hospital when he was 16 years old (G. S., J.H.H. U45942). Criscitiello and colleagues[83] described 2 OI patients, 43 and 47 years old, with dilatation of the aortic root and aortic regurgitation. A third OI patient, 50 years old, had a bicuspid

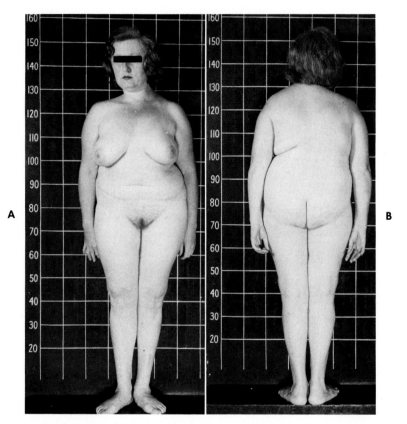

Fig. 8-14. J. G. (149692), 43 years old. In **A**, note the bulging calvarium with triangular facies. Flat feet and kyphoscoliosis are also evident in **A** and **B**. The x-ray film in **C** reveals the complex spinal deformity present in this patient. The bones are more radiolucent than is normal. The sclerae are deeply blue. Deafness has been present since at least the age of 25 years, and tinnitus has often been distressing. Scoliosis was first noted at the age of 13 years, and since the age of 16 years back pain has been a major complaint. The patient is, in general, loose-jointed with flat feet; the head of the humerus was dislocated on one occasion when she was thrown from a bicycle at the age of 7 years. A ganglion on the right wrist was described at one time. X-ray film of the skull shows characteristic decrease in the vertical dimension. A diastolic murmur at the left sternal border remains unexplained. An amazing feature of this case of undoubted osteogenesis imperfecta is the fact that *no* fractures have occurred in spite of appreciable trauma on several occasions. Follow-up (1971; 58 years of age): the patient had developed signs of "floppy mitral valve" (p. 128). The gallbladder, containing a large number of stones, was successfully removed.

aortic valve, fenestration of the pulmonic valve, and an aneurysm of the anterior leaflet of the mitral valve. Browell and Drake[52] described aortic stenosis and regurgitation in a 27-year-old woman with OI, but the presence of valvular cacification and a history of scarlet fever make a more common cause of aortic valve disease likely. Carey and associates[65] described aortic regurgitation in a man who had typical triad of OI and who died at the age of 32 years.

K. Y. (J.H.H. 594806), who has familial OI and has been under observation here all his life, developed aortic regurgitation at age 30 years[155a] and was found to have dilatation of the first part of the aorta. Scherlis[284a] has recent experience with two cases of aortic and mitral valve disease in association with osteogenesis imperfecta.

The following case of aortic regurgitation in OI has been studied by Galton[124]:

Case 1. R. H. L. (J.H.H. 1462391), a white male communications technologist, was born in 1929. During childhood he sustained "torn muscles" on several occasions and at the age of 31 years ruptured his Achilles tendon. However, he never fractured a bone. Although the patient's parents had no stigmata of OI, a sister and a cousin allegedly had blue sclerae, and all 3 of his children have unequivocal OI.

The patient has been known to have had a heart murmur since childhood. At the age of 41 years he noticed increasing dyspnea on exertion and increasingly easy fatigability. At age 42 aortic regurgitation and congestive heart failure were discovered. Aortograms showed dilatation of the aortic root and severe aortic regurgitation. In 1971 the aortic valve was replaced

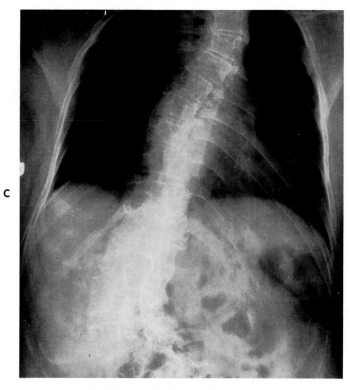

Fig. 8-14, cont'd. For legend see opposite page.

with a prosthetic valve. At operation the aortic regurgitation was found to be the result of dilatation of the aortic ring, with enlargement and thinning of the aortic cusps. Grossly and histologically no sign of acquired, i.e., rheumatic, disease was found.

Examination (April, 1972) showed height of 64¾ inches. The sclerae were blue, and all joints hypermobile. The heart sounds were dominated by those of the prosthetic valve. There was no diastolic murmur.

Minimal generalized osteoporosis was demonstrated by skeletal x-ray films.

We recently observed a 38-year-old man (R. R., 1410139) with severe classic OI and combined aortic and mitral regurgitation. No basis for his valvular defect, other than the connective tissue disorder, was evident. He died from subacute bacterial endocarditis; autopsy was not performed. Relevant here, are the histologic changes which have been observed in the valves as well as in the aortic tunica media.[262]

Heckman and Steinberg[153] described a 27-year-old man with osteogenesis imperfecta and congenital mitral regurgitation. In one of my patients (J. G., 149692), with severe S-type rotary scoliosis (Fig. 8-14), a faint early diastolic murmur was heard at the left sternal border over a period of several years. Subsequently, under observation, a loud late systolic semimusical murmur, introduced by a click and loudest at the apex, has developed. The auscultatory characteristics are those of the "floppy mitral valve" (p. 128). It is likely that the basophilic mucoid changes described histologically in the heart valves[262] are responsible for the clinical findings in these patients.

Severe spinal deformity may be followed by kyphoscoliotic cor pulmonale (e.g., C. B., 242806).

There are no pathognomonic chemical changes in the blood. Significant abnormalities of calcium and phosphorus do not occur. Alkaline phosphatase activity[310] is often increased as a result of multiple healing fractures. We have been unable to corroborate the report[127] that serum acid phosphatase activity is significantly increased in this disease. Jacobsen and colleagues[174] and Ginsberg[132] likewise found normal levels of serum acid phosphatase.

Siegel and co-workers[303] have described a 25-year-old man with OI and hemorrhagic diathesis manifested by epistaxes, hemoptyses, easy bruisability, and prolonged bleeding time. The Rumpel-Leede test was positive. A defect of the platelet was demonstrated by means of the thromboplastin generation test. There were multiple cases of OI in the family, but the only one available for study, a sister, did not show the abnormality. The authors suggested that the hemorrhagic diathesis was of the type described by Glanzmann[135] in 1918 as thrombasthenia. The cause of the capillary fragility was not clear, It was corrected by cortisone; however, this can be a nonspecific effect. Gautier and Guinard-Daniol[126] described a 13½-month-old patient with OI in whom defective clot retraction was demonstrated. The mother had blue sclerae with bone disease, abnormal prothrombin consumption test, and impaired clot retraction. The last two tests showed impairment in the father, also. Siegel and co-workers[303] suggest that these two mesenchymal defects (OI and platelet defect) are related and not simply coincidental.

Neurologic symptoms, particularly those of platybasia and of spinal cord compression, occur occasionally but are usually submerged by the other types of incapacitation from which these patients suffer. Backache and leg pains, which may have an element of nerve root compression in their causation, are of frequent occurrence. Neurologic deficits attributable to nerve root compression are less frequent. As with idiopathic varieties of platybasia (basilar impression), as well as that due to other bone-softening diseases such as Paget's disease, rickets, hyperparathyroidism, and sarcoid, four types of neurologic involvement should be sought[246]: (1) internal hydrocephalus; (2) bilateral, progressive cerebellar disturbance; (3) interference with the function of the lower cranial nerves; and (4) signs of spinal cord compression at the level of the foramen magnum. The impingement of the odontoid process of the axis on the brain stem is responsible for many of these manifestations. (Basilar impression in OI is discussed in references 167 and 333.)

Two methods are used to detect platybasia radiologically: Chamberlain's line (from the posterior end of the hard palate to the posterior lip of the foramen magnum) normally lies above the entirety of the cervical spine.[68] Such is not the case in platybasia. According to Bull's index,[56] the plane of the axis is normally parallel to that of the hard palate, whereas, in platybasia, the two planes make an acute angle with each other.

Bell[26] pictures the skeleton of a 12-year-old boy with marked skeletal changes of OI and with hydrocephalus. The skeleton is in the museum of the Royal College of Surgeons in London. Hydrocephalus developed in several of our patients with osteogenesis imperfecta congenita. (See Figs. 8-2 and 8-5B.)

Occasionally patients with OI have retarded intellect (e.g., S. V., H.L.H. 75237; R. F., 194765). Although arrested hydrocephalus may be the basis in some cases, others probably represent mere coincidence of OI and mental retardation on another basis. Most patients are of normal intelligence. Persons with OI known to me are a Ph.D. biochemist and a physician-anatomist.

Pregnancy has been reported in a number of women severely dwarfed and deformed as a result of OI.[27,57,94] Evans[103] reported the delivery by cesarean section of a normal infant from a woman with a supine height of only 27 inches. The patient shown in Fig. 8-11 was twice pregnant.

In severely affected women, pregnancy is not to be encouraged, not only because of the 50% chance of the child's being affected, but also because of adverse effects of the pregnant and the parturient[244] state on the skeleton. Deafness from otosclerosis often begins or is aggravated during pregnancy. (Some, like Nager,[240] doubt a relationship, however.) Because of the pelvic deformities of the disease, delivery may be mechanically very difficult.[88] One patient[220] has fractured her coccyx with each of the deliveries. There is a strikingly high incidence of breech presentation in cases of infants with OIC born of normal mothers.

Because of inactivity it is easy for victims of this disease to become obese. Obviously, obesity is to be avoided. In young patients, Fröhlich's syndrome is sometimes suspected without basis.

In OI, malformations of conventional type probably have no increased frequency. Navani and Sarzin,[242] in the autopsy of one infant with OI diagnosed antenatally, found atresia of the second part of the duodenum and wide foramen ovale and, in a second infant, a large atrial septal defect.

The wide variability in severity of OI, permitting long survival in some cases, is well illustrated by the 95-year-old woman reported by Stool and Sullivan,[327] by the 58-year-old man shown in Fig. 8-15, and by the severely deformed 54-year-old man reported by Scherr.[285]

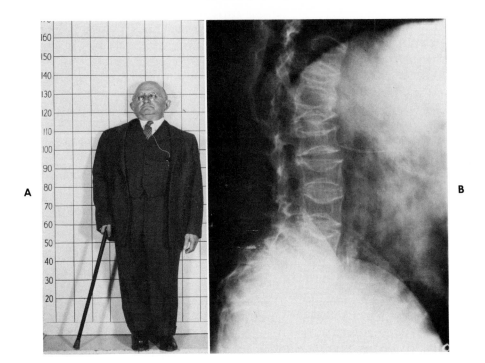

Fig. 8-15. I. L. (455357), white male born in 1902, was apparently a sporadic case of osteogenesis imperfecta. He was first seen at The Johns Hopkins Hospital for a fracture at 8 years of age. He had numerous fractures, necessitating admission thereafter. The diagnosis of OI was first made at the age of 21 years (1923). The last fracture occurred in 1932 (30 years of age). At the age of 45 years a bout of acute cholecystitis requiring cholecystectomy was withstood in a normal manner. Hypertension was first discovered then. Hearing defect was first noted in 1951 and a hearing aid was applied. The patient died of coronary occlusion at the age of 60 years. Examination in 1961 showed blue sclerae, deafness, characteristically shaped skull with overhang above the ears, and short stature, **A.** Profound osteoporosis of the spine was demonstrated, **B.**

A low frequency of malignancy in patients with OI has been claimed[216,276] but the evidence seems flimsy. In a family with OI in three generations, Gilchrist and Shore[129] described both acute lymphocytic leukemia and OI in 2 sisters. The association was probably coincidental.

Osteogenesis imperfecta in association with osteopoikilosis (p. 706) has been reported at least twice.[260] Association with arthrogryposis multiplex congenita has also been described.[298]

I have seen 2 unrelated males who have the combination of osteogenesis

Fig. 8-16. Osteogenesis imperfecta and panhypopituitarism. **A** to **C,** Overall appearance. Short trunk with kyphoscoliosis and chest deformity are results of OI. The short stature is the result of both OI and hypopituitarism. **D** and **E,** Face and head. The configuration of the head (occipital overhang, temporal bulge, triangular face, low-set and down-pointing ears), as well as the blue sclerae and embryotoxon, are typical of OI. The wrinkled, thickened skin is typical of hypopituitarism.

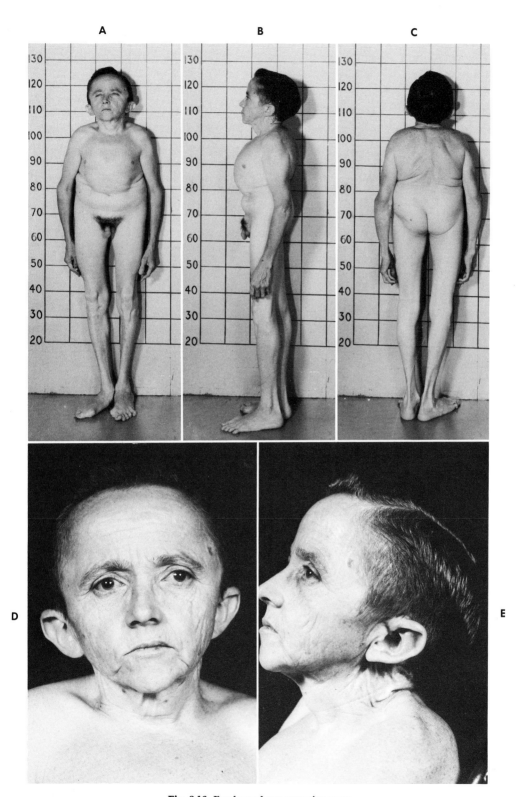

Fig. 8-16. For legend see opposite page.

imperfecta and panhypopituitarism. One of them is described in detail below. The association would seem more than coincidental. The only explanation that seem plausible is that the connective tissue defect permitted damage to the hypothalamopituitary axis at the time of birth. Intracranial hemorrhage is a hazard of birth in OI.

Case 2. R. F. S. (J.H.H. 1298366), born in 1927, was the product of an uncomplicated gestation and a breech delivery. Dislocation of the left knee, requiring casting, was present at birth. Weight was 6½ pounds, and length was 19 inches. The mother was 29 and the father was 36 years old. They denied blood relationship, being of different ethnic background. Two older brothers and a younger sister are normal and have normal offspring. No dwarfism, brittle bones, or other manifestations of OI were known in the family.

The patient was noted to be smaller than his peers when he entered school, and growth appeared to cease at the age of 16 years. No secondary sexual characteristics developed until he was 33 years of age, when scant pubic and axillary hair appeared; his genitalia remained infantile and he had no libido. In 1960 his physician prescribed thyroid, cortisone, and testosterone after finding the epiphyses unfused by x-ray examination. On that regimen he became more robust, vigorous, and energetic and enjoyed enlargement of the penis, with erections and emissions. The voice deepened only slightly, however, and no beard developed.

As a child the patient had loose-jointedness, which diminished as he became older, although he continued to have occasional minor subluxation in the shoulders or elbows. He never broke a bone, however, except for fractures of the left fourth and fifth fingers sustained in a childhood accident.

Examination (1968) showed a very small man with clinical features of both OI and panhypopituitarism (Fig. 8-16A to C). His height was 127.1 cm., span 138 cm., and US/LS value 0.73.

Signs of OI included relatively long, thin extremities with disproportionate dwarfism, oval head with marked bitemporal bulging and triangular face, protruding and downward-directed ears, slate-blue sclerae (Fig. 8-16D and E), short vertebral column including the neck, severe scoliosis, barrel chest with flared lower margins resting on the iliac crests, hyperextensible fingers, and mild hearing loss.

X-ray studies showed marked osteoporosis throughout the skeleton. The spine showed generalized platyspondyly and scoliosis. The bones of the limbs were thin relative to their lengths. No fractures were seen. The epiphyses were fused. Skull x-ray films showed osteoporosis, multiple Wormian bones, a normal sella turcica, and striking basilar invagination. Dental x-ray films showed partial obliteration of the pulp chambers of the molars and short, blunted roots, consistent with dentinogenesis imperfecta.

Signs of hypopituitarism included, in addition to his short stature, thickened, wrinkled, soft skin of the face, lack of beard and temporal hair recession, high-pitched voice, small penis, small left testis with right testis not identified, and scanty body hair. Basal plasma levels of growth hormone were zero, and no hormone was detectable after insulin hypoglycemia or arginine infusion.

Case 3. The second case[229] concerned a 19-year-old high school senior who sustained his first fractures in utero and had had many since that time. He was 99 cm. (39 inches) tall. The presence of both OI and hypopituitarism was indicated by clinical studies and was well substantiated by laboratory investigations.

Summary of clinical manifestations. Bell[26] provides entirely credible figures for the incidence of the several manifestations: among adult individuals "with blue sclerotics approximately 60% have an associated liability to fracture, approximately 60% have an associated otosclerosis, and 44% suffer from all three defects."

Prevalence and inheritance

Among the nine disorders under principal discussion in this book, osteogenesis imperfecta vies with the Marfan syndrome for first place as to incidence.

It was relatively easy to accumulate more than a hundred apparently unrelated propositi for purposes of this study.* Between 1920 and 1940, forty cases of OI were seen at the Mayo Clinic.[53] Of these patients, 11 had a story of the disease in other members of the family. Almost half of those with positive family histories had otosclerosis, whereas deafness occurred in only about one sixth of those without a positive family history, suggesting perhaps that the nonfamilial cases suffered from some other form of osteoporosis, such as idiopathic juvenile osteoporosis (p. 433).

There is no peculiar racial distribution of OI, cases having been described in Jews[220] and American Negroes,[137,220,351] and in natives of Japan,[184,241] China,[73] India,[150] Egypt,[12,13] and Russia,[350] as well as all the western European countries.

The evidence is overwhelming that OI is usually inherited as an autosomal dominant. Bell[26] found such to be the case for blue sclerae in 73 kinships with a total of 463 affected persons. In an analysis of 89 families with 1,000 individuals, of whom 515 were affected, Fuss[123] demonstrated autosomal dominance for the syndrome of bone fragility and blue sclerae. One of the best-studied pedigrees is that of a family of the eastern shore of Maryland, reported by Hills and McLanahan.[159] Twenty-seven of 51 members of five generations were affected. A number of other pedigrees with affected persons in five successive generations have been published. Scores of "dominant" pedigrees are on record.[80,155,178,189,264,265]

Seedroff,[294] after studying 55 kinships with 180 affected individuals, constructed a complicated schema based on the theories that each component of the syndrome is the result of a separate gene and that three separate genes control the bone fragility, with mutation in one, two, or three being responsible, respectively, for OIT levis, OIT gravis, and OIC. This complex schema is untenable because of the arguments against a multiple-gene basis of hereditary syndromes (Chapter 1) and because of the probability, on clinical and histopathologic grounds, that the three arbitrarily designated states are in fact different grades of severity of the same disorder of connective tissue.

Freda and co-workers[115] estimated the frequency of OIC to be about 1 in 40,000 births and quoted others as estimating the frequency as less than 1 in 60,000 births.

There have been advocates for the view that there is an entity called osteopsathyrosis idiopathica of Lobstein that is distinct from the triad of blue sclerae, deafness, and fragilitas ossium.[160,211] Some permit deafness in patients of the presumably distinct osteopsathyrosis group but insist that a main differentiating feature is the absence of blue sclerae. Holcomb[160] wrote as follows: "In the Davis family, whose history I have investigated, the tendency to break bones with abnormal frequency, especially in childhood, occurred in a number of persons in five generations of the family, but in no case was there the slightest indication of the blue sclera or progressive deafness."† This type of evidence does not necessarily indicate that a separate entity is involved, since it is clear that in a given family the individual components of a syndrome may display consider-

---

*Patients from Baltimore or Maryland and patients who have been seen at some time at The Johns Hopkins Hospital have been reported in several previous publications.[110 to 112,159,277,305]
†From Holcomb, D. Y.: J. Hered. **22:**105, 1931.

able independence in penetrance and expressivity. An alternative possibility is the existence of multiple alleles.

Seriki[296] reported 2 cases of like-sex twins, only one of whom had OIC. In each case 1 parent had blue sclerae, and in 1 case the parent was also short, with a relatively large head. Levin[209] described dizygotic twins discordant for OIC, in whom the diagnosis was made antenatally by a striking contrast in the state of skeletal calcification. Twins, both of whom were affected by OIC, have also been described.[108,258,288] One of the reports[288] is of further note because the father had blue sclerae and deafness but no apparent fragility of the bones; support for the identity of OIC and OIT is therefore provided. Others[150,274] have reported families in which one or more members were affected by the congenital form of OI and other members by the late form. Bierring[35] described OIC in mother and daughter.

"Skipped generations" have been described[80,160,376] in well-studied families. Because of the exceedingly wide range of expressivity, it is not surprising if manifestations in fundamentally affected persons are at times too mild to be recognized clinically. Smårs and associates[308,309] described an interesting family (Fig. 8-17) in which 4 of 6 children were affected but both parents could pass as unaffected. One of the affected children was proved by blood group data to be illegitimate, making recessive inheritance unlikely and also suggesting that the mother was heterozygous. In fact, the mother had had one fracture from falling from a bicycle and was slightly deaf in one ear.

Even with the excellent system for indexing hereditary diseases in Denmark, Seedorff[294] concluded that one is not justified in attempting to calculate the mutation rate for this anomaly. Furthermore, Seedorff could find no conclusive evidence that the parents in sporadic cases of osteogenesis imperfecta tend to be older, as is the case in achondroplasia.[234] In his group of cases of OIT, Seedorff[294] concluded that these individuals are 1.4 times more productive of children than their normal siblings. So far as perpetuating the disease is concerned, each affected individual produced, on the average, 0.75 affected children. If it were not for constantly occurring new cases on the basis of mutation, the disease would in time disappear. Seedorff estimated that in Denmark one infant with OIC is born each year.

Komai and associates[199] attempted a crude estimate of the mutation rate in

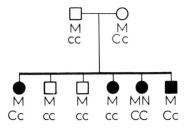

Fig. 8-17. Pedigree of family in which 4 sibs had osteogenesis imperfecta and both parents were seemingly unaffected. The blood group data indicate that the fifth child is not the progeny of the stated father. It is possible that the mother has the gene for OI, which is only very mildly expressed in her. (Redrawn from Smårs, G., Beckman, L., and Böök, J. A.: Acta Genet. **11:** 133, 1961.)

OI, assuming that all cases of OIC represent new dominant mutation; that the female preponderence in OIC is genuine; that 4 out of 5 affected male fetuses die before birth, whereas none of the affected female fetuses die in utero; and finally that the frequency of OIC is about 2 per 100,000 births. OIC cases represent by this estimate a mutation rate of 1.67×10^{-5} per gene per generation. Also, there is no reproduction in the severe form of OI tarda, which, according to Seedorff, is 2.14 times as frequent as OIC. In addition, the reduced effective fertility of late cases would bring the total estimate of the mutation rate to about 4×10^{-5} per gene per generation. In Westphalia, Germany, Schröder[287] estimated a mutation rate of 1×10^{-5} for OIT.

Accumulating experience suggests that in some cases osteogenesis imperfecta congenita may be an autosomal recessive disorder separate from the autosomal dominant one. Goldfarb and Ford[138] described OIC in 2 consecutive female sibs with normal parents and cited the description by Adatia[2] of another Indian family with 2 affected sibs. Chawla[69] observed OIC in 4 sibs with normal parents. A comparable experience is illustrated in Fig. 8-18. Awwaad and Reda[14]

Text continued on p. 427.

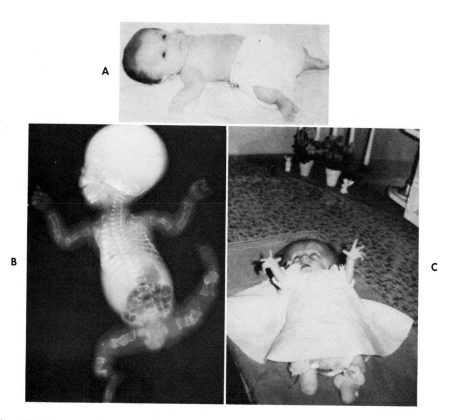

Fig. 8-18. Two cases of osteogenesis imperfecta congenita in offspring of ostensibly normal parents. **A** and **B,** Typical clinical and radiologic appearance in newborn infant. **C,** View at 10 months with development of hydrocephalus. A male sib with identical changes confirmed by x-ray examination died at the age of 2 days. Another sib is normal. The parents are not related. (From McKusick, V. A.: Medical genetics 1958-1960, St. Louis, 1961, The C. V. Mosby Co.)

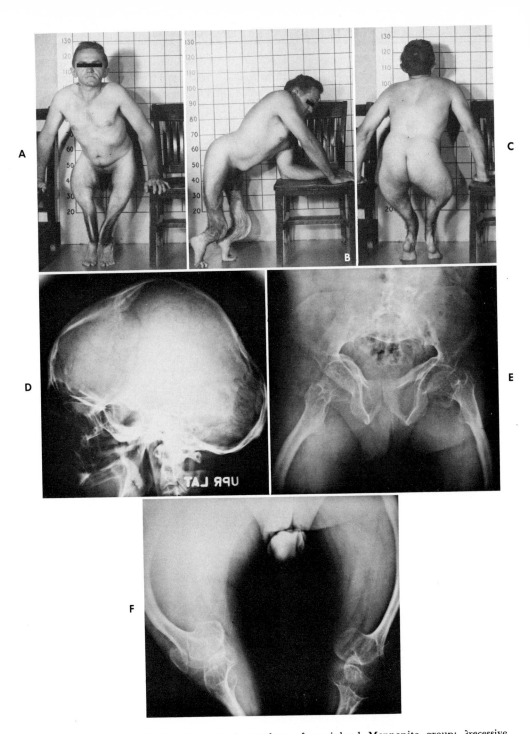

Fig. 8-19. Osteogenesis imperfecta in 3 members of an inbred Mennonite group; ?recessive inheritance.

    Case 1. S. H. (J.H.H. 1172142), born in 1937, believed that his first fracture occurred at the age of 6 months. Thereafter about thirty fractures occurred, most of them in the lower extremities and the last at 11 years of age. All teeth were removed at 20 years. He was deaf in the left ear, and the sclerae were faintly blue. **A** to **C,** Views of S. H. at the age of 28 years. **D,** Skull of S. H., showing many Wormian bones in the lambdoidal sutures and deformity of the calvarium typical of OI. **E,** Pelvis of S. H., showing acetabular protrusion. **F,** Legs of S. H., showing bowing and lateral rotation of the femurs, especially of the right. The bones are thin in the midshaft, with flared ends.

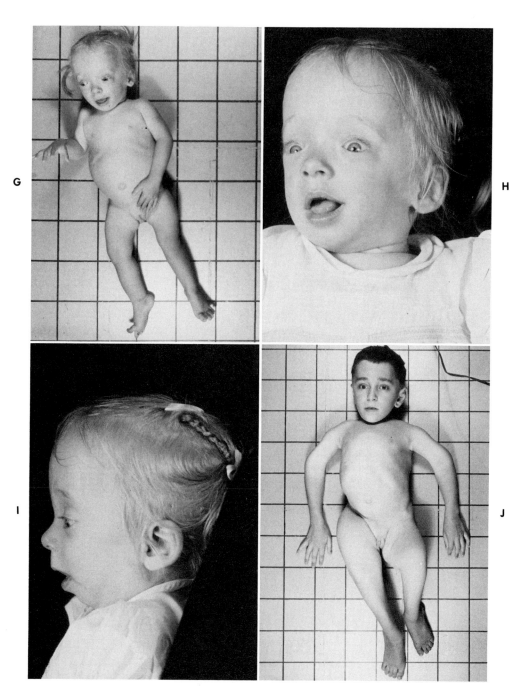

Fig. 8-19, cont'd

Case 2. G. H. (J.H.H. 1172146), daughter of S. H., was born in June, 1964, by breech delivery, which resulted in fracture of both femurs. Five more fractures of the femurs and a fracture of the left humerus occurred in the first fifteen months. At 15 months of age she showed a high forehead and a "setting sun" appearance of the eyes, resulting probably from deformity of the bony orbits, **G** to **I**.

Continued.

Fig. 8-19, cont'd

Case 3. I. H. Z. (J.H.H. 1172147), a distant cousin of the patients described in Cases 1 and 2, was born in 1954 and had his first known fracture at the age of 4 weeks. At least twenty-five fractures occurred before 11 years of age. The teeth were poor. Blue sclerae and severe myopia were present. **J** and **K,** General appearance of I. H. Z. X-ray films of the spine, **L** and **M,** showed marked osteoporosis, thin ribs, and deformed pelvis. Both humeri, **N,** were bowed. The pelvis, **O,** showed acetabular protrusion, a pseudoarthrosis of the left femur, and a malaligned, ununited fracture of the right femur. **P,** Both tibias and fibulas were thin and bowed, and the right fibula had a fracture. The skull of I. H. Z., **Q,** showed a high forehead and multiple Wormian bones in the lambdoid sutures. (The normally calcified teeth appeared abnormally dense because of the generalized osteoporosis.) **R,** The teeth are stunted and semitranslucent. As demonstrated by x-ray examination, **S,** some teeth show small or absent pulp canals.

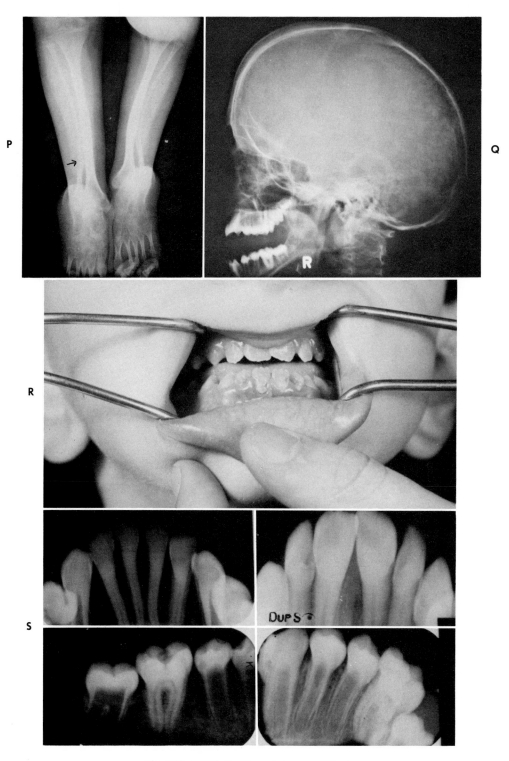

Fig. 8-19, cont'd. For legend see opposite page.

Continued.

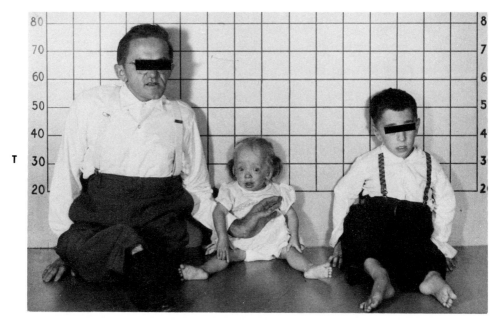

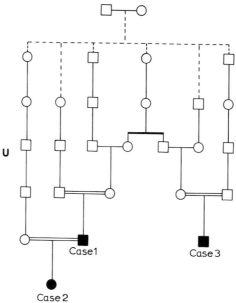

Fig. 8-19, cont'd

T, The three relatives are shown together. **U,** The relationship of the three is indicated. The wife of Case 1 (mother of Case 2) is thought to be heterozygous. All parents of the 3 affected persons probably trace their ancestry to Hans Huber (born in 1660). (**U** revised from Maloney, F. P.: Osteogenesis imperfecta of early onset in three members of an inbred group; ?recessive inheritance. Clinical delineation of birth defects. IV. Skeletal dysplasias, New York, 1969, The National Foundation–March of Dimes.)

described 2 cases of presumed OI in 1 sibship, offspring of consanguineous but unaffected parents. I am by no means convinced of the diagnosis in these 2 patients. The sclerae were described as normal. One of the sisters had fractures dating from infancy, and the other had never had fractures. The same doubt applies to the diagnosis of recessive osteoporosis reported by Chowers and associates[72] in a 19-year-old daughter and 14-year-old son of first-cousin Yemenite Jewish parents and in 3 daughters of second-cousin parents. No characteristic nonosseous features were described, and the patients had aminoaciduria. Remigio and Grinvalsky[262] reported a male and his female sib with the broad-boned type of OIC. One of the sibs had dislocated lenses, aortic coarctation, and basophilic mucoid histologic changes in the connective tissue of the heart valves and aorta. The other had less pronounced histologic changes of the same nature in the aorta. The form of osteogenesis imperfecta in the inbred Mennonite group described in Fig. 8-19 may be recessive also. As noted earlier two radiographic forms of OIC can be distinguished: a thick-boned type and a thin-boned type. The broad-boned type of OIC is illustrated in Figs 8-3 and 8-18 and by the sibs with OIC reported by Remigio and Grinvalsky[262]; the thin-boned type is shown in Fig. 8-5. It is not certain that these types represent fundamentally distinct forms since the radiologic appearance can change from one to the other with the passage of time. However, it will be of heuristic value to keep in mind the hypothesis that, at birth, recessive OIC is thick-boned and that OIC arising by dominant mutation is thin-boned. Hein[154] observed OIC in the offspring of a first-cousin marriage. Hanhart[148] described a recessive form of "osteopsathyrosis congenita." Meyer[231] described "atypical osteogenesis imperfecta" in 3 of the 11 offspring of incestuous mating between a mentally defective woman and her father. Manifestations were spontaneuos fractures, generalized osteoporosis, and Wormian bones in the region of the lamboidal sutures. Blue sclerae were absent. Mental retardation, requiring institutionalization, and microphthalmia were also present but appeared to be segregating independently in this sibship. Studying the same family, Berry[30] demonstrated cystinuria in the 3 sibs with atypical OI. Since arginine, ornithine, and lysine were also present and since other amino acids, glucose, and protein were not present in the urine in excess, the biochemical disorder seemed to be classic recessive cystinuria and not the Fanconi syndrome. Thus, these same 3 patients with atypical OI had cystinuria. Five of the 11 children mentioned above survived; the 2 without osteogenesis imperfecta and cystinuria are also mentally retarded.

The condition called "periosteal dysplasia of Porak and Durante" by French authors is probably the same as osteogenesis imperfecta, and several examples of recessive inheritance have been reported. Kaplan and Baldino,[182] described a case in an inbred, Arabic-speaking, polygamous sect called the Mozabites living in southern Algeria. Nine cases had occurred among the descendants of one marital couple, in a pattern supporting autosomal recessive inheritance (Fig. 8-20). The proband had bulging head and eyes, bent limbs (as in Fig. 8-2), slate-blue sclerae, mosaic skull bones, scoliosis, multiple fractures of ribs and bones of the extremities, and hernia. Reference was made to several other reported instances of apparent recessive inheritance, e.g., that by Glanzmann,[134] of an affected 9-year-old girl and her affected 4-month-old brother. Also, identity to Vrolik's type of osteogenesis imperfecta[349] (i.e., the congenital form) was suggested.

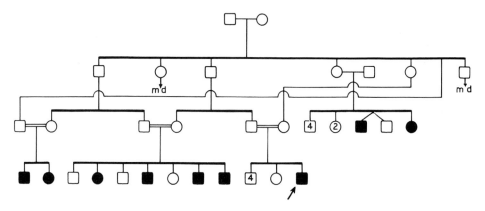

Fig. 8-20. Osteogenesis imperfecta congenita in kindred reported by Kaplan and Baldino.[182] **md,** Many descendants.

Consanguinity is not impressively frequent in the pedigrees of OI. Liber[211] reported on the offspring of a marriage of first-cousin children of first-cousin parents. The proband had bone disease and deafness. The mother "was short and squat, had a large skull, and was and apparently always had been almost totally deaf." A child of the proband had multiple fractures. Thus the consanguinity probably played no role. On the other hand, Komai and associates[199] made reference to the consanguineous mating of 2 individuals with only blue sclerae, resulting in a child with the full-blown syndrome.

Parental consanguinity has been noted in a few cases of OIC.[115,117,202] Rohwedder[270] observed OIC in the offspring of a brother-sister mating. In a thorough study of OI in Münster, Germany, comparable to the studies of Seedorff[294] in Denmark and Smårs[308] in Sweden, Schröder[287] adduced evidence for the existence of a recessive OIC. It is noteworthy that Seedorff found no "paternal age effect" (p. 149) in cases of OIC—a point against the alternative of new dominant mutation.

A recessive form of osteogenesis imperfecta must be rare, however. By a widespread search that made use of the records of this department and worked through the newsletter of the National Osteogenesis Imperfecta Foundation and other channels, Leonard[208] collected 13 sibships, each with 2 sibs with osteogenesis imperfecta. Both parents and all other relatives were ostensibly normal. One of the 26 affected persons, a male, had 4 normal children. No parental consanguinity was found in any of the 13 families. X-ray films were available for examination in 12 of the 26 patients. The changes were of the thick-bone type in 3 of the 12 cases, but most of the x-ray studies were made late. In 1 case there appeared to be a progression from an early thick-bone type of a later thin-boned type.

In a series studied in Kiel, Germany, Langness and Behnke[205] found 87 cases in 31 kindreds. Eighty cases were of the tarda, or Ekman-Lobstein, type; 8 of these 80 cases were sporadic, possibly new mutation cases, and 72 were distributed in 16 kindreds in an autosomal dominant pattern. The remaining 7 cases of the series were sporadic and of the congenital, or Vrolik, type; in 1 case the parents were related. In Westphalia, Germany, Schröder[287] found for OIT a frequency of 4.7 per 100,000 live births and for OIC a frequency of 2.6 per 100,000 live births and stillbirths combined.

The rarity of families in which recessive inheritance of OIC can be seriously considered forces me to conclude that most of the sporadic cases are the consequence of new dominant mutation.

From a review of the literature Ibsen[169,170] concluded that about 90% of cases have a dominant mode of inheritance, blue sclerae, and relatively favorable prognosis (OI tarda). A distinct, apparently recessive form, presents as OIC and usually leads to early death; this form is discussed above. A third entity, inherited as a dominant, has abnormality almost limited to the bones, there being normal sclerae and little or no otosclerosis, joint laxity, or capillary fragility. Such families were reported by Bender,[27] Bryan and Dimichele,[54] and Hurwitz and McSwiney,[167] as well as others such as Holcomb,[160] as noted above.

Confusion with hypophosphatasia (p. 842) must be avoided in any consideration of a recessive form of congenital OI.

In summary, an autosomal recessive disorder with all the features of OIC probably exists. However, this disorder probably accounts for only a small proportion of OIC cases. Therefore, the following statement relevant to genetic counseling is valid: "In the case of normal parents (i.e., without brittle bones and blue sclerae) who have one infant affected with OIC, the possibility of giving birth to a second affected child is almost negligible."*

Pathology[175,353,364]

Histologically, the cortical layer of the bones and the trabeculae of the spongiosa are thin. The periosteum may appear normal, but some have reported reduction in the number of subperiosteal osteoblasts. A peculiar, basophilic, periodic acid and Schiff—positive material has been found in place of osteoid. In other tissue, only argyrophilic reticulin fibers but—no mature collagen—are demonstrated. Histochemically, phosphatase activity is not demonstrably disturbed, epiphyseal cartilage appears to be completely normal,[112] and invasion of the regularly arranged cartilage cell columns by capillaries is normal. The metaphysis shows calcified cartilage but no true bone or osteoid. This calcified cartilage tends to fracture and fragment. Organic bone matrix fails to be deposited, and in its stead a peculiar basophilic material makes its appearance. As stated above, the material stains with periodic acid and leucofuchsin and, furthermore, is argyrophilic. Follis[110] suggests that it may represent immature bone matrix in the manner that reticulin, which it resembles in its staining properties, may represent immature collagen.

Swedish workers using recently developed biophysical techniques demonstrated disorganization of the collagen matrix.[29,100] The specific techniques they employed were microradiography, polarized light microscopy, and x-ray diffraction. Their findings are by no means inconsistent with those of Follis: ". . . in osteogenesis imperfecta the compact bone has a quite abnormal distribution of mineral salts and arrangement of organic fibers. . . . The immature fibrillar bone normally seen in the foetus and newborn infant resembles in several ways the

---

*From Freda, V. J., Vosburgh, G. J., and Di Liberti, C.: Obstet. Gynec. **18:**535, 1961.

tissue found in osteogenesis imperfecta. Normally this primary bone tissue is rapily replaced by secondary bone after birth, but in osteogenesis imperfecta this secondary bone tissue is not found."*

Osteoblasts and osteoclasts are usually present in normal numbers. Chemically, calcium and phosphorus are present in the bones in a normal ratio; the total content of bone salts is reduced, however. Ramser and colleagues[256,257] used rib biopsy and tetracycline labeling (with combined bright-field and fluorescence microscopy) to analyze the dynamics of bone growth. They concluded that the rate of bone formation is about three times the normal rate; yet the transverse dimension of the rib was less than half of the normal dimension. Howship's lacunae, thought to be sites of active bone resorption, were abundant. The reduced ability to lay down new bone was limited to the periosteal surfaces. Cortical endosteal lamellae and haversian systems seemed normal. An imbalance between the laying down of new bone and resorption in the modeling process was thought to be responsible for excessive metaphyseal "waisting," giving an abnormally abrupt metaphyseal flare. Diaphyseal buildup is defective, accounting for the slender shaft of the long bones, which may be of nearly normal length but is abnormally gracile.

In the skin, Follis[111] found absence of normal adult collagen fibers and substitution by argyrophilic fibers with other properties of reticulin. However, the shrinkage temperature of the skin was normal. In a patient with OIC who died shortly after birth, Haebara and colleagues[145] found abnormally thin, delicate connective tissue fibers in the periosteum, corium, sclera, and cornea. By electron microscopy, the collagen fibers had the following dimensions as compared with the normal:

	OIC	N
Periodicity of cross-striations	200 to 400 Å	640 to 700 Å
Thickness	400 Å	1000 Å

The abnormal connective tissue fibers were associated with irregular and granular calcification in bone. Chondroitin sulfate A and C were increased, at least relatively, in the matrix of epiphyseal cartilages.

Basophilic mucoid histologic changes were described in the connective tissues of the aorta and heart valves of 2 sibs dying with typical "broad-boned" OIC.[262] There is virtually no other information on the anatomic substrate of the cardiac valvular manifestations (p. 413) of OI.

In the eye, decreased thickness of the sclera was described as early as 1841 by von Ammon[347] and more recently by Buchanan,[55] Casanovas,[66] and Follis,[112] but normal thickness was found by Bronson[51] and Voigt.[346] Ruedemann[277] has found histologic changes in cornea and sclera fundamentally identical to those described by Follis[112] in the corium. Clearly, the blue coloration is the result of the brown-pigmented choroid's showing through the thin sclera.[354] The thin skin is reflected in the deficiency of measured collagen content, expressed per unit of surface area.[324]

In sections of the teeth, "clodlike" calcification of quite abnormal type is seen. Rushton[278] showed that peripheral pulp cells produce "precollagenous"

---

*From Engfeldt, B., Engstrom, A., and Zetterstrom, R.: J. Bone Joint Surg. **36-B**:654, 1954.

argyrophilic fibers but that these are not converted into collagen except in the immediate vicinity of blood vessels. These observations are in complete agreement with those of Follis, in bone, skin, and sclera.

The question whether the changes in the ear are histologically distinguishable from those of conventional otosclerosis has been much debated.[6,131,239,240,247,282] Some of the patients in whom the temporal bones have been studied may have had coincidental otosclerosis, but such cannot explain all of the deafness of OI. It seems most plausible to me that otosclerosis can have several different causes, one of which is OI.[168a] This is, then, a situation comparable to dentinogenesis imperfecta as an isolated abnormality and as part of OI.

In OIC the stapes has been found to be abnormal, its crura being fragile and incomplete, whereas the footplate and its surrounding tissue were normal.[146] Opheim[247] performed stapes mobilization in 5 ears of 4 patients. The crura of the stapes "were found to have degenerated into thin, fibrous threads in four." In the fifth the same anomaly may have been present. Sensorineural deafness has also been observed in OI.[247]

The fundamental defect

A generalized mesenchymal defect has been assumed for several decades. The histologic investigations of Follis (described above) appear to indicate that the fundamental difficulty may be in the maturation of collagen beyond the reticulin fiber stage. (This assumes that one can subscribe without reservation to the view that reticulin fibers are immature collagen fibers.[218] Even if this is not the case, it can be stated that the collagen fibers in OI are abnormal and resemble reticulin fibers in many respects.) As far as the bones are concerned, the disease must be considered a disorder of osteoblastic activity. Normal chondroblastic activity is suggested by the fact that growth and development of cartilage are normal.

Brown[52a] reported quantitative and qualitative differences in the collagen produced by fibroblasts cultured from patients with OI. The hydroxyproline-to-proline ratio was abnormally low, and the proportion of collagen extractable by neutral salt and weak acid solutions was abnormally high, when compared with collagen produced by fibroblasts from normal persons. The increased extractability suggests an abnormality of cross-linkage of collagen.

Giordano[133] in Milan, Italy, has been studying histochemical enzymatic reactions in OI. Caniggia and associates[62] claimed that the collagen in OI has an abnormally high proline content. Solomons and Styner[314] reported that bone collagen from OI patients inhibits calcification *in vitro*. Treatment of the collagen with pyrophosphatase in the presence of magnesium ion removed the inhibition. They found, furthermore, that serum and urinary pyrophosphate was elevated in OI patients and declined with administration of magnesium sulfate. By an isotope dilution method, using ^{32}P-labeled pyrophosphate, Russell and colleagues[279] could not demonstrate abnormality of inorganic pyrophosphate in osteogenesis imperfecta. Eleven patients, varying in age from 1 year to the late sixties were studied. They questioned the specificity of the method of assay used by Solomons and Styner.[314] Russell and colleagues[279] also could not confirm the claimed[314] increase in urinary excretion of pyrophosphate in OI.

Summer[330] studied serum levels of proline after oral administration of proline in 6 children with OIT and in one with OIC. Peak levels in the first hour were less high in the OI cases than in normal subjects. Elevated urinary excretion of hydroxyproline was found in 16 of 20 patients studied by Langness and Behnke.[204] The elevation was statistically significant in adults as well as in children. On the other hand, Goidanich and associates[142] found no elevation of urinary hydroxyproline in 3 OI patients. Langness and Behnke[203] also found elevation of plasma hyprotein, a high molecular weight, hydroxyproline-containing protein. A correlation was demonstrated between the level of plasma hyprotein and urinary hydroxyproline.

Chowers and colleagues[72] demonstrated aminoaciduria in 6 members of two families and postulated a renal tubular defect in OI. The affected persons had radiologic features consistent with osteogenesis imperfecta but not eye or ear abnormality, and inheritance was rather clearly autosomal recessive. It is likely that they were dealing with an entity related to the Fanconi syndrome and not with true OI. Brigham and Tourtellott[48] reported in brief an increased urinary excretion of glycine, serine, threonine, ethanolamine, and valine, with a reduced level of these substances in the plasma, and suggested a renal tubular defect in OI. A detailed report has not yet appeared.

Based on observations in 30 prepubertal patients with OI, Cropp et al.[85a] concluded that oral temperatures and heart and respiratory rates are elevated above normal and that body weight is abnormally low. They claim that obesity is rare in OI children despite good appetite in combination with inactivity. (I think obesity is not unusual in OI.) Serum thyroxine levels were, on the average, raised in their patients. Excessive sweating by OI children is a frequent observation. Humbert et al.[164] presented evidence of increased oxidative metabolism from the study of leukocytes in vitro. Studies were performed in the Warburg apparatus, and reduction of nitroblue tetrazolium was tested. Casting some doubt on the findings in OI patients was the further observation that about half the ostensibly unaffected relatives showed the same hypermetabolism. The majority of the probands can be expected to be heterozygotes, and penetrance cannot be expected to be so low as to account for the abnormal tests in a large number of clinically normal relatives. Brown et al.[52b] were unable to confirm any abnormality of the metabolism of leukocytes as gauged by reduction of nitroblue tetrazolium.

It has been claimed by Seedorff[294] that a condition in cattle called anosteoplasia congenita[171] is an identical disorder. In 1958 Coop[81] wrote as follows: "Osteogenesis imperfecta is a condition recognized with increased frequency in cats during the last eight years, especially in the Siamese and Burmese breeds."* It was thought that study of such animals could be very useful to the understanding of most OI in man. That the disease seemed to behave as an autosomal recessive in cats[162,163,307] might be an indication (p. 23) that its basic nature was different from that of the disease in man. (Hereditary spherocytosis in mice is recessive but in man is dominant.[235]) However, studying a kindred of Burmese cats, Scott and co-workers[292] showed that fractures did not develop after the diet was changed from horsemeat and ground beef heart to fish catfood, skim milk,

---

*From Coop, M. C.: J. Amer. Vet. Med. Ass. **132**:299, 1958.

and table scraps and that under these dietary circumstances even the offspring of two "homozygotes" had no skeletal abnormality. Riser[266] similarly concluded that "ostegenesis imperfecta" in cats is the result of calcium deficiency.

Calkins and associates[60] observed a disorder resembling osteogenesis imperfecta in the standard French poodle and in the Norwegian elkhound. The frequency of fractures diminished at puberty. Clinical differences from the disease in man were attributed to early weight bearing and rapid leg growth in dogs. A reduction in the net rate of collagen formation seemed to be present. Holmes and associates[161] described "osteogenesis imperfecta" in lambs.

Although such a suggestion must remain speculative at this stage, one wonders if there may not be synthesized, in osteogenesis imperfecta and possibly in some others of the hereditary disorders of connective tissue, an atypical species of fibrous connective tissue protein. Do the amino acid sequences of collagen, in OI, differ from those in the "normal" by a single amino acid substitution, comparable to the differences demonstrated in many hemoglobin variants? If there is indeed a recessive form of OIC (p. 429), an enzyme defect is likely to be found, rather than a structural change in a connective tissue protein, which on theoretical grounds (p. 23) is more likely in the dominantly inherited, usual form of OI.

Differential diagnosis

There are several reports[11,16,168,320,338] of a generalized disorder of connective tissue with features resembling osteogenesis imperfecta, but with enough differences to indicate that it is a distinct entity. It is characterized mainly by weak, thin cornea and sclera leading to blue sclerae, keratoglobus simulating buphthalmos but with normal intraocular pressure, and recurrent rupture (especially of the cornea) with minor trauma; however, proclivity to fracture of bones, dentinogenesis imperfecta, long hyperextensible fingers, and hernia are also described. Brothers and sisters have been affected, with both parents normal but consanguineous.[16,320,338] Autosomal recessive inheritance seems quite certain. Blue sclerae have been noted in relatives who may be heterozygous. This condition, which might be termed *fragilitas oculi,* has some features like those of the "ocular" form of the Ehlers-Danlos syndrome, the existence of which was suggested on p. 341. Bertelsen[32] probably described the same disorder, using the designation *dysgenesis mesodermalis corneae et sclerae.* He described an affected child whose parents were first cousins but clinically normal. Myopia, thin and large corneas, deep anterior chamber, and strikingly blue sclerae were present. The bones were normal.

Idiopathic juvenile osteoporosis (IJO)[10,91,173] consists of an acute attack of osteoporosis of varying severity that begins about two years before puberty and remits spontaneously in three to five years.[75,90] Treatment with sex hormones may be harmful by causing dwarfism from premature closure of epiphyses. In severe cases, a characteristic rarefaction of the metaphyses is demonstrated radiologically (Fig. 8-21). This rarefaction, as well as the negative family history, the normal sclerae and teeth, and the characteristic age of onset, distinguish this disorder from OI.

A distinctive disorder probably inherited as an autosomal recessive combines severe osteoporosis with ocular pseudoglioma. Opitz[248a] observed this syndrome

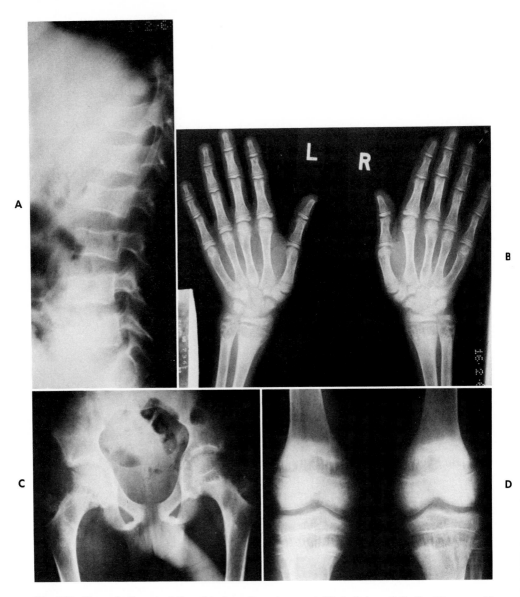

Fig. 8-21. X-ray findings in idiopathic juvenile osteoporosis.[190] **A,** Spine of C. G., 12 years old, showing flattened vertebral bodies. **B,** Wrists of C. G., showing rarefaction of the radial and ulnar metaphyses. **C,** Hips of C. G., showing rarefaction in the femoral necks. **D,** Knees of C. G., showing zones of metaphyseal rarefaction longer than that in the radius and ulna because of faster growth of the leg bones. (Courtesy Charles E. Dent and The National Foundation–March of Dimes.)

in 2 brothers and a sister. The following patient was studied by Bianchine and Murdoch[32a]:

Case 4. M. P. R. (J.H.H. 1105157), a white boy born in 1956, suffered multiple fractures beginning at the age of 3 years. He was the product of an uncomplicated pregnancy that was thought to have been full-term; however, his birth weight was only 5 pounds 10 ounces. Development was normal except that he did not walk until age 4 years.

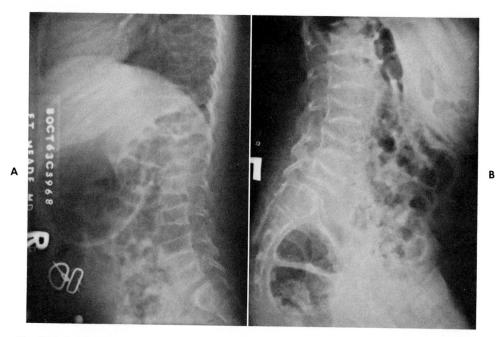

Fig. 8-22. Syndrome of osteoporosis and retinal pseudoglioma. See text for description of case of M. P. R. Lumbar spine at age 6 years, **A,** and at age 11 years, **B.** The vertebral bodies are flattened with concave end plates, and bone density is much reduced. Intervertebral disks are thick and biconvex.

At the age of 8 weeks the boy was noted to have lack of retinal reflex in each eye and retinoblastomas were suspected. Irradiation followed by bilateral enucleation was performed at age 3 to 4 months. The histopathologic diagnosis of pseudoglioma was made. The patient had normal hearing and intelligence.

Beginning at age 3 years the patient had many fractures involving hips, ankles, arms, and shoulders. The fractures resulted from minimal trauma, were relatively painless, and healed satisfactorily leaving slight outward bowing of the left humerus and anterior bowing of both tibias and femurs. Despite severe osteoporosis of the vertebrae with collapse of bodies known to have been present since at least 1962 (Fig. 8-22), the patient did not complain of back pain until 1967. During the next 18 months he had increasing incapacitation, an awkward waddling gait, stooped posture, and frequent complaints of pains in the ankles, knees, and hips.

Diet was always adequate; he was active until late in his course, and no steatorrhea or renal abnormalities were detected.

Both parents were 23 years old at the time of his birth. They were not related and were healthy as were 5 younger sibs. No relative had deafness, blue sclerae, or brittle bones.

Examination (August, 1968) showed an obese blind boy with limbs that were long relative to his trunk. X-ray films showed severe generalized osteoporosis. Hypercalciuria was marked, being about twice the normal. Serum calcium, phosphorus, alkaline phosphatase, and proteins were normal.

Familial protein intolerance,[222] also called dibasic aminoaciduria, is accompanied by fragile bones as demonstrated by x-ray studies, markedly decreased bone density. This rare disorder has been described mainly in Finns. It is inherited as an autosomal recessive. This or some disorder other than OI seems to have been present in the consanguineous cases of osteoporosis with aminoaciduria reported by Chowers and co-workers[72] as OI.

Caffey states that the mosaic phenomenon in the skull x-ray film occurs in

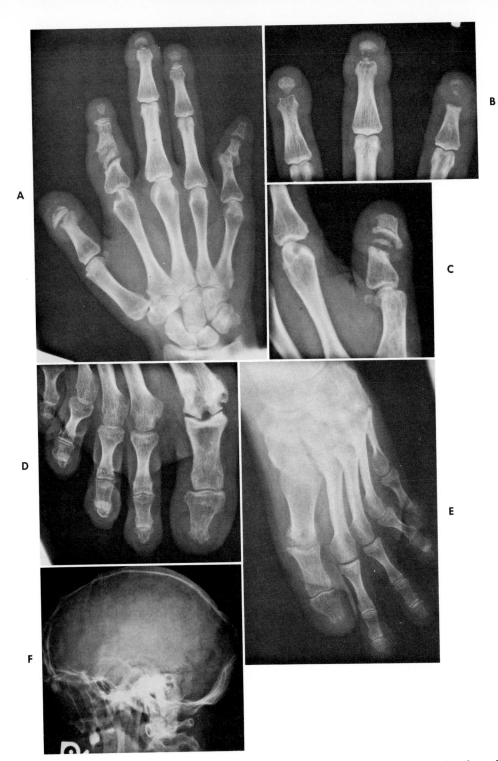

Fig. 8-23. Cheney syndrome. O. M. B., an Air Force sergeant, was 39 years old at the time of study in 1967. His fingers had, he said, always looked peculiar. He had sustained at least seven fractures of various bones. Physical examination showed short, clubbed distal phalanges of the fingers and toes, prominent occiput, and signs of pulmonary emphysema. **A** to **C**, X-ray films of the hands. **A**, Right hand showing acro-osteolysis. Fingers II and V are very short, and V is subluxated. Detail of acro-osteolysis in three fingers, **B**, and in left thumb, **C**.

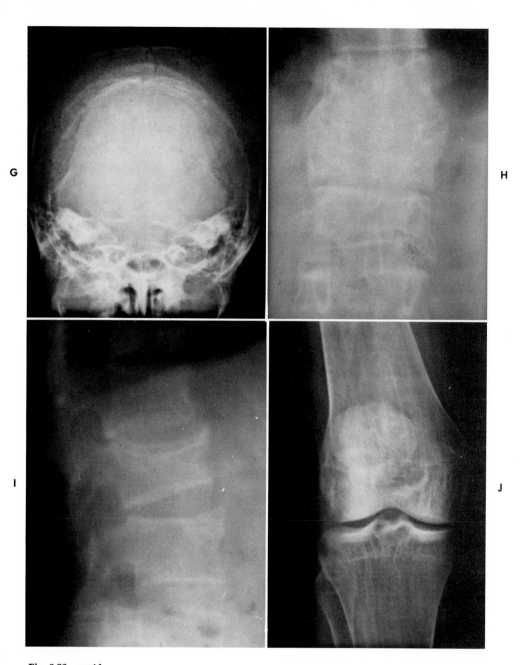

Fig. 8-23, cont'd

D and **E,** X-ray films of feet. **D,** Toes of right foot. Note osteolysis at ends of terminal phalanges and in the head of the first metatarsal. **E,** Left foot. Note short toes I and V, osteolysis on both sides of the first metatarsophalangeal joint, and terminal osteolysis of distal phalanges. **F** and **G,** X-ray films of skull, showing occipital bathycephaly, mild basilar impression, occipital Wormian bones, and straightened mandibular angle. **H** and **I,** X-ray films of spine. Osteoporosis, vertebral compression, and osteophyte formation are demonstrated. **J,** X-ray film of right knee. Osteoporosis and juxta-articular cystic change in the tibia are demonstrated. (**B** and **C** from Dorst, J. P., and McKusick, V. A.: Acro-osteolysis [Cheney syndrome]; clinical delineation of birth defects. III. Limb malformations, New York, 1969, The National Foundation–March of Dimes.)

only two conditions: osteogenesis imperfecta and cleidocranial dysostosis (see Fig. 43 of reference 58 and compare with Fig. 8-4 here). Pyknodysostosis,[221,225,227] a condition which in other ways simulates both osteogenesis imperfecta and cleidocranial dysostosis and from which Toulouse-Lautrec is now thought to have suffered (p. 820), should be added to the "causes" of multiple Wormian bones. Two other conditions that show multiple Wormian bones are Menkes kinky hair syndrome (p. 710), progeria (p. 727), and Cheney syndrome.

The *Cheney syndrome* resembles osteogenesis imperfecta in the occurrence of multiple Wormian bones, osteoporosis with tendency to fracture, basilar impression, and dominant (probably autosomal) inheritance. Distinctive features are acro-osteolysis and hypoplasia of the ramus of the mandible, as in pyknodysostosis. Cheney[70] described the condition in a woman and 4 of her 6 children. Dorst and I[93] described a patient whose radiologic findings are presented in Fig. 8-23.

Chowers and colleagues[72] described 6 cases, 5 of them familial, with radiologic features of osteogenesis imperfecta but no blue sclerae or deafness. Aminoaciduria and low serum uric acid levels were demonstrated by these patients. Because of these findings and rather clear autosomal recessive inheritance, the cases may be more accurately classified as a form of renal tubular defect related to the Fanconi syndrome.

Lifelong osteoporosis with codfish vertebrae and susceptibility to fracture occurs also in homocystinuria (Chapter 4) and might be confused with osteogenesis imperfecta.

As mentioned earlier (p. 429), hypophosphatasia (p. 842) must not be confused with osteogenesis imperfecta congenita. Blue sclerae occur in small children with hypophosphatasia (see the discussion of hypophosphatasia in Chapter 13). The newborn infant with this disorder has bowing of the legs and can look remarkably like the infant with OIC (compare illustration in reference 86a with Fig. 8-2).

Among the genetically determined skeletal disorders having osseous fragility as a feature is a newly recognized disorder, pyknodysostosis. The features are autosomal recessive inheritance, bone sclerosis with proneness to fracture, persistently wide cranial fontanelles, micrognathism with virtual absence of the ramus of the mandible, hypoplasia of the clavicles, and osteolysis in the terminal phalanges of the fingers. Some of the features resemble those of cleidocranial dysostosis, with which pyknodysostosis has sometimes been confused but which shows dominant inheritance. Maroteaux and Lamy[227] first described and named pyknodysostosis. Seedorff[294] suggested that Henri de Toulouse-Lautrec (1864-1901), a French painter, suffered from osteogenesis imperfecta. His appearance as displayed in photographs (Fig. 13-45) is certainly consistent. Particularly suggestive of OI are Lautrec's short legs; José Ferrer, when playing Lautrec in the motion picture *Moulin Rouge*, walked about on his knees. Review of available information has led Maroteaux and Lamy[225] to believe that Lautrec in fact suffered from pyknodysostosis. His parents were first cousins. The failure to grow dated from an early age. He was apparently already infirm, for he was using a stick when his first recognized fracture (of the left femur) occurred at 14 years of age from a fall as he tried to get out of a chair. The following year fracture of the right femur occurred when he slipped into a shallow ditch while on a walk. Photographs[237] do not suggest blue sclerae, and those showing him in swimming garb show no bowing deformity of the legs. Maroteaux and Lamy[225] conclude that photographs suggest micrognathia and they suggest further that Lautrec's perpetual wearing of a hat was prompted by an open anterior fontanelle!

Achondroplasia is a frequent misdiagnosis in these patients. Confusion regarding the diagnosis may occur at birth (see Fig. 8-2) or in later life. The patient described by Ruth[280] was diagnosed as having achondroplasia because of the big head and short limbs. At the age of about 50 years he was selling papers from a wheelchair. In discussion of a patient 53 years old (I. L., Sinai 70327), the following conclusion was stated: "In regard to the developmental anomaly of this patient: I believe he is an achondroplastic dwarf with typically well-built torso and relatively short spindly legs."

OI, a hereditary form of osteoporosis, is accompanied by blue sclerae. In other forms of osteoporosis, such as Cushing's syndrome, prolonged administration of adrenal steroids, and senile (or postmenopausal) osteoporosis, it is likely that the connective tissue defect is more extensive than merely involving the organic matrix of bone. I have (e.g., M. H., 738167) been impressed with the occurrence in isolated instances of blue sclerae in senile osteoporosis.

The presence of blue sclerae cannot, of course, as a rule be used as the only criterion for the diagnosis of OI. Evaluation is especially difficult in children, who normally have bluish sclerae.

Management

Medical therapy has been of doubtful benefit. As one might expect, many kinds of medication have been employed for this distressing and long-standing disorder—e.g., thymus extract.[293] Furthermore, because of difficulties in evaluating results, the variable course of the disease, and wishful thinking on the part of physicians and patients, overly enthusiastic reports have at times been forthcoming.

Muldowney[236] treated a 13-year-old girl with an anabolic steroid for eighteen months, during which time no further fractures occurred. Cattell and Clayton[67] concluded that anabolic steroids resulted in an apparent reduction in the incidence of fractures but no dramatic alleviation of the disease. "Side effects (mainly virilization) would preclude this use in all but the most severely affected boys."

Winterfeldt and co-workers[366] found high retention of ascorbic acid, decreased urinary excretion of hydroxyproline, and apparent decrease in the incidence of fractures in patients receiving high doses of vitamin C.

Fluoride, which is known to produce osteosclerosis, has been used.[253] Aeschlimann and colleagues[3] described treatment of an infant with severe OIC with 5 mg. of sodium fluoride a day from the ages of 1 month to 13 months. X-ray studies at the age of 21 days showed severe disorder of the thick-boned type. Clinically, including radiographically, improvement seemed to have occurred with reduction in the frequency of fractures. Strontium[300] has also been tested in one study[46] in which the author thought the results were favorable and rendered further study worthwhile.

Treatment with magnesium oxide, of which the rationale was presented on p. 431, is presently under trial.[314] Reduction in abnormally elevated serum pyrophosphate levels was observed in most cases, and a decrease in fracture rate was thought to parallel decrease in pyrophosphate. Decreased sweating was also noted during administration of magnesium oxide.[314] In the untreated disease, hypermetabolism, as indicated by elevated basal oxygen consumption and elevated basal temperature, has been claimed. Increased oxidative metabolism by leukocytes of patients with OI has also been claimed,[164] but the fact that seemingly unaffected relatives showed the same elevation vitiates the results.

A surgical procedure increasingly used for correcting the deformity of the legs and preventing further fractures and deformity[8,230,258a] is that developed by Sofield and colleagues[312] and graphically referred to as the "shish kebob" operation. The long bone is fragmented and the fragments are realigned; a rod is then placed in the medullary canal and threaded through the fragments. Williams[362] reported experience with the procedure. The youngest patient so treated was 10 months old. He recommended that medullary rodding should be performed when leg deformity begins even though replacement may be necessary approximately every three years to keep up with growth. Rodriguez and Wickstrom[268a] modified the procedure with the use of an extensible intramedullary device.

Kerr, a nurse, devised a posterior head splint to prevent head deformity in the infant with OI.

As in acquired forms of osteoporosis, it is highly important to avoid immobilization of the patient because of the further depletion of bone matrix occasioned thereby. It is doubtful that a high intake of calcium, phosphorus, and vitamin D is helpful, and the combination of these with immobilization may have dire effects: C. B. (J.H.H. 242806) developed large bladder stones and a *Proteus* infection of the urinary tract after immobilization for eleven weeks in a cast and a "bone-building diet" that included several quarts of milk a day and added calcium and vitamin D. The pinning and plating of fractures have much to recommend them because they reduce the necessity for immobilization.

Nonmedical resources. The National Osteogenesis Imperfecta Foundation, Inc., was incorporated August 21, 1970, under the laws of the State of Georgia, with Mr. Roy C. Burdette,* as president. A newsletter entitled *Breakthrough* is published quarterly under the editorship of Gemma Geisman†; it promises to be a valuable source of information and moral support for patients with osteogenesis imperfecta and their parents.

Give Every Day a Chance‡ is an intimate account of the trials and tribulations of a family with a child with osteogenesis imperfecta, as told by the mother, Beverly Plummer. The book has a happy ending in the child's triumph over her handicaps to the extent that she is able to attend college, drive an automobile, and enjoy a satisfactory social adjustment. The book is recommended reading for physicians who care for patients with osteogenesis imperfecta and similar chronic disorders of childhood. Unfortunately the experiences of this family with the medical profession were not always happy ones. The book jacket states that the impersonality of her treatment was matched only by the apathy and ignorance of doctors.

Letters to Polly: On the Gift of Affliction§ is a touching autobiographic and

---

*Address: 28 Maple Drive, Hogansville, G. A. 30230.
†Address: 632 Center St., Van Wert, Ohio 45891.
‡New York, 1970, G. P. Putnam's Sons.
§Grand Rapids, Mich., 1971, Wm. B. Eerdmans Publishing Co.

philosophic discourse by an affected father, clergyman Melvin Schoonover, to his affected daughter.

SUMMARY AND CONCLUSIONS

Osteogenesis imperfecta is a generalized disorder of connective tissue involving, in addition to bone, the skin, ligaments, tendons, fascia, sclera, and middle and inner ear. Although the most frequent functionally important manifestations are brittle bones and deafness, blue sclerae are a dramatic feature, and thin skin, loose-jointedness, and hernia occur as manifestations of a single basic defect.

An exceptionally wide range of expressivity has resulted in the description of several different syndromes, all of which may be but different expressions of a single type of connective tissue disorder, inherited as a Mendelian autosomal dominant. The existence of an infrequent autosomal recessive form presenting usually as osteogenesis imperfecta congenita is quite certain, however.

Studies to date are most consistent with the view that the basic defect is one which involves either the maturation of the collagen fiber beyond the stage of the argyrophilic, reticulin fiber or the synthesis of a different species of collagen with tinctorial resemblance to reticulin.

REFERENCES

1. Adair-Dighton, C. A.: Four generations of blue sclerotics, Ophthalmoscope 10:188, 1912.
2. Adatia, M. D.: J. Indian Med. Prof. 4:1810, 1957.
3. Aeschlimann, M. I., Grunt, J. A., and Crigler, J. F., Jr.: Effects of sodium fluoride on the clinical course and metabolic balance of an infant with osteogenesis imperfecta congenita, Metabolism 15:905, 1966.
4. Albright, F., and Reifenstein, E. C., Jr.: The parathyroid glands and metabolic bone disease; selected studies, Baltimore, 1948, The Williams & Wilkins Co., p. 150.
5. Alexander, J. B.: Fragilitas ossium associated with blue sclerotics in four generations, Brit. Med. J. 1:677, 1922.
6. Altmann, F.: The temporal bone in osteogenesis imperfecta congenita, Arch. Otolaryng. 75:486, 1962.
7. Angle, C. R.: Congenital bowing and angulation of the long bones, Pediatrics 13:193, 1954.
8. Anon.: Fragilitas ossium, J.A.M.A. 161:773, 1956.
9. Apert, E.: Les hommes de verre, Presse Méd. 36:805, 1928.
10. Archibald, R. M. (New York City): Personal communication.
11. Arkin, W.: Blue scleras with keratoglobus, Amer. J. Ophthal. 58:678, 1964.
12. Attiah, M. A. H.: Blue sclerotics, Bull. Ophthal. Soc. Egypt 26:96, 1933.
13. Attiah, M. A. H., and Sobhy Bey, M.: Blue sclerotics, Bull. Ophthal. Soc. Egypt 24:67, 1931.
14. Awwaad, S., and Reda, M.: Osteogenesis imperfecta; review of literature and report on three cases, Arch. Pediat. 77:280, 1960.
15. Axmann, E.: Merkwürdige Fragilität der Knochen ohne dyskrasische Ursache als krankhafte Eigenthümlichkeit dreier Geschwister, Ann. Ges. Heilk. (Karlsruhe) 4:58, 1831.
16. Badtke, G.: Ueber einen eigenartigen Fall von Keratokonus und blauen Skleren bei Geschwistern. Klin. Mbl. Augenheilk. 106:585, 1941.
17. Bain, A. D., and Barrett, H. S.: Congenital bowing of the long bones: report of a case, Arch. Dis. Child. 34:516, 1959.
18. Baker, S. L.: Hyperplastic callus simulating sarcoma in two cases of fragilitas ossium, J. Path. Bact. 58:609, 1946.
19. Bantz, W.: Ueber einen Fall von Osteogenesis imperfecta tarda mit gleichzeitger habitueller Schultergelenksluxation beiderseits, Zbl. Chir. 68:1726, 1941.
20. Bartter, F. C., and Bauer, W.: Fragilitas ossium. In Cecil, R. L., and Loeb, R. F.: Textbook of medicine, ed. 9, Philadelphia, 1955, W. B. Saunders Co., p. 1447.
21. Bauer, K. H.: Erbkonstitutionelle "Systemerkrankungen" und Mesenchym, Klin. Wschr. 2:624, 1923.

22. Bauer, K. H.: Ueber Identität und Wesen der sogenannten Osteopsathyrosis idiopathica und Osteogenesis imperfecta, Deutsch. Zschr. Chir. **160:**289, 1920.

23. Bauer, K. H.: Ueber Osteogenesis imperfecta, Deutsch. Zschr. Chir. **154:**166, 1920.

24. Becks, H.: Histologic study of tooth structure in osteogenesis imperfecta, Dent. Cosmos **73:**737, 1931.

25. Behr, C.: Keratokonus, blaue Sklera, habituelle Luxationen, Monatsbl. Augenheilk. **1:**281, 1913.

26. Bell, J.: Blue sclerotics and fragility of bone. Treasury of human inheritance., vol. 2, part III, Cambridge and London, 1928, University of London, Cambridge University Press.

27. Bender, S.: Pregnancy in a 31-inch (77.5 cm.) dwarf, Brit. Med. J. **5471:**1166, 1965.

28. Bergman, G.: The incremental pattern of the dentine in a case of osteogenesis imperfecta, Oral Surg. **13:**70, 1960.

29. Bergman, G., and Engfeldt, B.: Studies on mineralized dental tissues. IV. Biophysical studies in osteogenesis imperfecta, Acta Path. Microbiol. Scand. **35:**537, 1954.

30. Berry, H. K.: Cystinuria in mentally retarded siblings with atypical osteogenesis imperfecta, Amer. J. Dis. Child. **97:**196, 1950.

31. Bert, J. M.: Les formes de transition entre les syndromes familiaux de fragilité osseuse (type Lobstein) et de grande hyperlaxité-ligamentaire (type Morquio), Presse Méd. **50:**290, 1942.

32. Bertelsen, T. I.: Dysgenesis mesodermalis corneae et sclerae; rupture of both corneae in a patient with blue sclerae, Acta Ophthal. **46:**486, 1968.

32a. Bianchine, J. W., and Murdoch, J. L.: Juvenile osteoporosis (?) in a boy with bilateral enucleation of the eyes for pseudoglioma. In Bergsma, D., editor: Clinical delineation of birth defects. IV. Skeletal dysplasias, New York, 1969, The National Foundation–March of Dimes, pp. 225-226.

33. Biebl, E., and Streitmann, B.: Elastosis perforans bei einem Fall von Osteogenesis imperfecta, Z. Haut. Geschlechtskr. **35:**333, 1963.

34. Biering, A., and Iversen, T.: Osteogenesis imperfecta associated with Ehlers-Danlos syndrome, Acta Paediat. **44:**279, 1955.

35. Bierring, K.: Contribution to the perception of osteogenesis imperfecta congenita and osteopsathyrosis idiopathica as identical disorders, Acta Chir. Scand. **70:**481, 1933.

36. Bigler, M.: Ueber das gleichzeitige Vorkommen von Osteopsathyrose und blauer Verfärbung der Skleren bei Otosklerose, Arch. Ohr. Nas Kehlkopfheilk. **5:**233, 1923.

37. Bixler, D., Conneally, P. M., and Christen, A. G.: Dentinogenesis imperfecta; genetic variations in a six-generation family, J. Dent. Res. **48:**1196, 1969.

38. Blattner, R. J., Heyes, F., and Robinson, H. B. G.: Osteogenesis imperfecta and odontogenesis imperfecta (hereditary opalescent dentin), J. Dent. Res. **21:**325, 1942.

39. Blegvad, O., and Haxthausen, H.: Blue sclerotics and brittle bones, with macular atrophy of the skin and zonular cataract, Brit. Med. J. **2:**1071, 1921.

40. Blencke, A.: Ueber das gemeinsame Vorkommen von Knochembrüchigkeit mit blauen Skleren und Schwerhörigkeit, Zschr. Orthop. Chir. **45:**406, 1924.

41. Bonnet, P., and Wertheimer, C.: Un cas d'osteopsathyrose, Bull. Soc. Ophtal. Franc., p. 119, 1935.

42. Brenner, R. L., Smith, J. L., Cleveland, W. W., Bejar, R. L., and Lockhart, W. S., Jr.: Eye signs of hypophosphatasia, Arch. Ophthal. **81:**614, 1969.

43. Bretlau, P., and Balsley-Jorgensen, M.: Otosclerosis and osteogenesis imperfecta, Acta Otolaryng. **67:**269, 1969.

44. Bretlau, P., and Jorgensen, M. B.: Otosclerosis and osteogenesis imperfecta, Arch. Otolaryng. **90:**4, 1969.

45. Bretlau, P., Jorgensen, M. B., and Johansen, H.: Osteogenesis imperfecta; light and electron microscopic studies of the stapes, Acta Otolaryng. **69:**172, 1970.

46. Breuer, J.: Zur Therapie der Osteopsathyrosis mit blauen Skleren, Deutsch. Med. Wschr. **56:**1735, 1930.

47. Brickley, D. W.: Otosclerosis and blue scleras, Arch. Otolaryng. **46:**230, 1947.

48. Brigham, M. P., and Tourtellotte, C. D.: Amino acid changes in blood and urine in osteogenesis imperfecta (abstract), Fed. Proc. **21:**167, 1962.

49. Broca, A., and Herbinet: De l'osteopsathyrosis ou fragilité osseuse dite essentielle, Rev. Chir. **77:**284, 1905.

50. Bromer, R. S.: Rickets and infantile scurvy occurring in case of osteogenesis imperfecta, Amer. J. Roentgen. **55**:30, 1946.

51. Bronson, E.: On fragilitas ossium and its association with blue sclerotics and otosclerosis, Edinburgh Med. J. **18**:240, 1917.

52. Browell, J. N., Jr., and Drake, E. H.: Aortic valve lesions associated with osteogenesis imperfecta, Henry Ford Hosp. Med. Bull. **14**:245, 1966.

52a. Brown, D. M.: Collagen metabolism in fibroblasts from patients with osteogenesis imperfecta (abstract), Pediat. Res. **6**:394, 1972.

52b. Brown, D. M., Park, B. H., and Holmes, B. M.: Metabolic studies of leukocytes of patients with osteogenesis imperfecta, J. Pediat. **80**:221, 1972.

53. Bryan, R. S., Cain, J. C., and Lipscomb, P. R.: Hereditary osteogenesis imperfecta; a mother and son with their family tree, Mayo Clin. Proc. **31**:475, 1956.

54. Bryan, R. S., and Dimichele, J. D.: Osteogenesis imperfecta; report of six familial cases, U. S. Armed Forces Med. J. **10**:312, 1959.

55. Buchanan, L.: Case of congenital maldevelopment of the cornea and sclerotic, Trans. Ophthal. Soc. U. K. **23**:267, 1903.

56. Bull, J.: Paget's disease of the skull with platybasia, Proc. Roy. Soc. Med. **40**:85, 1946.

57. Burkhardt, H.: Schwangerschaft und Geburt bei einem Fall von Osteopoathyrosis Typ Lobstein, Zbl. Gynaek. **90**:990, 1968.

58. Caffey, J.: Pediatric x-ray diagnosis, ed. 2, Chicago, 1950, Year Book Medical Publishers, Inc., p. 41.

59. Caffey, J.: Prenatal bowing and thickening of the tubular bones with multiple cutaneous dimples in the arms and legs; a congenital syndrome of mechanical origin, Amer. J. Dis. Child. **74**:543, 1947.

60. Calkins, E., Kahn, D., and Diner, W. A.: Idiopathic familial osteoporosis in dogs; "osteogenesis imperfecta," Ann. N. Y. Acad. Sci. **64**:410, 1956.

61. Campbell, J. M.: Intrauterine osteogenesis imperfecta, Med. J. Aust. **1**:584, 1966.

62. Caniggia, A., Ravenni, G., and Del Giovane, L.: On the pathogenesis of fragilitas ossium hereditaria, Panminerva Med. **3**:67, 1961.

63. Caniggia, A., Stuart, C., and Guideri, R.: Fragilitas ossium hereditaria tarda (Eckman-Lobstein disease), Acta Med. Scand., supp, 340, p. 1, 1958.

64. Capdepont, C.: Dystrophie dentaire non encore décrite à type héréditaire et familial, Rev. Stomat. **12**:550; **13**:15, 1905-1906.

65. Carey, M. C., Fitzgerald, O., and McKiernan, E.: Osteogenesis imperfecta in twenty-three members of a kindred with heritable features contributed by a non-specific skeletal disorder, Quart. J. Med. **37**:437, 1968.

66. Casanovas, J.: Blue scleras and fragilitas ossium, Arch. Ophthal. Hispano-Amer. **34**:133, 1934.

67. Cattell, H. S., and Clayton, B.: Failure of anabolic steroids in the therapy of osteogenesis imperfecta; a clinical, metabolic, and biochemical study, J. Bone Joint Surg. **50-A**:123, 1968.

68. Chamberlain, W. E.: Basilar impression (platybasia); a bizarre developmental anomaly of the occipital bone and upper cervical spine, with striking and misleading neurologic manifestations, Yale J. Biol. Med. **11**:487, 1939.

69. Chawla, S.: Intrauterine osteogenesis imperfecta in four siblings, Brit. Med. J. **1**:99, 1964.

70. Cheney, W. D.: Acro-osteolysis, Amer. J. Roentgen. **94**:595, 1965.

71. Chont, L. K.: Osteogenesis imperfecta; report of 12 cases, Amer. J. Roentgen. **45**:850, 1941.

72. Chowers, I., Czaczkes, J. W., Ehrenfeld, E. N., and Landau, S.: Familial aminoaciduria in osteogenesis imperfecta, J.A.M.A. **181**:771, 1962.

73. Chu, H. I., Liu, S. H., Chen, K. C., Yü, T. F., Su, C. C., Wang, C. W., and Cheng, T. Y.: Osteogenesis imperfecta. II. Observations on the effect of vitamins C and D, and thyroid and pituitary preparations on the calcium, phosphorus and nitrogen metabolism, with a report of bone analysis, Chin. Med. J. **3** (supp.):539, 1940.

74. Cleminson, F. J.: Otosclerosis associated with blue sclerotics and osteogenesis imperfecta, Proc. Roy. Soc. Med. **20**:471, 1927.

75. Cloutier, M. D., Hayles, A. B., Riggs, B. L., Jowsey, J., and Bickel, W. H.: Juveline osteoporosis; report of a case, including a description of some metabolic and microradiographic studies, Pediatrics **40**:649, 1967.

76. Cocchi, U.: Hereditary diseases with bone changes. In Schinz, H. R.: Roentgen-diagnostics, New York, 1951, Grune & Stratton, Inc.

77. Colden, C.: Blaue Skleren mit eigenartigem ophthalmoskopischen Befund, Klin. Mbl. Augenheilk. **74**:360, 1925.

78. Committee on Otosclerosis, American Otological Society: Otosclerosis; a résumé of the literature to July, 1928, New York, 1929, Paul B. Hoeber, Inc., Medical Book Department of Harper & Row, Publishers.

79. Conlon, F. A.: Blue sclerotics; a note upon associated otosclerosis, Amer. J. Ophthal. **1** (series 3):726, 1918.

80. Conlon, F. A.: Five generations of blue sclerotics and associated osteoporosis, Boston Med. Surg. **169**:16, 1913.

81. Coop, M. C.: A treatment for osteogenesis imperfecta in kittens, J. Amer. Vet. Med. Ass. **132**:299, 1958.

82. Cornil, L., Berthier, J., and Sild, A.: Sur l'adjonction à osteopsathyrose hereditaire de deux nouveaux signes: tympans bleus et amyotrophie diffuse, Rev. Neurol. **67**:89, 1937.

83. Criscitiello, M. G., Ronan, J. A., Jr., Besterman, E. M. M., and Schoenwetter, W.: Cardiovascular abnormalities in osteogenesis imperfecta, Circulation **31**:255, 1965.

84. Cronental, R.: Ueber die Osteopsathyrosis hereditaria, Deutsch. Arch. Klin. Med. **174**:228, 1932.

85. Crooks, J.: Two unusual examples of osteogenesis imperfecta, Brit. Med. J. **1**:705, 1932.

85a. Cropp, G. J. A., and Myers, D. N.: Physiological evidence of hypermetabolism in osteogenesis imperfecta, Pediatrics **49**:375, 1972.

86. Crowe, F. W., Schull, W. J., and Neel, J. V.: A clinical pathological and genetic study of multiple neurofibromatosis, Springfield, Ill., 1956, Charles C Thomas, Publisher, p. 36.

86a. Currarino, G.: Hypophosphatasia, Amer. J. Roentgen. **78**:392, 1957.

87. Dalgaard, O.: Bilateral polycystic disease of the kidneys, Copenhagen, 1957, Ejnar Munksgaard Forlag.

88. Danelius, G.: Osteogenesis imperfecta intrauterin diagnostiziert, Arch. Gynaek. **154**:160, 1933.

89. Daubenspek, K.: Pseudoarthrosenbehandlung bei Osteopsathyrosis, Zbl. Chir. **67**:370, 1940.

90. Dent, C. E.: Idiopathic juvenile osteoporosis. In Bergsma, D., editor: Clinical delineation of birth defects. IV. Skeletal dysplasias, New York, 1969, National Foundation–March of Dimes, pp. 134-139.

91. Dent, C. E., and Friedman, M.: Idiopathic juvenile osteoporosis, Quart. J. Med. **34**:177, 1964.

92. Dessof, J.: Blue sclerotics, fragile bones and deafness, Arch. Ophthal. **12**:60, 1934.

93. Dorst, J. P., and McKusick, V. A.: Acro-osteolysis (Cheney syndrome); clinical delineation of birth defects. III. Limb malformations, New York, 1969, National Foundation–March of Dimes.

94. Dunham, C., and Spellacy, W.: Pregnancy in patients with osteogenesis imperfecta; a case report and a review of the literature, J. Lancet **87**:293, 1967.

95. Eddowes, A.: Dark sclerotics and fragilitas ossium, Brit. Med. J. **2**:222, 1900.

96. Ekman, O. J.: Dissertatio medica descriptionem et casus aliquot osteomalaciae sistens, Upsala, 1788.

97. Elefant, E., and Tošovsky, V.: Osteogenesis imperfecta congenita, Ann. Paediat. **202**:285, 1964.

98. Ellis, R. W. B.: Four cases of fragilitas ossium and blue sclerotics, Proc. Roy. Soc. Med. (Sect. Dis. Child.) **24**:1054, 1931.

99. Eltze, J., and Lennartz, K. J.: Callus luxurians bei Osteogenesis imperfecta unter dem Bilde eines Sarkoms, Z. Orthop. **106**:463, 1969.

100. Engfeldt, B., Engstrom, A., and Zetterstrom, R.: Biophysical studies of the bone tissue in osteogenesis imperfecta, J. Bone Joint Surg. **36-B**:654, 1954.

101. Epstein, C. J., Graham, C. B., and Hodgkin, W. E., et al.: Hereditary dysplasia of bone with kyphoscoliosis, contractures, and abnormally shaped ears, J. Pediat. **73**:379, 1968.

102. Estes, J. W.: Platelet size and function in the heritable disorders of connective tissue, Ann. Intern. Med. **68**:1237, 1968.

103. Evans, H. D.: Severe osteogenesis imperfecta with pregnancy; report of a case, Obstet. Gynec. **28**:394, 1966.

104. Evens, R. G., Pak, C. Y. C., Ashburn, W., and Bartler, F. C.: Clinical investigation in metabolic bone disease; quantitative measurements of bone mineral, Invest. Radiol. **4**:364, 1969.

105. Eyring, E. J., and Eisenberg, E.: Congenital hyperphosphatasia; a clinical, pathological, and biochemical study of two cases, J. Bone Joint Surg. **50-A**:1099, 1968.

106. Fairbank, T. A. T., and Baker, S. L.: Hyperplastic callus formation with or without evidence of fracture in osteogenesis imperfecta, with account of the histology, Brit. J. Surg. **36**:1, 1948.

107. Fairbank, Sir Thomas: An atlas of general affections of the skeleton, Baltimore, 1951, The Williams & Wilkins Co.

108. Faxén, N.: Case of twins with osteogenesis imperfecta, Acta Paediat. **14**:251, 1932.

109. Fineberg, N. L.: Rhinoplasty in osteogenesis imperfecta; case report, Eye Ear Nose Throat Monthly **44**:62, 1965.

110. Follis, R. H., Jr.: Histochemical studies on cartilage and bone. III. Osteogenesis imperfecta, Bull. Hopkins Hosp. **93**:386, 1953.

111. Follis, R. H., Jr.: Maldevelopment of the corium in the osteogenesis imperfecta syndrome, Bull. Hopkins Hosp. **93**:225, 1953.

112. Follis, R. H., Jr.: Osteogenesis imperfecta congenita; a connective tissue diathesis, J. Pediat. **41**:713, 1952.

113. Fraser, I.: Fragilitas ossium tarda, Brit. J. Surg. **22**:231, 1934.

114. Fraser, J. S.: Otosclerosis associated with fragilitas ossium and blue sclerotics; clinical report of 3 cases, Proc. Roy. Soc. Med. **12**:126, 1918.

115. Freda, V. J., Vosburgh, G. J., and Di Liberti, C.: Osteogenesis imperfecta congenita; a presentation of 16 cases and review of the literature, Obstet. Gynec. **18**:535, 1961.

116. Frerking, H. W., and Zink, O. C.: A case of osteogenesis imperfecta diagnosed in utero, Amer. J. Roentgen. **67**:103, 1952.

117. Freund, R., and Lehmacher, K.: Beitrag zur Vererbung der Osteogenesis imperfecta, Geburtsh. Frauenheilk. **14**:171, 1954.

118. Freytag, G. T.: Ueber blaue Sklera und Knochenbrüchigkeit, Klin. Mbl. Augenheilk. **66**:507, 1921.

119. Friedberg, C. K.: Zur Kenntnis des vererbbaren Syndroms: abnorme Knochenbrüchigkeit, blaue Skleren und Schwerhörigkeit, Klin. Wshr. **10**:830, 1931.

120. Friedenwald, J. S., and others: Ophthalmic pathology: an atlas and textbook, Philadelphia, 1952, W. B. Saunders Co.

121. Fulconis, H.: La fragilité osseuse congénitale (maladie de Durante), Paris, 1939, Masson et Cie.

122. Funk, P.: Beitrag zur Kenntnis der Osteopsathyrose (Typus Lobstein), Schweiz. Med. Wschr. **70**:473, 1940.

123. Fuss, H.: Die erbliche Osteopsathyrosis, Deutsch. Z. Chir. **245**:279, 1935.

124. Galton, B. B. (Wayne, N. J.): Personal communication, 1971.

125. Gardner, W. V., and Pfeiffer, C. A.: Influence of estrogen and androgens on the skeletal system, Physiol. Rev. **23**:139, 1954.

126. Gautier, P., and Guinard-Daniol, J.: Un cas de maladie de Lobstein associée à une thrombasthenie héréditaire et familial de Glanzmann, Bull. Soc. Méd. Hôp. Paris **68**:577, 1952.

127. Gebala, A.: Acid hyperphosphatasia in three families with osteogenesis imperfecta, Lancet **2**:1084, 1956.

128. Geipert, G.: Beitrag zur Erblichkeit der sog. Osteopsathyrosis, Z. Menschl. Vererb. Konstitutionsl. **19**:691, 1936.

129. Gilchrist, G. S., and Shore, N. A.: Familial leukemia and osteogenesis imperfecta, J. Pediat. **71**:115, 1967.

130. Gillanders, L. A.: Osteogenesis imperfecta diagnosed in utero, Brit. J. Radiol. **30**:500, 1957.

131. Gimplinger, E.: Blaue Verfärbung der Skleren und Herderkrankung der Labyrinthkapsel, Arch. Ohr. Nas. Kehlkopfheilk. **13**:345, 1925.

132. Ginsberg, D. M.: Normal serum acid phosphatase levels in osteogenesis imperfecta, Ann. Intern. Med. **56**:141, 1962.

133. Giordano, A.: Hereditary diseases of the osteo-cartilaginous system; comparative morphological basis, Acta Genet. 7:155, 1957.

134. Glanzmann, E.: Familiäre Osteogenesis imperfecta (Typus Vrolik) und ihre Behandlung mit Vitamin D-Stoss, Bull. Schweiz. Akad. Med. Wiss. 1:180, 1945.

135. Glanzmann, E.: Hereditäre hämorrhagische Thrombasthenie (ein Beitrag zur Pathologie des Blutplättchen), Jahrb. Kinderheilk. 88:113, 1918.

136. Glanzmann, E.: Osteogenesis imperfecta (Typus Vrolik) und Osteopsathyrosis idiopathica (Typus Lobstein), Schweiz. Med. Wschr. 66:1122, 1936.

137. Gleich, M.: Osteogenesis imperfecta tarda; report of 4 cases in one family, New York J. Med. 30:850, 1930.

138. Goldfarb, A. A., and Ford, D.: Osteogenesis imperfecta in consecutive siblings, J. Pediat. 44:264, 1954.

139. Gray, P. H. K.: A case of osteogenesis imperfecta, associated with dentinogenesis imperfecta, dating from antiquity, Clin. Radiol. 21:106, 1970.

140. Greenberg, E. I., and Faegenburg, D.: The antepartum diagnosis of osteogenesis imperfecta congenita: a report of two cases recognized in utero, J. Mount Sinai Hosp. N. Y. 31:90, 1964.

141. Guay, F. G., MacNab, I., and Yendt, E. R.: Primary hyperparathyroidism in osteogenesis imperfecta, Canad. Med. Ass. J. 98:960, 1968.

142. Goidanich, I. F., Lenzi, L., and Silva, E.: Urinary hydroxyproline excretion in normal subjects and in patients affected with primary disease of bone, Clin. Chim. Acta 11:35, 1965.

143. Gurlt, E.: Handbuch der Lehre von den Knochenbruchen, Berlin, 1862-1865, vol. 1, pp. 147-154.

144. Gutzeit, R.: Ueber blaue Sklera und Knochenbrüchigkeit, Klin. Mbl. Augenheilk. 68:771, 1922.

145. Haebara, H., Yamasaki, Y., and Kyogoku, M.: An autopsy case of osteogenesis imperfecta congenita; histochemical and electron microscopical studies, Acta Path. Jap. 19:377, 1969.

146. Hall, J. G., and Rohrt, T.: The stapes in osteogenesis imperfecta, Acta Otolaryng. 65:345, 1968.

147. Hanhart, E.: Ergebnisse der Erforschung von Erbkrankheiten und Missbildungen in der Schweiz, Arch. Klaus Stift. Vererbungsforsch. 18:632, 1943.

148. Hanhart, E.: Ueber eine neue Form von Osteopsathyrosis congenita mit einfachrezessivem Erbgang, sowie vier neue Sippen mit dominantem Erbgang und die Frage der Vererbung der sog. Osteogenesis imperfecta, Arch. Klaus Stift. Vererbungsforsch. 26:426, 1951.

149. Harlow, R. A.: A case of osteogenesis imperfecta diagnosed in utero, Brit. J. Clin. Pract. 22:446, 1968.

150. Harnett, W. L.: Two cases of osteogenesis imperfecta with blue sclerotics in natives of India, Brit. J. Surg. 22:269, 1934.

151. Hass, J.: Zur Kenntnis der Osteopsathyrosis idiopathica, Med. Klin. 15:1112, 1919.

152. Hatteland, K.: T. Norske Laegeforg. 77:75, 1957. Quoted in Brit. Med. J. 1:1172, 1957.

153. Heckman, B. A., and Steinberg, I.: Congenital heart disease (mitral regurgitation) in osteogenesis imperfecta, Amer. J. Roentgen. 103:601, 1968.

154. Hein, B. J.: Osteogenesis imperfecta with multiple fractures at birth: an investigation with special reference to heredity and blue sclera, J. Bone Joint Surg. 10:243, 1928.

155. Henley, F. A.: A case of congenital osteopsathyrosis with genealogical tree of the family, Brit. Med. J. 1:326, 1942.

155a. Heppner, R. L., Babitt, H. I., Bianchine, J. W., and Warbasse, J. R.: Aortic regurgitation and aneurysm of the sinus of Valsalva associated with osteogenesis imperfecta (submitted for publication).

156. Herndon, C. N.: Osteogenesis imperfecta; some clinical and genetic considerations, Clin. Orthop. 8:132, 1956.

157. Heys, F. M., Blattner, F. J., and Robinson, H. B. G.: Osteogenesis imperfecta and odontogenesis imperfecta: clinical and genetic aspects in eighteen families, J. Pediat. 56:234, 1960.

158. Hilgenfeldt, O.: Beitrag zum Krankheitsbilde der idiopathischen abnormen Knochenbrüchigkeit, Deutsch. Z. Chir. 238:433, 1933.

159. Hills, R. G., and McLanahan, S.: Brittle bones and blue scleras in five generations, Arch. Intern. Med. 59:41, 1937.

160. Holcomb, D. Y.: A fragile-boned family; hereditary fragilitas ossium, J. Hered. **22**:105, 1931.

161. Holmes, J. R., Baker, J. R., and Davies, E. T.: Osteogenesis imperfecta in lambs, Vet. Rec. **76**:980, 1964.

162. Holzworth, J.: Osteogenesis imperfecta, Vet. Bull. (Lederle) **15**:18, 1956.

163. Holzworth, J.: Disease conditions prominent in cats, Univ. Pennsylvania Bull. School Vet. Med., Veterinary Extension Quart. **58**:101, 1958.

164. Humbert, J. R., Solomons, C. C., and Ott, J. E.: Increased oxidative metabolism by leukocytes of patients with osteogenesis imperfecta and of their relatives, J. Pediat. **78**:648, 1971.

165. Hunter, D.: A case of osteogenesis imperfecta, Lancet **1**:9, 1927.

166. Hursey, R. J., Witkop, C. J., Jr., Miklashek, D., and Sackett, L. M.: Dentinogenesis imperfecta in a racial isolate with multiple hereditary defects, Oral Surg. **9**:641, 1956.

167. Hurwitz, L. J., and McSwiney, R. R.: Basilar impression and osteogenesis imperfecta in a family, Brain **83**:138, 1960.

168. Hyams, S. W., Kar, H., and Neumann, E.: Blue sclerae and keratoglobus; ocular signs of a systemic connective tissue disorder, Brit. J. Ophthal. **53**:53, 1969.

168a. Hyams, V. J. (Washington, D. C.): Personal communication, 1972.

169. Ibsen, K. H.: Distinct varieties of osteogenesis imperfecta, Clin. Orthop. **50**:279, 1967.

170. Ibsen, K. H.: Heterogeneity in osteogenesis imperfecta; clinical delineation of birth defects. IV. Skeletal dysplasias, New York, 1969, National Foundation–March of Dimes.

171. Inderbitzin, A.: Ueber Anosteoplasia congenita beim Kalbe, Virchow Arch. Path. Anat. **269**:665, 1928.

172. Ivancie, G. P.: Dentinogenesis imperfecta, Oral Surg. **7**:984, 1954.

173. Jackson, W. P. U.: Osteoporosis of unknown cause in younger people; idiopathic osteoporosis, J. Bone Joint Surg. **40-B**:420, 1958.

174. Jacobsen, J. G., Matienzo, J. A., Forbes, A. P., and Rourke, G. M.: Serum acid phosphatase in osteogenesis imperfecta, Metabolism **10**:483, 1961.

175. Jeckeln, E.: Systemgebundene mesenchymale Erschöpfung. Eine neue Bergriffsfassung der Osteogenesis imperfecta, Virchow Arch. Path. Anat. **280**:351, 1931.

176. Jelnes, K. T.: Osteogenesis imperfecta and otosclerosis, Ugeskr. Laeg. **111**:1262, 1949.

177. Jewell, F. C., and Lofstrom, L. E.: Osteogenic sarcoma occurring in fragilitas ossium, Radiology **34**:741, 1940.

178. Joachim, H., and Wasch, M. G.: Fragilitas ossium in five generations, Ann. Intern. Med. **7**:853, 1934.

179. Johansson, S.: Ein Fall von Osteogenesis imperfecta mit verbreiteten Gefassverkalkungen, Acta Radiol. **1**:17, 1921.

180. Johnson, W. A., and Karrer, M. C.: Osteogenesis imperfecta in pregnancy; report of a case, Obstet. Gynec. **10**:642, 1957.

181. Jornod, J., Rothlin, M., and Uehlinger, E.: Cardiovascular anomalies in Lobstein's disease, Schweiz. Med. Wschr. **98**:795, 1968.

182. Kaplan, M., and Baldino, C.: Dysplasie periostale paraissant familiale et transmise suivant le mode mendélien recessif, Arch. Franc. Pediat. **10**:943, 1953.

183. Kaplan, M., Laplane, R., Debray, P., and Lasfargues, F.: Sur l'hérédité de la dysplasie periostale complément à la communication de M. Kaplan et C. Baldino, Arch. Franç. Pédiat. **15**:1097, 1958.

184. Katsu, Y.: An instance of osteogenesis imperfecta congenita, Jap. J. Obstet. **16**:171, 1933.

185. Kaul, B.: Ein Abortivfall von Osteogenesis imperfecta congenita kombiniert mit Missbildungen der Blutgefasse (Osteoangiogenesis imperfecta), Frankfurt. Z. Path. **53**:289, 1939.

186. Keats, T. E.: Diffuse thickening of the calvarium in osteogenesis imperfecta, Radiology **69**:408, 1957.

187. Keats, T. E.: Diffuse thickening of the calvarium in osteogenesis imperfecta; further observations, Radiology **86**:97, 1966.

188. Keats, T. E., and Anast, G. S.: Circumscribed skeletal rarefactions in osteogenesis imperfecta, Amer. J. Roentgen. **84**:492, 1960.

189. Kellogg, C. S.: Osteogenesis imperfecta; study of five generations, Arch. Intern. Med. **80**:358, 1947.

190. Kersley, G. D.: Fragilitas ossium and allied conditions, St. Bartholomew's Hosp. Rep. **68**:159, 1935.

191. Key, J. A.: Brittle bones and blue sclerae (hereditary hypoplasia of the mesenchyme), Arch. Surg. **13**:523, 1926.

192. Khoo, F. Y.: Congenital pseudarthrosis of the tibia and its relation to fragilitas ossium, Amer. J. Dis. Child. **77**:201, 1949.

193. Kidd, F.: Case for diagnosis: imperfecta osteogenesis? Proc. Roy. Soc. Med. 4 (Clin. Sect.): 106, 1911.

194. Kienböch, R.: Über infantile Osteopsathyrose, Fortschr. Roentgenstr. **23**:122, 1915-1916.

195. Kingsley, H. J.: Elastosis perforans serpiginosa with osteogenesis imperfecta, Arch. Derm. **90**:453, 1964.

196. Kingsley, H. J.: Peculiarities in dermatology, case reports. II. Elastosis perforans serpiginosa associated with osteogenesis imperfecta, Cent. Afr. J. Med. **14**:176, 1968.

197. Klenerman, L., Ockenden, B. G., and Townsend, A. C.: Osteosarcoma occurring in osteogenesis imperfecta; report of two cases, J. Bone Joint Surg. **49-B**:314, 1967.

198. Knaggs, L.: Osteogenesis imperfecta, Brit. J. Surg. **11**:737, 1924.

199. Komai, T., Kunai, H., and Ozaki, Y.: A note on the genetics of van der Hoeve's syndrome, with special reference to a large Japanese kindred, Amer. J. Hum. Genet. **8**:110, 1956.

200. Krabbe, K. H.: La maladie de Henri de Toulouse-Lautrec, Acta Psychiat. Neurol. Scand. **108** (supp.):211, 1956.

201. Lamy, M.: L'infirmité de Toulouse-Lautrec, Presse Méd. **64**:249, 1956.

202. Langness, U., and Behnke, H.: Biochemische Untersuchungen zur Osteogenesis imperfecta, Deutsch. Med. Wschr. **95**:213, 1970.

203. Langness, U., and Behnke, H.: Collagen metabolites in plasma and urine in osteogenesis imperfecta, Metabolism **20**:456, 1971.

204. Langness, U., and Behnke, H.: Die Hydroxyprolinausscheidung im Urin bei der Osteogenesis imperfecta, Klin. Wschr. **44**:1294, 1966.

205. Langness, U., and Behnke, H.: Klinik und Genetik der Osteogenesis imperfecta, Deutsch. Med. Wschr. **95**:209, 1970.

206. Laurent, L. E., and Salenius, P.: Hyperplastic callus formation in osteogenesis imperfecta; report of a case simulating sarcoma, Acta Orthop. Scand. **38**:280, 1967.

207. Leicher, H., and Haas, E.: Labyrinthausfall bei Osteopsathyrosis, Z. Laryng. **36**:190, 1957.

208. Leonard, C. O. (Baltimore): Personal communication, 1971.

209. Levin, E. J.: Intrauterine osteogenesis imperfecta in one of a pair of twins, Amer. J. Roentgen. **93**:405, 1965.

210. Levin, E. J.: Osteogenesis imperfecta in the adult, Amer. J. Roentgen. **91**:973, 1964.

211. Liber, B.: Fragilitas ossium, J.A.M.A. **162**:700, 1956.

212. Lobeck, H.: Ein Beitrag zur Osteogenesis imperfecta, Frankfurt, 1938, A.M. Dissertation, p. 32, cited by Seedorff.[294]

213. Lobstein, J. G. C. F. M.: Lehrbuch der pathologischen Anatomie, Stuttgart, 1835, vol. 2, p. 179.

214. Looser, E.: Zur Kenntnis der Osteogenesis imperfecta congenita et tarda, Mitt. Grenzgeb. Med. Chir. **15**:161, 1906.

215. Lovett, R. W., and Nichols, H.: Osteogenesis imperfecta; with the report of a case, with autopsy and histological examination, Brit. Med. J. **2**:915, 1906.

216. Lynch, H. T., Lemon, H. M., and Krush, A. J.: A note on "cancer-susceptible" and "cancer-resistant" genotypes; implications for cancer detection and research, Nebraska Med. J. **51**:209, 1966.

217. Macgregor, A. G., and Harrison, R.: Congenital total color blindness associated with otosclerosis, Ann. Eugen. **15**:219, 1950.

218. McKinney, R.: Studies on fibers in tissue cultures. III. The development of reticulum into collagenous fibers in cultures of adult rabbit lymph nodes, Arch. Exp. Zellforsch. **9**:14, 1929.

219. McKusick, V. A.: Hereditary disorders of connective tissue, Bull. N. Y. Acad. Med. **35**:143, 1959.

220. McKusick, V. A.: Unpublished observations.

221. McKusick, V. A., and colleagues: Medical genetics 1963, J. Chronic Dis. **17**:1077, 1964.

222. Malmquist, J., Jagenburg, R., and Lindstedt, G.: Familial protein intolerance; possible nature of enzyme defect, New Eng. J. Med. **284**:997, 1971.

223. Maloney, F. P.: Osteogenesis imperfecta of early onset in three members of an inbred group; ?recessive inheritance. Clinical delineation of birth defects. IV. Skeletal dysplasias, New York, 1969, National Foundation–March of Dimes, pp. 219-224.

224. Manschot, W. A.: Ocular anomalies in osteogenesis imperfecta, Ophthalmologica **149**: 241, 1965.

225. Maroteaux, P., and Lamy, M.: The malady of Toulouse-Lautrec, J.A.M.A. **191**:715, 1965.

226. Maroteaux, P., and Lamy, M.: L'osteogenesis imperfecta et les difficultés de son diagnostic, Presse Méd. **73**:1535, 1965.

227. Maroteaux, P., and Lamy, M.: La pycnodysostose, Presse Méd. **70**:999, 1962.

228. Mehregan, A. H.: Elastosis perforans serpiginosa; a review of the literature and report of 11 cases, Arch. Derm. **97**:381, 1968.

229. Mengel, M. C.: Osteogenesis imperfecta and panhypopituitarism. In Bergsma, D., editor: Clinical delineation of birth defects. X. Endocrine system, Baltimore, 1971, The Williams & Wilkins Co.

230. Messinger, A. L., and Teal F.: Intramedullary nailing for correction of deformity in osteogenesis imperfecta, Clin. Orthop. **1**:221, 1955.

231. Meyer, H.: Atypical osteogenesis imperfecta; Lobstein's disease, Arch. Pediat. **72**:182, 1955.

231a. Milgram, J. W., Flick, M. R., and Engh, C. A.: Osteogenesis imperfecta. A histopathological case report. (To be published.)

232. Milne, M. D., Stanbury, S. W., and Thomson, A. E.: Observations on Fanconi syndrome and renal hyperchloraemic acidosis in adults, Quart. J. Med. **21**:61, 1952.

233. Monks, P. L.: Intrauterine osteogenesis imperfecta; report of a case associated with hydramnios and dystocia, Aust. New Zeal. J. Obstet. Gynaec. **8**:157, 1968.

234. Mørsch, E. T.: Chondrodystrophic dwarfs in Denmark. In Opera ex domo biologiae hereditarie humanae Universitatis Hafniensis, vol. 3, Copenhagen, 1941, Ejnar Munksgaard.

235. Motulsky, A., Heustis, R., and Anderson, R.: Hereditary spherocytosis in mouse and man, Acta Genet. (Basel) **6**:240, 1956.

236. Muldowney, F. P., O'Donovan, D. K., and Gallagher, J. E.: Bone formation in osteogenesis imperfecta; the effect of anabolic steroid therapy, J. Irish Med. Ass. **54**:132, 1964.

237. Murray, D., and Young, B. H.: Osteogenesis imperfecta treated by fixation with intramedullary rod, Southern Med. J. **53**:1142, 1960.

238. Mussio, T. J.: Osteogenesis imperfecta congenita: report of a case discovered in utero, Obstet. Gynec. **15**:361, 1960.

239. Nager, F. R.: Otosklerose bei infantiler Osteopsathyrosis und Blaufärbung der Skleren, Schweiz. Med. Wschr. **51**:660, 1921.

240. Nager, F. R.: Pathology of the labyrinthine capsule, and its cilnical significance. In Nelson loose-leaf medicine of the ear, New York, 1939, Thomas Nelson & Sons, p. 237.

240a. Nager, G. T. (Baltimore): Personal communication, June, 1972.

241. Naita, S.: Klinische und histologische Untersuchungen des Zahngewebes bei Osteogenesis imperfecta, etc., Mitt. Med. Fakült. Kais. Univ. Kyushu, Fukuoka. **9**:97, 1924. Ref. Zbl. Kinderheilk. **18**:822, 1925.

242. Navani, S. V., and Sarzin, B.: Intra-uterine osteogenesis imperfecta; review of the literature and a report of the radiological and necropsy findings in two cases, Brit. J. Radiol. **40**:449, 1967.

243. Nielsen, H. E.: Familial occurrence of osseus fragility, blue sclera and deafness, Nord. Med. **15**:2203, 1942.

244. Nordin, B. E., and Roper, A.: Post-pregnancy osteoporosis; a syndrome? Lancet **1**:431, 1955.

245. Noyes, F. B.: Hereditary anomaly in structure of dentin (abstract), J. Dent. Res. **15**:154, 1935.

246. O'Connell, J. E. A., and Turner, J. W. A.: Basilar impression of the skull, Brain **73**:405, 1950.

247. Opheim, O.: Loss of hearing following the syndrome of van der Hoeve–de Kleyn, Acta Otolaryng. **65**:337, 1968.

248. Ormerod, E. L.: An account of a case of mollities ossium, Brit. Med. J. **2**:735, 1859.

248a. Opitz, J. M. (Madison, Wis.): Personal communication, 1972.

249. Patterson, C. N., and Stone, H. B., III: Stapedectomy in van der Hoeve's syndrome, Laryngoscope **80**:544, 1970.

250. Pelner, L., and Cohen, J. N.: Osteogenesis imperfecta tarda, Amer. J. Roentgen. **61**:690, 1949.

251. Perruchot, H.: Toulouse-Lautrec (translated by Humphrey Hare), Cleveland and New York, 1960, The World Publishing Co.

252. Peters, A.: Blaue Sklera und Knochenbrüchigkeit, Klin. Mbl. Augenheilk. **51**:594, 1913.

253. Pierog, S. H., Fontana, V. J., and Ferrara, A.: Osteogenesis imperfecta; therapeutic challenge, New York J. Med. **69**:310, 1969.

254. Posner, A. C., and Goldman, J. A.: A case of osteogenesis imperfecta congenita diagnosed in utero, Amer. J. Obstet. Gynec. **73**:1143, 1957.

255. Puppel, E.: Osteogenesis imperfecta, Mschr. Geburtsh. Gyn. **82**:269, 1929.

256. Ramser, J. R., and Frost, H. M.: The study of a rib biopsy from a patient with osteogenesis imperfecta; a method using in vivo tetracycline labeling, Acta Orthop. Scand. **37**:229, 1966.

257. Ramser, J. R., Villanueva, A. R., and Pirok, D.: Tetracycline-based measurement of bone dynamics in 3 women with osteogenesis imperfecta, Clin. Orthop. **49**:151, 1966.

258. Rao, S., and Witkop, C. J.: Inherited defects in tooth structure. Clinical delineation of birth defects. XI. Orofacial structures, Baltimore, 1971, The Williams & Wilkins, Co.

258a. Rebouillat, J., Revelin, P., and Brault, A.: Le traitement chirurgical des ostéogénèses imparfaites par ostéotomies étagées et embrochage diaphysaires, Pediatrie **24**:411, 1969.

259. Reed, W. B., and Pidgeon, J. W.: Elastosis perforans serpiginosa with osteogenesis imperfecta, Arch. Derm. (Chicago) **89**:342, 1964.

260. Reid, J.: Congenital poikiloderma with osteogenesis imperfecta, Brit. J. Derm. **79**:243, 1967.

261. Relias, A., Sakellariou, G., Tsoitis, G., and Toubanaki, E.: Élastose perforante serpigineuse de Lutz-Miescher et osteogenesis imperfecta, Ann. Derm. Syph. **95**:491, 1968.

262. Remigio, P. A., and Grinvalsky, H. T.: Osteogenesis imperfecta congenita; association with conspicuous extraskeletal connective tissue dysplasia, Amer. J. Dis. Child. **119**:524, 1970.

263. Rennert, H., and Popella, E.: Abortive Fälle von Osteopsathyrose mit Marfan-Symptomatik, Med. Mschr. **9**:106, 1955.

264. Riddell, W. J. B.: A pedigree of blue sclerotics, brittle bones and deafness, with colour blindness, Ann. Eugen. **10**:1, 1955.

265. Rieseman, F. R., and Yater, W. M.: Osteogenesis imperfecta; its incidence and manifestations in seven families, Arch. Intern. Med. **67**:950, 1941.

266. Riser, W. H.: Juvenile osteoporosis (osteogenesis imperfecta)—a calcium deficiency, J. Amer. Vet. Med. Ass. **139**:117, 1961.

267. Roberts, E., and Schour, I.: Hereditary opalescent dentine—dentinogenesis imperfecta, Amer. J. Orthodont. **25**:267, 1939.

268. Robichon, J., and Germain, J. P.: Pathogenesis of osteogenesis imperfecta, Canad. Med. Ass. J. **99**:975, 1968.

268a. Rodriguez, R. P., Jr., and Wickstrom, J. K.: Osteogenesis imperfecta and a preliminary report on resurfacing of long bones with intramedullary fixation by an extensible intramedullary device, Southern Med. J. **64**:169, 1971.

269. Rogers, T. R.: Otosclerosis associated with blue sclerotics and fragilitas ossium, Proc. Roy. Soc. Med. **29**:1107, 1936.

270. Rohwedder, H. J.: Ein Beitrag zur Frage des Erbganges der Osteogenesis imperfecta Vrolik, Arch. Kinderheilk. **147**:256, 1953.

271. Rolleston, J. D.: Inherited syphilis and blue sclerotics, Ophthalmoscope **9**:321, 1911.

272. Root, A. W., Bongiovanni, A. M., and Eberlein, W. R.: Measurement of the kinetics of calcium metabolism in children and adolescents utilizing nonradioactive strontium, J. Clin. Endocr. **26**:537, 1966.

273. Ropes, M. W., Rossmeisl, E. C., and Bauer, W.: The effect of estrin medication in osteogenesis imperfecta, Conference on Metabolic Aspects of Convalescence, New York, 1946, Trans. 14th meeting, Josiah Macy Jr. Foundation, p. 87.

274. Rosenbaum, S.: Osteogenesis imperfecta and osteopsathyrosis; a contribution to the study of their identity and their pathogenesis, J. Pediat. **25**:161, 1944.

275. Rosenstock, H. A.: Osteogenesis imperfecta, J.A.M.A. **203**:740, 1968.

276. Rosenstock, H. A.: Osteogenesis imperfecta—biochemical cancer resistance, Texas Med. **66**:44, 1970.

277. Ruedemann, A. D., Jr.: Osteogenesis imperfecta congenita and blue sclerotics: a clinico-pathologic study, Arch. Ophthal. **49**:6, 1953.

278. Rushton, M. A.: The structure of the teeth in a late case of osteogenesis imperfecta, J. Path. Bact. **48**:591, 1939.

279. Russell, R. G. G., Bisaz, S., Donath, A., Morgan, D. B., and Fleisch, H.: Inorganic pyro-phosphate in plasma in normal persons and in patients with hypophosphatasia, osteo-genesis imperfecta and other disorders of bone, J. Clin. Invest. **50**:961, 1971.

280. Ruth, E. B.: Osteogenesis imperfecta; anatomic study of a case, Arch. Path. **36**:211, 1943.

281. Ruttin, E.: Ohrbefund bei Osteopsathyrose, Mschr. Ohrenheilk. **53**:305, 1919.

282. Ruttin, E.: Osteopsathyrose und Otosklerose, Arch. Ohr. Nas. Kehlkopfheilk. **3**:263, 1922.

283. Sargent, E. N., Turner, A. F., and Jacobson, G.: Superior marginal rib defects; an etiologic classification, Amer. J. Roentgen. **106**:491, 1969.

284. Sarma, V.: A case of intrauterine osteogenesis imperfecta, Brit. Med. J. **2**:1856, 1960.

284a. Scherlis, L. (Baltimore): Personal communication, 1972.

285. Scherr, D. D.: A severely deformed patient with osteogenesis imperfecta at the age of fifty-four, J. Bone Joint Surg. **46-A**:159, 1964.

286. Schmidt, M. B.: Die allgemeinen Entwicklüngshemmungen der Knochen, Ergebn. Allg. Path. **4**:612, 1897.

287. Schröder, G.: Osteogenesis imperfecta; eine klinisch-erbbiologische Untersuchung des Krankengutes in Westfalen. Schätzung der Mutationsraten für den Regrerungsbezirk Mün-ster (Westfalen), Z. Menschl. Vererb. Konstitutionsl. **37**:632, 1964.

288. Schultze, F.: Beitrag zur idiopathischen Osteopsathyrose, Arch. Klin. Chir. **47**:327, 1894.

289. Schulze, C.: Erbbedingte Strukturanomalien menschlicher Zähne, Munich and Berlin, 1956, Urban u. Schwarzenberg.

290. Schwarz, E.: Hypercallosis in osteogenesis imperfecta, Amer. J. Roentgen. **85**:645, 1961.

291. Scott, D., and Stiris, G.: Osteogenesis imperfecta tarda, a study of three families with special reference to scar formation, Acta Med. Scand. **145**:237, 1953.

292. Scott, P. P., McKusick, V. A., and McKusick, A. B.: The nature of "osteogenesis imperfecta" in cats; evidence that the disorder is primarily nutritional, not genetic, and therefore not analogous to the disease in man, J. Bone Joint Surg. **45-A**:125, 1963.

293. Second, E. W., Wilder, R. M., and Henderson, M. S.: Osteogenesis imperfecta tarda (os-teopsathyrosis) treated with thymus extract (Hanson), Proc. Mayo Clin. **11**:1, 1936.

294. Seedorff, K. S.: Osteogenesis imperfecta; a study of clinical features and heredity based on 55 Danish families comprising 180 affected persons, Copenhagen, 1949, Ejnar Munks-gaard.

295. Segrest, J. P., and Cunningham, L. W.: Variations in human urinary O-hydroxylysyl gly-coside levels and their relationship to collagen metabolism, J. Clin. Invest. **49**:1497, 1970.

296. Seriki, O.: Case report; osteogenesis imperfecta congenita in one of twins, Acta Paediat. Scand. **59**:340, 1970.

297. Shambaugh, G. E., Jr.: Fenestration operation for otosclerosis; experimental investigations and clinical observations in 2,100 operations over period of 10 years, Acta Otolaryng. **79** (supp.):1, 1949.

298. Sharma, N. L., and Anand, J. S.: Osteogenesis imperfecta with arthrogryposis multiplex congenita, J. Indian Med. Ass. **43**:124, 1964.

299. Shea, J.: Surgical treatment of the hearing loss associated with osteogenesis imperfecta, J. Laryng. **77**:679, 1963.

300. Shorr, E., and Carter, A. C.: The usefulness of strontium as an adjuvant to calcium in the remineralization of the skeleton in man, Bull. Hosp. Joint Dis. **13**:59, 1952.

301. Shrivastava, T. P., and Gupta, O. P.: Otosclerosis and osteogenesis imperfecta, J. Laryng. **83**:1195, 1969.

302. Shugrue, J. J., Rockwood, R., and Anderson, E. W.: Fragilitas ossium and deafness, Arch. Intern. Med. **39**:98, 1927.

303. Siegel, B. M., Friedman, I. A., and Schwartz, S. O.: Hemorrhagic disease in osteogenesis imperfecta; study of platelet functional defect, Amer. J. Med. **22**:315, 1957.

304. Simmons, C. C.: Osteogenesis imperfecta and idiopathic fragilitas ossium, Amer. Surg. **46**:179, 1907.

305. Simsky: Blue sclerotics, fragility of the bones and deafness, Amer. J. Ophthal. **9**:844, 1926.

306. Sisk, J. N.: Fragilitas ossium in twins, Wisconsin Med. J. **30**:273, 1931.

307. Skaggs, J. W., and Theobald, J. A.: Osteogenesis imperfecta in a kitten, J. Amer. Vet. Med. Ass. **130**:450, 1957.

308. Smårs, G.: Osteogenesis imperfecta in Sweden; clinical, genetic, epidemiological and socio-medical aspects, Stockholm, 1961, Svenska Bokförlaget.

309. Smårs, G., Beckman, L., and Böök, J. A.: Osteogenesis imperfecta and blood groups, Acta Genet. **11**:133, 1961.

310. Smith, O. N., and Mitchell, J. M.: The serum phosphatase in osteogenesis imperfecta, Amer. J. Med. Sci. **190**:765, 1935.

311. Snapper, I.: Medical clinics on bone diseases, ed. 2, New York, 1949, Interscience Publishers.

312. Sofield, H. A., and Millar, E. A.: Fragmentation, realignment, and intramedullary rod fixation of deformities of the long bones in children, J. Bone Joint Surg. **41-A**:1371, 1959.

313. Solomons, C. C., Millar, E. A., Hathaway, W. E., and Ott, J. E.: Osteogenesis imperfecta; new perspectives in diagnosis and treatment, in press, 1972.

314. Solomons, C. C., and Styner, J.: Osteogenesis imperfecta; effect of magnesium administration on pyrophosphate metabolism, Calcif. Tissue Res. **3**:318, 1969.

315. Spranger, J. (Kiel, Germany): Personal communication, Nov., 1970.

316. Spranger, J., Langer, L. O., and Maroteaux, P.: Increasing frequency of a syndrome of multiple osseous defects (letter), Lancet **2**:716, 1970.

317. Spurway, J.: Hereditary tendency to fracture, Brit. Med. J. **2**:844, 1896.

318. Stapes, P. P., Jr., and Riva, H. L.: Maternal osteogenesis imperfecta; report of two cases in sisters, Obstet. Gynec. **4**:557, 1954.

319. Stein, F. H.: Nogen tilfaelder av osteopsathyrosis idiopathica med nedarvning i 4 led, T. Norske Laegeforen. **47**:557, 1927. Cited by Seedorff.[294]

320. Stein, R., Lazar, M., and Adam, A.: Brittle cornea; a familial trait associated with blue sclera, Amer. J. Ophthal. **66**:67, 1968.

321. Steinbach, H. L.: The roentgen appearance of osteoporosis, Radiol. Clin. N. Amer. **2**:191, 1964.

322. Stenvers, H. W.: Röntgenologische Bemerkungen zur vorhergehenden Arbeit von J. van der Hoeve und A. de Kleyn, Arch. Ophthal. **95**:94, 1918.

323. Stephenson, S.: Blue sclerotics, Trans. Ophthal. Soc. U. K. **35**:274, 1915.

324. Stevenson, C. J., Bottoms, E., and Shuster, S.: Skin collagen in osteogenesis imperfecta, Lancet **1**:860, 1970.

325. Stilling, H.: Osteogenesis imperfecta, Virchow Arch. **115**:357, 1889.

326. Stobie, W.: The association of blue sclerotics with brittle bones and progressive deafness, Quart. J. Med. **17**:274, 1924.

327. Stool, N., and Sullivan, C. R.: Osteogenesis imperfecta in a 95-year-old woman, Proc. Mayo Clin. **34**:523, 1959.

328. Strach, E. H.: Hyperplastic callus formation in osteogenesis imperfecta; report of a case and review of the literature, J. Bone Joint Surg. **35-B**:417, 1953.

329. Strach, E.: Beobachtung von Fragilität der Knochen in der Jugend, ein Beitrag zu der Lehre von den Knochenkrankheiten, J. Pract. Arzneyk. Wundarzneyk. **25**:163, 1807.

330. Summer, G. K.: Oral proline tolerance in osteogenesis imperfecta, Science **134**:1527, 1961.

331. Summer, G. K., and Patton, W. C.: Intravenous proline tolerance in osteogenesis imperfecta, Metabolism **17**:46, 1968.

332. Sundberg, C. G.: Discussion of paper by G. Zander, Nord. Med. **1**:802, 1939. Quoted by Seedorff.[294]

333. Taylor, A. R., and Chakravorty, B. C.: Clinical syndromes associated with basilar impression, Arch. Neurol. **10**:475, 1964.

334. Terrien, F., Sainton, P., and Veil, P.: Deux cas de syndrome de van der Hoeve (oeil bleu; fragilité osseuse; surdité), Arch. Ophthal. **44**:293, 1927.

335. Terry, W. I.: Hereditary osteopsathyrosis, Trans. Amer. S. A. **36**:317, 1918.

336. Toit, S. N., and Weiss, C.: Congenital dislocation of hips associated with osteogenesis imperfecta in male siblings; a case report, Bull. Hosp. Joint Dis. 30:164, 1969.

337. Toto, P. D.: Osteogenesis imperfecta tarda with dentinogenesis imperfecta, Oral Surg. 6:772, 1953.

338. Tucker, D. P.: Blue sclerotics syndrome simulating buphthalmos, Amer. J. Ophthal. 47: 345, 1959.

339. Vallery-Radot, P., and Aris, P.: Osteopsathyrosis hereditaire, Bull. Soc. Pédiat. Paris 22:291, 1924.

340. Valvassori, G. E.: Tomographic findings in cochlear otosclerosis, Arch. Otolaryng. 89:377, 1969.

341. Van der Hoeve, J., and de Kleyn, A.: Blaue Sclerae, Knochenbrüchigkeit und Schwerhörigkeit, Arch. Ophthal. 95:81, 1918.

342. Vander Veer, E. A., and Dickinson, A. M.: Fragilitas ossium, Ann. Surg. 74:629, 1921.

343. Vaughan, J. H. (Richmond): Personal communication, 1956.

344. Villanueva, A. R., and Frost, H. M.: Bone formation in human osteogenesis imperfecta, measured by tetracycline bone labeling, Acta Orthop. Scand. 41:531, 1970.

345. Villanueva, A. R., Frost, H. M., and Ilnicki, L.: Cortical bone dynamics measured by means of tetracycline labeling in 21 cases of osteoporosis, J. Lab. Clin. Med. 68:599, 1966.

346. Voigt, O.: Ein Fall von Osteogenesis imperfecta, Freiburg, 1926, Dissertation. Cited by Seedorff.[294]

347. Von Ammon, F. A.: Klinische Darstellungen der angeborenen Krankheiten und Bildungsfehler des menschlichen Auges, Berlin, 1841, G. Reimer, p. 73.

348. Voorhoeve, N.: Blue sclerotics, in connection with other hereditary or congenital abnormalities, Lancet 2:740, 1918.

349. Vrolik, W.: Tabulae ad illustrandam embryogenesim hominis et mammalium, tam naturalem quam abnormem, Amstelodami, 1849.

350. Vyropaer, D.: Cited by Seedorff.[294]

351. Wagoner, G. W.: Idiopathic osteopsathyrosis, Ann. Surg. 80:115, 1924.

352. Watkyn-Thomas, F. W.: Diseases of the throat, nose and ear, Springfield, Ill., 1953, Charles C Thomas, Publisher, p. 612.

353. Weber, M.: Osteogenesis imperfecta congenita, a study of its histopathogenesis, Arch. Path. 9:984, 1930.

354. Weinmann, J. P., and Sicher, H.: Bone and bones, ed. 2, St. Louis, 1955, The C. V. Mosby Co.

355. Weinmann, J. P., Svoboda, J. F., and Woods, R. W.: Hereditary disturbances of enamel formation and calcification, J. Amer. Dent. Ass. 32:397, 1945.

356. Weller, S. V. D.: Hypophosphatasia with congenital dimples, Proc. Roy. Soc. Med. 52:637, 1959.

357. Wells, C.: Osteogenesis imperfecta from an Anglo-Saxon burial ground at Burgh Castle, Suffolk, Med. Hist. 9:88, 1965.

358. Welz, W. E., and Lieberman, B. L.: Report of a case of osteogenesis imperfecta in twins, Amer. J. Obstet. Gynec. 14:49, 1927.

359. Werner, R.: Mehrfaches Vorkommen einer Neigung zu Knochenbrüchen und Sarkomentwicklung in einer Familie, Z. Krebsforsch. 32:40, 1940.

360. White, C. A.: Osteogenesis imperfecta tarda and pregnancy; report of a case, Obstet. Gynec. 22:792, 1963.

361. Wiechmann, E., and Paal, H.: Zur Klinik der sogenannten blauen Skleren, München. Med. Wschr. 72:213, 1925.

362. Williams, P. F.: Fragmentation and rodding in osteogenesis imperfecta, J. Bone Joint Surg. 47-B:23, 1965.

363. Wilson, G. W., and Steinbecker, M.: Hereditary hypoplasia of dentine, J. Amer. Dent. Ass. 16:866, 1929.

364. Wilton, A.: Die Skelettveränderungen bei einem Spätfalle von Osteogenesis imperfecta nebst Erörterung der Entstehungsweise unter Berücksticktigung anderer Skelettkrankheiten, Virchow Arch. Path. 283:778, 1932.

365. Winter, G. R., and Maiocco, P. D.: Osteogenesis imperfecta and odontogenesis imperfecta, Oral Surg. 2:782, 1949.

366. Winterfeldt, E. A., Eyring, E. J., and Vivian, V. M.: Ascorbic-acid treatment for osteogenesis imperfecta (letter), Lancet 2:760, 1970.

367. Wirth, M.: Blaue Skleren und Knochenbrüchigkeit, Klin. Mbl. Augenheilk. **74**:505, 1925.

368. Witkop, C. (Bethesda, Md.): Personal communication.

369. Witkop, C. J.: Comment (on osteogenesis imperfecta). Clinical delineation of birth defects. IV. Skeletal dysplasias, New York, 1969, National Foundation–March of Dimes, pp. 143.

370. Witkop, C. J., Jr.: Hereditary defects in enamel and dentin, Acta Genet. **7**:236, 1957.

371. Wyatt, T. C., and McEachern, T. H.: Congenital bone dysplasia (osteogenesis imperfecta) associated with lesions of parathyroid glands, Amer. J. Dis. Child. **43**:403, 1932.

372. Wyllie, W. G., and Schlesinger, B.: Osteogenesis imperfecta presenting with delay in walking, two cases, Proc. Roy. Soc. Med. **42**:80, 1949.

373. Yeoman, P. M.: Multiple osteotomies and intramedullary fixation of the long bones in osteogenesis imperfecta, Proc. Roy. Soc. Med. **53**:946, 1960.

374. Young, B. K., and Gorstein, F.: Maternal osteogenesis imperfecta, Obstet. Gynec. **31**:461, 1968.

375. Zander, G. S. F.: Case of osteogenesis imperfecta tarda with platyspondylisis, Acta Radiol. **21**:53, 1940.

376. Zurhelle, E.: Osteogenesis imperfecta bei Mutter und Kind, Z. Geburtsh, Gynaek. **74**:942, 1913.

9 · Alkaptonuria

Historical note

Garrod[41] gave the following early history of alkaptonuria:

Until the early years of the nineteenth century no distinction was drawn in medical writings between urines which were black when passed and such as darkened on exposure to air, but it is difficult to suggest any other diagnosis than that of alkaptonuria for some cases referred to in works of the sixteenth and seventeenth centuries, such as that mentioned by G. A. Scribonius (in 1584) of a schoolboy who, although he enjoyed good health, continuously excreted black urine, and that cited by Schenck (in 1609) of a monk who exhibited a similar peculiarity and stated that he had done so all his life. The most interesting record of this kind is to be found in the work of Zacutus Lusitanus, published in 1649. The patient was a boy who passed black urine and who, at the age of fourteen years, was submitted to a drastic course of treatment which had for its aim the subduing of the fiery heat of his viscera which was supposed to bring about the condition in question by charring and blackening his bile. Among the measures prescribed were bleedings, purgation, baths, a cold and watery diet, and drugs galore. None of these had any obvious effect, and eventually the patient, who tired of the futile and superfluous therapy, resolved to let things take their natural course. None of the predicted evils ensued, he married, begat a large family, and lived a long and healthy life, always passing urine black as ink.*

In Slovakia, where alkaptonuria seems to be rather frequent—witness the large series reported by Červeňanský and colleagues[24]—the disease is said[24] to have been first recognized in 1775 in the medical thesis of Josephus Singer. In 1859 Boedeker[16] recognized that the reducing properties of the urine from a patient with alkaptonuria differed from those of urine containing glucose. Bismuth hydroxide was, for example, not reduced. Because of the avid uptake of oxygen in alkaline solutions, he gave the name alkaptonuria to the condition: ". . . in alkalischer Lösung bei gewöhnlicher Temperatur den Sauerstoff begierig zu verschlucken und nannte ihn danach Alcapton (freilich recht barbarisch zusammengesetzt aus dem arabischen *al kali* und dem griechischen καπτειν, begierig verschlucken)."† In 1861, Boedeker[17] spelled the name *alkaptonurie,*

---

*Knox called attention to this interesting historical note.
†From Boedeker, C.: Z. Rat. Med. 7:130, 1859. Translation: ". . . in alkaline solution at ordinary temperature avidly to absorb the oxygen and named it accordingly alcapton (admittedly somewhat barbarously compounded from the Arabic *al kali* and the Greek καπτειν, to suck up greedily)."

a practice that has been followed in the German literature. The French spell it *alcaptonurie,* and English writers use "c" and "k" interchangeably.

The morbid anatomy of ochronosis was described by Virchow[116] in 1866 on the basis of findings in a 67-year-old man. Although the gross coloration was gray to blue-black, an ochre color was observed microscopically—hence Virchow's designation *ochronosis.* Not until the early part of this century was the connection between ochronosis and alkaptonuria recognized—by Albrecht[3] in 1902 and by Osler[90] in 1904. Boedeker's patient[16,17] had severe pain in the lumbar spine "so severe that he lay mostly in bed and could take only a few steps." The development of severe arthritis in the course of alkaptonuria with ochronosis was emphasized by Gross and Allard[44] in 1907. The characteristic roentgenographic appearance of the spine in ochronosis was described by Söderbergh[108] in 1913.

The chemical structure of "alkapton" was established in 1891 by Wolkow and Baumann,[121] who identified it as 2, 5-dihydroxyphenylacetic acid and named it homogentisic acid because of its close structural similarity to gentisic acid (2, 5-dihydroxybenzoic acid).

Alkaptonuria is *par excellence* Garrod's disease.[25,42,57] Archibald Garrod (see frontispiece) greatly extended knowledge of the nature of the disorder and on the basis of these studies conceived the principle underlying most inborn errors of metabolism, the last being his terminology. As Beadle[10] pointed out in his Nobel lecture, the concept of one-gene—one-enzyme was essentially Garrod's. As Garrod[41] stated in 1908: "Of inborn errors of metabolism, alkaptonuria is that of which we know most, and from the study of which most has been learnt." In most research, following the lead of Wolkow and Baumann,[121] alkaptonuria had been viewed as a specific form of infection of the alimentary tract—a concept that was undoubtedly influenced by the thinking of the "bacteriology era" in which he worked—but Garrod[40] thought of alkaptonuria as an enzyme defect:

> We may further conceive that the splitting of the benzene ring in normal metabolism is the work of a special enzyme, [and] that in congenital alcaptonuria this enzyme is wanting. . . . The experiments of G. Embden and others upon perfusion of the liver suggest that organ as the most probable seat of the change.*

Garrod's contemporaries, such as Osler,[90] considered alkaptonuria to be a "freak" of metabolism, comparable to morphologic freaks, and to be of no pathologic importance. Indeed, it is likely that many of Garrod's contemporaries viewed his work in alkaptonuria as a harmless but practically noncontributory pastime. There is the tone of the *apologia* in Garrod's writings on the value of studying rare diseases (see quotation in the Preface). Clearly, Garrod was ahead of his time.

The juxtaposition of Garrod and Bateson and the rediscovery of Mendel's work were important factors in the development of the concept of inborn errors of metabolism. Bateson's *Mendel's Principles of Heredity* did much to acquaint the English-speaking world with "genetics," the term he applied to this field.[8] Because of the occurrence of affected sibs with normal parents and the high pro-

---

*From Garrod, A. E.: Lancet 2:1484, 1901.

portion of parents who are consanguineous, he suggested to Garrod that alkaptonuria is a recessively inherited disorder. In 1932 Hogben and colleagues[50] analyzed statistically the family data on alkaptonuria and supported the recessive hypothesis. There were, however, anomalous pedigrees in which alkaptonuria was transmitted through many successive generations, suggesting dominant inheritance, e.g., that of Pieter,[93] reported from Santo Domingo. However, the interpretation that the inheritance was quasidominant due to marriage, in successive generations, of affected homozygous persons with heterozygous carriers, in an inbred population, was demonstrated by restudy in the Dominican Republic by Milch.[78]

The question as to whether homogentisic acid is a normal metabolite which, in alkaptonuria, accumulates in unusual concentration behind an enzyme block (the view of Garrod), or whether it is an abnormal compound formed by an abnormal series of reactions, was resolved by 1928 in favor of the former view, by Neubauer[87] and by others.

In 1958 La Du and associates[61] succeeded in demonstrating deficiency of homogentisate oxidase in liver, as predicted by Garrod. The importance of ochronotic connective tissue changes in producing arthritis and cardiovascular pathology has become generally recognized only in the last few decades, although some contemporaries of Garrod[48,114] emphasized it. The pathogenesis of connective tissue alterations in alkaptonuria is the most recent chapter in the history of the disease.

Clinical manifestations

The phenotypic features of alkaptonuria are blackness of urine, pigmentation of cartilaginous and collagenous structures (ochronosis), and degenerative joint and vascular changes.

The urine turns dark on sitting. Darkening is hastened by alkalinization of the urine. Black diapers are sometimes the first clue to the presence of the disease. Washing with soap exaggerates the pigmentation of the diaper rather than removing it. Some patients never note black urine, the conditions for darkening apparently never being present. One patient first noted dark urine at age 93.[39] Garrod[40] observed that in the first hours after birth alkaptonuria may not be demonstrable although it appears in the second day of life and continues without interruption thereafter. It is probable that immaturity of the enzyme systems involved in tyrosine oxidation accounts for the failure of expression from the very beginning. As a reducing substance homogentisic acid produces a positive reaction in some urinary tests for glycosuria, such as that using Benedict's solution, but of course not in enzyme tests specific for glucose. The proper interpretation of an atypical test for reducing substance in the urine is the most frequent means of diagnosing alkaptonuria. A specific enzymatic method for quantitative determination of homogentisic acid in blood and urine is available.[100]

Pigmented prostatic calculi were described by Young[123] and by others and probably occur in all alkaptonuric men over 50 years of age. These calculi are usually calcified, as well, and evident by x-ray study. Enlargement of the stone-filled prostate may require prostatectomy.[15,51,58] Savastano and associates[99] described palpable prostatic calculi. Death in uremia from prostatic obstruction has been observed.[9,91] Apparently the alkalinity of the prostatic secretions promotes polymerization of homogentisic acid, and this pigment then affords a nidus for stone formation. Urinary calculi are also black in this disorder.[112]

Renal stones occur in ochronosis.[36,47,49,58,63,70,71,91] Deposition of pigment in the renal parenchyma occurs. Ochronotic nephropathy with ochronotic pigment casts is thought to occur[23,46] but cannot be considered fully documented. Patients with alkaptonuria who have renal failure due to an unrelated renal ab-

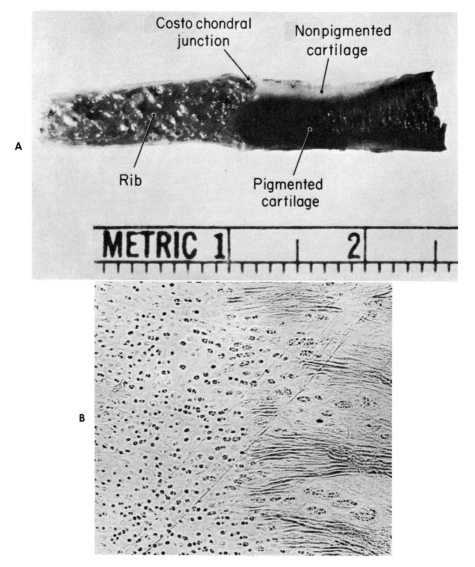

Fig. 9-1. A, Deeply pigmented costal cartilage in patient with alkaptonuria. Note that the periphery of the cartilage is not pigmented. **B,** Histologic appearance of cartilage from specimen shown in **A.** The pigmented area is on the right half. Sparsity of cells and artifactual streaks produced in sectioning, because of stiffness of the specimen, are evident. (Courtesy Dr. Robert A. Milch.)

normality show greatly aggravated ochronosis, e.g., the 11-year-old boy with polycystic kidneys reported by Arcangeli and co-workers.[5]

Ochronotic pigmentation of blue-black hue is most evident in the sclera and in ear cartilages, but pigmentation of many cartilaginous and collagenous structures is found at surgical operation or autopsy—e.g., costal cartilages (Fig. 9-1) and heart valves. Pigmentation does not become evident, as a rule, until the twenties or thirties. The scleral pigmentation is usually concentrated about midway between the corneal limbus and the inner and outer canthi, at the sites of insertion of the rectus muscles. Pigmentation of the cornea, concentrated peripherally at the three and nine o'clock positions, has been observed,[107] as well as pigmentation of the tarsal plates and eyelids. In one case[105] the pigmentation was mistaken for melanosarcoma and the eye was removed. Pigmentation of the nasal cartilages is sometimes evident at the tip of the nose. Pigmentation of the pinnae is best demonstrated by transillumination. The ear becomes stiff, also, so that it cannot be folded with the normal ease. Calcification and even ossification are radiographically demonstrable.[84,120] Other conditions accompanied by calcification of the ear cartilages include Addison's disease, diabetes mellitus, von Meyerborg's chondromalacia, cold hypersensitivity,[68] and diastrophic dwarfism.[69] The cerumen is jet black and the

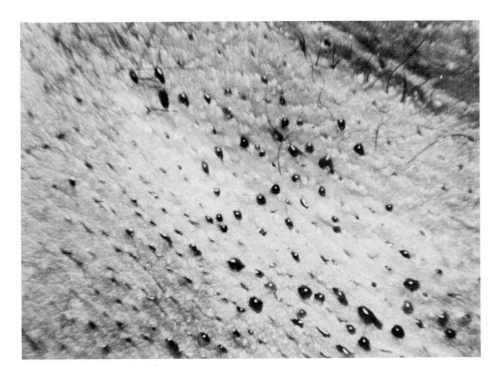

Fig. 9-2. Pigmentation of apocrine sweat in patient with ochronosis. Enlarged view of axilla, photographed 1 minute after stimulation with intradermal injection of epinephrine. Note darkly pigmented sweat around hair follicles. Clear eccrine sweat between hair follicles is less clearly demonstrated. Punch biopsy of skin in axillary area showed pigment outlining secretory tubules. (Courtesy Dr. Axel W. Hoke, U.S.P.H.S. Hospital, San Francisco.)

eardrum often shows steel-blue pigmentation. It is said[59] that pigmentation of tendons in the hand may be evident through the skin in some cases. The pigment is excreted in the sweat. Clothing in contact with the axilla may be stained, and the skin of the axillary and inguinal area, as well as the malar area of the face, may show brownish coloration. Hoke and colleagues[50a] showed that apocrine sweat stimulated by intradermal injection of epinephrine is bluish black (Fig. 9-2), whereas eccrine sweat stimulated by intradermal injection of acetylcholine is clear. They also demonstrated, by means of punch biopsy of the axillary area, pigment outlining apocrine coils and ducts. In one exceptional case a bluish gray discoloration of the fingernails was described.[38] Bluish discoloration of the teeth has been described,[101] as has extensive subcutaneous calcification in the legs.[19]

Ochronotic arthropathy was succinctly and graphically described by the late Joseph J. Bunim and his colleagues[88] in the following manner:

> The anatomic distribution and sequence of spinal and peripheral joint involvement in ochronosis are characteristic. The course is chronic and progressive, beginning early in the fourth decade with back pain and stiffness. During the ensuing ten years the knees become involved and later the shoulders and hips are affected. The patient becomes increasingly crippled and by sixty years of age may be totally disabled.
>
> Two acute manifestations may develop during the chronic course: herniation of the intervertebral discs and synovial effusion following negligible trauma. Acute rupture of a nucleus pulposus may be the first manifestation of ochronotic spondylosis. It occurs principally in males in early adult life. Articular structures in ochronosis seem to be vulnerable; pain and effusion may follow minor injuries. The friable articular cartilages are readily fragmented and embedded in the synovial lining with consequent effusion and pain.
>
> In males, joint involvement occurs more frequently, develops at an earlier age, and is of greater severity than in females. Ruptured discs are especially more common in males.*

These authors also provided a useful table in which the joint changes in males and females were compared (Table 9-1).

Low-back pain, limitation of motion in the lumbar spine, and symptoms of root pressure by extruded intervertebral disc[31,32,66] are matched by the x-ray finding of narrowing of the intervertebral space and collapse and calcification of the intervertebral discs of the lumbar spine (Fig. 9-3). The calcified discs present a spindle shape on lateral projection. Mueller and associates[84] and others[56] described a vacuum phenomenon. Joint spaces can be demonstrated by gas if traction is applied in order to produce a partial intra-articular vacuum— e.g., in the shoulder joint of children when the arms are raised above the head for chest x-ray studies or in the symphysis pubis in pregnant women at term. Intra-articular vacuum is a rather consistent finding in the ochronotic spine, being located, on lateral projection, anterior to the calcified disc. It is probably present in Fig. 9-3. Some degree of fusion of the vertebral bodies occurs. Unlike rheumatoid spondylitis, alkaptonuria is accompanied by little calcification of spinal ligaments. The radiographic findings are sufficiently typical that studies of Egyptian mummies[102,118] have led to the conclusion that certain of them are the bodies of persons with alkaptonuria.

---

*From O'Brien, W. M., La Du, B. N., and Bunim, J. J.: Amer. J. Med. **34**:813, 1963.

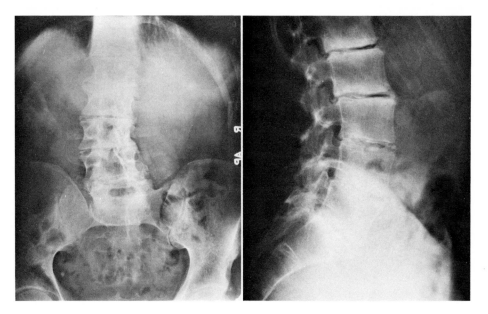

Fig. 9-3. Characteristic spinal changes of ochronotic arthropathy in 34-year-old man (R. S., 761270).

Table 9-1. Comparison of arthropathy in males and females*

Data	Males	Females
Number	116 cases	47 cases
Severity	Often severe	Usually mild
Spine	Onset in late thirties with loss of range of motion in lumbar and thoracic spine, loss in height	Onset in mid-forties, usually milder and more insidious course than in men
Disc rupture	Onset in late twenties, occurs in about 20%	Rare (4% or less)
Knee	Onset in early forties, often severe and disabling early in course with contracture and joint bodies	Onset in early fifties, usually milder than in men
Shoulder	Onset in early fifties, usually only loss in range of motion	Same as in men
Hip	Onset in early fifties with gradual progression—only occasionally severe	Onset in early fifties with gradual progression, frequently severe

*From O'Brien, W. M., La Du, B. N., and Bunim, J. J.: Amer. J. Med. **34:**813, 1963.

Large joints such as the hips and knees usually show degenerative changes by x-ray examination, with calcium deposits around the joint or present as loose bodies in the joint.[113] Frequently, ochronotic arthritis is of such severity as to keep the patient bedridden for many years. Severe pain over the symphysis pubis occurs rather frequently.[47,67,80,113] By x-ray film the pubic synchondrosis in such cases may present irregular sclerosis, narrowing, and destructive changes.[94,95] The shoulder joint sometimes shows degenerative changes of severity rarely seen in a non–weight-bearing joint except in syringomyelia and in this disorder. Suppurative arthritis was superimposed on ochronotic arthritis in one case.[23] Rupture of the Achilles tendon, which was found to be deeply pigmented, has been reported in at least two instances.[2,29]

A review[106] of case reports of alkaptonuria indicates a high frequency of cardiovascular abnormality. Generalized arteriosclerosis[27,39] and abnormalities of the heart valves, particularly calcific aortic stenosis, are frequent. Myocardial infarction is a common cause of death.[117]

Auditory impairment occurs in some cases. (See review by O'Brien and coworkers.[88]) Long-standing severe hoarseness,[43] fixed vocal cords, and pigmentation of the larynx observed by direct laryngoscopy[52] have been described.

The oldest individual with alkaptonuria was probably the one reported by Galdston and associates,[39] who died at 99 years of age. Perhaps because of this experience, one of the authors[110] stated that life expectancy is not reduced. I suspect that, in fact, average survivorship is appreciably decreased. A life-table analysis such as those given elsewhere for the Marfan syndrome (p. 354), homocystinuria (p. 240), and pseudoxanthoma elasticum (p. 492) should be made for alkaptonuria. Such an analysis would best be made on the basis of a large series of cases such as that collected in Czechoslovakia.[24]

Diagnosis

The demonstration of homogentisic acid in the urine establishes the diagnosis. Confirmation by demonstration of deficiency of homogentisic acid oxidase requires liver biopsy. Normal fibroblasts cultured from skin biopsies do not show homogentisic acid oxidase activity.[60] Hence, this method cannot be used in diagnosis, and presumably prenatal diagnosis by study of amniotic cells is also impossible.

The urine of affected patients turns dark promptly on addition of strong alkali.

Because of the reducing nature of homogentisic acid, a false-positive Benedict's test for glucose is produced. (A yellowish orange precipitate with black supernatant is formed.) Of course, the "dip stick" tests are specific for glucose. There is some virtue in continuing the use of Benedict's reagent for routine urine screening. Patients have been erroneously treated for diabetes.

Paradoxically, when both diabetes and alkaptonuria are present, glucose oxidase is inhibited, and the enzyme paper strips are likely to give a negative result.[33,85] Vitamin C, L-dopa, aspirin, and 5-hydroxyindoleacetic acid, as in carcinoid tumors, also interfere in the enzymic test.

Fishberg[35] pointed out that if a drop of alkalinized urine is dropped on sensitized photographic paper, the urine turns dark promptly. This can be done in full daylight. Bowcock[19] showed two photographic prints of the facial photograph of a patient, made from the same negative—one developed in the usual manner and the other developed in the patient's own urine.

A rapid semiquantitative method for homogentisic acid was developed by Kang and Gerald.[54]

Pathology

Coal-black pigmentary changes in the costal, laryngeal, and tracheal cartilages, as well as others, are striking in elderly alkaptonuric patients. Fibrous tissues such as tendons, ligaments, endocardium, and heart valves are likewise pigmented. Microscopically the pigment is found deposited both intracellularly and extracellularly and may be either granular or homogeneous. Ochronotic pigment can be distinguished histologically from melanin only with difficulty if at all.[28] Probably no patient with alkaptonuria escapes ochronosis, if survival to at least early adulthood occurs. Histopathologic changes in the eye were described by Rones[97] and by Allen and co-workers[4] and changes in the ear, by Brunner.[21]

Cardiovascular abnormalities have been observed in a high proportion of autopsied cases. In 1910 Beddard[11] found that of 11 persons with ochronosis, 8

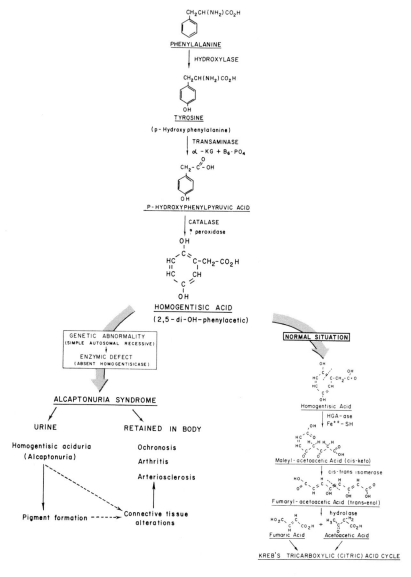

Fig. 9-4. Normal pathway for metabolism of tyrosine, and the defect in alkaptonuria. (Courtesy Dr. Robert A. Milch.)

had chronic mitral and aortic "valvulitis," 1 had aortic aneurysm, and 1 had aneurysm of the left ventricle. Generalized arteriosclerosis,[39] calcification of the heart valves, particularly calcific aortic stenosis, and calcified annulus fibrosus mitralis[63] have been noted. Many have suggested that ochronotic patients suffer accelerated arteriosclerosis. However, O'Brien and associates[88] from a review of reported cases, challenged this suggestion. The matter cannot be considered settled.

In one case[28] severe renal disease referred to as "ochronotic nephrosis" was observed, but it may have been a coincidental unrelated nephritis, since no similar case has been reported.

Basic defect and pathogenesis

Patients with alkaptonuria have been demonstrated to have a deficiency of homogentisic acid oxidase in liver[61] and in kidney.[126] (Normally this enzyme, which catalyzes the oxidative cleavage of homogentisic acid to maleyl-acetoacetic acid, is present only in these two tissues.) Because of the enzyme deficiency and

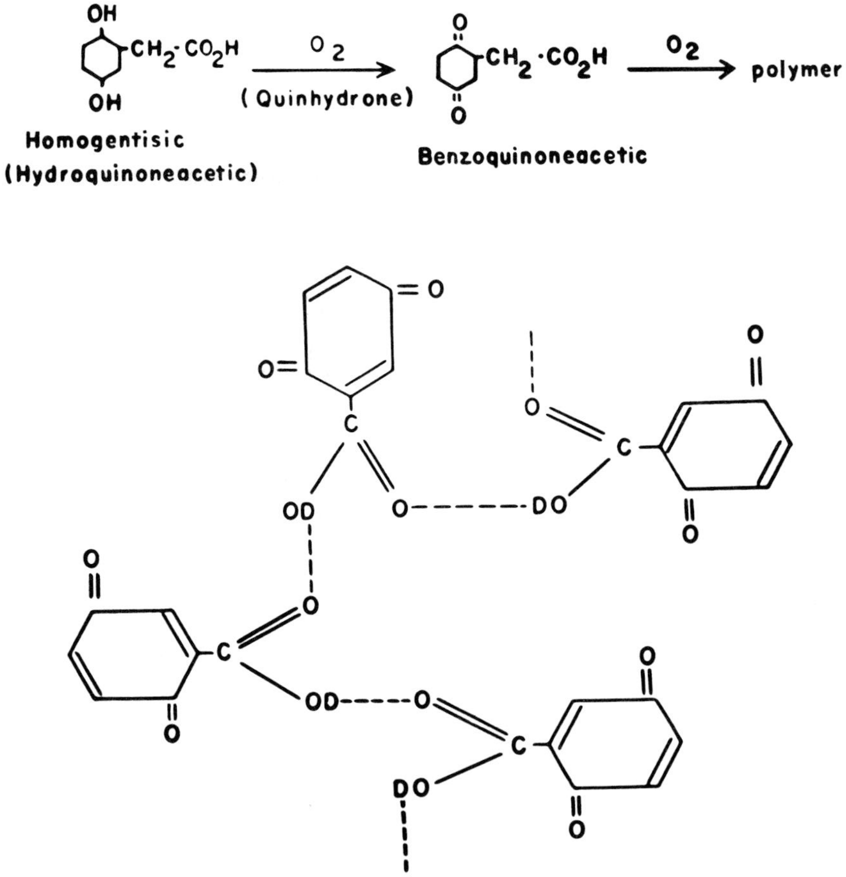

Fig. 9-5. Proposed conversion of homogentisic acid to a polymer by auto-oxidation (top). Proposed structure of the deuterium-labeled polymer, based on infrared spectrography (below). (Courtesy Dr. Robert A. Milch.[77])

the lack of an alternative pathway for the degradation of homogentisic acid, this substance, a normal intermediary in tyrosine metabolism (Fig. 9-4), is excreted in the urine. Whether enzyme protein lacking normal activity is present or no protein whatever is formed is not known. The level of homogentisic acid oxidase has not been measured in heterozygotes.

The alkaptonuric adult usually excretes from 4 to 8 grams of homogentisic acid a day.

Zannoni and co-workers[125] presented reasons for believing that benzoquinone-acetic acid, the quinone of homogentisic acid, is mainly responsible for the ochronotic pigmentation of connective tissue in alkaptonuria.

Milch[75,76] found that, although homogentisic acid does not bind to collagen, polymerized auto-oxidized homogentisic acid (HGA-OP) is bound to hide powder in solution. Furthermore, degradation of collagen by collagenase is interfered with appreciably when the collagen is treated with HGA-OP. Milch concluded: "Coupled with previous observations it is suggested that HGA-OP can act as a potent tanning agent for collagen. It is further suggested that ochronosis and degenerative joint disease observed in patients with alkaptonuria may possibly be explained by the *in vivo* occurrence of such a phenomenon."* (See Figs. 9-5 and 9-6.)

Moran and Yunis[82] produced clinical arthritis and typical joint changes of ochronosis by injecting homogentisic acid into the joints of rabbits. Alkaptonuria can be produced in animals such as the rat by giving a diet enriched with phenylalanine[92] or tyrosine.[14a,18] It also was observed[122] in rats with experimental tryptophan deficiency, the mechanism being unknown.

---

*From Milch, R. A.: Proc. Soc. Exp. Biol. Med. **107**:183, 1961.

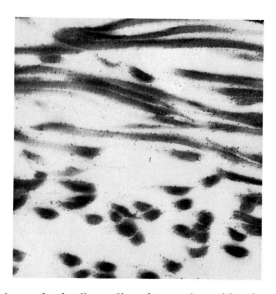

Fig. 9-6. Electron micrograph of collagen fibers from patient with ochronosis. The electron-dense ochronotic polymer is demonstrated as granules closely associated with, and presumably bound to, the collagen fibers. (Courtesy Dr. Robert A. Milch.)

Prevalence and inheritance

As shown in Table 9-2, autosomal recessive inheritance of alkaptonuria was demonstrated by the analysis of Hogben and associates,[50] who used alkaptonuria to test the so-called Lenz-Hogben, or *a priori,* method of segregation analysis. This method of testing the recessive hypothesis assumes complete, or truncate, ascertainment. The close agreement with the predictions of the recessive hypothesis supports the correctness of the assumption of complete ascertainment. Apparently the probability of ascertainment of a given family was not dependent on the number of sibs affected. The usual unaffected state of parents of affected sibships likewise supports the recessive hypothesis, as does also the rather high frequency of parental consanguinity.[81]

In Northern Ireland in 1957 Stevenson[111] found two families with alkaptonuria: a father and daughter, and a brother and sister. The population numbered about 1.4 million at that time. Dent is quoted[88] as estimating the phenotype frequency as 1 in 100,000. Like other recessive disorders—e.g., acatalasia, Tay-Sachs disease, familial Mediterranean fever, etc.—the frequency is not uniform; unusually high frequencies have been found in the Dominican Republic[47] and in Slovakia.[24,104,109a] (See Figs. 9-7 and 9-8.) In these areas in which there are high rates of inbreeding and of the occurrence of the defective gene, transmission of alkaptonuria through several generations creates a pedigree pattern simulating dominance.[56,72] This quasidominance is clearly the result of a high frequency of marriage between homozygous affected persons and heterozygous carriers. No evidence for the existence of a dominant form of alkaptonuria (or of more than one basically distinct recessive form) has been discovered.

The wide distribution of alkaptonuria is indicated by its description in Japanese,[2] Asiatic Indians,[86,98,103,115] American Negroes,[1] Filipinos,[89] a gypsy,[23] and the Bantu.[7] Furthermore, its antiquity is supported by the finding of typical ochronotic spondylosis in Egyptian mummies.[102,118]

In the study of Hogben and associates[50] it was noted that the reported cases

Table 9-2. Segregation analysis of alkaptonuria*

Sibship size	Number of sibships	Alkaptonuric members		Variance
		Observed	Expected	
1	5	5	5	0
2	8	10	9.14	0.97960
3	5	8	6.48	1.31485
4	2	4	2.93	0.84010
5	3	4	4.92	1.77534
6	3	8	5.47	2.32785
7	2	5	4.04	1.94048
8	3	5	6.67	3.51720
9	1	4	2.43	1.38020
10	1	2	2.65	1.59170
11	3	7	8.61	5.41590
14	1	4	3.56	2.44640
Total	37	66	61.90	23.52962

*From Hogben, L., Worrall, R. L., and Zieve, I.: Proc. Roy. Soc. Edinburgh **52**:264, 1932.

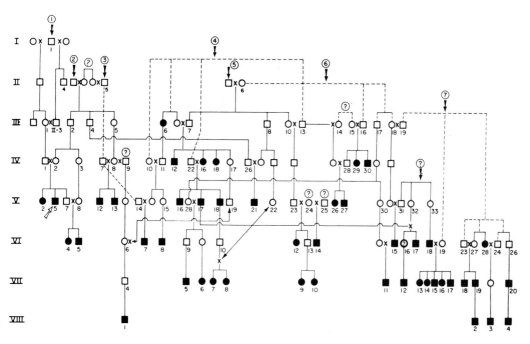

Fig. 9-7. Pedigree of inbred group in Dominican Republic with many cases of alkaptonuria, some in successive generations. (Courtesy Dr. Robert A. Milch.)

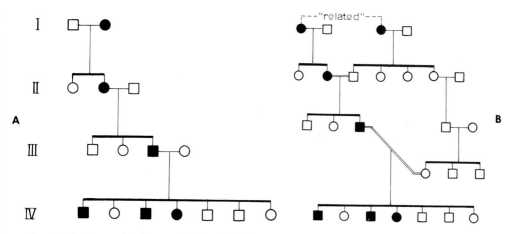

Fig. 9-8. Pedigree of Lebanese family with alkaptonuria. **A,** The pedigree suggests autosomal dominant inheritance. **B,** Consanguinity is indicated by the more complete pedigree. The spouses of the affected persons in the first, second, and third generations are presumably heterozygotes. (Based on data from Khachadurian, A., and Abu Feisal, K. A.: J. Chronic Dis. 7:455, 1958.)

included 100 males and 46 females. Since the proband was much more often a male, they concluded that the more frequent urine examination of males in connection with insurance, military service, and employment accounted for the distorted sex ratio. The explanation was supported by the finding that among infants slightly more females than males were detected. A higher frequency of arthritis in male alkaptonurics may contribute to the higher number of ascertained males. In the review of reported cases by O'Brien and co-workers[88] 60% of 520 patients were male.

Simple methods for recognizing heterozygotes—for use in genetic counseling, for example—are not available. Oral loading tests with homogentisic acid or tyrosine show no difference between the relatives of alkaptonurics and normal controls.[59,88]

Other considerations

Treatment with vitamins, brewer's yeast, tyrosinase, insulin, adrenocortical extract,[39] vitamin C,[83] vitamin B_{12},[37] cortisone,[14,124] and phenylbutazone[13] has no effect on alkaptonuria. Whether cortisone or vitamin C has any beneficial effects with regard to the ochronotic changes in connective tissue is not known. Possible benefit derived from vitamin C is suggested by the finding of Lustberg and co-workers[65] that ascorbic acid in high doses decreased binding of C^{14}-homogentisic acid in connective tissues of rats with experimental alkaptonuria. Long-term therapy in young patients with alkaptonuria is indicated. Thiouracil[24,30] was reported to relieve clinical symptoms but had no effect on the amount of homogentisic acid excreted in the urine.[121]

No one would question the desirability of preventive measures to avoid the crippling ochronotic arthropathy. Furthermore, survivorship of the alkaptonuric may be significantly reduced. Following the same rationale as in phenylketonuria, one would presume that a diet low in phenylalanine and tyrosine would be beneficial. Although it is known that the addition of L-tyrosine to the diet results in increase in the urinary output of homogentisic acid, to which it is converted to the extent of more than 50%,[121] there appear to be no observations on the effects of dietary restriction, either acute or chronic.

An excellent example of a phenocopy (a nongenetically produced phenotype resembling a gene-determined one) is provided by the ochronosis that develops after the prolonged use of carbolic acid dressings for chronic cutaneous ulcers.[11,12,20,34,48] Quinacrine (Atabrine),[64] after prolonged administration, also causes an ochronotic change with pigmentation (Fig. 9-9) in many of the same sites as in alkaptonuria, and probably with a comparable arthrosis.

In the differential diagnosis of alkaptonuria the several causes of black diapers must be considered.[26] Drummond and co-workers[30] described the "blue diaper syndrome" in two brothers. Hypercalcemia and nephrocalcinosis were features. A defect in intestinal transport of tryptophan led to excessive indole production by intestinal bacteria. Conversion of indican to indigo blue appeared to account for the staining of the diapers. The urine of patients receiving methyldopa (Aldomet) for hypertension becomes dark red and almost black when mixed with hypochlorite solution used in a proprietary lavatory cleanser.[22] The urine of patients receiving DOPA for Parkinsonism turns black with D, L-DOPA but not with L-DOPA.[6] The excretion of homogentisic acid when

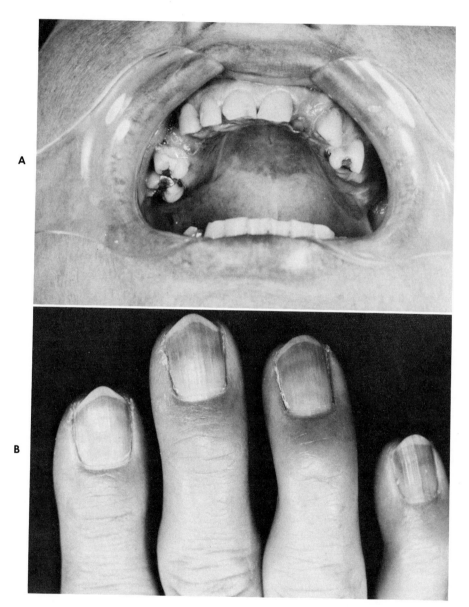

Fig. 9-9. Pigmentation of the hard palate, **A,** and fingernails, **B,** in G. E. (J.H.H. 463437), a 52-year-old woman who had received Atabrine intermittently for about twelve years in treatment for rheumatoid arthritis. The skin over the ankles, calves, malar areas of the face, and back was also pigmented. Under Wood's filter the fingernails fluoresced in nonpigmented areas. The sclerae and ears showed no pigmentation and the ears were supple. The urine contained no reducing substance.

D-DOPA is administered is probably the result of inefficiency of homogentisic acid oxidase in handling the D-isomer. Melanuria sometimes accompanies melanomas.[53]

Also to be considered in the differential diagnosis of alkaptonuria is apocrine chromhidrosis.[51a,99a] In this disorder colored sweat is secreted by the apocrine glands, which may be heterotopic as in so-called facial chromhidrosis. The pigment is a lipofuscin. Axillary chromhidrosis is not seen until after puberty, when apocrine secretory activity is activated; it occurs much more frequently among Negroes than among Caucasians. The appearance is the same as that shown in Fig. 9-2 in a patient with alkaptonuria.

Presumed spontaneous alkaptonuria in a rabbit[62] and ochronosis in cattle, dogs, and horses[71,96] have not been investigated biochemically and genetically for possible homology to the disease in man. La Du and co-workers[61] found that a generalized pigmentation of connective tissues in the silky bantam fowl is not due to alkaptonuria.

Several authors have pointed out that understanding the pathogenesis of joint changes in ochronosis may provide important clues for research in primary osteoarthritis and perhaps other types of arthritis. Evidence is now available indicating a significant genetic contribution to the pathogenesis of osteoarthritis in men[55] and in mice.[109] It is not unreasonable to suspect that a biochemical defect may be present in osteoarthritis.

As has been reviewed above, in alkaptonuria, excessive metabolites resulting from the failure of degradation of homogentisic acid appear to act as a crosslinking agent on mature collagen. A comparable role may be played by low molecular weight aliphatic aldehydes in producing many of the changes in connective tissue, such as aorta, with aging in nonalkaptonuric persons.[73,74]

SUMMARY

Like homocystinuria, alkaptonuria is an inborn error of metabolism, inherited as an autosomal recessive disorder, in which important connective tissue changes occur. The clinical manifestations are dark urine, urinary and prostatic calculi, pigmentation of connective tissues (especially cartilage), progressive arthropathy of characteristic type, and probably cardiovascular lesions, including valvular sclerosis and accelerated arteriosclerosis. The biochemical defect is a deficiency of homogentisic acid oxidase, an enzyme normally present in liver and kidney.

REFERENCES

1. Abbott, L. D., Jr., Mandeville, F. B., and Rein, W. J.: Complete roentgen and ophthalmologic examination for ochronosis in two alcaptonuric children, Virginia Med. Monthly **70:**615, 1943.
2. Abe, Y., Oshima, N., Hatanaka, R., Amako, T., and Hirohata, R.: Thirteen cases of alkaptonuria from one family tree with special reference to osteo-arthrosis alkaptonurica, J. Bone Joint Surg. **42-A:**817, 1960.
3. Albrecht, H.: Ueber Ochronose, Z. Heilk. **23:**366, 1902.
4. Allen, R. A., O'Malley, C., and Straatsma, B. R.: Ocular findings in hereditary ochronosis, Arch. Ophthal. **65:**657, 1961.
5. Arcangeli, A., Colloridi, V., and Chiarini, M.: Una eccezionale associazione morbosa congenita: rene policistico ed alcaptonuria con ochronose, Arch. Ital. Pediat. **20:**66, 1959.
6. Arras, M. J.: Metabolism of D- vs. L-DOPA, New Eng. J. Med. **282:**813, 1970.

7. Baldachin, B. J., and Rothman, W. T.: Alkaptonuric arthritis; report of a case in a Bantu, Cent. Afr. J. Med. **5**:287, 1959.

8. Bateson, W.: Mendel's principles of heredity, London, 1902, Cambridge University Press.

9. Bauer, O.: Ueber Steinbildungen in den Harnwegen bei Ochronose (Lithiasis ochronotica), Mitt. Grenzgeb. Med. Chir. **41**:451, 1929.

10. Beadle, G. W.: Genes and chemical reactions in neurospora, Science **129**:1715, 1959.

11. Beddard, A. P.: Ochronosis associated with carboluria, Quart. J. Med. **3**:329, 1910.

12. Beddard, A. P., and Plumtre, C. M.: A further note on ochronosis associated with carboluria, Quart. J. Med. **5**:505, 1912.

13. Biggs, T. G., Jr., and Cannon, E., Jr.: Ochronosis; report of a case, J. Louisiana Med. Soc. **105**:395, 1953.

14. Black, R. L.: Use of cortisone in alkaptonuria, J.A.M.A. **155**:968, 1954.

14a. Blivaiss, B. B., Rosenberg, E. F., Kutuzov, H., and Stoner, R.: Experimental ochronosis. Induction in rates by long-term feeding with L-tyrosine, Arch. Path. **82**:45, 1966.

15. Bluefarb, S. M.: Alkaptonuria and ochronosis, Quart. Bull. Northwest. Univ. Med. Schl. **32**:101, 1958.

16. Boedeker, C.: Ueber das Alcapton; ein neuer Beitrag zur Frage: welche Stoffe des Harns können Kupferreduction bewirken? Z. Rat. Med. **7**:130, 1859.

17. Boedeker, C.: Das Alkapton; ein Beitrag zur Frage: welche Stoffe des Harns können aus einer alkalischen Kupferoxydlösung Kupferoxydul reduciren? Ann. Chem. Pharm. **117**:98, 1861.

18. Bondurant, R. E., and Henry, J. B.: Pathogenesis of ochronosis in experimental alkaptonuria of the white rat, Lab. Invest. **14**:62, 1965.

19. Bowcock, L.: Alkaptonuria; a condition of unusual photographic interest, Med. Biol. Illus. **13**:273, 1963.

20. Brogren, N.: Case of exogenetic ochronosis from carbolic acid compresses, Acta Dermatovener. **32**:258, 1952.

21. Brunner, H.: Ueber die Verändergungen des Schläfenbeines bei der Ochronose, Mchr. Ohrenheilk. **63**:997, 1929.

22. Cardwell, J. B.: Red urine associated with methyldopa treatment (letter) Lancet **2**:326, 1969.

23. Case records of the Massachusetts General Hospital; Case 9-1966, New Eng. J. Med. **274**:454, 1966.

24. Červeňanský, J., Sitaj, Š., and Urbánek, T.: Alkaptonuria and ochronosis, J. Bone Joint Surg. **41-A**:1169, 1959.

25. Childs, B.: Sir Archibald Garrod's conception of chemical individuality, New Eng. J. Med. **282**:71, 1970.

26. Cone, T. E., Jr.: Diagnosis and treatment; some syndromes, diseases, and conditions associated with abnormal coloration of the urine or diaper, Pediatrics **41**:654, 1968.

27. Coodley, E. L., and Greco, A. J.: Clinical aspects of ochronosis, with report of a case, Amer. J. Med. **8**:816, 1950.

28. Cooper, J. A., and Moran, T. J.: Studies on ochronosis, Arch. Path. **64**:46, 1957.

29. DiFiore, J. A.: Ochronosis, Arthritis Rheum. **3**:359, 1960.

30. Drummond, K. N., Michael, A. F., Ulstrom, R. A., and Good, R. A.: The blue diaper syndrome: familial hypercalcemia with nephrocalcinosis and indicanuria; a new familial disease, with definition of the metabolic abnormality, Amer. J. Med. **37**:928, 1964.

31. Eisenberg, H.: Alkaptonuria, ochronosis, arthritis and ruptured intervertebral disk, Arch. Intern. Med. **86**:79, 1950.

32. Feild, J. R., Higley, G. B., Sr., and DeSaussure, R. L., Jr.: Ochronosis with ruptured lumbar disc; case report, J. Neurosurg. **20**:348, 1963.

33. Feldman, J. M., Kelley, W. N., and Lebovitz, H. E.: Inhibition of glucose oxidase paper tests by reducing metabolites, Diabetes **19**:337, 1970.

34. Fishberg, E. H.: Ueber die Carbolochronose, Virchow Arch. Path. Anat. **251**:376, 1924.

35. Fishberg, E. H.: The instantaneous diagnosis of alkaptonuria on a single drop of urine, J.A.M.A. **119**:882, 1942.

36. Fisher, R. G., and Williams, J.: Ochronosis associated with degeneration of an intervertebral disc, J. Neurosurg. **12**:403, 1955.

37. Flaschenräger, B., Halawani, A., and Nabeh, I.: Alkaptonurie und Vitamin B_{12}, Klin. Wschr. **32:**131, 1954.

38. Friderich, H., and Nikolowski, W.: Endogene Ochronose, Arch. Derm. Syph. **192:**273, 1951.

39. Galdston, M., Steele, J. M., and Dobriner, K.: Alcaptonuria and ochronosis with a report of three patients and metabolic studies in two, Amer. J. Med. **13:**432, 1952.

40. Garrod, A. E.: About alkaptonuria, Lancet **2:**1484, 1901.

41. Garrod, A. E.: The Croonian lectures on inborn errors of metabolism. Lecture II. Alkaptonuria, Lancet **2:**73, 1908.

42. Garrod, A. E.: Inborn errors of metabolism, London, 1909, Frowde, Hodder & Stoughton.

43. Gonnermann, R.: Kasuistischer Beitrag zur Ochronose, Beitr. Path. Anat. **100:**598, 1938.

44. Gross, O., and Allard, E.: Untersuchungen über Alkaptonuria, Z. Klin. Med. **64:**359, 1907.

45. Hammond, G., and Powers, H. W.: Alkaptonuric arthritis; report of a case, Lahey Clin. Bull. **11:**18, 1958.

46. Hao, J. U., and Patton, R. B.: Alcaptonuria and ochronosis with diabetes mellitus and mycosis fungoides; a case report, Henry Ford Hosp. Med. Bull. **17:**295, 1969.

47. Harrold, A. J.: Alkaptonuric arthritis, J. Bone Joint Surg. **38-B:**532, 1956.

48. Heile: Ueber die Ochronose und die durch Formol verursachte pseudo-ochronotische Färbung der Knorpel, Virchow Arch. **160:**148, 1900.

49. Hendel, H., and Ben-Assa, B. J.: Report about a Bedouin family affected by alkaptonuria (comprising two cases of uro-lithiasis), Ann. Paediat. **195:**77, 1960.

50. Hogben, L., Worrall, R. L., and Zieve, I.: The genetic basis of alkaptonuria, Proc. Roy. Soc. Edinburgh **52:**264, 1932.

50a. Hoke, A. W., Maibach, H. I., and Epstein, W. L.: Physiologic and histologic studies of chromidrosis due to ochronosis, presented to American Medical Association meeting, June 19, 1971.

51. Hollingsworth, R. P.: Homogentisic acid stone; a rare form of prostatic obstruction, Brit. J. Urol. **40:**546, 1968.

51a. Hurley, H. J., Jr.: Apocrine chromhidrosis. In Fitzpatrick, T. B., et al., editors: Dermatology in general medicine, New York, 1971, McGraw-Hill Book Co., pp. 388-390.

52. Janecek, M.: Osteoarthrosis ochronotica (alcaptonurica), Lek. Listy **2:**536, 1947.

53. Jeghers, H.: Pigmentation of the skin, New Eng. J. Med. **231:**88, 1944.

54. Kang, E. S., and Gerald, P. S.: Alcaptonuria; rapid semiquantitative determination of homogentisic acid in urine, J. Pediat. **76:**939, 1970.

55. Kellgren, J. H.: Osteoarthrosis in patients and populations, Brit. Med. J. **2:**1, 1961.

56. Khachadurian, A., and Abu Feisal, K.: Alkaptonuria; report of a family with seven cases appearing in four successive generations with metabolic studies in one patient, J. Chronic Dis. **7:**455, 1958.

57. Knox, W. E.: Sir Archibald Garrod's "Inborn errors of metabolism." II. Alkaptonuria, Amer. J. Hum. Genet. **10:**95, 1958.

58. Koonce, D. M.: Ochronosis: report of three cases in siblings, J. Tenn. Med. Ass. **51:**85, 1958.

59. La Du, B. N.: Alcaptonuria. In Stanbury, J. B., Wyngaarden, J. B., and Fredrickson, D. S., editors: The metabolic basis of inherited disease, New York, 1960, Blakiston Division, McGraw-Hill Book Co., Inc., pp. 394-427.

60. La Du, B. N. (New York): Personal communication, 1971.

61. La Du, B. N., Zannoni, V. G., Laster, L., and Seegmiller, J. E.: The nature of the defect in tyrosine metabolism in alcaptonuria, J. Biol. Chem. **230:**251, 1958.

62. Lewis, J. H.: Alcaptonuria in a rabbit, J. Biol. Chem. **70:**659, 1926.

63. Lichtenstein, L., and Kaplan, L.: Hereditary ochronosis; pathological changes observed in two necropsied cases, Amer. J. Path. **30:**99, 1954.

64. Ludwig, G. D., Toole, J. F., and Wood, J. C.: Ochronosis from quinacrine (Atabrine), Ann. Intern. Med. **59:**378, 1963.

65. Lustberg, T. J., Schulman, J. D., and Seegmiller, J. E.: Decreased binding of ^{14}C-homogentisic acid induced by ascorbic acid in connective tissue of rats with experimental alkaptonuria, Nature **228:**770, 1970.

66. McCollum, D. E., and Odom, G. L.: Alkaptonuria, ochronosis, and low-back pain; a case report, J. Bone Joint Surg. **47-A:**1389, 1965.

67. McKenzie, A. W., Owen, J. A., and Ramsay, J. H. R.: Two cases of alcaptonuria, Brit. Med. J. **2:**794, 1957.

68. McKusick, V. A., and Goodman, R. M.: Pinnal calcification; observations in systemic diseases not associated with disordered calcium metabolism, J.A.M.A. **179:**230, 1962.

69. McKusick, V. A., and Milch, R. A.: The clinical behavior of genetic disease; selected aspects, Clin. Orthop. **33:**22, 1964.

70. Manson-Bahr, P., and Ransford, O. N.: Some pigmentations of the skin occurring in patients from the tropics; carotinaemia, haemochromatosis and alkaptonuria, Trans. Roy. Soc. Trop. Med. Hyg. **32:**395, 1938.

71. Martin, W. J., Underdahl, L. O., and Mathieson, D. R.: Alkaptonuria; report of 3 cases, Proc. Mayo Clin. **27:**193, 1952.

72. Milch, R. A.: Direct inheritance of alcaptonuria, Metabolism **4:**513, 1955.

73. Milch, R. A.: Hydrothermal shrinkage of metabolite-treated aortae, J. Atheroscler. Res. **5:**215, 1965.

74. Milch, R. A.: Reaction of collagen–cross-linking aldehydes with phenylenediamines, Nature **205:**1108, 1965.

75. Milch, R. A.: Studies of alcaptonuria; binding of homogentisic acid solutions to hide powder collagen, Proc. Soc. Exp. Biol. Med. **106:**68, 1961.

76. Milch, R. A.: Studies of alcaptonuria; collagenase degradation of homogentisic–tanned hide powder collagen, Proc. Soc. Exp. Biol. Med. **107:**183, 1961.

77. Milch, R. A.: Studies of alcaptonuria; infra-red spectra of deuterated homogentistic acid solutions, Arthritis Rheum. **8:**1002, 1965.

78. Milch, R. A.: Studies of alcaptonuria; inheritance of 47 cases in eight highly inter-related Dominican kindreds, Amer. J. Hum. Genet. **12:**76, 1960.

79. Milch, R. A., and Robinson, R. A.: Studies of alcaptonuria; content and density of the water and solid phases of ochronotic cartilage, J. Chronic Dis. **12:**409, 1960.

80. Minno, A. M., and Rogers, J. A.: Ochronosis; report of a case, Ann. Intern. Med. **56:**179, 1957.

81. Molony, J., and Kelly, D. J.: Alkaptonuria, ochronosis, and ochronotic arthritis, J. Irish Med. Ass. **63:**22, 1970.

82. Moran, T. J., and Yunis, E. J.: Studies on ochronosis. II. Effects of injection of homogentisic acid and ochronotic pigment in experimental animals, Amer. J. Path. **40:**359, 1962.

83. Mosonyi, L.: A propos de l'alcaptonurie et de son traitement, Presse Méd. **47:**708, 1939.

84. Mueller, M. N., Sorensen, L. B., and Strandjord, N.: Alkaptonuria and ochronotic arthropathy, Med. Clin. N. Amer. **49:**101, 1965.

85. Naganna, B., Rajamma, M., and Rao, K. V.: On the failure of enzyme paper strips to detect glucose in certain abnormal urines, Clin. Chim. Acta **17:**219, 1967.

86. Natarajan, M.: Ochronotic arthritis (a report of three cases), Indian J. Surg. **22:**222, 1960.

87. Neubauer, O.: Intermediärer Eiweisstoffwechsel, Handb. Norm. Path. Physiol. **5:**671, 1928.

88. O'Brien, W. M., La Du, B. N., and Bunim, J. J.: Biochemical, pathologic and clinical aspects of alcaptonuria, ochronosis and ochronotic arthropathy; review of word literature (1584-1962), Amer. J. Med. **34:**813, 1963.

89. Oda, R. E.: Alkaptonuria; report of two cases in siblings, Amer. J. Dis. Child. **106:**301, 1963.

90. Osler, W.: Ochronosis: the pigmentation of cartilages, sclerotics and skin in alkaptonuria, Lancet **1:**10, 1904.

91. Pagan-Carlo, J., and Payzant, A. R.: Roentgenographic manifestations in a severe case of alcaptonuric osteoarthritis, Amer. J. Roentgen. **80:**635, 1958.

92. Papageorge, E., and Lewis, H. B.: Comparative studies of the metabolism of the amino acids. VII. Experimental alcaptonuria in the white rat, J. Biol. Chem. **123:**211, 1938.

93. Pieter, H.: Une famille d'alcaptonuriques, Presse Méd. **33:**1310, 1925.

94. Pomeranz, M. M., Friedman, L. J., and Tunick, I. S.: Roentgen findings in alcaptonuric ochronosis, Radiology **37:**295, 1941.

95. Poschl, M.: Röntgenbild und Röntgenbestrahlung bei der Arthrosis alkaptonurica, Fortschr. Roentgenst. **76:**97, 1952.

96. Poulsen, V.: Ueber Ochronose bei Menschen und Tieren, Beitr. Path. Anat. **48:**346, 1910.

97. Rones, B.: Ochronosis oculi in alkaptonuria, Amer. J. Ophthal. **49:**440, 1960.

97a. Roth, M., and Felgenhauer, W.-R.: Recherche de l'excretion d'acide homogentisique urinaire chez des heterozygotes pour l'alcaptonurie, Enzym. Biol. Clin. **9:**53, 1968.

98. Sarin, L. R., and Bhargava, R. K.: Alkaptonuria with ochronosis, J. Indian Med. Ass. **28**:481, 1957.

99. Savastano, A. A., Quigley, D. G., and Scala, M. E.: Spontaneous fractures associated with cortisone therapy in a patient with ochronosis, Amer. J. Orthop. Surg. **11**:116, 1969.

99a. Shelley, W. B., and Hurley, H. J., Jr.: Localized chromhidrosis; a survey, Arch. Derm. Syph. **69**:449, 1954.

100. Seegmiller, J. E., Zannoni, V. G., Laster, L., and La Du, B. N.: An enzymatic spectrophotometric method for the determination of homogentisic acid in plasma and urine, J. Biol. Chem. **236**:774, 1961.

101. Siekert, R. G., and Gibilisco, J. A.: Discoloration of the teeth in alkaptonuria (ochronosis) and Parkinsonism, Oral Surg. **29**:197, 1970.

102. Simon, G., and Zorab, P. A.: The radiographic changes in alkaptonuric arthritis, Brit. J. Radiol. **34**:384, 1961.

103. Sinha, H. K.: A case of alkaptonuria, Indian Med. Gaz. **65**:153, 1930.

104. Šiťaj, S., and Urbánek, T.: Alkaptonuria, Rev. Czech. Med. **2**:288, 1956.

105. Skinsnes, O. K.: Generalized ochronosis; report of an instance in which it was misdiagnosed as melanosarcoma, with resultant enucleation of an eye, Arch. Path. **45**:552, 1948.

106. Smith, H. P., and Smith, H. P., Jr.: Ochronosis; report of two cases, Ann. Intern. Med. **42**:171, 1955.

107. Smith, J. W.: Ochronosis of the sclera and cornea complicating alkaptonuria; review of the literature and report of four cases, J.A.M.A. **120**:1282, 1942.

108. Söderbergh, G.: Ueber Ostitis deformans ochronotica, Neur. Zbl. **32**:1362, 1913.

109. Sokoloff, L., Crittenden, L. B., Yamamoto, R. S., and Jay, G. E., Jr.: The genetics of degenerative joint disease in mice, Arthritis Rheum. **5**:531, 1962.

109a. Srsen, S. (Martin, Czechoslovakia): Personal communication, 1971.

110. Steele, J. M.: Alcaptonuria and ochronosis. In Beeson, P. B., and McDermott, W., editor: Cecil-Loeb textbook of medicine, ed. 11, Philadelphia, 1963, W. B. Saunders Co., pp. 1243-1244.

111. Stevenson, A. C. (Oxford): Personal communication.

112. Sussman, T.: Alkaptonuria, Proc. Roy. Soc. Med. **62**:485, 1969.

113. Sutro, C. J., and Anderson, M. E.: Alkaptonuric arthritis; cause for free intra-articular bodies, Surgery **22**:120, 1947.

114. Umber, G., and Burger, M.: Zur Klinik intermediarer Stoffwechselstörungen (Alkaptonurie mit Ochronose und Osteo-Arthritis deformans; Zystinurie), Deutsch. Med. Wschr. **39**:2337, 1913.

115. Vaishnava, S., and Pulimood, B. M.: Alkaptonuria, Indian J. Pediat. **25**:518, 1958.

116. Virchow, R.: Ein Fall von allgemeiner Ochronose der Knorpel und knorpelähnlichen Theile, Arch. Path. Anat. **37**:212, 1866.

117. Wagner, L. R., Knott, J. L., Machaffie, R. A., and Walsh, J. R.: Clinical and pathological findings in ochronosis, J. Clin. Path. **13**:22, 1960.

118. Wells, C., and Maxwell, B. M.: Alkaptonuria in an Egyptian mummy, Brit. J. Radiol. **35**:679, 1962.

119. White, A. G., Parker, J., and Block, F.: Studies in human alkaptonuria, J. Clin. Invest. **28**:140, 1949.

120. Wittenberg, J.: Gastrointestinal bleeding and arthropathy, J.A.M.A. **195**:1048, 1966.

121. Wolkow, M., and Baumann, E.: Ueber das Wesen der Alkaptonurie, Z. Physiol. Chem. **15**:228, 1891.

122. Woodford, V. R., Quan, L., and Cutts, F.: Experimental alkaptonuria in the rat induced by tryptophan deficiency, Canad. J. Biochem. **45**:791, 1967.

123. Young, H. H.: Calculi of the prostate associated with ochronosis and alkaptonuria, J. Urol. **51**:48, 1944.

124. Yules, J. H.: Ochronotic arthritis; report of a case, Bull. New Eng. Med. Center **16**:168, 1954.

125. Zannoni, V. G., Malawista, S. E., and La Du, B. N.: Studies on Ochronosis. II. Studies on benzoquinoneacetic acid, a probable intermediate in the connective tissue pigmentation of alkaptonuria, Arthritis Rheum. **5**:547, 1962.

126. Zannoni, V. G., Seegmiller, J. E., and La Du, B. N.: Nature of the defect in alkaptonuria, Nature, (London) **193**:952, 1962.

10 · Pseudoxanthoma elasticum

Historical note

The first description of the skin changes occurring in pseudoxanthoma elasti-cum is that by Rigal[144] in 1881, and the first autopsy report was provided by Balzer[9] in 1884. Because of the yellow and elevated appearance of the skin lesions, the disorder was grouped with the xanthomatoses by Rigal and Balzer and by Chauffard.[28] The disease was identified as a separate and nonxanthoma-tous entity by Darier[36] in 1896.

In 1889 Chauffard,* at a meeting of the Société Médicale des Hôpitaux in Paris, described a patient destined to occupy a prominent role in the history of this disease. His case was separately reported, during the next fifteen years, by Besnier and Doyon[17]; by Darier,[36] who established the histopathology and offered the name *pseudoxanthoma elasticum* with the alternative *elastorrhexis;* and by Hallopeau and Laffitte,[71] who described dramatic changes in the fundus oculi. The patient's well-documented story is of further interest because it demonstrates the typical features of the syndrome from which he suffered: changes in the skin, repeated massive gastrointestinal hemorrhages, weak peripheral pulses, and failing vision. Chauffard's description[27] follows†:

> This is a man of 35 years. . . . At 24 years of age, while doing his military service in New Caledonia, he suffered a large hematemesis. This accident repeated itself sev-eral times (at ages 26, 31, and 33). This summer he was admitted to the Hôtel Dieu for a hematemesis.
>
> In 1880 L. was discharged and returned to France; and it was shortly afterward, he states, when he noted the beginning of his skin affection. . . . The xanthomatous erup-tion is composed of a series of evolving groups, perfectly symmetrical and confined exclusively to the several flexural folds—the base of the neck, the two axillary creases, the folds of the elbows, the anterior abdominal wall, especially just below the umbili-cus, the two inguinal triangles, the inferior aspect of the penis, around the anus, the two popliteal fossae. . . . The center of the group is formed by an almost confluent ag-glomeration of intradermal plaques, soft to the touch, projecting to some extent like papules, separated by small folds of skin. Their coloration is rather pale, resembling

---

*Anatole Chauffard (1855-1932), an internist, is better known for his discovery (with Min-kowski) of congenital hemolytic icterus (1900), now more generally called hereditary sphero-cytosis, and of the increased osmotic fragility of the erythrocytes in this condition (1907).[3]
†Translation mine.

475

that of fresh buttter or yellow chamois; the size of the largest plaque is scarcely greater than that of a pea. . . . If one retracts both lips, one sees that the mucosa of the inner aspect is involved. It demonstrates a cluster of small, yellowish intramucosal nodules, resting on a richly vascular background traversed by numerous dilated and tortuous capillaries. . . . In February there developed an unusual phenomenon, of which there is today scarcely any trace remaining. The peripheral zone of the eruptive groups in the skin was traversed by rather large, violaceous rose networks that were not elevated and formed a congestive halo around the yellow plaques. . . . Today traces of this perinodular hyperemia remain only in the pectoral regions, on the anterior extension of the axillary groups. . . .

The pulse is feeble and compressible and gives with the sphygomometer of Verdin a tension of 650, rather than of 750, the average normal figure.

In August, 1896, at the Third International Dermatologic Congress in London, Darier[36] reported histologic studies on the skin of Chauffard's patient. By 1903, this patient had developed amblyopia; and Hallopeau and Laffitte[71] reported that there was "chorioretinitis of the central region, involving the macula, with secondary atrophy of the optic disc."

Although Hallopeau and Laffitte in 1903 speculated that there might be some connection between the changes in the skin and those in the fundus oculi of

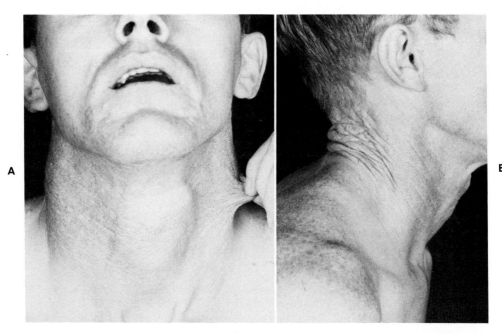

Fig. 10-1. C. T. (582989), a 32-year-old man. **A** and **B,** The skin is lax, rigid, and grooved, with a yellowish tint. **C,** Angioid streaks and proliferative changes in fundus oculi. **D,** Calcification of deep femoral artery (photograph retouched). **E,** Calcification of posterior tibial artery (photograph retouched). **F,** Histologic changes in the skin. Elastic tissue stain. (×50.) **G,** Same as in **F.** (×125.) The skin of the neck, axillae, and groin is involved. Both second toes have a congenital flexion deformity ("hammertoe"). Beginning at the age of 30 years, the patient has had about ten massive gastrointestinal hemorrhages necessitating hospitalization and transfusion. No bleeding site has ever been identified. X-ray film of the lungs reveals peculiar nodular densities diffusely distributed throughout both lung fields. (**B** from McKusick, V. A.: Bull. N. Y. Acad. Med. **35:**143, 1959.)

Chauffard's patient, it was not until 1929 that the relationship of angioid streaks and pseudoxanthoma elasticum was established by Ester Grönblad,[66] an ophthalmologist, and James Strandberg,[170] a dermatologist, both of Stockholm. Angioid streaks had been described by Doyne[41] in 1889, and the name was assigned by Knapp[95] in 1892. Knapp thought angioid streaks had a vascular basis. Their origin as a result of crazing of Bruch's membrane was first suggested by Kofler[96] in 1917.

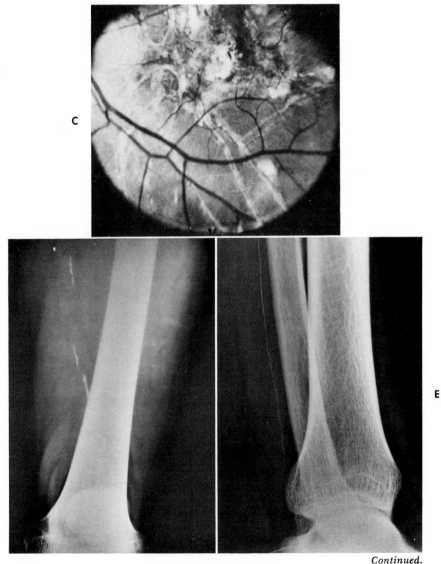

Continued.

Fig. 10-1, cont'd. For legend see opposite page.

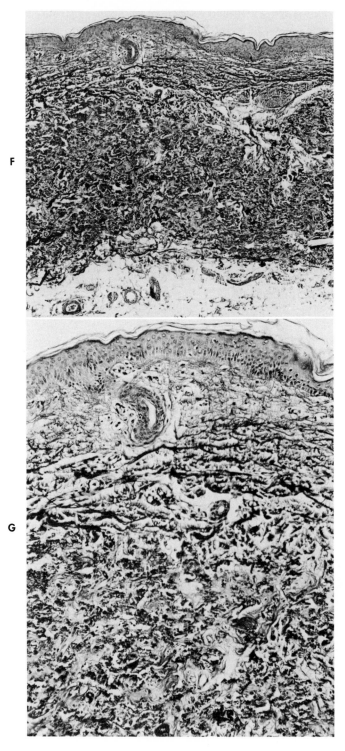

Fig. 10-1, cont'd. For legend see p. 476.

Involvement of the peripheral arteries in this syndrome and the physiologic consequences thereof have been studied in the last twenty-five years by Carlborg,[23] Van Embden Andres,[186] Scheie and Freeman,[153] Urbach and Wolfram,[185] Prick,[89,141] Guenther,[67] Wolff and associates,[197] and Goodman and colleagues,[64] among others. Gastrointestinal hemorrhage was emphasized by several of these authors and particularly by Revell and Carey[143] in 1948. During the early 1950's the suggestion that this disease is an abnormality of collagen fibers rather than elastic fibers was advanced by Hannay,[72] who used standard histologic techniques, and by Tunbridge and collaborators,[184] who used electron microscopy. Return to the view that the elastic fiber is primarily involved came from the work of Rodnan and associates,[146] Fisher and co-workers,[48] Goodman and colleagues,[64] and others.

Pseudoxanthoma elasticum is the name usually given this syndrome. With the renewed evidence that the elastic fiber is the main site of abnormality, "elasticum" seems accurate, and the skin and arterial changes certainly justify the designation "pseudoxanthoma." In our present understanding, Touraine's term *élastorrhexie systématisée*[182] is an appropriate term, although a change is not proposed, especially since a term similar to it (systemic elastolysis) is used for cutis laxa (p. 372). The only eponym that has been applied to this syndrome at all frequently, Grönblad-Strandberg, is not easily remembered or spoken and has not attained wide use. The abbreviation PXE is the term that will be used frequently in this presentation to refer to the entire syndrome.

Clinical manifestations

Clinical expression of PXE is found mainly in three areas: the skin, the eye, and the cardiovascular system. Because of the widespread involvement of the muscular arteries, hemorrhagic symptoms referable to virtually every organ system may occur. The following descriptions are based in part on more than 25 cases observed at The Johns Hopkins Hospital.

Skin and mucosa. The changes in the skin (Figs. 10-1*A* and 10-2) are often not recognizable clinically before the second decade of life or later. The face, neck, axillary folds, cubital areas, inguinal folds, and periumbilical area are particularly prone to involvement. The skin in the perioral area, including the creases of the skin, another zone of particular wear and tear, is likely to show changes. (It is of note that senile "elastotic degeneration" [see below] occurs frequently in the same area, as indicated by the frequency with which this histologic change is seen in specimens of lip carcinoma. Surgical pathologists and skin pathologists become very familiar with senile elastosis because of its frequency in specimens with neoplasms of the skin in older individuals.) The skin becomes thickened and grooved like coarse-grained Moroccan leather. The areas between the grooves, diamond-shaped, rectangular, and polygonal, are elevated and yellowish. *Cutis rhomboidalis nuchae* and *la peau citréine,* although terms more often used for conditions distinct from PXE, would be appropriate for the changes seen in some of these patients.[176] "Crepelike" skin[129] and "plucked chicken" skin[127] are other suggested descriptions. The skin in the involved areas becomes lax, redundant, and relatively inelastic. In girls the cosmetically undesirable changes in the skin, especially that of the neck, are often occasion for consulting a physician. Exaggeration of the nasolabial folds and chin creases

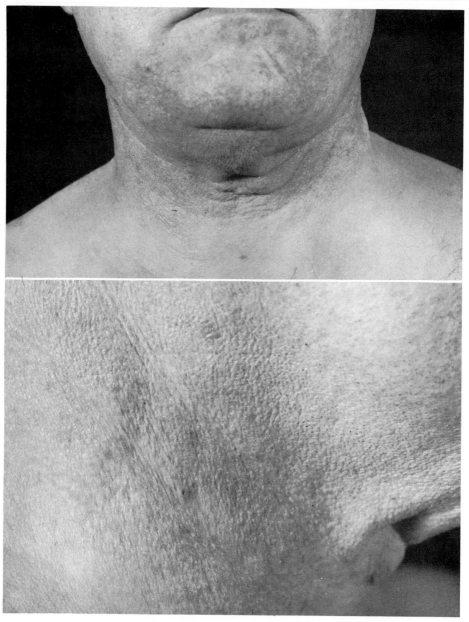

Fig. 10-2. P. J. G. (J.H.H. 721600), 45 years old, had a severe gastrointestinal hemorrhage at the age of 34 years. No basis was discovered and there was no recurrence. He was told at that time that he had hemorrhage in the right eye. For several years, especially in winter, he noted cramping and fatigability of the legs. At the age of 44 years there was onset of progressive failure of vision. There are no similar abnormalities in the family. Examination revealed only minimal changes in the skin of the neck. The skin would have been passed as normal were it not for the rest of the clinical picture. The skin elsewhere was normal except possibly for slightly increased looseness in flexure areas. Both fundi showed large areas of old hemorrhage and fibrosis in the macular area, typical angioid streaks, and hyaline bodies near the optic discs. No pulses were palpable in the legs below the femorals. Blood pressure and electrocardiogram were normal. The aorta was moderately tortuous, and serum cholesterol was 355 mg./100 ml. (Patient seen through courtesy of Dr. J. R. Krevans.)

is often striking (Fig. 10-3) and may create a "hound dog" appearance of the face. Profound laxity of skin in the neck, axillary folds, and abdominal wall is observed in some. Striking lesions in the inguinal triangles and on the penis occur in some patients (Fig. 10-4).

The soft[59] or hard[124] palate often shows changes grossly and histologically identical to those in the skin; the inner aspect of the lips and the buccal mucosa are commonly affected areas[129] (Fig. 10-5). At times the mucosa of the rectum and vagina is affected.[23] By gastroscopy a majority of PXE patients show linear or nodular submucosal lesions that are yellow in color and similar to the xanthoma-like skin lesions.[29,64]

In some patients the cutaneous changes are exceedingly mild despite advanced ocular and arterial changes (Fig. 10-2). Van Embden Andres[186] described 4 patients with only minimal clinical but typical histologic changes in the skin. In 2 other cases of his, there were no clinically detectable changes in the skin; yet there were positive findings on biopsy. Goodman and colleagues[64] described similar experiences; see Fig. 10-3. Rubbing or stretching of the skin may make the lesions more evident.[129] Sometimes the patients report expressing "matter"

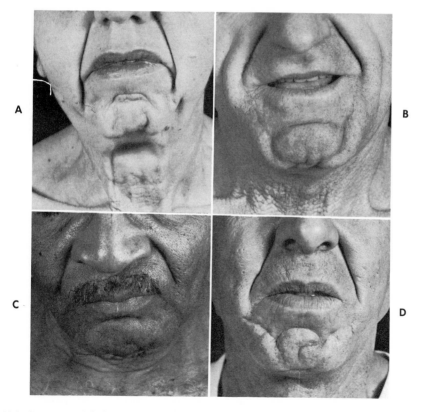

Fig. 10-3. Accentuated facial folds and creases in 4 patients with PXE. Those shown in **A, B,** and **D** are sibs. (From Goodman, R. M., Smith, E. W., Paton, D., Bergman, R. A., Siegel, C. L., Ottesen, O. E., Shelley, W. M., Pusch, A. L., and McKusick, V. A.: Medicine **42:**297, 1963.)

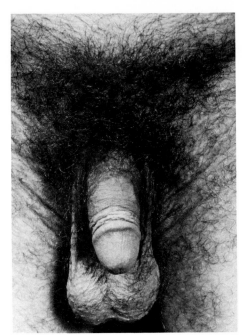

Fig. 10-4. Skin lesions of the lower abdomen, femoral triangles, and penis in a 33-year-old man (C. G., 456025). (From Goodman, R. M., Smith, E. W., Paton, D., Bergman, R. A., Siegel, C. L., Ottesen, O. E., Shelley, W. M., Pusch, A. L., and McKusick, V. A.: Medicine **42:**297, 1963.)

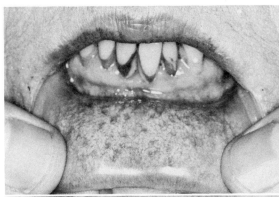

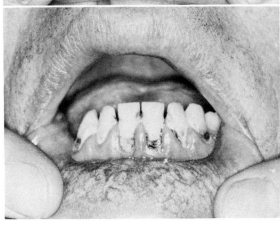

Fig. 10-5. Lesions of the labial mucosa.

from the nodular lesions of the neck and about the chin. In Gold's case[63] ulceration and drainage of the skin lesions occurred. Suppuration and ulceration of PXE lesions were described by Heyl[78] in the Cape colored of South Africa. Poor personal hygiene may have been responsible for this complication.

In addition to the classic features, some patients have localized skin changes of a different type on the neck, axilla, or anterior abdominal wall. These changes consist of large (3 by 4 cm.) circinate plaques of closely grouped, hyperkeratotic papules, 1 to 2 mm. in size. A hyperkeratotic cap can be dislodged to leave a small, bloody depression. This lesion[160] is termed reactive perforating elastoma (elastoma perforans serpiginosa, Miescher's elastoma, etc.). It occurs not only in PXE,[120,156] but also in other heritable disorders of connective tissue—Marfan syndrome, Ehlers-Danlos syndrome, and osteogenesis imperfecta.

The skin changes about the neck were noted at birth by the mother of one patient. In others they have been noted in early childhood. In some patients no remarkable peculiarity is evident to the patient until the changes are pointed out by the physician consulted because of failing vision or gastrointestinal hemorrhage.

Calcification in the middle and deeper layers of the dermis is identifiable by radiographic techniques (Fig. 10-6). In 3 of 10 patients who were appropriately studied, Goodman and colleagues[64] found calcinosis cutis. Knuckle pads have been described on the thumb in PXE[165] but it is unlikely that they were more than coincidental.

The eye. The characteristic changes in the eye are demonstrated by fundu-

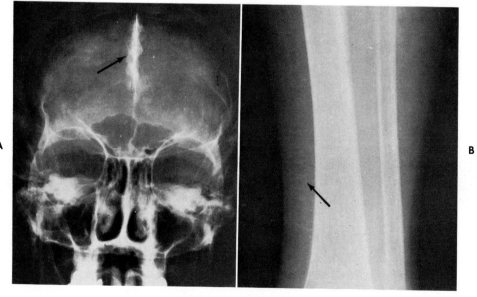

Fig. 10-6. Calcification of the falx cerebri, **A,** and of the skin, **B,** in D. G. (757257), 54-year-old white female (shown also in Fig. 10-15). (From Goodman, R. M., Smith, E. W., Paton, D., Bergman, R. A., Siegel, C. L., Ottesen, O. E., Shelley, W. M., Pusch, A. L., and McKusick, V. A.: Medicine 42:297, 1963.)

scopic examination and consist of angioid streaking of the fundus. (Fig. 10-1*C*). These streaks are red, brownish, or gray and are four or five times wider than veins but resemble vessels in the manner in which they course over the fundus.[194] That the streaks lack pigmentation can be demonstrated by applying sufficient pressure to the eye to occlude the retinal artery. Pallor of the avascular retina produced by this maneuver decreases visible contrasts and in many patients leads to virtual disappearance of the streaks. That the streaks are cracks in a membrane beneath the retina is clinically substantiated by observation of their tapering and their complementary zigzag borders. They always underlie the retinal vessels. In later stages the streaks are bordered by proliferating scar tissue and retinal pigment epithelium, producing cuffing of the type shown (Figs. 10-7 to 10-9). Electroretinography usually shows no abnormality until late stages. Fundus photographs after injection of fluorescein[164] yield clear demonstrations of angioid streaks and other changes of PXE.

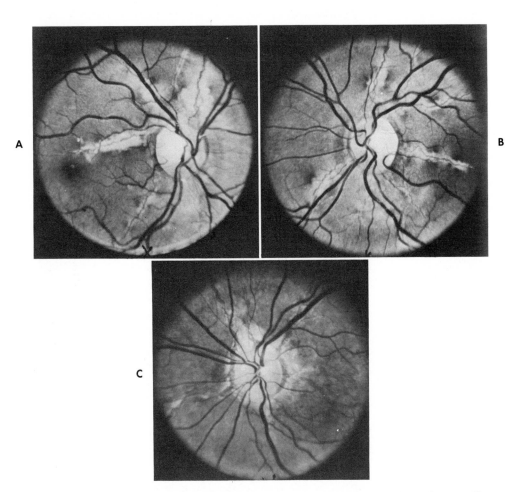

Fig. 10-7. Fundus photographs in PXE. Angioid streaks in typical configuration. Fibrous cuffing accompanying the streaks is especially striking in **A.** Note that the streaks underlie the blood vessels. In **C,** increased visibility of choroidal vessels is demonstrated.

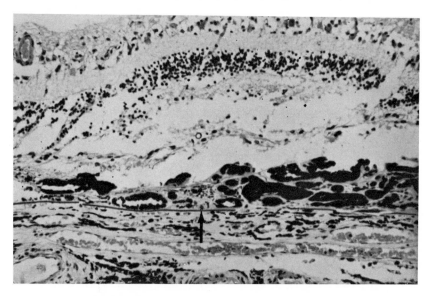

Fig. 10-8. Histopathology of angioid streaks. Bruch's membrane is indicated by the arrow. Breaks are shown in the right of the picture. (Courtesy Dr. David Paton.)

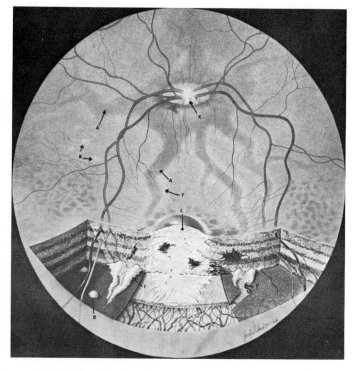

Fig. 10-9. Diagram correlating the funduscopic and histologic features of the eye in PXE. **A,** Angioid streaks; **B,** *Drusen* of Bruch's membrane; **C,** mound of vascularized scar tissue at the macula; **X,** hyaline body of the optic disc; **Y,** fibrous tissue cuffing an angioid streak. In the lower part of the diagram the retina is shown in cross section and between two angioid streaks. Bruch's membrane and the choriocapillaris have been cut away, showing the pattern of underlying choroidal vessels. (Courtesy Dr. David Paton.)

The angioid streaks are probably not present at birth but, like the skin changes, they usually develop in the second decade or later. They may be the only ocular sign of PXE for many years. The development of hemorrhage and the appearance of chorioretinal scarring are ominous signs. Although complete blindness does not occur, macular involvement frequently results in diminution of visual acuity to 20/200, 20/400, or the ability to see fingers at a few feet. When chorioretinal scarring and accompanying retinal pigment proliferation are extensive, angioid streaks may be obscured, although indistinct remnants of streaks usually persist at the periphery of such scars.

In some cases the occurrence of retinal hemorrhage can be related to trauma such as, for example, that sustained in one patient by high diving and in another by a blow from a tennis ball.[147] White or yellowish dots referred to as colloid bodies, or *Drüsen,* are described[197] and were present in the vicinity of the discs in the patient whose skin changes are demonstrated in Fig. 10-2.

Some patients show only pigmentary mottling of the fundus.[64,158] This change is interpreted as the earliest manifestation of alteration in Bruch's membrane.

Although angioid streaks are the ocular hallmark of PXE, not infrequently only a less specific central chorioretinitis is present.[15,186] This may have been the case with Chauffard's famous patient.[71] Like the hemorrhages, the central chorioretinitis is a grave threat to vision because of involvement of the macular areas. Anderson[2] described a family in which PXE of the skin was associated with choroidal sclerosis in 4 males. The choroidal sclerosis alone was present in a fifth male. Short angioid streaks seem evident in certain of the illustrations; however, one author reported observations of a single patient spanning thirty-six years.[202] Atrophy of the choroid and sclerosis of choroidal vessels were present in the late stages. Funduscopic findings in heterozygotes are discussed on p. 502.

The cardiovascular system. Clinically the arterial involvement is expressed by pulse changes and symptoms of arterial insufficiency in the extremities, by x-ray evidence of premature medial calcification of peripheral arteries, by symptoms of coronary insufficiency, by hemorrhage in one or more of many different areas, and by hypertension.

Weakness or absence of pulses in the extremities is a frequent finding. Fatigability or frank intermittent claudication may occur in the legs. The development of these manifestations by the third decade or earlier and the involvement of the arms as well as the legs aid in the differentiation of these changes from those of ordinary arteriosclerosis. In Fig. 10-1D and E are given examples of arterial calcification that began to develop at least as early as the latter part of the third decade of life. Calcification as early as the age of 9 years has been described[197]; in this child, intermittent claudication, loss of pulsations in the distal arteries of the limbs, calcification of the arteries, and repeated attacks of melena (see Case 3, below) were present. A brother, 25 years of age, had similar symptoms.

The radial and/or ulnar pulses are sometimes absent in PXE. Substituting for these pulses may be an arterial pulsation in an anomalous position near the middle of the volar surface of the wrist. Although ischemic symptoms are rather unusual in the upper extremities—especially when considered in relation to the high frequency of drastic angiographic changes—easy fatigability of the arms, in washing clothes, for example,[33] and ischemic resorption of the terminal phalan-

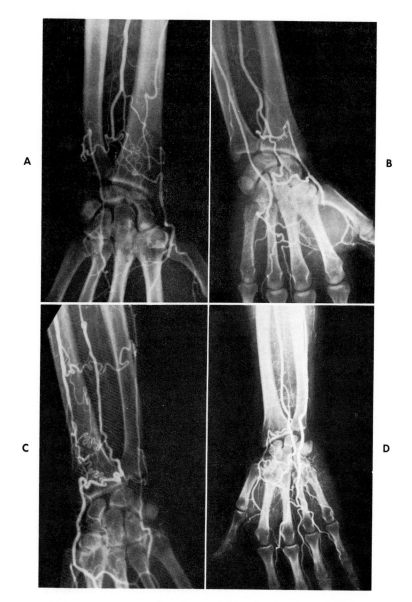

Fig. 10-10. Findings of brachial arteriography in PXE. **A,** Obstruction of both the radial and the ulnar artery, with refilling from a dilated interosseous artery, in J. C. (279288), 65-year-old Negro male. **B,** Obstruction of the radial artery, with refilling from the interosseous, in C. G. (456025), 33-year-old white male. **C,** Occlusion, narrowing, and irregularity of the main arteries in the forearm, with marked collateral formation, in R. T. (1022161), 54-year-old white female. **D,** Occlusion of the radial artery in D. W. (1023639), 50-year-old white female.

geal tufts, as well as the necessity for surgical amputation of digits,[83] have been reported. Bäfverstedt and Lund[6] found no abnormality of the brachial arteriogram in a 9-year-old child with PXE. Carlborg and co-workers[24] found narrowing of arteries in the forearm in 1 of 4 cases studied. Goodman and colleagues[64] found drastic changes in the brachial arteriograms of 6 patients, of whom the youngest was 33 years old at the time of study. In all, the radial and/or ulnar arteries were occluded or markedly narrowed. The interosseous arteries were little, if at all, affected and had undergone dilatation. In cases of occluded radial and ulnar arteries, terminal collaterals from the interosseous arteries provided apparently adequate filling of the arterial system in the hand. These changes are illustrated in Figs. 10-10 and 10-11. Selective diminution of blood supply to one finger was pictured by James and associates.[83]

Reduced pulse wave velocity in the arteries of the extremities was found in most cases of PXE.[23,186] The pulse wave was, furthermore, of reduced amplitude and plateau configuration. The dicrotic notch may be lost. The peak is attained more slowly than normal.[6,157] The fact that the 9-year-old child studied by Bäfverstedt and Lund[6] showed these changes in the pulse curves, despite normal arteriograms, suggests that occlusive changes are not essential to the alterations in the pulse curves.

Angina pectoris,[53] electrocardiographic changes compatible with myocardial ischemia, radiographic evidence of coronary artery calcification,[129] and myocardial infarction[129] are observed in patients with PXE and leave little doubt that the coronary arteries are involved in this disorder. In one patient (N. G., 1136343) with substernal pain and nonspecific electrocardiographic changes, an electrocardiographic exercise test was negative, and coronary arteriograms showed no definite abnormality. Levine[104a] described to me a girl who had onset of angina

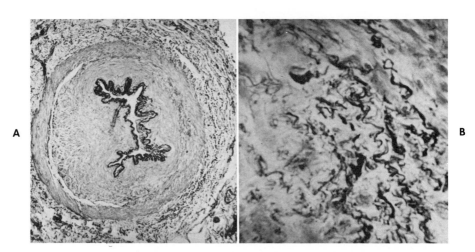

Fig. 10-11. Biopsy of radial artery in R. T. (1022161), 54-year-old white female with PXE. The lumen is almost completely occluded due to marked fibrous proliferation in the media. The intima is delicate and the internal elastic membrane appears normal. Elastic fibers in the region of the external elastic membrane are ruptured and irregular. The cleft shown laterally is an artifact of sectioning; it probably occurred in a weakened part of the wall. **A,** Verhoeff stain (× 100.) **B,** Region of external elastic membrane, Verhoeff stain. (×600.)

pectoris at the age of 11 years. Coronary arteriograms at the age of 18 years showed three vessel disease. A triple graft was performed at 19 years of age with highly satisfying results.

Hemorrhages constitute the major medical problem in most cases of PXE that come to the attention of the internist. Gastrointestinal hemorrhage is common[88] and may be fatal.[69,181] It may occur from a lesion such as peptic ulcer or hiatal hernia, which per se can produce hemorrhage, but in most cases of PXE the source of bleeding is not evident on clinical study. In cases of peptic ulcer, the arterial disease plays a strong contributory role to hemorrhages, similar to that of arteriosclerosis and primary amyloid disease. Superficial ulceration has been discovered by gastroscopy[109] or on gastrectomy.[88] Hemorrhage from the jejunum has been described.[151] In my own experience, gastrointestinal bleeding in PXE has occurred as early as 6½ years of age. (Fig. 10-12), and hematemesis at 3 years[188] and at 12 years[62] has been reported. In cases of gastrointestinal hemorrhage, the physician should almost automatically look for the skin changes of this syndrome, just as one should look for Kayser-Fleischer rings in patients with liver disease, and for cutaneous telangiectasia in these same patients with gastrointestinal hemorrhage. Some patients visit many different clinics, seeking

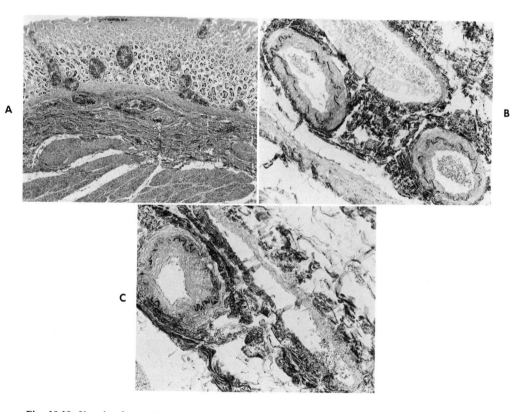

Fig. 10-12. Vessels of gastrointestinal tract in N. C. (p. 509). **A,** Dilated gastric mucosal vessels, some of which are probably ruptured. **B** and **C,** Submucosal vessels showing rupture of elastic membranes and surrounding reaction.

the cause of bleeding. Some have repeated abdominal explorations and repair of some lesion, such as hiatal hernia, which may or may not be incidental. The reports of massive gastrointestinal hemorrhage during pregnancy in 3 women with PXE[111,198] suggest that pregnancy has an aggravating influence. Nellen and Jacobson[129] noted flushing of the skin lesions with each episode of hematemesis. (See p. 476 for a description of perinodular hyperemia in Chauffard's patient.)

In addition to gastrointestinal bleeding, the types of hemorrhage by location include subarachnoid, retinal, renal, uterine,[186] bladder, and nasal. Spontaneous hemarthroses occur.[186] Excessive bleeding from cuts of the skin does not seem to be a problem, although hemorrhages in the skin lesions have been described[55,116]. Foerster's patient[51] sought medical advice because of purpura on the legs and, later, on the left forearm. At the age of 16 years, one of the patients in my series (R. E. H., J.H.H. 193470) had a severe illness diagnosed as "black (hemorrhagic) measles." It is possible that the connective tissue disease was responsible for the hemorrhagic manifestations of the measles. Subarachnoid hemorrhage is commonly a cause of death.

Hypertension is frequent in PXE and in some cases has been convincingly shown to be the result of vascular disease, of the PXE type, in the renal vessels. The occurrence of hypertension is unfortunate because of its aggravating influence on the tendency to hemorrhage. In one patient,[38] 29 years old, intracranial "berry" aneurysm occurred in association with skin changes and angioid streaks. Scheie and Hogan[154] had a similar case. Another patient (E. W., J.H.H. 69818), seen in the past in The Johns Hopkins Hospital and twice reported,[82,143] died of cerebral hemorrhage at the age of 43 years. Severe hypertension and pronounced albuminuria were persistently present in the last few years of life. Cerebrovascular accident in a 40-year-old man has been reported.[98] Rosenheim[148] told me of a case of PXE in a teen-ager, with severe hypertension and with calcification of both renal arteries. Parker and colleagues[133] reported 2 sisters with PXE in whom the presenting manifestation was hypertension, at 10 years of age in one and at 6 in the other. Farreras-Valenti and co-workers[44] described "unilateral renal hypertension" associated with an angiomatous change in the posterior branch of the right renal artery in a 27-year-old man with severe hypertension. Right nephrectomy resulted in cure. Bardsley and Koehler[11] observed the same type of angiomatous change in the abdominal viscera in 2 patients with PXE. In one it involved an intrahepatic artery and the splenic artery above the left kidney.

Second to gastrointestinal hemorrhage, abdominal angina resulting from celiac artery stenosis is probably the most frequent abdominal complaint in PXE. The symptoms consist usually of pain coming on 40 to 45 minutes after eating. Gallbladder disease is often mistakenly suspected.

Calcification in peripheral arteries (both arms and legs) has been determined radiologically by a number of observers, including Sanbacka-Holström,[152] Zentmayer,[202] Silvers,[158] Silvers and Wolfe,[159] Carlborg,[23] Scheie and Freeman,[153] Wolff and associates,[197] and Goodman and associates.[64] Both medial and intimal calcification can be demonstrated (Fig. 10-13). Calcification, probably also of vascular location, is sometimes demonstrated in the choroid plexus[154,186] on skull x-ray film. It was demonstrated in the siphon of the internal carotid artery in a 30-year-old patient of this series and in reported cases.[154,202] In a 31-year-old

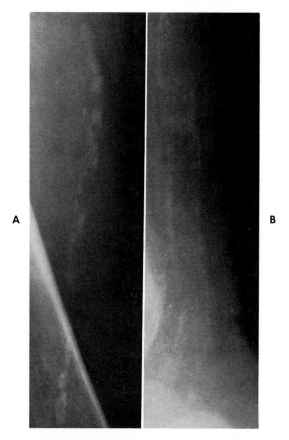

Fig. 10-13. Arterial calcification. **A,** The femoral artery of C. T. (1022514), 52-year-old man, shows intimal (dense patches) and medial (fine mottling) calcification. **B,** The radial artery of D. C. (863132), 58-year-old man, shows medial calcification. (From Goodman, R. M., Smith, E. W., Paton, D., Bergman, R. A., Siegel, C. L., Ottesen, O. E., Shelley, W. M., Pusch, A. L., and McKusick, V. A.: Medicine 42:297, 1963.)

European woman living in South Africa, Nellen and Jacobson[129] demonstrated calcification of the coronary arteries radiographically. Calcification of the falx cerebri and of the pineal body was also present. (See Fig. 10-6 for another example of calcification of the falx cerebri.) A 34-year-old brother with skin lesions had coronary thrombosis. Scheie and Hogan[154] described a case of PXE with "bilateral calcified carotid artery aneurysms." Hypercholesterolemia is not a necessary factor in the premature vascular change, although its presence probably exaggerates pathologic alterations. We had one patient (J. C., 279228) with typical cutaneous and fundal changes of PXE and equally typical Leriche syndrome (thrombotic obliteration of the bifurcation of the aorta) for which successful homografting was performed (autopsy Case 5 below). In another patient, a 48-year-old woman (Fig. 10-15), there is extensive calcification in the abdominal aorta. Both manifestations may bear no relation to the PXE. Lieberman[107] described extensive calcification in the great vessels and, at autopsy, well-advanced occlusive changes in the aortic arch and its branches—the aortic arch syndrome. Others[121,122] described the same case. The father of the patient had failing vision and died at 50 years of age of heart failure. The patient showed features that suggested the tumoral calcinosis syndrome (p. 503), specifically elevation of serum phosphorus and particularly extensive calcification and ossification.

Dilatation of the aorta has been remarked on in several of the cases. This was the case, for instance in the 30-year-old patient of Joffe and Joffe[84] and in the 35-year-old normotensive patient of Marchionini and Turgut.[117] Whether this finding bears a direct relationship to the fundamental defect is unclear. Case 9 of Carlborg[23] demonstrated marked dilatation (phlebectasia) of the jugular veins.

Other features. Joint manifestations are conspicuously absent in PXE. Sairanen and colleagues[150] reported polyarthritis beginning at the age of 65 years in a man with PXE but it may have been coincidental. The report of elevated immunoglobulins (gamma G and gamma A) in 8 patients with PXE requires confirmation.[85] Psychiatric disorders seem to occur with abnormally high frequency in these patients. Whether they can be explained on the basis of cerebro-

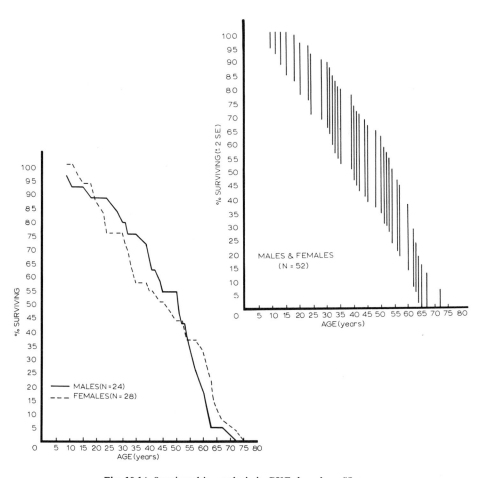

Fig. 10-14. Survivorship analysis in PXE, based on 52 cases.

vascular change is difficult to state. Certainly the high incidence of neurologic abnormalities is attributable to the vascular disease and hypertension. The nature of the neurologic abnormalities will not be discussed in detail because they are highly variable; yet per se they are not unlike what one customarily encounters with advanced arteriosclerosis and/or hypertension. The unusual feature is the relatively early age at which the neurologic accidents and deterioration occur.

Prognosis

In some patients death occurs at an early age from the occlusive or hemorrhagic manifestations of arterial involvement in PXE—e.g., patient N. C. (Case 3, p. 509), who died at the age of 13 years. Others fare remarkably well, as illustrated by the patients B. J. (Case 4) and J. C. (Case 5), who died at the ages of 72 and 74 years, respectively, of causes probably unrelated to the generalized connective tissue disorder. A life-table type of analysis of survivorship in 52 cases from the records of this department is shown in Fig. 10-14.

Pathology

In the skin, the characteristic changes occur in the deeper and middle zones of the corium (Fig. 10-1F). Large aggregations of material with the staining property of elastic fibers dominate the field. This material is granular for the most part, but in places rodlike structures are seen. Tuberculoid areas with giant cells[180,191] occur in the area of degeneration. (See Fig. 2-C in reference 20.) Calcification of the degenerated material occurs to a pronounced degree. This was established by Finnerud and Nomland,[47] using the von Kossa stain, and by Lobitz and Osterberg,[108] using microincineration. Actual bone formation is claimed.[13] Goodman and colleagues[64] have presented evidence that calcium deposition in elastic fibers is the earliest demonstrable histopathologic change in PXE. Elastic fibers surrounding sweat glands may, for example, show early changes. Later the elastic fibers become fragmented. (See Figs. 10-11 and 10-16.) Exposure of the tissue section to collagenase does not alter the appearance of the foci of calcified elastic fibers. Elastase, however, removes many of the elastic fiber ends that project from the edge of large concretions. Densely calcified fibers are usually not affected by elastase treatment.

Most histologic studies of the eye[18,56,69,94,187] have shown basophilia and tears in the lamina elastica of Bruch's membrane. (Benedict[14] and Law[100] failed to find them, however.) No primary abnormality is observed in the inner cuticular layer of Bruch's membrane.[123] Most observers, furthermore, have found advanced sclerotic changes in the choroidal vessels. When tears are present in Bruch's membrane, scar tissue tends to occupy the breaks or extend through beneath the pigment epithelium.[36] The breaks correspond to the streaks seen on funduscopic examination. Basophilia of the lamina elastica is encountered not infrequently in the eyes of older individuals; it occurs more regularly and at a younger age in PXE. Descemet's membrane of the cornea has chemical, physical, and tinctorial resemblances to the lamina elastica of Bruch's membrane. However, clinical or histologic evidence of involvement of the cornea has apparently not been observed in PXE.

Gross and histologic studies of the cardiovascular system are few. In the orig-

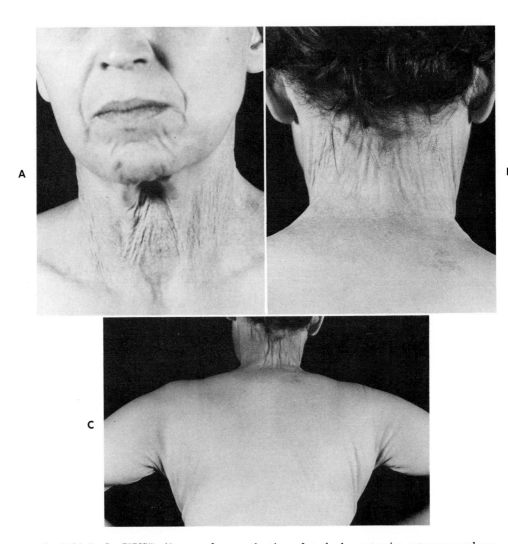

Fig. 10-15. D. G. (757275), 48 years of age at the time of study, has extensive cutaneous and mucosal changes and fundus changes. In her early twenties several massive hematemeses occurred, for which gastric resection was performed. It may be significant that the skin changes first appeared after measles at the age of 3 years. No pulses were palpable in the feet. X-ray films showed extensive calcification in the abdominal aorta. In this patient the diagnosis might be suspected from the chest x-ray film, which showed folds of redundant skin in both axillary areas. This patient had congenital short thumbs (short terminal phalanx), probably as an independent hereditary anomaly. Stecher[166] suggested that the abnormality is inherited as a recessive, although numerous other studies have proposed dominant inheritance. **A** and **B,** Changes in the skin of the neck. **C,** The neck and axillae. **D,** The anterior abdominal wall. **E** and **F,** The neck before and after plastic surgical repair.

inal case of Balzer[9] whitish thickening of the endocardium of the right atrium was described, as well as plaques of the same description on the pericardium and on the ventricular endocardium. Histologically, degeneration, thought to involve elastic elements, was demonstrated at these sites and in the walls of the pulmonary alveoli. (I have observed identical findings in 2 of 5 autopsied cases described in detail below, as did also Carlborg and colleagues.[24]) In Prick's case[89,141] the patient had hypertension and died at the age of 45 years of a cerebrovascular accident. Histologic changes interpreted as degeneration of elastic fibers were described in the coronary, renal, pancreatic, uterine, cutaneous, and mesenteric arteries, as well as in the splenic trabeculae, hepatic veins, and Bruch's membrane of the eye. In the patient of Urbach and Wolfram,[185] a 49-year-old man who died with a Korsakoff type of psychosis and who had widening of the

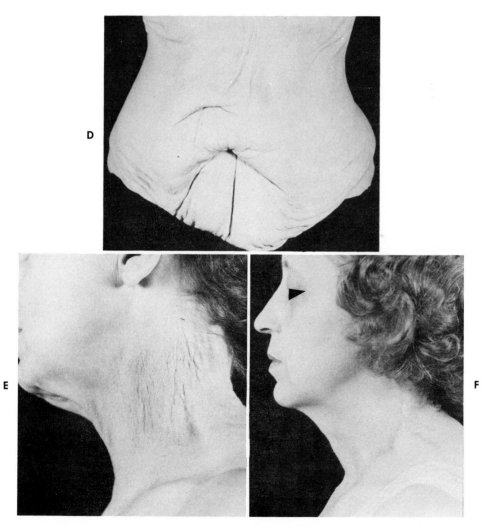

Fig. 10-15, cont'd. For legend see opposite page.

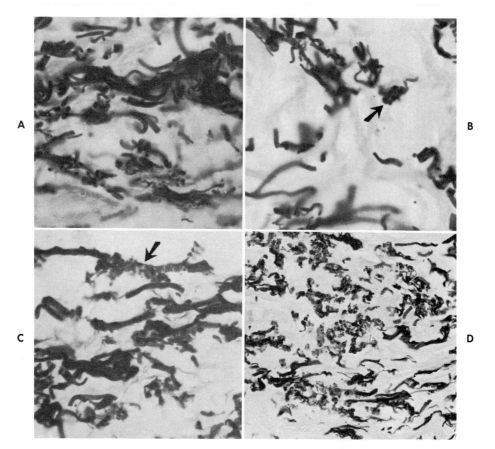

Fig. 10-16. Elastic fibers in skin. **A,** Normal. **B,** The arrow indicates a focus of altered elastic tissue in the skin of a patient with PXE. **C,** More extensive granular degenerative change in PXE. **D,** Advanced elastic tissue change in PXE.

aorta, as seen by x-ray examination, identical histologic changes were found in the brachial, cutaneous, and cerebral arteries and in Bruch's membrane. They also described and illustrated histologic changes in the aorta, which are, in my opinion, probably merely those seen in the senile aorta, sometimes even at the age of 49 years. Coffman and Sommers[31] thought there were specific aortic changes in their patient. Furthermore, these authors attributed valvular disease to PXE; mitral stenosis in one individual was thought to have this basis.

Carlborg[23] recorded autopsy observations made by another physician without particular knowledge of, or attention to, this syndrome. Klein[94] also reported an autopsied case. Five other autopsied cases are described below.

In the original case, Balzer[9] described degenerative changes involving presumably the elastic fibers in the walls of the pulmonary alveoli. However, the patient was a 49-year-old stonemason who died of extensive pulmonary tuberculosis, which may have been responsible for any changes observed in the lungs. Furthermore, in the autopsied cases of Prick[141] and of Urbach and Wolfram,[185] no abnormality of pulmonary elastic tissue was found. One can only speculate about the possible basis of a miliary mottling of one lung field described in x-ray examination of one patient[197] and observed in both lung fields of one of my patients. (C. T., J.H.H. 582989). It is possible that repeated small interstitial hemorrhages with resultant hemosiderosis are responsible. Calcification in small vessels is another possible explanation. In this same patient, there are no evidences of pulmonary hypertension, and studies of pulmonary function show no definite abnormality. In patients studied by Van Embden Andres,[186] no abnormality of residual air volume, maximum breathing capacity, or vital capacity was discovered.

In thyroid arteries removed during thyroidectomy, there were described[89] abnormalities of the type seen at autopsy in small coronary arteries in Case 1 on p. 504. Scheie and Freeman[153] biopsied the ulnar artery in one case and described "elastic tissue degeneration" with compensatory muscular hypertrophy. Identical findings were reported by Goodman and colleagues,[64] as shown in Fig. 10-13. The tunica intima was found to be delicate. The lumen was almost completely obliterated as a result of the medial process. Without illustration, Kaplan and Hartman[88] described degeneration of elastic elements, especially internal elastic lamella, in the vessels of the stomach removed in a 23-year-old white woman because of gastrointestinal bleeding. Beadlike microaneurysms were also present. Woo and Chandler[198] and Flatley and colleagues[49] reported similar findings. In one case of Revell and Carey[143] there were changes demonstrated in the peritonsillar tissues.

Many of the patients have advanced and premature arterial changes indistinguishable from ordinary atherosclerosis and arteriosclerosis. By producing changes in the tunica media, PXE probably sets the stage for the development of intimal changes, unusually early in life and to an unusually severe degree.

The basic defect

Whether PXE is a dystrophy of elastic fibers or of collagen fibers has been much debated. Certainly the degenerate material that develops in the skin has certain tinctorial characteristics of elastic fibers. The accumulated evidence now indicates that the defect is indeed one primarily of the elastic fiber, as proposed in 1896 by Darier.[36]

The reasons for thinking that PXE is an abiotrophy of collagenous rather than elastic fibers were as follows[72,186]: (1) Normally the skin contains relatively few elastic fibers. Elastin makes up only about 2% of the dry weight of skin.[46] Collagen, on the other hand, constitutes about 72%. The few elastic fibers present are concentrated immediately beneath the epidermis and serve, according to one view,[46] a principal function of attaching the epidermis to the corium. (A defect in these fibers[177] may be responsible for the lesions of epidermolysis bullosa. This point is moot, however.) The lesions of PXE are located in the deeper layers of the corium and are more extensive than can be accounted for on the basis of the normal amount of elastic fibers in the skin. The skin of the soles and palms is more liberally supplied with elastic fibers, but PXE lesions do not occur there ordinarily. (2) The arteries predominantly involved are the so-called muscular arteries, the tunica media of which contains collagenous fibers but little elastic tissue. (3) The tunica elastica interna of these vessels (except in one report[88]) remains intact. (4) Except for their orceinophilia, most of the abnormal fibers resemble collagen fibers more than elastic fibers, because of their width. (5) Electron microscopic studies[184] reveal that the dystrophic fibers, although abnormal in other respects, have the characteristic 640 A periodicity of collagen. It appears, then, that in PXE the collagen may undergo dystrophic chemical or physicochemical changes, with resulting acquisition of the tinctorial characteristics of elastic fibers. (6) There has been no acceptable clinical or pathologic evidence of abnormality arising from a defect of elastic tissue in the lungs or aorta. (See p. 496 for possible contradictions to this statement.)

Gillman and co-workers[90] make important observations on what appears to be a rather widely occurring phenomenon. This they term "elastotic degeneration of collagen fibers." Irradiation, trauma, and aging (Fig. 10-17) appear to be responsible. In addition to degeneration of existing collagen fibers, the authors admit the possibility that there may be a disturbance of formation of new collagen fibers, resulting in simulation of elastic fibers. By means of a battery of many staining procedures, they showed that there are distinct differences between "normal" elastic fibers of skin and arteries and "elastotically degenerated" collagen fibers at the same site. Although no studies of PXE were made, the important observations of the South African group are probably pertinent in connection with this hereditary syndrome: "elastotic degeneration" of collagen can occur on either an acquired or a hereditary basis. In both, fragmentation and calcification occur. Gillman and colleagues[90] maintain that Mallory's phosphotungstic acid–hematoxylin stain differentiates the presumed degenerated collagen of PXE from normal elastic fibers.

Tunbridge and co-workers[184] noted that enzymatic digestion of skin increases "elastic staining" and results in an increase in amorphous material. Keech and Reed,[90] working in the same group, using electron microscopy, conclude that by a variety of means, physical, chemical, and enzymatic, one can produce so-called "moth-eaten" fibers (MEF) from either collagenous or

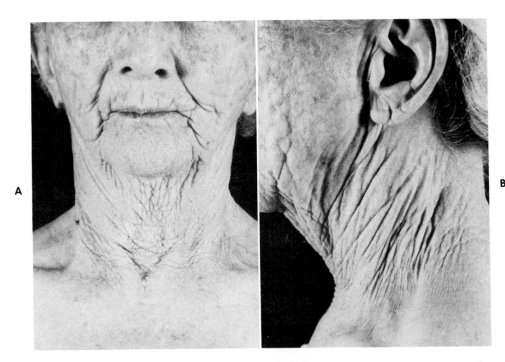

Fig. 10-17. Senile elastosis. A. H. (775457), 73-year-old female, was admitted because of bleeding from the lower bowel. The changes in the skin, **A** and **B**, resemble those of PXE but differ in the relative absence of changes in the axillae, **D**. The changes on the hands, **C**, are more striking than those usually seen in PXE. There were no angioid streaks in the fundi, and the peripheral arteries showed very little calcification. The histologic appearance, **E** and **F**, probably is distinct from that in PXE. Note that there is very little granular material. In **E** is presented the results of hematoxylin and eosin stain of the skin biopsy. Note the broad ribbons of connective tissue fibers, suggesting fragmented collagen. In **F** is presented the orcein stain of the same tissue. Both are at ×100 magnification. The cause of the lower bowel bleeding has not been identified.

elastic fibers, that MEF represent an intermediate form, and finally that "collagen and elastin are not two separate and distinct entities but are probably intimately associated *in vivo.*" (See also references 21 and 91.)

The view that collagen is the source of the degenerated material has been challenged, and the earlier "elastic theory" has been defended by Rodnan and associates[146] and by Moran and Lansing,[125] who in histochemical studies, studies by elastase digestion and microincineration, and examinations by fluorescence and electron microscopy concluded that there is a striking resemblance to elastic tissue in the following respects: brilliant autofluorescence, lack of periodicity in ultrastructure, liability to elastase, inhibition of affinity for elastic tissue dyes

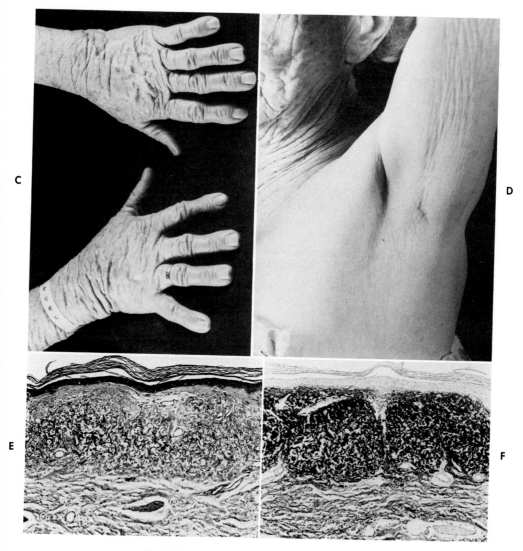

Fig. 10-17, cont'd. For legend see opposite page.

following methylation, and strong proclivity to calcium incrustation. Other electron microscopic studies also support the elastic theory.[75,80]

Calcification of the elastic fibers has been viewed as a secondary phenomenon comparable to the calcification of degenerated tissues occurring in chronic inflammation, atherosclerosis, hematomas, etc. Goodman and colleagues,[64] after finding that calcium accretion on elastic fibers is the earliest demonstrable histologic change, proposed that deposition of calcium may lead to brittleness and subsequent fracture of elastic fibers. A similar sequence of events has been proposed in the case of Bruch's membrane and the development of angioid streaks. If this view of the pathogenesis is accurate, the question of the nature of the basic defect resolves itself into the question of what causes the increased affinity of the elastic fibers for calcium. Smith and associates[162] concluded that an increase of acid mucopolysaccharides, particularly hyaluronic acid and to some extent chondroitin sulfate B, is involved in the calcification process. Johnson and Helwig[86] also concluded that hyaluronic acid coats the elastic fiber and is implicated in calcification.

Findlay[46] reported that the enzyme elastase removes the degenerate material from sections of skin from PXE patients. An earlier objection was that elastase is not entirely specific; for example, it is said[70] to dissolve mucoproteins, behaving, therefore, fundamentally as a mucase. Furthermore, other studies[10] with elastase indicate some effects on normal collagen. More recently, elastase has been purified, and it has been demonstrated[106,149] that elastase digestion is relatively specific for elastic tissue.

The argument that elastic fiber normally present is insufficient to account for the relatively large amount of degenerate material is disputed by Moran and Lansing,[125] who feel that there are sufficient elastic fibers in the deeper layers of the corium and further suggest that proliferation of elastic fibers may occur in this disease. They point to the occurrence of macrophages and giant cells[131,180] as a characteristic more of degenerate elastic fiber than of collagen. A similar reaction in the lung, presumably to degenerated elastic tissue, described by Walford and Kaplan,[189] was referred to by Moran and Lansing, who state also that there is "a definite increase in collagenous tissue in the involved areas." They suggest that it would be easy, under these circumstances, to conclude that all fibers have the electron microscopic characteristics of collagen, simply through inaccurate selection of the fields of study.

Potentially very important observations have been made by Weidman and associates,[190] Pautrier,[136] and Lever[104]: young asymptomatic individuals may show in the skin abundant, irregularly branching, thick, nonfragmented fibers with the tinctorial characteristics of elastic fibers. The implication has been that these individuals would subsequently develop typical PXE and/or that they are members of kinships containing other definite cases. However, to my knowledge, this implication has not been borne out except possibly in one patient of Van Embden Andres,[186] who had central chorioretinitis of the type seen in PXE, and, by skin biopsy, "hyperplasia of elastic fibers without elastorrhexis." If it is further confirmed that these individuals with what Weidman calls "juvenile elastoma" do indeed represent instances of predegenerative PXE, it would means that a unique type of connective tissue fiber is produced in these persons and undergoes degeneration with physiologic stresses. It would mean, furthermore, that the efforts to relate the basic defect to collagen or to elastica are pointless.

I find it difficult to believe that these cases of Weidman and others are related to PXE, mainly because there should be identifiable, in one and the same individual, areas of as yet nondegenerate "elastoma" and other areas of typical PXE.

The pathogenesis of the angioid streaks has been considered to be unsettled.[35] The theory propounded by Kofler[96] in 1917 is that breaks in Bruch's membrane explain this finding. After reviewing the matter, Cowper[35] concluded that the original view (that the primary difficulty is a degeneration and sclerosis of the choroidal arteries, with secondary changes in the retina and in Bruch's membrane) seems more consistent with the known facts. When the other conditions in which angioid streaks occur (p. 504) are considered, as well as the histologic findings of breaks in Bruch's membrane, Kofler's theory seems almost certainly the correct one. Adelung[1] demonstrated that the lines of force within the eye, resulting from pull of the intrinsic and extrinsic ocular muscles on the relatively fixed site of the optic nerve, have the same configuration as the peripapillary interlacement and radial extensions of angioid streaks. Such forces, acting on a weakened Bruch's membrane, undoubtedly account for the distribution of angioid streaks.

As mentioned on p. 23, recessive inheritance suggests an enzyme defect. Possibly some as yet unidentified metabolic defect in some way damages the elastic fibers so that degeneration occurs, or perhaps some enzyme important to the integrity of the elastic fiber protein or a substance closely associated with it may be deficient.

PXE is one of the conditions associated with metachromasia of fibroblasts.[25] The significance of this observation in relation to the nature of the basic defect is unknown.

Whatever the nature of the basic defect, the clinical behavior of PXE is that of an abiotrophy. The predominant involvement of areas of the skin exposed to maximum wear and tear, such as flexion folds, belt line,[15] pressure points, etc., is striking. Szymanski and Caro[172] describe a lesion at a site of trauma. No clinical or pathologic changes in the joints have been encountered. (Gold[63] described Still's disease in a child with PXE, but the association may have been a coincidence.)

Prevalence and inheritance

PXE probably occurs quite generally without particular racial distribution. The 4 autopsied patients at the Johns Hopkins Hospital were Negroes, and several Negro patients with PXE have been reported.[54,121] In addition to being described in natives of many European countries, including Turkey,[117] PXE has been observed in Japanese.[130]

Some indication of the frequency of PXE is provided by the fact that 125 cases of associated skin and fundus changes and 68 cases of skin changes alone had been described prior to 1940.[176] Several hundred cases have by now been reported. Berlyne and colleagues[16] estimated the frequency to be between 1 in 160,000 and 1 in one million persons. It is my impression that it occurs more frequently than 1 in 160,000.

Tabulations of cases of PXE in the literature show a preponderance of females.[30,42,182] Since women are more prone to seek medical advice, especially regarding a cosmetic problem created by the skin involvement, the female preponderance may be factitious. A review of 106 cases from the Mayo Clinic showed a 1 to 1.2 ratio of males to females.[35] Within this group there were 32 cases with only angioid streaks; the ratio in this group was 2.2 to 1, males to females.

Increased frequency of parental consanguinity,[74,118,124,179,186] the occurrence of multiple affected sibs, both males and females, and the rarity of the disorder in successive generations[31,81,117,167] suggest autosomal recessive inheritance. The occasional observation of affected parent and child may be explained by marriage of the affected homozygous parent with a heterozygote or by occasional manifestation in a heterozygous person. Wise[196] found about twenty examples of parent-child affection—a frequency too high, in his opinion, to mean anything other than the existence of a dominant form. In most of the twenty families mother and child were affected, but father-to-son transmission was noted by Berlyne and co-workers[17] and by Weve.[192] Gills and Paton[61] described 2 brothers with mottling of the fundus and skin changes of PXE. The mother had no skin changes clinically or histologically but did show similar mottled changes of the fundus. It may be significant that affection in no more than two generations has only rarely been reported.[22] If a dominant form of PXE exists, one would expect some families to have affected members in three or more generations. This may indicate that the two-generation families result from either (1) quasi-dominance (mating of homozygote with heterozygote) or (2) occasional expression in the heterozygote.

Extensive studies in the U.K. by Pope[140a] established beyond reasonable doubt that there is genetic heterogeneity in PXE with which phenotypic heterogeneity can be correlated. In a series of 180 cases, he observed several 3-generation families. At least one autosomal dominant form of PXE is quite clear, and more than one autosomal recessive form may exist.

Berlyne and colleagues[16] thought that in given sibships affected persons are usually either all males or all females. On this basis they proposed that the mode of inheritance is that of partial sex linkage, as would be observed if the responsible gene were located on a homologous segment of the X and Y chromosomes. Cytologic and genetic evidence would suggest, however, that this mechanism of inheritance does not exist in man.[114] Furthermore, in our personal experience, several sibships have had affected members of both sexes.

The occasional instance of affected parent and child (e.g., reference 132) may have resulted because the unaffected parent was heterozygous.

Berlyne and colleagues[16] reported that persons presumed to be heterozygous for the PXE gene had an abnormally prominent choroidal vascular pattern and suggested that this resulted from atrophy of the choriocapillaris. In family members studied by Goodman and colleagues[64] and in those patients with early ocular involvement the choroidal vessels were not unusually prominent, although they were prominent in some patients with advanced changes (Fig. 10-7). Since the choriocapillaris lies below Bruch's membrane, any increased density in the latter structure in early stages of PXE as a possible heterozygous manifestation should render the choroidal vascular layer *less* visible. The increased visibility of these vessels in later stages of PXE is readily accounted for by damage to, and atrophy of, the pigment epithelium of the retina.

Miscellaneous considerations

There is no definitive treatment for this disorder. Tocopherol (vitamin E) was said[169] to effect dramatic improvement in the skin and eyes of one patient.

Others[4,150] also claim improvement. No beneficial effect was observed in one patient studied. Adrenocortical steroids have been used in several patients. In one patient (N. G., 1136343) the treatment was continued for over a year. Although the results are difficult to evaluate, no clear benefit has been noted. Although the reactive process in the skin, eye, and arteries might be reduced by such treatment, the chronic, indeed lifelong, nature of the disease process makes steroid therapy impractical. Good cosmetic effects have been reported by plastic surgeons,[28,139] who have removed the loose, excess skin around the neck, which may be distressingly unsightly, especially in women. In Fig. 10-15*E* and *F* are demonstrated the changes in the skin of a patient in whom plastic surgery was performed.

It seems conceivable that a funduscopic picture indistinguishable from that of the angioid streaks seen with PXE may occur on other bases than this particular genetic one. For example, angioid streaks are encountered in association with Paget's disease.[126] However, PXE is the most common basis for the finding. Scholz[155] stated that, previous to 1941, 59% of 139 cases of streaks had the skin condition. On the other hand, in a series collected from the literature, Goedbloed[62] found 57 cases with skin involvement among 67 with streaks, and Sanbacka-Holström[152] found 87 out of 100 cases. Not only may angioid streaks occur with either PXE or Paget's disease, but also there are a few adequately documented instances of the occurrence of changes in the skin, fundus oculi, and bones of the same individual. Woodcock[199] described a 54-year-old white man with bilateral angioid streaks, skin changes of PXE in the axillae, and Paget's disease as manifested by cephalic enlargement, bowing of the legs, spontaneous fractures, renal calculi, and characteristic radiologic changes. Sanbacka-Holström[152] refers in passing to such a patient, and there are loose references to the coincidence of the three manifestations in textbooks and reviews. Shaffer and colleagues[157] have described a 58-year-old woman with angioid streaks and evidences of Paget's disease from the age of 40 years. The only skin lesion was an "elliptical lemon-yellow plaque 1.0 cm. long on the left posterior axillary fold." The histology was typical of PXE. One sister had mild Paget's disease. Larmande and Margaillan[99] had a case of combined disease. Dr. David Paton[135] tells me of 2 patients he has studied, in whom there is association of PXE skin changes, angioid streaks, calcification in peripheral vessels, and Paget's disease of bone.

There may be reason (Chapter 12) to think that there is no fundamental relationship between PXE and at least one common variety of Paget's disease. One reason is that Paget's disease usually behaves like an autosomal dominant. Furthermore, it is more frequent in men. In Paget's disease, as in PXE, calcification occurs in the media of arteries. Calcium deposition in Bruch's membrane is probably responsible for the development of angioid streaks in this condition.

Tumoral calcinosis, hyperphosphatemia, and angioid streaks constitute a well-established syndrome.[115] Familial cases have been reported by Baldursson and colleagues,[8] Barton and Reeves,[12] Harkess and Peters,[73] Thomson and Tanner,[178] McPhaul and Engel,[115] and Ghormley.[58] In a family reported by McPhaul and Engel,[115] 2 brothers were affected, and in a second family the proband's grandfather was thought to have tumoral calcinosis and was related to a family with PXE. Dodge and colleagues[1,39] described 3 sibs with heterotopic calcification, hyperphosphatemia, unresponsiveness to parathyroid hormone, and elevated renal tubular maximum for phosphate resorption. From Beirut, Najjar and colleagues[128] described 2 sibs who demonstrated periarticular calcified masses, elevated serum phosphorus, normal serum calcium, calcified vessels, and skin changes of PXE. The parents may have been related. An aunt was said to have heterotopic calcification. I suspect that this disorder is distinct from ordinary PXE but with many similar features, e.g., changes of skin and eyes. In a review of the radiologic findings of PXE, James and associates[83] pictured a large calcified mass in the region of the elbow. This patient had, I suspect, the tumoral calcinosis syndrome and not true PXE.

The occurrence of angioid streaks in this condition is consistent with the view that a brittle state resulting from calcium (or iron) deposition is responsible for the angioid streaks of PXE, Paget's disease, and sickle cell anemia. Angioid streaks have been observed in one patient with familial hyperphosphatemia and metastatic calcification,[115] in a patient with idiopathic thrombocytopenic purpura,[201] and in several instances of lead poisoning.[37] Depositions in Bruch's membrane may account for the development of cracks in these disorders also. Angioid streaks have also been observed[7] in so-called juvenile Paget's disease, which is an autosomal recessive disorder fundamentally distinct from ordinary Paget's disease and goes by other designations,[113] such as osteoectasia with macrocranium, hyperostosis corticalis deformans juvenilis, and congenital idiopathic hyperphosphatasia.

Rather numerous cases of sickle cell disease with angioid streaks have been described. Skin changes of PXE were present in at least 3 cases.[57,64,171] In those cases of sickle cell anemia with only angioid streaks, it is likely that deposition of iron renders Bruch's membrane brittle.

Clinically, the skin changes in "senile elastosis" (Fig. 10-17) are somewhat similar to those of PXE.[161] *Actinic elastosis* is the term recommended by the American Dermatological Association, inasmuch as age and senility probably are not primary factors. Clinical differences from PXE include involvement of the hands in actinic elastosis and sparing of the axillae and other unexposed areas commonly affected in PXE. The histologic appearance in actinic elastosis is different, being characterized by diffuse involvement in the superficial parts of the corium, less intense basophilia of the connective tissue fibers, and, usually, absence of fragmentation of the involved fibers into granular material. Percival and associates[137] concluded that this condition is a dystrophy of collagen. However, Smith and associates[161] concluded that the electron microscopic features, enzyme susceptibilities, and amino acid composition indicate an increase in elastic fibers. There is, however, a decrease in collagen, mainly in the insoluble fraction.

In the differential diagnosis of PXE, vitamin D intoxication must also be considered. A few years ago I saw a 15-year-old girl (P. Y., 856728) who had a hard, elevated, nodular eruption in the axillary folds, in the antecubital area, around the intertriginous areas of the hips, and on the flexor aspects of the knees. Biopsy of the skin lesions showed changes considered compatible with severely calcified PXE. No angioid streaks were noted. Self-administration of excessive vitamin D seemed to be responsible. There were nephrotoxic effects as well.

Case reports, with autopsy observations

Case 1. R. K. (J.H.H. 156572), a Negro male born in 1891, died in 1954 from accidental mercury poisoning.

The family history was largely unknown. He had no children.

About 1932 the patient was found to have a positive serologic test for syphilis, and treatment with arsenicals, mercury, and bismuth was given at another hospital where he had gone because of failing vision. He was first seen at this hospital in 1938 because of continuing dimming of vision. He had worn spectacles for about six years with no apparent staying of the visual failure in spite of several changes. Bilaterally the entire macular area was the site of atrophy and scarring. The vessels were normal. Running out from each disc in all directions were wide, branching, brownish streaks. About the neck he was noted to have many linear 4 or 5 mm. yellowish papules about 1 mm. thick. These were arranged parallel to the clavicle and coalesced in many areas to form short streaks several centimeters in length. The diagnosis of PXE with angioid streaks was made and confirmed by skin biopsy (Skin Path. No. 9606). On general examination the patient was noted to have an arcus senilis bilaterally. The blood pressure was 170/90 mm. Hg. No pulse change or circulatory abnormality in the legs or elsewhere was detected by history or examination.

The patient was visited in his home several times late in 1953 but refused to come to the hospital for investigation of the connective tissue disorder. He was now almost completely blind. For many years he had been suffering from intermittent swelling and pain of the proximal interphalangeal joints. He had also had much pain in the tibial and calf areas, as well as the knees. He had developed ulcerations of the pretibial area and made a practice of soaking them with bichloride of mercury solution. He took Dolcin, a proprietary analgesic, for his aches and pains. Several years previously he had been told that he had diabetes mellitus.

About 6 A.M. on Jan. 11, 1954, the patient intended to take Dolcin tablets for relief of pains in both shins and, because of his faulty vision, took three tablets of bichloride of mercury instead. He first noted burning of his mouth and thereafter pain in the mid-epigastrium, accompanied by the vomiting first of a large amount of clear yellow fluid and later of bright red blood of unknown quantity. Severe persistent bloody diarrhea followed. He was seen by his family physician, who could record no blood pressure and sent him to the hospital, where he arrived about eight hours after the accidental ingestion of mercury.

The patient had been noted to be easily confused in recent years, and therefore the exact details of the history of the final days of life are not entirely certain.

Physical examination revealed the skin of the neck, axillae, inguinal areas, and anterior abdominal wall to be nodular and leathery. It was strikingly inelastic, but this may have been in part the result of dehydration. All interphalangeal joints showed fusiform enlargement, and nodules were located around the knuckles. The heart showed a loud blowing apical systolic murmur and rather numerous extrasystoles. Femoral pulses were present, but none could be felt in the popliteal fossae or feet. There were two large depigmented scars with some unhealed and scabbed areas on both pretibial prominences.

The patient was virtually anuric throughout his hospital stay and died on the sixth hospital day. The diagnosis of mercury poisoning was corroborated by the finding of 6 mg. Hg^{++} per 20 ml. of stomach fluid taken at admission. Death occurred despite the use of BAL and supportive measures.

Autopsy (No. 24837) was performed ten hours after death by Dr. H. M. Hill. (In spite of the delay, fibroblasts grew out in tissue culture from explants of skin and of aortic adventitia.) The body weighed 50 kilograms and measured 168 cm. in length. The changes in the skin and joints and the juxta-articular nodules were observed as during the clinical examination.

The heart weighed 325 grams and did not appear to be enlarged. A most impressive finding was thickening of the endocardium of the right atrium. This was somewhat yellowish, and over the trabecular ridges there were peculiar nodular thickenings. The posterior leaflet of the tricuspid valve had a smooth, thickened, firm, rolled edge without excrescenses. The aortic leaflet of the mitral valve was similarly thickened at the edge, and there was marked calcific change at its attachment. The coronary ostia were normal, but everywhere the coronary arteries were exceedingly sclerotic and calcified, with reduction of their caliber to little more than a pinpoint.

The aorta was of normal caliber, with only minimal atherosclerosis in the abdominal portion and normal elasticity by gross test. There were marked calcification and narrowing of the femoral, popliteal, and posterior tibial arteries. These changes were particularly striking at areas of bending, such as in the popliteal fossae. The posterior tibial arteries were exceedingly beaded. The vessels at the base of the brain were sclerotic. Grossly and histologically there were characteristic changes of mercury poisoning in the kidney and gastrointestinal tract.

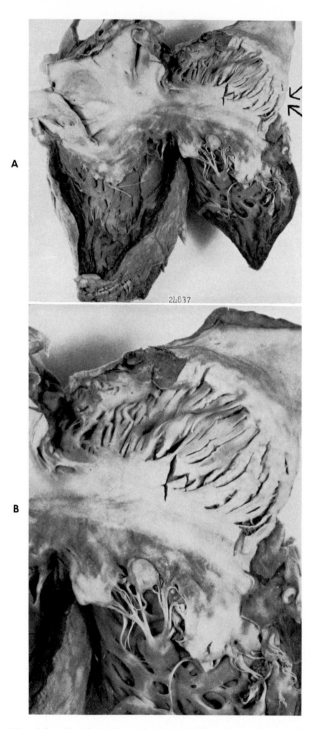

Fig. 10-18. A, The right side of the heart in Case I. There is an abnormal, pearly thickening of the endocardium, with yellowish, irregularly nodular lesions in the area indicated by the arrows. The latter lesions look not unlike those in the skin. **B,** Enlarged view of part of heart shown in **A.**

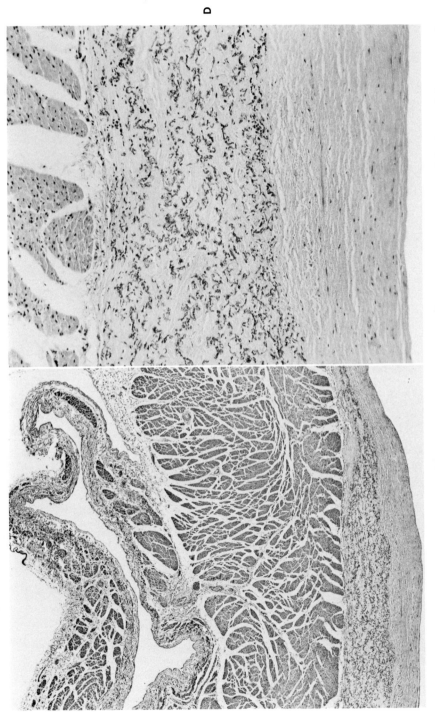

Fig. 10-18, cont'd. C, Wall of right atrium. (Hematoxylin and eosin stain; × 25.) On the endocardial surface (below) one of the opaque elevated plaques is seen in section. On the epicardial surface a branch of a cardiac vein is seen. **D,** Enlarged view of one part of the field in C. (Hematoxylin and eosin stain; ×100.) Striking similarity to the changes in the skin is evident. (See Fig. 10-1F and G.)

Continued.

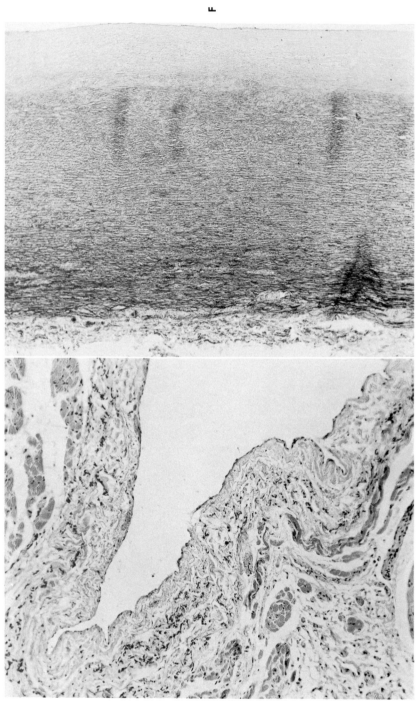

Fig. 10-18, cont'd. E, Enlarged view of another part of the field in **C** to show the changes in the wall of the vein, which again are identical to those in the skin and endocardium. (Hematoxylin and eosin stain; ×100.) **F,** Elastic fiber stain of aorta. The intima (on right) is thickened, but the media shows no striking disorganization. (×50.)

Histologically, the corium, the sclera, and the subendocardial area of the right atrium showed the same changes which previously have been frequently described in the skin of patients with PXE. Faintly basophilic (by hematoxylin and eosin stain), fragmented material was concentrated most heavily in the mid-dermis. Present in great abundance in the clinically involved areas and present sparsely elsewhere, it had the tinctorial characteristics of elastic tissue. The popliteal and coronary arteries showed marked medial and intimal sclerosis and calcification. As demonstrated in Fig. 10-18C, branches of the coronary sinus near the right atrium showed changes in the tunica media comparable to those in the atrial endocardium and corium. Small arteries showed similar changes.

Comment. Of particular interest are the histologic changes in the endocardium of the right atrium and in the sclera. Neither site normally demonstrates more than a very sparse distribution of elastic fibers. The deforming arthropathy is likewise of special note. The manifestation has not been commented on previously in cases of PXE, except for the patient with Still's disease reported by Gold.[63] Unfortunately, no histologic studies of either joint structures or juxta-articular nodules were performed.

Case 2. C. J. (J.H.H. 292168), a Negro woman born in 1896, was seen here on several occasions in 1943 and died at the hospital on Jan. 1, 1944.

Her mother died of a stroke at the age of 48 years. The patient had 4 brothers: 2 died in childhood and 1 shortly after discharge from the Army in World War I; the other was living and well. The patient had 16 children, of whom 7 were living in 1943. No other instance of PXE is known to have occurred in the family. However, the family has not been traced and studied with this point specifically in mind.

The patient's eyesight had always been poor but had become worse in the last years of life. She noted tarry stools on several occasions and complained at times of epigastric burning. Early in 1943 she developed anginal symptoms for the first time.

Examinations revealed a blood pressure of 190/110 mm. Hg. There was evidence of marked weight loss (about 50 pounds in one year). The skin everywhere was very loose, due in part to PXE. The neck veins were full and dilated but not the arm veins. The heart was enlarged to the left anterior axillary line. The patient was so debilitated that carcinoma was suspected. Directly above the umbilicus there was a plaque of smooth skin containing small, hard, elevated nodular areas. Histologically (Skin Path. No. 5157) there were changes typical of PXE. The fundi showed no angioid streaking, but there were fairly marked hypertensive and sclerotic changes in the arteries, many hemorrhages, and in the macula area many yellow shiny plaques.

Total serum protein was 8.3 gm/100 ml., of which 5.5 gm./100 ml. was globulin. Hemoglobulin was 10.5 gm./100 ml. Electrocardiogram revealed left axis deviation, left ventricular strain pattern, and prolonged A-V conduction. On chest x-ray examination, calcification in superficial vessels in the left axilla was demonstrated. The aorta was dilated and tortuous. On barium swallow the esophagus was relaxed and tortuous. Gastric analysis revealed normal acidity.

After four months away from the hospital, during which time she had become steadily weaker, the patient was brought back to the hospital with massive leg edema and ascites and with Cheyne-Stokes breathing. She died two hours later.

Autopsy (No. 18717) revealed marked generalized arteriosclerosis, arteriosclerotic and arteriolosclerotic nephritis with Kimmelstiel-Wilson lesions of glomeruli, and coronary sclerosis with myocardial scarring. In addition, there were tuberculous peritonitis and caseous obstructon of the thoracic duct with chylous ascites. The aorta was atheromatous, with a few ulcerations.

Comment. Hyperglobulinemia was probably due to tuberculosis. It is of interest that Kimmelstiel-Wilson lesions occurred in this nondiabetic individual. In general, premature and severe arteriosclerosis dominated the clinical picture and the findings at autopsy. What relation there may have been between the skin changes and the vascular disease is unclear. In general, however, this patient demonstrates the early and rapidly progressive dissolution of the vascular system characteristic of patients with PXE.

Case 3. N. C. was 13 years old at the time of death from gastrointestinal hemorrhage. Hematemeses and/or melena had occurred repeatedly during the previous 6½ years, necessitating nine hospital admissions. Death occurred in 1945. The diagnosis was always in doubt clinically. At autopsy, too, the precise diagnosis was not made. PXE was first diagnosed in the brother, R. C., then (1957) 35 years old, on the basis of typical skin and eye changes and a history of gastrointestinal hemorrhage at the age of 15 years. On review of the medical records of the proband (N. C.), it was found that on a hospital admission four years before death it was noted that "over the cervical region is a raised pebbly eruption." Later it was recorded that "over the neck, chest, abdomen, and flexor surfaces of the arm there were elevated, small white papules, some discrete, others confluent, which appear like scar tissue." On one occasion the diagnosis of PXE, along with other possibilities, was suggested by a dermatologist, but the total picture was not put together. An ophthalmologist commented as follows: "The eyegrounds are essentially negative. Over a broad area temporally from the fovea in both eyes, there is a peculiar light brown mottling. The patient's brother is said to have this too and also the same sort of bleeding."

Histologic studies showed striking focal or segmental vascular changes, especially in the stomach and small intestine, but also to some extent in many other organs, including the heart, pancreas, kidney, and brain. In some vessels there was fragmentation of the elastica, with deposition of collagenous material between it and the lumen, as well as loss of muscle (Fig. 10-12*A*). In the walls of some vessels, there was material which in part stained brilliantly red with picro-Mallory dye, like "fibrinoid." Mucosal vessels in the stomach and intestine were widely dilated and exceedingly thin walled (Fig. 10-12*B* and *C*). The wall of the atrium showed dense elastosis of the endocardium (Fig. 10-18*C* and *D*) of the type seen in Case 1 and reported in several instances in the literature.[9,24]

Case 4. B. J. (J.H.H. 1018324), a Negro woman, is remarkable for the fact that she survived to the age of over 70 years despite the presence of two serious disorders: sickle cell anemia and pseudoxanthoma elasticum. Her date of birth was placed variously as 1892, 1893, and 1896. She died in 1968. Charache and Richardson[26] described her case, when she was 66

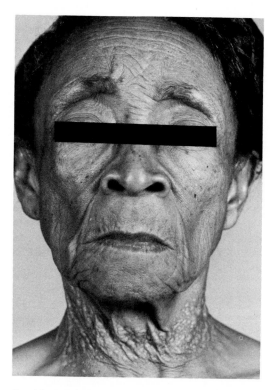

Fig. 10-19. B. J. (Case 4), with sickle cell anemia and pseudoxanthoma elasticum. Note the typical skin lesions about the neck.

years old, as a remarkable instance of prolonged survival in sickle cell anemia. She was also included in the series of PXE patients studied by Goodman and associates.[64]

In 1912, about the time of Herrick's original description[77] of sickle cell anemia, the patient was admitted to this hospital twice for chills, fever, and "pains all over." Similar pains had occurred episodically since her early childhood. At that time she was pale, the heart was enlarged, and the spleen was palpable. The hemoglobin was recorded as 46% of normal, as determined by the Sahli technique.

She had noted yellowish spots on her neck since adolescence (Fig. 10-19). None of her relatives showed similar lesions.

At the age of 23 years she became pregnant but aborted spontaneously in the fourth month. Menstrual periods, which began at the age of 18 years, ceased at the age of 38 after an "appendectomy" at another hospital.

In 1946, she was first recognized to have sickle cell anemia and was given her first transfusion. At the age of 61 years she was hospitalized for dyspnea, cough, and pedal edema. Occult blood was found in the stools but x-ray examination of the gastrointestinal tract showed

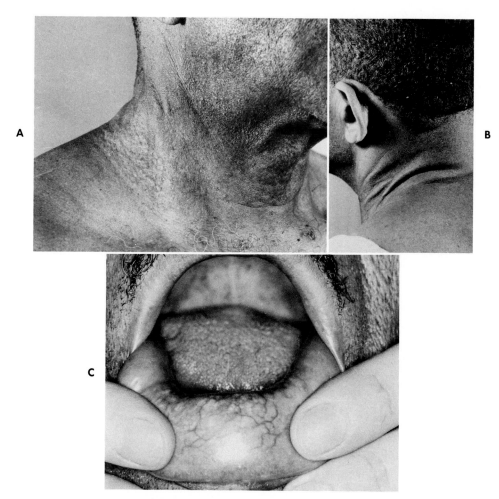

Fig. 10-20. J. C. (Case 5), with PXE and malignant histiocytosis. Note the typical changes in the skin of the neck, **A** and **B**, and in the labial mucosa, **C**.

no abnormalities. During the next five years exertional dyspnea recurred, angina pectoris developed, and she was forced to stop work as a domestic.

In 1962 the patient was admitted to the hospital for acute pain and swelling of the left ankle. At that time she showed numerous yellow-brown, waxy nodules on the skin of the neck and axillae, as well as in the umbilical and inguinal areas. No angioid streaks were found in the fundi; however, several whitish linear marks were noted near the disc and were thought to represent an abnormality of Bruch's membrane. No macular change was noted, but chorioretinal atrophy was present. The heart was markedly enlarged, with a loud, blowing apical systolic murmur. The liver was enlarged, but the spleen was not felt. Peripheral pulses were normal. The left ankle was warm and tender.

The hematocrit was 19%. Sickle cell preparations were strongly positive. Electrophoresis showed only hemoglobin S and a very small amount of fetal hemoglobin. Hemoglobin "fingerprints" were characteristic of pure hemoglobin S. Biopsy of a skin nodule showed changes characteristic of PXE. During a period when the patient was receiving hydrochlorothiazide, the serum uric acid was 10.5 mg./100 ml. and the urea nitrogen was 37 mg./100ml. The pain in the left ankle subsided spontaneously but recurred at least twice in the next few months.

By x-ray examination, calcification was visualized in the falx cerebri, in the tunica media and intima of the femoral arteries, and in the aorta. A right brachial arteriogram showed marked narrowing of the ulnar artery. The deep volar arch was unusually dilated and there was tortuosity of the digital arteries, with obstruction of the digital artery to the third finger. A right femoral arteriogram showed no evidence of obstruction. The posterior tibial artery was narrow in its entire length and, at the level of the ankle, formed collaterals with the peroneal artery.

The patient died of cardiac and renal failure in 1968.

Autopsy (Baltimore City Hospitals 22400) showed atrophy of the spleen (weight, 7.3 grams), sickle cell nephropathy, and multiple calcium bilirubinate stones in the gallbladder. The heart was enlarged, but changes in the endocardium and pericardium, such as occurred in Case 1, were not observed.

Case 5. J. C. (J.H.H. 279288), a Negro male born in 1896, was first recognized as having PXE when he presented in 1955 with the Leriche syndrome (thrombotic obliteration of the terminal aorta). An aortic homograft was installed at that time with excellent results. Subtotal thyroidectomy was performed for thyroid adenoma in 1956. In 1959 giddiness on standing led to the diagnosis of basilar insufficiency.

During the last ten years of his life the patient suffered from frequent indolent inflammations (small inguinal abscess, proctitis, rectal fistula, otitis media, pansinusitis, proctitis), was chronically anemic (hematocrit 17% to 29%), had mild leukocytosis with monocytes in the range of 22% to 34%, and showed hyperglobulinemia and splenomegaly. In 1970 the number of monocytes increased, and young-appearing cells on blood smear supported the diagnosis of chronic monocytic leukemia. In May, 1970, a severe nosebleed necessitated blood transfusion. The terminal illness was a stormy one, with semicoma and other grave neurologic signs and symptoms. A fibrinogen level of 100 mg./100 ml. and a platelet count of 9000 indicated the presence of a consumptive coagulopathy. Bone marrow aspirate showed numerous giant histiocytes phagocytizing white and red blood cells. The diagnosis of malignant histiocytosis was made on the basis of this finding. Gram-negative septicemia developed terminally.

Autopsy (37335) confirmed the clinical diagnosis of malignant histiocytosis. Changes of PXE were found in the skin and eyes. Arteriosclerosis was generalized and severe. The aortic graft was intact and showed less atherosclerosis than the rest of the aorta. The heart was dilated. Microscopically the endocardium (site not specified) was described as thickened and showing abundant elastic tissue with fragmentation. It was felt that the myeloproliferative disorder and PXE were unrelated.

SUMMARY AND CONCLUSIONS

The clinical manifestations of pseudoxanthoma elasticum include (1) characteristic skin changes, occurring especially in areas of wear and tear; (2) angioid streaks of the fundus oculi; and (3) hemorrhage, symptoms of ischemia, and hypertension, resulting from arterial degeneration. Gastrointestinal hemorrhage is the complication of most importance to the internist.

Evidence on the nature of the basic defect is reviewed, and it is concluded that the elastic fiber is primarily involved in this abnormality, which behaves as an abiotrophy.

Descriptions of 5 autopsied cases are added to the meager information available on the state of tissues other than the skin and eye. In 3 cases, changes unique to PXE were demonstrated in the endocardium of the right atrium and in the coronary vessels.

Pseudoxanthoma elasticum is inherited as an autosomal recessive in the largest number of instances, but at least one autosomal dominant form exists.

REFERENCES

1. Adelung, J. C.: Zur Genese der Angioid Streakes (Knapp), Klin. Mbl. Augenheilk. **119**:241, 1951.
2. Anderson, B.: Familial central and peripapillary choroidal sclerosis associated with familial pseudoxanthoma elasticum, Trans. Amer. Ophthal. Soc. **46**:326, 1948.
3. Anon.: Obituary of A. Chauffard, Bull. Soc. Franc. Hist. Méd. **26**:402, 1932.
4. Ayres, S., Jr.: Discussion of paper of Shaffer et al.,[157] Arch. Derm. Syph. **76**:632, 1957.
5. Ayres, S., Jr., and Mihan, R.: Pseudoxanthoma elasticum, Arch. Derm. **100**:119, 1969.
6. Bäfverstedt, B., and Lund, F.: Pseudoxanthoma elasticum and vascular disturbances with special reference to a case in a nine-year-old child, Acta Dermatovener. **35**:438, 1955.
7. Bakwin, H., Golden, A., and Fox, S.: Familial osteoectasis with macrocranium, Amer. J. Roentgen. **91**:609, 1964.
8. Baldursson, H., Evans, E. B., Dodge, W. F., and Jackson, W. T.: Tumoral calcinosis with hyperphosphatemia; a report of a family with incidence in four siblings, J. Bone Joint Surg. **51-A**:913, 1969.
9. Balzer, F.: Récherches sur les charactères anatomiques du xanthélasma, Arch. Physiol. 4 (series 3):65, 1884.
10. Banga, I.: Thermal contraction of collagen and its dissolution with elastase, Nature **172**:1099, 1953.
11. Bardsley, J. L., and Koehler, P. R.: Pseudoxanthoma elasticum; angiographic manifestations in abdominal vessels, Radiology **93**:559, 1969.
12. Barton, D. L., and Reeves, R. J.: Tumoral calcinosis; report of three cases and review of the literature, Amer. J. Roentgen. **86**:351, 1961.
13. Beeson, B. B.: Pseudoxanthoma elasticum (Darier) associated with formation of bone, Arch. Derm. Syph. **34**:729, 1936.
14. Benedict, W. L.: The pathology of angioid streaks in the fundus oculi, J.A.M.A. **109**:475, 1937.
15. Benedict, W. L., and Montgomery, H.: Pseudoxanthoma elasticum and angioid streaks, Amer. J. Ophthal. **18**:205, 1935.
16. Berlyne, G. M., Bulmer, H. G., and Platt, R.: The genetics of pseudoxanthoma elasticum, Quart. J. Med. **30**:201, 1961.
17. Besnier, E., and Doyon, P. A. A.: Annotations et appendices en traité des maladies de la Peau, de Kaposi, ed. 2, 1891, p. 336. Cited by Darier.[97]
18. Böck, J.: Zur Klinik und Anatomie der gefässähnlichen Streifen im Augenhintergrund, Z. Augenheilk. **95**:1, 1938.
19. Britten, M. J.: Unusual traumatic retinal haemorrhages associated with angioid streaks, Brit. J. Ophthal. **50**:540, 1966.
20. Bronner, A.: Considérations sur la syndrome de Groenblad et Strandberg, Bull. Soc. Franc. Derm. Syph. **61**:78, 1954.
21. Burton, D., Hall, D. A., Keech, M. K., Reed, R., Sax, H., Tunbridge, R. E., and Wood, M. J.: Apparent transformation of collagen fibrils into elastin, Nature **176**:966, 1955.
22. Cahill, J. B.: Pseudoxanthoma elasticum, Aust. J. Derm. **4**:28, 1957.
23. Carlborg, U.: Study of circulatory disturbances, pulse wave velocity and pressure pulses in larger arteries in cases of pseudoxanthoma elasticum and angioid streaks; a contribution to the knowledge of the function of the elastic tissue and the smooth muscles in larger arteries, Acta Med. Scand., supp. 151, pp. 1-209, 1944.
24. Carlborg, U., Ejrup, B., Grönblad, E., and Lund, F.: Vascular studies in pseudoxanthoma elasticum and angioid streaks, Acta Med. Scand. **350**:1, 1959.

25. Cartwright, E., Danks, D. M., and Jack, I.: Metachromatic fibroblasts in pseudoxanthoma elasticum and Marfan's syndrome, Lancet 1:533, 1969.
26. Charache, S., and Richardson, S. N.: Prolonged survival of a patient with sickle cell anemia, Arch. Intern. Med. 113:844, 1964.
27. Chauffard, A.: Xanthélasma disséminé et symétrique sans insuffisance hépatique, Bull. Soc. Méd. Hôp. Paris 6 (series 3):412, 1889.
28. Chikelair, G. F.: Pseudoxanthoma elasticum treated surgically, Plast. Reconstr. Surg. 12: 152, 1953.
29. Cocco, A. E., Grayer, D. I., Walker, B. A., and Marryn, L. J.: The stomach in pseuxanthoma elasticum, J.A.M.A. 210:2381, 1969.
30. Cockayne, E. A.: Inherited abnormalities of the skin and its appendages, London, 1933, Oxford University Press and Humphrey Milford, pp. 319-321.
31. Coffman, J. D., and Sommers, S. C.: Familial pseudoxanthoma elasticum and valvular heart disease, Circulation 19:242, 1959.
32. Collier, M.: Generalized elastorrhexia and corneal dystrophies in 2 sisters, Bull. Soc. Ophtal. Franç. 65:301, 1965.
33. Collomb, H., Graveline, J., and Diop, M.: Systemic elastorrhexis in a sicklemia patient, Bull. Soc. Med. Afr. Noire Lang. Franç. 10:597, 1965.
34. Connor, P. J., Juergens, J. L., Perry, H. O., Hollenhorst, R. W., and Edwards, J. E.: Pseudoxanthoma elasticum and angioid streaks; a review of 106 cases, Amer. J. Med. 30:537, 1961.
35. Cowper, A. R.: Angioid streaks; tears in Bruch's membrane or pigmented choroidal vessels? Arch. Ophthal. 51:762, 1954.
36. Darier, J.: Pseudoxanthoma elasticum, Mschr. Prakt. Derm. 23:609, 1896.
37. DeSimone, S., and DeConcilliis, U.: Strie angioidi della retina (considerazioni cliniche e patogenetiche), Arch. Ottal. 62:161, 1958.
38. Dixon, J. M.: Angioid streaks and pseudoxanthoma elasticum with aneurysm of the internal carotid artery, Amer. J. Ophthal. 34:1322, 1951.
39. Dodge, W. F., Travis, L. B., and Assemi, M.: Familial heterotopic calcification and hyperphosphatemia unresponsive to parathyroid extracts (abstract), J. Pediat. 67:944, 1965.
40. Donaldson, D. D.: Angioid streaks, Arch. Ophthal. 72:264, 1964.
41. Doyne, R. W.: Choroidal and retinal changes; the result of blows on the eyes, Trans. Ophthal. Soc. U. K. 9:129, 1889.
42. Eddy, D. D., and Farber, E. M.: Pseudoxanthoma elasticum. Internal manifestations; a report of cases and a statistical review of the literature, Arch. Derm. 86:729, 1962.
43. Edwards, H.: Haematemesis due to pseudoxanthoma elasticum, Gastroenterologia 89:345, 1958.
44. Farreras-Valenti, P., Rozman, C., Jurado-Grau, J., del Rio, G., and Elizalde, C.: Grönblad-Strandberg-Touraine syndrome with systemic hypertension due to unilateral renal angioma; cure of hypertension after nephrectomy, Amer. J. Med. 39:355, 1965.
45. Felsher, Z.: Collagen, reticulin, and elastin. In Rothman, S.: Physiology and biochemistry of the skin, Chicago, 1954, The University of Chicago Press, p. 391 ff.
46. Findlay, G. H.: On elastosis and the elastic dystrophies of the skin, Brit. J. Derm. Syph. 66:16, 1954.
47. Finnerud, C. W., and Nomland, R.: Pseudoxanthoma elasticum; proof of calcification of elastic tissue; occurrence with and without angioid streaks of the retina, Arch. Derm. Syph. 35:653, 1937.
48. Fisher, E. R., Rodnan, G. P., and Lansing, A. I.: Identification of the anatomic defect in pseudoxanthoma elasticum, Amer. J. Path. 34:977,1958.
49. Flatley, F. J., Atwell, M. E., and McEvoy, R. K.: Pseudoxanthoma elasticum with gastric hemorrhage, Arch. Intern. Med. 112:352, 1963.
50. Fleischmajer, R., and Lara, J. V.: Actinic elastosis and pseudoxanthoma elasticum, Dermatologica 133:366, 1966.
51. Foerster, O. H.: Transactions of the Dermatological Conference of the Mississippi Valley, Arch. Derm. Syph. 30:280, 1934.
52. Fontan, P., Mérand, A., and Pfister, R.: Syndrome de Groenblad-Strandberg, Bull. Soc. Franc. Derm. Syph. 62:101, 1955.
53. Fountain, R. B., and Bett, D.: Pseudoxanthoma elasticum, Proc. Roy. Soc. Med. 58:1091, 1965.

54. Fountain, R. B., and Scott, O. L.: Pseudoxanthoma elasticum, Proc. Roy. Soc. Med. **58:** 1091, 1965.

55. Franceschetti, A., and Roulet, E. L.: Le syndrome de Groenblad et Strandberg (striés angioïdes de la rétine et pseudoxanthome élastique) et ses rapport avec les affections du mésenchyme, Arch. Ophtal. (Paris) **53:**401, 1936.

56. Friedenwald, J. S., and others: Ophthalmic pathology; an atlas and textbook, Philadelphia, 1952, W. B. Saunders Co.

57. Geereats, W. J., and Guerry, D.: Angioid streaks and sickle cell disease, Amer. J. Ophthal. **50:**213, 1960.

58. Ghormley, R. K.: Multiple calcified bursae and calcified cysts in soft tissues, Trans. West. Surg. Ass. **51:**292, 1942.

59. Giesen, H.: Beitrag zur Kasuistik des Pseudoxanthoma elasticum, Inaugural dissertation, Erlangen, 1936.

60. Gillman, T., Penn., J., Bronks, D., and Roux, M.: Abnormal elastic fibers; appearance in cutaneous carcinoma, irradiation injuries, and arterial and other degenerative connective tissue lesions in man, Arch. Path. **59:**733, 1955.

61. Gills, J. P., Jr., and Paton, D.: Mottled fundus oculi in pseudoxanthoma elasticum; a report on two siblings, Arch. Ophthal. **73:**792, 1965.

62. Goedbloed, J.: Syndrome of Groenblad and Strandberg; angioid streaks in the fundus oculi, associated with pseudoxanthoma elasticum, Arch. Ophthal. **19:**1, 1938.

63. Gold, S. C.: Still's disease with pseudoxanthoma elasticum, Proc. Roy. Soc. Med. **50:**473, 1957.

64. Goodman, R. M., Smith, E. W., Paton, D., Bergman, R. A., Siegel, C. L., Ottesen, O. E., Shelley, W. M., Pusch, A. L., and McKusick, V. A.: Pseudoxanthoma elasticum, a clinical and histopathological study, Medicine **42:**297, 1963.

65. Grant, A. K., and Aldor, T. A.: Haemorrhage into the upper part of the gastrointestinal tract in three patients with heritable disorders of connective tissue, Aust. Ann. Med. **16:** 75, 1967.

66. Grönblad, E.: Angioid Streakes—Pseudoxanthoma elasticum; vorläufige Mitteilung, Acta Ophthal. **7:**329, 1929.

67. Guenther, E.: Untersuchungen über den Pulsverlauf in den grösseren distalen Arterien der Extremitäten in einigen Fällen von Pseudoxanthoma elasticum cum angioid streakes (Grönblad-Strandbergs Syndrom), Acta Med. Scand. **123:**482, 1946.

68. Haber, H.: Histological report on a case shown by Dr. Fenner at the Royal Society of Medicine, Proc. Roy. Soc. Med. (Sect. Derm.) **42:**136, 1949.

69. Hagedoorn, A.: Angioid streaks, Arch. Ophthal. **21:**746, 935, 1939.

70. Hall, D. A., Reed, R., and Tunbridge, R. E.: Structure of elastic tissue, Nature **170:**264, 1952.

71. Hallopeau and Laffitte: Nouvelle note sur un cas de pseudo-xanthome élastique, Ann. Derm. Syph. (Paris) **4:**595, 1903.

72. Hannay, P. W.: Some clinical and histopathological notes on pseudoxanthoma elasticum, Brit. J. Derm. **63:**92, 1951.

73. Harkess, J. W., and Peters, H. J.: Tumoral calcinosis; a report of six cases, J. Bone Joint Surg. **49-A:**721, 1967.

74. Hartung, H.: Ueber familiäre angioide Pigmentstreifenbildung des Augenhintergrundes, Klin. Mbl. Augenheilk. **88:**43, 1932.

75. Hashimoto, K., and Dibella, R. J.: Electron microscopic studies of normal and abnormal elastic fibers of the skin, J. Invest. Derm. **48:**405, 1967.

76. Hermann, H.: Das Grönblad-Strandberg-Syndrom in erbbiologischer Betrachtung, Z. Haut. Geschlechtskr. **20:**314, 1956.

77. Herrick, J. B.: Peculiar elongated and sickle-shaped red corpuscles in a case of severe anemia, Arch. Intern. Med. **6:**517, 1910.

78. Heyl, T.: Pseudoxanthoma elasticum with granulomatous skin lesions, Arch. Derm. **96:**528, 1967.

79. Hoffmann, D.: Kardiovaskuläre Erkrankunkgen beim Strandberg-Grönblad-Syndrom, Z. Menschl. Vererb. Konstitutionsl. **33:**389, 1956.

80. Huang, S. N., Steele, H. D., and Kumar, G.: Ultrastructural changes of elastic fibers in pseudoxanthoma elasticum; a study of histogenesis, Arch. Path. **83:**108, 1967.

81. Hubler, W. R.: Two cases of pseudoxanthoma elasticum, Arch. Derm. Syph. **50:**51, 1944.

82. Jacoby, M. W.: Pseudoxanthoma elasticum and angioid streaks; report of a case, Arch. Ophthal. 11:828, 1934.

83. James, A. E., Jr., Eaton, S. B., and Blazek, J. V.: Roentgen findings in pseudoxanthoma elasticum (PXE), Amer. J. Roentgen. 106:642, 1969.

84. Joffe, E., and Joffe, M.: Zur Aetiologie des Pseudoxanthoma elasticum (Darier), Arch. Derm. u. Syph. 165:713, 1932.

85. Johnson, G. J., and Bloch, K. J.: Immunoglobulin levels in retinal vascular abnormalities and pseudoxanthoma elasticum, Arch. Ophthal. 81:322, 1969.

86. Johnson, W. C., and Helwig, E. B.: Histopathology of the acid mucopolysaccharides of skin in normal and in certain pathologic conditions, Amer. J. Clin. Path. 40:123, 1963.

87. Jones, J. W., Alden, H. S., and Bishop, E. L.: Pseudoxanthoma elasticum; report of five cases illustrating its association with angioid streaks of the retina, Arch. Derm. Syph. 27:423, 1933.

88. Kaplan, L., and Hartman, S. W.: Elastica disease; case of Grönblad-Strandberg syndrome with gastrointestinal hemorrhage, Arch. Intern. Med. 94:489, 1954.

89. Kat, W., and Prick, J. J. G.: A case of pseudoxanthoma elasticum with anatomico-pathological irregularities of the thyroid arteries, Psychiat. Neurol. (Basel) 44:417, 1940.

90. Keech, M. K., and Reed, R.: Enzymatic elucidation of the relationship between collagen and elastin; an electron-microscopic study, Ann. Rheum. Dis. 16:35, 1957.

91. Keech, M. K., Reed, R., and Wood, M. J.: Further observations on the transformation of collagen fibrils into "elastin" and electron-microscopic studies, J. Path. Bact. 71:477, 1956.

92. Kennedy, C. B.: Discussion of paper of Shaffer et al.,[157] Arch. Derm. Syph. 76:631, 1957.

93. Kissmeyer, A., and With, C.: Clinical and histological studies on the pathological changes in the elastic tissue of the skin, Brit. J. Derm. 34:175, 1922.

94. Klein, B. A.: Angioid streaks; a clinical and histopathologic study, Amer. J. Ophthal. 30:955, 1947.

95. Knapp, H.: On the formation of dark angioid streaks as an unusual metamorphosis of retinal hemorrhage, Arch. Ophthal. 21:289, 1892.

96. Kofler, A.: Beitrag zur Kenntnis der Angioid Streakes (Knapp), Arch. Augenheilk. 82:134, 1917.

97. Kupfer, C.: Personal communication.

98. Kutty, P. K., and Sadasivan, P. B.: Pseudoxanthoma elasticum, J. Indian Med. Ass. 44:200, 1965.

99. Larmande, A., and Margaillan, A.: Maladie de Paget et syndrome de Groenblad-Strandberg, Bull. Soc. Franc. Ophtal. 70:206, 1957.

100. Law, F. W.: A contribution to the pathology of angioid streaks, Trans. Ophthal. Soc. U. K. 58:191, 1938.

101. Laymon, C. W.: Cutaneous manifestations of some internal diseases, J. Lancet 85:394, 1965.

102. Leblanc, J. V.: Pseudoxanthoma elasticum; a review with case reports of two sisters, J. Arkansas Med. Soc. 60:327, 1964.

103. Lee, M. M. C.: Physical and structural age changes in human skin, Anat. Rec. 129:473, 1957.

104. Lever, W. F.: Histopathology of the skin, ed. 2, Philadelphia, 1949, J. B. Lippincott Co., p. 56.

104a. Levine, H. J. (Boston): Personal communication, 1972.

105. Levy, G., and Brewer, R. L.: Pseudoxanthoma elasticum; report of a case, Amer. J. Med. 26:157, 1959.

106. Lewis, U. J., Williams, D. E., and Brink, N. G.: Pancreatic elastase; purification, properties and function, J. Biol. Chem. 222:705, 1956.

107. Lieberman, A.: The case of the rocky ripples, J. Indiana Med. Ass. 62:804, 1969.

108. Lobitz, W., and Osterberg, A. E.: Pseudoxanthoma elasticum; microincineration, J. Invest. Derm. 15:297, 1950.

109. Loria, P. R., Kennedy, C. B., Freeman, J. A., and Henington, V. M.: Pseudoxanthoma elasticum (Groenblad-Strandberg syndrome). A clinical, light- and electron-microscope study, Arch. Derm. Syph. 76:609, 1957.

110. Lynch, F. W.: Elastic tissue in fetal skin, Arch. Derm. Syph. 29:57, 1934.

111. McCaughey, R. S., Alexander, L. C., and Morrish, J. A.: The Grönblad-Strandberg syn-

drome; a report of three cases presenting with massive gastrointestinal hemorrhage during pregnancy, Gastroenterology **31**:156, 1956.

112. McKusick, V. A.: Hereditary disorders of connective tissue, Bull. N. Y. Acad. Med. **35**:143, 1959.

113. McKusick, V. A.: Mendelian inheritance in man; catalogs of autosomal dominant, autosomal recessive, and X-linked phenotypes, ed. 3, Baltimore, 1971, The Johns Hopkins Press.

114. McKusick, V. A.: On the X chromosome of man, Quart. Rev. Biol. **37**:69, 1962, Also AIBS monograph, Washington, D. C., 1964.

115. McPhaul, J. J., Jr., and Engel, F. L.: Heterotopic calcification, hyperphosphatemia and angioid streaks of the retina, Amer. J. Med. **31**:488, 1961.

116. Marchesani, O., and Wirz, F.: Die Pigment-streifenerkrankung der Netzhaut—das Pseudoxanthoma elasticum der Haut—eine Systemerkrankung, Arch. Augenheilk. **104**:522, 1931.

117. Marchionini, A., and Turgut, K.: Ueber Pseudoxanthoma elasticum hereditarium, Derm. Wschr. **114**:145, 1942.

118. Matras, A.: Pseudoxanthoma elasticum, Zbl. Haut- Geschl.-Kr. **50**:280, 1935.

119. Mehregan, A. H.: Elastase and dermal elastoses, J. Invest. Derm. **45**:404, 1965.

120. Mehregan, A. H.: Elastosis perforans serpiginosa; a review of the literature and report of 11 cases, Arch. Derm. **97**:381, 1968.

121. Messis, C. P., and Budzilovich, G. N.: Pseudoxanthoma elasticum; report of an autopsied case with cerebral involvement, Neurology **20**:703, 1970.

122. Milstoc, M.: An unusual anatomo-pathologic aspect of a case with pseudoxanthoma elasticum, Dis. Chest **55**:431, 1969.

122a. Mitsudo, S. M.: Chronic idiopathic hyperphosphatasia associated with pseudoxanthoma elasticum, J. Bone Joint Surg. **53-A**:303, 1971.

123. Mitchell, A.: Angioid streaks, Boston Med. Quart. **15**:22, 1964.

124. Miyake, H., Tanaka, J., Izawa, Y., and Hayakawa, R.: A new finding in oral cavity in pseudoxanthoma elasticum, Nagoya J. Med. Sci. **29**:251, 1967.

125. Moran, T. J., and Lansing, A. I.: Studies on the nature of the abnormal fibers in pseudoxanthoma elasticum, Arch. Path. **65**:688, 1958.

126. Morrison, W. H.: Osteitis deformans with angioid streaks, Arch. Ophthal. **26**:79, 1941.

127. Moschella, S. L., Greenbaum, C. H., and Fleischmajer, R.: Pseudoxanthoma elasticum, Arch. Derm. **96**:97, 1967.

128. Najjar, S. S., Farah, F. S., Kurban, A. K., Melhem, R. E., and Khatchadourian, A. K.: Tumoral calcinosis and pseudoxanthoma elasticum, J. Pediat. **72**:243, 1968.

129. Nellen, M., and Jacobson, M.: Pseudoxanthoma elasticum (Grönblad-Strandberg disease) with coronary artery calcification, S. Afr. Med. J. **32**:649, 1958.

130. Ohno, T.: Ueber Pseudoxanthoma elasticum und dessen Histologie, Arch. Derm. Syph. **149**:420, 1925.

131. Ormsby, O. S., and Montgomery, H.: Diseases of the skin, ed. 8, Philadelphia, 1954, Lea & Febiger, p. 747.

132. Osbourn, R. A., and Olivo, M. A.: Pseudoxanthoma elasticum in mother and daughter, Arch. Derm. Syph. **63**:661, 1951.

133. Parker, J. C., Friedman, A. E., Kien, S., Levin, S., and Bartter, F. C.: Pseudoxanthoma elasticum and hypertension, New Eng. J. Med. **271**:1204, 1964.

134. Paton, D.: Angioid streaks and sickle cell anemia, Arch. Ophthal. **62**:852, 1959.

135. Paton, D.: Personal communication.

136. Pautrier, L. M.: A propos de deux affections d'élastine du revêtement cutané, témoins d'affections généralisées de l'élastine de tout l'organisme, Arch. Belg. Derm. Syph. **4**:259, 1948.

137. Percival, G. H., Hannay, P. W., and Duthie, D. A.: Fibrous changes in the dermis, with special reference to senile elastosis, Brit. J. Derm. **61**:269, 1949.

138. Percival, S. P.: Angioid streaks and elastorrhexis, Brit. J. Ophthal. **52**:297, 1968.

139. Pickrell, K. L., Kelley, J. W., and Marzoni, F. A.: The plastic surgical treatment of pseudoxanthoma elasticum, Plast. Reconstr. Surg. **3**:700, 1948.

140. Poliner, I. J.: Pseudoxanthoma elasticum and gastrointestinal bleeding, J. Maine Med. Ass. **58**:76, 1967.

140a. Pope, M. (Liverpool and Baltimore): Personal communication, 1972.

141. Prick, J. J. G.: Pontine pseudobulbar-paralyse bei Pseudoxanthoma elasticum; eine klinische anatomische Studie, Doctoral thesis, Maastricht, 1938.

142. Reinertson, R. P., and Farber, E. M.: Pseudoxanthoma elasticum with gastrointestinal bleeding, Calif. Med. **83**:94, 1955.

143. Revell, S. T. R., Jr., and Carey, T. N.: Pseudoxanthoma elasticum as a disseminated disease, Southern Med. J. **41**:782, 1948.

144. Rigal, D.: Observation pour servir à l'histoire de la chéloide diffuse xanthélasmique, Ann. Derm. Syph. **2**:491, 1881.

145. Rizzuli, A. B.; Angioid streaks with PXE; a case followed with fundus photograph over a period of 27 years, Amer. J. Ophthal. **40**:387, 1955.

146. Rodnan, G. P., Fisher, E. R., and Warren, J. E.: Pseudoxanthoma elasticum; clinical findings and identification of the anatomic defect (abstract), Clin. Res. **6**:236, 1958.

147. Rosen, E.: Fundus in pseudoxanthoma elasticum, Amer. J. Ophthal. **66**:236, 1968.

148. Rosenheim, M. (London): Personal communication.

149. Rosenthal, T. B., and Lansing, A. I.: Isolation and assay of elastase from prancreatin (abstract), Anat. Rec. **124**:356, 1956.

150. Sairanen, E., Itkonen, A., and Kangas, S.: Pseudoxanthoma elasticum (PXE) and joint manifestations, Acta Rheum. Scand. **16**:130, 1970.

151. Sames, C. P.: Pseudoxanthoma elasticum: severe melaena from the jejunum treated by resection, Proc. Roy. Soc. Med. **54**:519, 1961.

152. Sanbacka-Holström, I.: Das Grönblad-Strandbergische Syndrome; Pseudoxanthoma elasticum—angioid streaks—Gefässveränderungen, Acta Dermatovener. **20**:684, 1939.

153. Scheie, H. G., and Freeman, N. E.: Vascular disease associated with angioid streaks of the retina and pseudoxanthoma elasticum, Arch. Ophthal. **35**:3, 1946.

154. Scheie, H. G., and Hogan, T. F., Jr.: Angioid streaks and generalized arterial disease, Arch. Ophthal. **57**:855, 1957.

155. Scholz, R. O.: Angioid streaks, Arch. Ophthal. **26**:677, 1941.

156. Schutt, D.: Pseudoxanthoma elasticum and elastosis perforans serpiginosa, Arch. Derm. **91**:151, 1965.

157. Shaffer, B., Copelan, H. W., and Beerman, H.: Pseudoxanthoma elasticum; a cutaneous manifestation of a systemic disease; report of a case of Paget's disease and a case of calcinosis with arteriosclerosis as manifestations of this syndrome. Arch. Derm. Syph. **76**:622, 1957.

158. Silvers, S.: Pseudoxanthoma elasticum with angioid streaks of retina, Arch. Derm. Syph. **42**:155, 1940.

159. Silvers, S. H., and Wolfe, H. E.: Pseudoxanthoma elasticum with angioid streaks; the syndrome of Groenblad and Strandberg, Arch. Derm. Syph. **45**:1142, 1942.

160. Smith, E. W., Malak, J., Goodman, R. M., and McKusick, V. A.: Reactive perforating elastoma; a feature of certain genetic disorders, Bull. Hopkins Hosp. **11**:235, 1962.

161. Smith, J. G., Jr., Davidson, E. A., and Clark, R. D.: Dermal elastin in actinic elastosis and pseudoxanthoma elasticum, Nature **195**:716, 1962.

162. Smith, J. G., Jr., Davidson, E. A., and Taylor, R. W.: Cutaneous acid mucopolysaccharides in pseudoxanthoma elasticum, J. Invest. Derm. **43**:429, 1964.

163. Smith, J. G., Jr., Sams, W. M., Jr., Davidson, E. A., and Clark, R. D.: Pseudoxanthoma elasticum; histochemical and biochemical alterations, Arch. Derm. **86**:741, 1962.

164. Smith, J. L., Gass, J. D., and Justice, J., Jr.: Fluorescein fundus photography of angioid streaks, Brit. J. Ophthal. **48**:517, 1964.

165. Stankler, L.: Pseudoxanthoma elasticum with a knuckle pad on the thumb, Acta Dermatovener. **47**:263, 1967.

166. Stecher, R. M.: The physical characteristics and heredity of short thumbs, Acta Genet. (Basel) **7**:217, 1957.

167. Stegmaier, O. C.: Pseudoxanthoma elasticum associated with angioid streaks of the retina, Arch. Derm. Syph. **70**:530, 1954.

168. Storsteen, K. A., and Janes, J. M.: Arteriography and vascular studies in Paget's disease of the bone, J.A.M.A. **154**:472, 1954.

169. Stout, O. M.: Pseudoxanthoma elasticum with retinal angioid streaking, decidedly improved on tocopherol therapy, Arch. Derm. Syph. **63**:510, 1951.

170. Strandberg, J.: Pseudoxanthoma elasticum, Z. Haut Geschlechtskr. **31**:689, 1929.

171. Suerig, K. C., and Siefert, F. E.: Pseudoxanthoma elasticum and sickle cell anemia, Arch. Intern. Med. **113:**135, 1964.

172. Szymanski, F. J., and Caro, M. R.: Pseudoxanthoma elasticum; review of its relationship to internal diseases and report of an unusual case, Arch. Derm. **71:**184, 1955.

173. Tanenbaum, H. L., and de Margerie, J.: Sudden bilateral loss of central vision in pseudoxanthoma elasticum; fluorescence photography of the ocular lesions, Canad. J. Ophthal. **1:**221, 1966.

174. Tannenhein, V.: Zur Kenntnis des Pseudoxanthoma elasticum (Darier), Wein. Klin. Wschr. **14:**1038, 1901.

175. Teller, H., and Vester, G.: Elektronenmikroskopiche Untersuchungsergebnisse an der kollagenen Interzellularsubstanz des Koriums beim Pseudoxanthoma elasticum, Derm. Wschr. **136:**1373, 1957.

176. Témine, P.: Contribution à l'étude de l'élastorrhexie systématisée, Paris thesis, Paris, 1940, Jouve & Cie.

177. Terry, T. S.: Angioid streaks and osteitis deformans, Trans. Amer. Ophthal. Soc. **32:**555, 1934.

178. Thomson, J. E. M., and Tanner, F. J.: Tumoral calcinosis, J. Bone Joint Surg. **31-A:**32, 1949.

179. Throne, B., and Goodman, H.: Pseudoxanthoma elasticum, Arch. Derm. Syph. **6:**419, 1921.

180. Tominaga, B., Harada, S., and Hashimoto, T.: A case of pseudoxanthoma elasticum with tuberculoid granulation tissue, Arch. Derm. Syph. **30:**864, 1934.

181. Touraine, A.: L'elastorrhexie systématisée, Bull. Soc. Franc. Derm. Syph. **47:**255, 1940.

182. Touraine, A.: L'élastorrhexie systématisée, Presse Méd. **49:**361, 1941.

183. Touraine, A., and James: Pseudoxanthome élastique (élastorrhexis), Bull. Soc. Franc. Derm. Syph. **47:**217, 1940.

184. Tunbridge, R. E., Tattersall, R. N., Hall, D. A., Astbury, W. T., and Reed, R.: The fibrous structure of normal and abnormal skin, Clin. Sci. **11:**315, 1952.

185. Urbach, E., and Wolfram, S.: Ueber Veränderungen des elastischen Gewebes bei einem autoptisch untersuchten Fälle von Groenblad-Strandbergschem Syndrom, Arch. Derm. u. Syph. **176:**167, 1938.

185a. Van Balen, A. T., and Houtsmuller, A. J.: Syndrome of Groenblad-Strandberg-Touraine, Ophthalmologica **149:**246, 1965.

186. Van Embden Andres, G. H.: Afwijkingen, aan de inwendige organen bij Pseudoxanthoma elasticum en Angioide Stregpen, Groningen, 1952.

187. Verhoeff, F. H.: Histological findings in a case of angioid streaks, Brit. J. Ophthal. **32:**531, 1948.

188. Vickers, H. R.: Discussion, Proc. Roy. Soc. Med. **58:**1093, 1965.

189. Walford, R. L., and Kaplan, L.: Pulmonary fibrosis and giant-cell reaction with altered elastic tissue; endogenous "pneumoconiosis," Arch. Path. **63:**75, 1957.

190. Weidman, F. D., Anderson, N. P., and Ayres, S.: Juvenile elastoma, Arch. Derm. Syph. **28:**183, 1933.

191. Welti, M. H.: Pseudoxanthoma elasticum (Darier) in Verbindung mit einer tuberculoiden Granulationsbildung, Arch. Derm. u. Syph. **163:**427, 1931.

192. Weve, H. J. M.: Demonstrationem Niederländische Ophthalmologische Gesellschaften, 1933, Klin. Mbl. Augenheilk. **92:**538, 1934.

193. Whitecomb, F. F., Jr., and Brown, C. H.: Pseudoxanthoma elasticum; report of twelve cases; massive gastrointestinal hemorrhage in one patient, Ann. Intern. Med. **56:**834, 1962.

194. Wilmer, W. H.: Atlas fundus oculi, New York, 1934, The Macmillan Co., plate 92.

195. Winer, L. H.: Elastic fibers in unusual dermatoses, Arch. Derm. Syph. **71:**338, 1955.

196. Wise, D.: Hereditary disorders of connective tissue. In Gottron, H. A., and Schnyder, U. W., editors: Vererbung von Hautkrankheiten, Berlin, 1966, Julius Springer Verlag, pp. 467-532.

197. Wolff, H. H., Stokes, J., and Schlesinger, B.: Vascular abnormalities associated with pseudoxanthoma elasticum, Arch. Dis. Child. **27:**82, 1952.

198. Woo, J. C., Jr., and Chandler, F. W.: Pseudoxanthoma elasticum with gastric hemorrhage; report of a case, Ann. Intern. Med. **49:**215, 1958.

199. Woodcock, C. W.: Transactions of the Cleveland Dermatological Society, Arch. Derm. Syph. **65:**623, 1952.

200. Woringer, F.: Sur deux aspects histologiques différents de pseudoxanthome élastique, Bull. Soc. Franc. Derm. Syph. **61**:80, 1954.

200a. Yaghmai, I., and Mirbod, P.: Tumoral calcinosis, Amer. J. Roentgen. **111**:573, 1971.

201. Yatzkan, D. N.: Angioid streaks of the fundus, Amer. J. Ophthal. **43**:219, 1957.

202. Zentmayer, W.: Angioid streaks of the fundus oculi observed over a period of thirty-six years; report of a case, Arch. Ophthal. **35**:541, 1946.

11 · The mucopolysaccharidoses*

Historical note

The disorder (or group of disorders) now called, among other names, the Hurler syndrome is said by Henderson[197] to have been recognized in 3 sibs by John Thompson of Edinburgh between about 1900 and 1913.† Berkhan's case,[27] reported in 1907, may have been the Hurler syndrome. The first definitive description was that of Charles H. Hunter,‡ whose report appeared in the *Proceedings of the Royal Society of Medicine* in 1917, while he was serving in England as a major in the Canadian Army Medical Corps. This beautifully detailed and descriptive report concerned 2 brothers, 10 and 8 years of age, respectively, who were admitted to the Winnipeg General Hospital in 1915. The habitus was typically dwarfed. Deafness, widely spaced teeth, short neck, protuberant abdomen with hepatosplenomegaly, inguinal hernias, short, broad, thick, stiff hands, semiflexed knees, and noisy respiration were present. "The face [was] very large, of deep burnt-red colour, as after much exposure, with a tinge of cyanosis in cheeks and lips. . . . In the younger child, over strips of skin 1½ in. wide, extending from the angles of both scapulae parallel to the ribs forward to the mid-axillary lines, these are pinhead elevations, grouped closely and regularly, smooth of surface, normal in colour . . . ." The elder boy had cardiomegaly and "a distinct diastolic murmur audible in the third and fourth left interspaces close to the sternum . . .; at the apex, a systolic murmur was conducted towards the axilla." Twelve illustrations, including many x-ray films demonstrating typical changes (such as "shoe-shaped" sella turcica), were presented by Hunter. The boys appeared to be normally intelligent; clouding of the cornea was not observed; the spine was straight, with loss of the normal contour, but there was no gibbus. We have been able to obtain follow-up information (Fig. 11-1). Hunter's patients clearly suffered from the X-linked mucopolysaccharidosis now called MPS II.

---

*A detailed discussion of mucopolysaccharide metabolism and of the mucopolysaccharidoses was provided by Dorfman and Matalon.[117a]

†Of the 9 children of James McLeod, 3 had the Hurler syndrome[554]: John (1895-1905), Charles (1905-1909), and Jane (1911-1918).

‡Hunter was later Professor of Medicine in the University of Manitoba, Winnipeg. He died March 18, 1955, at the age of 82 years (Canad. Med. Ass. J. 72:712, 1955).

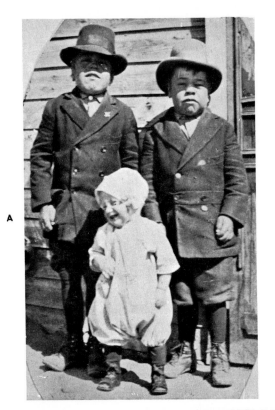

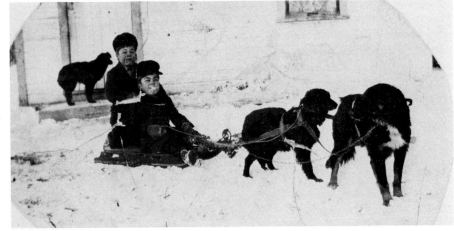

Fig. 11-1. Photographs of the patients Hunter described in 1917.[218] The younger brother (G. B. C., born in 1907) died in 1918 of pneumonia, and the elder one (R. W. C., born in 1904) died in 1920 of "dropsy." The youngest sibling in **A** was apparently unaffected. The characteristic facies and clawhand deformity are evident. These brothers are thought to have had the X-linked recessive form of mucopolysaccharidosis (MPS II). (Photographs and follow-up information courtesy Dr. Nancy Gemmell and Dr. L. G. Bell, University of Manitoba, Winnipeg.)

In 1919 Gertrud Hurler of Munich[219] published cases at the suggestion of Professor Meinhard von Pfaundler,[417] who was chief of the University Clinic of Pediatrics and who had presented 2 patients with this syndrome to the Munich Society for Pediatrics on June 27 of the same year. The patients of Hurler and Pfaundler were infants; gibbus was present, as were corneal clouding and retardation of intellect. They probably suffered from the autosomal recessive form of the disease, referred to below as MPS I.

It is surprising that Hunter's beautiful publication received, compared to Hurler's, relatively little attention. Subsequently, even in the English-speaking medical world, it was principally Hurler's paper that was referred to and the names of Hurler and Pfaundler that became most firmly associated with the syndrome. (A similar situation exists in connection with the Morquio syndrome, which was described in England by Brailsford slightly earlier than by Morquio of Montevideo.)

The first case from the United States was that reported by Putnam and Pelkan[426] in 1925 under the title "Scaphocephaly with Malformations of the Skeleton and Other Tissues." The nosography of the Hurler syndrome has now advanced to the point where the limits of the syndrome and its several clinical and pathologic features are reasonably well described, although mildly affected persons are still difficult to identify with certainty except by chemical test (p. 629). A tabular survey of the cases reported up to 1950 was presented by Jervis.[233] Emanuel[130] estimated that over 200 cases had been reported, by 1954.

In 1952, Brante[41] classified the Hurler syndrome as a mucopolysaccharidosis (he also suggested this term), after he isolated dermatan sulfate from the liver of 2 patients with the Hurler syndrome. Brown[44] isolated heparan sulfate from the liver of a similar patient. Discovery of mucopolysacchariduria by Dorfman and Lorincz[116] and by Meyer and colleagues[360] firmly established the nature of the disease.

Van Hoof and Hers, in Louvain, Belgium, suggested that the electron microscopic findings[542] and the natural history of the mucopolysaccharidoses are consistent with their being "lysosomal diseases."[199,200] In the first edition of *Heritable Disorders of Connective Tissue* (1956), I wrote:

> Tissue culture of fibroblasts is possibly one of the more promising, although as yet unexplored, techniques for the study of heritable disorders of connective tissue. (In general, tissue culture has been too little used in physiologic genetics.) . . . In connection with the heritable disorders of connective tissue, the first objective of tissue culture studies should be the in vitro replication of the morphologic abnormalities. In . . . the Hurler syndrome one can with justification anticipate success in demonstrating morphologic abnormality, . . . i.e., the "gargoyle cell." . . . If the initial morphologic studies are consonant with the view that a fibroblast strain growing in the test tube represents the original donor's disease "in pure culture," then intensive studies should be undertaken of the chemical characteristics.

The prediction was fulfilled by the demonstration by Danes and Bearn[88] that fibroblasts show cytoplasmic metachromasia, i.e., the "gargoyle cell" does exist in culture; and by the work of Neufeld and colleagues indicating that cells from several of the mucopolysaccharidoses have a defect in the degradation of mucopolysaccharides[153] and that a diffusible factor produced by normal cells or by cells from a different mucopolysaccharidosis corrects this metabolic defect *in vitro*.[154]

Table 11-1. The genetic mucopolysaccharidoses (as classified in 1966)

MPS	Clinical	Genetic	Biochemical
I (Hurler syndrome)	Early clouding of cornea, grave manifestations	Autosomal recessive	Dermatan sulfate Heparan sulfate
II (Hunter syndrome)	No clouding of cornea, milder course	X-linked recessive	Dermatan sulfate Heparan sulfate
III (Sanfilippo syndrome)	Mild somatic, severe central nervous system effects	Autosomal recessive	Heparan sulfate
IV (Morquio syndrome)	Severe bone changes of distinctive types, cloudy cornea, intellect $+/-$, aortic regurgitation	Autosomal recessive	Keratan sulfate
V (Scheie syndrome)	Stiff joints, coarse facies, cloudy cornea, normal intellect, aortic regurgitation	Autosomal recessive	Dermatan sulfate Heparan sulfate
VI (Maroteaux-Lamy syndrome)	Severe osseous and corneal change, normal intellect	Autosomal recessive	Dermatan sulfate

Although males with clinical features which we now recognize as typical of the X-linked form were reported by many workers, beginning with the brothers described by Hunter, the earliest pedigree clearly indicating X-linked inheritance was published in 1942 by Wolff,[566] who did not comment on sex-linkage, however. In 1946 Njå[388] in Norway presented an X-linked pedigree, specifically proposed this mode of inheritance, and emphasized lack of corneal clouding as a hallmark of the X-linked cases. He can be forgiven for having overlooked Wolff's publication (in *Laryngoscope* during World War II) in making the statement that "this type of heredity in gargoylism has not been described previously."

Many different names have been suggested for the group of disorders we now term mucopolysaccharidoses. Most are now of historic interest only. Husler[220] suggested the term "dysostosis multiplex." Ellis and co-workers,[127] Cockayne[69] and other English authors used the term "gargoylism."* Washington[552] suggested "lipochondrodystrophy," believing this disorder to be one of lipid metabolism. This term is used by the *Cumulated Index Medicus*. However, it is a misnomer, as indicated by present evidence bearing on the basic defect of the disease. This is another instance demonstrating the desirability of using noncommittal terms such as eponyms in connection with syndromes in which the basic defect is as yet unknown.

By 1965 (as reflected in the third edition of *Heritable Disorders of Connective Tissue*) six distinct mucopolysaccharidoses had been differentiated by com-

---

*This term seems unnecessarily cruel in view of the facts that the intellect may be little impaired and that survival to adulthood is not infrequent. It is scarcely a diagnosis that can be cited to a parent, for example. Families sometimes raise legitimate objections to such statements (all too frequent in the literature) as these: "He is a typical gargoyle" or "There are three gargoyles in this family."

Table 11-2. The genetic mucopolysaccharidoses (as classified in 1972)

Designation	Clinical features	Genetics	Excessive urinary MPS	Substance deficient
MPS I H — Hurler syndrome	Early clouding of cornea, grave manifestations, death usually before age 10	Homozygous for MPS IH gene	Dermatan sulfate Heparan sulfate	α-L-iduronidase (formerly called Hurler corrective factor)
MPS I S — Scheie syndrome	Stiff joints, cloudy cornea, aortic regurgitation, normal intelligence, ?normal life-span	Homozygosity for MPS IS gene	Dermatan sulfate Heparan sulfate	α-L-iduronidase
MPS I H/S — Hurler-Scheie compound	Phenotype intermediate between Hurler and Scheie	Genetic compound of MPS I H and I S genes	Dermatan sulfate Heparan sulfate	α-L-iduronidase
MPS II A — Hunter syndrome, severe	No clouding of cornea, milder course than in MPS IH but death usually before age 15 years	Hemizygous for X-linked gene	Dermatan sulfate Heparan sulfate	Hunter corrective factor
MPS II B — Hunter syndrome, mild	Survival to 30's to 50's, fair intelligence	Hemizygous for X-linked allele for mild form	Dermatan sulfate Heparan sulfate	Hunter corrective factor
MPS III A — Sanfilippo syndrome A	Identical phenotype:	Homozygous for Sanfilippo A gene	Heparan sulfate	Heparan sulfate sulfatase
MPS III B — Sanfilippo syndrome B	Mild somatic, severe central nervous system effects	Homozygous for Sanfilippo B (at different locus)	Heparan sulfate	N-acetyl-α-D-glucosaminidase
MPS IV — Morquio syndrome (probably more than one allelic form)	Severe bone changes of distinctive type, cloudy cornea, aortic regurgitation	Homozygous for Morquio gene	Keratan sulfate	Unknown
MPS V — Vacant				
MPS VI A — Maroteaux-Lamy syndrome, classic form	Severe osseous and corneal change, normal intellect	Homozygous for M-L gene	Dermatan sulfate	Maroteaux-Lamy corrective factor
MPS VI B — Maroteaux-Lamy syndrome, mild form	Severe osseous and corneal change, normal intellect	Homozygous for allele at M-L locus	Dermatan sulfate	Maroteaux-Lamy corrective factor
MPS VII — β-glucuronidase deficiency (more than one allelic form?)	Hepatosplenomegaly, dysostosis multiplex, white cell inclusions, mental retardation	Homozygous for mutant gene at beta-glucuronidase locus	Dermatan sulfate	β-glucuronidase

bined clinical, genetic, and biochemical study. These six were designated MPS I through MPS VI, as shown in Table 11-1. The Hurler syndrome, as the prototype mucopolysaccharidosis, was termed MPS I. The X-linked disorder, Hunter syndrome, was labelled MPS II. MPS III (Sanfilippo syndrome), MPS V (Scheie syndrome), and MPS VI (Maroteaux-Lamy syndrome) had previously been considered "Hurler variants." MPS IV (Morquio syndrome) was, by 1965, known to have a characteristic mucopolysacchariduria as well as distinctive skeletal features.

The nosology of the mucopolysaccharidoses has been greatly influenced since 1968 by the work of Neufeld and her colleagues on specific corrective factors that could, by studies of fibroblasts *in vitro*, be shown to be deficient in various ones of these disorders. Some surprises were forthcoming, e.g., that the Hurler syndrome and the Scheie syndrome, although clinically very different, have deficiency of the same corrective factor[558] and that two phenotypically indistinguishable forms of the Sanfilippo syndrome can be identified by mutual cross-correction of the metabolic defect exhibited by cultured fibroblasts.[262b] In 1972, using

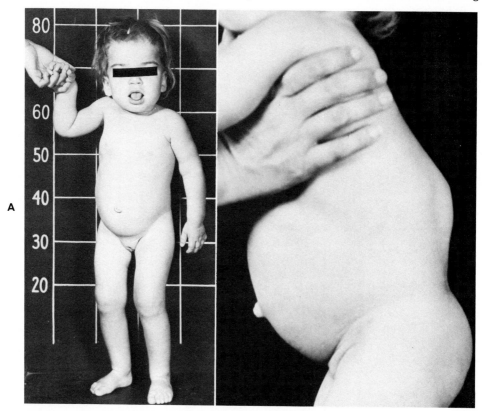

Fig. 11-2. Thirty-four-month-old child (S. S., B3747). **The child is mentally retarded. The liver** and spleen are enlarged, the corneas cloudy, and the teeth short, abnormally formed, and late in appearing. The fingers show flexion contractures, as do other joints to a slight extent. There is constant nasal congestion, so that the patient is a mouth-breather. Most of these features are evident in **A.** In **B** the lower dorsal, upper lumbar gibbus is evident. The skeletal basis for this appearance is shown by the x-ray film of the spine in **C.** Note the lumbar kyphos, beaking of the second lumbar vertebra, concavity of the anterior margins of the other vertebrae, the saber-shaped ribs, and hepatosplenomegaly.

the test substrate phenyl-L-iduronide prepared by Bernard Weissman and his colleagues,[555a] Matalon and Dorfman[34ia] and Bach and colleagues[15a] showed that the Hurler syndrome has a deficiency of α-L-iduronidase. These and other advances have permitted the revised classification given in Table 11-2. My colleagues and I[321a,321b] postulated allelism at the MPS I, II, and VI loci and presented cases that satisfy the criteria for a genetic compound (p. 553) at the MPS I locus.

Beta-glucuronidase deficiency has been tentatively labelled as MPS VII (p. 627). The Dyggve-Melchior-Claussen disorder, for which this designation was previously suggested,[117a,316] is now thought not to be a mucopolysaccharidosis (p. 610).

The use of plasma infusions in the attempted treatment of mucopolysaccharidoses was initiated by DiFerrante and colleagues[110] on the rationale that normal plasma contains corrective factors. Their first report appeared in 1971.

A number of conditions that have clinical and/or biochemical features resembling those of the mucopolysaccharidoses have been delineated. These in-

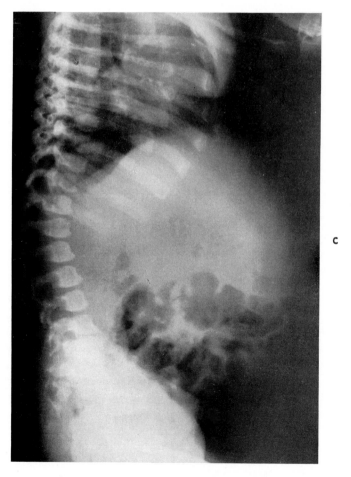

C

Fig. 11-2, cont'd. For legend see opposite page.

clude the conditions that combine features of the mucopolysaccharidoses and the sphingolipidoses and that have been called mucolipidosis I, mucolipidosis II, and mucolipidosis III by Spranger and Wiedemann.[497] These three disorders were initially called, respectively, lipomucopolysaccharidosis, I-cell disease, and pseudo-Hurler polydystrophy. Additional Hurler-like conditions are generalized gangliosidosis, fucosidosis, mannosidosis, and other disorders discussed later in this chapter.

A note on nomenclature

The now preferred chemical term for the mucopolysaccharides is *glycosaminoglycans* (p. 46). However, *mucopolysaccharidosis* is not likely to be replaced as the generic designation for the entities discussed here. Furthermore, the familiar and therefore easier term mucopolysaccharide will be used here. Nonetheless, usage has developed to the point that it seems appropriate to use the new terms for the individual mucopolysaccharides:

Old term	New term
Chondroitin sulfate B	Dermatan sulfate
Heparitin sulfate	Heparan sulfate
Keratosulfate	Keratan sulfate
Chondroitin sulfate A	Chrondroitin-4-sulfate
Chondroitin sulfate C	Chondroitin-6-sulfate

MUCOPOLYSACCHARIDOSIS I H (MPS I H, HURLER SYNDROME)

As the prototype mucopolysaccharidosis, MPS I H will be described in especially full detail. This severe disorder leads to death before the age of 10 years in most cases. Clouding of the cornea develops in all cases. When MPS I is used without the qualifying letter *H*, the Hurler syndrome will be meant.

Clinical manifestations

This form of the disease becomes clinically evident in infancy or early childhood. Of the six mucopolysaccharidoses, it produces death at the earliest age, on the average. The infant usually develops normally for a few months (indeed, the patient often is unusually large in the first year of life[286]) and then progressively deteriorates mentally and physically. Lumbar gibbus, stiff joints, chest deformity, or rhinitis may first prompt the parents to seek medical advice. Dwarfing is accompanied by radiologic changes in the skeleton that are more or less typical of this specific entity (Figs. 11-2C and 11-4). Progressive clouding of the cornea occurs in all cases and may conceal retinal degeneration that is occurring concurrently. The liver and spleen are enlarged (Fig. 11-5) as a result of mucopolysaccharide deposits. The usual causes of death, which in most cases occurs before 10 years of age, are respiratory infection and cardiac failure. The anatomic basis for the cardiac features is the deposition of mucopolysaccharide in the tunica intima of the coronary arteries (Fig. 11-6B to D) and in the heart valves.

Mental development, which appears to be normal for the first year or so of life, shows regression thereafter. Hydrocephalus may be obvious, and even in those cases in which it develops more slowly, so that the skull sutures close, internal hydrocephalus (Fig. 11-6A), probably the result of meningeal deposits, is a frequent finding at autopsy.

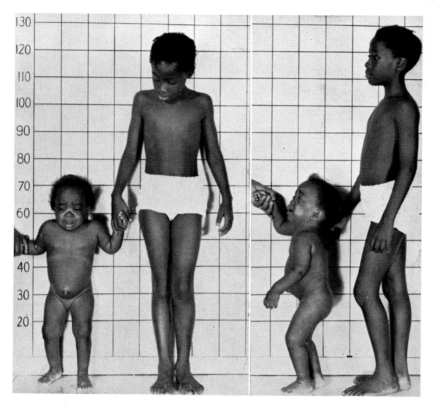

Fig. 11-3. The Hurler syndrome. On the left of each view: C. D. (B41371), 2½ years of age, is a member of the only Negro family with the Hurler syndrome I have seen. The head is large and the facies characteristic of the Hurler syndrome. The elbows, shoulders, knees, and other joints show reduced mobility, preventing full extension. The hands are short, and the terminal phalanges cannot be fully extended. Both the liver and the spleen are enlarged. Nasal breathing is obstructed by a continuous mucopurulent discharge. Both corneas are clouded. Of 6 children, 3—2 boys and this girl—have been affected with the autosomal recessive form of the Hurler syndrome. A normal 8-year-old sister is also shown here. The 2 other affected children died at the ages of 3 and 4 years. (From McKusick, V. A.: Bull. N. Y. Acad. Med. 35:143, 1959.)

The line along which development occurs in these patients is so similar from patient to patient that—as in the Marfan syndrome, myotonic dystrophy, mongolism, and some other conditions—the patients, even though unrelated, tend to resemble each other more than their unaffected siblings.

The head is large and bulging, and there are often prominent scalp veins in the case of small children. The bridge of the nose is flattened, creating a saddle appearance. The tip of the nose is broad with wide nostrils. Hypertelorism is usual. The skull is often scaphocephalic,* i.e., shaped like the keel of a boat, seemingly as a result of premature closure of the sagittal and frontal sutures, with

---

*There is usually no difficulty in distinguishing the Hurler syndrome from the specific conditions given the generic names *acrocephaly* and *scaphocephaly*,[414] although in the earlier days of the nosography of Hurler's syndrome such confusion did occur.[234]

hyperostosis in those areas. This hyperostosis often creates a longitudinal (sagittal) ridge, which may cross the forehead. Radiologic changes in the sella turcica, in the form of unusual length and depth and an anterior "pocketing" (Figs. 11-4B and 11-11E), are striking. This type of sella turcica was called "shoe-shaped" by Ullrich,[533] who found in other cases a shallow "shell-shaped" or a deeper "bowl-shaped" fossa. Neuhauser and colleagues[384] described the radiologic and autopsy features of arachnoid cysts in patients with the Hurler syndrome. (Such cysts were observed also in the Scheie syndrome (MPS I S) but not in the Hunter or Sanfilippo syndromes (MPS II and MPS III). A favored location for cyst development was anterior to the sella turcica. Erosion of the body of the sphenoid bone and of the anterior clinoids resulted. Yuhl and Schmitz[571] seem to have been first to describe large anomalous occipital channels, i.e., enlarged occipital emissary veins, in a case of "Hurler's syndrome" with normal intracranial pressure. From this finding and a normal patient with the radiologic finding, they concluded that enlargement of these veins is not a sign of increased intracranial

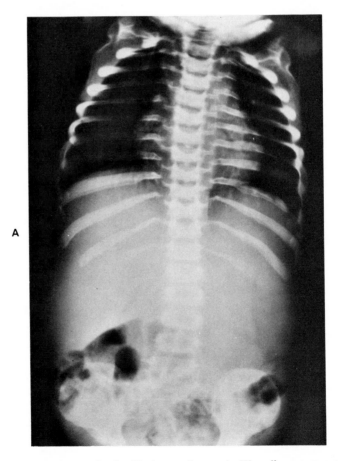

Fig. 11-4. Radiologic changes in the Hurler syndrome. **A,** The ribs are unusually broad and spatulate, with narrow vertebral ends giving them an oarlike shape. Note the evidence of hepatosplenomegaly.

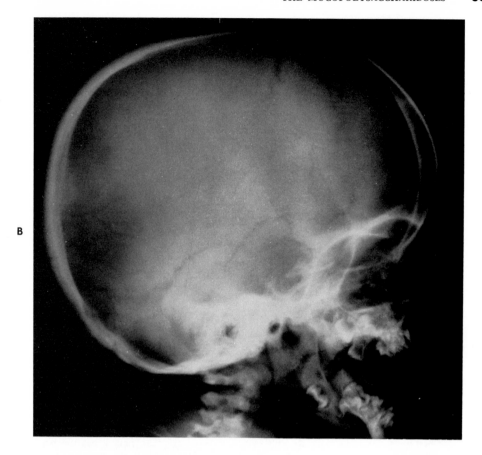

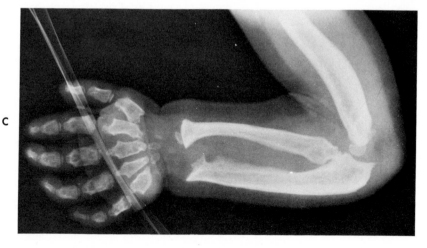

Fig. 11-4, cont'd. B, The calvaria is relatively large and is devoid of the usual digital markings. The sutures are fused prematurely, and the mastoids are small and airless. The anterior pocketing of the sella turcica ("shoe-shaped" sella) is highly characteristic. **C,** The long bones are abnormally short and broad. The hand is clawed and its bones are strikingly abnormal in configuration. Their shape is virtually pathognomonic of the Hurler syndrome. Furthermore, pronounced abnormality in the region of the paranasal sinuses is evident.

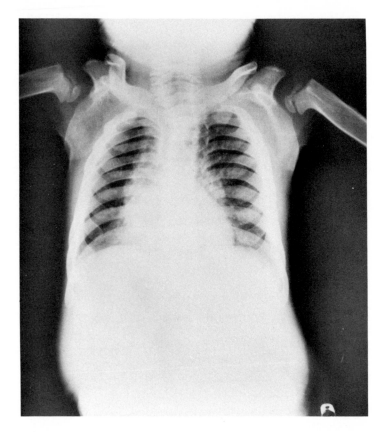

Fig. 11-5. Chest x-ray film of G. V. D., Jr. (B2188), 4½ years of age. This patient has the Hurler syndrome in entirely typical form. He reached a peak of intellectual development at about 2 years and has deteriorated since then. Gibbus was noted at 1 year. Thick skin, lanugo, "shoe-shaped" sella turcica, and ground-glass corneas are present. Hydrocele and right inguinal hernia were treated surgically at the age of 1½ years. The central infiltrations of the lungs were present in an unchanged form for at least 6 months. Tuberculin skin tests were negative. The changes are believed to be the result of chronic bronchopneumonia. However, interstitial pulmonary infiltration as part of the disease and analogous to the infiltrations elsewhere cannot be excluded. The opacification of the upper abdomen by hepatosplenomegaly, the broad ribs, the varus deformity of the proximal ends of the humeri, and the deformed scapulae, which are elevated because of the stiff shoulder joints, are evident.

pressure. Enormous optic foramina are often demonstrable by special radiographic views.[282a]

The shape of lips, which are large and patulous, the apathetic facies, the open mouth, and, frequently, the enlarged tongue, may lead to a false diagnosis of cretinism. In general, the facial features are coarse and ugly. The teeth are usually small, stubby, widely spaced, and malformed. In many of the cases there is hypertrophy both of the bony alveolar ridges and of the overlying gums.[77] An actual bone cyst of the alveolar ridge was present in one of Caffey's cases.[49] Chronic "rhinitis" with noisy mouth breathing is virtually universal in this group of patients. X-ray films of the skull and face usually show marked deformities, which may be responsible for the nasal manifestations. The inferior surface of the sphenoid bone approximates the back of the hard palate, narrowing the nasopharyngeal airway. A mass of adenoid tissue often obliterates the remaining air shadow.

The neck is exceedingly short, so that the head appears to rest directly on the thorax, which is deformed. There is usually a flaring of the lower rib cage, probably due in part to the hepatosplenomegaly. Kyphosis with gibbus in the lower thoracic and upper lumbar area is likely to be present. Myelograms in one case revealed partial obstruction of the spinal canal at the level of the gibbus. Radiologic examination usually shows wedge-shaped deformity of the vertebral body at the apex of the gibbus. This vertebra often has an anterior hooklike projection, so-called beaking of the vertebra. In some instances this beaking appears to be caused by anterior herniation of the nucleus pulposus,[23] with pressure atrophy of the upper anterior margin of the subjacent vertebral body (usually the second lumbar). (See Fig. 11-2C and reference 49.) The gibbus is often the first observed abnormality. When the infant begins to sit, he is likely to assume a posture like a cat's sitting (Fig. 11-2B), the "cat-back deformity." Swischuk[513] proposed a plausible common denominator for the beaked, notched, or hooked vertebra that occurs characteristically at the upper lumbar level or thoracolumbar junction, not only in the Hurler syndrome, but also in cretinism, achondroplasia, and various conditions of abnormal hypotonia and laxity. He maintained that the beaked vertebra is the result, not of primary hypoplasia of the vertebral body, but rather of damage caused by the hyperflexion at the thoracolumbar junction which occurs in the hypotonic child with sitting. The occurrence of the same lesion after acute traumatic hyperflexion supports his hypothesis. A similar finding occurs in generalized gangliosidosis.

The hands are usually broad, with stubby fingers.[485] The fifth fingers are often bent radially, and, in general, there is likely to be at least partial flexion contracture of the fingers as well as of the larger joints. The terminal phalangeal bones are often hypoplastic, as can be demonstrated both by x-ray examination and clinically. Clawhand is present in most patients more than a few years old. (See Figs. 11-1, 11-11, and 11-14.) This deformity results from stiffening of the phalangeal joints, with incapacity for full extension.

Limitation in extensibility of joints is usually striking.[219] This feature may be due in part to deformity of the joint surfaces but is more likely the result of changes in the tendons and ligaments surrounding the joints. Thus patients often find it necessary to walk on their toes, especially if they have been in bed for extended periods. A deformity of the wrist may superficially suggest rickets. However, the stiff joints (along with many other features) help distinguish the Hurler syndrome[211]; the joints in rickets are more limber than normal. The limitation of motion of joints seems to extend to the thorax, which often is relatively fixed in position.[130]

In addition to the radiologic changes already described in the skull and in the vertebral column, the bones of the limbs are abnormal in appearance. Caffey[49] pointed out that metaphyseal changes are mild and that the predominant change involves the diaphyses. The tubular bones show a swelling of the shaft due to expansion of the medullary cavity. The cortex may be thinned. Changes tend to be more striking in the bones of the upper than in the lower limbs. A curious narrowing of the proximal third of the femora to a caliber less than half that of normal has been noted.[49] The phalangeal bones are short and misshapen, with wide shafts and constricted ends (Fig. 11-4C). The ribs are characteristically broad, saber-shaped, or spatulate (Figs. 11-4A and 11-5). The vertebral ends of the ribs are unusually narrow, particularly by comparison with the remainder of the rib. (The radiologic changes in most of the conditions discussed in this chapter have been fully detailed by Grossman and Dorst.[184])

Genu valgum, coxa valga, pes planus, and other deformities occur frequently. Deformity of the sternum has been said[222] not to be a feature; however, congenital deformity of one type or another has been seen (Fig. 11-11).[248] "Funnel chest" was present in one of Hurler's cases[233] and in one of mine.

The abdomen is protuberant, due in part to hepatosplenomegaly, in part to

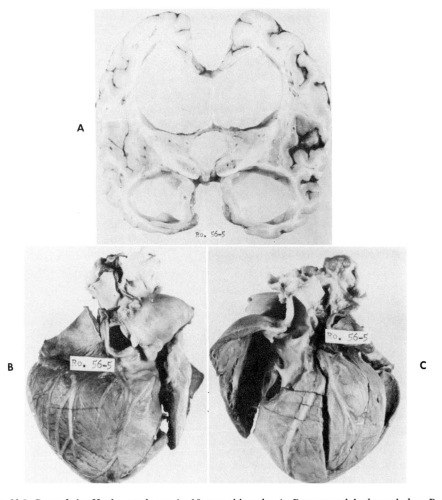

Fig. 11-6. Case of the Hurler syndrome in 10-year-old male. **A,** Pronounced hydrocephalus. Possibly involvement of the meninges is responsible. **B** and **C,** Two views of the heart. The coronaries are obviously thickened.

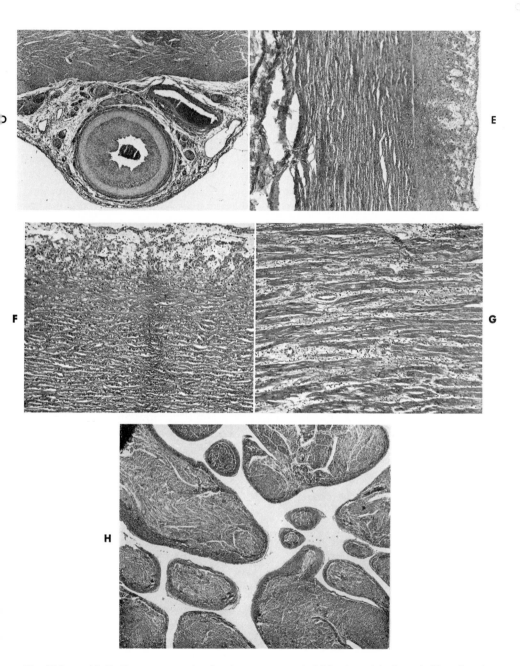

Fig. 11-6, cont'd. D, Coronary arteries showing pronounced thickening of intima. (×30; reduced ⅝.) **E,** Section of pulmonary artery showing enormous thickening of intima. (×67; reduced ⅝.) **F,** Section of aorta showing, in addition to intimal deposit, inclusion-laden connective tissue cells between the elastic lamellae. **G,** Section of myocardium showing infiltration of connective tissue cells laden with inclusion material. (×100; reduced ⅝.) **H,** Endocardial thickening surrounding the carneous trabeculae of the ventricle is evident. (×30; reduced ⅓.)

the defect of the supporting tissues. Both liver and spleen may be so large that their lower borders dip into the pelvis. One patient developed pancytopenia and epistaxes, possibly on the basis of hypersplenism.[485] Lindsay[290] described an abnormal hippuric acid test in one patient and, in another, prolonged elevation of galactose in the blood after intravenous injection. The number of patients tested was not stated. Although no systematic study has been made, the impression is given that surprisingly little functional impairment results from the marked gross and histologic involvement of the liver.

McCormick[312] reported fatal rupture of the stomach in a 6-year-old boy who had suffered from repeated episodes of gastric dilatation. Diastasis recti and umbilical hernia are almost invariable, and inguinal hernia is frequent. Engel[134] described scrotal hernias the size of a child's head. Bilateral hydrocele is also seen.[195]

In most of the cases the entire surface of the body, including both trunk and limbs, is covered by fine, lanugo-like fuzz. In older patients, too, hairiness is quite striking, especially over the arms and hands (Fig. 11-11*B* and *C*); it is a feature of all the mucopolysaccharidoses. Nodular thickening of the skin, of the type described later under MPS II (Fig. 11-12*A*), may be unusual in MPS I H.

No consistent endocrine abnormality is clinically detectable, in spite of the histologic evidence of cellular deposits in most glands of internal secretion. Thyroid enlargement without dysfunction has been described and is probably related to the histologic infiltration referred to. Hypoglycemia from hepatic involvement is thought to be a risk but has not actually been demonstrated, to my knowledge. The deformity of the sella turcica is part of the disorder of bone and not a result of enlargement of the pituitary.

Clouding of the cornea develops in all cases of MPS I. The cornea usually has merely a steamy appearance in earlier stages. On inspection this feature is most apparent if light is shined on the cornea from the side. Slit-lamp examination confirms the finding. The opacities are located in the medial and deeper layers of the cornea. The epithelium and endothelium are spared. Other ocular abnormalities such as buphthalmos[96] and megalocornea[28,127,233,366] have been described. There may be a retinal element in visual impairment, since histopathologic changes in the retina have been described,[291] and the electroretinogram is diminished or "extinguished" in many cases.[167]

Mental retardation is a conspicuous feature of all cases of MPS I H. Hydrocephalus may occur in severely affected infants.[10,290] Some patients may show simple dilatation of the ventricles, secondary to cortical atrophy.[533] There is true internal hydrocephalus in some cases; the ventricular dilatation is too marked to be accounted for on the basis of cortical atrophy alone (Fig. 11-6*A*). The mental deterioration is likely to be progressive, resembling juvenile amaurotic idiocy in this respect.[233] There may be accompanying neurologic signs such as motor paralysis, increase in muscular tone, and the Babinski sign.

One would presume that deafness is, in the main, secondary to the bone disease, as in osteogenesis imperfecta. In a 16-month-old child and a 2-year-old child studied by Dr. William G. Hardy of The Johns Hopkins Hearing and Speech Clinic, the deafness was of the conductive type, and in a 3-year-old patient hearing was unimpaired. Because of the deformity of the nasopharynx, these patients probably have more than the average susceptibility to middle ear infection. Furthermore, the ossicles have shown deformity with limitation of joint motion as in other joints and bones.[566] Therefore, a conductive element in the deafness of some patients is to be expected.

Nasal congestion, noisy mouth breathing, and frequent upper respiratory infections occur in essentially all patients with the Hurler syndrome. The malformation of the facial and nasal bones is probably in large part responsible. Ellis and associates[127] commented on this feature. Most other writers have also emphasized it and considered malformation of the nasopharynx to be its basis. The teeth tend to be small and widely spaced in the mucopolysaccharidoses. Dentigerous cysts have been described.[59]

Murmurs also were described by Meyer and Okner,[366] Engel,[134] and others. Ashby and co-workers[10] described "congenital heart disease" as the cause of death at 9 years of age in one child and in a 19-year-old patient who died suddenly. Mouth breathing and dyspnea resulting from thoracic deformity and restriction of expansion[130] (which may be very striking), abnormality of the bronchial cartilages, and, finally, frequent attacks of bronchitis and pneumonia make it difficult to determine that part of the dyspnea which has a cardiac basis. The best specific descriptions of the cardiovascular aspects of the Hurler syndrome are those of Lindsay[290] and Emanuel.[130] Emanuel described in 2 brothers cardiac signs he interpreted as being those of pulmonary hypertension. In one, cardiac catheterization demonstrated a much elevated pulmonary artery pressure (88/50 mm. Hg). The peripheral arteries of the arms were described as thickened in a $6\frac{1}{2}$-year-old child,[291] and there was hypertension (132/100 mm. Hg). Some of the above cases were probably instances of MPS II (p. 556). Catheterization and angiocardiographic studies were reported by Krovetz and associates,[264] who demonstrated increased total systemic, total pulmonary, and pulmonary arterial resistance in patients with the Hurler syndrome.

What was interpreted as angina pectoris occurred[77] as early as $4\frac{3}{4}$ years of age in a child who died at the age of 7 years. The extensive occlusive disease of the coronary arteries discovered at autopsy in this child suggests that it is the basis of sudden death in many of these patients (Fig. 11-6).

Lindsay[290] stated that systolic murmurs along the left sternal border were so striking in these patients that 4 of 16 were suspected of having an interventricular septal defect. There was a similar clinical experience in the group of cases at The Johns Hopkins Hospital. The experience with other heritable disorders of connective tissue, specifically the Marfan and Ehlers-Danlos syndromes, in which cardiac malformations of the conventional types occur with predictably increased frequency, suggests that the same might occur in the Hurler syndrome. Pathologic studies have not corroborated this suspicion (see below). Although some cardiovascular abnormality was present in the great majority of patients who have died, all the changes have been of a specific type, as described later.

Krovetz and associates[264] found that the dosage of premedication required for cardiac catheterization in patients with the Hurler syndrome was two or three times greater than that usually required, and others[109] have commented on the relative resistance to sedation.

The clinical diagnosis is corroborated biochemically by identifying excessive mucopolysaccharide in the urine and by finding metachromatic granules in the circulating lymphocytes or bone marrow cells. Methods for these tests are detailed later (p. 629). The last courts of appeal in the diagnosis of the Hurler syndrome are the Neufeld type of co-cultivation experiment (p. 635) using standard reference cell lines and, as the artificial substrate for the assay becomes available, test for the specific deficiency of α-L-iduronidase.

The following narrative by an intelligent and observing father outlines the evolution of the Hurler syndrome up to the age of about 4 years:

My impression is that her most difficult period was roughly that of her first to second year. Deafness appeared, so far as we could tell, shortly after her first birthday, becoming complete by about 16 to 18 months of age. Around this time the more pronounced abdominal swelling also began to show, and she was sick much of the time. Nights were very difficult for her and everyone during this time, and until a bit beyond 2 years of age, she would cry for hours, perhaps in pain. On the other hand, she has seemed to be a bit less sensitive to outside pain than the other children. After the crying spells began to diminish, her personality became more buoyant. During the last year or more, *angelic* would scarcely be too strong a word. She radiates love and affection and thoughtfulness, coupled with a good sense of humor. Her motor skills have kept up remarkably well; she ate with a spoon before 1 year and has kept it up with normal increase in proficiency; she was diaper-trained by about 2½ years and bed-trained by about 3¼ years, with no unusual effort; although the gait is a bit awkward because of underdevelopment of leg muscles and a very large abdomen, she loves to run and dance and slide and swing. Picture books are great favorites; animals are adored, as are dolls and cuddly toys, toward which she is quite maternal. Vision seems still acute, although cloudiness is apparent in the cornea. She dresses and undresses herself as far as her build permits and is almost fastidious about putting away clothes, hanging things up, removing dishes to the sink after eating, etc. (this behavior pronounced since 3 years of age). Simple cutout jigsaw puzzles she handles well. She understands gestures and expressions perfectly and uses them herself for very efficient communication. During April and May of this year (at the age of 3¾ years) she was a day pupil at a nursery school for the deaf. Since September she has been a Monday to Friday boarding pupil at a state institution for deaf children. Here a very capable teacher seems to be making progress with lip reading and vocalization instruction. Other than the direct Hurler's symptoms, her general health has been reasonably good: chickenpox, several periods of respiratory infection each year; and occasional (every six weeks or so?) flash fevers to about 103° F., which are over in a few hours, leaving her worn out for a day. Her teeth have never developed fully, even now being little more than widely separated stumps; however, she can handle, and seems to enjoy, practically any kind of food.

My wife and I feel that, at least until quite recently, her intelligence has been essentially normal. She usually learns new patterns of action, or placement of objects, or play, after only one or two repetitions—unless something arouses the stubbornness, of which she has a powerful streak. She watches the other children playing, with close comprehension of their actions and antics, often either joining or copying, nearly always enjoying. She knows all the clothing in the house, often bringing the appropriate items, in proper order, to those of us getting dressed. In driving, she will often back-seat drive, telling me which turns to take, by murmurs and gestures, even when we are several miles from home but headed for it. She sets great store on the proper way of doing things! Her sleep is now peaceful, 11 hours a night and usually an hour's nap; even when she is tired her personality holds up cheerfully. When hurt in any way she usually cries but little; however, the offended member *must* be kissed to make the hurt go away.

It is possible that her rate of development is slowing down; she is learning, or at least responding, among the slowest members of her eighteen-pupil nursery class. Also, recently there has been pronounced increase in the swelling. Our local pediatrician believes that the liver is almost entirely responsible for the more than double normal girth, and that x-ray treatment might offer her a palliative. Should the swelling become much greater, walking will become extremely difficult. Difficulties with respiratory disease might have been too much for her system already, before modern drugs; except for a couple of summer months, there is a constant nasal discharge of varying rate of flow. Her circulation seems to have its troubles, in that lips and fingernails are often very blue.

As further illustration, the following 2 patients, brothers, are described in detail:

Case 1. P. H. (J.H.H. 818143), the product of a normal pregnancy, is the elder son of unrelated healthy parents. He was considered a healthy baby, and initial development was uneventful, but a gibbus of the thoracolumbar spine and pectus excavatum were noted at 3 months of age. No specific diagnosis was made until the age of 13 months, when the patient already exhibited many of the classic features of the autosomal recessive Hurler syndrome. He stood at 9 months but walking was poor, partly, the parents feel, because corneal clouding was already dimming vision. Other Hurler features at the age of 13 months included the "gargoyle facies" and broad, short, stubby fingers with clawhand deformity. Most of the other joints also showed early limitation of movement, with flexion contractures in some. The abdomen was prominent, though without hernias, and the lower thoracic cage was flared; the neck was short and thick, and there was a pronounced sagittal ridge. The teeth were widely spaced and poorly formed, and respirations were noisy. Deafness was marked, although there was no evidence of past otitis media.

By 21 months, progression of the disease was obvious, with marked impairment of intellect and enlargement of the head, and the child had ceased to walk. Attempts at toilet training had been unsuccessful. Gross motor and neurosensory functions were normal and there were no heart murmurs. While showing severe deafness to pure tones of 2,000 and 4,000 cycles per second at 80 to 90 decibels, the child babbled in a relatively normal fashion, indicating that at one time hearing must have been nearly normal.

Laboratory studies at 21 months yielded normal results and included routine hematology, urinalysis, fasting blood sugar, total cholesterol, calcium, phosphorus, albumin and globulin, and alkaline phosphatase. Reilly bodies were not found in the peripheral leukocytes. An electrocardiogram and lumbar puncture were normal, but an electroencephalogram showed mild diffuse abnormalities. An intravenous infusion of glucose showed a diabetic pattern, but there were no other diabetic stigmata. Glucagon stimulation and an insulin tolerance test were normal.

X-ray films at this time showed slight cardiac enlargement. The long bones showed shortening and widening of the shafts with lack of tubulation. The distal ends of the radii and humeri showed abnormalities in angulation and configuration. The skull was enlarged, with prominence of the frontal and parietal bones, and in the lateral view the sella turcica showed the typical slipper shape. The spinal x-ray films revealed angulation between L1 and L2, with beaking along the anterior surfaces of these vertebrae. The pelvis was wide, with large, shallow, angulated acetabular shelves; coxa valga was present. The metacarpals and phalanges showed shortening and broadening, with the proximal ends pointed, whereas the ribs were broad and spatulate.

Urinary studies of mucopolysaccharide excretion were performed at the ages of 5 and 7 years. On both occasions considerable amounts of both dermatan sulfate and heparan sulfate were found.

The patient, now 7 years of age, is completely bedfast, exhibiting huge hydrocephalus, with an open anterior fontanelle. Undoubtedly this is playing a large part in the general picture, particularly as a cause of the extreme apathy. The facial features have become progressively gross, and the corneas are opaque to the extent that the pupils cannot be visualized. Estimates of the hepatomegaly, over the years, have varied from 3 to 8 cm. and of the splenomegaly, from 0 to 2 cm. below the costal margin. At no time has there been evidence of valvular heart damage.

Follow-up. This patient died at the age of 10 years.

Case 2. M. H. (J.H.H. 1038296), the younger and only sib of Case 1, was noted at birth to have a curved back and a depression of the front of the chest. Despite this deformity he was considered to be a normal baby until, between the ages of 6 and 12 months, his facial features were noted to be taking on appearances similar to those of his brother. He walked at 2 years and learned to utter a few syllables; true speech, however, was never attained. From an early

Table 11-3. Two brothers with the Hurler syndrome (MPS I H)

Case 1* P. H. (J.H.H. 818143) 5 years	Case 2* M. H. (J.H.H. 1038296) 4 years
Weight, 40 pounds	Weight, 42 pounds
Length, 36½ inches; chest, 23 inches	Length, 39 inches; chest, 24 inches
Head circumference, 27 inches (hydrocephalic)	Head circumference, 21½ inches
Severe mental retardation	Mental retardation
Unable to sit or talk; deaf	Able to walk but not talk; deaf
Typical Hurler facies	Same
Edema of eyelids	Same
Widely spaced teeth	Same
Corneal opacity	Same
Low-set ears	Same
Lanugo	Same
Hands and feet wide, with clawhand	Same
Cool lower extremities	Warm lower extremities
Slight lumbar gibbus	Large lumbar gibbus
Stiff joints	Moderately stiff joints
Pectus excavatum	More severe pectus excavatum
Rhonchi	Same
Liver edge 3 cm. below costal margin	Same
No palpable spleen	Spleen tip 2 cm. below costal margin
No hernia	Surgical repair of inguinal hernias
Decreased femoral pulses	Pulses normal
Uncircumcised	Circumcised

*The patients died at the ages of 10 and 12 years, respectively.

age respirations were noisy, and bilateral inguinal hernias were repaired at 6 weeks and 7 months, respectively.

By the age of 4 years mental retardation was severe, and examination revealed most of the signs of Hurler syndrome. These are tabulated and compared to those of his brother in Table 11-3. X-ray films at this time were also classic. The spine showed vertebral changes, affecting D12, L1, and L2 in particular, and there was anterior "beaking." The bones of the upper extremity were thickened and short, particularly the metacarpals, which showed "pointing" at both proximal and distal ends. The skull was somewhat enlarged, with hyperostosis of the sagittal suture, and the sella turcica was elongated. The pelvis showed shallow acetabula and there was coxa valga. The ribs were typically broad and spatulate with coarse trabeculations.

Urinary studies at the age of 4 years revealed increased excretion of mucopolysaccharide, composed of a large fraction of dermatan sulfate and a smaller heparan sulfate fraction. Routine study of a peripheral blood film revealed no abnormality.

At the age of 5, the boy described as Case 2 has deteriorated further and has ceased to walk, preferring to crawl. His eyesight is poor due to corneal opacities, and his mental function approaches the imbecile level.

Peripheral blood smears were taken from both boys and stained with toluidine blue. Definite metachromatic granules were seen in the cytoplasm of 18% of the lymphocytes of Case 1 and in 10% of those of Case 2.

Follow-up. This patient died at the age of 12 years.

Pathology

The first autopsy in a case of MPS I H was reported by Tuthill,[531] an American working in Munich, who examined one of Hurler's original cases. At least 40 autopsies had been reported when a count was made in 1965: many individual case reports,[10,22,105,130,180,198,236,257,263,326,368,466,485,507,508,531,533,536,552] 2 by Jervis,[233] 8 by Lindsay and co-workers,[291] and so on. Jackson[222] and others have reported on biopsies of the liver.

Abnormalities have been identified in, among other sites, cartilage, fasciae, tendons, periosteum, blood vessels, heart valves, meninges, and cornea. All these tissues may contain cells that are thought to be of the fibroblast line and are distended with large amounts of deposited material. They are appropriately called "clear cells" by Millman and Whittick,[368] but perhaps it would be preferable to use the more specific designation "gargoyle cells."[521] In addition, collagen in many of these areas has been said to look abnormal in a poorly defined way. Collagen fibers are described by some (e.g., reference 290) as swollen, homogeneous, and lacking in their normal fibrillary characteristics. Material presumably identical to that in the fibroblasts balloons the nerve cells of both the central nervous system and the peripheral ganglia, the nerve cells in the nuclear layer of the retina,[291] the Kupffer cells of the liver, the parenchymal cells of the liver, the reticulum cells of the spleen and lymph nodes, and the epithelial cells of several endocrine organs such as the pituitary[263] and testis. Mental retardation and hepatosplenomegaly are explained by these deposits.

Enlargement and vacuolization of the chondrocytes and osteocytes, as well as of the periosteal cells, are described[34,291] and probably are intimately related to the skeletal malformation.

In the heart, in persons dying after a few years of life, the aortic and mitral valves almost invariably have shown some degree of nodular thickening,[130,291] as well as changes in the chordae tendineae.[34] Functionally both stenosis and regurgitation can result. In the case of Smith and co-workers[485] the histologic picture in the heart valves was dominated by the presence of "gargoyle cells." These cells have also been seen in the coronary arteries.[74,291,326] Grossly[130] even in young individuals the coronary arteries may "stand out like white cords." Virtually complete occlusion may result from the extensive intimal deposits.[77,98] The aorta[326] and pulmonary artery[130] may also show intimal deposits, presumably of the same material that forms the vacuoles of the cells of various organs. The myocardial cells may show marked ballooning by vacuoles (see photomicrograph, reference 32). Patchy thickening of the endocardium and epicardium is described.[130,291,508] Of the peripheral arteries, changes have been described in those of the brain, spleen, pancreas, and kidney, as well as in the mesenteric, carotid, radial, and anterior tibial arteries.

Emanuel[130] was able to find 32 autopsy reports, with specific description of the heart provided in 26. (Some were undoubtedly instances of MPS II.) Of the 26 patients, 22 had cardiovascular abnormalities (85%). In 15 patients the mitral valve was deformed, in 9 the aortic, in 7 the tricuspid, and in 2 the pulmonary. In 3 (including Emanuel's case) all four valves, the epicardium, the endocardium, the coronary arteries, and the aorta and pulmonary artery were involved.[291,508]

It is of note that the order of incidence of involvement of the heart valves—mitral, aortic, tricuspid, pulmonary—is precisely as in rheumatic fever. In both situations at least two prominent factors are probably operating: the metabolic aberration (in one case acquired, in the other inherited) and the hemo-

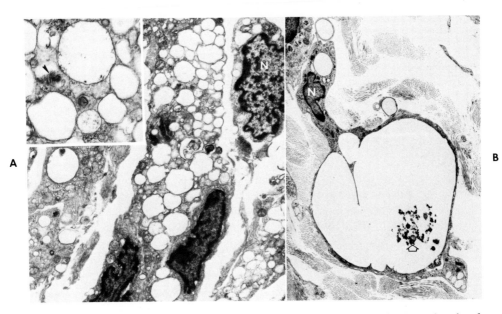

Fig. 11-7. A, Electron micrograph of the thickened skin from a 4-year-old Caucasian female (C. M., J.H.H. 1315339) with the Hurler syndrome (MPS I H). The connective tissue cells of the dermis are markedly vacuolated. Inset: The intracellular vacuoles are limited by a single-unit membrane and have predominantly clear-to-fine granular contents with occasional membranous lamellar inclusions (arrow). There are no collections of abnormal extracellular material. **N,** Nucleus (×7100; inset, ×21,000). **B,** Electron micrograph of conjunctival connective tissue from a 4-year-old Caucasian female (C. M., J.H.H. 1315339) with the Hurler syndrome (MPS I H) and corneal clouding. The ballooned histiocyte is a striking example of the "gargoyle" cell, in which a single immense storage vacuole (measuring approximately 14 mμ in diameter) has displaced the nucleus, **N,** and other cytoplasmic components. Electron-dense lipoid globules (arrow) are evident within the intracellular vacuole, but no abnormal extracellular accumulations are present in the collagenous stroma. (×5000.) (Courtesy Kenneth R. Kenyon and Harry A. Quigley, Baltimore, Md.)

dynamic stresses. The peak pressures* sustained by the four valves in the position of closure are in the same sequence as the incidence of valve involvement: mitral, 120 mm. Hg; aortic, 80 mm. Hg; tricuspid, 25 mm. Hg; pulmonary, 12 mm. Hg.

Vanace and co-workers[539] described advanced mitral stenosis in a boy who died at the age of 5½ years. No clouding of the cornea was noted, but slit-lamp examination was not done. (As indicated on p. 640, it has been suggested that this patient had a "new" type of mucopolysaccharidosis called geleophysic dwarfism.) Lagunoff and associates[269] studied the mitral valve in one case and concluded that two types of cells are present—one containing glycolipid and one containing acid mucopolysaccharide.

Okada and colleagues[411] found involvement of the conduction system by increased fibrous tissue in the 2 cases they studied.

A conventional type of congenital malformation of the heart has been thought

---

*All values here are approximations.

clinically to be present in some patients seen at this hospital. Seemingly, however, no such malformation has been revealed by any of the pathologic studies.

Abnormality of the tracheobronchial cartilages together with that of the upper airways may be responsible for the susceptibility to respiratory infection in these patients. Bronchopneumonia is a frequent cause of death.[233]

Kobayashi[258] demonstrated granules of acid mucopolysaccharide in the epithelial cells of the glomeruli of 3 patients. He discussed their relationship to the mucopolysacchariduria and the Reilly granules. Cole and associates[70] illustrate a histologic section of skin that was interpreted as showing "marked fragmentation of collagen fibers and mucinous degeneration."

Vacuolated cells (Fig. 11-7) have been described in Bowman's membrane by Berliner[28] and by others. Lindsay and co-workers[291] described highly metachromatic granules in the cornea. The literature on the corneal histopathology was reviewed by Scheie and co-workers,[463] with the addition of information from several cases. The basal layer of the epithelium shows edema, cytoplasmic vacuolization, and metachromatic cytoplasmic granules. Bowman's membrane is replaced in part by large cells with vacuolated cytoplasm and metachromatic cytoplasmic granules. Corneal corpuscles in the stroma likewise contain metachromatic granules. Conjunctival biopsy may be positive in all cases with corneal clouding and has been recommended[463] as a simple diagnostic procedure. The connective tissue of the conjunctiva shows monocytes with toluidine blue–positive granules in the cytoplasm. (These corneal and conjunctival findings are also present in MPS I S,[427] MPS IV, and MPS VI.[247] Conjunctival biopsy provides useful material for electron microscopy.) Mailer[328] found optic atrophy in a patient who died at the age of 20 months and suggested that increased intracranial pressure was a causative factor.

The skin of the fingers was shown by Hambrick and Scheie[188] to be useful for biopsy in MPS I:

> The characteristic cellular lesion of Hurler's was present within the skin from all sites, clinically normal or abnormal. This consisted of a peculiar, granular vacuolization of the cytoplasm of epithelial cells and fibrocytes of the dermis. The degree of involvement of the epidermis may be quite extensive, particularly in the skin of the involved fingers.*

The granules have metachromatic tinctorial properties and are positive for stains relatively specific for mucopolysaccharides.

Extensive changes in the leptomeninges were described by Magee.[326] The coincidence of subdural hematoma in his case makes these changes difficult to interpret. However, others report extensive changes in the meninges.[98,180,453] Millman and Whittick[368] found thickening of the leptomeninges over the cerebral hemispheres and "clear cells" histologically. In Njå's[388] Case 2, an instance of MPS II, there was hydrocephalus with "thickened and milky leptomeninges." The hydrocephalus[453] may be the result of interference with drainage, produced by the deposits characteristic of the disease.[181] The frequency of hydrocephalus (Fig. 11-6*A*) has been underestimated. It is probably an important factor in the cerebral impairment in these patients.

---

*From Hambrick, G. W., and Scheie, H. G.: Arch. Derm. **85**:455, 1962.

Neuhauser and colleagues[384] described the autopsy features of arachnoid cysts. Although they are situated predominantly in the area anterior to the sella turcica, they are also found below the cerebellum. The cysts are apparently related to leptomeningeal fibrosis. No ill effects of the cysts *per se* have been noted. There has been no evidence of damage to the pituitary, hypothalamus, or visual tracts. However, the cysts may contribute to difficulties in cerebrospinal fluid flow and therefore to the hydrocephalus.

Greenfield and associates[181] describe the central nervous system changes as being predominantly a distention of the nerve cells of the cerebral cortex with little or no defect of myelination. A peculiar feature of the Hurler syndrome is "the presence in the centrum semiovale and medullary cores of the gyri of greatly enlarged perivascular spaces."

Formalin or alcohol dissolves the vacuolar material.[34] Some reported failures[98,291,507] to stain the material in postmortem tissues may have their bases in this fact. Dioxane-dinitrophenol fixative has been useful[291] in preserving the deposited material. In the study of mucopolysaccharides in the tissues of cases of mucopolysaccharidosis, the best method, in the opinion of Haust and Landing,[193] is to cut frozen sections of unstained tissue and then fix in a 1:1 mixture of tetrahydrofuran and acetone. In their view, lead acetate is a poor fixative because it preserves mucopolysaccharide poorly and interferes with metachromatic staining. Scheie and associates[463] found that absolute alcohol, Carnoy's solution, trichloroacetic acid, acridine, and lead acetate, in descending order, gave the best preservation of mucopolysaccharides in skin biopsies.

Some have reported that the intracellular deposits take conventional fat stains.[32,191,531] Most, however, have found that the vacuoles do not stain as fat, or that they stain atypically.[485] Analyses of hepatic and splenic tissue for fat reveal no increase.[198,507,521] The material may stain with periodic acid–Schiff's reagent (PAS) or with Best's carmine. It displays striking metachromasia.[536] Bishton and colleagues[34] suggest that even if precautions are taken to prevent solution of the material deposited in the liver, one cannot expect satisfactory staining of "heparin-type" polysaccharides by the periodic acid–Schiff technique. They recommend use of toluidine blue as a stain in these cases.

Histochemical studies led Lindsay and collaborators[291] to suspect that the storage material is glycoprotein. Brante[41] isolated a material, polysaccharide in nature, having 0.9% sulfur, 27% hexosamine, and 26% glucuronic acid, containing no fatty acids by hydrolysis, and representing 10% of the dry weight of the liver. Uzman[536] described two storage materials isolated from the liver and spleen of these patients: (1) a complex polysaccharide containing glucose, galactose, hexosamines, and sulfate, soluble in water and formaldehyde but insoluble in other organic solvents, and staining metachromatically with toluidine blue; (2) a glycolipid, soluble in water and ethanol but not in other organic solvents, and containing fatty acids, sphingosine, neuraminic acid, hexuronic acid, hexosamines, glucose, and galactose. Uzman refers to these two storage materials as fractions P and S, respectively. Stacey and Baker[499] reported the presence of sulfated polysaccharide fractions as well as of nonsulfated fractions, the latter somewhat related to blood group–specific substances. Brown[44] has proposed a possible molecular structure of the material he isolated in large amounts from the liver of patients with the Hurler syndrome and has referred to it as an oligosaccharide.

By his evidence the material is composed exclusively of D-glucosamine and D-glucuronic acid units combined in glycosidic linkage. The material in point may be identical to the type of mucopolysaccharide called heparan sulfate by Meyer.[356] Meyer and colleagues[360] found large amounts of heparan sulfate in the liver of one patient.

Dawson[98] thought that the deposits in the brain consisted of phospholipid, although those elsewhere seemed to be mucopolysaccharide. Uzman[536] did not study brain. Meyer[358] found that mucopolysaccharide (both dermatan sulfate and heparan sulfate) was deposited in the brain in appreciable amounts.

There has accumulated in the last decade an extensive literature on the electron microscopic changes in the liver[51,52,194,243,267,295,542] and to a lesser extent in other tissues[119,539a] in the Hurler syndrome. These findings, together with the general natural history of the Hurler syndrome, led to the characterization of this and related disorders as lysosomal diseases.[200] The same changes are found in noncultivated (i.e., *in situ*) fibroblasts and macrophages of skin[100] and conjunctiva[245] and in cultured skin fibroblasts.[17] "Membranous cytoplasmic bodies" were also described in ganglion and satellite cells of intramural plexi of the rectal wall obtained by biopsy[129] in a patient with the Hunter syndrome (MPS II) and probably would be found also in MPS I. (The changes at the last site were thought to be causally related to chronic diarrhea in the Hunter syndrome[129]; diarrhea has also been described in MPS VI [p. 611].)

The fundamental defect

Excessive urinary excretion of dermatan sulfate and heparan sulfate[116,360] in patients with MPS I H indicate that a defect in mucopolysaccharide metabolism is the basic fault. (Mucopolysaccharides are also elevated in the plasma of these patients.[50,455]) Although theories of abnormality in substances other than mucopolysaccharides had been proposed previously,[70,106,127,291,507,508,552] and although excessive synthesis or some other disturbance[360] of mucopolysaccharides has been postulated more recently, present evidence indicates that the Hurler syndrome results from a defect in the degradation of mucopolysaccharides. As discussed in detail on p. 635, α-L-iduronidase is deficient in the Hurler syndrome.[15a,347a] The explanation for the fact that two mucopolysaccharides appear in the urine in MPS I is indicated diagrammatically in Fig. 11-8: both dermatan sulfate and heparan sulfate have iduronide as a component of their polysaccharide side-chains. Iduronidase is a lysosomal enzyme with a pH optimum of about 3.5[555a]

Prevalence and inheritance

Several cases of MPS I H in Negroes have been reported,[14,115,136,165,230,272,509,524] and we have observed a Negro family with 3 affected members (Fig. 11-3). The syndrome has been reported in Caucasians, in Chinese,[62,134] in Oriental Indians,[182,350] and in Egyptians.[13] It has been plausibly suggested[8] that the Hurler syndrome has an unusually high frequency in the province of L'Aquila in Italy. Although only 0.6% of the population of Italy lives in that province, at least 7 cases have been reported, as compared with about 50 cases in the entire Italian medical literature.

MPS I H displays features of inheritance consistent with an autosomal recessive trait.[187] Parental consanguinity[38,187] is frequent, and affection of multiple sibs

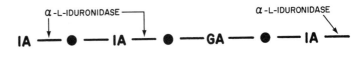

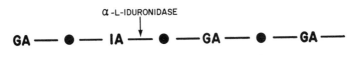

DERMATAN SULFATE

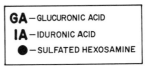

HEPARAN SULFATE

GA — GLUCURONIC ACID
IA — IDURONIC ACID
● — SULFATED HEXOSAMINE

Fig. 11-8. Schematic representation of polysaccharide side-chains of dermatan sulfate and heparan sulfate to show sites of degradative action of α-L-iduronidase and explaining the urinary excretion of two mucopolysaccharides in the Hurler and Scheie syndromes. (After a diagram of Dr. E. F. Neufeld.)

of both sexes without the occurrence of affected individuals in the preceding generation ("familial" characteristics) is often the case. There are no well-documented descriptions of skeletal deformities or other abnormalities in close relatives of patients to suggest that partial expression of the trait in the heterozygous state may occur. Concordance in identical twin sisters has been described.[390] Craig[77] described the disorder in a twin brother and sister.

In 1950, Jervis[233] reviewed the information on 103 families described in the literature. When the ratio of affected to unaffected sibs was corrected by the method of Bernstein and that of Lenz, no statistically significant disagreement with the expected 1:3 ratio was obtained. (Jervis did not recognize the possibility of a second genotype, the sex-linked recessive form—see below. If sex is not taken into account, a sex-linked recessive disorder will fulfill satisfactorily certain of the criteria for an autosomal recessive trait: both parents are phenotypically normal and one fourth of all children are affected. In the group analyzed by Jervis there were 93 affected males and 52 affected females. Halperin and Curtis[187] had earlier analyzed 40 published sibships with similar conclusions supporting autosomal recessive inheritance. The patient they pictured as a typical case almost certainly had the Hunter syndrome, as did also several of the reported families involved in their analysis.) Cousin marriages were *known* to have occurred in 11 of the 103 families and probably actually occurred in more. Using Hogben's formula, Jervis calculated that a 10% consanguinity rate would correspond to a phenotype frequency of 1 in 40,000. In British Columbia, Lowry and Renwick[305] estimated the frequency to be about 1 in 100,000, an entirely plausible value.[491a]

Management

The following discussion is relevant to others of the mucopolysaccharidoses.

No definitive treatment for the mucopolysaccharidoses is known, but several new approaches are under trial. Hurler,[219] in one of her original cases,[222] observed that desiccated thyroid, although having no measurable effect, produced subjective improvement in the patient. We have observed the same phenomenon (Fig. 11-11). Large doses of prednisone had no effect on urinary excretion of mucopolysaccharide.[186]

Supplemental vitamin A in the form of vitamin A alcohol was tried in patients with the Hurler and Hunter syndromes on the basis of vitamin A effects in clearing metachromasia in fibroblasts cultured from these patients.[29,86] No substantiated benefit could be observed in the patients, and possible harm can be done by aggravation of hydrocephalus.[163,374]

Vitamin C exaggerates the formation of mucopolysaccharides by fibroblasts in culture.[461] For this reason a scorbutigenic diet was tried in patients with the Hurler syndrome. Although there was no unequivocal improvement, the patient seemed unusually resistant to the development of scurvy, perhaps because of a low vitamin C requirement.[101]

Plasma infusions have been used by DiFerrante and co-workers[110] with apparent benefit. The rationale was the supply of the Neufeld correction factor. Correction of metachromasia by addition of normal plasma to cultured fibroblasts of MPS patients had been demonstrated.[208] However, Neufeld[383] states that assays for correction factor in blood show a low level of activity. Thus other mechanisms may be involved, in addition to simply supplying the correction factor. Knudsen and associates[256] transfused lymphocytes into a patient with the Hunter syndrome and observed striking clinical improvement as well as a rise in mucopolysaccharides, particularly partially degraded ones, in the urine.

DiFerrante and colleagues[110] also found that plasma infusion was followed by a decreased excretion of urinary acid mucopolysaccharides (AMPS) of relatively high molecular weight and an increased excretion of presumed products of degradation. They described the clinical changes as follows:

> Thus far, two patients with Hurler's syndrome and five with Hunter's syndrome have been treated. All the patients were hyperactive and difficult to manage prior to the infusion but became quiet and almost "sedated" during and after the infusion. Striking changes occurred in the skin; thick and cold before infusion, it became soft and warm and somewhat elastic during and after the infusion. The "claw hands" of a Hunter patient could be extended almost completely; the cold, rigid, and poorly vascularized extremities of a Hurler patient improved dramatically. The improved behavior of several patients lasted from a few weeks to about one month, to return abruptly to that observed prior to the infusion. It was frequently reported that during the "remission" period, the children would entertain themselves to some extent and show more attention to their environment.*

---

*From DiFerrante, N., Nichols, B. L., Donnelly, P. V., Neri, G., Hrgovcic, R., and Berglund, R. K.: Proc. Nat. Acad. Sci. **68**:303, 1971.

The long-term effectiveness of plasma therapy and its mode of action are not yet established. An objective way to demonstrate its effectiveness[321b] is by scanning of the reticuloendothelial system with technetium-99 colloidal sulfur.[108a,220a] Before plasma infusions very little uptake is observed, an expression of the well-known defect in this condition,[231] whereas after the infusions uptake returns to or toward normal. Repeat infusions have been necessary each 4 to 6 weeks. Even if replacement of enzyme is the mechanism of the improvement, improvement for several weeks might be expected in a lysosomal storage disease; accumulation is reduced and time is needed for reaccumulation. Complications of therapy, possibly immunologic in nature, have not been proved.[220a] Final evaluation of therapy is not yet available.

Crocker[80,80a] has discussed general problems in the management of patients with mucopolysaccharidoses and the impact of the disorder on the family.

Corneal transplants. Rosen and associates[448] performed penetrating keratoplasty on 2 patients with presumed Hurler's syndrome. Since they were 13 and 15 years old at the time of report and one was specifically described as of normal intelligence, the disorder may have been MPS VI (Maroteaux-Lamy syndrome). The transplant remained clear for three and two years, respectively, after operation. The older patient remained blind despite the surgical procedure, seemingly because of optic atrophy.

In cases of MPS I S reported by Scheie and colleagues[463] transplants became opacified, suggesting that the corneal clouding in this mucopolysaccharidosis and perhaps in the others as well is a consequence of deposition of mucopolysaccharide. It is possible that the opacification was a graft reaction, however, because it occurred within a few weeks after surgery. Lahdensuu[271] of Helsinki noted opacification of corneal transplants in 1 of 4 sibs who were labeled "Pfaundler-Hurlerschen Krankheit" but, as noted earlier, more likely suffered from MPS I S or VI.

In a case of MPS I H King[249] performed a lamellar corneal graft in one eye and a penetrating graft in the other. Whereas the first resulted in improved vision, the second never healed, with resulting loss of all vision. Lamellar grafts may therefore be the treatment of choice. Results are, of course, limited not only by severity of the generalized disease but also by the progressive retinal degeneration, which is now recognized as a feature of these disorders.

MUCOPOLYSACCHARIDOSIS I S (FORMERLY MPS V, SCHEIE SYNDROME)

This condition was described by Scheie and colleagues[463] as a variant of the Hurler syndrome, which indeed further studies show it to be. The same enzyme, α-L-iduronidase, is deficient in the Hurler and Scheie syndromes, and they are presumably allelic, like SS and CC diseases among the hemoglobinopathies.

MPS I, Scheie type, is characterized by major clouding of the cornea, deformity of the hands, and aortic valve involvement, with few other somatic effects and with normal intelligence.

Although formerly the Scheie syndrome was designated MPS V because it was thought to be quite distinct from other mucopolysaccharidoses, studies of its basic nature (see below) necessitated its reclassification as a type of MPS I. To avoid confusion, the numerical designation MPS V will not be reassigned. (In the field of blood-clotting factors, the designation factor VI has not been

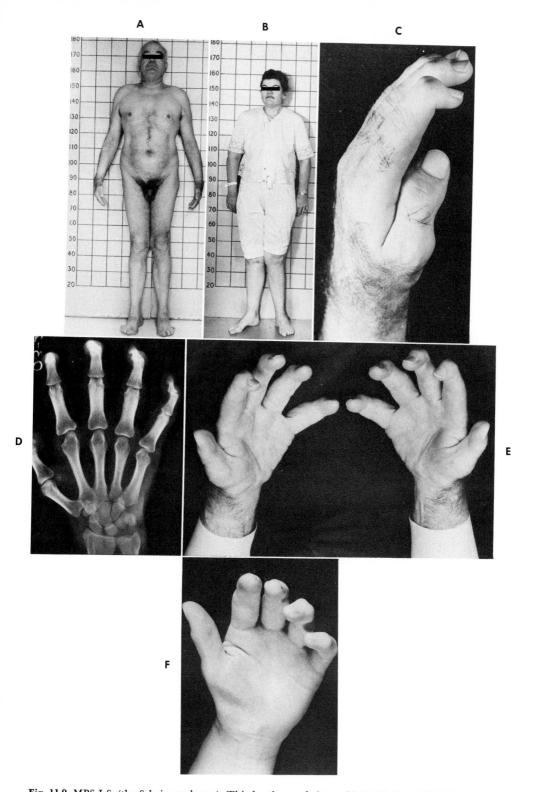

Fig. 11-9. MPS I S (the Scheie syndrome). This brother and sister (M. E. McC. and M. McC.) are described in detail in the text. **A** and **B,** General appearance. Hypertrichosis, genu valgum, misshapen foot, and "broad-mouthed" facies are noteworthy features. **C,** Clawhand in brother. **D,** X-ray film of hand in **C. E** and **F,** Atrophy of abducens pollicis brevis muscle, due to carpal tunnel compression of the median nerve, in brother, **E,** and in sister, **F.** See Plate 1*C,* for corneal clouding in the brother.

used after the demonstration that the factor tentatively so designated was not *bona fide*.) Undoubtedly, some writers will continue to use MPS V meaning Scheie syndrome.

Clinical manifestations

The intellect is impaired little or not at all. Scheie's patients were of "near genius" intelligence, and one of ours (Case 3, below) is an attorney of more than average intelligence. Stiff joints, clawhand deformity, excessive body hair, and "retinitis pigmentosa" occur, as in MPS II; however, corneal clouding, which is not evident grossly in MPS II, is a striking feature of MPS V. The clouding is most dense peripherally in some patients, although in others, particularly in the earlier stages, involvement is uniform. Both sibs reported below (Cases 3 and 4) developed glaucoma, at the ages of 51 and 40 years, respectively. Corneal grafts become opacified.[271,463] Stature is usually in the normal or low-normal range. The facies is characteristically "broad-mouthed." Median nerve compression in the carpal tunnel ("carpal tunnel syndrome") is frequently present.

It is clear from the patients we have studied that aortic valve disease is a feature of the syndrome. Most have aortic regurgitation. One patient 55 years of age, however, has remained asymptomatic in this respect. (See Case 3.) Experience is still too limited to know to what extent life-span is abbreviated in this disorder.

Psychosis was a feature in 2 (Cases 4 and 5) of the 4 adults we have studied. The following 2 patients are brother and sister (Fig. 11-9*A* and *B*):

Case 3. M. E. McC. (1050314), the proband, is a white male attorney, born in 1917. Deformed feet and stiff fingers were noted at 7 years of age. He was considered the most intelligent member of his family and more intelligent than his unaffected brother. He was class valedictorian in high school, for example. Progressive difficulty with night vison began at the age of 27 years, with restriction of the fields of vision in daylight. "Steamy corneas" were first noted by his ophthalmologist, at age 13 years.* Right inguinal herniorrhaphy was performed at 42 years of age. Hearing deficit was noted in the right ear at 46 years. Intellect may have deteriorated somewhat in recent years.

The findings, when the patient was investigated in 1962 and again in 1964, included height of 175 cm. (68%₀ inches); short neck and coarse features, with broad mouth and jaw and fleshy tongue; stiff, clawlike hands with carpal tunnel syndrome and stiff wrists; short feet with high arches and overlapping fifth toe; marked clouding of the cornea, more dense peripherally; extensive retinitis pigmentosa bilaterally; and the diastolic murmur of aortic regurgitation (blood pressures, 145/65 mm. Hg). The aortic second sound was exceptionally ringing. The distal phalanges were flexed at about 90 degrees with the rest of the fingers but could be straightened passively. The wrists could not be extended beyond the neutral position. He could not supinate the forearms more than about 60 degrees. Except for the foot abnormalities, all other peripheral joints had normal range of motion. The liver was palpable and probably somewhat enlarged.

X-ray films showed spatulate ribs, and cystic and other changes in the bones of the wrists and hands.

The presence of carpal tunnel syndrome was indicated by numbness of the fingers supplied by the median nerve, marked wasting of the abducens pollicis brevis muscle, and characteristic nerve conduction changes†: stimulation at the elbow evoked no thumb movement or muscle action potential. Antidromic sensory velocity (stimulating at the wrist and recording at the elbow) was estimated at 26.8 M./sec. as compared with a velocity of 63.6 M./sec. in the unaffected ulnar nerve.

The hearing loss was largely limited to the right ear, and audiologic findings suggested a

---

*Courtesy of the late Dr. Harvey B. Searcy, Tuscaloosa, Ala.

†These studies were performed by Dr. Michael P. McQuillan, The Johns Hopkins Hospital.

cochlear location of the lesion. The electroretinogram was almost completely extinguished, consistent with neuroepithelial degeneration.

The urine showed 48 to 63 mg./L. of mucopolysaccharide, which was dermatan sulfate and heparan sulfate in the proportion of 3:1.[238] Bone marrow and circulating leukocytes showed no definite mucopolysaccharide inclusions.

Follow-up (1971). This patient developed bilateral narrow- or closed-angle glaucoma at the age of 51 years.

Case 4. M. McC. (1119314), white female, sister of M. E. McC., was born in 1930. Stiff hands and wrists and deformed feet were first noted at the age of 5 years. As early as 7 years of age an appearance suggesting mongolism was noted by her ophthalmologist. Clouding of the cornea was first noted by him at about 20 years of age. She was regarded by her parents as a slow learner. However, she succeeded in completing a four-year college course, of which the last year was spent in a Southern teachers' college. She attempted to teach school but had a "nervous breakdown" for which she was hospitalized and given electroshock therapy. Other treatments have been necessary since that time. She cares for her aged parents. She has noted numbness and anesthesia of the fingers.

Physical examination in 1964 showed height of 160.5 cm. (63½ inches), the same facial characteristics as in her brother (Fig. 11-9*A*), and similar hand and foot deformities, which were less severe, however (Fig. 11-9*B*). There was bilateral genu valgum. Grossly the corneal clouding seemed more diffuse than in the brother; however, slit-lamp examination showed possible peripheral concentration. The fundi showed retinal pigmentation and the electroretinogram was almost completely extinguished. The heart had a harsh systolic murmur with characteristics of aortic stenosis. The abducens pollicis brevis muscle was strikingly atrophied.

In the peripheral blood approximately 1% to 3% of the lymphocytes showed indistinct, poorly formed metachromatic granules in the cytoplasm. The Rebuck skin window demonstrated metachromatic inclusions in macrophages. The urine contained 131 mg./L. of mucopolysaccharide, which was dermatan sulfate and heparan sulfate in the proportion of about 3:1.[238]

No other similarly affected persons are known in this family. One other sib is completely normal. Interestingly, he is slightly shorter than the affected brother, M. E. McC., and in the past has been considered less competent intellectually.

Follow-up (1971). This patient developed narrow- or closed-angle glaucoma at the age of 40 years. From the age of 23 years she had been night-blind, a development consistent with the pigmentary degeneration of the retina which she and her brother demonstrate.

Cases 5 and 6. Through the courtesy of Dr. Scheie it was possible to examine the brother and sister (T. L. and R. L.) in whom he described the entity to which we assign his name. The facial resemblance to the cases reported here and shown in Fig. 11-9 was so striking that they could all pass for sibs. Other clinical features were also similar. It is specifically to be noted that both of Scheie's patients—a male, 33 years, and his sister, 31 years—have aortic regurgitation. The brother has had a psychotic episode. Leukocyte studies reveal no obvious metachromatic granules. Urine mucopolysaccharide analyses show both dermatan sulfate and heparan sulfate in a proportion of about 2:1.[238] (See follow-up by Constantopoulos et al.[71a]) R. L. has a healthy son born in 1965.

Pathology

The skin[188] and the cornea and conjunctiva[463] show the same histologic changes observed in MPS I H (p. 541). In those instances in which the carpal tunnel has been explored for relief of nerve compression,[553] an excess of collagenous tissue has been found. No autopsy observations are available. The nature of the aortic valve lesion is not known, but presumably the changes are like those in other mucopolysaccharidoses. Electron microscopic studies of conjunctiva and skin[427] showed multiple vacuolations in fibroblasts and in conjunctival epithelial cells. Inclusions were single membrane limited, contained a granulofibrillar material, and were associated with the Golgi bodies. Skin epithelium was normal.

The fundamental defect

Patients with the Scheie syndrome excrete excessive amounts of dermatan sulfate and heparan sulfate in the urine. Although the total amount excreted is not as great in adults as it is in children with the Hurler syndrome, the proportions of the two mucopolysaccharides is about 70:30 as in MPS I H.[238] (Kaplan[238] presented data on cases 16 to 19 in his Tables VII and VIII.) Thus the patients with the Scheie syndrome resemble those with the Hurler syndrome in the pattern of mucopolysacchariduria, Kaplan's mixed mucopolysacchariduria type B.

The Hurler and Scheie syndromes, despite the striking clinical differences, show identity by the Neufeld method of mixed fibroblast culture,[558] are both corrected by Hurler factor,[18a] and show deficiency of the same enzyme, α-L-iduronidase.[15a] These findings have led to the reclassification of the Hurler and Scheie syndromes as subtypes of MPS I.

That deficiency of the same enzyme should result in differing clinical pictures is no longer surprising because the same phenomenon has been demonstrated in the case of the infantile and adult forms of metachromatic leukodystrophy, the classic and juvenile forms of Tay-Sachs disease, the infantile and visceral forms of the Niemann-Pick disease, three forms of Gaucher disease, and so on. In some of these disorders, differences in the kinetics of the mutant enzyme in the two or more different forms can be demonstrated. Such may be found in comparisons of α-L-iduronidase in the Hurler and Scheie syndromes and may provide an explanation for the clinical differences.

Prevalence and inheritance

In British Columbia, Lowry and Renwick estimated that the frequency of the Scheie syndrome is 1 in 500,000 births, a plausible value.

MPS I S is inherited as an autosomal recessive disorder. Both Scheie and colleagues[463] and we[322] have observed an affected brother and sister. The female patient of Scheie and colleagues[463] has a son, now (1972) 7 years old, who appears to be normal.

It is entirely possible, indeed likely, that the Hurler and Scheie syndromes are produced by homozygosity for different genes at one and the same locus, that which determines the structure of α-L-iduronidase. (If α-L-iduronidase has two or more structurally different subunits, it is possible that the mutations responsible for the two conditions are at different loci.) If the two are allelic states, then the Hurler syndrome might be compared to sickle cell anemia, a severe disorder, and the Scheie syndrome to Hb CC disease, a mild disorder.

Features distinguishing the Scheie syndrome from MPS VI (see below) are normal or near-normal height, well-formed tubular bones, and hypoplastic or cystic changes of the carpal bones and the proximal portions of the metacarpals. Normal intelligence and corneal opacities are features of both.

In the view of Rampini,[430] cases of the Scheie syndrome were described in at least 7 reports,[131,244,262,389,423,465,533] in addition to the cases of Scheie and colleagues[463] and of my colleagues and me[322] (Cases 3 and 4, above). One case reported by Murray[378] and accepted as the Scheie syndrome by Rampini[430] is in fact an instance of the Hunter syndrome. (See p. 561.) Like Rampini,[430] Spranger[490] concluded that the disorder in the patients reported by Schinz and Furtwängler[465] and by others[209,467] was MPS V, or the Scheie syndrome. However, it is much more likely, in my opinion, that that family had pseudo-Hurler polydystrophy, or mucolipidosis III (p. 652).

It is possible that Case 4 in Watson-Jones' report on Léri's pleonosteosis had, in fact, the Scheie syndrome. The patient had joint stiffness and the carpal tunnel syndrome. Confirmation of the presence of corneal clouding (for which corneal transplant had been recommended) was provided to me in 1971 by Dr. C. E. C. Wells of Cardiff. The patient, born in 1926, was a highly intelligent and educated man who until the summer of 1971 led an active life in forestry and was an avid sailor. In 1971 he underwent surgery for spinal cord compression at multiple levels. One analysis for mucopolysaccharide in the urine had been negative. It is possible, therefore, that the disorder in this patient is mucolipidosis III (pseudo-Hurler polydystrophy) or some other condition not the Scheie syndrome. Against ML III (p. 652) are the normal intelligence and stature (about 65 inches) and the relative sparing of the shoulders in the joint stiffness.

MUCOPOLYSACCHARIDOSIS I H/I S (THE HURLER-SCHEIE COMPOUND)

As stated earlier, fibroblasts from Hurler and Scheie patients, when mixed, fail to show mutual correction of the metabolic defect as evidenced by metachromasia and handling of ^{35}S-labeled substances.[558] Clinically, the Hurler and Scheie syndromes are clearly distinct entities. The easiest explanation for the findings may be allelism (p. 25); the same degradative enzyme may be altered, but the mutation occurred at different sites in the cistron determining that enzyme or a different change at the same site. As a consequence the enzyme molecule would be altered in different ways, the functional properties of the two mutant enzymes would be expected to differ, and the clinical manifestations also might differ. (Of course, the mutation could be in the same codon, i.e., at the same site in the cistron. If this is the case, the Hurler and Scheie syndromes would be analogous to Hb SS and Hb CC diseases among the hemoglobinopathies, and the Hurler-Scheie compound would be analogous to Hb SC disease, which has a phenotype distinct from, although bearing some similarities to, Hb SS and Hb CC diseases.)

In the absence of consanguinity, and given a frequency of 1 in 200 for the gene for the Hurler syndrome (q_H) and 1 in 200 for the gene for the Scheie syndrome (q_S), the frequency of each syndrome (q_H^2) and q_S^2) should be 1 in 40,000. The compound disorder (in which an individual has the Hurler gene on one chromosome and the Scheie gene on the other chromosome) would be expected to occur in a frequency of 1 in 20,000 (2 $q_H q_S$). An individual with a compound disorder might be expected to have an intermediate phenotype. Parental consanguinity should not be increased in the case of the compound disorder.

On clinical grounds the disorder in the patient described below was tentatively labeled as the Maroteaux-Lamy syndrome. However, unlike the patients with MPS VI shown in Fig. 11-34, the fibroblasts of this patient did not show cross-correction with those of a Hurler patient or with those of a Scheie patient.[383] The phenotype is probably consistent with the suggestion that she represents a compound of the Hurler and Scheie genes, these being alleles.

Case 7. P. S. (J.H.H. 889799), a white female born in 1950, represents a sporadic case. The parents were not known to be related. An older sister was normal.

The patient's infancy was marked by neonatal pneumonia and persistent feeding difficulties. Physical developmental milestones lagged. She attended public school through the sixth grade and received home tutoring thereafter. Her performance deteriorated coincident with progressive physical impairment. Beginning at the age of 10 years, she frequently experienced momentary loss of vision and at the age of 15 years became totally blind. Four weeks prior to the development of blindness she had experienced facial hemiparalysis and inability to speak or walk. She later regained these functions. Hearing steadily declined. Severe frontal headaches and a constant clear rhinorrhea began at about the age of 14 years. At 19 years of age she was still able to get about, write, and make handicrafts despite severe physical and sensory handicaps. Beginning sometime in her late teens, the patient experienced intermittent rhinorrhea, which was subsequently identified as cerebrospinal fluid.

The diagnosis of the Hurler syndrome was suggested at 18 months of age because of hypertelorism, mild kyphosis, enlarged wrists, cardiomegaly, hepatosplenomegaly, and umbilical hernia. Skeletal x-ray studies at 3 years showed only mild changes of mucopolysaccharidosis. By 9 years

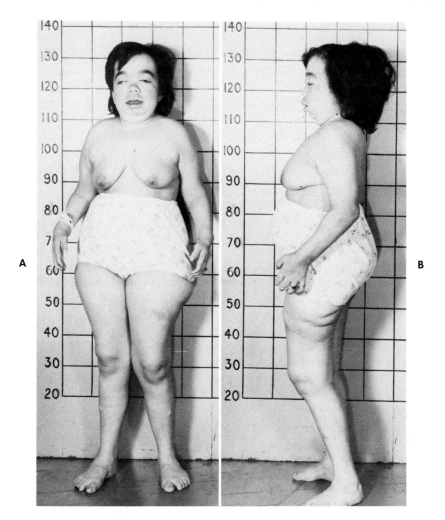

Fig. 11-10. The Hurler/Scheie compound heterozygote? See discussion of **P. S.** (Case 7) in text. **A** and **B,** Note short stature, abnormal facies and joint contractures. **C,** X-ray of skull, showing multiple oval radiolucencies in the frontal and parietal parts of the calvaria, extraordinarily extensive destruction in the region of the sella turcica and cribiform plate, sclerotic mastoids, hypoplastic mandibular head and ramus, and impaction of second molars with large follicular cysts. **D,** X-ray of head, showing clawing, sloping of distal radius and ulna toward each other, small carpal bones, and wide middle phalanges.

of age, she was described as having grotesque facies, mild mental retardation, corneal clouding, enlarged tongue, hepatosplenomegly, generalized limitation of joint mobility, and clawhand deformity.

Examination (1969) showed a short (135 cm.) girl weighing 47 kg. (Fig. 11-10). The head circumference measured 55 cm. The facies was characterized by prominent forehead, depressed nasal bridge, anteverted nostrils, ocular proptosis with esotropia and corneal clouding, and thick lips. The tongue was enlarged, and 24 widely spaced teeth were present. A systolic murmur was heard at the left lower sternal border. The abdomen was protuberant, with right inguinal and umbilical herniorrhaphy scars. A hernia in the right inguinal area measured 3 cm. The liver extended 12 cm. and the spleen 5 cm. below their respective costal margins. The breast and vulva showed adult development and the vaginal mucosa showed estrogen effects. Pubic and axillary hair was scant, however. Decreased mobility was evident in all joints. The hands were broad with short, clawlike fingers. There was mild scoliosis.

By means of psychologic testing designed to take account of her visual and auditory handicaps, Dr. Henry J. Mark estimated her maximal mental performance, primarily verbal skills, at an I.Q. equivalent of 63.

X-ray findings included mild cortical thickening of the skull with multiple small radiolucent areas and a diffusely enlarged sella turcica (Fig. 11-10C). Body section roentgenograms, made with the polytome, and a carotid arteriogram showed changes suggesting an anterior encephalocele extending through the cribriform plate into the posterior nasal cavity and protruding into the anterior part of the nasopharynx. (This was thought to be related to the patient's rhinorrhea.) Thoracolumbar scoliosis was present and the vertebral bodies were variably deformed. The long bones of the upper limbs were short and broad, with metaphyseal and epiphyseal deformities. The carpal bones were hypoplastic and the metacarpals were short and broad with proximal tapering (Fig. 11-10D). Similar but milder changes were present in the lower limbs.

Further investigations confirmed the theory that the rhinorrhea was cerebrospinal fluid. Electroencephalogram suggested severe cerebral disturbance involving primarily the frontal lobes. Echoencephalogram demonstrated enlargement of the lateral ventricles, as did also the

C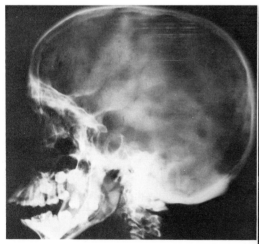

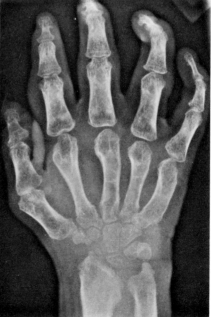 D

Fig. 11-10, cont'd. For legend see opposite page.

carotid arteriogram. A cystic white mass was visualized in the left nasal fossa. Plasma thryoxine (4.1 mg./100 ml), I^{131} uptake, and urinary 17-hydroxycorticosteroids were normal. A flat 17-hydroxycorticosteroid response to metyrapone (Metopirone) suggested abnormality of the pituitary-adrenal axis. Urinary 17-ketosteroids were markedly reduced.

Urinary screening for mucopolysaccharides by toluidine blue, CTAB, and acid albumin turbidity methods gave strongly positive results. Urinary excretion of acid mucopolysaccharides was 215 mg./24 hr. Dermatan sulfate accounted for 80% of the AMPS, the remainder being heparan sulfate.

The patient lacked the striking metachromatic inclusions seen in patients with MPS VI (p. 633).

We[321a,321b] have 6 other patients in whom the clinical picture and results of fibroblast studies are consistent with the compound Hurler/Scheie condition. Two are sisters, one of whom had a pregnancy artificially terminated[301] (p. 618). In addition Neufeld[383] found that cultured fibroblasts from the brother and sister reported by Horton and Schimke[210] have the corrective characteristics of the Hurler and Scheie syndromes and show deficiency of α-L-iduronidase. The intermediate phenotype, in combination with the enzymatic studies, suggest that these cases may also be examples of the mixed heterozygote.

MUCOPOLYSACCHARIDOSIS II (MPS II, HUNTER SYNDROME)

MPS II is distinguished from MPS I H clinically by lack of corneal clouding and longer survival, genetically by X-linked recessive inheritance, and biochemically by a different pattern of mucopolysaccharide excretion in the urine and deficiency of a different corrective factor. At least two presumably allelic forms of MPS II can be distinguished on the basis of length of survival and severity of neurologic involvement.

Clinical manifestations

Usually MPS II is in all respects less severe than MPS I H. But here, as in MPS I H, leading features are stiff joints (with, for example, clawhand), dwarfing, hepatosplenomegaly, and gross facial appearance, which is responsible for the designation "gargoylism." However, mental deterioration progresses at a slower rate, lumbar gibbus does not occur, and progressive deafness is a frequent feature. Nodular skin lesions are sometimes present on the posterior thorax or arms. Clouding of the cornea of clinically evident degree has not been observed*; this is the clearest difference between MPS I and MPS II. In older patients with MPS II, slight corneal clouding may be evident on the slit-lamp examination, but the involvement is minimal. Indeed, mucopolysaccharide deposits in the cornea are demonstrable histologically in adult cases of MPS II.[171] (The features distinguishing MPS I and MPS II are outlined in Table 11-4.) Atypical retinitis pigmentosa occurs in cases of MPS II.[206] Some of the oldest survivors in the kindred (Fig. 11-15) reported by Beebe and Formel[22] are blind as a result of the retinal changes.[132]

Retinal degeneration of pigmentary type has often escaped attention in other

---

*The only possible exception to this statement is represented by 1 of 12 affected males in a kindred report by van Pelt.[543,544] The patient was a 3¼-year-old boy who was said to have "weakly positive" corneal clouding. However, van Pelt did not examine the patient personally, slit-lamp examination was not done, and by the time of report the patient had died as a result of complications of surgery for umbilical hernia.

mucopolysaccharidoses, in large part because of the difficulties in observing the changes in the presence of corneal clouding. Changes of this type were found in the case of MPS II shown in Fig. 11-11. They were observed, furthermore, in cases of MPS III and MPS I S described here. The electroretinogram was strikingly abnormal, being "nearly extinguished" in some. Franceschetti and co-workers[146] gave a full review of the retinal changes in the mucopolysaccharidoses, together with personal observations. It is clear from the electroretinograms,[167] as well as from histologic studies, that retinal changes occur in MPS types I H, I S, II, and III.[441]

The patient often survives to his thirties; the oldest known patient with MPS II died at the age of 60 years.[132] There appear to be two classes of MPS II cases as to age at death. In one group (MPS IIA) death usually occurs before age 15 years; the second group (MPS IIB) is the variety that is compatible with survival to the fifties or later. As noted on p. 574, these may be allelic forms, i.e., may be caused by different mutations at the same X-linked locus.

Adult Hunter patients tend to have a "high coloration" or "rosy cheeks." F. Parkes Weber, in a discussion of Hunter's historic paper,[218] noted that a "remarkable feature" of these individuals "is a 'precociously plethoric' appearance of their faces," like "that of a middle-aged farmer who is fond of malt liquor, and whose work naturally exposes him much to the weather." The voice of the patients is somewhat hoarse.

Beebe[21] suggested that Washington Irving's description of the "odd-looking" personages in "Rip Van Winkle" who played at ninepins in their hideaway in the Catskills were drawn from real life—that is, from the cases of the Hunter syndrome which existed in that area and have been described by Beebe and Formel.[22] (See Fig. 11-15.)

Changes in the head of the femur with precocious osteoarthritis are usually present in older patients. The foot is of the pes cavus type. The fifth toe is often overlapping. Hooper's patient[206] was operated on for talipes equinovarus at the age of 17 years. The roentgenographic abnormalities in patients with the Hunter syndrome are similar to those in patients with the Hurler syndrome but tend to be less severe. Involvement of the pelvis and spine, in particular, are less striking in the Hunter syndrome. Many of the patients do not have either a gibbus, or a beaked, notched, or hooked vertebra. Occasional Hunter syndrome patients have fairly severe bony abnormalities, however, which are indistinguishable from those of Hurler syndrome patients with milder bony changes. The bony abnormalities in the two conditions thus form a continuum, which is covered by the term *dysostosis multiplex*.

Changes in the skin[282] in the form of grooving and either ridged[70] or nodular[7] thickening, especially over the upper arms and thorax, have been described. In two of the reports[7,70] the changes were strikingly similar, especially as to location—"symmetrically distributed in an area of about 6 by 10 cm., extending from the angle of the scapula towards the axillary line." (See Fig. 11-12A.) This distribution is probably the characteristic one.[185] Hypertrichosis is usually striking.

The occurrence of papilledema in these patients (Figs. 11-11 and 11-14) has suggested hydrocephalus, or at least increased intracranial pressure. The patient shown in Fig. 11-11 retained the fundus picture of "papilledema" for at least ten years. Optic atrophy was described in 2 sibs by Davis and Currier.[96] Consistent with the development of atypical retinitis pigmentosa,[206] the electroretinogram becomes "extinguished."[167]

Mental regression occurs more rapidly in type A, or the severe form, of MPS II (p. 574). In the mild form, type B, it is usual for mathematical ability to be better preserved than verbal ability.

Petit mal seizures developed in the patient shown in Fig. 11-11. The deaf-

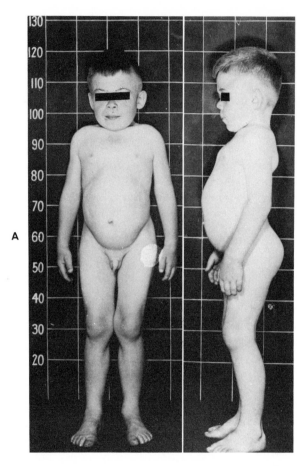

Fig. 11-11. Typical case of the Hunter syndrome, or MPS II (I. S. 204375). **A,** At the age of 10 years. This patient, 22 years old in **B,** had dysostosis multiplex, deafness, "chronic rhinitis," exertional dyspnea, hepatomegaly, restricted joint mobility, hydrocele, and hernia, but no splenomegaly or corneal opacification. Mentality was retarded. The patient graduated from high school because of courtesy promotions. He read voluminously, especially Ellery Queen novels! No inclusions could be demonstrated in the white cells. The testes were small and soft. However, the patient shaved daily and erections and nocturnal emissions occurred. Vision was 20/100 in the right eye, 20/30 in the left. A startling finding was bilateral papilledema, probably long-standing, with "bone corpuscle" pigmentary degeneration of both fundi, especially the right. A peculiar feature was the subjective response to administration of thyroid extract (p. 547). The patient died at 32 years of age. Autopsy showed cerebral atrophy with internal hydrocephalus, extensive involvement of the heart valves, and, in the cornea (which was not grossly cloudy but had a "deep haze" on biomicroscopy), accumulations of material with the staining properties of mucopolysaccharide.

ness in this patient, when tested at 24 years of age, appeared to be of the perceptive type.

Despite long-standing hepatosplenomegaly, manifestations of hepatic dysfunction are usually minimal. In a 29-year-old patient[485] with fairly marked hepatosplenomegaly, cephalin flocculation, thymol turbidity, serum protein levels, prothrombin time, and Bromsulphalein excretion were all unequivocally normal.

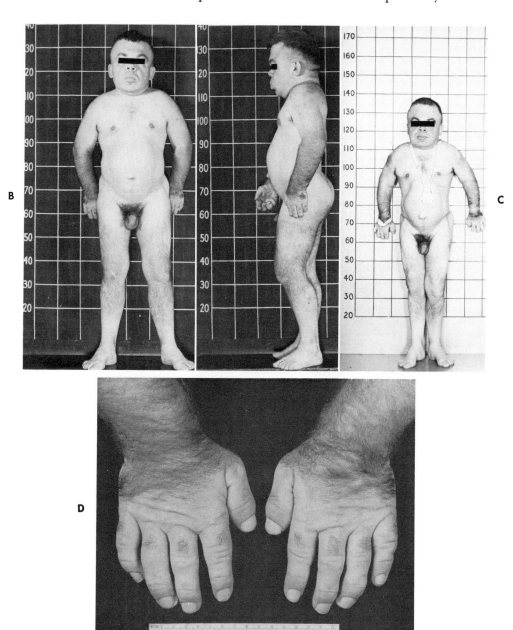

Fig. 11-11. cont'd. C, Same patient as in **A** and **B,** at the age of 30 years. **D,** Hands of same patient.

Continued.

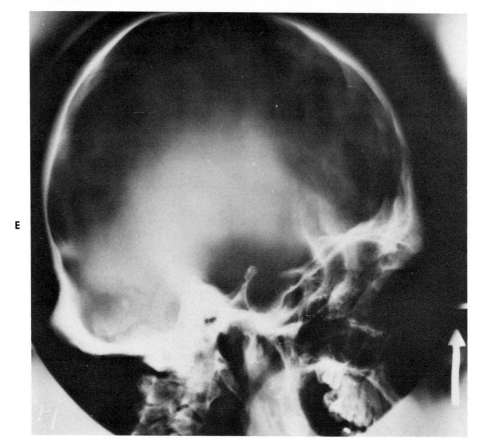

E

Fig. 11-11, cont'd. E, Lateral radiograph of skull. The sella turcica is large, with mild anterior pocketing. There are obvious frontal and occipital areas of hyperostosis. The mastoids are unaerated and more dense than normal.

Chronic intermittent diarrhea is a frequent complaint of patients with the Hunter syndrome.[129]

In Hunter's historic report[218] he remarked on the occurrence in one of his patients of cardiomegaly and both systolic and diastolic murmurs. As noted on p. 522, follow-up suggests that one and possibly both brothers died cardiac deaths at ages 11 and 16. Pulmonary hypertension is frequent in patients with MPS II (Fig. 11-13).

Death from "heart failure" (either congestive or coronary artery in type) often occurs before the age of 20 years. Of the patients described by Smith and associates,[485] one died at the age of 28 years and another was "reasonably well" at 29 years of age. Hooper[206] described a 37-year-old patient who was still living. In 2 of his other patients, death occurred at 20 and 30 years of age, respectively. The oldest patient in my series is now 34 years old, and another died at 32 years. (See Fig. 11-11 for the latter patient.) Beebe and Formel[22] described 9 well-documented cases of the Hurler syndrome in one family. Five had died at an age in excess of 40 years. There were 4 survivors—45, 43, 17, and 14 years of age, respec-

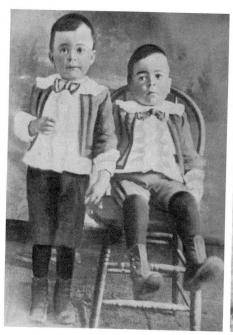

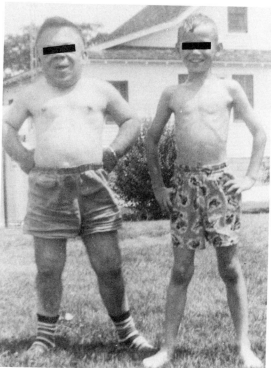

F   G

Fig. 11-11, cont'd. F, Two uncles of the patient. Both probably had the Hurler syndrome. **G,** The propositus (on left), 22 years of age, and his unaffected brother (on right), 8 years of age.

Two maternal uncles, **F,** had the Hunter syndrome with characteristic skeletal features, deafness, and symptoms of cardiac incompetence. They died at the ages of 12 and 17 years, one having been found dead in bed. The patient's parents are normal and he has two normal siblings. A young nephew of the patient may have the disease; I have not had an opportunity to examine the child but the descriptions are suggestive.

The possible occurrence in 4 males in three generations is consistent with, and at least mildly indicative of, inheritance of the trait as a sex-linked recessive. Lamy and associates[274] have also presented a pedigree with affected males in three generations.

Meyer[358] was able to demonstrate relatively large amounts of dermatan sulfate and heparan sulfate in the urine of the propositus. No chemical difference from the autosomal recessive form of the disease was demonstrated by these studies.

tively. Follow-up[132] showed that one affected male had died at the age of 61 years and one was still living at that same age. (See Fig. 11-15.)

Murray[378] described a 43-year-old patient with MPS II and marked respiratory disability. The man had sufficient intelligence to do defense work during World War II and to work as a flagman on construction jobs thereafter. Clinical features were stunting of growth, limitation of joint mobility, deafness, coarse facies, short neck, kyphoscoliosis with mild pectus excavatum, hernias, hepatosplenomegaly, and pallor of the optic discs with visual impairment. Deformity of

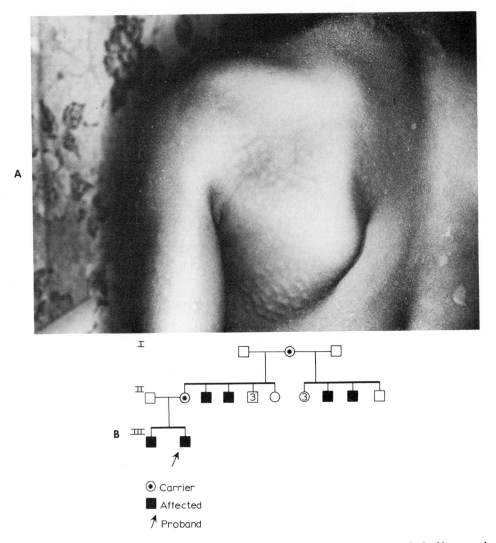

Carrier

Affected

Proband

Fig. 11-12. The Hunter syndrome in a Negro family. **A,** Pebbly skin over scapula in Negro male with Hunter syndrome. Both this patient, 16 years old, and his brother, 26 years old, have aortic regurgitation. **B,** The pedigree.

the larynx and nasopharynx and enlargement of the tongue seemed to be responsible for airway obstruction. This impression was supported by the marked relief afforded by tracheostomy, which the patient had for over ten years. Kyphoscoliosis, restriction of chest movement, upper airway obstruction, chronic respiratory infection, and abnormalities of diffusion from parenchymal involvement in the basic process are mechanisms in the respiratory disability of the mucopolysaccharidoses. In 1971, Murray's patient[378] was still alive at the age of 55 years.[242] His condition had remained remarkably stable over the previous fifteen years. Surgical revision of the tracheostomy had been required several times, and he suctioned his own trachea daily. Digitalis and a diuretic were taken daily. He had

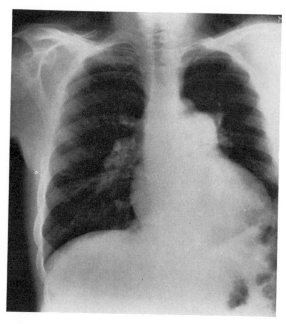

Fig. 11-13. MPS II. Chest x-ray film in W. B. (see text), 33-year-old patient with severe pulmonary hypertension.

prostatic hypertrophy and degenerative arthritis of the right knee. Two nephews may have the same disorder.

Case 8. W. B. (605145), age 33 years, has typical clinical and chemical features of MPS II. As is often the case in X-linked recessive states in which affected males do not have children, the family history is negative.

Skeletal features common to several of the mucopolysaccharidoses are demonstrated by clinical and x-ray examination. However, he is 66 inches tall—an unusual height in this disease (Fig. 11-13). His parents are tall and he has had exceptionally good care throughout his life. Although intellect is clearly affected, the impairment is not uniform. He attended a top-notch private school, and although he did not graduate, he received advanced instruction in economics. He works in his father's stock exchange office and reads the *Wall Street Journal*.

Hernias were repaired at the ages of 6 and 14 years. Splenectomy for suspected Banti's disease was performed at 8 years of age and operations for knock-knees at 12 and 14 years. A hearing aid has been worn from 7 years of age.

Episodic faintness beginning about 29 years of age was interpreted as due to hypoglycemia and was helped by a high-protein diet. The mild breathlessness present for most of his life he attributed to limitation in chest expansion. Several episodes of heart failure were precipitated by respiratory infections.

Examination revealed the facial features of "gargoylism," some limitation of motion in all joints, clawhand deformity and peculiar, highly arched feet, with the fifth toe overlapping the side of the foot. By slit-lamp view the cornea showed a slight haze, deep in the stroma and more pronounced in the lower third. By direct inspection, however, the corneas were perfectly clear. The second sound in the pulmonary area was markedly accentuated. The liver was five fingerbreadths below the right costal margin.

Laboratory studies showed bilirubin of 1.4 mg./100 ml., 30% BSP retention in 45 minutes, glucose tolerance tests with glucose levels of 32 and 46 mg./100 ml. at 4 and 5 hours, respectively, and uric acid consistently above 7 mg./100 ml.

Chest x-ray films showed prominent pulmonary arteries and generalized enlargement of the heart (Fig. 11-13). Cardiac catheterization showed pulmonary artery pressure to be 109/45 mm.

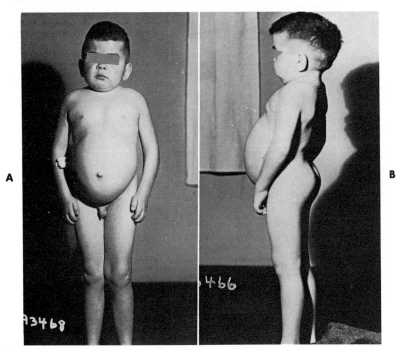

Fig. 11-14. J. M. J. (U53195, 10 years old, was noted to have a short neck and large head at birth, had frequent colds and trouble in breathing because of a "low bridge" of the nose, and had noted limitation of joint movement. However, he had always done well in school and was in the fifth grade. In a school examination he was found to "need glasses," and papilledema was discovered by the ophthalmologist consulted. There had been no headache or vomiting and no impairment of vision so far as the patient was concerned. Examination revealed, in addition to the features obvious in the photographs, the liver to be enlarged 4 cm. below the right costal margin and the spleen 2 cm. below the left; limitation of motion of the elbows, wrists, toes (which were fixed in a position of partial flexion like the fingers), ankles, knees, and spine; height of 44½ inches; papilledema of about 2.5 diopters. Dr. Walter E. Dandy performed ventriculograms which showed "symmetrically dilated ventricles and large third ventricle, aqueduct of Sylvius, and fourth ventricle, and air in all the cisternae, including chiasmatis and interpeduncularis, and, curiously, the large main trunks of the subarachnoid spaces but no air in the branches. The main trunks were terminated in large bulbous ends. It was, therefore, communicating hydrocephalus with congenital absence of the terminal branches of the subarachnoid space." (The quotation is from Dr. Dandy's operative note.) Choroid plexectomy was performed in an effort to relieve the hydrocephalus. Histologically, the excised choroid plexus appeared atrophic. The patient died two weeks after operation, of an infectious complication. Autopsy was not performed. This patient resembles closely the one pictured in Fig. 11-8A, who also had papilledema that has, however, not been progressive. The photographs, **A** and **B,** demonstrate the general skeletal changes, prominent abdomen, and clawhand deformity. In **C** and **D** is displayed the bilateral papilledema.

Hg, with moderate elevation of end-diastolic pressure in the right ventricle and mild elevation in the left ventricle. Electrocardiogram showed the changes of right ventricular hypertrophy. Respiratory function studies showed marked reduction in vital capacity (37% of predicted) and, by spirogram, there was evidence of moderate airway obstruction. Isoproterenol (Isuprel) produced no change.

Both dermatan sulfate and heparan sulfate were present in the urine in excess. In the circulating blood, 20% of the lymphocytes had metachromatic granules in the cytoplasm when stained with toluidine blue.

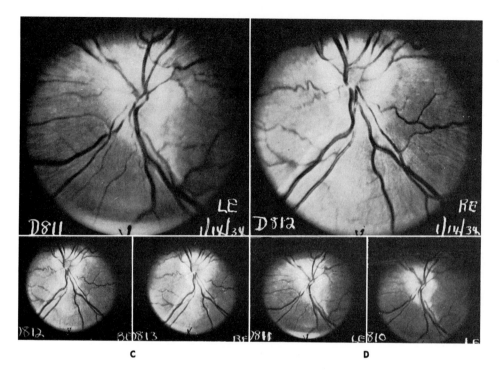

Fig. 11-14, cont'd. For legend see opposite page.

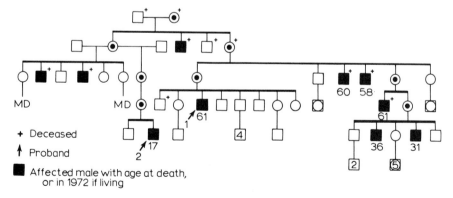

Fig. 11-15. MPS II, type B. Updated (1972) pedigree of kindred reported by Beebe and Formel[22] and previously (1962) updated by A. E. H. Emery (Fig. 9-11, p. 356, *Heritable Disorders of Connective Tissue*, 1966). Arrow 1 indicates Emery's proband and arrow 2 our proband, 17 years of age in 1972. The family demonstrated the difficulties in tracing an X-linked trait; the surname of affected persons is likely to be different for each affected sibship. The man who died at 61 and the one now living at 61 represent the longest survival known to me. MD = many descendants, all apparently unaffected.

Case 9. W. P. W. (J.H.H. 1404524) is a member of a kindred in which at least 6 other males have had the Hunter syndrome (see pedigree, Fig. 11-16*A*). An affected member was reported by Smith and colleagues in 1952.[485] The disorder is relatively mild in this family, with survival to 37 years of age in one instance. Intelligence is well preserved until late. One affected male, the earliest shown in the pedigree, is said to have been a judge in Scotland.

Umbilical hernia was noted in W. P. W. when he was a baby, and joint stiffness had its onset at about the age of 3 years. He did well in school, especially in mathematics and spelling, even though he was handicapped in writing because of his hand deformity. At 11 years of age he was diagnosed as having the Hunter syndrome and evaluated together with his maternal cousin, J. B. Puberty began at 13 years of age. He was graduated from college and has been a civilian overseas employee of the army as an accountant. His voice was always deep and husky. He had many episodes of otitis media. His hearing was diminished from childhood, but a hearing aid improved his hearing somewhat. At the age of 26 years he married a Korean woman.

Examination (1970) showed a height of 58 inches (Fig. 11-16*B* and *C*). The facies was coarse, with very prominent supraorbital ridges (Fig. 11-16*D*), large lips, and a striking flush of the cheeks and forehead. The head was large for the rest of the body. The margins of the optic discs were blurred, and venous pulsations were absent. The corneas were clear (Fig. 11-17); no retinal pigmentary change was seen. I heard a short early diastolic murmur of presumed aortic origin. The liver was felt 8 cm. below the right costal margin. The spleen was not palpable. Normal external genitalia and bilateral indirect inguinal hernias were demonstrated. Motion was limited in all joints. He could not extend the elbows beyond 120 degrees or raise his arms above 90 degrees. The hands were clawed, with atrophy of the thenar eminence, which is indicative of carpal tunnel compression.

Semen analysis showed a normal count (30 million/ml.) with reduced (10%) motile forms. Studies included urine mucopolysaccharide fractionation.

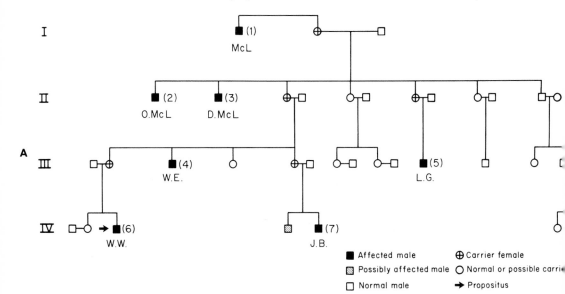

Fig. 11-16. The Hunter syndrome in W. P. W. (J.H.H. 1404524) (see text). **A**, Pedigree. **B** and **C**, Stiff joints, clawhand deformity, coarse facies, and short stature are evident. **D**, Very prominent supercilliary ridges are demonstrated. **E**, Lateral x-ray view of the skull, showing brachycephaly and prominent superciliary ridge. **F**, Lateral x-ray view of spine, showing hypoplasia and recessing of the second lumbar vertebra. **G**. X-ray view of the pelvis, showing bilateral narrowing in the area above the acetabulum, irregularity of the acetabulum, flattened femoral heads, and relatively large femoral trochanters with a medial spine on the greater trochanter. **H**, X-ray view of hand and wrist, showing hypoplasia or absence of the proximal row of carpal bones and lipping on the proximal ends of the middle and distal phalanges. (Patient studied through courtesy of Dr. G. L. Bilbrey.[288a])

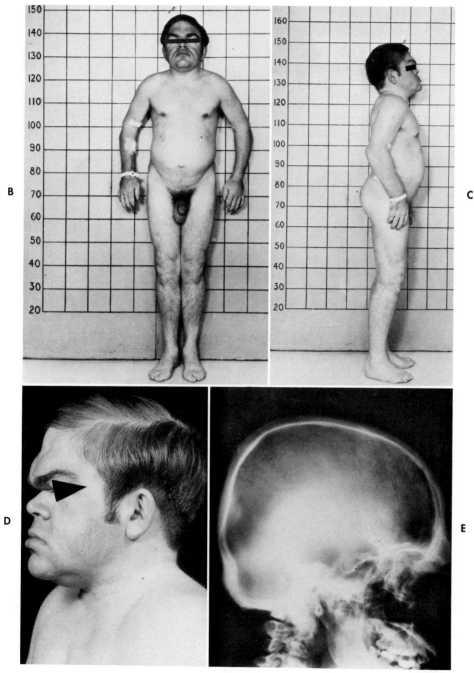

Continued.

Fig. 11-16, cont'd. For legend see opposite page.

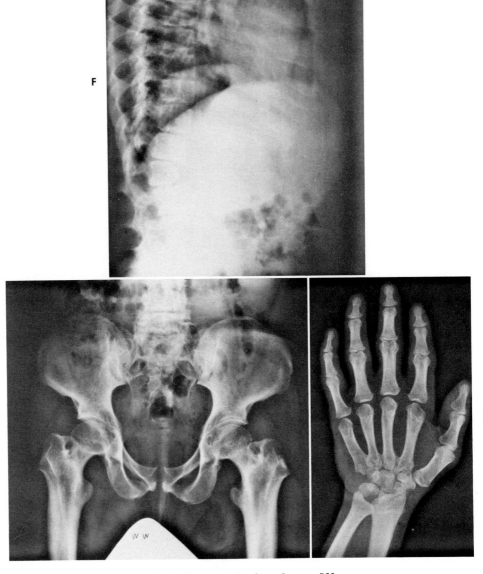

Fig. 11-16, cont'd. For legend see p. 566.

Pathology

In general the changes are identical to those described for MPS I. Histologically, even the cornea may show qualitatively the same changes as in MPS I, even though clouding is not evident grossly (Fig. 11-11). Goldberg and Duke[171] described the histologic findings in the eye in the patient pictured in Fig. 11-8. Although the cornea had been free of clouding and deposition of abnormal mucopolysaccharides was minimal in the stroma, heavy concentrations were found in the endothelium of the cornea, in the epithelial structures of the iris

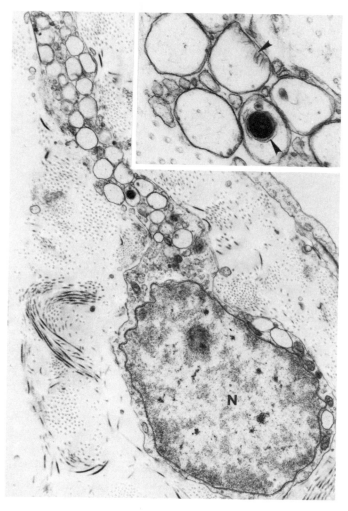

Fig. 11-17. Electron micrograph of the conjunctival connective tissue from a 26-year-old Caucasian male (W. P. W., J.H.H. 1404524) with the Hunter syndrome (MPS II) and clear corneas. Within the stromal fibroblasts, numerous small storage vacuoles (averaging approx. 0.5 mμ in diameter) do not distort the cellular architecture as they do in MPS I. Inset: These vacuoles are limited by a single-unit membrane, contain fine granular material or membranous lamellar inclusions (arrows), and are thought to represent lysosomes containing acid mucopolysaccharide and glycolipid. (**N**, nucleus; ×11,000; inset, ×33,000.) (Courtesy Kenneth R. Kenyon and Harry A. Quigley, Baltimore, Md.)

and ciliary body, and in the sclera (which was markedly thickened). Pigmentary degeneration of the retina was demonstrated, thus confirming histologically the findings of clinical examination.

It has been claimed[491a] that there is a histopathologic difference between the two forms of MPS II, the severe (type A in my terminology) and the mild (type B). Type A patients, who demonstrate relatively early neurologic deterioration and death before age 15 years, have much more neuronal storage than do type B patients, who are significantly older at death.

Multiple abnormalities of the middle and inner ear were discovered in one twice-reported case.[485,566]

The fundamental defect

Patients with MPS II excrete excessive amounts of dermatan sulfate and heparan sulfate in the urine. Maroteaux[333] followed up on the work of Knecht and Dorfman,[254] who showed that two types of heparan sulfate can be identified in normal and in Hurler tissues by the characteristic pattern of elution from ion-exchange resin by NaCl solutions of different strengths. He found that even though the proportion of total heparan sulfate to dermatan sulfate was not clearly different in the Hurler and the Hunter syndromes, the proportion of the two types of heparan sulfate did serve to distinguish the two disorders in individual patients. On the other hand, Terry and Linker,[520] Kaplan,[238] and Gordon and Haust[177] could distinguish MPS I and MPS II by the proportions of dermatan sulfate and heparan sulfate, which were about 70:30 in both the Hurler and the Scheie varieties of MPS I and about equal (50:50) in MPS II.

The basic defect in this and other mucopolysaccharidoses is discussed in detail on p. 634. As indicated later, severe (type A) and mild (type B) forms of MPS II can be distinguished clinically and presumably represent allelic forms, since the same corrective factor is deficient in the two. Although some of the physical and biologic properties of the Hunter corrective factor are known, its precise enzymatic function has not yet been identified.

Prevalence and inheritance

Although no patient with the Hunter syndrome reproduces (with a single known exception noted later), and therefore the progeny test is lacking, there can be no question that the Hunter syndrome is X-linked. Demonstration[90] of the Lyon phenomenon by the culture of clones of two types from mothers of affected males (p. 10) and the failure to find abnormality in the fathers are conclusive evidence of X-linked recessive inheritance. Berg and associates[25] concluded that the locus for Xm, an X-linked polymorphic macroglobulin of blood, is sufficiently close to the Xg blood group locus that linkage is demonstrable in family studies. This is, of course, strong support for X-linkage.

In the case of an X-linked trait which is of such a nature that the affected males do not reproduce, it can be shown that one third of the cases arise by new mutation in the X chromosome given to the affected son by his mother and that two thirds are inherited from the mother through an X chromosome in which the mutation occurred in an early generation.[317] Even if the mutation occurred in the maternal grandfather or grandmother, no second case might occur in the family. Thus, a typical X-linked pedigree pattern is expected in only a minority of cases. There are, nonetheless, numerous reports of an X-linked pedigree pattern for the Hunter syndrome,[22,55,82,206,308,368,388,519,543,544,566] and in many other instances[70,105,130,218,234,308,309] this theory of inheritance is consonant with the known facts. Njå[388] first proposed that cases without corneal opacity are most likely to show X-linked recessive inheritance. Lamy's analysis[274] corroborated Njå's suggestion. Whereas about 90% of all reported patients with "gargoylism" had cloudy cornea, only about 60% of male patients showed the sign.

In the report of Beebe and Formel[22] 9 cases were described, occurring in four generations of a family of Dutch extraction that has resided in the Catskill Mountains for about 250 years. Of 19 males, 9 were affected. Of 16 female sibs of affected males, none was affected. All 9 affected males were related through their mothers, who were presumably carriers. Furthermore, they were all descended from the same female ancestor, who was almost certainly likewise a carrier or who perhaps started the disease (by mutation), just as Queen Victoria probably initiated hemophilia[503] in the royal houses of Europe. Five other females could be identified as carriers by reason of affected brothers and sons. Six females had borne only normal children. (See Fig. 11-15.)

Most of the patients with "gargoylism" who survived beyond the age of 20 years were male. In Jervis' survey,[233] which concerned "gargoylism" generally and probably included cases of MPS I, MPS II, and MPS III, of which only MPS II is X-linked, the sex was stated in 145 cases. Of these, 93 (64%) were male. Of 112 sibships, 65 could, by reason of the fact that all affected individuals were male, represent the hypothesized sex-linked variety of the disease. There were 27 sibships with more than 1 affected individual; of these, 12 had only males affected, 4 had only females affected, and in 11 both males and females were affected. The average age of the affected individuals in the sibships with more than 1 affected individual, all males, was 6.65 years. The comparable value for the sibships containing both male and female affected individuals was 10.02 years. Although this appears to contradict the rough impression that the patients with the sex-linked variety are older when they come to medical attention and when they die, it must be remembered that these collected sibships may contain some in which the trait was inherited as an autosomal recessive; these may weigh down the average. It is likely that some females with the Sanfilippo syndrome (MPS III), an autosomal recessive, survive beyond the age of 20 years.

In one instance, illustrated in Figs. 11-18 and 11-19, a man with the Hunter syndrome of mild type comparable to that in the man described above in Case 4 was a successful marine engineer and had a son as well as a daughter who, of course, was necessarily a carrier and proved it by producing 2 affected sons.[109] This instance of reproduction by a patient with the Hunter syndrome is the only one known to me. The marine engineer died at the age of 57 years. His affected grandsons were subjects of the initial studies of the effects of plasma infusions.[110]

Parents of the subjects with the Hunter syndrome (and the other five mucopolysaccharidoses) have invariably been unaffected. Study of urinary mucopolysaccharides has provided no sure method for identifying the heterozygous female.[55] Study of skin fibroblasts may, however, be such a method. In skin fibroblasts from males with the Hunter syndrome, Danes and Bearn[88] have demonstrated intracellular accumulation of mucopolysaccharides, by staining with toluidine blue. In the fibroblasts of mothers in such cases a proportion of cells have a normal appearance with this stain, whereas the remainder show mucopolysaccharide accumulations identical to those in the hemizygous affected males.[419] The fathers show no abnormality. The observations provide strong proof of X-linked inheritance; they also support the Lyon hypothesis (p. 10). The heterozygous female shows no abnormality, probably because her normal cells "correct" those with defective metabolism, as can be shown by *in vitro* mixture of normal and abnormal cells.[154]

Assuming that the mutation rates for the Hurler syndrome and the Hunter syndrome are the same, one would predict that the Hunter syndrome at birth would be one and one-half times more frequent than the Hurler syndrome.[318] This conclusion is derived as follows:

Since persons affected with either syndrome do not reproduce, the mutation rate for the autosomal disorder (μ_1) is q_1^2 and the mutation rate for the X-linked disorder (μ_2) is $\frac{1}{3} q_1$, where q_1 and q_2 are, respectively, the frequencies of the autosomal (MPS I) and X-linked (MPS II) genes. Mutation rates are gametic rates. Since two mutant genes are lost with each person affected by an autosomal recessive, the mutation rate at equilibrium equals the frequency of affected persons (q_1^2). Since one third of the mutant genes are lost in each person affected by the X-linked recessive condition, the mutation rate, at equilibrium, is equal to $3 q_2$. Since the premise was that the mutation rates for the two disorders are the same, $q_1^2 = \frac{1}{3} q_2$. The frequency of an X-linked gene (e.g., q_2) is also the phenotype frequency in males. Thus, the expression $q_1^2 = \frac{1}{3} q_2$ says that the

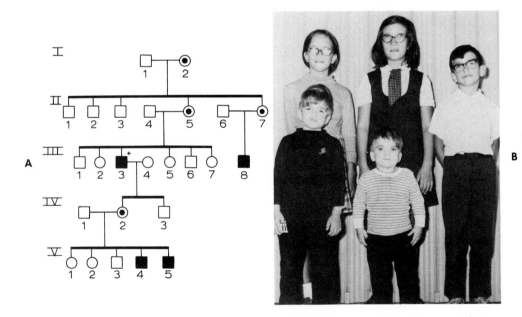

Fig. 11-18. Reproduction in the Hunter syndrome. **A,** Pedigree. **B,** The probands (V 4 and V 5), who were treated with plasma infusions by DiFerrante and colleagues,[110] are shown here with their 3 older sibs. (From DiFerrante, N., and Nichols, B. L.: Johns Hopkins Med. J. **130:**325, 1972.)

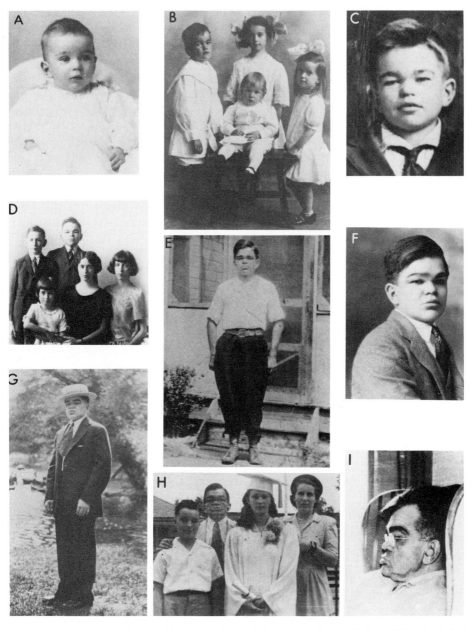

Fig. 11-19. Reproduction in the Hunter syndrome. The maternal grandfather (III$_3$, R. M. W.) of the probands (Fig. 11-15) is shown at the age of 8 or 9 months, **A**; 8 years (first on left in **B**); 14 years, **C**; 16 years (behind in **D**); 18 years, **E**; 20 years, **F**; 23 years, **G**; 45 years (with his wife, carrier daughter and son), **H**; and 53 years, **I**. He died at 57 years of age. All views, except possibly **A**, show characteristic facial features; the hearing aid is evident in **H** and **I**. (From Di Ferrante, N., and Nichols, B. L.: Johns Hopkins Med. J. **130**:325, 1972.)

Hunter phenotype frequency in males is three times the frequency of the Hurler syndrome. Without regard to sex, the frequency of the Hunter syndrome at birth is one and one-half times the frequency of the Hurler syndrome.

The predicted relative frequency of Hurler and Hunter cases is a figure on incidence at birth. Since the survival of Hunter cases is greater than that of Hurler cases, the prevalence should show an even greater excess of Hunter cases.

Consanguinity does not influence the 1.5:1 ratio under conditions of equilibrium. When the level of consanguinity increases, the relative proportion of Hurler cases increases; when the level of consanguinity decreases, as has been the case in the last few decades, the frequency of Hurler cases will decrease, until a new equilibrium is achieved. Consanguinity has no influence on the frequency of the X-linked recessive.

I am told[491] that a registry in Westphalia, West Germany, showed about one and one-half times as many Hurler cases as Hunter cases, the opposite of prediction. Similarly, Lowry and Renwick,[305] in a registry of handicapped children and adults in British Columbia, found 6 cases of the Hurler syndrome and 4 cases of the Hunter syndrome among 606,157 live births in the period of 1952 to 1968. Thus the incidence figure for the Hurler syndrome is 1 per 100,000 births, and for the Hunter syndrome, 0.66 per 100,000 births. This relative frequency, like that in Westphalia, is the opposite of the predicted figure. The incidence figures are probably underestimates, and the underestimation may be greater in the case of the Hunter syndrome than in the Hurler syndrome.

One expects no particular ethnic concentration of cases of an X-linked recessive such as MPS II. I recall seeing no Negro cases, however, until 1971, when I saw the family illustrated in Fig. 11-9. An affected Vietnamese boy has been reported.[107]

The possibility of two or more distinct forms of X-linked mucopolysaccharidosis is suggested by families in which affected males consistently fare rather well and by other families in which relatively early deterioration and death occur. Neufeld[383] has found only one X-linked form by her cross-correction methods. (Danes and Bearn[85] used the same approach of mixing cultures to demonstrate cross-correction of metachromasia. As yet unexplained is their finding of mutual cross-correction of two groups of X-linked mucopolysaccharidosis and a third presumed X-linked type that did not cross-correct the autosomal recessive Hurler syndrome.)

The clearest clinical delineation of the two forms of the Hunter syndrome is that provided by Spranger[517b] who refers to them as the juvenile and late forms. The kindreds of Cunningham,[55] Njå,[214] and van Pelt[292] among others fall into the juvenile or severe group, whereas those of Beebe and Formel,[15] Smith et al.,[261] and others fall into the mild or late group. Spranger[517b] further pointed out that neuronal storage is marked in the severe type and lacking (or at least inconspicuous) in the late form.

We[321a] prefer to call these severe and mild forms and use the letters A and B for them, respectively. Since the same corrective factor is functionally deficient in the two forms, they are presumably allelic. (As in all examples of inferred allelism, it is possible that if the corrective factor has two different subunits, each under separate genetic control, the two forms of the disease are nonallelic.)

MUCOPOLYSACCHARIDOSIS III (MPS III, SANFILIPPO SYNDROME, POLYDYSTROPHIC OLIGOPHRENIA, HEPARANSULFATURIA)

Although inherited as an autosomal recessive, as is MPS I, MPS III is distinct clinically and biochemically from MPS I and MPS II.[334] Two biochemically different forms of MPS III, Sanfilippo syndromes A and B, are indistinguishable clinically.

Clinical manifestations

In brief the clinical characteristics are severe mental retardation and relatively less severe somatic changes.[456] Intellect deteriorates so that by school age, mental retardation is evident and by the teens, outspoken. Because good bodily strength is combined with severe mental defect, management is often a problem. Clouding of the cornea does not occur. (In the patients of Sanfilippo and associates[456] corneal changes were detected in 1 of 5 patients subjected to slit-lamp examination.) Hepatosplenomegaly is only slight or moderate. Stiffness of all joints occurs, as in MPS I and MPS II, but is less severe. Dwarfing also is only moderate, and radiologically the skeleton shows only a mild degree of dysostosis multiplex. In the patients with MPS III who have severe bone changes, the abnormalities may be indistinguishable from those in patients with mild bone changes of the Hunter syndrome. In some other patients with MPS III the roentgen findings closely approach normal. MPS III thus represents the mildest portion of the dysostosis multiplex continuum, with MPS I representing a severe portion and MPS II the moderate portion. (The most severe changes of dysostosis multiplex occur in I-cell disease, or mucolipidosis II.) There is, however, one fairly specific roentgen finding in many patients with MPS III—increased thickness and density of the posterior portion of the calvaria. Spranger and associates[495] emphasized the occurrence of "ovoid dysplasia" (i.e., a biconvex configuration) of the dorsolumbar vertebral bodies, a feature that has been uncommon in the patients my colleagues and I have seen. The ribs are moderately thickened.

Cardiac abnormalities have not been described in these patients. This disorder is probably compatible with survival to the third or fourth decade in some instances. However, in 2 reported cases[551] the patients died at the ages of 27 months and 4 years, respectively, and another also died at 4 years.[102] The patient described in Case 10, below, died at 20 years.

In MPS III, metachromatic inclusions in the circulating lymphocytes are distinguished by their coarseness, relative sparsity, and restricted distribution in the cytoplasm. Gasser and Buhot cells (p. 633) are found in the bone marrow.[495]

As noted on p. 582, two clinically indistinguishable forms of the Sanfilippo syndrome are found to have different enzyme deficiencies. Fig. 11-20 presents the case of the Sanfilippo syndrome A, which Neufeld and colleagues[262a] first studied. The following two sibs had Sanfilippo syndrome B, as demonstrated enzymatically by O'Brien[398a] in one of them.

Case 10. D. F. (799359), born July 20, 1947, was first seen in February, 1958 (Fig. 11-21*A*). The parents are apparently unrelated. Both are of German ancestry, but several generations separate them from the ancestors who immigrated to this country. For the first four years of life the boy was not considered abnormal. In the latter part of his fourth year an increase in aggressive behavior was noted. Thereafter, agitation increased markedly. He started school at 6

Text continued on p. 580.

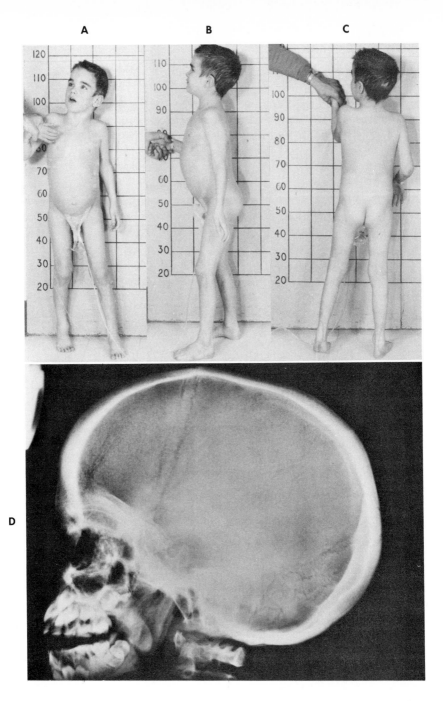

Fig. 11-20. MPS III A (Sanfilippo syndrome A). A. B. (J.H.H. 1309884) was born in 1962 of non-consanguineous parents. Frequent colds and chronically "stuffy nose" has been present essentially all his life. Mental retardation was first noted at about 2 years of age, when he was evaluated for behavior problems. At about age 3 years he suffered an electric burn when he put an extension cord in his mouth. The parents date his regression from that time. He lost speech and toilet training. At the age of 4½ years the diagnosis of Sanfilippo syndrome was made on the basis of excessive mucopolysacchariduria, predominantly heparan sulfate, and metachromatic granules of the lymphocytes. His fibroblasts were used in the cross-correction studies of Fratantoni, Hall, and Neufeld published in 1968.[153],[154] Behavior problems necessitated institutionalization.

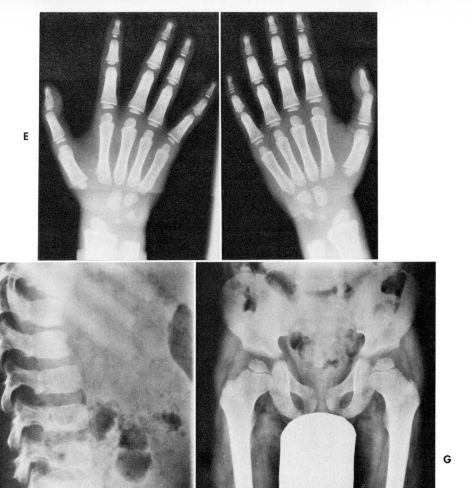

Fig. 11-20, cont'd. Examination at age 9, **A** to **C**, showed a hyperactive, speechless, severely retarded boy. Mild hypertrichosis was noted over the trunk. The corneas were clear. The liver and spleen were enlarged to about 3 fingerbreadths below the rib margins. A small umbilical hernia and bilateral inguinal hernias were present. The back showed mild low thoracic gibbus and increased lumbar lordosis. The boy walked with difficulty. The legs showed loss of muscle mass. The joints of the fingers were somewhat stiff and the fingers were tapering.

X-ray films taken at the age of 9 years are sampled in **D** to **F**. The entire cranial vault is thickened, as are the orbital plates; the mastoids are underdeveloped and sclerotic **D**. The lower spine **F** shows hypoplasia of the bodies of vertebrae T12 and L1, and the latter is mildly hooked. The hands **E** show delay in development of the carpal bones, a mild notch at the proximal end of metacarpal V, and somewhat coarse trabecular architecture of the tubular bones. The view of the pelvis and femurs **G** is notable for its normality. There is mild coxa valga, and the capital epiphyses are somewhat small.

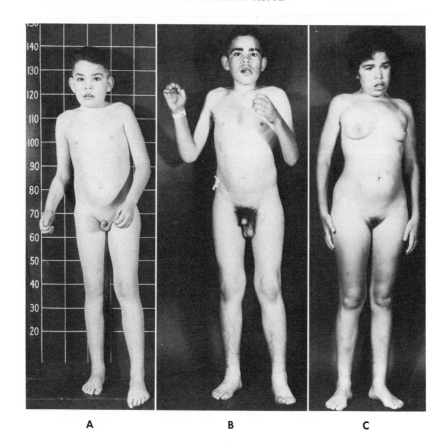

A   B   C

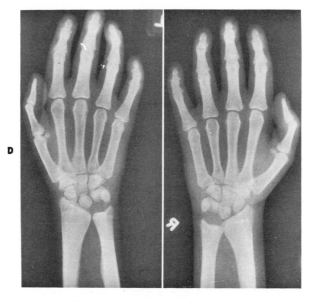

D

Fig. 11-21. For legend see opposite page.

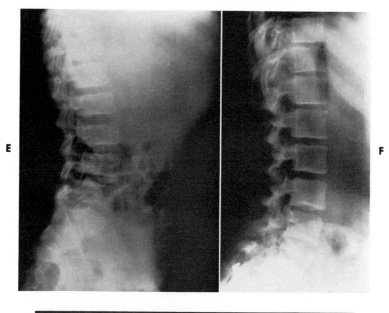

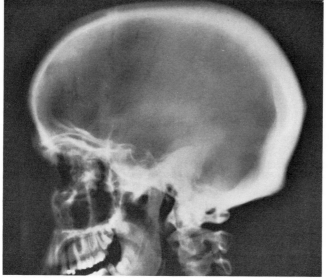

Continued.

Fig. 11-21. MPS III B (the Sanfilippo syndrome B). The brother and sister (D. F. and M. F.) are described in detail in the text. **A,** D. F., 10 years old. **B,** D. F., 16 years old. **C,** M. F., 15 years old. **D,** Hands in M. F. at 15 years old. Mild clawhand deformities with slight loss of modeling of the metacarpals and proximal phalanges are demonstrated. **E,** Spine in D. F., 16 years old. Minimal changes are present at the anterior surfaces of the lumbar vertebrae. **F,** Spine in M. F., 15 years old. Other than possible straightening of the vertebral column, no abnormalities are seen. **G,** Skull in M. F., 15 years old. Thickening of the calvaria, especially in the posterior parietal and occipital areas, is striking. Mastoids are sclerotic but the sella turcica is normal, as is usual in cases of MPS III. **H,** Pelvis and hips in D. F., 16 years old. The greater trochanters are large and hooked. The pelvis shows some narrowing above the acetabulum on each side. (**A** to **G** from McKusick, V. A., Kaplan, D., Wise, D., Hanley, W. B., Suddarth, S. B., Sevick, M. E., and Maumenee, A. E.: Medicine 44:445, 1965.)

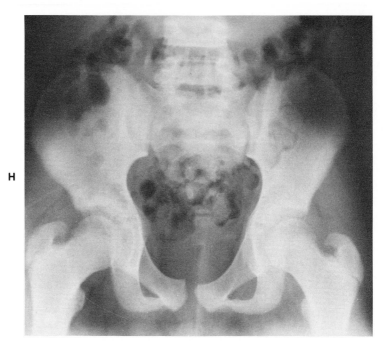

H

Fig. 11-21, cont'd. For legend see p. 579.

years of age but was able to attend only about six weeks because he would not sit still in class or follow instructions. His speaking ability deteriorated rapidly in the seventh and eighth years. The patient was at that time noted to have a "potbelly." At the age of 9 years, as part of his agitated behavior, he acquired the habit of clapping his hands as he walked around and of pounding the walls with the flat of the hands. The diagnosis of the Hurler syndrome was first made at the age of 10 years.

The appearance in 1958 is well illustrated by Fig. 11-21*A*. All features are consistent with mild Hurler syndrome: coarse facial features, short neck, mild clawhand deformity, and prominent abdomen. He was of normal height, however, and had no enlargement of the liver and spleen. Examination of the eyes under anesthesia showed no abnormality. X-ray films showed the long bones of the extremities and the ribs to be somewhat enlarged. The vertebrae were judged normal. Dr. Karl Meyer of Columbia University found mucopolysaccharide in the urine, 36 mg./L., most of which was heparan sulfate; there was no dermatan sulfate.

At the age of 12 years the patient stopped talking altogether and made only animal-like sounds. He also became totally incontinent, requiring the wearing of diapers. A stiff manner of walking was noted and the patient stopped growing. At the age of 14 years a left inguinal hernia was repaired but it recurred six months later. "Curling of the fingers" and inability to extend the elbows fully were noted at the age of 15 years. During that year also, puberty occurred, with development of pubic hair and a deeper voice and enlargement of the phallus. He was always a mouth breather and had frequent respiratory infections. Whereas the first teeth were normal, the second teeth were widely and irregularly spaced and small. During the fifteenth year, severe generalized seizures had their onset.

Examination at the age of 16 years showed an agitated, severely retarded boy (Fig. 11-21*B*). Fine lanugo-like hair covered the back and buttocks. The bridge of the nose was depressed, the nares were patulous, and the lips were large. The mouth was held open constantly. The neck was strikingly short and thick. The liver edge was 4 cm. below the right costal margin. The spleen was not felt. The elbows and fingers could not be fully extended. No cardiac abnormality was detected by physical examination, electrocardiogram, or chest x-ray study.

X-ray films showed a thickened calvaria and distal tapering of the radius and ulna bilaterally. Again the cornea was clear by slit-lamp examination.

In 1963 the patient was found to excrete heparan sulfate, 123 mg./L., in the urine. (Urine volumes were, however, rather small. Three days were required to collect about 1 liter.)

Follow-up. This patient died in a state institution at the age of 20 years. From studies of his liver, O'Brien[398a] demonstrated deficiency of N-acetyl-α-D-glucosaminidase (p. 582). Thus this is a case of type B Sanfilippo syndrome (see later).

Case 11. M. F. (1084542), born July 25, 1948, was first seen in August, 1963, at the age of 15 years (Fig. 11-21*C*). She was more intelligent than her brother, used some words and phrases, and was toilet-trained. Menses began at the age of 12 years.

The patient began school at 6 years and for two years apparently performed satisfactorily. In her third year she began to be inattentive and agitated and refused to sit still in class. She became excited and aggressive when with other children. Hearing loss was first noted at 7 years of age and was progressive thereafter. At 10 or 11 years of age, limitation of motion of the elbows and fingers were noted. Speech deteriorated, and repetition of words or phrases when she was agitated became a feature. She would bite her fingernails until bleeding occurred.

The permanent teeth were late in developing and were irregularly spaced. Unlike her brother, she would sit quietly and watch television. She was a mouth breather and snored.

Examination revealed, as in the brother, depressed nasal bridge, patulous lips, crowded, irregular teeth, short neck, enlargement of the liver 3 cm. below the costal margin, and limitation in extension of the elbows and fingers. Unlike the brother, she had a flat abdomen. The skin showed lanugo-like hair generally. Examination of the eyes (including slit-lamp examination) and heart revealed no abnormality.

When the patient was studied in 1963, heparan sulfate was excreted in the urine in large amounts—about 83 mg./L. (As in the brother, urine volumes were small and about three days were required for collection of 1 liter.)

In the brother and sister, 20% and 28%, respectively, of the peripheral lymphocytes contained metachromatic granules on staining with toluidine blue.

The father (H. F. F. 1084513) and the mother (S. F., 1084544) showed no abnormality in the physical examination, skeletal x-ray films, or urine mucopolysaccharide excretion. The mother has no other children.

Pathology

The findings in several autopsies have been reported.[102,551] Electron microscopic studies were reported by Dodion and colleagues[111] and by Wallace and associates.[551] As noted above, the patients studied by Wallace and associates died at the ages of 27 months and 4 years, respectively. In the younger child the spleen weighed 60 grams (normal, 37 grams). Heparan sulfate was identified in the brain. Histochemically, lipid was shown in neurons and metachromatic material in macrophages. By electron microscopy, neurons were shown to have lipid cytosomes like those in Tay-Sachs disease, and these bodies showed alkaline phophatase activity indicating lysosomal origin. Parenchymal and Kupffer cells of the liver, rectal mucosa cells, and cells of the distal convoluted and collecting tubules of the kidney showed metachromatic inclusions positive histochemically for acid mucopolysaccharide and acid phosphatase. (Haust et al.,[192a] in a case that seemed to qualify otherwise for classification as MPS III, described unusual "mitochondrial crystalloids.") The patient studied by Dekaban and Patton[102] was 4 years old at the time of death. They found that layers II and IV of the cerebral cortex were more severely affected than layers III and V and suggested that a relation exists between this fact and the early and severe mental deterioration in the face of the relatively good preservation of motor function that characterizes MPS III.

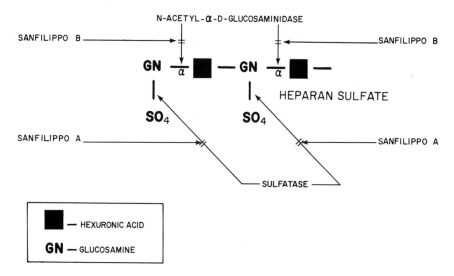

Fig. 11-22. Diagrammatic representation of the polysaccharide side-chains of heparan sulfate to show sites of action of heparan sulfate sulfatase (deficient in Sanfilippo syndrome A) and of N-acetyl-α-D-glucosaminidase (deficient in Sanfilippo syndrome B). (After a diagram of Dr. E. F. Neufeld.)

The fundamental defect

Patients with MPS III excrete large amounts of heparan sulfate in the urine. Almost only this mucopolysaccharide is excreted in excess. See p. 635 for further discussion of the basic defect. Cross-correction studies in fibroblasts indicate the existence of two clinically indistinguishable forms of heparan-sulfate–excreting mucopolysaccharidosis,[262b] arbitrarily designated types A and B. The enzyme deficient in Sanfilippo syndrome A is heparan sulfate sulfatase.[262a] That deficient in Sanfilippo syndrome B is N-acetyl-α-D-glucosaminidase.[398a] Having had an opportunity to study the same patients in whom Neufeld and O'Brien established the enzymes deficient in the two forms, I conclude that the two forms are completely indistinguishable phenotypically. Fig. 11-22 represents schematically the site of the metabolic defect in Sanfilippo syndromes A and B.

Prevalence and inheritance

MPS III is inherited as an autosomal recessive disorder. Males and females are affected with about equal frequency. The parents are normal but in some instances consanguineous.[334,495] An estimate of frequency is even more of a guess than in the cases of MPS I and MPS II. Some patients are probably institutionalized and not recognized as cases of the Hurler syndrome because of the relatively inconspicuous somatic features. The disorder may occur appreciably more often than in "one out of every 100,000 to 200,000 people," as estimated by Terry and Linker.[520] It may be one half to one third as frequent as the Hurler and Hunter syndromes combined.[406] Thus, Langer[277] had 23 Hurler-Hunter cases and 9 Sanfilippo cases. Kaplan[238] had 15 cases of MPS III as compared with 12 of MPS II, 11 of MPS I, and 8 of MPS VI. MPS III has been reported in American Negroes.[476]

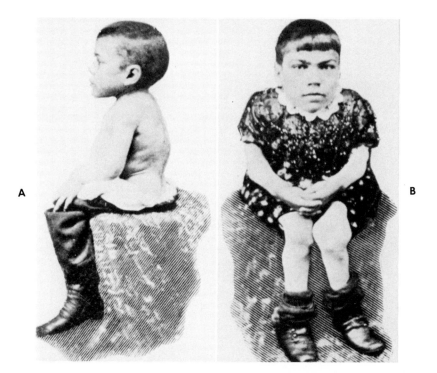

Fig. 11-23. MPS IV (the Morquio syndrome). Brother, **A**, and sister, **B**, in a French-Canadian family reported by Osler in 1897, Laberge[260a] has followed these patients and shown their probable relationship to other cases of the Morquio syndrome in French Canadians of eastern Quebec Province. (From Osler, W.: Trans. Cong. Amer. Phys. 4:169, 1897.)

MUCOPOLYSACCHARIDOSIS IV (MPS IV, MORQUIO SYNDROME, KERATANSULFATURIA)

Probable cases of the Morquio syndrome were reported as cases of achondroplasia by Osler[413] (Fig. 11-23) and by Voisin and Voisin.[546] Simultaneously and independently in 1929, Morquio[373]* of Uruguay, and Brailsford[40] of Birmingham, England, gave definitive descriptions. Thereafter the disorder became known as the Morquio syndrome or, less frequently, as the Morquio-Brailsford syndrome. Other designations used in the literature included chondro-osteodystrophy and eccentro-osteochondrodysplasia.

---

*Morquio (Fig. 11-24) was born in Montevideo, Uruguay, in 1867 and was graduated in medicine there in 1892. He studied pediatrics at the *Hôpital des enfants malades* in Paris from 1893 to 1894. In 1899 he was appointed professor of pediatrics at Montevideo and continued in that post until his death in 1935.[380]

Morquio's patients[372,373] affected with the disease that bears his name were of Swedish extraction. Their parents were first cousins. Of 5 children, only the first, a male, was unaffected. The second, Maria, born in 1913, was described in the initial report in 1929[373]; she died of pulmonary complications in the 1930's. The third child, Arturo, born in 1915, died of the same cause in 1939. The fourth, Julio (Fig. 11-25), born in 1917, is still living (1971) at the age of 54 years! He has corneal clouding but is said to have no sign of cardiac abnormality. The fifth child, Carlos, was born in 1919 and died of pulmonary complications. (I am indebted to Dr. Horacio Cardoso of Montevideo for the above information.) Maroteaux and Lamy[341a] obtained confirmation of the presence of corneal clouding.

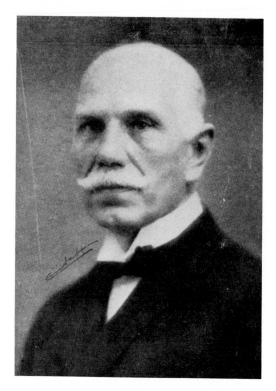

Fig. 11-24. Professor Luis Morquio (1867-1935).

In the 1950's other features of this disorder, in addition to merely the orthopedic ones, began to come to attention. During a thirty-year period after the publication of Morquio's and Brailsford's descriptions, a wide variety of cases found their way into the literature under the Morquio sobriquet.[422,432,482] Many of these, with our increased knowledge of hereditary skeletal disease, are not now considered to have been the same disorder as that described by Morquio. Cases pigeonholed with the Morquio syndrome include what we would now classify as X-linked spondyloepiphyseal dysplasia,[223] multiple epiphyseal dysplasia,[486] diastrophic dwarfism,[273,324] metatropic dwarfism,[343,367] parastremmatic dwarfism,[279,432] spondyloepiphyseal dysplasia congenita,[92,494] or other entities.[48,196,450] Robinow[444] included under the "Morquio syndrome" a considerable number of entities clearly distinct from that described by Morquio and Brailsford and stated that inheritance could be dominant, recessive, or X-linked. Partly because of the "trash-can" state of the nosography of the Morquio syndrome, it was proposed, when corneal abnormalities were discovered in the Morquio syndrome, that a new entity was involved, deserving a new name. Wiedemann,[557] followed by Zellweger and colleagues,[574] gave the name Morquio-Ullrich syndrome to the disorder in cases having the typical skeletal features described by Morquio and Brailsford but also with corneal changes

It is plausible to suggest,[339,445] however, that the patients reported by Morquio and by Brailsford suffered from the form of spondyloepiphyseal dys-

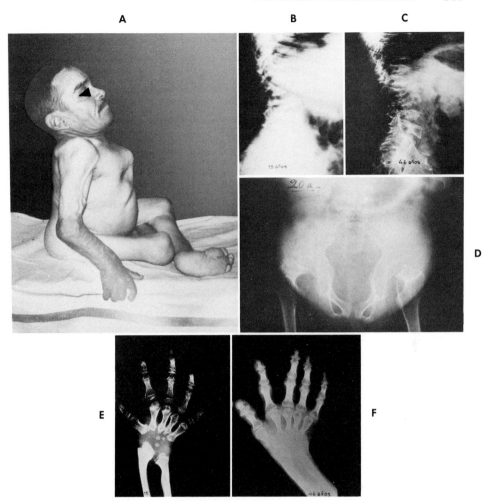

Fig. 11-25. Surviving patient of Morquio with the Morquio syndrome. **A,** Appearance at 53 years of age. **B** and **C,** X-ray views of lateral spine at 15 and 46 years, respectively. **D,** Pelvis at 20 years of age. **E** and **F,** X-ray views of hand at 15 and 46 years, respectively.

plasia in which we now recognize extraskeletal features such as corneal clouding and aortic valve damage. It is this entity which we have proposed to call simply the *Morquio syndrome*. Additional justification for considering it a distinct disorder, and a mucopolysaccharidosis, comes from identification of a characteristic mucopolysacchariduria—namely, excessive keratan sulfate—and fibroblast metachromasia. Certainly heterogeneity remains. Two reasonably clear forms of the Morquio syndrome can, in my opinion, be distinguished: a keratan-sulfate–excreting form and a non-keratan-sulfate–excreting form.

Clinical manifestations

Differences of the Morquio syndrome (MPS IV) from MPS I will be emphasized. The MPS IV patients are strikingly dwarfed (Fig. 11-26), and in older

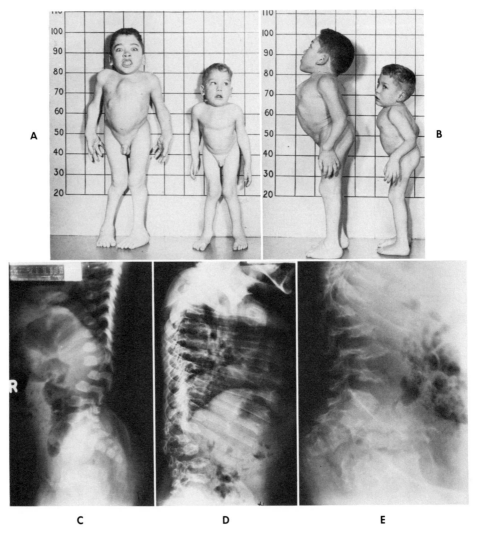

Fig. 11-26. MPS IV (the Morquio syndrome). These brothers (J. G. and M. G.) are described in detail in the text. **A**, and **B**, General appearance. **C** to **E**, Spine in J. G. at the ages of 13 months, 8 years, and 15 years, respectively. The early changes are indistinguishable from those of MPS I (cf. Fig. 11-2C). Marked osteoporosis and platyspondyly are later developments. **F** and **G**, Hands in J. G., 15 years old, **F**, and in M. G., 5 years old, **G**. Osteoporosis and abnormal shapes of all bones are demonstrated. Carpal bones ossify late and are small and severely misshapen. The shafts of the metacarpals and phalanges are relatively normally constructed (cf. Fig. 11-4C). **H**, Spinal curvature in M. G., 5 years old. **I**, Left hip in M. G., 5 years old See Plate 1B for corneal clouding in older boy. (From McKusick, V. A., Kaplan, D., Wise, D., Hanley, W. B., Suddarth, S. B., Sevick, M. E., and Maumenee, A. E.: Medicine 44:445, 1965.)

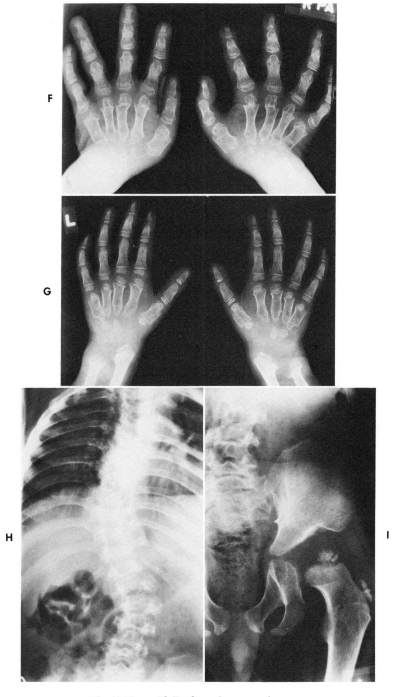

Fig. 11-26, cont'd. For legend see opposite page.

children the skeletal findings are quite distinctive. In the first year or two of life, however, the lumbar spine may show beaking similar to that of the Hurler syndrome; for other reasons, as well, MPS I and MPS IV are difficult to distinguish, at that stage, by any means except the urinary pattern of mucopolysaccharide excretion. This point is well illustrated by the cases described below. See also Fig. 5 of Robins and co-workers.[445] Later, the radiologic changes in MPS IV are different from those of MPS I, flat vertebrae being particularly characteristic of MPS IV. All the bones become markedly osteoporotic.

Abnormalities are not evident at birth, and psychomotor development is normal in the first year, although roentgenographic abnormalities may be detectable at that time.[445] In the second or third year of life, awkward gait, retarded growth, knock-knees, sternal bulging, flaring of the rib cage, flat feet, prominent joints, or dorsal kyphosis, or some combination of these anomalies, usually brings the child to medical attention. With advancing age all these deformities are exaggerated and growth is severely deficient. Growth slows remarkably after the age of 5 or 6 years. The fact is implied by the heights of the brothers, 15 and 5 years old, shown in Fig. 11-26A and B. In my experience, patients with MPS IV achieve a maximal height of 85 to 100 cm., usually by 7 or 8 years of age.

The wrists are enlarged and the hands misshapen. However, the joints are usually not stiff. Indeed some, such as the wrists, may be hyperextensible. A barrel chest with pigeon breast ("sternal kyphos") is surmounted by a short neck. The stance is semi-crouching (Fig. 11-26). Knock-knees are usual. The facies is characteristic, with broad mouth, prominent maxilla, short nose, and widely spaced teeth. The corneas become diffusely opacified,[548] but this process progresses more slowly than in MPS I. Clouding obvious to the unaided eye is usually not evident until after the age of 10 years. Grossly it has the appearance of a filmy haze rather than of ground glass, as seen in MPS I and MPS V. Hernia probably occurs with increased frequency; inguinal hernia was present in Brailsford's case.[40] The skin[178] is loose, thickened, tough, and inelastic, particularly over the limbs, and telangiectasia has been found, particularly on the face and limbs.

Neurologic symptoms frequently result from spinal cord and medullary compression. Spastic paraplegia is frequent (Plate I*A*), and respiratory paralysis occurs in late stages.[6] High spinal cord compression related to hypoplasia of the odontoid is a major complication of the Morquio syndrome.[37,123,204,278] Five of 6 adults reported by Langer and Carey[278] had long tract signs referable to abnormality at the upper cervical area. Ligamentous laxity comparable to that evident at the wrists contributes to the spinal cord compression. A usual history[259] is that by 7 or 8 years of age the child manifests decreasing physical endurance and increasing difficulty walking through snow and upstairs; increasingly he asks to be carried. He may complain that his legs "buckle under him." He shows severe genu valgum, which is blamed for the symptoms. Osteotomies for leg straightening fail to relieve the symptoms. Neurologic manifestations may be minimal. The parents resign themselves to a progressively deteriorating, chair-ridden state. Sometimes the story is that the legs are useless when he first gets up in the morning. As pointed out by Kopits,[259] the level of physical endurance is one of the best indications of the state of the atlantoaxial area. Odontoid aplasia or marked hypoplasia is probably present in all cases of MPS IV, and all patients sooner or later develop serious spinal compression from atlantoaxial subluxation. Intelligence is normal or only mildly impaired. Progressive deafness has its onset usually in the teens and is present in almost all patients who survive to the third decade or later.[295] Audiologic studies indicate that the deafness is neurosensory (see Case 10, below).

In our series[322] aortic regurgitation was present in 3 teen-age patients from three unrelated families. Two affected brothers known to us (E. J. J. and R. E. J.) died at the ages of 37 and 40 years; both had aortic regurgitation.*

Garn and Hurme[161] described abnormality of both the deciduous and the permanent teeth in 3 sibs out of 9. The 6 unaffected sibs had normal dental enamel. The evidence of defect consisted of thinness of enamel, shown by x-ray film, tendency of the enamel to fracture and flake off, and a dull grayish appearance of the crowns of the teeth. The diagnosis of MPS IV was supported by the description of corneal opacities in a follow-up report.[444] The molars have sharp, pointed cusps. Because of the thin enamel, the teeth are vulnerable to caries, a feature noted by Brailsford[40] in his 4-year-old patient.

Cases reported by Ruggles[451] by Whiteside[556] and by Gasteiger and Liebenam[162] were probably also instances of MPS IV.

A characteristic radiologic feature of MPS IV is universal platyspondyly. In the early stages the thoracic vertebrae are ovoid in shape. Growth in height of the vertebrae is slow between the ages of 2 and 6 years, and an anterior projection, or tongue, develops during this stage. In the adult the vertebral bodies are flattened and rectangular, with wide disc spaces. The odontoid process is hypoplastic or absent. Flaring of the ilia is particularly striking because of narrowing above the acetabula. In the early years the femoral capital epiphyses are normal or only slightly flattened. However, progressive flattening and fragmentation, with coxa valga, develop. In the adolescent and adult the femoral heads frequently disappear, resulting in erosion and widening of the femoral necks. The carpal centers are small and retarded in development. The distal ends of the radius and ulna are inclined toward each other, and the metaphyses are wide and irregular. The long bones are short and poorly tubulated, especially in the upper limbs. Spatulate ribs, a bulging sternum, often with an almost horizontal upper part, and dorsal kyphosis are also evident roentgenographically.

Cases 12 and 13. The patients shown in Fig. 11-26 were 5 and 15 years old at the time of this study. However, x-ray films covering the entire life-span were available for review. Five sibs were normal. Another sib, male, died at 33 hours. He may have been affected. The father and mother were of English and English-Irish ancestry, respectively, and were not known to be related.

The elder brother had clubbed feet at birth. The diagnosis of Morquio syndrome was made at the age of 13 months. In the younger brother the diagnosis was made at birth because his facial appearance was like his brother's and because motion at the elbows was limited. An inguinal hernia was repaired at the age of 14 months in the younger brother.

A diffuse corneal haze was noted when the elder brother, then 8 years old, was first seen by an ophthalmologist. Examination four years later showed little change.

The findings of the physical and radiologic examinations are well shown in Fig. 11-26. Intelligence was normal. The older brother (15 years old) had lax wrists, the murmur of aortic regurgitation, and diffuse grayish clouding of the cornea bilaterally. Slit-lamp examination showed the corneal changes to be primarily in the posterior stroma and to be uniformly distributed.

---

*Information courtesy Dr. John J. Rick, Coldwater, Mich.

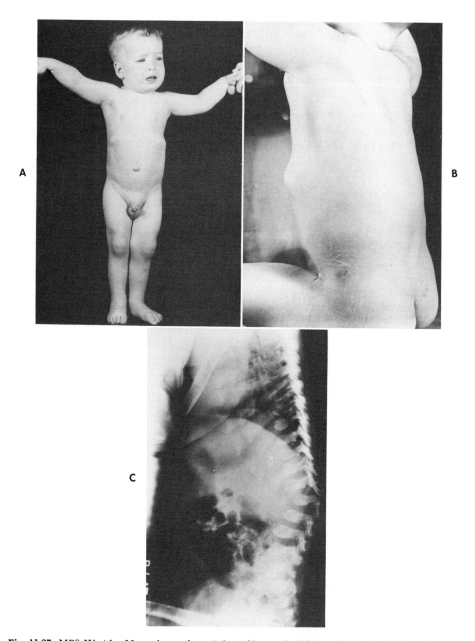

Fig. 11-27. MPS IV (the Morquio syndrome) in a 21-month-old boy, J. J., described in detail in the text. **A,** General appearance. **B,** Lumbar gibbus and flared lower ribs are demonstrated. **C,** X-ray view of the spine. As in Fig. 11-21*C,* the findings are identical to those of MPS I. **D,** Hands. The shape of the metacarpal and carpal bones is distinctive and quite different from that in MPS I (cf. Fig. 11-4*C*). **E,** Feet. (From McKusick, V. A., Kaplan, D., Wise, D., Hanley, W. B., Suddarth, S. B., Sevick, M. E., and Maumenee, A. E.: Medicine 44:445, 1965.)

The 5-year-old brother had slight but definite clouding of the cornea, demonstrable by slit lamp only. A granular appearance of the fundus in the macular area was observed. Urine from only the younger brother has been studied so far, and 60 to 70 mg./L. of keratan sulfate was found. Peripheral blood films for both boys revealed no lymphocytic metachromatic granules, but the majority of the polymorphonuclear leukocytes showed varying numbers of small clusters of clearly defined metachromatic granules within the cytoplasm, i.e., Reilly granulation.

Follow-up. The younger brother died unexpected in his sleep at the age of 7 years. The elder brother died at the age of 21 years after being confined to a wheelchair for several years because of tetraparesis.

Case 14. J. J. (1106668) is the only child of parents who are not known to be related. No similarly affected persons are known in the family of either parent.

The child was first studied at the age of 21 months (Fig. 11-27) because of skeletal abnormalities, which had been noted first at the age of 4 months: flaring of the lower rib cage and a lump on the lumbar spine. Mental and physical development had been normal, otherwise. His first tooth erupted at the age of 4 months, and he stood with support at 8 months, walked at 17 months, and spoke two-word sentences at 19 months. At the age of 6 weeks he had been hospitalized for two weeks with vomiting, jaundice, and mild enlargement of the liver. Neonatal hepatitis was diagnosed. A right hydrocele was found at that time.

Main features of the examination at the age of 21 months are shown in the illustrations. The flaring of the lower ribs and the lumbar gibbus are striking. The hands are stubby and less extensive than one would expect for a child of this age. The liver was palapted 3 cm. below the right costal margin, the tip of the spleen was palpable, and a small umbilical hernia and right hydrocele were present.

The child was initially thought to show a typical instance of the Hurler syndrome.

Significant investigations included the following: Slit-lamp examination revealed fine gray stippling in the corneal stroma bilaterally, most marked in the periphery, X-ray films showed a gibbus at Ll, a slight reduction in height of the vertebral bodies, and an anteroinferior lipping of the lumbar vertebral bodies. The metacarpals and phalanges showed swelling of the shafts, with tapering distally. Carpal ossification was delayed, and the bones were small and severely misshapen. The metacarpals and phalanges were short and wide with, however, relatively normal constriction in their diaphyses. Coxa valga was present. No lymphocyte inclusions were found in the peripheral blood but, as in the previous 2 cases, the cytoplasm of approximately 50% of the polymorphonuclear leukocytes contained clusters of small but clearly defined metachromatic granules.

On study of the urine, 92.7 mg./L. of acid mucopolysaccharide was recovered, most of it

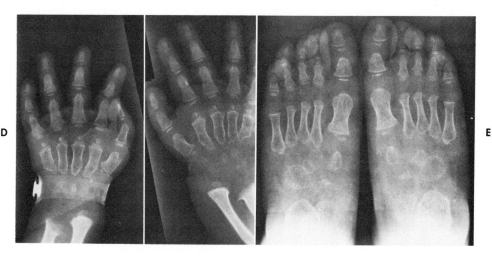

Fig. 11-27, cont'd. For legend see opposite page.

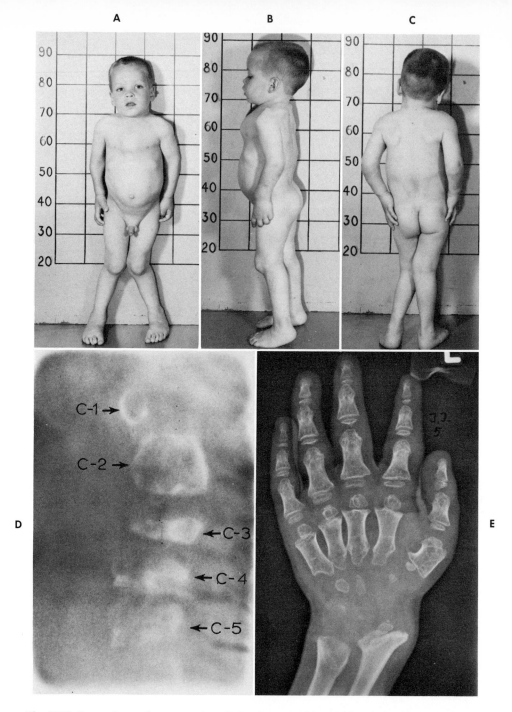

Fig. 11-28. Later observations on patient J. J., shown in Fig. 11-22 and described in the text. **A** to **C**, Appearance at 6 years of age. Genu valgum and pectus carinatum are striking, and lumbar gibbus is still evident. **D**, Tomographic view (at the age of 5½ years) of the upper cervical spine to demonstrate absence of the odontoid process. **E**, X-ray view of hand at the age of 5½ years. The carpal bones are delayed in their development. The distal ends of the radius and ulna and the bones of the hand are expanded and deformed. **F**, X-ray view of feet at 5½ years of age. **G**, X-ray view of legs at 5½ years. **H** and **I**, Appearance at 7 years. The knee deformity has been partially corrected. Hirsutism of the legs is marked. **J**, X-ray view of pelvis and femora at the age of 8½ years. **K** and **L**, X-ray views of the spine at the age of 8½ years. Characteristic changes of MPS IV are now fully developed.

being keratan sulfate. A second study two months after the first yielded similar results. The cetyltrimethylammonium bromide screening test[440,441] was strongly positive.

For later observations on this patient, see Fig. 11-28.

Case 15. J. M. S. (J.H.H. 1328788), born in 1938, is one of the oldest patients with the keratan-sulfate–excreting form of the Morquio syndrome I have seen (Fig. 11-29). Since the excessive mucopolysacchariduria is absent in adults with MPS IV, the diagnosis is based on clinical grounds.

There is no history of a similar disorder in the family, and the parents are not related. A brother and 2 sisters are normal. At birth she weighed 9 pounds and measured 20 inches. Development was considered normal until the age of 2 years, when she fell from a hayloft. Thereafter she grew little. At the age of 7 years surgical procedures for leg straightening were performed. By 20 years of age the corneas were noted to be grossly cloudy. Hearing began to fail when she was in her twenties. At 30 years of age a hearing aid was fitted with good results. She wore complete dentures from the age of 22 years. Examination revealed marked dwarfism (height, 34 inches) with kyphoscoliosis, short neck, protruding sternum, hyperextensible and unstable joints, mild hirsutism, and long tract signs in both the arms and the legs, presumably related to the demonstrable aplasia of the odontoid process and C1-2 laxity. The poor stability at the wrists made it difficult for her to continue the handiwork that was her main pasttime. Casts applied to the wrists greatly improved hand function, and surgical fusion of the wrists was considered but not performed. Breast development was normal. (Menses began at the age of 15 years.) Intelligence was apparently normal.

Tests indicated bilateral neurosensory hearing loss.

X-ray studies showed severe genu valgum, dislocation of both hips with no femoral heads and short, broad, eburnated femoral necks, marked generalized platyspondyly, and characteristic deformity of the ribs, sternum, and hands.

Pathology

An autopsy has been reported by Einhorn and colleagues[124]; and bone biopsies were presented by Aegerter and Kirkpatrick,[2] by Shelling,[478] and by Anderson and colleagues.[6] Zellweger and colleagues[574] found Reilly granules in the leukocytes of their cases. These granules may be absent in early stages, however.

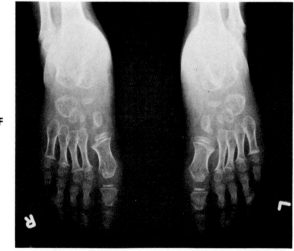

F

Continued.

Fig. 11-28, cont'd. For legend see opposite page.

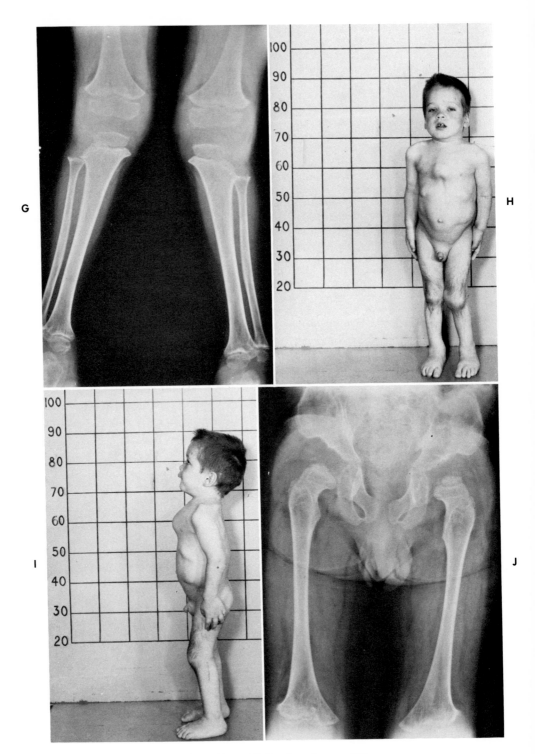

Fig. 11-28, cont'd. For legend see p. 592.

K

L

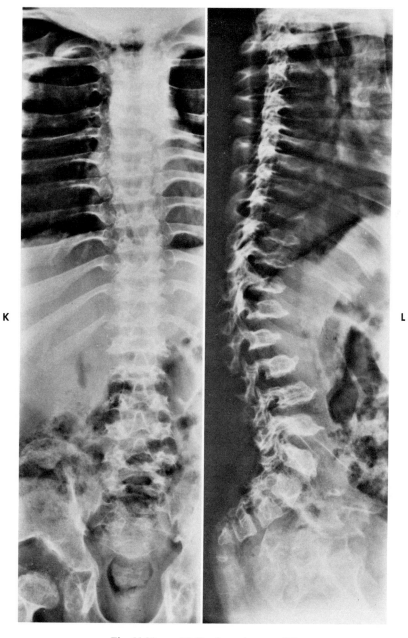

Fig. 11-28, cont'd. For legend see p. 592.

(See reference 464.) Tondeur and Loeb[529] studied the ultrastructure of the liver in 2 children with keratan-sulfate–excreting Morquio syndrome. The Kupffer cells contained membrane-bound inclusions. Much fewer and smaller inclusions were found in hepatic cells. Schenk and Haggerty[464] demonstrated accumulation of acid mucopolysaccharide in chondrocytes. Bona and colleagues[390] studied cartilage histologically.

Prognosis

At least until the last decade or so, a majority of patients with MPS IV probably died before the age of 20 years. In part the deaths were due to cardiorespiratory failure in the face of respiratory infection. However, many died suddenly, in their sleep, for example, possibly as a result of acute atlantoaxial subluxation. Respiratory arrest during induction of surgical anesthesia may have the same basis. Manipulation of the head for intubation is a dangerous matter. Surgical fusion of the upper cervical spine (see below) should be a life-prolonging measure in this disorder.

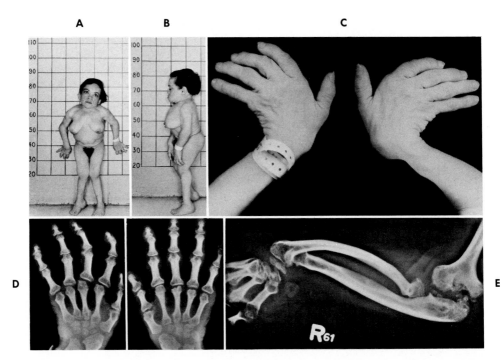

Fig. 11-29. MPS IV in 33-year-old woman. **A** and **B,** Note marked dwarfing and skeletal deformities typical of MPS IV. **C,** Marked ulnar deviation of the hands related to instability of the wrists. **D,** X-ray views of the hands and wrist show relatively short ulnas, contributing to the ulnar deviation, small carpal bones, and typical deformity of the hand bones. On the left, the second and third fingers are subluxated at the metacarpophalangeal joint. **E,** X-ray view of the right forearm, showing marked bowing of the radius and many loose osseous bodies in the region of the elbow. **F** and **G,** X-ray views of the spine showing typical platyspondyly in severe form. **H,** No femoral heads can be identified, although the largest of the loose bodies in the region of the left acetabulum may be a remnant. The hips are dislocated. The constriction above the acetabulum is typical of MPS IV. **I,** Marked genu valgum is demonstrated.

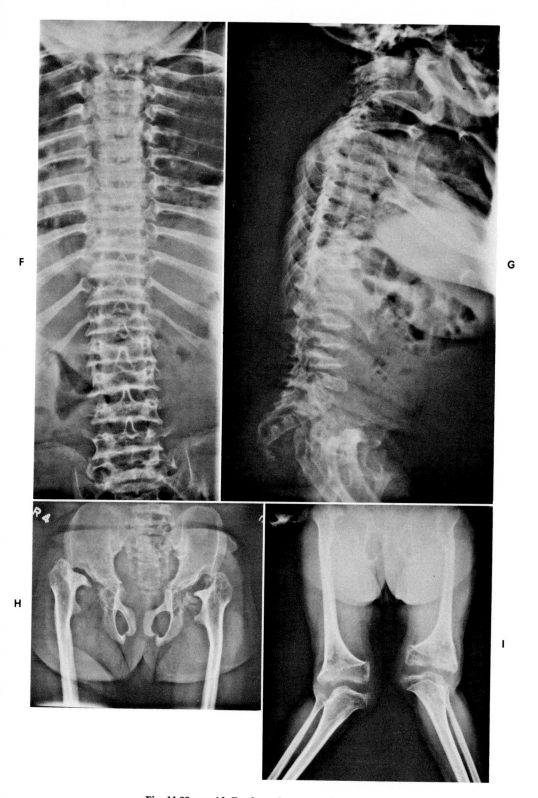

Fig. 11-29, cont'd. For legend see opposite page.

Although the prognosis is in general poor, I have studied 8 cases of the Morquio syndrome in persons age 21 years or older. All are female except the youngest, age 21. Of the others, 2 are 33, 2 are 32, and 1 each is 30, 28, and 24 years old. One remarkable woman with MPS IV has had two children both of whom at ages 8 and 7 are appreciably taller than she.

It appears that females fare better than males, perhaps because females generally lead a more sheltered, less active life than do males and are therefore under less risk of the complications of atlantoaxial subluxation. The better prognosis in females seems to be borne out by two affected brother-sister pairs. In each pair the brother has died, whereas the sister (P. P., 1429793; C. S. H., 1460074) is living at an age well beyond that at which the brother died. To be sure, Morquio's patient, who is still surviving at age 55 years, is male (Fig. 11-25).

The fundamental defect

Patients with the Morquio syndrome excrete excessive amounts of keratan sulfate in the urine.[18,339,340,416,502] This excretion is about two or three times normal excretion. The keratansulfaturia diminishes, however, as the patient becomes older and in the adult may not be excessive.[54,292,341a] (Even though the total excretion of mucopolysaccharides may not be outside the normal range in adults with MPS IV, keratan sulfate excretion may be elevated.)

Keratan-sulfate excretion is relatively high in normal infants and children, falling to low levels after 20 years of age. (The excretion of uronic acid–containing mucopolysaccharide is also increased somewhat in MPS IV.[295] This increase may not be unexpected, since keratan sulfate is part of the same protein complex as chondroitin-6-sulfate and may be excreted as such.[238]) Keratan sulfate precipitates with cetyltrimethylammonium bromide (CTAB), thus giving a positive screening test by this method (p. 629). Keratan sulfate is more difficult to quantitate than the uronic-acid–containing mucopolysaccharides, which can be measured specifically by analysis of microsamples for constituent monosaccharide units. For keratan sulfate, isolation on a preparative scale is necessary. (For details, see references 240 and 292.)

The abnormally thin dental enamel occurring in MPS IV may not be surprising in view of the conclusions of Weill and Tassin,[555] on the basis of staining with toluidine blue and alcian blue, that the enamel matrix is relatively rich in acid mucopolysaccharides. Wislocki and Sognnaes[562] demonstrated toluidine-blue metachromasia in the developing enamel. Some of the metachromasia remained after hyaluronidase digestion, suggesting the presence of some highly sulfated acid mucopolysaccharides. Others were removed by the enzyme and presumably represent chondroitin-4- and chondroitin-6-sulfates. Clark and associates[64] determined hexosamines in acid-glycosaminoglycan fractions isolated from human teeth.

Metachromatic granules in fibroblasts of patients with the Morquio syndrome were simultaneously and independently discovered by Fraccaro and colleagues[144] and by Danes and co-workers.[84] Magrini and associates[327] showed a strict parallelism between S[35]-labeling and metachromasia. They further suggested the existence of heterogeneity in the Morquio syndrome on the basis of 2 affected sisters whose fibroblasts were negative by both criteria despite visceral involvement and excess keratan sulfate in the urine.

Robins and associates[445] concluded that one group of patients with the Morquio syndrome excrete, during childhood at least, excessive amounts of chondroitin-4-sulfate in the urine. The clinical characterization of this group will be important.

Differential diagnosis

The Morquio syndrome as defined here is a form of spondyloepiphyseal dysplasia (SED). The differential diagnosis includes other types of SED, such as the X-linked form, which are discussed in Chapter 13.

There appears to exist a form of Morquio syndrome very similar to the keratan-sulfate–excreting form but characterized by lesser severity of both the skeletal and the extraskeletal features and by no excessive mucopolysacchariduria. This condition might be termed the *non-keratan-sulfate–excreting Morquio syndrome*,[394] or Morquio syndrome type II. The following is a description of the family on which I base the claim for a distinct form.

Case 16. E. M. J. (J.H.H. 695487), the white female proband, was born in 1945. Her case was presented as representative of the Morquio syndrome in the second edition of this monograph (p. 271, 1960). Since that time 3 affected cousins (Cases 17, 18, and 19) have come to attention. (See the pedigree detailed in Fig. 11-30*A*).

No abnormality was noted by her parents until the age of 6 years, by which time increased anteroposterior diameter of the chest, genu valgum, and enlarged knees and knuckles were evident. Radiographic studies at the age of 10 years showed generalized platyspondyly and severe changes in the femoral heads.

The patient married and in 1964 was delivered of a normal son by cesarean section.

Physical examination in 1967 (Fig. 11-30*C*) showed a height of 45 inches, a short neck, a barrel chest with protuberant upper sternum, genu valgum, and flat feet. The joints, especially the wrists, were hyperextensible but not to the degree observed in the usual Morquio syndrome. Slit-lamp examination showed a stromal haze in the posterior part of the cornea and punctate zonular cataracts bilaterally. The heart and lungs were normal and the liver and spleen were not enlarged. Genitalia and secondary sex characteristics were normal. Her intelligence was above average.

Radiographic studies are shown in Fig. 11-30*D* to *F*.

Case 17. L. B. (J.H.H. 1238045), a white male born March 12, 1952, is a cousin of E. M. J. He was considered normal by his parents until the age of 6 years, when flat feet were noted.

Examination (1967) showed a height of 49 inches, short neck, barrel chest, lumbar gibbus, hypermobility of the wrists, flat feet, and bilateral genu valgum with external rotation of the right tibia (Fig. 11-30*G* and *H*). The hips were fully mobile.

Radiographic findings are described in Fig. 11-30*I* to *L*.

Case 18. R. B., brother of Case 12, was born in 1953. As in his brother, the first abnormality noted was flat feet at about 6 years of age.

In 1967 (Fig. 11-30*M* and *N*) height was 45½ inches; other findings were similar to those in the brother. Although the hips had a full range of motion, the knees showed flexion contractures.

Selected radiographic views are shown in Fig. 11-30*O* to *Q*.

Case 19. C. B., sister of Cases 17 and 18, was born in July, 1963. When she was seen in May, 1968, it was evident that she was affected. Height was 39 inches, the wrists were enlarged and hypermobile, and flat feet and genu valgum on the right were noted. Further investigations were not permitted.

These 4 patients are members of an inbred kindred which has lived in the peninsula counties of southern Maryland for 200 to 250 years. The original cases of the Crigler-Najjar syndrome were described in this kindred,[79] and several other rare recessive disorders, including Seckel's bird-headed dwarfism,[323] metachromatic leukodystrophy, homocystinuria, and Friedreich's ataxia, have been observed. The patient reported by Norum[395] probably has SED congenita. He had manifestations of chronic compression myelopathy dating from the first month of life—specifically, attacks of rapid respirations, follower by apnea, vomiting, and "rolling up" of the eyes. At 4 years of age, after a fall, he developed acute quadriplegia. Atlantoaxial subluxation secondary to hypoplasia of the odontoid process was demonstrated and successfully treated with posterior cervical fusion, by Kopits and Robinson.[260]

Danes and Grossman[92] had at least 2 patients in their Group 1A (Cases 11 and 12) who probably represented this syndrome, i.e., non-keratan-sulfate–excreting

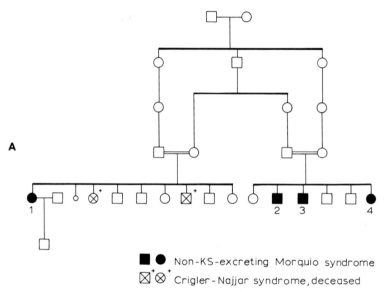

■ ● Non-KS-excreting Morquio syndrome

⊠⁺⊗⁺ Crigler-Najjar syndrome, deceased

Fig. 11-30. Non-keratan-sulfate–excreting Morquio snydrome. **A,** Pedigree. **B** and **C,** E. M. J. (Case 16) at the ages of 13 years and 22 years, respectively. **D,** At the age of 10 years, the spine and pelvis of E. M. J. show platyspondylisis and strikingly defective ossification of the femoral capital epiphyses. **E** and **F,** Radiographically the hands in E. M. J. at 10 and 18 years, respectively, show hypoplasia of the carpal bones and inclination of the distal ends of the radius and ulna toward each other. There is a lateral defect in the proximal end of the fifth metacarpal. **G** and **H,** L. B. (Case 17) at the age of 14 years. **I,** Hands in L. B. at 14 years. As in his cousin, as shown in **E,** the ulnas are short, with hypoplastic distal epiphyses. The distal radial epiphyses are triangular. The carpal bones are hypoplastic. Indeed, the minute navicular bone appears to be in the process of being incorporated into the radial epiphysis. **J,** The frontal x-ray film of the upper cervical spine in L. B. at the age of 14 years shows that the axis and atlas are separated by an unusually wide disc. Their end-plates slope laterally to an excessive degree. The odontoid process is hypoplastic, and the posterior arch of the atlas is unfused. **K** and **L,** These two views of the spine in L. B. show flat vertebrae with wavy, irregular end-plates and flattening particularly of the anterior portions. The intervertebral discs are widened. The ribs are relatively long and thin. **M** and **N,** R. B. (Case 18) at the age of 13 years. **O,** Pelvis at 13 years of age. The femoral necks are wider than the femoral shafts, and ossification of the flattened capital epiphyses is limited to multiple small dots. The acetabula are enlarged superiorly, extending to the anterioinferior iliac spines. **P** and **Q,** Arms and right leg in R. B. at 13 years. Irregularly formed, thin epiphyses are demonstrated. The tarsal bones are small and irregular, and the foot is flat.

Morquio syndrome. They showed no clouding of the corneas, metachromatic inclusions in circulating leukocytes, or excessive mucopolysacchariduria. However, their skeletal x-ray studies showed changes like those shown here, and their fibroblasts showed cytoplasmic metachromasia. The uronic acid content of fibroblasts was not elevated, but the hexose content showed a marked increase above normal.

Rubin[450] referred to the Morquio syndrome as spondyloepiphyseal dysplasia congenita, an inappropriate term since abnormality is not evident at birth. Furthermore, *SED congenita* is the designation now used for a specific skeletal dysplasia (Fig. 11-31) inherited as an autosomal dominant disorder.[494,496] The skeletal abnormality is evident at birth. Other differences from the Morquio syndrome include lack of corneal and dental changes, relative sparing of epiphyses in the distal parts of the limbs, including the hands and feet, and occurrence of retinal detachment. Major changes involve the spine and proximal epiphyses. The hands, for example, are normal. Clubbed feet and cleft palate are

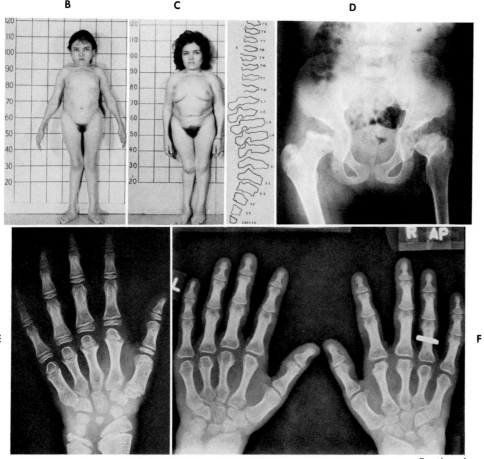

Continued.

Fig. 11-30, cont'd. For legend see opposite page.

rather frequent.[151] Moderately flat, or dishlike, face is the result of underdevelopment of the facial bones. The head is normal in size and because of a very short neck seems to rest directly on the shoulders. The chest is barrel-shaped, with pectus carinatum. The normal thoracic kyphosis and lumbar lordosis are exaggerated. Scoliosis develops during late childhood and adolescence. The limbs are relatively long. Intelligence is normal. Adult height is variable (37 to 52 inches).

Over half the patients with SED congenita have high-grade myopia and/or retinal detachment.[151,443] Areas of peripheral retinal degeneration have been ob-

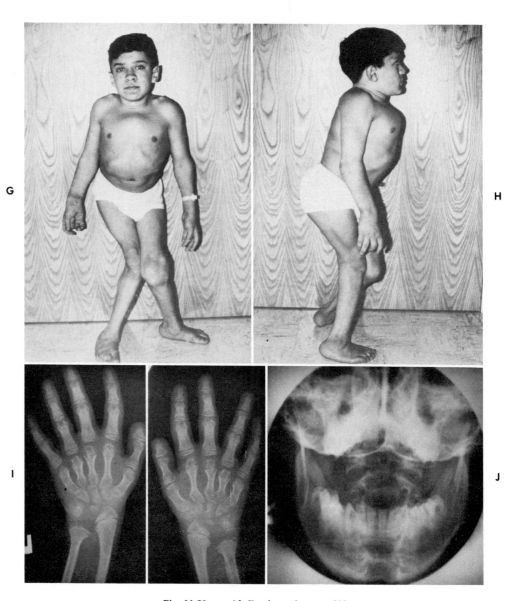

Fig. 11-30, cont'd. For legend see p. 600.

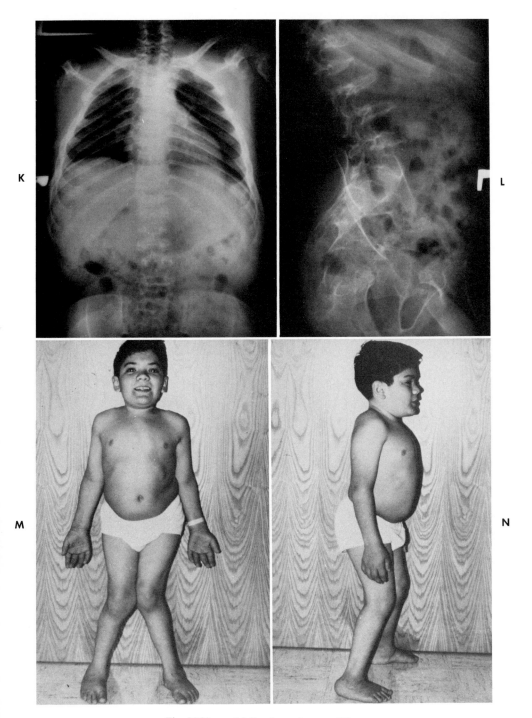

Fig. 11-30, cont'd. For legend see p. 600.

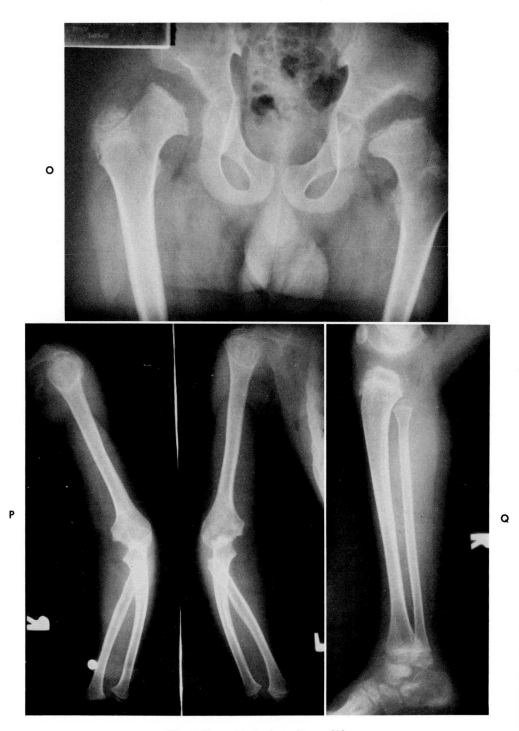

Fig. 11-30, cont'd. For legend see p. 600.

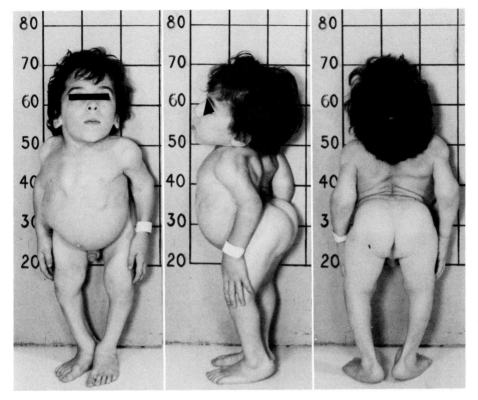

Fig. 11-31. Spondyloepiphyseal dysplasia congenita in 11-year-old boy.

served to precede detachment, which occurs in the absence of myopia in some cases. Odontoid hypoplasia, with its attendant neurologic complications, occurs in this condition as in MPS IV.

Metachromatic inclusions were observed in peripheral lymphocytes of some patients.[496]

In the early years, the striking roentgenographic finding is retarded ossification of the pubic bones, knee epiphyses, and calcanei and tali. The ossification centers of the femoral heads develop very slowly. Early the vertebral bodies are ovoid or pear shaped; later they are irregular and flat, with narrow disc spaces. Changes in the hands are minor, the most frequent being accessory epiphyses.

SED congenita was first delineated by Spranger and Wiedemann[496] in 1966. In 1970 Spranger and Langer[494] were able to collect 19 cases from the literature and add 29 cases from their own experience. The importance of the ocular complications in terms of frequency and severity is reflected by the fact that the attention of Fraser and colleagues[151] was drawn to this disorder in the course of their studies of severe visual handicap of childhood in England. Although most cases are sporadic, several instances of parent-to-child transmission[151] and raised paternal age of sporadic cases[491] speak for autosomal dominant inheritance.

Cases reported as the Morquio syndrome but considered SED congenita by Spranger and Langer[494] included those of Freeman,[156] Meyer and Brennemann,[355] and several others.

Metatropic dwarfism is another recently delineated skeletal dysplasia that was often labeled Morquio's disease in the past. Maroteaux, Spranger, and Wiedemann[343] pointed out the characteristic features and gave the name, which refers to the change in body proportions with aging: at birth the long, narrow torso with relatively short limbs suggests achondroplasia. Later, rapidly progressing scoliosis results in short-trunk dwarfism suggesting the Morquio syndrome. Some patients have over the sacrum a double fold of skin that resembles a tail.

Roentgenographically the pelvis has a peculiar battle-ax (or halberd) configuration due to the peculiar shape of the iliac alae. In the limbs, the bones show a striking dumbbell or trumpet appearance because of markedly exaggerated metaphyseal widening.

The mode of inheritance (one assumes the disorder is Mendelian) of metatropic dwarfism is not fully established. The cases of 2 brothers who probably had this condition have been reported[367]—as examples of the Morquio syndrome.

We have seen 2 patients (N. D., 1321613; L. G., 1223071) with many features like those of metatropic dwarfism but with some differences. Since these patients resemble the one reported by Kniest,[255] the disorder might be called metatropic dwarfism II, or the Kniest syndrome.

The following case is one that was labeled Morquio's disease in life but was recognized as metatropic dwarfism from the roentgenographic features by Bailey and colleagues[15]:

Case 20. R. A. W. was born in 1945. Birth weight was 7 pounds. Although her length is not known, she was short. The parents were not related and no other dwarfism was known in the family. The father and mother were 27 and 23 years old, respectively, at her birth.

Shortly after birth a "lump" was noted in the midlumbar area. At 14 months, a back brace was prescribed for kyphoscoliosis. At the age of 2½ years the patient was unable to stand; yet she spoke as well as other children her age. Extension at the elbows and both flexion and extension at the knees were limited (Fig. 11-32A and B).

The patient never was able to walk alone. Kyphoscoliosis increased, and she developed dyspnea, which eventually troubled her even at rest. She died at 11 years of age of a respiratory infection. No autopsy was performed.

The x-ray changes spanning eight years are demonstrated in Fig. 11-32C to N. Cardinal features are severe kyphoscoliosis and short limb bones with metaphyseal flaring. Anterior beaking of the proximal tibia is noteworthy, as well as hyperostoses on the diaphyses of the femur, radius, and ulna.

A reported instance of the "Morquio syndrome" in father and daughter[432] is now known to represent a newly delineated disorder, *parastremmatic dwarfism*.[279] The designation, invented by Langer and colleagues,[279] comes from the Greek for "distorted limb". Severe dwarfism, kyphoscoliosis, distortion and bowing of the limbs, and contracture of large joints are features. Roentgenographic studies show platyspondylisis and striking changes in the epiphyses and metaphyses that in some ways resemble those of Jansen's metaphyseal dysostosis. The evidence for autosomal dominant inheritance is transmission from father to daughter, with similar severity in both,[432] and increased age of the normal fathers of sporadic cases. In the one known familial instance the daughter inherited not only parastremmatic dwarfism from the father but also osteogenesis imperfecta from the mother. The father, a presumed new mutation for parastremmatic dwarfism, was the last-born of 11 children.

Among the children from an uncle-niece marriage in Greenland, Dyggve and

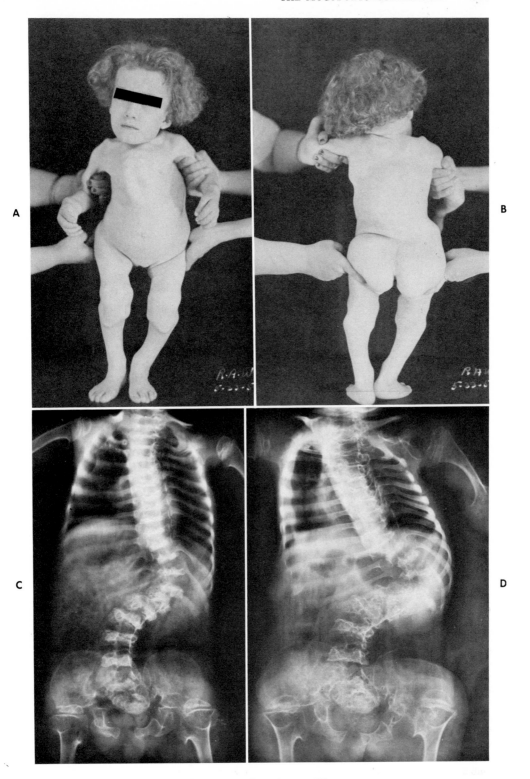

Fig. 11-32. For legend see p. 608.

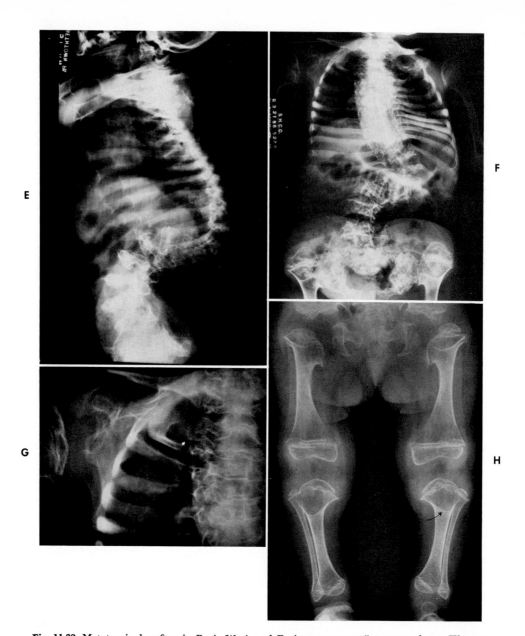

Fig. 11-32. Metatropic dwarfism in R. A. W. **A** and **B,** Appearance at 5½ years of age. The protuberance below the knees corresponds to the tibial heads shown in Fig. 11-32*H* and *I*. **C,** Frontal
view of the spine at 2½ years. **D** and **E,** Frontal and lateral views of the spine at 5½ years of
age. **F,** Frontal view of spine at 10½ years. **G,** Shoulder at 10½ years. The medial end of the
clavicle is broad, whereas the lateral portion is unusually narrow. **H** and **I,** Frontal and lateral
views of lower limbs at 2½ years of age. The metaphyses are flared, especially at the knees. The
arrows indicate a beak on the anterior surface of the proximal tibia. **J,** At 10½ years of age,
x-ray appearance of legs. The femoral heads and necks are just beginning to ossify (upper
arrow). Hyperostoses project medially from the diaphysis of each femur (lower arrow). **K** and
L, Right upper limb at the age of 2½ years. The metaphyses flare markedly. At the distal
humerus the flaring is so marked that an exostosis is simulated. **M,** Wrist and hand at 7½
years. The hand bones are square. Carpal ossification is markedly delayed. Well-formed hyperostoses project into the interosseous space from both the radius and the ulna (arrows). **N,** Upper
limb at 10½ years of age.

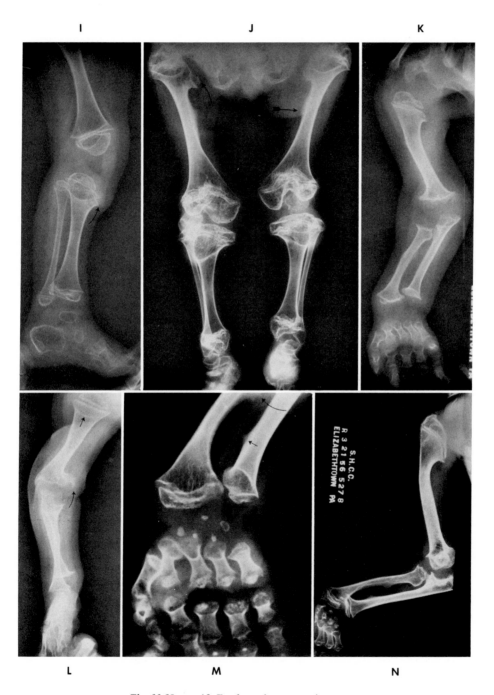

Fig. 11-32, cont'd. For legend see opposite page.

co-workers[121] found 3 with a condition resembling the Hurler syndrome and the Morquio syndrome in some respects. The fingers were clawed, with limitation of extension. The patients were mentally retarded and dwarfed. The spine showed generalized platyspondyly. Irregularities of the iliac crest gave an appearance of a lace border around it. These workers[66] concluded that excessive mucopolysaccharides in the form of dermatan sulfate and altered hyaluronic acid, and not keratan sulfate, were being excreted in the urine. A patient (Family 121, Plate XII) pictured by Hobaek[204] probably had the same condition. Although the original authors[121] labeled the disorder "Morquio-Ullrich's disease," it is clearly a separate entity. Four patients referred to Linker and associates[292] as having Morquio syndrome had this condition instead. Recent electron microscopic studies[442a] suggest that this may, in fact, not be a lysosomal storage disease and therefore not a mucopolysaccharidosis as here defined.

Prevalence and inheritance

The Morquio syndrome is inherited as an autosomal recessive disorder (Fig. 11-33). Morquio[372,373] described 4 affected sibs whose normal parents were first cousins. It appears to be quite rare, probably no more frequent than 1 in 40,000 births.

It is entirely possible, indeed very likely, that allelic forms of MPS IV exist. I would not be surprised to discover, for example, that the non-keratan-sulfate–excreting Morquio syndrome is allelic with classic MPS IV. Until the basic defect is known in the two, no basis for conclusion about allelism will be available.

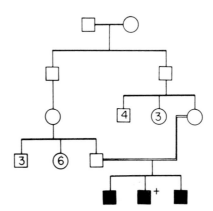

Fig. 11-33. MPS IV (the Morquio syndrome) in all 3 offspring (black squares) of the marriage of first cousins once removed. The second son, the proband, indicated by the cross, died suddenly at 9 years of age with acute breathlessness attributed to heart failure. The surviving sons were 21 and 16 years old at the time of study. Both appeared normal at birth. In the older son, spinal curvature was noted as the first abnormality at the age of 2 years. In the younger, the disorder was anticipated and spinal curvature and prominent chest were detected by the age of 8 months. In both, examination revealed skeletal features typical of the Morquio syndrome. Their heights were 40 inches and 37 inches. The wrists were excessively mobile. Both had diffusely cloudy corneas. Respiratory movements were restricted in both, and the younger had the murmur of aortic regurgitation. Both had mildly spastic legs with sustained ankle clonus and extensor plantar response. The younger had difficulty in initiating micturition. The elder surviving brother is shown in Plate 1A.

Management

Orthopedic surgery is the main approach. The genu valgum is corrected by means of tibiofibular osteotomies. Surgery on the upper cervical spine, as developed by Kopits and Robinson,[260] can be lifesaving and is indicated in most patients. Decompression by resecting of spinal lamellae is not beneficial because the compression is anterior, and the procedure may be harmful. Posterior spinal fusion has been developed as a satisfactory procedure. A special halo brace fixation is used for immobilization before, during, and after surgery.[261] As pointed out earlier (p. 588), the patients grow little after the age of 7 or 8 years. Hence, alignment osteotomies of the lower limbs performed at about 7 years of age do not have to be repeated. Kopits and Robinson[260] have performed bilateral varus osteotomies of the tibias and posterior fusion of C 1-2 during a single hospitalization.

The instability of the wrists is a serious impediment to use of the hands. Special wrist splints have been used with some success.

MUCOPOLYSACCHARIDOSIS VI (MPS VI, MAROTEAUX-LAMY SYNDROME, POLYDYSTROPHIC DWARFISM)

MPS VI is a condition that was first delineated on clinical and chemical grounds by Maroteaux, Lamy, and their colleagues.[338,342] It is characterized by clinical features like those of MPS I H, including dwarfism, but is distinguished from the other mucopolysaccharidoses, except MPS I S and IV, by retention of normal intelligence, at least until the late stages of the disorder, and/or by a preponderant urinary excretion of dermatan sulfate. The greater severity of "dysostosis multiplex" and of the other somatic features and the more limited survivorship in MPS VI distinguish it from MPS I S.

Clinical manifestations

Abnormality, namely growth retardation, is first noted at the age of 2 or 3 years. Stunting of both the trunk and the limbs is usually present, as well as genu valgum, lumbar kyphosis, and anterior sternal protrusion. The face is abnormal, as shown in Fig. 11-34A. Although the facial features are not pathognomonic and are not as striking as in MPS I, they suggest that the patient's ailment falls in the category of mucopolysaccharidoses. Restriction of articular movement is present, as in several of the other entities. The carpal tunnel syndrome (Fig. 11-35C) contributes to the hand deformity in this syndrome, as in MPS II and IV and in mucolipidosis III (pseudo–Hurler polydystrophy). In 2 affected sisters,[493] the subcutaneous tissues of the volar surface of the second to fourth fingers were thickened, as in Dupuytren's contracture. Some patients have come to medical attention as supposed examples of bilateral Perthes' disease.[493]

Serious cardiac abnormality, with murmurs indicative of valvular involvement, has developed in 2 of the sibs shown in Figs. 11-34 and 11-35.[266] The clinical characteristics (except for the later onset of heart failure) and the pathogenetic mechanisms are identical to those in MPS I.

Frequent episodes of diarrhea, requiring hospitalization, occurred in some cases.[493] Inguinal hernias frequently required surgical repair in the first years of life.[493] The liver is consistently enlarged in patients over the age of 6 years, and the spleen is enlarged in about half the cases.

Growth is severely retarded and in many patients seems virtually to stop after the age of 7 or 8 years. The ultimate height ranges from 107 to 138 cm., a point of differentiation from the Scheie syndrome (MPS I S), in which height is probably always over 144 cm.

Deafness is present in some patients and may be due in part to recurrent

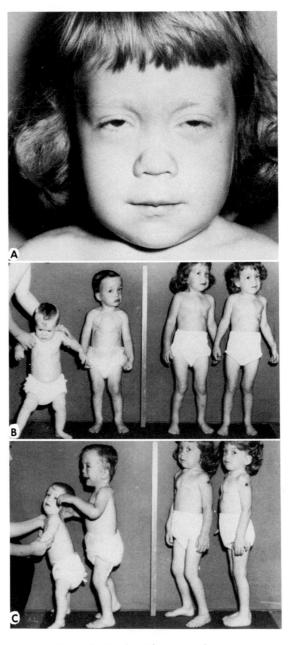

Fig. 11-34. For legend see opposite page.

otitis media. Corneal opacities develop fairly early. The cornea is increased in thickness, especially at its periphery, where clouding is most dense.

Neurologic complications include hydrocephalus and spastic paraplegia from atlantoaxial subluxation consequent to hypoplasia of the odontoid process. The youngest of the sibs shown in Figs. 11-34 and 11-35 developed acute signs of

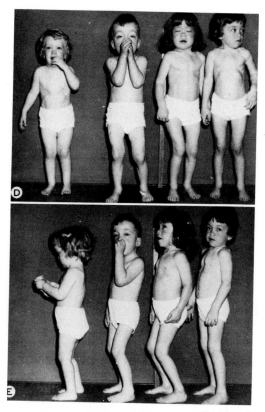

Continued.

Fig. 11-34. MPS VI (the Maroteaux-Lamy syndrome). The 4 sibs shown in this series of photographs are described in detail in the text. **A,** Facial appearance in the proband, K. S., 5½ years old. **B** and **C,** Four affected sibs. Left to right: L. S., 6 months old; S. S., 2½ years old; K. S., 5¼ years old; D. S., 4 years old; **D** and **E,** Four affected sibs, in order of age, 2 years after views shown in **B** and **C.** The progressive changes are particularly striking in the 2 youngest children. Semiflexion at the knees is evident. **F,** Clawhand deformity in proband, K. S., 5½ years old. **G,** Hands and forearms in D. S. The radius and ulna are short, thickened, and somewhat bowed. The metacarpals and phalanges have an abnormal configuration. **H,** Spine in L. S., 2½ years old. **I,** Spine in D. S., 4 years old. In this and the preceding figure, beaking and posterior displacement of the D12 and L1 vertebrae are evident. The ribs are abnormally broad and short. **J,** Skull in L. S., showing shoe-shaped sella turcica, sclerotic mastoids, fused lambdoidal sutures, and a fine, ground-glass appearance of the calvaria. The face is relatively small, the teeth are quite irregular, and the cervical vertebrae are small and irregular. **K,** Pelvis and hips in K. S., 5½ years old. Note irregularity of the epiphyseal ossification centers, coxa valga, and oblique acetabular roofs. (From McKusick, V. A., Kaplan, D., Wise, D., Hanley, W. B., Suddarth, S. B., Sevick, M. E., and Maumenee, A. E.: Medicine 44:445 1965.)

increased intracranial pressure and required shunt.[173] She and her oldest sister have marked "long tract signs" and demonstrable subluxation of C1 on C2. Vitamin A in excess is known to cause increased intracranial pressure[163,373]; in this and other mucopolysaccharidoses, it might aggravate a preexisting tendency to hydrocephalus. However, unlike 2 of her older sibs, the patient had not received treatment with vitamin A alcohol (retinol).

In one patient, T. H., a male now (1972) 18 years old, bilateral papilledema with progressively failing vision is apparently due to increased intracranial pres-

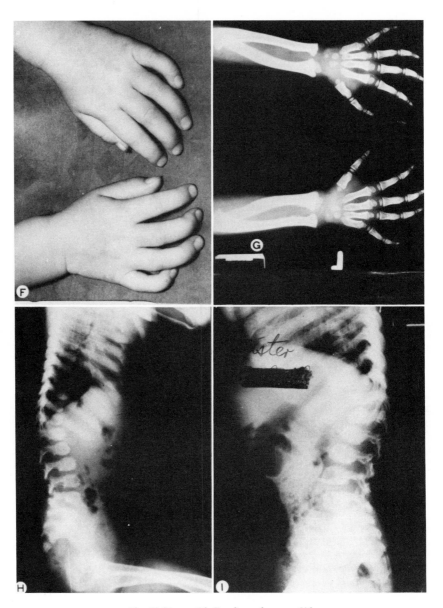

Fig. 11-34, cont'd. For legend see p. 613.

sure. Complete lack of development of secondary sexual characteristics and an unusual degree of dwarfing suggest that function of the anterior pituitary may be compromised.

Points of central importance to the differentiation from MPS I H and MPS I S are, respectively, (1) that intellectual development is normal and (2) that the osseous abnormality is severe.

The osseous abnormality as revealed by roentgenography is quite variable in severity, rivaling that in MPS I in the most severely affected patients. The diaphyses of the long bones are, however, usually less swollen than in MPS I. Even when they are as swollen as in MPS I, there is a localized constriction of many metaphyses not seen in the Hurler syndrome. This constriction is partic-

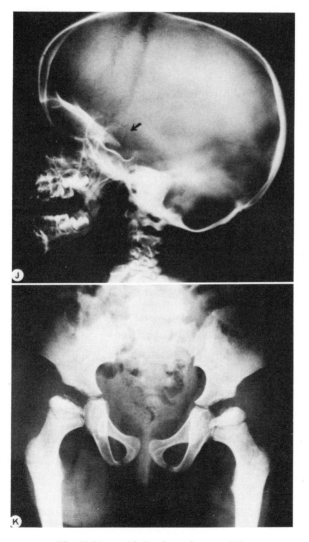

Fig. 11-34, cont'd. For legend see p. 613.

ularly striking in the surgical neck of the humerus, where it pairs with marked varus deformity to give the upper humerus a hatchetlike appearance. At the elbows and wrists the epiphyses and metaphyses may be quite irregular, a finding more suggestive of MPS IV than of MPS I. The proximal one third of the humerus usually is bowed anteriorly. The radius and ulna may be bowed, and their distal surfaces usually slope toward each other.

As in all the mucopolysaccharidoses, the long bones below the hips are less affected than in the upper limbs.[184] Although the tibial shaft may be quite swollen, the femur is usually normally or excessively constricted, and the epiphyses are more regular. In the 4 affected sibs to be described (cases 21 to 24), the epiphyseal plates were wide, especially in the hands, where the appearance was reminiscent of metaphyseal chondrodysplasia (formerly termed metaphyseal dysostosis, p. 787). Moreover, oval radiolucencies permeated the tibial and distal femoral metaphyses. They may represent residual islands of cartilage. Such abnormalities of the epiphyseal plates and metaphyses are encountered in approximately one fourth of the patients with MPS VI.

The odontoid process is hypoplastic. In some patients the vertebral bodies show little change. In most, the superior and inferior margins are convex, and in some patients the anterior and posterior margins are also concave. Hypoplasia and beaking of L1 and L2 are common. While the involved vertebra usually is recessed, little or no gibbus results.

The narrowing of the vertebral ends of the ribs may extend considerably farther laterally than in MPS I, so that the ribs have the shape more of canoe paddles than of oars. Frequently the medial thirds of the clavicles are distended. The remainder is relatively narrow and bowed superiorly, and the ends are pointed and directed inferiorly at the shoulders. The scapulae are small and high, with hypoplastic glenoid fossae.

Changes in the pelvis are striking. The iliac wings flare above constricted bodies. Acetabula are small, with oblique roofs. Ossification of the femoral head is irregular in most patients, leading to the diagnosis of bilateral Legg-Perthes disease in some. The femoral necks tend to be long, excessively constricted, and turned outward.

The degree of involvement of the short bones of the hands and feet is especially variable. They may be almost unaffected. More commonly, the ends of the shafts are widened and the metacarpal bases pointed. When the diaphyses are constricted, the appearance is suggestive of MPS IV. In some patients the shafts are more swollen than the ends, and making a distinction from MPS I is impossible.

Frequently the skull is severely involved and cannot be distinguished from that in a patient with MPS I. The emissary vessels are likely to be particularly numerous and wide, particularly in the region of the torcular Herophili in such patients. In others, skull involvement is much milder.

Although many of the roentgenographic findings are similar to those in other mucopolysaccharidoses, in many cases of MPS VI the metaphyseal constriction and the appearance of the shoulders, pelvis, hips, and knees permit a reasonably certain diagnosis on roentgenologic grounds alone.

Worth[569] pictured a number of examples of dental changes similar to those shown in Fig. 11-35O to R. The only patients whose clinical photographs he provided (sibs Linda and Thomas C., 11 and 10 years of age) appear to have had the Maroteaux-Lamy syndrome. He pointed out that Reilly and Lindsay[436] commented on "dentigerous cysts" and that others[59,127] pictured or described the same phenomenon.

Of the six major mucopolysaccharidoses, cytoplasmic inclusions are most striking in MPS VI. With proper staining and search, coarse and fine granulations can be found in 90% to 100% of granulocytes and in up to 50% of lymphocytes.[493]

A male patient reported by Young and associates[570] almost certainly represents this entity. Although somatic features, including corneal clouding, were striking, the patient was of average intelligence throughout life. Hydrocephalus was treated by ventriculoatrial shunt at 16 years of age. He died of heart failure and carbon dioxide retention at 23 years. Autopsy showed thickened leptomeninges but no storage material in neuronal cells.

The 4 sibs described below as Cases 21 to 24 (Figs. 11-34 and 11-35) have the Maroteaux-Lamy syndrome:

Cases 21 to 24. The eldest, K. S. (J.H.H. 1214199), a daughter of apparently unrelated parents, had been noted since infancy to have noisy breathing, a wobbly gait, and stiff joints. Hip pain, beginning at about 5 years of age, prompted medical attention. Mental development has progressed normally and she remains in the highest section of her class. The gross facies is shown in Fig. 11-34*A*, and the broad hands with stubby fingers and flexion contractures are seen in Fig. 11-34*F*. Other evident features are an elongated large head, corneal cloudiness, macroglossia, lower dorsal kyphosis, and a prominent sternum. Examination showed hepatosplenomegaly and a vibratory systolic murmur. The roentgenograms showed severe dysostosis multiplex with most of the features described above.

After these features were pointed out to the parents, they suggested that all 4 of their children might be affected. Their similarities are illustrated in Fig. 11-34. There are also noteworthy differences: the features of D. S. have remained fine and her corneal opacities are only faintly visible; S. S. has a head size that is disproportionately large. The skeletal changes are illustrated in Fig. 11-34*G* to *K*.

The 2 older girls (now 6 and 8 years of age) are performing superiorly in the first and third grades despite recurrent catarrhal otitis with intermittent gross hearing loss, recurrent and persistent bronchitis, increased deformity and stiffness of the fingers in K. S., and the need for a body jacket in D. S. to prevent progressive scoliosis. Both have systolic murmurs, prominent second sounds, and normal blood pressures. K. S. may have early clubbing of the fingers. Adenoidectomy and tonsillectomy helped the noisy respirations but apparently not the recurrent otitis and bronchitis.

S. S. has changed the most during 2½ years of observation. His head size has increased only from 52.5 to 54 cm., but his eyes are much more prominent and grossly cloudy. He limps, with apparent shortening of the right limb, and has much louder breathing and more frequent otitis media and bronchitis. There is a persistent small umbilical hernia, and he had an inguinal hernia repaired in infancy. Both S. S. and L. S. have developed soft systolic murmurs with a prominent second sound. Both have grown 6 to 7 inches, speak well, and are toilet-trained.

L. S., the youngest of these children, developed hydrocephalus and papilledema in 1969 at the age of 7 years 9 months, and a ventriculojugular shunt was installed.[173]

Progressive changes in these 4 sibs are detailed in Fig. 11-35.

No abnormality of the electroretinogram was detected.[167]

All 4 children show Reilly granulations of the polymorphonuclear leukocytes and metachromatic cytoplasmic inclusions in 10% to 25% of lymphocytes. Large amounts of mucopolysaccharide, almost exclusively dermatan sulfate, were identified in the urine. Values, expressed as milligrams per liter, were as follows: K. S., age 7½ years, 250 mg.; D. S., age 6. 185 mg.; S. S., age 4½, 90 mg.; and L. S., age 2½, 180 mg.

Prognosis

A patient reported by Spranger and colleagues[493] died at 25 years of age of progressive heart failure; her sister, one year older, was still alive. Lorincz[301] observed sisters, 15 and 20 years old, thought to have MPS VI. The 20-year-old became pregnant out of wedlock. The fetus, necessarily heterozygous, was aborted. However, studies by Dr. Elizabeth Neufeld indicated that this is α-L-iduronidase deficiency, presumably Hurler-Scheie compound (p. 556). (As indicated elsewhere [p. 571], a male with the Hunter syndrome had a child, a woman with MPS IV has had 2 children, and a female with the non-keratan-sulfate–excreting Morquio syndrome [Fig. 11-30B to F], which I consider distinct from MPS IV, also had a child. Females with MPS I S might be expected to have children, and one such instance is known to me [p. 551].)

Pathology

No information is available on cases in which the diagnosis of MPS VI is certain.

The fundamental defect

The urinary excretion of acid mucopolysaccharides is increased twofold to fifteenfold. Dermatan sulfate accounts for 70% to 95% of the excreted mucopolysaccharide. The remainder has the characteristics of heparan sulfate.

Neufeld[383] found that the fibroblasts from the children pictured in Fig. 11-34 are biochemically distinguishable from the Hurler fibroblasts, although the abnormality in their cells was only marginally corrected by secretions from other cell lines. Correction did occur in the MPS VI cells with a factor which is

---

Fig. 11-35. Later observations on 4 sibs with MPS VI shown in Fig. 11-34 and described in text. **A** and **B**, Appearance in 1967, at the ages of 11, 10, 8, and 7 years (left to right). **C**, Clawhand in K. S., with atrophy of abductor pollicis brevis muscle (arrow), indicating compression of medial nerve in carpal tunnel. **D**, X-ray view of hands in S. S., 8 years old. **E** to **H**, Skull x-ray films: in K. S. at the age of 10 years **E**; in D. S. at 10 years **F**; in S. S. at 8 years **G**; and in L. S. at 6 years (**H** and **I**). In all except L. S. **H**, where the coronal suture is open but narrow, the calvarial sutures are fused. All the skulls are dolichocephalic, suggesting that the sagittal suture closed first. In all 4 sibs, large irregular occipital radiolucencies are demonstrated. **F**, In D. S. the radiolucencies are almost certainly caused by large deposits of mucopolysaccharide within the calvaria. In the other 3, the defects are probably also due to deposit of mucopolysaccharide but could represent large emissary vessels. In each child the tuberculum sellae turcicae is eroded and the chiasmatic sulcus greatly enlarged, presumably because of an adjacent dural or arachnoid cyst. **J**, Spine in K. S., 10 years old. The two lowest thoracic vertebrae are shorter than the others and mildly recessed. **K**, Spine in D. S., 9 years old. The changes are more severe than in K. S. Vertebral bodies T12 and L1 are short and recessed, with resulting gibbus. The lumbar pedicles are long. **L**, Pelvis and hips in K. S., 11 years old. The femoral capital epiphyses are flat, with large, cystlike radiolucencies and surrounding sclerosis, and the femoral necks are narrow. The acetabula are shallow with oblique roofs. **M** and **N**, Distal femur **M** and tibia **N** in D. S. and L. S., respectively, show irregular longitudinal radiolucent and radiodense bands of the metaphyses with minimal cupping. **O** to **R**, Teeth in K. S., at 10 years of age **O**; D. S., 9 years **P**; S. S. 7 years **Q**; and L. S. 6 years **R**. The height of the mandible is reduced. Eruption of permanent dentition is retarded, and several teeth are displaced toward the inferior border of the mandible. In several places the lower border is nearly penetrated by the roots of teeth. **S** and **T**, The 4 sibs at the ages of 14, 9, 13, and 11 years (left to right).

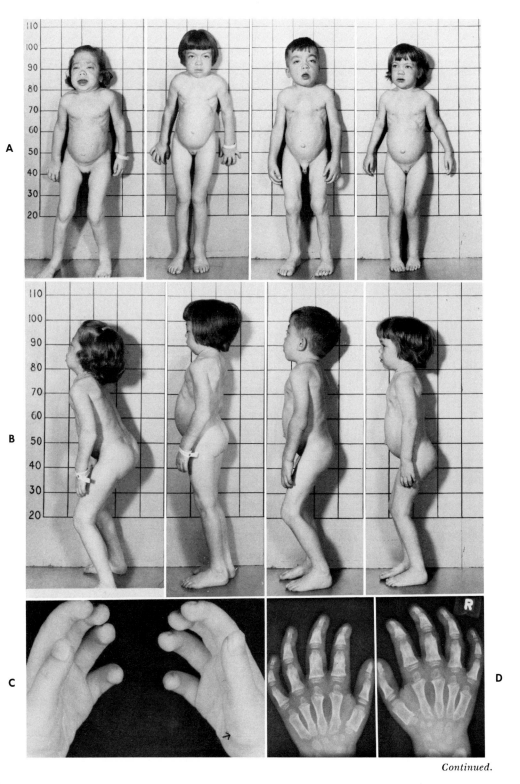

Continued.

Fig. 11-35. For legend see opposite page.

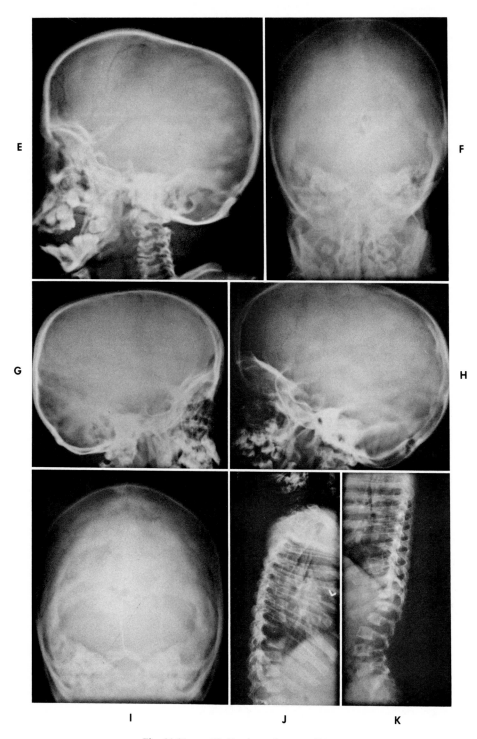

Fig. 11-35, cont'd. For legend see p. 618.

present in urine and is different and separable from all the other correction factors.

Prevalence and inheritance

Although no worthwhile estimates are available, in part because the Maroteaux-Lamy syndrome has only recently been delineated, the disorder must be

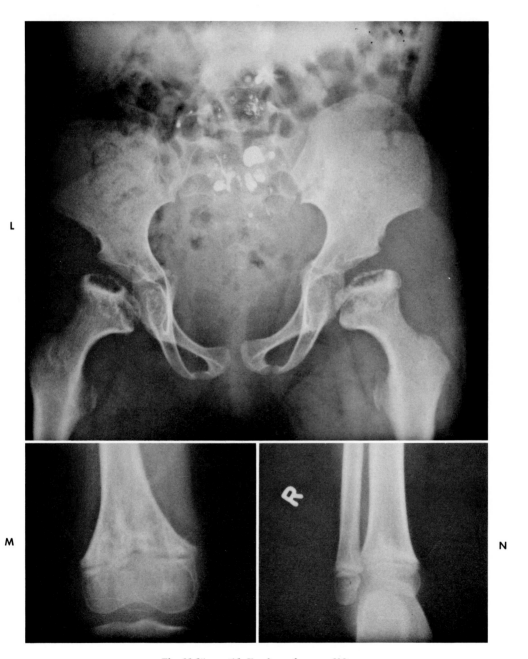

Fig. 11-35, cont'd. For legend see p. 618.

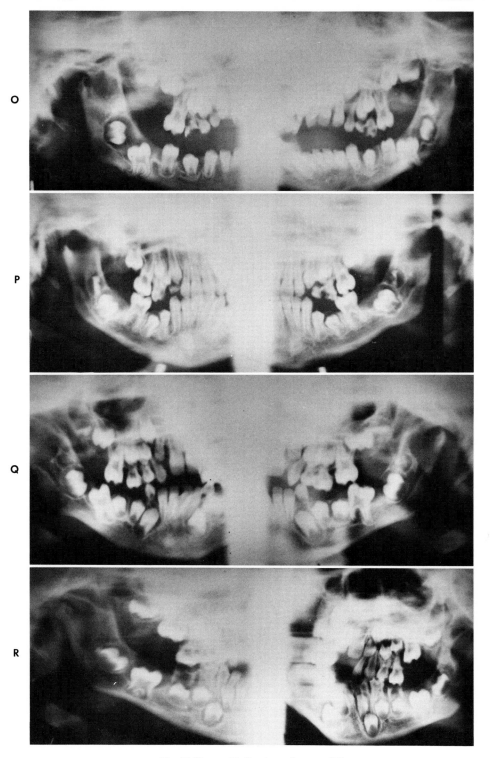

Fig. 11-35, cont'd. For legend see p. 618.

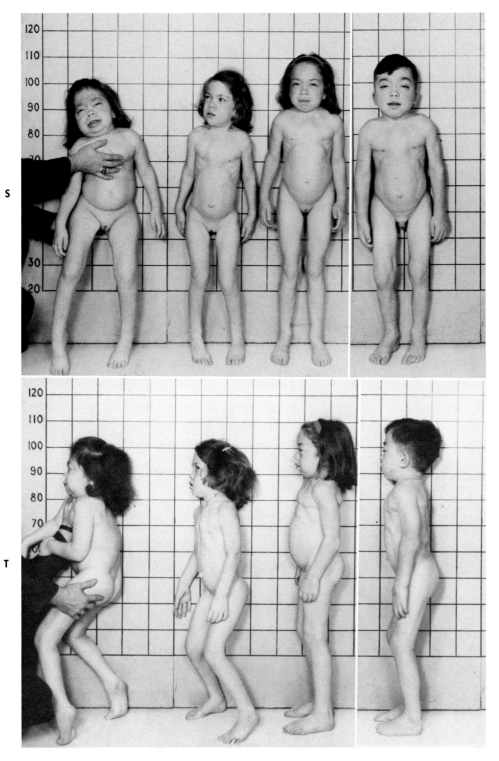

Fig. 11-35, cont'd. For legend see p. 618.

quite rare. Spranger and associates[493] tabulated the cases of 9 males and 10 females. In addition to the originally described cases,[342] MPS VI has been specifically reported by Fallis and co-workers[138] and by Segni and collaborators,[474] and several patients reported in the past are thought to have had this disorder.[292,431,458,570] Two sibs reported in 1953 by Ullrich and Wiedemann[534] are now known to have this syndrome.[493] The diagnosis of the Maroteaux-Lamy syndrome can be entertained in a number of other reported cases.[126,234,291,390,500]

Inheritance is clearly autosomal recessive. Sibships with 2 or more affected members have been reported several times. The parents have been normal in all cases; they were consanguineous in at least four out of thirteen families.[481] (See Fig. 11-36.)

All 4 sibs of the family described above (Cases 21 to 24; Figs. 11-34 and 11-35) were affected. Of 4-sib families whose parents are both heterozygous for the Maroteaux-Lamy gene (and this intercross mating must be no more frequent than 1 in 10,000), only 1/256 would be expected to have all 4 sibs affected. Of all 4-sib families ascertainable by the presence in them of at least 1 affected child,

$$\frac{(\frac{1}{4})^4}{1 - (\frac{3}{4})^4}, \text{ or } \frac{1}{175},$$

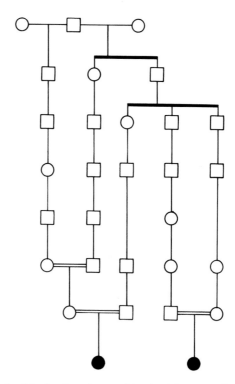

Fig. 11-36. Distant relationship in 2 patients with the Maroteaux-Lamy syndrome and consanguinity of the parents in each case. (Redrawn from Spranger, J. W., Koch, F., McKusick, V. A., Natzschka, J., Wiedemann, H. R., and Zellweger, H.: Helv. Paediat. Acta **25:**337, 1970.)

would be expected to have all 4 children affected. The parents of the S. children were indeed unlucky!

On clinical grounds Spranger and colleagues[493] and others[431] have raised the question of heterogeneity in the Maroteaux-Lamy syndrome. The difference resides mainly in the severity of radiologic changes, especially in the bones of the hand. Some of the patients labeled clinically as suffering from the Maroteaux-Lamy syndrome, leading to suspicions of genetic heterogeneity, may in fact be affected by a distinct entity or a "compound" disorder. (See Fig. 11-10.) Some patients thought to represent the Hurler/Scheie compound (p. 553) were earlier considered to have MPS VI.

An allelic form of MPS VI?

Case 25. The patient shown in Fig. 11-37 (P. B., J.H.H. 1268002) was born in 1942. He was treated for bilateral Legg-Perthes disease between age 8 and 12 years. Bilateral inguinal hernias were repaired at age 20. Mild stiffness of the hands and corneal clouding were first noted at the age of about 20 years. He completed high school. At age 30 he showed short stature (61 inches as compared with about 6 feet in several of his 6 sibs), clouding of the corneas most dense peripherally and posteriorly (Fig. 11-37C), and mild joint stiffness limited mainly to the hands, which also showed signs typical of carpal tunnel syndrome. He had no pigmentary changes in the retina and no night blindness. A grade III/VI systolic ejection murmur was heard loudest at the left sternal border. This had been heard at age 24 during an examination for employment but had been heard at the age of 8 years when he was thought to have rheumatic fever because of it, combined with stiffness in his legs.

He was of normal intelligence and worked as an automotive mechanic. He is not married.

Leukocytes showed striking metachromatic inclusions like those seen in classic Maroteaux-Lamy syndrome. Screening tests for excessive mucopolysacchariduria were negative. He excreted about 12 mg./L. of mucopolysaccharide (Dr. David Kaplan). Dr. J. W. Spranger determined that although urinary mucopolysaccharides were within normal limits, an abnormal amount of dermatan sulfate (78% of the total) was present.

Radiologic changes in the pelvis (Fig. 11-37D) consisted of shallow acetabula with femoral heads of about normal size extending beyond the acetabular margins. The left femoral head was flattened with irregular ossification. There was generalized platyspondyly, with decreased width of the vertebral discs (Fig. 11-37E), sparing the cervical spine. The carpal bones (Fig. 11-37F), especially the proximal row, were somewhat smaller than average. The metacarpal and phalangeal bones were normal in appearance. Slight clawhand deformity seemed to be due exclusively to soft tissue changes.

Clinically the Scheie syndrome comes to mind, but patients with that disorder are not as short as this patient (compare Fig. 11-9 with Fig. 11-37), have less skeletal change, in the spine for example, and have pigmentary retinal changes. Furthermore, the striking cytoplasmic inclusions and almost exclusive urinary excretion of dermatan sulfate suggest MPS VI. However, the patient's disorder is much milder than that seen in any patient with MPS VI.

That the patient shown in Fig. 11-37 indeed has a form, presumably allelic, of MPS VI is indicated by the findings of Neufeld[383] that fibroblasts of P. B. are corrected by semipurified Maroteaux-Lamy corrective factor and show cross-correction with fibroblasts from the other mucopolysaccharidoses, notably those of the Scheie syndrome.[321b]

Tentatively we propose to call the classic Maroteaux-Lamy syndrome MPS VI A and the mild variant (which I have thus far seen only in P. B.) MPS VI B.

The same disorder was probably present in the patient of Glober and associates,[169] whose sister was said to be identically affected. That man, 44 years

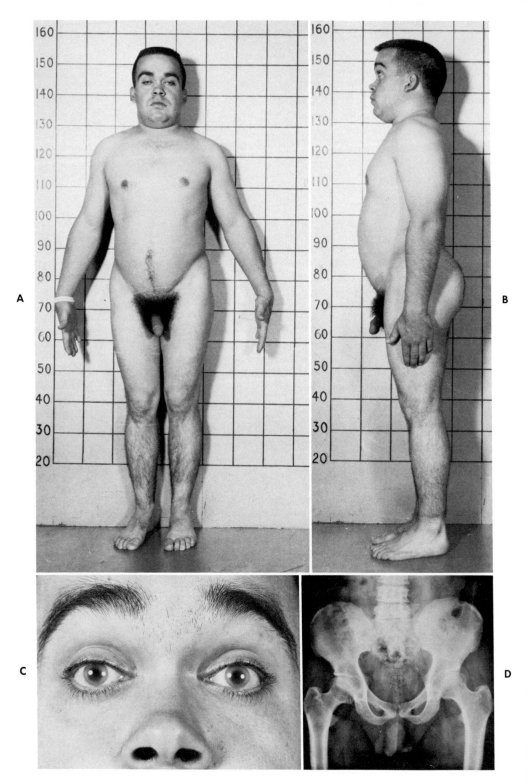

Fig. 11-37. Mucopolysaccharidosis, type VI B.

old at death, was a merchant marine, 62 inches tall. At the age of 30 years he had had a left hip prosthesis inserted for presumed Legg-Perthes disease. The corneas were cloudy. Dorfman's screening test (acid bovine albumin) for mucopolysaccharides was negative, but cytoplasmic inclusions were found in blood cells. Severe cardiac changes led to the patient's death. At autopsy the heart showed a markedly thickened aortic valve with partial fusion of the posterior and left cusps and advanced calcification that extended into the ventricular endocardium.[169] Fibrous thickening of less severe degree was found in the myocardium adjacent to the aortic valve, embedded in a matrix of homogeneous eosinophilic material and creating a cartilage-like picture.

MUCOPOLYSACCHARIDOSIS VII
(β-GLUCURONIDASE DEFICIENCY)

Two unrelated patients with β-glucuronidase deficiency have been recognized.[20a,484a] The basic defect of this disorder, its mode of inheritance, and potential therapy were discovered at a time when only one case was known—a record probably matched only by oroticaciduria.

The first reported patient, C. R., a Negro male, was investigated by Dr. William S. Sly and his colleagues in St. Louis.* The parents were apparently unrelated. When he was seen at the age of 7 weeks for metatarsus adductus, genetic consultation was requested because of unusual facies. Hepatosplenomegaly, umbilical hernia, diastasis recti, small thoracolumbar gibbus, and puffy hands and feet were noted. Circulating and bone marrow granulocytes showed striking metachromatic granules.

During the next two years the child grew along the 75th percentile but his gibbus increased. He acquired a short-trunk appearance with an asymmetric

*I am endebted to Dr. William S. Sly for prepublication information on this patient.

E

F

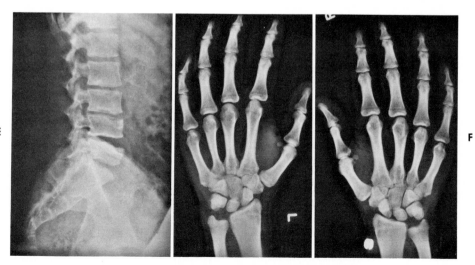

Fig. 11-37, cont'd. For legend see opposite page.

bulge of the left anterior chest. An increase in the anteroposterior dimension of the chest was probably caused by chronic pulmonary infection. Bilateral inguinal hernias appeared and required repair. No mental retardation or corneal clouding was noted. His main clinical problem was chronic pneumonitis. Pulmonary infections were associated by moderate leukocytosis with granulocytes always demonstrating striking granulation.

Between age 2 and 3 mental and physical development slowed, and his sister, a year younger, appeared to be catching up with him.

Radiographic findings included expansion of the ribs, underdevelopment of the anterior portion of the T12 vertebral body and the anterosuperior portions of T10 and 11 and L1-4, and medullary expansion in the proximal humeri and to some extent in other tubular bones.

In the early stages, the ribs showed a "double contour." Minimal periosteal new bone formation was present in each tibia.

Mucopolysaccharides in the urine were within normal limits or at the most minimally elevated.

In the Neufeld system[186a] cultured skin fibroblasts from this patient accumulated abnormal levels of $^{35}SO_4$-labelled mucopolysaccharide like patients with classic mucopolysaccharidoses. Furthermore, very low levels of β-glucuronidase were found, whereas other lysosomal enzymes were normal or elevated.[186a] That the deficiency of β-glucuronidase was responsible for the abnormal accumulation of the radioactive label was supported by the fact that the metabolic abnormality of the fibroblasts was corrected by partially purified β-glucuronidase from calf liver.[186a]

The patient's circulating white cells showed a very low level of β-glucuronidase, whereas both parents and several maternal relatives showed levels about 50% of normal—evidence for autosomal recessive inheritance.[484a] Other lysosomal enzymes were not abnormal in heterozygotes. (The level of β-galactosidase was 40% to 50% of control values in the proband and his father but normal in all others, both those with normal and those with intermediate levels of β-glucuronidase. Presumably the proband and his father were by chance heterozygotes for generalized G_{M1}-gangliosidosis.

The second patient, a white female born of nonconsanguineous parents, was 14 months old at the time of study by DiFerrante's group in Houston, Texas.[20a] Differences from the first case are evident in the clinical picture and probably also in the biochemical features. She showed "neonatal hepatitis" and thereafter progressed to severe mental, motor, and growth retardation, with hepatosplenomegaly, massive ascites, inguinal hernias, thoracolumbar gibbus, corneal clouding, metachromatic inclusions of granulocytes, and radiographic changes like those of mucopolysaccharidoses.

The ratio of high molecular weight to low molecular weight mucopolysaccharides (measured as hexuronic acid) was 1.4:1.8 (normal 0.06:0.10). The ratio was particularly high for dermatan sulfate, indicating defective degradation of this mucopolysaccharide.[20a]

Cultured skin fibroblasts showed an abnormal accumulation of ^{35}S in mucopolysaccharide. When 4-methylumbelliferyl-β-D-glucuronide was used as substrate, β-glucuronidase activity was consistently absent, whereas it was variable with p-nitrophenyl glucuronide as the substrate.[20a] The findings were taken to mean that β-glucuronidase was structurally abnormal with altered substrate recognition. On further study,[20b] however, no inconsistency of the assays using p-nitrophenol glucuronide was found. Furthermore, the *in vitro* findings in fibroblasts of the Texas patient were identical to those in Sly's patient when studied in parallel.[20b] Other lysosomal enzymes showed normal or high activity.[20a]

Comments. That the clinical (but not the biochemical) picture in the two cases is different is not impossible with deficiency of the same enzyme. We may be dealing here with two allelic forms of β-glucuronidase deficiency comparable to the Hurler and Scheie syndromes, presumably allelic varieties of MPS I. The Houston case is more severely affected than the St. Louis, but the presence of a congenital infection in addition to the inborn error of metabolism may account for part of the clinical picture in the Texas case.

Relative deficiency of β-glucuronidase is known in mice. In 1950 Morrow and his colleagues[374a] found that the C3H line has only 5% to 10% as much enzyme in the liver as do other lines. In the hands of Paigen[413a,413b] and others, this enzyme system has been useful in elucidating many aspects of biochemical genetics in a mammal. These aspects include the genetics of enzyme realization (the set of processes acting to produce the final phenotypic characteristics of the enzyme, such as catalytic properties, intracellular localization, tissue distribution, regulation of synthesis, and breakdown). However, the deficiency, perhaps because it is not marked, has no evident pathologic consequences in the C3H mouse.

Although several other disorders have been "waiting in the wings" for the role of MPS VII, β-glucuronidase deficiency would seem to have strongest claim to it because the enzymatic defect has been demonstrated. In 1969 I[316] suggested that the disorder first described by Dyggve, Melchior, and Claussen[121] be tentatively designated MPS VII, and the suggestion was followed by Dorfman and Matalon.[117a] Most recent evidence indicates, however, that this disorder is not a mucopolysaccharidosis (p. 610).

DIAGNOSIS OF THE MUCOPOLYSACCHARIDOSES

The amount of mucopolysaccharides excreted normally in the urine ranges from 3 to 15 mg./24 hr.[442] Chondroitin-4-sulfate comprises about 80% of the excreted mucopolysaccharide, with dermatan sulfate and heparan sulfate accounting, in about equal parts, for the remainder.[293]

Simple tests for excessive acid mucopolysaccharides in the urine have been devised by Dorfman, using the turbidity produced with acidified bovine serum albumin,[58,118] and by Berry and Spinanger,[30] using metachromasia produced with toluidine blue.* Another simple procedure, the cetyltrimethylammonium bro-

---

*The following is the simplified "filter paper test" devised by Berry and Spinanger[29,30]: Place 5, 10, and 25 μl. of urine as separate spots on a piece of Whatman No. 1 filter paper. Use a micropipette to add 5 μl. at a time, allowing each increment to dry before adding another. Dip paper in an aqueous solution of 0.04 toluidine blue (buffered at pH 2.0) for about 1 minute, drain, and rinse in 95% ethanol. (The toluidine blue solution is prepared by dissolving 30 mg. of dye in 100 ml. of Coleman certified buffer solution, pH 2.0.) Berman and colleagues[28a] have devised a seemingly reliable spot test using commercially produced (Ames Co.) "MPS test-papers" impregnated with Azure A.

mide test* of urine, adapted from Meyer's preparative method for mucopolysac-charides,[363,396] has also proved useful.[61,440,441] A procedure requiring preliminary dialysis of urine and based on Dische's carbazole reaction for uronic acid was proposed by Segni and co-workers.[475] Dorfman[114] urges caution in use of the screening tests in infants and young children because mucopolysaccharide excretion may normally be greater early in life.

A simple form of the Dorfman test[118] consists of adding 4 drops of a 20% bovine albumin solution to an inch of urine in a 12.7 mm. test tube. The contents of the tube are mixed, and 10% acetic acid is added drop by drop. A positive test is indicated by a dense white precipitate. Since the reaction is sensitive to variations in salt concentration, pH, protein concentration, and other factors, some have preferred a more complex but standardized procedure[113,115] which involves dialysis of the urine specimen and determination of optical density.

Lagunoff and Warren[270] showed that the nitrous acid reaction for N-sulfated hexosamines is useful for detecting and measuring heparan sulfate. Only DNA interferes significantly by reacting chromogenically. Matalon and co-workers[349] used the method for direct assay of heparan sulfate in the amniotic fluid for prenatal diagnosis of the Hurler syndrome. Lorincz and West[303] have preliminary experience with a promising microspectrophotofluorometric technique. Cells from the amniotic fluid are vitally stained with acridine orange and observed immediately. The cytoplasm of cells stains metachromatically if abnormal amounts of acid mucopolysaccharide are present.

Since the report of Reilly in 1941,[435] the demonstration of metachromatic granules in circulating polymorphonuclear leukocytes and in bone marrow cells has been used by many workers as a diagnostic approach.[231,449] Although the bone marrow was more often positive (Plate 1), Reilly granulation† (of the circulating polymorphs) was frequently not demonstrable.[441] However, Muir and co-workers[376] demonstrated a good correlation between the lymphocytic findings and the urinary excretion of mucopolysaccharide in the Hurler syndrome.

The method used to demonstrate metachromatic granules in the cytoplasm of circulating lymphocytes is that of Muir and co-workers.[376] The toluidine blue stain after methyl alcohol fixation has been found[322] completely satisfactory and, in contrast to the May-Grünwald stain which the above workers also used, is specific for mucopolysaccharide. (See Fig. 11-38, Plate 1D to G, and Plate 2.)

We[322] have found no metachromatic granules in the cytoplasm of lymphocytes from normal persons or in patients with a variety of disorders such as

---

*The following is the CTAB test as used by Renuart[441]: The reagent consists of a 5% solution of cetyltrimethylammonium bromide (hexadecyltrimethylammonium bromide) in one molar buffer, pH 6.0. One milliliter of CTAB reagent is added to 5 ml. of clean, fresh urine at room temperature. (Any cold urine gives a positive test.) The mixture is agitated by swirling and then allowed to stand at room temperature for 30 minutes. Increased urinary mucopolysaccharide concentration is indicated by a heavy, flocculent precipitate. The reaction is almost immediate in cases of MPS I, but may be more delayed and less striking in others of the mucopolysaccharidoses. A control urine should be tested simultaneously. In addition to a chilled urine, pyuria can produce a false positive test.

†Reilly granulations are probably indistinguishable from the Alder granulations of the polymorphonuclear leukocytes, which occur as a dominantly inherited trait without associated manifestations.[3,235,563]

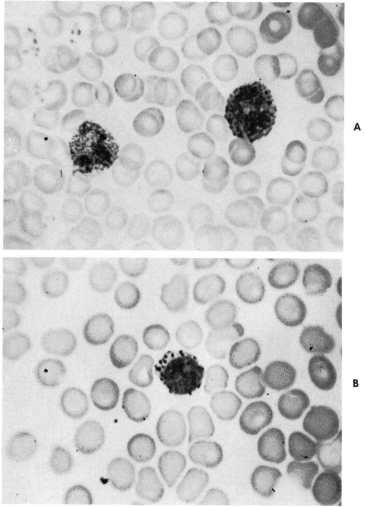

A

B

Continued.

Fig. 11-38. Cytoplasmic inclusions in the Hurler syndrome. **A,** Peripheral blood. The lighter cell is a polymorphonuclear leukocyte of the type described by Reilly[435] (type I polymorph). There are small lilac-staining granules of relatively uniform size in the cytoplasm. The darker cell, which superficially resembles a basophil, has large lilac-blue granules of nonuniform size (type II polymorph). **B,** Peripheral blood. Lymphocyte with lilac and blue granules. **C,** Bone marrow myelocytes. The darker cell in the center is probably the precursor of the type II polymorph in the peripheral blood. The other two cells with lilac granules are probably the precursors of the similar cells in the peripheral blood (type I polymorph). The patient was a 3½-year-old boy with typical manifestations of the Hurler syndrome. The total white cell count was 17,400/cu. mm. with the following differential:

$$28\% \text{ type I polymorph}$$
$$6\% \text{ type II polymorph}$$
$$55\% \text{ lymphocytes without granules}$$
$$9\% \text{ lymphocytes with granules}$$
$$2\% \text{ monocytes}$$
$$\overline{100\%}$$

Formalin was found to dissolve the granules. After basic lead acetate fixation the granules were stained by toluidine blue. (Wright-Giemsa stain; ×1,600; reduced ¼.) (Courtesy Dr. Ralph L. Engle, Jr., New York City.)

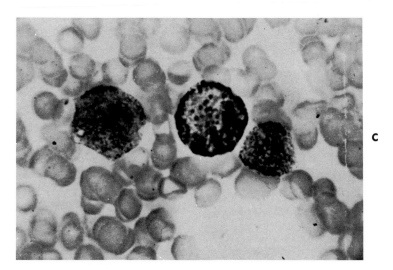

Fig. 11-38, cont'd. For legend see p. 631.

achondroplasia, the Marfan syndrome, and multiple epiphyseal dysplasia. Occasionally, however, isolated clusters of a few very small, clearly defined pink granules have been found in the cytoplasm of polymorphonuclear leukocytes from normal persons.

The circulating leukocytes were studied[322] in 8 cases of MPS I, 2 of MPS II, and 5 of MPS III. In all, obvious metachromatic granules were found in 10% to 60% of the lymphocytes, thus confirming the findings of Muir and associates.[376] On the other hand, Reilly granulations have been found infrequently and with no apparent relation to one or more of the entities. They were present in only 1 case of the Sanfilippo syndrome (MPS III). Possibly the appearance of Reilly granulations depends on a quantitative phenomenon, but it may well be that other, unrecognized factors are involved.

In 4 cases of the Morquio syndrome (MPS IV), scattered irregular aggregations of metachromatic granules, distinct from Reilly granules, have been noted in the cytoplasm of the majority of the polymorphs. Possibly this difference in form reflects the fact that in the Morquio syndrome it is a different mucopolysaccharide, namely keratan sulfate, which accumulates.

Plate 1. **A**, MPS IV (the Morquio syndrome). The elder surviving brother in the kindred diagrammed in Fig. 11-33. There are signs of spastic paraplegia. **B**, MPS IV (the Morquio syndrome). Steamy corneal clouding in elder brother pictured in Fig. 11-26. **C**, MPS I S (the Scheie syndrome). Corneal clouding, most dense peripherally, in male shown in Fig. 11-9. **D** to **G**, Inclusions in white blood cells. **D**, Specific lymphocytic inclusions, in case of MPS III. **E**, Reilly granulations of polymorphonuclear leukocytes, in case of MPS III. **F**, Metachromatic cytoplasmic inclusions in macrophage in bone marrow of case of MPS II, shown also in Fig. 11-11. **G**, Metachromatic granules in cytoplasm of inflammatory cells elicited by the Rebuck skin window technique in a case of MPS II, also shown in Fig. 11-11. (From McKusick, V. A., Kaplan, D., Wise, D., Hanley, W. B., Suddarth, S. B., Sevick, M. E., and Maumenee, A. E.: Medicine 44:445, 1965.)

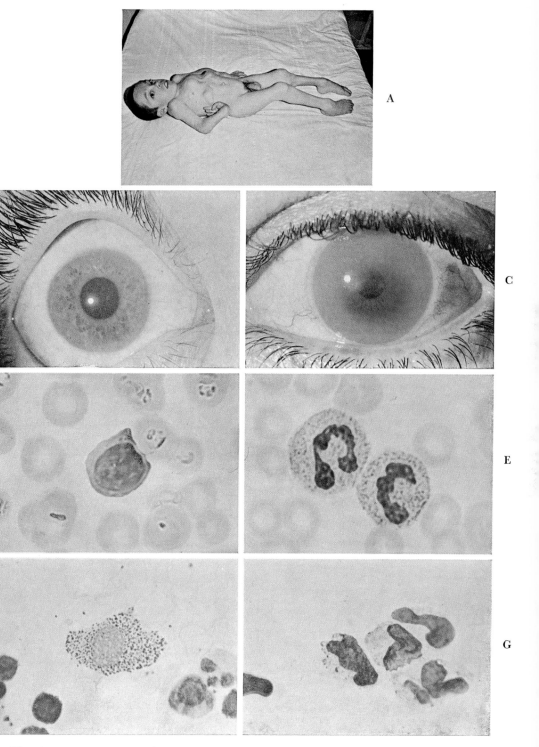

Plate 1. For legend see opposite page.

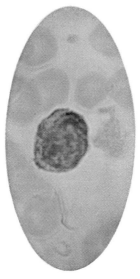

Plate 2. Metachromatically staining cytoplasmic inclusions in a circulating lymphocyte. Stained with toluidine blue. (From J.A.M.A., Jan. 18, 1965.)

In 4 cases of the Scheie syndrome (MPS I S) lymphocytic granules either have been absent or have been present in a very ill-defined form in only a small proportion of cells; this probably represents a quantitative phenomenon, since patients in these cases excrete less mucopolysaccharide than do those in cases of MPS types I, II, and III. Reilly granulations of the polmorphs were found in none of the 4 subjects.

Two types of inclusion cells have been identified in the bone marrow in the mucopolysaccharidoses. The Gasser cell is a reticulum cell with fine, densely distributed inclusions. The Buhot cell is a plasma cell with large inclusions of variable size and shape surrounded by a clear area.

Pearson and Lorincz[415] demonstrated mucopolysaccharide granules in bone marrow cells of 17 of 18 consecutive patients with "the Hurler syndrome" seen in a two-year period. The patient without such findings was a 7-year-old boy thought to have the X-linked form (MPS II). Presumably, the other cases were MPS I. Some X-linked cases do show bone marrow inclusions, however, as we were able to demonstrate (Plate 1F) in the 31-year-old male shown in Fig. 11-8. All 12 patients studied by Jermain and associates[231] showed granulated bone marrow cells that they considered to be phagocytic clasmatocytes.

Hansen[189a] found the May-Grünwald-Giemsa stain preferable to either Wright's stain or toluidine blue. MPS I and II are indistinguishable hematologically. Inclusions may be found in neutrophils, monocytes, and lymphocytes. The *diffuse* distribution of granules throughout the cytoplasm of the lymphocyte is characteristic. In the bone marrow reticulum cells contain inclusions, these being the "Gasser cells." In MPS III, granules are clustered in restricted areas of the cytoplasm of lymphocytes. The color of the inclusions is unusually reddish. In the bone marrow, a striking phenomenon is seen in plasma cells, which are increased in number and often in size. The inclusions are highly polymorphic and often enclosed in a large vacuole. These are the "Buhot cells."

The peripheral blood and bone marrow show unimpressive, although definitely abnormal, metachromatic inclusions in both MPS IV and MPS V (MPS I S). However, MPS VI makes up for them with the most striking inclusions of all. Especially the neutrophils are choked with coarse, closely packed granules. These are the cells described by Alder and by Reilly.

The mucolipidoses, including the G_{M1}-gangliosidoses, also have hematologic changes, as reviewed by Hansen.[189a]

With the Rebuck skin window technique[433,463] one can detect metachromatic granules in both macrophages and polymorphonuclear leukocytes.[42] (See Plate 1G.)

Definitive differential diagnosis sometimes requires refined studies of urinary mucopolysaccharides with precise identification of the substance (s) excreted. For example, in young children with MPS IV the differentiation from MPS I may be possible only by identifying the mucopolysaccharide present in excess in the urine as keratan sulfate.

Elevated plasma levels of acid mucopolysaccharide in the Hurler syndrome were found by Sanfilippo and Good,[455] using the Bollet method, and by Calatroni.[50]

DiFerrante and his colleagues[20a,110] have made heavy use of the ratio between high molecular weight MPS and low molecular weight MPS in the urine. Since the former is raised and the latter reduced in the mucopolysaccharidoses, the ratio is particularly useful in discriminating patients from normals and in evaluating the effects of therapy. The ratio appears to reflect the degradative defect that underlies the mucopolysaccharidoses.

Both the Hurler and the Hunter syndromes have been diagnosed antenatally[155] in cases of mothers who had given birth to an affected child in a previous pregnancy. Fratantoni and colleagues[155] made use of ^{35}S kinetics and cytoplasmic metachromasia of amniotic cells. Matalon and associates[349] at first thought that elevated mucopolysaccharide content of the amniotic fluid is a valid diagnostic method. They found that normal fluid had about 0.02 mg/ml. (range 0.006 to 0.035) of mucopolysaccharides in the second trimester of pregnancy. The fluid from a fourteen-week pregnancy which subsequently produced a baby with the Hurler syndrome contained 0.087 mg/ml. Furthermore, whereas the mucopolysaccharide of pooled normal amniotic fluid was about 80% hyaluronic acid and 13% dermatan sulfate, the Hurler fluid was 63% heparan sulfate. The authors pointed out that the increased heparan sulfate could be detected directly in both the amniotic fluid and the urine of the newborn child by the nitrous acid reaction for N-sulfated hexosamines.[268] Danes and co-workers[94] showed that the mucopolysaccharide content of amniotic fluid, as reflected by uronic acid, decreases progressively during pregnancy, being relatively high in the early stages.

In a later publication Matalon et al.[348a] concluded that direct chemical study of the amniotic fluid is *not* a reliable method for prenatal diagnosis of mucopolysaccharidoses. Study of cultured amniotic cells is necessary. This conclusion is consistent with that arrived at in connection with almost all other inborn errors of metabolism: study of the fluid and uncultured cells cannot be made the basis of prenatal diagnosis.

BASIC DEFECTS IN THE GENETIC MUCOPOLYSACCHARIDOSES

That the disorders discussed here involve a defect in mucopolysaccharide metabolism was suspected in 1952 by Brante[41] on the basis of the nature of the stored material. The supposition was given strong support by the demonstration by Dorfman and Lorincz[116] and by Meyer and associates[360] of excess mucopolysacchariduria. The acid mucopolysaccharides excreted in the urine in excess in the mucopolysaccharidoses are of lower molecular weight than those found in normal urine,[66] indicating partial degradation.

In the early 1960's Hers[199] developed the concept of lysosomal diseases, and he and others amassed evidence in the next few years that the Hurler syndrome satisfied the criteria. The archetypic lysosomal disease was glycogenosis type II (acid maltase deficiency). The characteristics of a lysosomal disease are as follows:

1. Storage of material occurs, as is demonstrated in the mucopolysaccharidoses.

2. The storage material is heterogeneous since the degradative enzymes are not strictly specific. This feature is demonstrated by the predominant deposition of ganglioside in the brain and the predominant mucopolysaccharide deposition in the liver in MPS I, and perhaps by the excessive urinary excretion of *two* mucopolysaccharides in MPS I and MPS II.

3. Deposition is vacuolar, i.e., is membrane bound, which is demonstrated in the mucopolysaccharidoses by electron microscopy, as noted above.

4. Several tissues are affected, which is obviously true in the mucopolysaccharidoses.

5. The disease is progressive, which is also true in the mucopolysaccharidoses.

6. Replacement therapy by getting missing enzyme into lysosomes by means of endocytosis is at least theoretically possible and has some proof in the case of glycogenosis type II[281] and Fabry's disease.[331] As will be pointed out below, the correction factors, the absence of which is demonstrated in studies of fibroblasts from patients with the mucopolysaccharidoses, may be agents for use in replacement therapy of the Hurler syndrome and other mucopolysaccharidoses.

Support for the idea that the Hurler syndrome and related disorders are lysosomal diseases was provided by the electron microscopic studies of Van Hoof and Hers[540] published in 1965: accumulation of material occurred in membranous structures with the characteristics of lysosomes. (See Figs. 11-7 and 11-17 for comparable findings in two of our patients.) To say that a disorder is a lysosmal disease is equivalent to concluding that the defect is in degradation. This was, however, not promptly appreciated; for example, writers at that time including myself (see 1966 edition of this monograph) discussed excessive synthesis of mucopolysaccharide as the basic defect.

About the same time (1965) Danes and Bearn[88] demonstrated a morphologic abnormality, cytoplasmic metachromasia, in the cultured fibroblasts from patients with mucopolysaccharidoses. In 1968, Fratantoni, Hall, and Neufeld[153] provided definitive proof of a degradative defect: cultured fibroblasts accumulated excessive amounts of $^{35}SO_4$-labelled mucopolysaccharide (Fig. 11-39A), and washout of the radioactive label occurred abnormally slowly when the fibroblasts were placed in "cold" medium (Fig. 11-39B).

Fratantoni, Hall, and Neufeld[154] also did seminal experiments mixing fibroblasts from patients of different clinical type and demonstrated mutual correction of the metabolic defects (Fig. 11-39). They could show that the medium in which cells of a different MPS type or normal cells had grown would also correct the metabolic defect, as would also the urine from normal persons. These observations indicated the existence of diffusible substances that are produced by fibroblasts, which are essential to the normal degradation of mucopolysaccharides and one or another of which is deficient in each of the mucopolysaccharidoses. (Only the Morquio syndrome, MPS IV, has not yet yielded to this type of study.) The factor deficient in each clinical syndrome was termed the corrective factor for that condition: Hurler corrective factor, Hunter corrective factor, etc. Their nature as proteins and some of their physical properties were delineated,[18a,18b,56,56a] and for some their specific enzymatic properties have been identified.

Surprises coming from the Neufeld approach included the discoveries that (1) the Hurler and Scheie syndromes, although clinically quite different, behave the same,[18a,558] i.e., have deficiency of the same corrective factor (p. 552) and (2) the clinical picture of the Sanfilippo syndrome can be produced by either of two different deficiences (p. 582).

The enzymatic nature of the corrective factors, where known, are given in Table 11-2: the Hurler corrective factor is a α-L-iduronidase,[15a] the Sanfilippo A corrective factor is heparan sulfate sulfatase,[262a] and the Sanfilippo B corrective

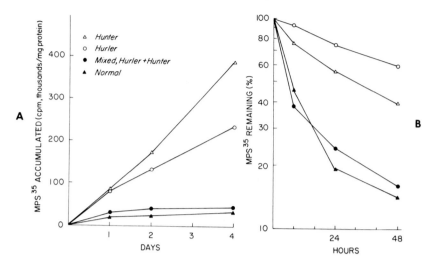

Fig. 11-39. Experiments indicating defect in the degradation of mucopolysaccharides in the Hurler, Hunter, and Sanfilippo syndromes and correction of the defect when normal cells or cells of a different mucopolysaccharidoses are co-cultivated with cells of the given type. **A,** Excessive accumulation of label in disease fibroblasts. **B,** Retarded washout of label in disease fibroblasts. (Courtesy Dr. Elizabeth F. Neufeld.)

factor is N-acetyl-α-D-glucosamidase.[398a] The corrective factor in MPS VII, β-glucuronidase deficiency, is of course β-glucuronidase.

The distinctness of the several corrective factors is indicated by their approximate molecular weights[383]:

Factor	Molecular weight
Sanfilippo B corrective factor	300,000
Sanfilippo A corrective factor	112,000
Hunter corrective factor	112,000
Hurler-Scheie corrective factor	84,000
Maroteaux-Lamy corrective factor	71,000

OTHER GENETIC MUCOPOLYSACCHARIDOSES?

It is more than likely that the six entities described earlier in this chapter are not the only genetic defects of mucopolysaccharide metabolism. The following discussion concerns conditions in which such a disturbance is suspected.

Lahdensuu[271] described 4 affected sibs, 3 girls and a boy, the oldest being 19 years of age, with joint contractures, corneal clouding that was most dense in the periphery, coarse facies, bony changes, and normal intelligence. The carpal bones were small with irregular contours. Corneal transplants became opacified. Again, these cases resemble most closely the cases of the Scheie syndrome but may represent the Maroteaux-Lamy syndrome, as was suggested by Maroteaux and colleagues.[338] Mucolipidosis III (p. 652) is yet another possibility.

Abul-Haj and co-workers[1] proposed that Farber's lipogranulomatosis (Fig. 11-40) is a mucopolysaccharidosis. This disorder is characterized by onset in the first weeks of life and the following features: irritability, hoarse cry, nodular, erythematous swellings of the wrists and other sites, particularly those subject to trauma, and severe motor and mental retardation. Death occurs by 2 years of age. The histologic appearance of the nodules is granulomatous. In the nervous system both neurons and glial cells are swollen, with stored material having the characteristics of a nonsulfonated acid mucopolysaccharide.[1] Bierman and colleagues[31] confirmed Abul-Haj's suggestion by demonstrating increased tissue and urinary mucopolysaccharide, mainly dermatan sulfate.

Autosomal recessive inheritance is likely. Two of Farber's patients were sibs.[139]

Puretič and colleagues[424] described a newly recognized form of connective tissue disorder in an 11-year-old boy. Three sibs died in infancy with painful flexural contractures of the elbows, shoulder joints, and knees, which developed at about 3 months of age. Other features included deformity of the skull and face, stunted growth, osteolysis of the terminal phalanges, and multiple subcutaneous nodules. Ishikawa and Hori[221] reported cases and suggested the designation *systemic hyalinosis,* which has the disadvantage of possible confusion with lipoid proteinosis, which is also called *hyalinosis cutis et mucosae* (p. 640).

The case reported by Rocher and Pesme[446] as an instance of "pleonosteosis (Léri's disease) with opalescent corneas" was probably MPS I S or MPS VI. As pointed out by Rukavina and colleagues,[452] others of the reported cases of Léri's pleonosteosis were probably in fact instances of a mucopolysaccharidosis, especially MPS I S or MPS II. True Léri's disease[284,553] is a rare entity characterized by dominant inheritance, flexion contractures of the fingers, enlarged thumbs and first toes, limited joint motion, short stature, mongoloid facies, and normal intelligence. The hand looks like that in mucopolysaccharidoses, but fixed finger flexion occurs only at the first interphalangeal joint. Carpal tunnel syndrome is said[553] to occur in Léri's pleonosteosis, as in MPS V (Fig. 11-9E and F). However, it is likely that Watson-Jones' patient with this complication (his Case 4) indeed had MPS I S; only his first family appears to have had Léri's pleonosteosis with dominant inheritance. "Pleonosteosis," the term suggested by Léri because he thought overproduction of bone was the nature of the disorder, is a misnomer because the main abnormality seems to reside in ligaments. Mucopolysaccharide metabolism has apparently not been studied.

François' syndrome (dermo-chondro-corneal dystrophy) is characterized[147, 149,229] by skeletal deformity of the hands and feet, "xanthomatous" nodules on the pinnae, dorsal surface of the metacarpophalangeal and interphalangeal joints, posterior surface of the elbows, nose, etc., and by corneal dystrophy. Mucopolysaccharide metabolism has apparently not been studied in this disorder. A hypercholesterolemic phase has been identified,[437] suggesting that this disorder is a derangement of lipid metabolism. Inheritance is almost certainly autosomal recessive.

The genetic determination of macular corneal dystrophy is clearly established.[351,549] Autosomal recessive inheritance has been observed. On the basis of 9 cases of macular corneal dystrophy Klintworth and Vogel[252] concluded that this disorder is a localized acid mucopolysaccharide storage disease of the corneal fibroblast. The cutaneous fibroblasts of one patient were structurally unaltered, and the urine did not contain an excess of acid mucopolysaccharide. No entirely adequate autopsy studies excluding systemic abnormality have been reported.[251] Electron microscopic studies[427] showed no abnormality of skin or bulbar conjunctiva in 4 patients. Similar studies of the corneal fibroblasts[252] showed that the vacuoles in macular corneal dystrophy are a direct extension of rough endoplasmic reticulum. Thus the defect in mucopolysaccharide metabolism is probably at an earlier stage than that in the classic mucopolysaccharidoses.

In the third edition of this monograph (1966, p. 386, legend), I raised the question of whether Maumenee's congenital hereditary corneal dystrophy is a localized mucopolysaccharidosis. This theory has been disproved by the work of

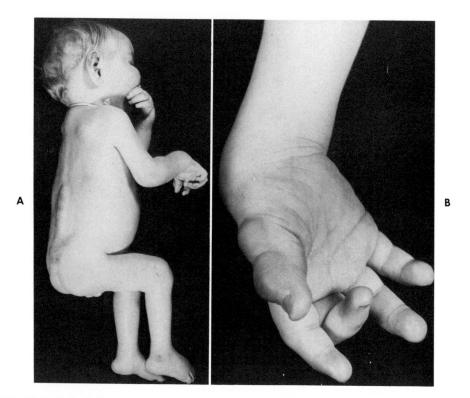

Fig. 11-40. Farber's lipogranulomatosis. J. R. C. (J.H.H. 932852), 5 months old at the time of these photographs, was apparently well until the age of 10 weeks. Thereafter, hoarseness, stridor, and the joint and skin changes demonstrated here developed. Motor and intellectual development was severely retarded. Persistent neutrophilic leukocytosis (15,000 to 20,000/cu. mm.) was a feature. X-ray films showed joint destruction. He died at the age of 20 months. In addition to the changes shown in the photographs, nodular thickenings of the heart valves, especially the aortic and mitral, were found. Histologically the nodular lesions at many sites showed polymorphous granulomatous infiltration, with vacuolated cells. The spleen, lymph nodes, and bone marrow were minimally involved and the liver not at all. The intestinal changes resembled those of Whipple's disease. In the central nervous system both neuronal and glial cells were ballooned by cytoplasmic storage material. The additional finding of gliosis and granuloma formation distinguished it from Tay-Sachs or Niemann-Pick disease. (The above patient was referred to by Ford[142] and was reported in detail by Abul-Haj and colleagues.[1] Radiographic features of this case were presented by Schultze and Lang.[465]) **A,** General appearance. Note swellings over pressure points such as the spine and ischial tuberosities. **B,** Swellings of the thumb and wrist. **C,** Biopsy of granuloma showing ballooned cells. (Hematoxylin and eosin; ×430.) A biopsied lymph node showed cells of the same type. **D** and **E,** PAS-positive inclusion material in cells of lymph node. (PAS stain; **D,** ×380; **E,** ×1400.)

Kenyon and Maumenee[245a] which suggests that this disorder is a primary endothelial dystrophy with stromal edema and corneal clouding as effects thereof.

A chrondroitin-4-sulfate mucopolysaccharidosis was reported by Thompson and co-workers.[527,528] The patient was a 48-year-old woman who showed short stature (height, 56½ inches), mental retardation, pectus carinatum, short fourth metacarpal, congenital dislocation of the hip, clouding of the cornea at the periphery, auscultatory signs of aortic and mitral valve disease, hepatomegaly, deafness, and increased height of lumbar vertebrae with degenerative changes at the margins. Circulating leukocytes showed basophilic granulations. Over

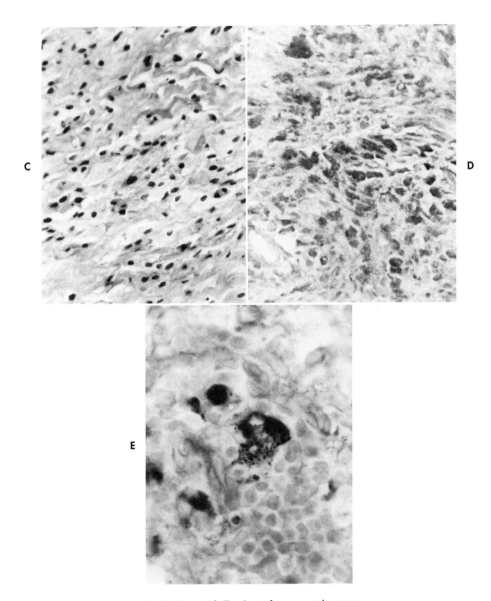

Fig. 11-40, cont'd. For legend see opposite page.

50 mg. of mucopolysaccharide were excreted per 24 hours, and most of this amount was chrondroitin-4-sulfate.

Philippart and Sugarman[418] also described a patient with increased excreation of chrondroitin-4-sulfate. The clinical features in the 12-year-old Negro girl included progressive painful limitation of joint motion, hepatosplenomegaly, diffuse anterior peripheral haze of the cornea, slight beaking of the first lumbar vertebra, shallow acetabula, and a large sella turcica. Intelligence was normal, and granulation of the leukocytes was not found.

From a long experience at the Mayo Clinic with many affected members of one kindred, and Stickler and co-workers[505,506] described an autosomal dominant disorder consisting of progressive myopia beginning in the first decade of life and resulting in retinal detachment and blindness. Affected persons also exhibited premature degenerative changes in various joints, with abnormal epiphyseal development and joint hypermobility in some. Vertebral abnormalities and hearing deficit are other features. A justification for mentioning it here is that a probable case was reported by David in 1953 as "polytopen enchondralen Dysostose Typ Pfaundler-Hurler."[95]

Winchester and colleagues[560,561] described a "new" mucopolysaccharidosis *sine* mucopolysacchariduria. Severe and progressive deforming arthritis, simulating juvenile rheumatoid arthritis, coarse facies, and peripheral corneal opacities were the features. Two sisters, the offspring of first-cousin parents, were affected. The evidence that this is a disorder of mucopolysaccharide metabolism consisted of increased metachromasia of fibroblasts with increased intracellular uronic acid. Beals[20] has observed what appears to be the same disorder. From electron microscopic studies of material from a family with several affected sibs, Rimoin and his colleagues[492a] concluded that this is not a lysosomal storage disease and therefore probably not a mucopolysaccharidosis.

Szabo and associates[515] described a 13-year-old boy with skeletal abnormalities, large round white deposits in the retina, and granulation of circulating leukocytes. Large amounts of dermatan sulfate, heparan sulfate, and another, unidentified mucopolysaccharide, perhaps hyaluronic acid sulfate, were excreted in the urine.

Moynahan[375] suggested that "hyalinosis cutis et mucosae (lipoid proteinosis),￼" an autosomal recessive disorder, is a genetic mucopolysaccharidosis. Spranger[491] found no abnormality of urinary excretion of mucopolysaccharides in a 25-year-old patient (A. E., J.H.H. 1371970).

Esterly and McKusick[137] described a "stiff skin syndrome" in 4 persons in two unrelated families. Very firm skin and limitation of joint motion were features. Histochemically, the dermis showed abnormal amounts of hyaluronidase-digestible acid mucopolysaccharide. Fibroblasts cultured from 1 patient showed a marked increase in cytoplasmic metachromatic material. None of the patients excreted excessive amounts of mucopolysaccharide in the urine. A genetically determined abnormality of mucopolysaccharide metabolism was postulated. Pichler[419] probably described the same condition in a father and 2 children, under the designation "hereditary contractures with sclerodermatoid changes of the skin."

Spranger and colleagues[492] described a "new" clinical syndrome they called "geleophysic dwarfism" because of the unusual but pleasant and happy facial

appearance and the short stature. Other features included a dysostosis-multiplex–
like bone dysplasia affecting particularly the hands and feet and focal accumulation of mucopolysaccharides in the liver and perhaps in cardiovascular tissues.
They suggested that the patient of Vanace and co-workers[539] had this condition,
which they presumed to have autosomal recessive inheritance and a "focal" mucopolysaccharidosis. This patient was a 5½-year-old child who died with severe
cardiac involvement.

"Acquired" disturbances in mucopolysaccharide metabolism do not concern
us here. For example, Ultmann and colleagues[535] described a 58-year-old man
with systemic mastocytosis, in whose urine Dr. Karl Meyer of Columbia University found 24 mg./L./day of a mucopolysaccharide identified as heparan sulfate.
We found no excess mucopolysacchariduria in a 68-year-old man with long-
standing severe systemic mastocytosis. Zimmer and associates[577] found normal
24-hour urine mucopolysaccharide excretion in 21 patients with mastocytosis,
and in 7 patients studied in this way serum mucopolysaccharides were not increased.

DIFFERENTIAL DIAGNOSIS

The differentiation of the mucopolysaccharidoses has been discussed *in
extenso* already and is summarized in Table 11-4. Some simulating conditions
are discussed, furthermore, in the section on other possible genetic mucopolysaccharidoses, above.

It is worthwhile mentioning the simulation of the changes in the lumbar
spine, as well as some of the other features of MPS I, by *congenital hypothyroidism*.[514] I had the opportunity to see one such case (C. D., U.S.P.H.S. 235041).
Modern methods for the laboratory diagnosis of hypothyroidism easily resolve
the problem of differentiation.

The mucolipidoses

Table 11-4 intends to demonstrate, the group of mucolipidosis as defined
by Spranger and Wiedemann[497] show phenotypic and biochemical features overlapping those of the mucopolysaccharidoses on the one hand, and of the
sphingolipidoses on the other. This group includes three disorders specifically
termed mucolipidosis by Spranger and Wiedemann.[497] It includes the Hurler-
like conditions, fucosidosis and mannosidosis, and the Austin type of metachromatic leukodystrophy which is accompanied by mucopolysacchariduria and is
referred to here as Austin's juvenile sulfatidosis. Perhaps Farber's lipogranulomatosis (p. 636) should be included.

In the interpretation of Spranger and Wiedemann,[497] the mucolipidoses also
include the G_{M1}-gangliosidoses, types I and II. In the young infant, type I, now
generally known as *generalized gangliosidosis,* is particularly likely to occasion
confusion with the Hurler syndrome, but appreciation of the fact that roentgenographic features evolve much earlier in this condition allows easy clinical differentiation, and specific laboratory tests are now available for confirming the
diagnosis. In retrospect, patients in whom Caffey[49] described prenatal and neonatal bone lesions of Hurler syndrome appear to have suffered from this condition (or perhaps I-cell disease; see below.) The disorder has been variously
called "Hurler variant,"[76] "pseudo-Hurler disease," "Tay-Sachs disease with vis-

Table 11-4. Characterization and classification of three categories of lysosomal storage disorders*

Mucopolysaccharidoses	Mucolipidoses	Sphingolipidoses
Characterization		
MPS-type dysmorphism	MPS-type dysmorphism	No MPS features
Dysostosis multiplex	Dysostosis multiplex	No dysostosis multiplex
Abnormal mucopolysac- chariduria	Normal mucopolysac- chariduria†	Normal mucopolysac- chariduria
Visceral storage of mucopolysaccharides	Visceral storage of mucopolysaccharides, glycolipids, and/or sphingolipids	Visceral storage of glycolipids and/or sphingolipids
Classification		
MPS I H (Hurler)	G_{M1}-gangliosidosis I (neurovisceral lipidosis)	Tay-Sachs disease and other G_{M2} gangliosidoses
MPS I S (Scheie)	Juvenile sulfatidosis, Austin type	Fabry's disease
MPS I H/MPS I S		
MPS II (Hunter)	G_{M1}-gangliosidosis II	Niemann-Pick disease and other sphingomyelinoses
MPS III (Sanfilippo A and B)	Fucosidosis	Infantile metachromatic leukodystrophy and other sulfatidoses
MPS IV (Morquio)	Mannosidosis	Gaucher's disease and other cerebrosidoses
MPS VI (Maroteaux-Lamy)	ML I (lipomucopoly- saccharidosis)	Lactosyl ceramidosis
MPS VII (β-glycuronidase deficiency)	ML II (I-cell disease) ML III (pseudo–Hurler polydystrophy) Farber's disease	

*Modified from Spranger, J., and Wiedemann, H. R.: Humangenetik **9**:113, 1970.
†Except in juvenile sulfatidosis, Austin type, and possibly in the G_{M1}-gangliosidoses.

ceral involvement,"[393] and "neurovisceral lipidosis."[276] Features resembling the mucopolysaccharidoses include bone changes (e.g., beaked lumbar vertebra), hepatosplenomegaly, and corneal clouding. Those suggesting a sphingolipidosis include large head, early and progressive neurologic deterioration, and cherry-red spot of the macula. O'Brien and associates[400] introduced the term generalized gangliosidosis because small but excessive amounts of G_{M1}-gangliosides were found in the liver and spleen in accompaniment with large excesses in the brain.

Scott and colleagues[471] reported high accumulations of a mucopolysaccharide in the liver and spleen and suggested a relationship to the genetic mucopolysaccharidoses. Suzuki[511] tentatively identified the mucopolysaccharide as keratan sulfate.

Okada and O'Brien[410] discovered deficiency of β-galactosidase in generalized

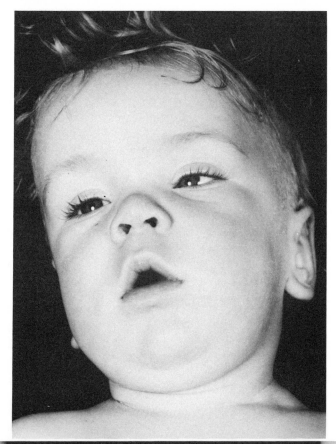

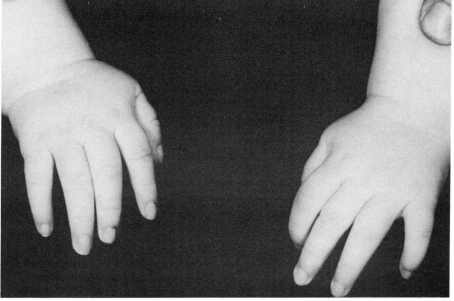

Fig. 11-41. Generalized gangliosidosis in J. F. Y. (see text).

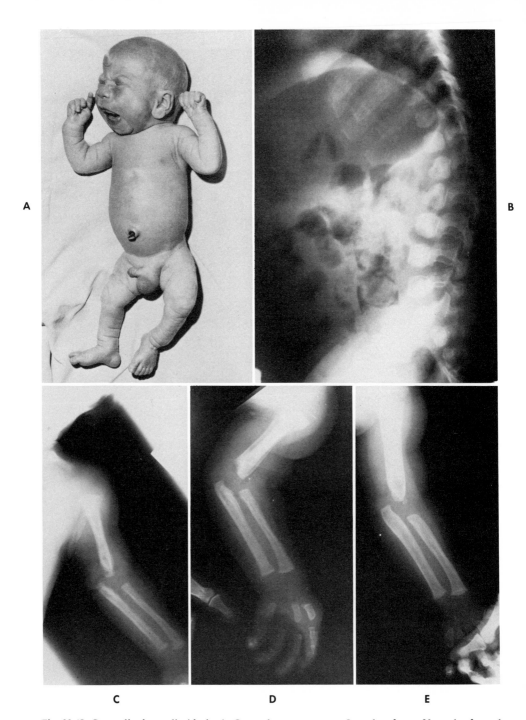

Fig. 11-42. Generalized gangliosidosis. **A,** General appearance at 2 weeks of age. Note the frontal bossing, depressed nasal bridge, wide upper lip, maxillary hyperplasia, and prominent wrists and ankles. **B,** Spinal deformity at 7 months of age. The vertebral bodies are hypoplastic, with beaking of L1 and L2 producing lumbar kyphosis. **C** to **E,** Upper limb at the ages of 2 weeks, 2 months, and 7 months, respectively, in patient shown in **B.** Note "pinching off" of end of humerus, **E,** midshaft widening, and, in **D,** periosteal cloaking, which subsequently became less striking. **F,** Liver β-galactosidase activity for ganglioside G_{M1} in normal 3-year-old boy ("normal"),

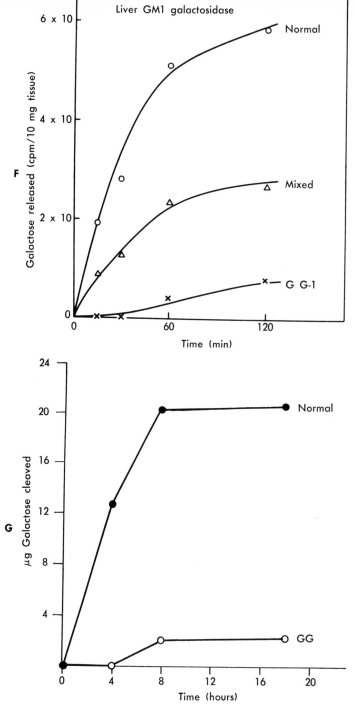

in 8-month-old patient with generalized gangliosidosis ("G G-1"), and in mixture of equal portions of the two ("mixed"). **G,** Cleavage of galactose from keratan sulfate by β-galactosidase prepared from equivalent amounts of normal (above) and generalized gangliosidosis (**GG**) liver tissue. (**A** from Scott, C. R., Lagunoff, D., and Trump, B. F.: J. Pediat. **71:**357, 1967; **B** to **E** courtesy G. Mitchell and A. Berne, Syracuse, N. Y., from O'Brien, J.: J. Pediat. **75:**167, 1969; **F** from Okada, S., and O'Brien, J. S.: Science **160:**1002, 1968; **G** from MacBrinn, M. C., Okada, S., Ho, M. W., Hu, C. C., and O'Brien, J. S.: Science **163:**946, 1969. Copyright 1968 and 1969 by the American Association for the Advancement of Science.)

gangliosidosis. Normally this enzyme is responsible for the breakdown of G_{M1} ganglioside by cleavage of the terminal galactose from the molecule. The same group[310] further demonstrated that the same enzyme is able to break down keratan sulfate, the stored mucopolysaccharide, by galactose cleavage.

Another form of generalized gangliosidosis, called type II or the juvenile form[399] because of later onset, has much less in the way of skeletal and visceral change but the same generalized accumulation of G_{M1}-ganglioside and of a keratan sulfate.[565] Whereas all β-galactosidase isoenzymes are deficient in the classic type I generalized gangliosidosis, only isoenzymes B and C are deficient in type II. The following case report is illustrative of generalized gangliosidosis:

Case 26. J. F. Y. (1302628), a white male born in 1968, at birth had marked scrotal edema, and at 24 hours of age the hands and feet were noted to be edematous. At 6 weeks of age psychomotor retardation, a systolic murmur, hepatosplenomegaly, and mild peripheral edema were described. He was first seen at this hospital at the age of 6 months (Fig. 11-41). In addition to all the features noted above, he showed a large head (far above the 97th percentile), marked hypotonia, coarse facial features with a broad nasal bridge, corneal clouding, a cherry-red spot of each macula. Laboratory studies showed intermittent, mild mucopolysacchariduria, electrocardiographic evidence of left ventricular hypertrophy, large foam cells in the bone marrow, and reduced activity of β-galactosidase in white blood cells, cultured fibroblasts, and urine.[523] X-ray studies showed cardiomegaly, spatulate ribs, beaking of a lumbar vertebra, and thickening of the midshaft of the humerus. The child died of bronchopneumonia at the age of 12 months. The diagnosis of generalized gangliosidosis was confirmed by demonstration of accumulation of G_{M1} ganglioside in the brain and deficiency of β-galactosidase activity in brain and liver. In studies of the eyes, Emery and collaborators[133] demonstrated storage of mucopolysaccharide in the cornea and of ganglioside in retinal ganglion cells.

Three members of the mucolipidosis group are specifically labeled mucolipidosis I, II, and III by Spranger and Wiedemann.[497]

Mucolipidosis I (formerly lipomucopolysaccharidosis[520]) is characterized by mild Hurler-like manifestations with moderate progressive mental retardation, the skeletal changes of dysostosis multiplex, no excess mucopolysacchariduria, and peculiar inclusions in cultured fibroblasts. The birefringent cytoplasmic inclusions in cultured fibroblasts are PAS and Sudan black positive. Matalon and co-workers[344] demonstrated that they stain metachromatically with toluidine blue after treatment with chloroform-methanol. Thus, storage of both AMPS and glycolipids is indicated. Storage is in lysosomes.[157] Unlike MPS I, II, and III, β-galactosidase levels are normal. Spranger and Wiedemann[497] observed 3 affected sibs, and parental consanguinity in one instance. They suggested that the sibs described by Pincus and associates[420] had this disorder, as did also a patient reported by Sanfilippo and colleagues.[457]

Mucolipidosis II (I-cell disease) is a Hurler-like disorder with severe clinical and radiologic features, striking fibroblast inclusions (hence "I-cell" for "inclusion-cell"), and no excess mucopolysacchariduria. Congenital dislocation of the hips, thoracic deformities, hernia, and hyperplastic gums are evident soon after birth. X-ray studies show that the bones undergo changes of dysostosis multiplex similar to, but more severe than, those of MPS I. Retarded psychomotor development, clear corneas, and restricted joint mobility are other features. Leroy and co-workers[286,287] first delineated the disorder. Few cases have been reported thus far.[306] Affected sibs, both male and female, have been observed more than once, and the parents of one of the patients of Spranger and Wiedemann[497] were first

Fig. 11-43. Mucolipidosis II (I-cell disease). The patient shown here was C. McK., a 25-month-old boy. The parents were of different ethnic stock. Peculiar facies and a right inguinal hernia were noted at birth. At the age of 2 months bilateral inguinal herniorrhaphies were performed without difficulty. Bony abnormalities such as severe metatarsus adductus and tibial torsion were noted at that time. The initial diagnosis was Caffey's disease, presumably because of periosteal cuffing, demonstrated on skeletal x-ray films.

At 6 months of age, abnormal facies was again noted, as well as hypertrophied gums and a triangular-shaped head. The liver and spleen were not enlarged. X-ray findings were thought to be consistent with the Hurler syndrome, which was felt to be the diagnosis, although the urine was negative for mucopolysaccharides.

Beginning at the age of 7 months the child had frequent episodes of otitis media complicated by febrile convulsions. He never achieved most of the usual milestones except for holding up his head. At 25 months of age he was unable to sit or roll over.

Examination at 25 months showed a child with severe psychomotor retardation. He was able to distinguish his mother from a stranger. The facies and skull shape are demonstrated in **A.** Note the marked gum hypertrophy. Marked lumbar gibbus, **B,** and limitation of both extension and flexion in all joints were present. The ears were relatively small and were thickened and very firm. Bones of the limbs were thick and the wrists particularly broad. The fingers were broad and tapering, **C.** The lower limbs showed marked flexion contractures at the hips and tibial torsion. The liver extended 5 cm. below the right costal margin, and the tip of the spleen was just palpable.

Laboratory investigations showed large metachromatic granules within vacuoles in the cytoplasm of lymphocytes. Alkaline phosphatase was greatly elevated (156 I.U.); LDH, SGOT, and SGPT were each somewhat elevated. The urine showed no excess of mucopolysaccharides, arylsulfatase A and β-galactosidase were elevated.

X-ray films showed that the cranial vault was increased in thickness; scaphocephaly and infantile sella turcica were demonstrated. The spine showed hypoplasia of the odontoid process, thoracolumbar gibbus with beaked L1, and immaturity of the vertebral bodies. The ribs were broad, tapering at the vertebral ends, as in the Hurler syndrome. The pelvic inlet was severely constricted, with acetabular protrusion, external rotation of ischial and pubic bones, and narrow iliac bases. Long, narrow femoral neck and broad, laterally bowed femoral shaft were present bilaterally. In the arms the bones were very short, with broad diaphyses. The hands showed bullet-shaped proximal phalanges, and proximal pointing of the metacarpals with marked widening at the distal ends. In brief, the changes were those of severe dysostosis multiplex.

Very mild corneal clouding was demonstrated by slit-lamp examination only.

D and **E,** X-ray films of arms and pelvis at 6 months of age. **F** to **O,** X-ray studies at 25 months: **F,** Skull; **G,** chest; **H,** upper arm; **I,** hands; **J** and **K,** frontal and lateral views of lower half of spine; **L,** pelvis; **M,** femora; **N,** knees and legs; **O,** feet.

(I am indebted to Dr. Charles I. Scott and Dr. Judith A. Sensenbrenner for clinical information on this patient and for permission to include the account here.)

P, Electron micrograph of the thickened skin from same patient. The epithelial cells, **E,** of the epidermis are ultrastructurally unremarkable. However, in the superficial dermis, numerous vacuole-distended histiocytes are present. The intracytoplasmic vacuoles are limited by single membranes and have heterogeneous contents. Inset: Membranous lamellar inclusions (arrows) are more commonly observed in I-cell disease than in the mucopolysaccharidoses. No abnormal accumulations of extracellular material are apparent. **N,** Nucleus; **M,** mitochondria. ($\times$8,500; inset, $\times$33,000). (Courtesy Drs. K. R. Kenyon and H. A. Quigley, Baltimore, Md.)

Q, Electron micrograph of the enlarged liver from a 25-month-old Caucasian male (C. McK., J.H.H. 1402575) with I-cell disease (mucolipidosis type II). The hepatic parenchymal cells are ultrastructurally unaffected and, in particular, are not vacuolated. In the reticuloendothelial cells of the sinusoids and portal areas, however, membrane-limited intracytoplasmic vacuoles with granular, lipoid, or membranous lamellar inclusions (inset arrows) are prominent. **N,** Nucleus; **M,** mitochondria; **E,** vascular endothelium. ($\times$16,000; inset, $\times$40,000). (**P** and **Q** courtesy Dr. K. R. Kenyon and Dr. H. A. Quigley, Baltimore, Md.)

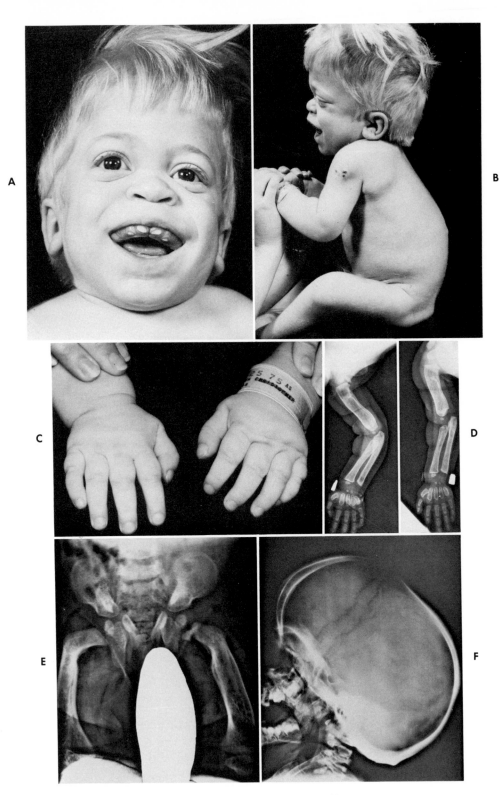

Fig. 11-43. For legend see p. 647.

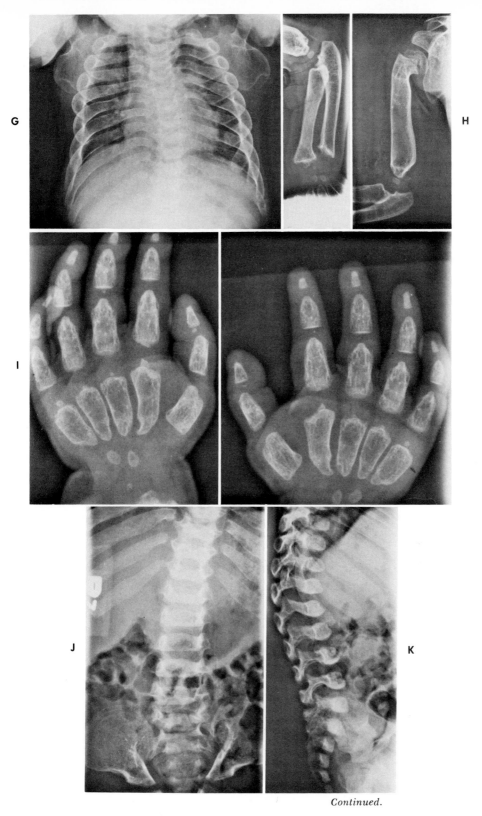

Continued.

Fig. 11-43, cont'd. For legend see p. 647.

cousins. Thus, this disorder, like the two other mucolipidoses, appears to have autosomal recessive inheritance. Abnormal inclusions were found in the fibroblasts of some heterozygotes.[287]

Subepithelial connective tissue is hypercellular, and the numerous histiocytes and fibroblasts are extensively vacuolated.[247] Electron microscopy shows that the inclusions are single membrane limited and consist of fibrillogranular and membranous lamellar material. Schwann cells and the axonal processes of peripheral nerves and vascular perithelial cells show similar changes. The inclusions appear

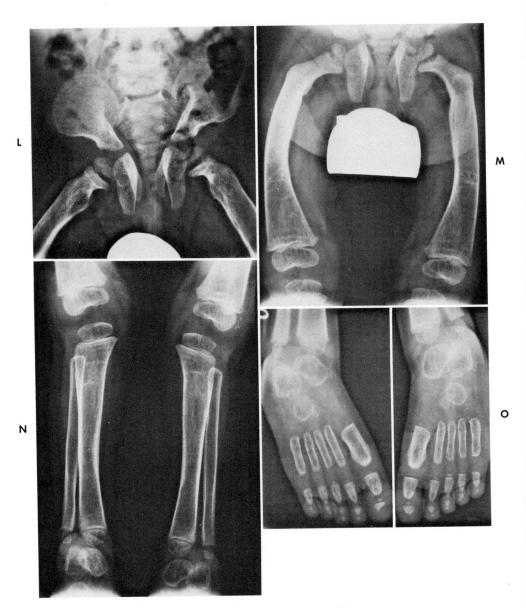

Fig. 11-43, cont'd. For legend see p. 647.

to be derived from lysosomes. As shown by electron microscopy, the I-cell inclusions are filled with osmophilic membranous material, whereas MPS I and MPS II are empty. The lipid content of I-cells is three times that of normal.[189] Weismann and associates[559] found high levels of lysosomal enzymes in the medium of cultured fibroblasts and postulated "leaky lysosomes." Hickman and Neufeld postulated defective hydrolases that do not enter lysosomes. The following case report is illustrative.

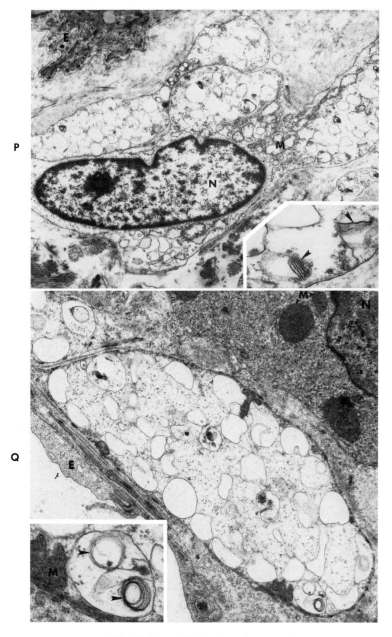

Fig. 11-43, cont'd. For legend see p. 647.

Case 27. C. McK. (J.H.H. 1402575), a white male born in 1968, was first studied in this hospital at the age of 25 months (Fig. 11-43). Coarse facies and inguinal hernias were noted at birth. Psychomotor development was very slow. The coarse features and gingival hyperplasia are indicated in Fig. 11-43*A*. The liver was enlarged to 8 cm. below the right costal margin, and the spleen tip was palpable. Everywhere the skin was smooth, tight, and thickened. Both corneas were symmetrically increased in size to 12.5 mm. in diameter. Although the corneas were grossly clear, slit-lamp examination revealed fine, diffuse stromal granularity. No macular cherry-red spot and no retinal pigmentary changes were found. All joints showed limitation of motion, and a pronounced thoracolumbar gibbus was present. He was unable to sit or roll over.

Mucolipidosis III (pseudo–Hurler polydystrophy). Under the designation "pseudopolydystrophie de Hurler," Maroteaux and Lamy[341] in 1966 described 4 cases with many of the features of the Hurler syndrome but a much slower clinical evolution and no mucopolysacchariduria. They pointed out that the same disorder was probably present in a patient listed among "cases defying classification" by my colleagues and me.[322] The sibs reported by Steinbach and collaborators[501] presumably had this condition. The children usually present at the age of about 3 years, with stiffness of joints as the main complaint. Coarse facies and short stature are features. The cornea shows a fine, ground-glass clouding. Aortic valve disease, often resulting in regurgitation, is present in most. Hypoplasia of the odontoid process was noted in at least one case. In the bone marrow Maroteaux and Lamy[341] found cells reminiscent of those in the Hurler syndrome, but the vacuoles were empty. Danes[83] found cytoplasmic metachromasia with toluidine blue and alcian blue in the cultured skin fibroblasts of several of our patients. Spranger and Wiedemann's classification[497] of pseudo–Hurler polydystrophy as a mucolipidosis is supported by electromicroscopic studies.[426] Fibroblasts of the conjunctiva show cytoplasmic vacuolization which is delimited by a single membrane. (Metachromasia on light microscopic observation of specimens stained with toluidine blue and alcian blue suggests that the vacuoles contain acid mucopolysaccharides.) In addition, a rather large amount of membranous lamellar material similar to that seen in fibroblasts from the sphingolipidoses is demonstrated by electron microscopy. Its appearance is consistent with its representing glycolipid of sphingolipid. It appears to emerge from the Golgi apparatus. No abnormality was visualized in the conjunctival fibroblasts of the presumptively heterozygous parents.[426] I have observed two families each with affected brother and sister, and in addition three families each with a single case. A detailed account of the radiologic changes is given elsewhere.[354a] These cases are described below in the order in which they came to my attention:

Case 28. B. W. (J.H.H. 873524), a white female born in 1954, was the offspring of normal unrelated parents. Pregnancy and delivery were normal. A single sib, a sister two years older, is normal. At the age of about 30 months, painless stiffness of the shoulders, elbows, and fingers was first noted. By the age of 3 years, claw deformity of the terminal phalanges was evident (Fig. 11-44).

When B. W. was first seen at this hospital at the age of 5 years, the facies was noted to be coarse, and limitation of motion in all joints was evident. There was no hepatosplenomegaly. A basilar diastolic murmur was first heard at the age of about 7½ years. At 8½ years of age corneal clouding was detected by slit-lamp examination. Genu valgum was then evident also; I.Q. was estimated at 74.

At the age of 13 years carpal tunnel decompression was performed bilaterally, with successful relief of the previously existing symptoms and signs of median nerve entrapment.

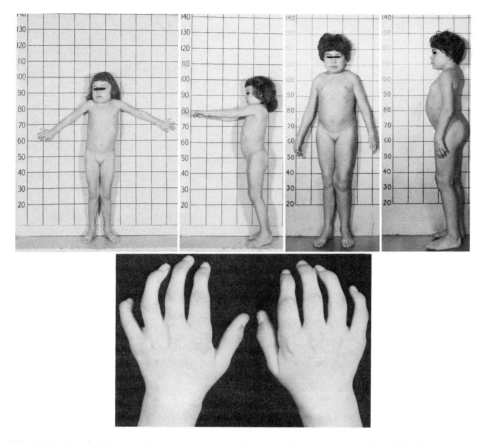

Fig. 11-44. Pseudo-Hurler polydystrophy (mucolipidosis III) in B. W. (J.H.H. 873524). Top left, at age 6 years. The arms are maximally raised. Top right, at age 13 years. Below, hands at age 13 years.

At the age of 16½ years the patient was 53¼ inches tall. She had been in special education throughout most of her schooling. Intelligence tests had shown only slow deterioration at the most. The facies was coarse with mild synophrys, broad mouth, and widely spaced, stubby teeth. The corneas showed faint clouding to the naked eye. By slit-lamp examination the clouding was seen to be situated mainly in the posterior third of the cornea, which was involved uniformly, centrally, and peripherally. The cornea was increased in thickness by about one and one-half times that of normal. The fundi were normal.

A grade II/VI murmur of aortic regurgitation was audible at the left sternal border. The liver was palpable 3 cm. below the right costal margin; the spleen was not felt.

The skin had a thickened feel generally. There was no hirsutism. All joints were stiff, although with persistently applied passive pressure, almost full extension of some joints was possible. The hands were clawed. Striking knuckle pads were present.

The urine has always been negative for mucopolysaccharides. However, Dr. B. S. Danes found that the fibroblasts of the patient and of both parents showed cytoplasmic metachromasia.

Case 29. R. W. (J.H.H. 1243588), a white male born in 1956, was first noted to have stiffness in the hands at the age of 18 months. This began as a "curling" of the fourth fingers and slowly progressed to involve the others. Slowly the stiffness extended to all joints, causing an awkward gait, limited ability to run, and difficulties with daily routines such as tying shoes and using eating utensils. Hand surgery at the ages of 2½ and 4 years had little benefit.

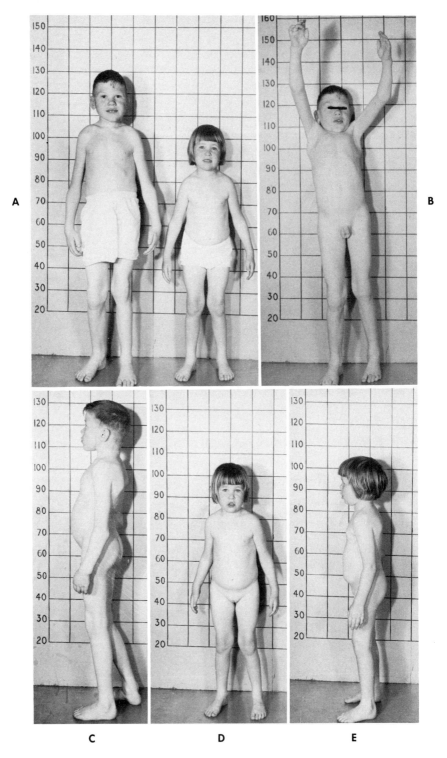

Fig. 11-45. For legend see opposite page.

In school R. W. did somewhat poorly; he repeated the fourth grade because of difficulty in both reading and arithmetic.

The parents were not related. A sister, born in 1959, was normal, whereas a sister born in 1961 (Case 30) had the same disorder.

Examination (1970) showed a height of 56½ inches. The facies was characterized mainly by prominent superciliary ridges. Although grossly clear, the corneas showed, by means of slit-lamp examination, clouding in the posterior third. An early aortic diastolic murmur was audible. The hands were clawed. The range of motion of all joints was reduced. The feet showed high arches, and the fourth toes were curled under the third toes.

Dr. B. S. Danes found that this patient and his sister (Case 30) show cytoplasmic metachromasia of fibroblasts, but those of both parents are, in this instance, nonmetachromatic. In all 4 the urine shows no excessive mucopolysacchariduria.

Case 30. C. W. (J.H.H. 1243591), the sister of R. W. (Case 29), born in 1961, was noted to have minimal stiffness of the hands and a poor grip as early as 13 months of age, since the parents were alerted by the disorder in the older sib. As in the other cases, the stiffness slowly progressed to involve other joints but has never been as severe or limiting as it was in her brother at the same age.

At 9 years of age she was 47½ inches tall. She seemed intelligent and the facies was not definitely abnormal. Although clinically clear, the corneas showed increased thickness and general-

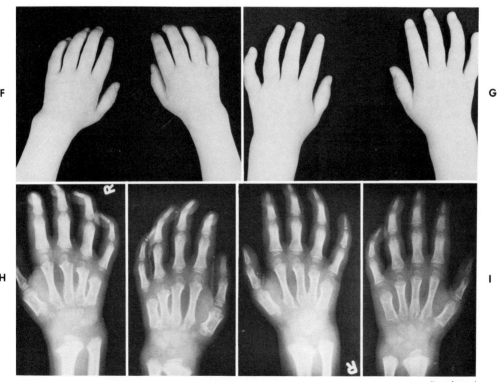

Continued.

Fig. 11-45. Pseudo-Hurler polydystrophy (mucolipidosis III) in brother (R. W.) and sister (C. W.). **A,** Sibs together. **B,** Brother showing maximal elevation of arms. **C,** Brother, lateral view. **D** and **E,** Sister. **F** and **G,** Photographs of hands of brother and sister, respectively. **H** and **I,** X-ray views of hands of brother and sister, respectively. **J** and **K,** Lateral views of spine of brother and sister, respectively. **L** and **M,** X-ray views of pelvis of brother and sister, respectively. Note the difference in severity in the 2 sibs.

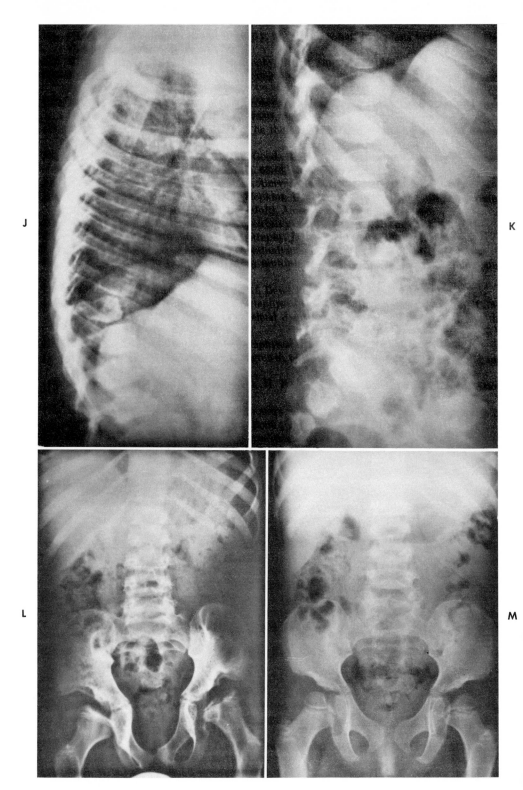

Fig. 11-45, cont'd. For legend see p. 655.

ized clouding. Hirsutism was not present. All joints showed decreased range of motion, especially the shoulders and those of the hands, which were clawed. The skin of the hands was tight and shiny. (See Fig. 11-45 for illustration of this pair of sibs.)

Case 31. J. S. (J.H.H. 1337061), a white male born in 1955, was born of parents who are both of Swedish extraction but are not known to be related. He and his sister (Case 32) are the only children.

No abnormality of development was noted until the patient was 7½ years old, when he began to limp slightly and swing out his legs in walking. He also complained of knee pain and fatigued easily. After x-ray studies, bilateral Legg-Perthes disease was diagnosed, and he was treated with bed rest for fourteen months. He was an honor roll student.

Examination (1969) showed a height of 142.3 cm. He was an intelligent-appearing boy with no signs of puberty. He walked with a stiff-hip gait, showed generalized joint stiffness, and had clawhand deformities. The facies suggested that of the mucopolysaccharidoses, i.e., was similar to that in the other patient in this series. The corneas were grossly somewhat cloudy, and by slit-lamp examination, a fine haze, heaviest in the periphery and in the posterior part of the stroma, was seen. The nose was broad and flat, and the mouth was broad. The neck was short. The chest had an increased anteroposterior dimension, with protuberance of the lower half of the sternum. A soft early diastolic murmur, presumably of aortic origin, was heard at the left sternal border. The second heart sound had an unusual "wooden" quality. The heart was not enlarged, nor were the liver and spleen.

The skin had a firm texture. There was no hirsutism.

The patient could not raise the arms much above the level of the shoulders. The knees appeared somewhat enlarged. Despite the clawhand deformity he could make a full fist. Mild dorsal kyphosis and severe lumbar lordosis were present.

No excessive mucopolysacchariduria or metachromatic inclusion of leukoctyes was demonstrated. Cytoplasmic metachromasia of fibroblasts was demonstrated by Dr. B. S. Danes.

X-ray studies of the skull showed a deep posterior fossa with probable mild basilar invagination. Calvarial thickness and the sella turcica were normal. Prominent radiolucencies were seen at the torcular Herophili. The vertebrae were generally somewhat flat, with minimal irregularity of the end-plates. The disc spaces appeared to be relatively wide. Mild deficiency of the anterior positions of the tenth and twelfth thoracic vertebrae led to a mild gibbus with its apex at T-11. The pelvis showed moderately flared iliac wings and somewhat sloping acetabular roofs. The femoral heads were poorly mineralized, and the necks were long and in coxa valga position. All long-bone metaphyses were irregular, with vertical bands of radiolucency and sclerosis. Most epiphyses were narrowed. The distal tibial epiphysis sloped because of narrowing laterally. The tubular bones of the bands were relatively wide and the metacarpals showed some proximal pointing. Fifth-finger clinodactyly resulted from hypoplasia of the middle phalanx. The distal end of the ulna, but not that of the radius, was sloping.

Case 32. L. S. (J.H.H. 1340582), the sister of J. S. (Case 31), was born in 1956. Development was normal and she has been an honor student. A small umbilical hernia was repaired at the age of 3 years. Spectacles were fitted at 9 years, and mild left-sided conductive deafness was discovered at the age of 11 years. Menarche occurred at 13 years of age. Until seen by my associate Dr. Charles I. Scott, she had been considered normal by her family.

Examination (1969) showed facies and corneal clouding like her brother's. The nose had a broad, low bridge. The mouth was also broad with somewhat thick lips. Minimal pectus carinatum and a grade II/VI systolic ejection aortic murmur were found on chest examination. The skin was generally thick. All joints showed reduced mobility, but the limitation was less marked than in the brother. It was most marked in the elbows and wrists and in the hands, where flexion contractions produced mild clawhand deformity. Lumbar lordosis was somewhat increased. In addition to bilateral pes planus, the left fourth and fifth toes were short and recessed.

Laboratory findings, as in the brother, included alcianophilia of the fibroblasts. Osseous changes were similar to those in her brother but less severe.

Case 33. M. R. (J.H.H. 1339982), a white male born in 1965 of nonconsaguineous parents, first came to medical attention at the age of 3 years because of limitation of joint mobility, especially in the upper limbs. A diagnosis of the Hunter syndrome was made.

Examination in 1969 showed mild generalized hirsutism, somewhat coarse facial features, and a peculiar gait and stance from generalized joint stiffness (Fig. 11-46). The hands had a claw

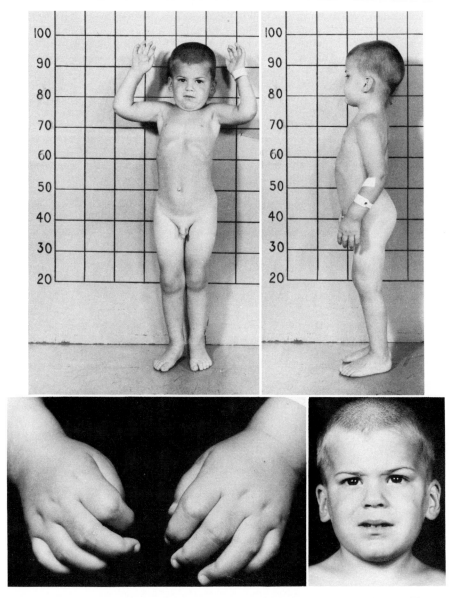

Fig. 11-46. Pseudo-Hurler polydystrophy (mucolipidosis III) in M. R., 4 years old.

deformity with fusiform fingers and firm skin. He was unable to make a tight fist. There was fine clouding of the posterior part of the corneal stroma. Urinary mucopolysaccharides were not increased. Radiographic findings were qualitatively like those of the Hurler syndrome but less severe; on the other hand, they were more severe than those in any of the other patients. Great variability in the severity of x-ray changes in ML III is indicated by the marked differences even in the same family, as indicated by comparisons of the two pairs of sibs.[354a] Specifically, the cervical vertebrae were flat, with a bullet configuration; the thoracic and lumbar vertebral bodies had unusually convex superior and inferior endplates; the iliac wings flared with oblique acetabular roofs; coxa valga with small femoral necks was present; the carpal bones were small and poorly ossified; the metacarpals were wide with pointed bases, and the phalanges were short and wide.

In February, 1972, he was reevaluated because of recent decline in visual acuity. He continued in having problems getting in and out of cars and with dressing and other manual tasks. The major new finding was mild papilledema, starlike discoloration of the retina about the macula. Opening pressure on lumbar puncture was 320 mm. H_2O. By April, 1972, visual loss had increased slightly, he complained of occasional dizziness, and the parents were aware of increased irritability. A lumbar cysternogram was normal, although the opening pressure was 350 mm. H_2O. Pneumoencephalogram under anesthesia showed an initial pressure of 360 mm. H_2O but normal sized ventricles and no evident obstruction. Cerebral arteriograms by the brachial route showed no abnormality. It was assumed that meningeal infiltration with defective resorption of cerebrospinal fluid was responsible for the elevated pressure.

Palliative glycerol therapy was instituted with clearing of the edema of the right nerve head after 8 days but no change on the left.

Case 34. My seventh patient* with the pseudo–Hurler polydystrophy is the oldest. B. S. (J.H.H. 1469509) was born in 1947 of nonconsanguineous parents. No similar condition was known in the family.

A right inguinal hernia was discovered in the neonatal period and repaired at the age of 6 weeks. Spectacles were worn from the age of 3 years for hypermetropia and strabismus. At the age of 4 years, the diagnosis of the Hurler syndrome was made because it was noted that his joints, particularly the shoulders, were stiff and the facies were coarse, suggesting that condition. Urinary excretion of mucopolysaccharide was always within normal limits, however.

All joints, including those of the fingers, became increasingly stiff. He was a slow learner in school. IQ was estimated to be 58. He attended special school until age 19. At the age of 18 years he had tendon release operations on the hips and knees. From about age 10 years he had increasing pain in the legs, hips, and occasionally the shoulders.

From the age of about 24 years, he suffered from occasional bouts of tachycardia.

Examination (1972) showed (Fig. 11-47) height 157 cm. and coarse facial features with heavy supraorbital ridges, thick lips, wide nose, and low anterior hair line. Although corneal clouding was not evident on direct inspection, slit-lamp inspection showed clouding, as well as left internal strabismus. He walked in a stiff manner. The shoulders were sloping, and movement of the shoulders in all directions was severely limited. The fingers were stiff, resulting in clawhand deformity. Hollowing of the thenar eminence bilaterally suggested carpal tunnel compression, which was confirmed by positive Tinel sign. All other joints such as the hips, knees, elbows, and so on had limited motion.

The anterior thorax showed a mild pigeon-breast deformity. Aortic systolic and diastolic murmur, each of about II/VI intensity, were heard.

Results of investigations in 1972 were all consistent with the diagnosis of ML III, including the findings of radiography. Cultured skin fibroblasts showed striking cytoplasmic inclusions as in other cases.

Gorlin[177a] is convinced that the disorder in the patient reported by Langer, Kronenberg, and him[280] is pseudo–Hurler polydystrophy. If so, this is the oldest known case, 67 years of age in 1972. The patient excreted an excess of an unidentified glycoprotein in the urine.

After seeing the seventh case of ML III described above (Case 34), I consider it virtually certain that this was the disorder in the family which was thrice reported many years ago.[209,465,467] Langer, Kronenberg, and Gorlin[280] had suggested that their patient had the same disorder as Schinz and Fürtwängler's family.[465]

In 1928, Schinz and Furtwängler[465] of Zurich described a sibship of 11, the offspring of a first-cousin marriage, in which a man then 29 years old and 3 of his sisters were identically affected by a disorder in which the most striking feature was stiff joints. Flexion deformity and reduced mobility in the fingers and toes

---

*Studied through the courtesy of Dr. Charles W. Reynolds, Akron, Ohio.

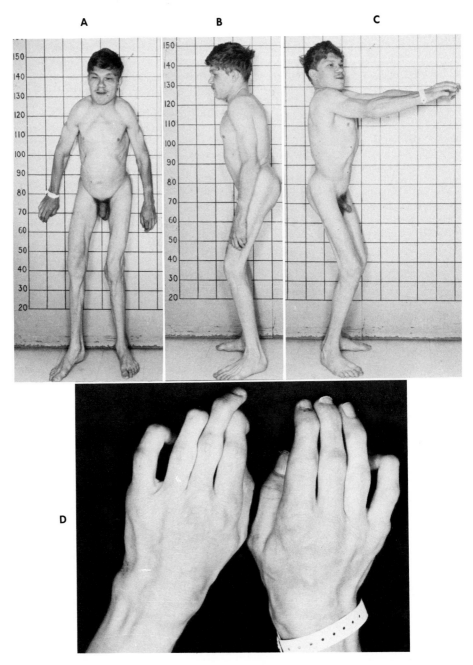

Fig. 11-47. Mucolipidosis III (pseudo-Hurler polydystrophy) in B. S., 25 years old at the time these pictures were taken. See text, Case 34.

were combined with limited mobility in the ankles, wrists, knees, elbows, hips, shoulders, and spine. The face was described as red, with somewhat prominent forehead, broad nose, and fleshy ("fleischig") tongue. Umbilical hernia was present in the brother, whose eyes were said then to be normal. He worked as a bookkeeper and was considered to be of normal intelligence. Height was 156 cm. (61⅖ inches). X-ray films in this man showed thick skull, shortened posterior cranial fossa, and prominent external and internal occipital protuberances. A striking feature was extensive disturbance in the development of (or a destruction of) the carpal and tarsal bones. (See Fig. 11-48C.)

In 1934 Horsch[209] described a sister from the same sibship. The features were identical, including those in the carpal and tarsal bones. The brother described in the earlier report[465] was restudied; cysts in the head of the humerus and in the epiphyses of the radius were described. Cysts were also observed in the digital epiphyses of these patients, and secondary subluxation of the phalanges was noted.

In 1938 Schmidt,[467] an ophthalmologist in Freiburg, Germany, where the family lived, reported corneal abnormality in the same 4 sibs:

> Both corneas appear finely clouded in their totality. Slit-lamp examination shows that the diffuse clouding is composed of numerous very fine gray specks which are located mainly in the middle parenchymal layers. In the deep and superficial portions they are less numerous. A difference is noted between the center and periphery of the cornea, the granules being coarser in the center than at the periphery. They are grayish white in color. Otherwise the cornea has no alteration. The surface is smooth and fluorescein-negative. No defect in Descemet's membrane is detected. Surface sensibility is reduced. The other reflecting media, the iris and the fundus of the eye are free of pathologic changes.*

The family lived in Eigeltingen in southwest Germany. All affected sibs are now (1972) deceased (information from Prof. P. E. Becker, Göttingen).

Scharf[462] described an isolated case similar to the patients of Schinz and others; the parents were first cousins. The only other plausible possibility is MPS I S. However, the short stature and stiffness in large joints, especially the shoulders, points more to ML III.

Juvenile sulfatidosis with mucopolysacchariduria is a very rare Hurler-like disorder that has been reported in only a few cases.[12,522] It is also called the Austin type of metachromatic leukodystrophy. Slowly progressive neurologic deterioration begins in the second year of life, and death occurs in the early teens. The facies has mild Hurler-like features, but the corneas are not clouded and there is no hepatosplenomegaly. Growth failure develops and the patients are short of stature. Peripheral nerve biopsy shows metachromatic degeneration of myelin. In contradistinction to the classic type of metachromatic leukodystrophy, in which only arylsulfatase A is absent, all three arylsulfatases, A, B, and C, are deficient in the Austin type of metachromatic leukodystrophy. Autosomal recessive inheritance is likely.

In a child with clinical features suggesting the Hurler syndrome, Öckerman and Hultberg[402,404,407] found normal urinary excretion of mucopolysaccharides but increased amounts of mannose-containing compounds in tissues, accompanied by deficiency of α-mannosidase. This condition, called mannosidosis, is another

---

*Translation from Schmidt, R.: Klin. Mbl. Augenheilk. **100**:616, 1938.

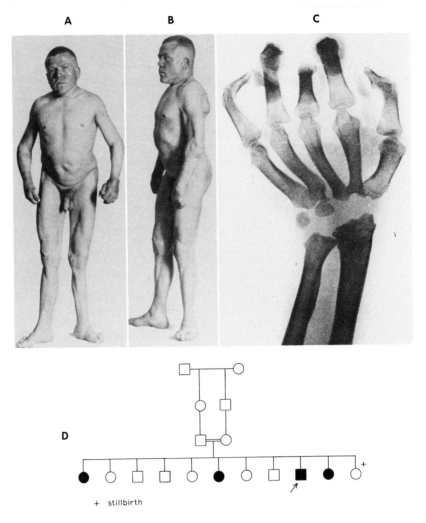

Fig. 11-48. Family reported by Schinz and Furtwängler and by others.[209,465,467] Diagnosis: probably ML III, or pseudo Hurler polydystrophy. **A** and **B**, General appearance. **C**, X-ray film of the hand. Both wrists showed more drastic changes than in any of the cases reported here. **D**, The pedigree. Born in 1897, the proband, J. W., died in 1964 (information obtained by Prof. P. E. Becker, Göttingen).

lysosomal disease which, like generalized gangliosidosis, I-cell disease, and others, simulates the Hurler syndrome in some respects. Mannosidosis has been discovered in cattle.[205a,234a]

In patients with clinical features somewhat suggesting MPS I, described by Durand and associates,[120a] Van Hoof and Hers[541] found deficiency of α-fucosidase activity in the liver. Durand and associates found accumulation of fucose in all tissue and suggested the term fucosidosis.[120] Dawson and Spranger[97] demonstrated that glycosphingolipid is present in high concentration in the liver. The clinical features were those of progressive cerebral degeneration, dementia, and loss of muscle strength, followed by intense spasticity, decorticate rigidity, progressive emaciation, thick skin, excessive sweating, cardiomegaly, and death in 2 sibs reported by Durand and colleagues[120a] at 3 years 9 months and 5 years 2 months. Lymphocytes showed cytoplasmic vacuoles.

In a 9-year-old child with an unusual skeletal dysplasia labeled as spondylo-metaphyseoepiphyseal dysplasia, Schafer and collaborators[459] found deficiency of α-L-fucosidase in fibroblasts cultured from the skin. The patient showed no extraskeletal features. Thus the phenotype was quite different from that in fucosidosis, which also has deficiency of α-L-fucosidase. This does not indicate that deficiency of fucosidase is not the "cause" of both these disorders, since different isoenzymes may be involved. The relationship of this patient's abnormality to that in 4 patients observed by my colleagues and me[377] is under study. Patel and colleagues[414a] described yet another phenotype with deficiency of α-L-fucosidase. Their patient survived to age 16 years, and from age 4 angiokeratoma had been present as in Fabry disease. Unlike Fabry disease, severe mental retardation was present.

The biochemical basis of phenotype

Why do mental retardation, corneal clouding, stiff joints, and aortic regurgitation occur in some and not in others of the six mucopolysaccharidoses? To a considerable extent the presence or absence of these extraskeletal features is a matter of degree. All six entities may show them at some stage. The relation between heparan sulfate and mental retardation is most suggestive of a clinical-chemical correlation. In our experience heparan sulfate is absent in MPS V and MPS VI, in which mental retardation is mild at the most, and is excreted in large amounts in MPS III, in which the clinical picture is dominated by mental retardation. However, the biochemical findings of Terry and Linker[520] are in disagreement with ours and would not indicate a particular association between heparan sulfate excretion and mental retardation.

Stiff joints and the carpal tunnel syndrome imply involvement of collagen. Several observations made by using *in vitro* systems suggest that mucopolysaccharides exert an influence on collagen fiber formation.[381,567] The role of mucopolysaccharide-protein complexes in the rigidity of hyaline cartilage is demonstrated by the drooping ears of rabbits injected with papain.[526] The absence of stiff joints in the Morquio syndrome (limitation of motion may result from joint deformity in this entity) is unique among the six types of MPS. The marked bone rarefaction of Morquio syndrome may bear some relationship to the observation that mucopolysaccharides inhibit nucleation of apatite crystals by collagen fibrils.[385]

Meyer and associates[364] reported that injection of certain acid mucopolysaccharides stimulates the regrowth of hair of shaved areas in rabbits. The findings are of obvious note in connection with the excessive growth of body hair, which is characteristic of all six mucopolysaccharidoses with the probable exception of MPS IV.

As pointed out earlier, hydrocephalus from meningeal involvement in undoubtedly a factor in the progressive impairment of intellect. Furthermore, a biochemical mechanism common to connective tissue and brain may be faulty. Just as in phenylketonuria and galactosemia, the details of how the normal biochemical and functional status of the brain is disturbed in the Hurler syndrome are unknown.

The manner in which abnormal deposits occur in the tunica intima and elsewhere is reminiscent of the handling in rabbits of methylcellulose and pectin[212,213] both of which are macromolecular carbohydrates. Hueper[212] observed ballooning of cells in the liver, spleen, kidney, arterial intima, bone marrow, and anterior pituitary when pectin was administered intravenously in rabbits and dogs. However, "no lesion was found in the cerebral parenchyma, the vascular system of the brain or the choroid plexus."

Although AMPS deposition is found in the cornea in the Hunter syndrome,[171] the amount is much less than that in the mucopolysaccharidoses with clinically significant corneal clouding (MPS I, V, and VI). The mechanism of corneal clouding in the mucopolysaccharidoses is thought to be consistent[247] with the theory[174] that loss of corneal transparency is the result of light scattering that occurs if the collagenous stromal lamellae are separated by distances exceeding 2000 Å, as, for example, by vacuole-ballooned keratocytes or extracellular pools of AMPS.

As in other lysosomal disorders, the storage material in the mucopolysaccharidoses is heterogeneous. Gangliosides accumulate intracellularly in the brain and contribute to the progressive mental deterioration. To what extent occlusion of cerebral vessels through progressive intimal accumulations plays a role is unclear.

Possibly relevant to the cerebral involvement in several of the mucopolysaccharidoses is the finding that glial cell tumors of either rat[1150] or man,[1170] when grown in tissue culture, produce heparan sulfate.

An animal homolog?

The clinical, biochemical, and pathologic features of snorter dwarfism of Hereford cattle[530] have been studied by Lorincz and colleagues[297,298,302,304] as a possible animal homolog of the Hurler syndrome. The disorder is inherited as an autosomal recessive. Clinical features include short nose with labored breathing (from which the term "snorter" is derived), rounded forehead, widely spaced eyes, large tongue, short neck, hydrocephalus, beaked lumbar vertebrae, dwarfism, rough hair, and thickened hide. The abnormalities are progressive. Differences from MPS I include absence of corneal clouding, significant hepatosplenomegaly, characteristic changes in the long bones, and typical "gargoyle" cells in the liver and other tissues. Mucopolysacchariduria was demonstrated by Lorincz and confirmed by McIlwain and Eveleth.[314] Tyler and co-workers,[532] on the other hand, recovered only chondroitin-4-sulfate, and no dermatan sulfate or heparan sulfate. They concluded that this difference and the absence of gargoyle cells from the tissues make it unlikely that the bovine disease is comparable to gargoylism in man. (See also Mayes and associates.[354])

SUMMARY

As presented in Table 11-2 (p. 525), six major classes of genetic mucopolysaccharidoses can be recognized. The main criterion for this group of disorders has been the presence of excessive mucopolysacchariduria. To this can now be added, for all six classes except MPS IV (the Morquio syndrome), demonstrable impairment in the degradation of acid mucopolysaccharides as indicated by the accumulation of radioactive sulfate by cultured fibroblasts. For the same five classes of mucopolysaccharidoses, deficiency of a specific "corrective factor" can be demonstrated; indeed, for the Sanfilippo syndrome (MPS III) two separate corrective factors can be identified in different cases that are phenotypically identical.

The genetic mucopolysaccharidoses are lysosomal diseases, and the corrective factors are lysosomal enzymes. The enzymatic nature of the corrective factor deficient in the Hunter syndrome (MPS II) and of that deficient in the Maroteaux-Lamy syndrome (MPS VI) has not yet been demonstrated.

The enzyme deficient in the Hurler syndrome is α-L-iduronidase. The same enzyme is deficient in the Scheie syndrome even though the phenotype is rather different. These conditions are probably allelic, and for this reason new designations of MPS I H for the Hurler syndrome and MPS I S for the Scheie syndrome have been used. To avoid confusion, the designation MPS V (formerly used for the Scheie syndrome) should not be assigned to a different mucopolysaccharidosis.

Distinctive, presumably allelic, severe and mild forms of MPS II and of MPS VI can be recognized. Although the two forms of each disorder are clinically clearly different—almost as different as the Hurler and Scheie syndromes—the same corrective factor is deficient in each of the two forms. Genetic compounds ("mixed heterozygotes") of the MPS IH/IS type may occur.

The two clinically indistinguishable forms of the Sanfilippo syndrome, arbitrarily designated A and B, show deficiency, respectively, of heparan sulfate sulfatase and N-acetyl-α-D-glucosaminidase.

MPS VII is the designation assigned to β-glucuronidase deficiency. Although experience is limited to two cases, there may be more than one allelic form of β-glucuronidase deficiency.

Several disorders resemble the genetic mucopolysaccharidoses clinically and to some extent metabolically. A particularly instructive one of these is pseudo–Hurler polydystrophy, or mucolipidosis III.

Therapy of the genetic mucopolysaccharidoses by enzyme replacement is promising.

REFERENCES

1. Abul-Haj, S. K., Martz, D. G., Douglas, W. F., and Geppert, L. J.: Farber's disease; report of a case, with observations on its histogenesis and notes on the nature of the stored material, J. Pediat. **61**:221, 1962.
2. Aegerter, E. E., and Kirkpatrick, J. A., Jr.: Orthopaedic diseases; physiology, pathology and radiology, Philadelphia, 1958, W. B. Saunders Co., p. 99.
3. Aleu, F. P., Terry, R. D., and Zellweger, H.: Electron microscopy of two cerebral biopsies in gargoylism, J. Neuropath. Exp. Neurol. **24**:304. 1965.
4. Allansmith, M., and Senz, E.: Chondrodystrophia congenita punctata (Conradi's disease), Amer. J. Dis. Child. **100**:109, 1960.
5. Anderson, B., Hoffman, P., and Meyer, K.: A serine-linked peptide of chondroitin sulfate, Biochim. Biophys. Acta **74**:309, 1963.
6. Anderson, C. E., Crane, J. T., Harper, H. A., and Hunter, T. W.: Morquio's disease and dysplasia epiphysalis multiplex, J. Bone Joint Surg. **44-A**:295, 1962.
7. Andersson, B., and Tandberg, O.: Lipochondrodystrophy (gargoylism, Hurler syndrome) with specific cutaneous deposits, Acta Paediat. **41**:162, 1952.
8. Andreassi, A., and Andreassi, A.: A proposito di un caso di gargoilismo: esiste nella provincia de l'Aquila un "focolaio" di tale forma morbosa? Minerva Pediat. **21**:1077, 1969.

9. Asboe-Hansen, G.: Bullous diffuse mastocytosis with urinary hyaluronate excretion, Acta Dermatovener, **42**:211, 1962.

10. Ashby, W. R., Stewart, R. M., and Watkins, J. H.: Chondro-osteo-dystrophy of the Hurler type (gargoylism); a pathological study, Brain **60**:149, 1937.

11. Astaldi, G., and Strosselli, E.: Histochemische Untersuchungen an den Leukoblasten und Leukocyten der konstitutionellen Alderschen Anomalie, Schweiz. Med. Wschr. **88**:989, 1958.

12. Austin, J. H.: Metachromatic leukodystrophy. In Carter, C. C., editor: Medical aspects of mental retardation, Springfield, Ill., 1965, Charles C Thomas, Publisher.

13. Awwaad, S.: Dysostosis multiplex; review of literature and report of two cases with unusual manifestations, Arch. Pediat. **78**:184, 1961.

14. Aycock, E. K., and Paul, J. R., Jr.: Gargoylism; a report of two cases in Negroes, J. S. Carolina Med. Ass. **53**:128, 1957.

15. Bailey, J. A., III, Dorst, J. P., and Saunderson, R. W., Jr.: Metatropic dwarfism, recognized retrospectively from the roentgenographic features. In Bergsma, D., editor: Clinical delineation of birth defects, New York, 1969, National Foundation—March of Dimes, p. 376.

15a. Bach, G., Friedman, R., Weissmann, B., and Neufeld, E. F.: The defect in the Hurler and Scheie syndromes: deficiency of α-L-iduronidase, Proc. Nat. Acad. Sci. **69**:2048, 1972.

16. Barnett, E. J.: Morquio's disease, J. Pediat. **2**:651, 1933.

17. Bartman, J., and Blanc, W. A.: Fibroblast cultures in Hurler's and Hunter's syndromes; an ultrastructural study, Arch. Path. **89**:279, 1970.

18. Bartman, J., Mandelbaum, I. M., and Gregoire, P. E.: Mucopolysaccharides of serum and urine in a case of Morquio's disease, Rev. Franç. Étude Clin. Biol. **8**:250, 1963.

18a. Barton, R. W., and Neufeld, E. F.: The Hurler corrective factor: purification and some properties, J. Biol. Chem. **246**:7773, 1971.

18b. Barton, R. W., and Neufeld, E. F.: A distinct biochemical deficit in the Maroteaux-Lamy syndrome (mucopolysaccharidosis VI), J. Pediat. **80**:114-116, 1972.

19. Bartsacos, C. S., Moser, H.. and Neufeld, E. F. (Boston and Bethesda): Personal communication, 1971.

20. Beals, R. K. (Portland Ore.): Personal communication, 1971.

20a. Beaudet, A. L., DiFerrante, N., Nichols, B., and Ferry, G. D.: β-glucuronidase deficiency: altered enzyme substrate recognition (abstract), Amer. J. Hum. Genet. **24**:25a, 1972.

20b. Beaudet, A. L. (Houston, Texas): Personal communication, Oct., 1972.

21. Beebe, R. T.: Hunter's syndrome; gargoyles—Washington Irving—"Rip Van Winkle," Bull. Hist. Med. **44**:582, 1970.

22. Beebe, R. T., and Formel, P. F.: Gargoylism: sex-linked transmission in nine males, Trans. Amer. Clin. Climat. Ass. **66**:199, 1954.

23. Begg, A. C.: Nuclear herniations of the intervertebral disc; their radiological manifestations and significance, J. Bont Joint Surg. **36-B**:180, 1954.

24. Beradinelli, W.: Gargoylisme chez un petit noir, Presse Méd. **64**:1757, 1956.

25. Berg, K., Danes, B. S., and Bearn, A. G.: The linkage relation of the loci for the Xm serum system and the X-linked form of Hurler's syndrome (Hunter's syndrome), Amer. J. Hum. Genet. **20**:398, 1968.

26. Berggård, I., and Bearn, A. G.: The Hurler syndrome; a biochemical and clinical study, Amer. J. Med. **39**:221, 1965.

27. Berkham, O.: Zwei Fälle von Skaphokephalie, Arch. Anthrop. **34**:8, 1907.

28. Berliner, M. L.: Lipin keratitis of Hurler's syndrome (gargoylism or dysostosis multiplex); clinical and pathologic report, Arch. Ophthal. **22**:97, 1939.

28a. Berman, E. R., Vered, J., and Bach, G.: A reliable spot test for mucopolysaccharidoses, Clin. Chem. **17**:886, 1971.

29. Berry, H. K.: Procedures for testing urine specimens dried on filter paper, Clin. Chem. **5**:603, 1959.

30. Berry, H. K., and Spinanger, J.: A paper spot test useful in study of Hurler's syndrome, J. Lab. Clin. Med. **55**:136, 1960.

31. Bierman, S. M., Edgington, T., and Newcomer, V. D.: Farber's disease; a disorder of mucopolysaccharide metabolism with articular, respiratory, and neurologic manifestations, Arthritis Rheum. **9**:620, 1966.

32. Bindschedler, J. J.: Polydystrophie du type Hurler chez un frére et une soeur, Bull. Soc. Pédiat. Paris **36**:571, 1938.

33. Binswanger, E., and Ullrich, O.: Ueber die Dysostosis multiplex (Typus Hurler) und ihre Beziehungen zu anderen Konstitutionsanomalien, Z. Kinderheilk. **54**:699, 1933.

34. Bishton, R. L., Norman, R. M., and Tingey, A.: The pathology and chemistry of a case of gargoylism, J. Clin. Path. **9**:305, 1956.

35. Bitter, T., Muir, H., Mittwoch, U., and Scott, J. D.: A contribution to the differential diagnosis of Hurler's disease and forms of Morquio's syndrome, J. Bone Joint Surg. **48-B:** 637, 1966.

36. Blattner, R. J.: Hurler's syndrome, J. Pediat. **69**:313, 1966.

37. Blaw, M. E., and Langer, L. O.: Spinal cord compression in Morquio-Brailsford disease, J. Pediat. **74**:593, 1969.

38. Böcker, E.: Zur Erblichkeit der Dysostosis multiplex, Z. Kinderheilk. **63**:688, 1943.

39. Boldt, L.: Beitrag zur Dysostosis multiplex (von Pfaundler-Hurler), Z. Kinderheilk. **63**:679, 1943.

39a. Bona, C., Stanescu, V., and Ionescu, V.: Histochemical studies of growing human cartilage in Morquio's disease, J. Pathol. **103**:134, 1971.

40. Brailsford, J. F.: Chondro-osteo-dystrophy, roentgenographic and clinical features of child with dislocation of vertebrae, Amer. J. Surg. **7**:404, 1929; The radiology of bones and joints, ed. 5, Baltimore, 1953, The Williams & Wilkins Co.

41. Brante, G.: Gargoylism: a mucopolysaccharidosis, Scand. J. Clin. Lab. Invest. **4**:43, 1952.

42. Bridge, E. M., and Holt, L. E., Jr.: Glycogen storage disease; observations on the pathologic physiology of two cases of the hepatic form of the disease, J. Pediat. **27**:299, 1945.

43. Brown, D. H. (St. Louis): Personal communication.

44. Brown, D. H.: Tissue storage of mucopolysaccharides in Hurler-Pfaundler's disease, Proc. Nat. Acad. Sci. **43**:783, 1957.

45. Brown, D. O.: Morquio's disease, Med. J. Aust. **1**:598, 1933.

46. Burke, E. C., and Teller, W. M.: Snorter dwarfism in cattle related to gargoylism in children, J. Amer. Vet. Med. Ass. **139**:1211, 1961.

47. Burrows, E. H.: The so-called J-sella, Brit. J. Radiol. **37**:661, 1964.

48. Butterworth, T., and Strean, L. P.: Clinical genodermatoses, Baltimore, 1962, The Williams & Wilkins Co.

49. Caffey, J.: Gargoylism (Hunter-Hurler disease, dysostosis multiplex, lipochondrodystrophy); prenatal and neonatal bone lesions and their early postnatal evaluation, Amer. J. Roentgen. **67**:715, 1952.

50. Calatroni, A., Donnelly, P. V., and DiFerrante, N.: The glycosaminoglycans of human plasma, J. Clin. Invest. **48**:332, 1969.

51. Callahan, W. P., Hackett, R. L., and Lorincz, A. E.: New observations by light microscopy on liver histology in the Hurler's syndrome; a needle biopsy study of 11 patients utilizing plastic-embedded tissue, Arch. Path. **83**:507, 1967.

52. Callahan, W. P., and Lorincz, A. E.: Hepatic ultrastructure in the Hurler syndrome, Amer. J. Path. **48**:277, 1966.

53. Cameron, J. M., and Gardiner, T. B.: Atypical familial osteochondrodystrophy, Brit. J. Radiol. **36**:135, 1963.

54. Campailla, E., and Martinelli, B.: Morquio's disease: modification of mucopolysachariduria with advancing age; report of three cases. Clinical delineation of birth defects. IV. Skeletal dysplasias, New York, 1969, National Foundation–March of Dimes, pp. 172-173.

55. Campbell, T. N., and Fried, M.: Urinary mucopolysaccharide excretion in the sex-linked form of the Hurler syndrome, Proc. Soc. Exp. Biol Med. **108**:529, 1961.

56. Cantz, M., Chrambach, A., and Neufeld, E. F.: Characterization of the factor deficient in the Hunter syndrome by polyacrylamide gel electrophoresis, Biochem. Biophys. Res. Commun. **39**:936, 1970.

56a. Cantz, M., Chrambach, A., Bach, A., and Neufeld, E. F.: The Hunter corrective factor: purification and preliminary characterization, J. Biol. Chem. **247**:5456, 1972.

57. Carlisle, J. W., and Good, R. A.: The inflammatory cycle—a method of study in Hurler's disease, Amer. J. Dis. Child. **99**:193, 1960.

58. Carter, C. H., Wan, A. T., and Carpenter, D. G.: Commonly used tests in the detection of Hurler's syndrome, J. Pediat. **73**:217, 1968.

59. Cawson, R. A.: The oral changes in gargoylism, Proc. Roy. Soc. Med. **55**:1066, 1962.

60. Chadwick, D. L.: In Fishbein, M., editor: First Inter-American Conference on Congenital Defects, Philadelphia, 1963, J. B. Lippincott Co., p. 147.
61. Chadwick, D. L. (Los Angeles): Personal communication, 1964.
62. Chou, Yi-Che: Ocular signs in gargoylism, Clin. Med. J. 78:130, 1959.
63. Cifonelli, J. A., and Dorfman, A.: The uronic acid of heparin, Biochem. Biophys. Res. Commun. 7:41, 1962.
64. Clark, R. D., Smith, J. D., Jr., and Davidson, E. A.: Hexosamine and acid glycosaminoglycans in human teeth, Biochim. Biophys. Acta 101:267, 1965.
65. Clausen, J. Dyggve, H. V., and Melchior, J. C.: Chemical studies in gargoylism, Arch. Dis. Child. 42:62, 1967.
66. Clausen, J., Dyggve, H. V., and Melchoir, J. C.: Mucopolysaccharidosis: paper electrophoretic and infra-red analysis of the urine in gargoylism and Morquio-Ullrich's disease, Arch. Dis. Child. 38:364, 1963.
67. Cocchi, U.: Hereditary diseases with bone changes. In Schinz, H. R., Baensch, W. E., Friedl, E., and Uehlinger, E.: Roentgen-diagnostics, New York, 1951, Grune & Stratton, Inc., p. 728.
68. Cocchi, U.: Polytope erbliche enchondrale Dysostosen, Fortschr. Roentgenstr. 72:435, 1950.
69. Cockayne, E. A.: Gargoylism (chondro-osteodystrophy, hepatosplenomegaly, deafness in two brothers), Proc. Roy. Soc. Med. 30:104, 1936.
70. Cole, H. N., Jr., Irving, R. C., Lund, H. Z., Mercer, R. D., and Schneider, R. W.: Gargoylism with cutaneous manifestations, Arch. Derm. Syph. 66:371, 1952.
71. Constantopoulos, G.: Hunter-Hurler syndrome; gel filtration and dialysis of urinary acid mucopolysaccharides, Nature 220:583, 1968.
71a. Constantopoulos, G., Dekaban, A. S., and Scheie, H. G.: Heterogeneity of disorders in patients with corneal clouding, normal intellect, and mucopolysaccharidosis, Am. J. Ophthal. 72:1106, 1971.
72. Coran, A. G., and Eraklis, A. J.: Inguinal hernia in the Hurler-Hunter syndrome, Surgery 61:302, 1967.
73. Cordes, F. C., and Hogan, J. J.: Dysostosis multiplex (Hurler's disease); lipocondrodystrophy; gargoylism; report of ocular findings in five cases with a review of the literature, Arch. Ophthal. 27:637, 1942.
74. Cottier, H.: Infantile kardiovaskuläre Sklerose bei Gargoylismus, Schweiz. Z. Allg. Path. 20:745, 1957.
75. Coward, N. R., and Nemir, R. L.: Familial osseous dystrophy (Morquio's disease), Amer. J. Dis. Child. 46:213, 1933.
76. Craig, J. M., Clark, J. T., and Banker, B. Q.: Metabolic neurovisceral disorder with accumulations of an unidentified subtsance: variant of Hurler's syndrome? Amer. J. Dis. Child. 98:577, 1959.
77. Craig, W. S.: Gargoylism in a twin brother and sister, Arch. Dis. Child. 29:293, 1954.
78. Crawford, T.: Morquio's disease, Arch. Dis. Child. 14:70, 1939.
79. Crigler, J. F., Jr., and Najjar, V. A.: Congenital familial nonhemolytic jaundice with kernicterus, Pediatrics 10:169, 1952.
80. Crocker, A. C.: Therapeutic trials in the inborn errors; an attempt to modify Hurler's syndrome, Pediatrics 42:887, 1968.
80a. Crocker, A. C., and Cullinane, M. M.: Families under stress: the diagnosis of Hurler's syndrome, Postgrad. Med. 51:223, 1972.
81. Crome, L.: Epiloia and endocardial fibro-elastosis, Arch. Dis. Child. 29:136, 1954.
82. Cunningham, R. C.: A contribution to the genetics of gargoylism, J. Neurol. Neurosurg. Psychiat. 17:191, 1954.
83. Danes, B. S. (New York): Personal communication.
84. Danes, B. S., and Bearn, A. G.: Cellular metachromasia; a genetic marker for studying the mucopolysaccharidoses, Lancet 1:241, 1967.
85. Danes, B. S., and Bearn, A. G.: Correction of cellular metachromasia in cultured fibroblasts in several inherited mucopolysaccharidoses, Proc. Nat. Acad. Sci. 67:357, 1970.
86. Danes, B. S., and Bearn, A. G.: The effect of retinol (vitamin A alcohol) on urinary excretion of mucopolysaccharides in the Hurler syndrome, Lancet 1:1029, 1967.
87. Danes, B. S., and Bearn, A. G.: A genetic cell marker in cystic fibrosis of the pancreas, Lencet 1:1061, 1968.

88. Danes, B. S., and Bearn, A. G.: Hurler's syndrome; demonstration of an inherited disorder of connective tissue in cell culture, Science **149**:987, 1965.

89. Danes, B. S., and Bearn, A. G.: Hurler's syndrome; effect of retinol (vitamin A alcohol) on cellular mucopolysaccharides in cultured human skin fibroblasts, J. Exp. Med. **124**:1181, 1966.

90. Danes, B. S., and Bearn, A. G.: Hurler's syndrome; a genetic study in cell culture, J. Exp. Med. **123**:1, 1966.

91. Danes, B. S., and Bearn, A. G.: Hurler's syndrome; a genetic study of clones in cell culture, with particular reference to the Lyon hypothesis, J. Exp. Med. **126**:509, 1967.

92. Danes, B. S., and Grossman, H.: Bone dysplasias, including Morquio's syndrome studied in skin fibroblast cultures, Amer. J. Med. **47**:708, 1969.

93. Danes, B. S., Scott, J. E., and Bearn, A. G.: Further studies on metachromasia in cultured human fibroblasts; staining of glycosaminoglycans (mucopolysaccharides) by Alcian blue in salt solutions, J. Exp. Med. **132**:765, 1970.

94. Danes, B. S., Queenan, J. T., Gadow, E. C., and Cederquist, L. L.: Antenatal diagnosis of mucopolysaccharidoses (letter), Lancet **1**:946, 1970.

95. David, B.: Ueber einen dominanten Erbgang bei einer polytopen enchondralen Dysostose Typ Pfaundler-Hurler, Z. Orthop. **84**:657, 1954.

96. Davis, D. B., and Currier, F. P.: Morquio's disease; report of two cases, J.A.M.A. **102**:2173, 1934.

97. Dawson, G., and Spranger, J. W.: Fucosidosis; a glycosphingolipidosis (letter), New Eng. J. Med. **285**:122, 1971.

98. Dawson, I. M.: The histology and histochemistry of gargoylism, J. Path. Bact. **67**:587, 1954.

99. Debré, R., Marie, J., and Thieffry, S.: La polydystrophie de Hurler; le "gargoylisme" d'Ellis (á l'occasion des trois observations nouvelles), Sem. Hôp. Paris **22**:309, 1946.

100. DeCloux, R. J., and Friederici, H. H. R.: Ultra-structural studies of the skin in Hurler's syndrome, Arch. Path. **88**:350, 1969.

101. DeJong, B. P., Robertson, W. V., and Schafer, I. A.: Failure to induce scurvy by ascorbic acid depletion in a patient with Hurler's syndrome, Pediatrics **42**:889, 1968.

102. Dekaban, A. S., and Patton, V. M.: Hurler's and Sanfilippo's variants of mucopolysaccharidosis, Arch. Path. **91**:434, 1971.

103. Dekaban, A. S., and Rennert, O.: Histological, histochemical and chemical studies in Hurler's disease, J. Neuropath. Exp. Neurol. **26**:127, 1967.

104. Dekaban, A. S., and Zelson, J.: Studies in the Hunter-Hurler's syndrome, Trans. Amer. Neurol. Ass. **93**:75, 1968.

105. De Lange, C.: Dysostosis multiplex of the Hurler type (gargoylism), Psychiat. Neurol. (Basel) **1-2**:2, 1942.

106. De Lange, C., Gerlings, P. G., de Kleyn, A., and Lettinga, T. W.: Some remarks on gargoylism, Acta Paediat. **31**:398, 1944.

107. Delorme, G., Montagnac, A., Tessier, J. P., Caillé, J. M., and Bellet, M.: Maladie de Hurler; à propos d'un cas (forme récessive liée au sexe), Ann. Radiol. **11**:599, 1968.

108. Denny, W., and Dutton, G.: Simple urine test for gargoylism, Brit. Med. J. **1**:1555, 1962.

108a. De Rudder, B.: Ueber "Phosphatiddiathese" und ihr Verhältnis zur Dysostosis multiplex und Dysostosis Morquio, Z. Kinderheilk. **63**:407, 1942.

108b. Dibos, P. E., Judisch, J. M., Spaulding, M. B., Wagner, H. V., Jr., and McIntyre, P. A.: Scanning the reticuloendothelial system (RES) in hematological diseases, Johns Hopkins Med. J. **130**:68, 1972.

109. DiFerrante, N. (Houston, Texas): Personal communication, 1971.

109a. DiFerrante, N., and Nichols, B. L.: A case of the Hunter syndrome with progeny, Johns Hopkins Med. J. **130**:325, 1972.

110. DiFerrante, N., Nichols, B. L., Donnelly, P. V., Neri, G., Hrgovcic, R., and Berglund, R. K.: Induced degradation of glycosaminoglycans in Hurler's and Hunter's syndromes by plasma infusion, Proc. Nat. Acad. Sci. **68**:303, 1971.

111. Dodion, J., Resibois, A., Loeb, H., and Crémer, N.: Étude d'un cas d'oligophrénie polydystrophique (mucopolysaccharidose H.S.). Path. Europ. **1**:50, 1966.

112. Dorfman, A.: The Hurler syndrome. In Fishbein, M., editor: First Inter-American Conference on Congenital Defects, Philadelphia, 1963, J. B. Lippincott Co., pp. 41-52; also 146-149.

113. Dorfman, A.: In Stanbury, J. B., Wyngaarden, J. B., and Fredrickson, D. S., editors: The metabolic basis of inherited disease, ed. 2, New York, 1966, McGraw-Hill Book Co.

114. Dorfman, A.: Metabolism of acid mucopolysaccharides, Biophys. J. 4 (supp.):155, 1964.

115. Dorfman, A.: Studies on the biochemistry of connective tissue, Pediatrics 22:576, 1958.

115a. Dorfman, A., and Ho, P. L.: Synthesis of acid mucopolysaccharides by glial tumor cells in tissue culture, Proc. Nat. Acad. Sci. 66:495, 1970.

116. Dorfman, A., and Lorincz, A. E.: Occurrence of urinary acid mucopolysaccharides in the Hurler syndrome, Proc. Nat. Acad. Sci. 43:443, 1957.

117. Dorfman, A., and Matalon, R.: The Hurler and Hunter syndromes, Amer. J. Med. 47: 691, 1969.

117a. Dorfman, A., and Matalon, R.: The mucopolysaccharidoses. In Stanbury, J. B., Wyngaarden, J. B., and Frederickson, D. S., (editors): The metabolic basis of inherited disease, ed. 3, New York, 1972, McGraw-Hill Book Co., pp. 1218-1272.

118. Dorfman, A., and Ott, M. L.: A turbidimetric method for the assay of hyaluronidase, J. Biol. Chem. 172:367, 1948.

119. Duckett, S., Christian, J. C., Thompson, J. N., and Drew, A. L.: The ultrastructure of metachromatic bodies in cultured fibroblasts in Hunter's syndrome, Develop. Med. Child Neurol. 11:764, 1969.

120. Durand, P., and Borrone, C.: Fucosidosis and mannosidosis; glycoprotein and glycosylceramide storage diseases, Helv. Paediat. Acta 26:19, 1971.

120a. Durand, P., Borrone, C., and Della Cella, G.: Fucosidosis, J. Pediat. 75:665, 1969.

121. Dyggve, H. V., Melchior, J. C., and Clausen, J.: Morquio-Ullrich's disease; an inborn error of metabolism? Arch. Dis. Child. 37:525, 1962.

122. Eichenberger, K.: Kann die Dysostosis Morquio als selbständiges Krankheitsbild vom Gargolyismus abgetrennt werden? Ann. Paediat. 182:107, 1954.

123. Einhorn, N. H., Moore, J. R., Ostrum, H. W., and Rountree, L. G.: Osteochondrodystrophia deformans (Morquio's disease); report of three cases, Amer. J. Dis. Child. 61:776, 1941.

124. Einhorn, N. H., Moore, J. R., and Rountree, L. G.: Osteochondrodystrophia deformans (Morquio's disease); observations at autopsy in one case, Amer. J. Dis. Child. 72:536, 1946.

125. Ek, J. I.: Cerebral lesions in arthrogryposis multiplex congenita, Acta Paediat. 47:302, 1958.

126. Ellis, R. W. B.: Gargoylism (chondro-osteodystrophy, corneal opacities, hepatosplenomegaly and mental deficiency), Proc. Roy. Soc. Med. 30:158, 1936.

127. Ellis, R. W. B., Sheldon, W., and Capon, N. B.: Gargoylism (chondro-osteo-dystrophy, corneal opacities, hepatosplenomegaly and mental deficiency), Quart. J. Med. 5:119, 1936.

128. Ellman, P.: A rare primary osseous dystrophy, Brit. J. Child. Dis. 30:188, 1933.

129. Elsner, B.: Ultrastructure of the rectal wall in Hunter's syndrome, Gastroenterology 58:856, 1970.

130. Emanuel, R. W.: Gargoylism with cardiovascular involvement in two brothers, Brit. Heart J. 16:417, 1954.

131. Emerit, I., Maroteaux, P., and Vernant, P.: Deux observations de mucopolysaccharidose avec atteinte cardio-vasculaire, Arch. Franç. Pédiat. 23:1075, 1966.

132. Emery, A. E. H.: Unpublished observations on the kindred reported by Beebe and Formel,[22] supplemented by personal observations in 1972.

133. Emery, J. M., Green, W. R., Wyllie, R. G., and Howell, R. R.: G_{M1}-gangliosidosis; ocular and pathological manifestations, Arch. Ophthal. 85:177, 1971.

134. Engel, D.: Dysostosis multiplex (Pfaundler-Hurler syndrome), two cases, Arch. Dis. Child. 14:217, 1939.

135. Engle, R. L., Jr. (New York City): Personal communication.

136. Epps, R. P., and Scott, R. B.: Gargoylism (Hurler's syndrome; lipochondrodystrophy dysostosis multiplex); report of 2 cases in Negro children, J. Pediat. 52:182, 1958.

137. Esterly, N. B., and McKusick, V. A.: Stiff-skin syndrome, Pediatrics 47:360, 1971.

138. Fallis, N., Barnes, F. L., and DiFerrante, N.: A case of polydystophic dwarfism with urinary excretion of dermatan sulfate and heparan sulfate, J. Clin. Endocr. 28:26, 1968.

139. Farber, S., Cohen, J., and Uzman, L. L.: Lipogranulomatosis, a new lipo-glyco-protein "storage" disease, J. Mount Sinai Hosp., N. Y. 24:816, 1957.

140. Fluharty, A. L., Porter, M. T., Lassila, E. L.: Trammell, J. Carrel, R. E., and Kihara, H.: Acid glycosidases in mucopolysaccharidoses fibroblasts, Biochem. Med. 4:110, 1970.

141. Foley, K. M., Danes, B. S., and Bearn, A. G.: White blood cell cultures in genetic studies on the human mucopolysaccharidoses, Science **164**:424, 1969.
142. Ford, F. R.: Diseases of the nervous system in infancy, childhood and adolescence, ed. 4, Springfield, Ill., 1960, Charles C Thomas, Publisher, p. 828.
143. Ford, N., Silverman, F. N., and Kozlowski, K.: Spondylo-epiphyseal dysplasia (pseudo-achondroplastic type), Amer. J. Roentgen. **86**:462, 1961.
144. Fraccaro, M., Mannini, A., Lenzi, L., Magrini, V., Perona, P., and Sartori, E.: Morquio's disease; metachromatic granules in cultured fibroblasts, Lancet **1**:508, 1967.
145. Franceschetti, A., and Forni, S.: The heredo-familial degenerations of the cornea, Acta 16th Internat. Cong. Ophthal. London, July 17-22, 1950, pp. 157-193.
146. Franceschetti, A., François, J., and Babel, J.: Les hérédodégénéréscences chorio-rétiniennes (dégénéréscences tapeto-rétiniennes), vol. 2, Paris, 1963, Masson et Cie, pp. 998-1000.
147. François, J.: Dystrophie dermo-chondro-cornéenne familiale, Ann. Oculist (Paris) **182**:409, 1949.
148. François, J.: Dystrophie dermo-chondro-cornéenne familiale, Bull. Acad. Roy. Med. Belg. **14**:135, 1949.
149. François, J., and Detrait, C.: Dystrophie dermo-chondro-cornéenne familiale, Ann. Paediat. **174**:145, 1950.
150. François, J., and Rabaey, M.: Examen histochimique de la dystrophie cornéenne et étude de l'hérédité dans un cas de gargloylisme (maladie de Hurler), Ann. Oculist (Paris) **185**:784, 1952.
151. Fraser, G. R.: Friedmann, A. I., Maroteaux, P., Glen-Bott, A. M., and Mittwoch, U.: Dysplasia spondyloepiphysaria congenita and related generalised skeletal dysplasias among children with severe visual handicaps, Arch. Dis. Child. **44**:490, 1969.
152. Fratantoni, J. C., Hall, C. W., and Neufeld, E. F.: The defect in Hurler and Hunter syndromes. II. Deficiency of specific factors involved in mucopolysaccharide degradation, Proc. Nat. Acad. Sci. **64**:360, 1969.
153. Fratantoni, J. C., Hall, C. W., and Neufeld, E. F.: The defect in Hurler's and Hunter's syndromes; faulty degradation of mucopolysaccharide, Proc. Nat. Acad. Sci. **60**:699, 1968.
154. Fratantoni, J. C., Hall, C. W., and Neufeld, E. F.: Hurler and Hunter syndromes; mutual correction of the defect in cultured fibroblasts, Science **162**:570, 1968.
155. Fratantoni, J. C., Neufeld, E. F., Uhlendorf, B. W., and Jacobson, C. B.: Intrauterine diagnosis of the Hurler and Hunter syndromes, New Eng. J. Med. **280**:686, 1969.
156. Freeman, J.: Morquio's disease, Amer. J. Dis. Child. **55**:343, 1938.
157. Freitag, F., Blümcke, S., and Spranger, J.: Hepatic ultrastructure in mucolipidosis I (muco-polysaccharidosis), Virchow Arch, Abt. B Zellpath. **7**:189, 1971.
158. Freitag, F., Küchemann, K., Blümcke, S., and Spranger, J.: Hepatic ultrastructure in fucosidosis, Virchow Arch. Abt. B Zellpath. **7**:99, 1971.
159. Gardner, D. G.: Metachromatic cells in the gingiva in Hurler's syndrome, Oral Surg. **26**:782, 1968.
159a. Gardner, D. G.: The oral manifestations of Hurler's syndrome, Oral Surg. **32**:46, 1971.
160. Garn, S. M. (Yellow Springs, Ohio): Personal communication.
161. Garn, S. M., and Hurme, V. O.: Dental defects in three siblings afflicted with Morquio's disease, Brit. Dent. J. **93**:210, 1952.
162. Gasteiger, H., and Liebenam, L.: Beitrag zur Dysostosis multiplex unter besonderer Berüchsichtigung des Augenbefundes, Klin. Mbl. Augenheilk. **99**:333, 1937.
163. Gerber, A., Raab, A. P., and Sobel, A. E.: Vitamin A poisoning in adults with description of a case, Amer. J. Med. **16**:729, 1954.
164. Gerich, J. E.: Hunter's syndrome; beta-galactosidase deficiency in skin, New Eng. J. Med. **280**:799, 1969.
165. Gilbert, E. F., and Guin, G. H.: Gargoylism; a review, including two occurrences in the American Negro, J. Dis. Child. **95**:69, 1958.
166. Gills, J. P., Hobson, R., and Hanley, W. B.: Electroretinography and fundus oculi findings in Hurler's disease and allied mucopolysaccharidoses, Arch. Ophthal. **74**:596, 1965.
167. Gills, J. P., Hobson, R., Hanley, W. B., and McKusick, V. A.: Hurler's disease and allied mucopolysaccharidoses, Arch. Ophthal. **74**:596, 1965.
168. Glegg, R. E., Eidinger, D., and Leblond, C. P.: Some carbohydrate components of reticular fibers, Science **118**:614, 1953.

169. Glober, G. A., Tanaka, K. R., Turner, J. A., and Liu, C. K.: Mucopolysaccharidosis, an unusual cause of cardiac valvular disease, Amer. J. Cardiol. **22**:133, 1968.

170. Goidanich, I. F., and Lenzi, L.: Morquio-Ullrich disease; a new mucopolysaccharidosis, J. Bone Joint Surg. **46-A**:734, 1964.

171. Goldberg, M. F., and Duke, J. R.: Ocular histopathology in Hunter's syndrome; systemic mucopolysaccharidosis, type II, Arch. Ophthal. **77**:503, 1967.

172. Goldberg, M. F., Maumenee, A. E., and McKusick, V. A.: Corneal dystrophies associated with abnormalities of mucopolysaccharide metabolism, Arch. Ophthal. **74**:516, 1965.

173. Goldberg, M. F., Scott, C. I., and McKusick, V. A.: Hydrocephalus and papilledema in the Maroteaux-Lamy syndrome (mucopolysaccharidosis, type VI), Amer. J. Ophthal. **69**: 969, 1970.

174. Goldman, J. N., Benedek, G. B., Dohlman, C. H., and Kravitt, B.: Structural alterations affecting transparency in swollen human corneas, Invest. Ophthal. **7**:501, 1968.

175. Gonatas, N. K.: A generalized disorder of nervous system, skeletal muscle and heart resembling Refsum's disease and Hurler's syndrome. II. Ultrastructure, Amer. J. Med. **42**:169, 1967.

176. Gordon, B. A., and Feleki, V.: Acid hydrolases in the serum and liver in mucopolysaccharidoses type I and II, Clin. Biochem. **3**:193, 1970.

177. Gordon, B. A., and Haust, M. D.: The mucopolysaccharidoses, types I, II, and III; urinary findings in 23 cases, Clin. Biochem. **3**:203, 1970.

177a. Gorlin, R. J. (Minneapolis): Personal communication, 1972.

178. Greaves, M. W., and Inman, P. M.: Cutaneous changes in the Morquio syndrome, Brit. J. Derm. **81**:29, 1969.

179. Grebe, H.: Die Chrondrodysplasia, ihre Klinik, Differentialdiagnose und Erbpathologie, Habilitationsschrift, Frankfurt, 1942. Cited by Ullrich and Wiedemann.[534]

180. Green, M. A.: Gargoylism (lipochondrodystrophy), J. Neuropath. Exp. Neurol. **7**:399, 1948.

181. Greenfield, J. G., and others: Neuropathology, London, 1958, Edward Arnold & Co., p. 468.

182. Griffiths, S. B., and Findlay, M., Gargoylism; clinical, radiological and haematological features in two siblings, Arch. Dis. Child. **32**:229, 1958.

183. Grossman, H., and Danes, B. S.: Neurovisceral storage disease; roentgenographic features and mode of inheritance, Amer. J. Roentgen. **103**:149, 1968.

184. Grossman, H., and Dorst, J. P.: The mucopolysaccharidoses. In Kaufmann, H., editor: Progress in pediatric radiology, vol. IV, Chicago, 1972, Year Book Medical Publishers.

185. Grumbach, M. M. (New York City): Personal communication.

186. Grumbach, M. M., and Meyer, K.: Urinary excretion and tissue storage of sulfated mucopolysaccharides in Hurler's syndrome, Amer. J. Dis. Child. **96**:467, 1958.

186a. Hall, C. W., Cantz, M., and Neufeld, E. F.: A β-glucuronidase deficiency mucopolysaccharidosis: studies in cultured fibroblasts, Arch. Biochem. Biophys. (in press).

187. Halperin, S. L., and Curtis, G. M.: The genetics of gargoylism, Amer. J. Ment. Defic. **46**:298,

188. Hambrick, G. W., and Scheie, H. G.: Studies of the skin in Hurler's syndrome: mucopolysaccharidosis, Arch. Derm. **85**:455, 1962.

189. Hanai, J., Leroy, J., and O'Brien, J. S.: Ultrastructure of cultured fibroblasts in I-cell disease, Amer. J. Dis. Child. **122**:34, 1971.

189a. Hansen, H. G.: Hematologic studies in mucopolysaccharidoses and mucolipidoses. In Bergsma, D., editor: Clinical delineation of birth defects. XIV. Blood, Baltimore, 1972, The Williams & Wilkins Co.

190. Harvey, R. M.: Hurler-Pfaundler syndrome (gargoylism); review of the literature with report of an additional case, Amer. J. Roentgen. **48**:732, 1942.

191. Hässler, E.: Die Beziehungen der Hurlerschen Krankheit (Dysostosis multiplex-dysostotische Idiotie-Gargolismus) zum Kretinismus, Mschr. Kinderheilk. **86**:96, 1941.

192. Haust, M. D.: Mitochondrial budding and morphogenesis of cytoplasmic vacuoles in hepatocytes of children with the Hurler syndrome and Sanfilippo disease, Exp. Molec. Path. **9**:242, 1968.

192a. Haust, M. D., Gordon, B. A., Bryans, A. M., Wollin, D. G., and Binnington, V.: Heparitin sulfate mucopolysaccharidosis (Sanfilippo disease): a case study with ultrastructural, biochemical, and radiological findings, Pediat. Res. **5**:137, 1971.

193. Haust, M. D., and Landing, B. H.: Histochemical studies in Hurler's disease; a new method for localization of acid mucopolysaccharide, and an analysis of lead acetate "fixation," J. Histochem. Cytochem. **9**:79, 1961.

194. Haust, M. D.: Orizaga, M., Bryans, A. M., and Frank, H. F.: The fine structure of liver in children with Hurler's syndrome, Exp. Molec. Path. **10**:141, 1969.

195. Helmholtz, H. F., and Harrington, E. R.: Syndrome characterized by congenital clouding of the cornea and by other anomalies, Amer. J. Dis. Child. **41**:793, 1931.

196. Helwig-Larsen, H. F., and Mørch, E. T.: Genetic aspects of osteochondrodystrophy; Silfver-skiöld's and Morquio's syndromes, Acta Path. Microbiol. Scand. **22**:335, 1945.

197. Henderson, J. L.: Gargoylism; review of principal features with report of five cases, Arch. Dis. Child. **15**:215, 1940.

198. Henderson, J. L., MacGregory, A. R., Thannhauser, S. J., and Holden, R.: Pathology and biochemistry of gargoylism; report of three cases with review of literature, Arch. Dis. Child. **27**:230, 1952.

199. Hers, H. G.: Inborn lysosomal diseases, Gastroenterology **48**:625, 1965.

200. Hers, H. G., and Van Hoof, F.: The genetic pathology of lysosomes, Progr. Liver Dis. **3**:185, 1970.

201. Hessburg, P. C.: Hurler's disease, Henry Ford Hosp. Med. Bull. **10**:419, 1962.

201a. Hickman, S., and Neufeld, E. F.: A hypothesis for I-cell disease: defective hydrolases that do not enter lysosomes, Biochem. Biophys. Res. Commun. (in press, 1972).

202. Hillman, J. W., and Johnson, J. T. H.: Arthrogryposis multiplex congenita in twins, J. Bone Joint Surg. **34-A**:211, 1952.

203. Ho, M. W., and O'Brien, J. S.: Hurler's syndrome; deficiency of a specific beta galactosidase isoenzyme, Science **165**:611, 1969.

204. Hobaek, A.: Problems of hereditary chondrodysplasias, Oslo, 1961, Oslo University Press.

205. Hochheim, W., Körner, H., and Liebe, S.: Beitrag zur den polytopen, erblichen, enchon-dralen Dysostosen, Arch. Orthop. Unfallchir. **47**:463, 1955.

205a. Hocking, J. D., Jolly, R. D., and Batt, R. D.: Deficiency of α-mannosidase in Angus cattle, Biochem. J. **128**:69, 1972.

206. Hooper, J. M. D.: Unusual case of gargoylism, Guy's Hosp. Rep. **101**:222, 1952.

207. Horrigan, W. D., and Baker, D. H.: Gargoylism; a review of the roentgen skull changes with description of a new finding, Amer. J. Roentgen. **86**:473, 1961.

208. Hors-Cayla, M. C., Maroteaux, P., and deGrouchy, J.: Fibroblastes en culture au cours de mucopolysaccharidoses; influence du sérum sur la métachromasie, Ann. Génét. **11**:265, 1968.

209. Horsch, K.: Ueber hereditäre degenerative Osteoarthropathie, Arch. Orthop. Unfallchir. **34**:536, 1934.

210. Horton, W. A., and Schimke, R. N.: A new mucopolysaccharidosis, J. Pediat. **77**:252, 1970.

211. Hubeny, M. J., and Delano, R. J.: Dysostosis multiplex, Amer. J. Roentgen. **46**:336, 1941.

212. Hueper, W. C.: Experimental studies in cardiovascular pathology; pectin atheromatosis and thesaurosis in rabbits and in dogs, Arch. Path. **34**:883, 1942.

213. Hueper, W. C.: Macromolecular substances as pathogenic agents, Arch. Path. **33**:267, 1942.

214. Hultberg, B., and Öckerman, P. A.: Properties of 4-methylumbelliferyl-beta-galactosidase activities in human liver, Scand. J. Clin. Lab. Invest. **23**:213, 1969.

215. Hultberg, B., Öckerman, P. A., and Dahlqvist, A.: Gargoylism; hydrolysis of beta-galactosides and tissue accumulation of galactose- and mannose-containing compounds, J. Clin. Invest. **49**:216, 1970.

216. Hultberg, B., Öckerman, P. A., and Eriksson, O.: Urinary amino acids in storage disorders; mucopolysaccharidosis; Gaucher's disease and metachromatic leucodystrophy, Metabolism **18**:713, 1969.

217. Humbel, R., Marchal, C., and Fall, M.: Differential diagnosis of mucopolysaccharidosis by means of thin-layer chromatography of urinary acidic glycosaminoglycans, Helv. Paediat. Acta **24**:648, 1969.

218. Hunter, C.: A rare disease in two brothers, Proc. Roy. Soc. Med. **10**:104, 1917.

219. Hurler, G.: Ueber einen Typ multipler Abartungen, vorwiegend am Skelettsystem, Z. Kin-derheilk. **24**:220, 1919.

220. Husler, J.: Handbuch der Kinderheilkunde, ed. 4, vol. 1, p. 651.

220a. Hussels, I. E. (Baltimore): Personal communication, 1972.

221. Ishikawa, H., and Hori, Y.: Systematisierte Hyalinose in Zusammenhang mit Epidermolysis bullosa polydystrophica und Hyalinosis cutis et mucosae, Arch. Klin. Exp. Derm. **218**: 30, 1964.

222. Jackson, W. P. U.: Clinical features, diagnosis and osseous lesions of gargoylism exempli-fied in 3 siblings, Arch. Dis. Child. **26**:549, 1951.

223. Jacobsen, A. W.: Hereditary osteochondrodystrophia deformans; a family with twenty members affected in five generations, J.A.M.A. 113:121, 1939.

224. Jacobson, L., and Kibel, M. A.: Hurler's syndrome; a clinical report on two cases, Central Afr. J. Med. 4:193, 1958.

225. James, T.: Multiple congenital articular rigidities; a review of the literature with report of 2 cases, Edinburgh Med. J. 58:565, 1951.

226. Jeanloz, R. W.: The nomenclature of mucopolysaccharides, Arthritis Rheum. 3:233, 1960.

227. Jelke, H.: Gargoylism. II. Post-mortem findings in an earlier published case, Ann. Paediat. 184:101, 1955.

228. Jelke, H.: Gargoylism; report of a case, Ann. Paediat. 177:355, 1951.

229. Jensen, W. J.: Dermo-chondro-corneal dystrophy, Acta Ophthal. 36:71, 1958.

230. Jermain, L. F., Rohn, R. J., and Bond, W. H.: Studies on the role of the reticuloendothelial system in Hurler's disease, Clin. Res. 7:216, 1959.

231. Jermain, L. F., Rohn, R. J., and Bond, W. H.: Studies on the role of the reticuloendothelial system in Hurler's disease, Amer. J. Med. Sci. 239:612, 1960.

232. Jervis, G. A.: Familial mental deficiency akin to amaurotic idiocy and gargoylism, Arch. Neur. Psychiat. 47:943, 1942.

233. Jervis, G. A.: Gargoylism: study of 10 cases with emphasis on the formes frustes, Arch. Neur. Psychiat. 63:681, 1950.

234. Jewesbury, R. C., and Spence, J. C.: Two cases: (1) oyxcephaly and (2) acrocephaly, with other congenital deformities, Proc. Roy. Soc. Med. 14:27, 1921.

234a. Jolly, R. D. (Massey University, Palmerston North, New Zealand): Personal communication, 1972.

235. Jordans, G. H. W.: Hereditary granulation anomaly of leucocytes (Alder), Acta Med. Scand. 129:348, 1947.

236. Josephy, H.: Lipoidosis of the brain combined with glycogenosis of the liver, J. Neuropath. Exp. Neurol. 8:214, 1949.

237. Julius, R., Aylsworth, A., and Rennert, O.: Hunter-Hurler syndrome; a prototype for the study of storage disease, J. Florida Med. Ass. 57:23, 1970.

238. Kaplan, D.: Classification of the mucopolysaccharidoses based on the pattern of mucopolysacchariduria, Amer. J. Med. 47:721, 1969.

239. Kaplan, D., and Fisher, B.: The effect of methylprednisolone on mucopolysaccharides of rabbit vitreous humor and costal cartilage, Biochem. Biophys. Acta 93:102, 1962.

240. Kaplan, D., McKusick, V. A., Trebach, S., and Lazarus, R.: Keratosulfate–chondroitin sulfate peptide from normal urine and from urine of patients with Morquio syndrome (mucopolysaccharidosis IV), J. Lab. Clin. Med. 71:48, 1968.

241. Kaplan, D., and Meyer, K.: The fate of injected mucopolysaccharides, J. Clin. Invest. 41:741, 1962.

242. Kattus, A. A. (Los Angeles): Personal communication, 1971.

243. Kelemen, G.: Hurler's syndrome and the hearing organ, J. Laryng. 80:791, 1966.

244. Kennealy, E. V.: The ocular manifestations of gargoylism, Amer. J. Ophthal. 36:663, 1953.

245. Kenyon, K. R. (Baltimore): Personal communication, 1971.

245a. Kenyon, K. R., and Maumenee, A. E.: The histological and ultrastructural pathology of congenital hereditary corneal dystrophy: a case report, Invest. Ophthal. 7:475, 1968.

246. Kenyon, K. R., and Sensenbrenner, J. A.: Mucolipidosis II (I-cell disease): ultrastructural observations of conjunctiva and skin, Invest. Ophthal. 10:555, 1971.

247. Kenyon, K. R., Topping, T. M., Green, W. R., and Maumenee, A. E.: Ocular pathology of the Maroteaux-Lamy syndrome; a histologic and ultrastructure report of two cases, Am. J. Ophthal. 73:718, 1972.

248. Kibel, M., and Jacobson, L. (Southern Rhodesia): Personal communication.

249. King, J. H., Jr. (Washington, D. C.): Personal communication, 1964.

250. Kjellman, B., Gamstorp, I., Brun, A., Öckerman, P. A., and Palmgren, B.: Mannosidosis; a clinical and histopathologic study, J. Pediat. 75:366, 1969.

251. Klintworth, G. K.: Current concepts on the ultrastructural pathogenesis of macular and lattice corneal dystrophies. In Bergsma, D., editor: Clinical delineation of birth defects. VIII. The eye, Baltimore, 1971, The Williams & Wilkins Co., pp. 27-31.

252. Klintworth, G. K., and Vogel, F. S.: Macular corneal dystrophy; an inherited acid mucopolysaccharide storage disease of the corneal fibroblast, Amer. J. Path. 45:565, 1964.

253. Knecht, J., Cifonelli, J. A., and Dorfman, A.: Structural studies on heparitin sulfate of normal and Hurler tissues, J. Biol. Chem. **242**:4652, 1967.

254. Knecht, J., and Dorfman, A.: Structure of heparitin sulfate in tissues of the Hurler syndrome, Biochem. Biophys. Res. Commun. **21**:509, 1965.

255. Kniest, W.: Zur Abgrenzung der Dysostosis enchondralis von der Chondrodystrophie, Z. Kinderheilk. **70**:633, 1952.

256. Knudsen, A. G., Jr., DiFerrante, N., and Curtis, J. E.: The effect of leukocyte transfusion in a child with mucopolysaccharidosis II, Proc. Nat. Acad. Sci. **68**:820, 1971.

257. Kny, W.: Zur Kenntnis der Dysostosis multiplex Typ Pfaundler-Hurler, Z. Kinderheilk. **63**:366, 1942.

258. Kobayashi, N.: Acid mucopolysaccharide granules in the glomerular epithelium in gargoylism, Amer. J. Path. **35**:591, 1959.

259. Kopits, S. E. (Baltimore): Personal communication, 1971.

260. Kopits, S. E., and Robinson, R. A. (Baltimore): Personal communication, 1971.

261. Kopits, S. E., and Steingass, M. H.: Experience with the "halo-cast" in small children, Surg. Clin. N. Amer. **50**:935, 1970.

262. Koskenoja, M., and Suvanto, E.: Gargoylism, Acta Ophthal. **37**:324, 1959.

262a. Kresse, H., and Neufeld, E. F.: The Sanfilippo A corrective factor. Purification and mode of action, J. Biol. Chem. **247**:2164, 1972.

262b. Kresse, H., Wiesmann, U., Cantz, M., Hall, C. W., and Neufeld, E. F.: Biochemical heterogeneity of the Sanfilippo syndrome: preliminary characterization of two deficient factors, Biochem. Biophys. Res. Commun. **42**:892, 1971.

263. Kressler, R. J., and Aegerter, E. E.: Hurler's syndrome (gargoylism); summary of literature and report of case with autopsy findings, J. Pediat. **12**:579, 1938.

264. Krovetz, L. J., Lorincz, A. E., and Schiebler, G. L.: Cardiovascular manifestations of the Hurler syndrome; hemodynamic and angiocardiographic observations in 15 patients, Circulation **31**:132, 1965.

265. Krovetz, L. J., McLoughlin, T. G., and Schiebler, G. L.: Left ventricular function in children studied by increasing peripheral resistance with angiotensin, Circulation **37**:729, 1968.

266. Krovetz, L. J., and Schiebler, G. L.: Cardiovascular manifestations of the genetic mucopolysaccharidoses. In Bergsma, D., editor: Clinical delineation of birth defects. XIII. Cardiovascular system, Baltimore, 1972, The Williams & Wilkins Co.

266a. Laberge, C. (Quebec): Personal communication, 1972.

267. Lagunoff, D., and Gritzka, T. L.: The site of mucopolysaccharide accumulation in Hurler's syndrome; an electron microscopic and histochemical study, Lab. Invest. **15**:1578, 1966.

268. Lagunoff, D., Pritzl, P., and Scott, C. R.: Urinary N-sulfate glycosaminoglycan excretion in children normal and abnormal values, Proc. Soc. Exp. Biol. Med. **126**:34, 1967.

269. Lagunoff, D., Ross, R., and Benditt, E. P.: Histochemical and electron microscopic study in a case of Hurler's syndrome, Amer. J. Path. **41**:273, 1962.

270. Lagunoff, D., and Warren, G.: Determination of 2-deoxy-2-sulfoaminohexose content of mucopolysaccharides, Arch. Biochem. **99**:396, 1962.

271. Lahdensuu, S.: Fälle der sogenannten Pfaundler-Hurlersche Krankheit (Dysostosis multiplex), Mschr. Kinderheilk. **92**:340, 1943.

272. Lahey, M. E., Lomas, R. D., and Worth, T. C.: Lipochondrodystrophy (gargoylism), J. Pediat. **31**:220, 1947.

273. Lamy, M., and Maroteaux, P.: La nanisme diastrophique, Presse Méd. **68**:1977, 1960.

274. Lamy, M., Maroteaux, P., and Bader, J. P.: Étude génétique du gargoylisme, J. Génét. Hum. **6**:156, 1957.

275. Lamy, M., Maroteaux, P., and Frézal, J.: Les chondrodystrophies genotypiques; définition et limites, Sem. Hôp. Paris **34**:1675, 1958.

276. Landing, B. H., Silverman, F. N., Craig, J. M., Jacoby, M. D., Lahey, M. E., and Chadwick, D. L.: Familial neurovisceral lipidosis, Amer. J. Dis. Child. **108**:503, 1964.

277. Langer, L. O.: The radiographic manifestations of the HS-mucopolysaccharidosis of Sanfilippo, with discussion of this condition in relation to the other mucopolysaccharidoses and a classification of these fundamentally similar entities, Ann. Radiol. **7**:315, 1964.

278. Langer, L. O., and Carey, L. S.: The roentgenographic features of the KS-mucopolysaccharidosis of Morquio (Morquio-Brailsford's disease), Amer. J. Roentgen. **97**:1, 1966.

279. Langer, L. O., Petersen, D., and Spranger, J.: An unusual bone dysplasia; parastremmatic dwarfism, Amer. J. Roentgen. **110**:550, 1970.

280. Langer, L. O., Jr., Kronenberg, R. S., and Gorlin, R. J.: A case simulating Hurler syndrome of unusual longevity, without abnormal mucopolysacchariduria; a proposed classification of the various forms of the syndrome and similar diseases, Amer. J. Med. **40**:448, 1966.

281. Lauer, R. M., Mascarinas, T., Racela, A. S., and Diehl, A. M.: Administration of a mixture of fungal glycosidases to a patient with type II glycogenosis (Pompe's disease), Pediatrics **42**:672, 1968.

282. Lausecker, H.: Zur Symptomatologie der Dysostosis multiplex (Pfaundler-Hurler), Hautarzt **5**:538, 1954.

282a. Leonidas, J. (Kansas City, Mo.): Personal communication via Dr. John P. Dorst, 1972.

283. Léri, A.: Une maladie congénitale et héréditaire de l'ossification; la pléonostéose familiale, Bull. Soc. Méd. Hôp. Paris **45**:1228, 1921.

284. Léri, A.: Pléonostéose familiale (dystrophie osseuse genéraliseé, congénitale et héréditaire), Presse Méd. **2**:13, 1922.

285. Leroy, J. G., and Crocker, A. C.: Clinical definition of the Hurler-Hunter phenotypes; a review of 50 patients, Amer. J. Dis. Child. **112**:518, 1966.

286. Leroy, J. G., and DeMars, R. I.: Mutant enzymatic and cytological phenotypes in cultured human fibroblasts, Science **157**:804, 1967.

287. Leroy, J. G., DeMars, R. I., and Opitz, J. M.: I-cell disease. In Bergsma, D., editor: The clinical delineation of birth defects. IV. Skeletal dysplasias. New York, 1969 National Foundation–March of Dimes, pp. 174-185.

288. Levin, S.: A specific skin lesion in gargoylism, Amer. J. Dis. Child. **99**:444, 1960.

288a. Lichtenstein, J. R., Bilbrey, G. L., and McKusick, V. A.: Probable genetic heterogeneity within mucopolysaccharidosis II. Report of a family with the mild form, Johns Hopkins Med. J. **131**: Dec., 1972.

289. Liebenam, L.: Beitrag zur Dysostosis multiplex, Deutsch. Z. Kinderheilk. **59**:91, 1938.

290. Lindsay, S.: The cardiovascular system in gargoylism, Brit. Heart J. **12**:17, 1950.

291. Lindsay, S., Reilly, W. A., Gotham, Th. J., and Skahen, R.: Gargoylism. II. Study of pathologic lesions and clinical review of twelve cases, Amer. J. Dis. Child. **76**:239, 1948.

292. Linker, A., Evans, L. R., and Langer, L. O.: Morquio's disease and mucopolysaccharide excretion, J. Pediat. **77**:1039, 1970.

293. Linker, A., and Terry, K. D.: Urinary acid mucopolysaccharides in normal man and in Hurler's syndrome, Proc. Soc. Exp. Biol. Med. **11**:743, 1963.

294. Lipton, E. L., and Morgenstern, S. H.: Arthrogryposis multiplex congenita in identical twins, Amer. J. Dis. Child. **89**:233, 1955.

295. Loeb, H., Jonniaux, G., Resibois, A., Cremer, N., Dodion, J., Tondeur, M., Gregoire, P. E., Richard, J., and Cieters, P.: Biochemical and ultrastructural studies in Hurler's syndrome, J. Pediat. **73**:860, 1968.

296. Lorincz, A. E.: Acid mucopolysaccharides in the Hurler syndrome, Fed. Proc. **17**:266, 1958.

297. Lorincz, A. E.: Heritable disorders of acid mucopolysaccharide metabolism in humans and in snorter dwarf cattle, Ann. N. Y. Acad. Sci. **91**:644, 1961.

298. Lorincz, A. E.: Hurler's syndrome in man and snorter dwarfism in cattle; heritable disorders of connective tissue acid mucopolysaccharide metabolism, Clin. Orthop. **33**:104, 1964.

299. Lorincz, A. E.: Mucopolysacchariduria in children with hereditary arthro-osteo-onychodysplasia (abstract), Fed. Proc. **21**:173, 1962.

300. Lorincz, A. E. (Chicago): Personal communication.

301. Lorincz, A. E. (Birmingham, Ala.): Personal communication, 1971.

302. Lorincz, A. E.: "Snorter" dwarf cattle, a naturally occurring heritable disorder of acid mucopolysaccharide metabolism which resembles the Hurler syndrome, Amer. J. Dis. Child. **100**:488, 1960.

303. Lorincz, A. E., and West, S. S. (Birmingham, Ala.): Personal communication, 1971

304. Lorincz, A. E., and colleagues: Mucopolysaccharidosis in snorter dwarf cattle, J. Anim. Sci. **19**:1216, 1960.

305. Lowry, R. B., and Renwick, D. H. G.: The relative frequency of the Hurler and Hunter syndromes (letter), New Eng. J. Med. **284**:221, 1971.

306. Luchsinger, U., Buhler, E. M., Menes, K., and Hirt, H. R.: I-cell disease, New Eng. J. Med. **282**:1374, 1970.

307. Lundquist, A., and Ockerman, P. A.: Fine-needle aspiration biopsy of human liver for enzymatic diagnosis of glycogen storage disease and gargoylism, Acta Paediat. Scand. 59:293, 1970.

308. Lunström, R.: Gargoylism; three cases, Nord. Med. 33:41, 1947.

309. Lurie, L. A., and Levy, S.: Gargoylism, Amer. J. Med. Sci. 207:184, 1944.

310. MacBrinn, M. C., Okada, S., Ho, M. W., Hu, C. C., and O'Brien, J. S.: Generalized gangliosidosis; impaired cleavage of galactose from a mucopolysaccharide and a glycoprotein, Science 163:946, 1969.

311. MacBrinn, M., Okada, S., Woollacott, M., Patel, V., Wan Ho, M., Tappel, A. L., and O'Brien, J. S.: Beta-galactosidase deficiency in the Hurler syndrome, New Eng. J. Med. 281:338, 1969.

312. McCormick, W. F.: Rupture of the stomach in children; review of the literature and a report of seven cases, Arch. Path. 67:416, 1959.

313. MacGillivray, R. C.: Gargoylism (Hurler disease), J. Ment. Sci. 98:687, 1952.

314. McIlwain, P., and Eveleth, D. F.: Urinary mucopolysaccharides of dwarf cattle, Vet. Med. 57:508, 1962.

315. McKusick, V. A.: Hereditary disorders of connective tissue, Bull. N. Y. Acad. Med. 35:143, 1959.

316. McKusick, V. A.: The nosology of the mucopolysaccharidoses, Amer. J. Med. 47:730, 1969.

317. McKusick, V. A.: On the X chromosome of man, Quart. Rev. Biol. 37:69, 1962; also Washington, D. C., AIBS, 1964.

318. McKusick, V. A.: The relative frequency of the Hurler and Hunter syndromes, New Eng. J. Med. 283:853, 1970.

319. McKusick, V. A., and colleagues: Medical genetics 1958-1960, St. Louis, 1961, The C. V. Mosby Co., Figs. 64 and 65, pp. 476-479.

320. McKusick, V. A., Egeland, J. A., Eldridge, R., and Krusen, D. E.: Dwarfism in the Amish. I. The Ellis–van Creveld syndrome, Bull. Hopkins Hosp. 115:306, 1964.

321. McKusick, V. A., Eldridge, R., Hostetler, J. A., and Ruanguit, U.: Dwarfism in the Amish. II. Cartilage-hair hypoplasia, Bull. Hopkins Hosp. 116:285, 1965.

321a. McKusick, V. A., Howell, R. R., Hussels, I. E., Neufeld, E. F., and Stevenson, R.: Allelism, non-allelism and genetic compounds among the mucopolysaccharidoses: hypotheses, Lancet 1:993, 1972.

321b. McKusick, V. A., Howell, R. R., Hussels, I. E., Neufeld, E. F., and Stevenson, R.: Allelism, non-allelism and genetic compounds among the mucopolysaccharidoses. Corrective factors in nosology, genetics and therapy, Trans. Assoc. Amer. Phys. (in press, 1972).

322. McKusick, V. A., Kaplan, D., Wise, D., Hanley, W. B., Suddarth, S. B., Sevick, M. E., and Maumenee, A. E.: The genetic mucopolysaccharidoses, Medicine 44:445, 1965.

323. McKusick, V. A., Mahloudji, M., Abbott, M. H., Lindenberg, R., and Kepas, D.: Seckel's bird-headed dwarfism, New Eng. J. Med. 277:279, 1967.

324. McKusick, V. A., and Milch, R. A.: The clinical behavior of genetic disease; selected aspects, Clin. Orthop. 33:22, 1964.

325. Madsen, J. A., and Linker, A.: Vitamin A and mucopolysaccharidosis; a clinical and biochemical evaluation, J. Pediat. 75:843, 1969.

326. Magee, K. R.: Leptomeningeal changes associated with lipochondrodystrophy (gargoylism), Arch. Neur. Psychiat. 63:282, 1950.

327. Magrini, U., Fraccaro, M., and Tiepolo, L., and colleagues: Mucopolysaccharidoses; autoradiographic study of sulphate-35S uptake by cultured fibroblasts, Ann. Hum. Genet. 31:231, 1968.

328. Mailer, C.: Gargoylism associated with optic atrophy, Canad. J. Ophthal. 4:266, 1969.

329. Manley, G., and Hawksworth, J.: Diagnosis of Hurler's syndrome in the hospital laboratory and the determination of its genetic type, Arch. Dis. Child. 41:91, 1966.

330. Manley, G., and Williams, U.: Urinary excretion of glycosaminoglycans in the various forms of gargoylism, J. Clin. Path. 22:67, 1969.

331. Mapes, C. A., Anderson, R. L., Sweeley, C. C., Desnick, R. J., and Krivit, W.: Enzyme replacement in Fabry's disease, an inborn error of metabolism, Science 169:987, 1970.

332. Marchal, C., Grignon, G., Humbel, R., Vidaillret, M., Fall, M., Grignon, M., Pierson, M., and Neimann, N.: Mucopolysaccharidose sans mucopolysacchariduric, Ann. Pediat. 15:606, 1968.

333. Maroteaux, P.: Différenciation biochemique des maladies de Hurler et de Hunter par fractionnement de l'héparitine sulfate, Rev. Europ. Etud. Clin. Biol. **15**:203, 1970.

334. Maroteaux, P., Frézal, J., Tahbaz-Zaden, and Lamy, M.: Une observation familiale d'oligophrénie polydystrophique, J. Génét. Hum. **15**:93, 1966.

335. Maroteaux, P., Hors-Cayla, M. C., and Pont, J.: La mucolipidose de type II, Presse Méd. **78**:179, 1970.

336. Maroteaux, P., and Lamy, M.: Achondroplasia in man and animals, Clin. Orthop. **33**:91, 1964.

337. Maroteaux, P., and Lamy, M.: Les dysplasies spondylo-épiphysaires génotypiques, Sem. Hôp. Paris **34**:1685, 1958.

338. Maroteaux, P., and Lamy, M.: Hurler's disease, Morquio's disease, and related mucopolysaccharidoses, J. Pediat. **67**:312, 1965.

339. Maroteaux, P., and Lamy, M.: La maladie de Morquio; étude clinique, radiologique et biologique, Presse Méd. **71**:2091, 1963.

340. Maroteaux, P., and Lamy, M.: Opacités cornéennes et trouble metabolique dans la maladie de Morquio, Rev. Franc. Étud. Clin. Biol. **6**:481, 1961.

341. Maroteaux, P., and Lamy, M.: La pseudopolydystrophie de Hurler, Presse Méd. **74**:2889, 1966.

341a. Maroteaux, P., and Lamy, M.: Studying the mucopolysaccharidoses (letter), Lancet **2**:510, 1967.

342. Maroteaux, P., Lévêque, B., Marie, J., and Lamy, M.: Une nouvelle dysostose avec elimination urinaire de chondroitine-sulfate B, Presse Méd. **71**:1849, 1963.

343. Maroteaux, P., Spranger, J., and Wiedemann, H. R.: Der metatropische Zwergwuchs, Arch. Kinderheilk. **173**:211, 1966.

343a. Matalon, R., Cifonelli, J. A., and Dorfman, A.: α-L-iduronidase in cultured human fibroblasts and liver, Biochem. Biophys. Res. Commun. **42**:340, 1971.

344. Matalon, R., Cifonelli, J. A., Zellweger, H., and Dorfman, A.: Lipid abnormalities in a variant of the Hurler syndrome, Proc. Nat. Acad. Sci. **59**:1097, 1968.

345. Matalon, R., and Dorfman, A.: Acid mucopolysaccharides in cultured fibroblasts of cystic fibrosis of the pancreas, Biochem. Biophys. Res. Commun. **33**:954, 1958.

346. Matalon, R., and Dorfman, A.: Acid mucopolysaccharides in cultured human fibroblasts, Lancet **2**:838, 1969.

347. Matalon, R., and Dorfman, A.: Hurler's syndrome; biosynthesis of acid mucopolysaccharides in tissue culture, Proc. Nat. Acad. Sci. **56**:1310, 1966.

347a. Matalon, R., and Dorfman, A.: Hurler's syndrome, an α-L-iduronidase deficiency, Biochem. Biophys. Res. Commun. **47**:959, 1972.

348. Matalon, R., and Dorfman, A.: The structure of acid mucopolysaccharides produced by Hurler fibroblasts in tissue culture, Proc. Nat. Acad. Sci. **60**:179, 1968.

348a. Matalon, R., Dorfman, A. and Nadler, H. L.: A chemical method for the antenatal diagnosis of mucopolysaccharidoses (letter), Lancet **1**:798, 1972.

349. Matalon, R., Dorfman, A., Nadler, H. L., and Jacobson, C. B.: A chemical method for the antenatal diagnosis of mucopolysaccharidoses, Lancet **1**:83, 1970.

350. Mathur, P. S.: Gargoylism, Indian J. Pediat. **24**:372, 1957.

351. Maumenee, A. E.: Congenital hereditary corneal dystrophy, Amer. J. Ophthal. **50**:1114, 1960.

352. Mauri, C., and Soldati, M.: Les caracteristiques cytochimiques des granulations cellulaires de Alder. Definition de la dysostose enchondrale multiple en tant que polysaccharidose, Schweiz. Med. Wschr. **88**:992, 1958.

353. Mayes, J. S., and Hansen, R. G.: Mucopolysaccharide excretion in patients with Hurler's syndrome, their families, and normal man, Proc. Soc. Exp. Biol. Med. **122**:927, 1966.

354. Mayes, J. S., Hansen, R. G., Gregory, P. W., and Tyler, W. S.: Mucopolysaccharide excretion in dwarf and normal cattle, J. Anim. Sci. **23**:833, 1964.

354a. Melhem, R., Dorst, J. P., Scott, C. I., Jr., and McKusick, V. A.: Roentgen findings in mucolipidosis III (pseudo-Hurler polydystrophy), Radiology (in press, 1973).

355. Meyer, H. F., and Brennemann, J.: A rare osseous dystrophy (Morquio), Amer. J. Dis. Child. **43**:123, 1932.

356. Meyer, K.: Abstracts of 130th Amer. Chem. Soc. Meetings, Sept., 1956, p. 150.

357. Meyer, K.: Chemistry of ground substance. In Asboe-Hansen, G., editor: Connective tissue in health and disease, Copenhagen, 1954, Ejnar Munksgaard, p. 54.

358. Meyer, K. (New York City): Personal communication.

359. Meyer, K., Davidson, E., Linker, A., and Hoffman, P.: The acid mucopolysaccharides of connective tissue, Biochim Biophys. Acta 21:506, 1956.

360. Meyer, K., Grumbach, M. M., Linker, A., and Hoffman, P.: Excretion of sulfated mucopoly-saccharides in gargoylism (Hurler's syndrome), Proc. Soc. Exp. Biol. Med. 97:275, 1958.

361. Meyer, K., and Hoffman, P.: Hurler's syndrome, Arth. Rheum. 4:552, 1961.

362. Meyer, K., Hoffman, P., and Linker, A.: Chondroitin sulfate B and heparitin sulfate (Abstract), Ann. Rheum. Dis. 16:129, 1957.

363. Meyer, K., Hoffman, P., Linker, A., Grumbach, M. M., and Sampson, P.: Sulfated muco-polysaccharides of urine and organs in gargoylism (Hurler's syndrome). II. Additional studies, Proc. Soc. Exp. Biol. Med. 102:587, 1959.

364. Meyer, K., Kaplan, D., and Steigleder, G. K.: Effect of acid mucopolysaccharides on hair growth in the rabbit, Proc. Soc. Exp. Biol. Med. 108:59, 1961.

365. Meyer, K., Linker, A., Davidson, E. A., and Weissman, B.: The mucopolysaccharides of bovine cornea, J. Biol. Chem. 205:611, 1953.

366. Meyer, S. J., and Okner, H. B.: Dysostosis multiplex with special reference to ocular findings, Amer. J. Ophthal. 22:713, 1939.

367. Michail, J., Matsoukas, J., Theodorou, S., and Houliaras, K.: Maladie de Morquio (ostéochondrodystrophie polyépiphysaire déformante) chez deux frères, Helv. Paediat. Acta 11:403, 1956.

368. Millman, G., and Whittick, J. W.: A sex-linked variant of gargoylism, J. Neurol. Neurosurg. Psychiat. 15:253, 1952.

369. Mittwoch, V.: Nuclear segmentation of the neutrophils in heterozygous carriers of gargoylism, Nature 193:1209, 1962.

370. Mittwoch, V. (London): Personal communication, 1964.

371. Moore, W. T., and Federman, D. D.: Familial dwarfism and "stiff joints"; report of a kindred, Arch. Intern. Med. 115:398, 1965.

372. Morquio, L.: Sur une forme de dystrophie osseuse familiale, Arch. Méd. d'Enf. 38:5, 1935.

373. Morquio, L.: Sur une forme de dystrophie osseuse familiale, Bull. Soc. Pédiat. de Paris 27:145, 1929.

374. Morrice, G., Jr., Havener, W. H., and Kapetansky, F.: Vitamin A intoxication as a cause of pseudotumor cerebri, J.A.M.A. 173:1802, 1960.

374a. Morrow, A. G., Greenspan, E. M., and Carroll, D. M.: Comparative studies of liver glu-curonidase activity in inbred mice, J. Nat. Cancer Inst. 10:1199, 1950.

375. Moynahan, E. J.: Hyalinosis cutis et mucosae (lipoid proteinosis); demonstration of a new disorder of mucopolysaccharidosis metabolism, Proc. Roy. Soc. Med. 59:1125, 1966.

376. Muir, H., Mittwoch, V., and Bitter, T.: The diagnostic value of isolated urinary mucopoly-saccharides and of lymphocytic inclusions in gargoylism, Arch. Dis. Child. 38:358, 1963.

377. Murdoch, J. L., and Walker, B. A.: A "new" form of spondylometaphyseal dysplasia. In Bergsma, D., editor: Clinical delineation of birth defects. IV. Skeletal dysplasias, New York, 1969, National Foundation–March of Dimes,

378. Murray, J. F.: Pulmonary disability in the Hurler syndrome (lipochondrodystrophy); a study of two cases, New Eng. J. Med. 261:378, 1959.

379. Naidoo, D.: Gargoylism (Hurler's disease); neuropathological report, J. Ment. Sci. 99:74, 1953.

380. Nécrologie (L. Morquio), Arch. Méd. Enf. 38:579, 1935.

381. Nemeth-Csoka, M.: Untersuchungen über die kollagen Fasern. I. Ueber die submicroscop-ische Struktur der in vitro präzipitierten kollagen Fasern und die stabilisierende Rolle der sauren Mukopolysaccharide, Acta Histochem. 9:282, 1960.

382. Neufeld, E. F., and Fratantoni, J. C.: Inborn errors of mucopolysaccharide metabolism, Science 169:141, 1970.

383. Neufeld, E. F. (Bethesda, Md.): Personal communications, 1971 and 1972.

384. Neuhauser, E. B., Griscom, N. T., Gilles, P. H., and collaborators: Arachnoid cysts in the Hurler-Hunter syndrome, Ann. Radiol. 11:453, 1968.

385. Neuman, W. F.: Chemical dynamics of bone mineral. In Rodahl, K., Nicholson, J. T., and Brown, E. M., editors: Bone as a tissue, New York, 1960, McGraw-Hill Book Co., Inc.

386. Newell, F. W., and Koistinen, A.: Lipochondrodystrophy (gargoylism); pathologic findings in five eyes of three patients, Arch. Ophthal. 53:45, 1955.

387. Nisbet, N. W., and Cupit, B. F.: Gargoylism; report of a case, Brit. J. Surg. **41:**404, 1954.

388. Njå, A.: A sex-linked type of gargoylism, Acta Paediat. **33:**267, 1946.

389. Noller, F.: Dysostosis multiplex (Hurler) und verwandte Krankheitsbilder, Deutsch. Z. Chir. **258:**259, 1943.

390. Nonne, M.: Familiäres Verkommen (3 Geschwister) einer Kombination von imperfekter Chondrodystrophie mit imperfekten Myxoedema infantile, Deutsch. Z. Nervenheilk. **833:** 263, 1925.

391. Norman, A. P.: Gargoylism, Practitioner **202:**409, 1969.

392. Norman, R. M., Tingey, A. H., Newman, C. G. H., and Ward, S. P.: Tay-Sachs disease with visceral involvement and its relation to gargoylism, Arch. Dis. Child. **39:**634, 1964.

393. Norman, R. M., Urich, H., and Tingey, A. H.: Tay-Sachs disease with visceral involvement and its relationship to Niemann-Pick's disease, J. Path. Bact. **78:**709, 1959.

394. Norum, R. A.: Nonkeratosulfate-excreting Morquio syndrome. In Bergsma, D., editor: Clinical delineation of birth defects. IV. Skeletal dysplasias, New York, 1969, National Foundation–March of Dimes.

395. Norum, R. A.: Spondyloepiphyseal dysplasia with quadriplegia from atlantoaxial subluxation. In Bergsma, D., editor: Clinical delineation of birth defects. IV. Skeletal dysplasias, New York, 1969, National Foundation–March of Dimes, pp. 319-321.

396. O'Brien, D., and Ibbott, F. A., editors: Laboratory manual of pediatric micro- and ultra-micro-biochemical techniques, ed. 3, New York, 1962, Harper & Row, Publishers.

397. O'Brien, J.: Generalized gangliosidosis, J. Pediat. **75:**167, 1969.

398. O'Brien, J. S.: Five gangliosidoses (letter), Lancet **2:**805, 1969.

398a. O'Brien, J. S.: Sanfilippo syndrome: profound deficiency of alpha-acetylglucosaminidase activity in organs and skin fibroblasts from type B patients, Proc. Nat. Acad. Sci. **69:**1720, 1972.

399. O'Brien, J. S., Okada, S., Ho, M. W., Fillerup, D. L., Veath, M. L., and Adams, K.: Ganglioside storage diseases, Fed. Proc. **30:**956, 1971.

400. O'Brien, J. S., Stern, M. B., Landing, B. H., O'Brien, J. K., and Donnell, G. N.: Generalized gangliosidosis; another inborn error of ganglioside metabolism? (abstract), J. Pediat. **67:**949, 1965; also Amer. J. Dis. Child. **109:**338, 1965.

401. Öckerman, P. A.: Acid hydrolases in skin and plasma in gargoylism, Clin. Chim. Acta **20:**1, 1968.

402. Öckerman, P. A.: Deficiency of beta-galactosidase and alpha-mannosidase; primary enzyme defects in gargoylism and a new generalized disease, Acta Paediat. Scand. **177:**35, 1967.

403. Öckerman, P. A.: Diseases of glycoprotein storage, Lancet **1:**734, 1969.

404. Öckerman, P. A.: A generalized storage disorder resembling Hurler's syndrome, Lancet **2:** 239, 1967.

405. Öckerman, P. A.: Lysosomal acid hydrolases in the liver in gargoylism; deficiency of 4-methylumbelliferyl-beta-galatcosidase, Scand. J. Clin. Lab. Invest. **22:**142, 1968.

406. Öckerman, P. A.: Mannosidosis; isolation of oligosaccharide storage material from brain, J. Pediat. **75:**360, 1969.

407. Öckerman, P. A.. and Hultberg, B.: Fractionation of 4-methylumbelliferyl-β-galactosidase activities in liver in gargoylism, Scand. J. Clin. Lab. Invest. **22:**199, 1968.

408. Öckerman, P. A., Hultberg, B., and Eriksson, O.: Enzyme patterns in tissues and body fluids in mucopolysaccharidoses, Clin. Chim. Acta **25:**97, 1969.

409. Öckerman, P. A., and Kohlin, P.: Glycosidases in skin and plasma in Hunter's syndrome; abnormality of a beta-galactosidase in skin, Acta Paediat. Scand. **57:**281, 1968.

410. Okada, S., and O'Brine, J. S.: Generalized gangliosidosis; β-galactosidase deficiency, Science **160:**1002, 1968.

411. Okada, R., Rosenthal, I. M., Scaravelli, G., and Lev, M.: A histopathologic study of the heart in gargoylism, Arch. Path. **84:**20, 1967.

412. Onisawa, J., and Lee, T. Y.: Increased urinary excretion of chondroitin sulfate A and C in Hunter's syndrome, Biochem. Biophys. Acta **208:**144, 1970.

413. Osler, W.: Sporadic cretinism in America, Trans. Cong. Amer. Phys. **4:**169, 1897.

413a. Paigen, K.: The genetic control of enzyme realization during differentiation. In Fishbein, M., editor: Congenital malformations, New York, 1963, Int. Med. Congress, pp. 181-190.

413b. Paigen, K.: The genetics of enzyme realization. In Rechcigl, M., editor: Enzyme synthesis and degradation in mammalian systems, Basel, 1971, S. Karger AG, pp. 1-46.

414. Park, E. A., and Powers, G. F.: Acrocephaly and scaphocephaly with symmetrically distributed malformations of the extremities, Amer. J. Dis. Child. **20:**235, 1920.

414a. Patel, V., Watanabe, I., and Zeman, W.: Deficiency of α-L-fucosidase, Science **176:**426, 1972.

415. Pearson, H. A., and Lorincz, A. E.: A characteristic bone marrow finding in the Hurler syndrome, Pediatrics **34:**280, 1964.

416. Pedrini, V., Lenuzzi, L., and Zambotti, V.: Isolation and identification of keratosulfate in urine of patients affected by Morquio-Ullrich disease, Proc. Soc. Exp. Biol. Med. **110:**847, 1962.

417. Pfaundler, M.: Demonstrationen über einen Typus kindlicher Dysostose, Jahrb. Kinderheilk. **92:**420, 1920.

418. Philippart, M., and Sugarman, G. I.: Chondroitin-4-sulphate mucopolysaccharidosis; a new variant of Hurler's syndrome (letter), Lancet **2:**854, 1969.

419. Pichler, E.: Hereditäre Kontrakturen mit sclerodermieartigen Hautveränderungen, Z. Kinderheilk. **104:**349, 1968.

420. Pincus, J. H., Rossi, J. P., and Daroff, R. B.: Delayed development of disturbed mucopolysaccharide metabolism in a Hurler variant, Arch. Neurol. **16:**244, 1967.

421. Pinsky, L., Callahan, J. W., and Wolfe, L. S.: Fucosidosis, Lancet **2:**1080, 1968.

422. Pohl, J. F.: Osteodystrophy (Morquio's disease); progressive kyphosis from congenital wedge-shaped vertebrae, J. Bone Joint Surg. **21:**187, 1939.

423. Poulet, J.: Maladie de Hurler authentique avec intelligence normale chez une adulte et ses deux germains. Sem. Hôp. Paris **119:**457, 1968.

424. Puretič, S., Puretič, B., Fiser-Herman, M., and Adamčić, M.: A unique form of mesenchymal dysplasia, Brit. J. Derm. **74:**8, 1962.

425. Putnam, M. C., and Pelkan, K. F.: Scaphocephaly with malformations of skeleton and other tissues, Amer. J. Dis. Child. **29:**51, 1925.

426. Quigley, H. A., and Goldberg, M. F.: Conjunctival ultrastructure in mucolipidosis III (pseudo-Hurler polydystrophy), Invest. Ophthal. **10:**568, 1971.

427. Quigley, H. A., and Goldberg. M. F.: Scheie syndrome and macular corneal dystrophy; an ultrastructural comparison of conjunctiva and skin, Arch. Ophthal. **85:**553, 1971.

428. Quinton, B. A., Sly, W. S., McAlister, W. H., Rimoin, D. L., Hall, C. W., and Neufeld, E. F.: β-glucuronidase deficiency; a new mucopolysaccharide storage disease (abstract), Proc. Soc. Pediat. Res., 1971.

429. Rainer, S., and Böök, J. A.: Genetics and blood morphology in amaurotic idiocy, Lancet **1:**1077, 1958.

430. Rampini, S.: Der Spät-Hurler, Schweiz. Med. Wschr. **99:**1769, 1969.

431. Rampini, S., and Maroteaux, P.: Ein ungewöhnliche Phänotyp des Hurler-Syndrome, Helv. Paediat. Acta **21:**376, 1966.

432. Rask, M. R.: Morquio-Brailsford osteochondrodystrophy and osteogenesis imperfecta; report of a patient with both conditions, J. Bone Joint Surg. **45-A:**561, 1963.

433. Rebuck, J., and Crowley, J.: A method of studying leukocyte functions in vivo, Ann. N. Y. Acad. Sci. **59:**757, 1955.

434. Reilly, W. A.: An atypical familial endocrinopathy in males with a syndrome of other defects, Endocrinology **19:**639, 1935.

435. Reilly, W. A.: The granules in the leucocytes in gargoylism, Amer. J. Dis. Child. **62:**489, 1941.

436. Reilly, W. A., and Lindsay, S.: Gargoylism, Amer. J. Dis. Child. **75:**595, 1948.

437. Remky, H., and Engelbrecht, G.: Dystrophia dermo-chondro-cornealis (French), Klin. Mbl. Augenheilk. **151:**319, 1967.

438. Rennert, O. M.: Disk electrophoresis of acid mucopolysaccharides, Nature **213:**1133, 1967.

439. Rennert, O. M., and Dekaban, A. S.: Amino acid metabolism in patients with Hurler's syndrome, Metabolism **15:**429, 1966.

440. Renuart, A. W. (Butner, N. C.): Personal communication.

441. Renuart, A. W.: Screening procedures in mentally retarded and/or neurologically abnormal children, Unpublished paper.

442. Rich, C., Di Ferrante, N., and Archibald, R. M.: Acid mucopolysaccharide excretion in the urine of children, J. Lab. Clin. Med. **50:**686. 1957.

442a. Rimoin, D. L. (Torrance, Calif.): Personal communication, 1972.

443. Roaf, R., Longmore, J. B., and Forrester, R. M.: A childhood syndrome of bone dysplasia, retinal detachment and deafness, Develop. Med. Child. Neurol. **9:**464, 1967.

444. Robinow, M.: Morquio's disease, Clin. Orthop. **11:**138, 1958.

445. Robins, M. M., Stevens, H. F., and Linker, A.: Morquio's disease; an abnormality of mucopolysaccharide metabolism, J. Pediat. **62:**881, 1963.

446. Rocher, H.-L., and Pesme, P.: Un cas de pléonostéose (maladie de Léri) avec cornées opalescentes, J. Méd. Bordeaux **123:**121, 1946.

447. Rose, J. R., Hawke, W. A., and Brown, A.: Gargoylism, Arch. Dis. Child. **16:**71, 1941.

448. Rosen, D. A., Haust, M. D., Yamashite, T., and Bryans, A. M.: Keratoplasty and electron microscopy of the cornea in systemic mucopolysaccharidosis (Hurler's disease), Canad. J. Ophthal. **3:**218, 1968.

449. Royer, P.: La cellule de Buhot et le diagnostic du gargoylisme, Sang **30:**37, 1959.

450. Rubin, P.: Dynamic classification of bone dysplasia, Chicago, 1964, Year Book Medical Publishers, Inc.

451. Ruggles, H. C.: Dwarfism due to disordered epiphyseal development, Amer. J. Roentgen. **25:**91, 1931.

452. Rukavina, J. G., Falls, H. F., Holt, J. F., and Block, W. G.: Léri's plenosteosis; a study of a family with review of the literature, J. Bone Joint Surg. **41-AA:**397, 1959.

453. Russell, D. S.: Observations on the pathology of hydrocephalus; special report series, Med. Res. Counc. No. 265, London, 1948, p. 52.

454. Salam, M., and Idriss, H.: Infantile amaurotic family idiocy and gargoylism in siblings, Pediatrics **34:**658, 1964.

455. Sanfilippo, S. J., and Good, R. A.: A laboratory study of the Hurler syndrome (Abstract), Amer. J. Dis. Child. **102:**140, 1964.

456. Sanfilippo, S. J., Podosin, R., Langer, L. O., Jr., and Good, R. A.: Mental retardation associated with acid mucopolysacchariduria (heparitin sulfate type), J. Pediat. **63:**837, 1963.

457. Sanfilippo, S. J., Yunis, J., and Worthen, H. G.: An unusual storage disease resembling the Hurler-Hunter syndrome, Amer. J. Dis. Child. **104:**553, 1962.

458. Sarrouy, C., Farouz, S., Roche, M. T., Sabatini, R., Vaillaud, J. D., and Revol, A.: A propos d'une nouvelle observation de maladie de Hurler, Presse Méd. **73:**3219, 1965.

459. Schafer, I. A., Powell, D. W., and Sullivan, J. C.: Lysosomal bone disease (abstract), Pediat. Res. **5:**391, 1971.

460. Schafer, I. A., Sullivan, J. C., Svejcar, J., Fofoed, J., and Robertson, W. Van B.: Study of the Hurler syndrome using cell culture: definition of the biochemical phenotype and the effects of ascorbic acid on the mutant cell, J. Clin. Invest. **47:**321, 1968.

461. Schafer, I. A., Sullivan, J. C., Svejcar, J., Kofoed, J., and Robertson, W. V.: Vitamin C–induced increase of dermatan sulfate in cultured Hurler's fibroblasts, Science **153:**1008, 1966.

462. Scharf, J.: Ein Beitrag zur Kenntnis der Dysostosis multiplex (Hurler) unter besonderer Berücksichtigung der Erbverhältnisse, Gräefe Arch. Ophthal. **143:**477, 1941.

463. Scheie, H. G., Hambrick, G. W., Jr., and Barness, L. A.: A newly recognized forme fruste of Hurler's disease (gargoylism), Amer. J. Ophthal. **53:**753, 1962.

464. Schenk, E. A., and Haggerty, J.: Morquio's disease, a radiologic and morphologic study, Pediatrics **34:**839, 1964.

465. Schinz, H. R., and Furtwängler, A.: Zur Kenntnis einer hereditären Osteoarthropathie mit rezessivem Erbgang, Deutsch. Z. Chir. **207:**398, 1928.

466. Schmidt, M. B.: Die anatomischen Veränderungen des Skeletts bei der Hurlerschen Krankheit, Zbl. Allg. Path. **79:**113, 1942.

467. Schmidt, R.: Eine bischer nicht beschriebene Form familiäres Hornhautentartung in Verbindung mit Osteoarthropathie, Klin. Mbl. Augenheilk. **100:**616, 1938.

468. Schultze, G., and Lang, E. K.: Disseminated lipogranulomatosis; report of a case, Radiology **74:**428, 1960.

469. Schwarz, H., and Gagne, R.: A case of gargoylism, Canad. Med. Ass. J. **66:**375, 1952.

470. Scott, C. R. (Seattle): Personal communication, 1971.

471. Scott, C. R., Lagunoff, D., and Trump, B. F.: Familial neurovisceral lipidosis, J. Pediat. **71:**357, 1967.

472. Scott, J. E., and Dorling, J.: Differential staining of acid glycosaminoglycans (mucopolysaccharides) by Alcian blue in salt solutions, Histochemie **5:**221, 1965.

473. Sears, H. R., and Maddox, J. K.: A case of Hurler's disease, Med. J. Aust. **1:**488, 1945.

474. Segni, G., Borvelli, A., Tortolo, G., Polidori, G., and Posri, B.: Mucopolisaccaridosis atipica (sindrome di Hurler con chondroitinsulfaturia B), Minerva Pediat. **21**:1943, 1969.

475. Segni, G., Romano, C., and Tortorolo, G.: Diagnostic test for gargoylism (letter), Lancet **2**:420, 1964.

476. Shands, A. R., Raney, R. B., and Brashear, H. R.: Handbook of orthopaedic surgery, ed. 7, St. Louis, 1967, The C. V. Mosby Co.

477. Shelling, D. H.: Osteochondrodystrophia deformans (Morquio's disease). In Brennemann's practice of pediatrics, vol. 4, Hagerstown, Md., 1948, W. F. Prior Co., Inc., chap. 29.

478. Shelling, D. H.: In McQuarrie, I., and Kelley, V. C., editors: Brennemann's practice of pediatrics, Hagerstown, Md., 1959, W. F. Prior Co., Inc., chap. 29.

479. Shy, G. M., Silberberg, D. H., Appel, S. H., Mishkin, M. M., and Godfrey, E. H.: A generalized disorder of nervous system, skeletal muscle and heart resembling Refsum's disease and Hurler's syndrome. I. Clinical, pathologic and biochemical characteristics, Amer. J. Med. **42**:163, 1967.

479a. Silberberg, R., Rimoin, D. L., and Rosenthal, R.: Ultrastructure of cartilage in mucopolysaccharidoses I (the Hurler syndrome) and III (the Sanfilippo syndrome), J. Pediat. (in press, 1972).

480. Singer, H. S., and Schafer, I. A.: White-cell beta-galactosidase activity, New Eng. J. Med. **282**:571, 1970.

481. Singh, M., and Bachawat, B. K.: The distribution and variation with age of different uronic-acid–containing mucopolysaccharides in brain, J. Neurochem. **12**:519, 1965.

482. Singh, S., Petrie, J. G., and Pirozynski, W. J.: Clinicopathological review of ten cases of Morquio's disease, Canad. J. Surg. **5**:404, 1962.

483. Sjolin, S., and Skoog, T.: The clawhand in gargoylism; its pathology and treatment, Acta Paediat. **41**:563, 1952.

484. Slot, G., and Burgess, G. L.: Gargoylism, Proc. Roy. Soc. Med. **31**:1113, 1937.

484a. Sly, W. S., Quinton, B. A., McAlister, W. H., and Rimoin, D. L.: Isolated β-glucuronidase deficiency: clinical report of a new mucopolysaccharidosis, J. Pediat. (in press, 1972).

485. Smith, E. B., Hempelmann, T. C., Moore, S., and Barr, D. P.: Gargoylism (dysostosis multiplex); two adult cases with one autopsy, Ann. Intern. Med. **36**:652, 1952.

486. Smith, R., and McCort, J. J.: Osteochondrodystrophy (Morquio-Brailsford type); occurrence in three siblings, Calif. Med. **88**:55, 1959.

487. Solomon, L.: Heridtary multiple exostosis, Amer. J. Hum. Genet. **16**:351, 1964.

488. Sorsby, A.: Hereditary affections of the retina and choroid, Acta Genet. Med. (Roma) **13**:20, 1964.

489. Spranger, J. W.: Biochemical definition of the mucopolysaccharidoses, Z. Kinderheilk. **108**: 17, 1970.

490. Spranger, J. W.: The genetic mucopolysaccharidoses. In Bergsma, D., editor: Clinical delineation of birth defects. IV. Skeletal dysplasias, New York, 1969, National Foundation–March of Dimes.

491. Spranger, J. W. (Madison, Wis.): Personal communication, 1970.

491a. Spranger, J. W.: The systemic mucopolysaccharidoses, Ergebn. Inn. Med. Kinderheilk. **32**:165, 1972.

492. Spranger, J. W., Filbert, E. F., Tuffli, G. A., Rossiter, F. P., and Opitz, J. M.: Geleophysic dwarfism; a "focal" mucopolysaccharidosis? (letter), Lancet **2**:97, 1971.

493. Spranger, J. W., Koch, F., McKusick, V. A., Natzschka, J., Wiedemann, H. R., and Zellweger, H.: Mucopolysaccharidosis VI (Maroteaux-Lamy's disease), Helv. Paediat. Acta **25**: 337, 1970.

494. Spranger, J. W., and Langer, L. O., Jr.: Spondyloepiphyseal dysplasia congenita, Radiology **94**:313, 1970.

494a. Spranger, J. W., Schuster, W., and Freitag, F.: Chondroitin-4-sulfate mucopolysaccharidosis, Helv. Paediat. Acta **26**:387, 1971.

495. Spranger, J. W., Teller, W., Kosenow, W., Murken, J., and Eckert-Huseman, E.: Die HS-mucopolysaccharidose von Sanfilippo (polydystrophie oligophrenie); Bericht über 10 patienten, Z. Kinderheilk. **101**:71, 1967.

496. Spranger, J. W., and Wiedemann, H. R.: Dysplasia spondyloepiphysaria congenita, Helvet. Paediat. Acta **21**:598, 1966.

497. Spranger, J. W., and Wiedemann, H. R.: The genetic mucolipidoses; diagnosis and differential diagnosis, Humangenetik **9:**113, 1970.

498. Spranger, J. W., Wiedemann, H. R., Tolksdorf, M., Graucob, E., and Caesar, R.: Lipomucopolysaccharidose, eine neue Speicherkrankheit, Z. Kinderheilk. **103:**285, 1968.

499. Stacey, M., and Baker, S. A.: Chemical analysis of tissue polysaccharides, J. Clin. Path. **9:** 314, 1956 (appendix to paper of Bishton et al.[34]).

500. Steen, R. E.: A family consisting of three cases of Hunter's polydystrophy (gargoylism) with cardiac lesions (abstract), Brit. Heart J. **19:**585, 1957; Hunter's polydystrophy (gargoylism) with cardiac lesions and some formes frustes, Brit. Heart J. **21:**269, 1959.

501. Steinbach, H. L., Preger, L., Williams, H. E., and Cohen, P.: The Hurler syndrome without abnormal mucopolysacchariduria, Radiology **90:**472, 1968.

502. Steiness, I.: Acid mucopolysaccharides in urine in gargoylism, Pediatrics **27:**112, 1961.

503. Stern, C.: Principles of human genetics, San Francisco, 1950, W. H. Freeman & Co., Publishers, p. 406.

504. Stern, W. G.: Arthrogryposis multiplex congenita, J.A.M.A. **81:**1507, 1923.

505. Stickler, G. B., Belau, P. G., Farrell, F. J., Jones, J. D., Pugh, D G., Steinberg, A G., and Ward, L. E.: Hereditary progressive arthro-ophthalmopathy, Mayo Clin. Proc. **40:**433, 1965.

506. Stickler, G. B., and Pugh, D. G.: Hereditary progressive arthro-ophthalmopathy. II. Additional observations on vertebral abnormalities, a hearing defect, and a report of a similar case, Mayo Clin. Proc. **42:**495, 1967.

507. Straus, R., Merliss, R., and Reiser, R.: Gargoylism; review of the literature and report of the sixth autopsied case with chemical studies, Amer. J. Clin. Path. **17:**671, 1947.

508. Strauss, L.: The pathology of gargoylism; report of a case and review of the literature, Amer. J. Path. **24:**855, 1948.

509. Strauss, L., and Platt, R.: Endocardial sclerosis in infancy associated with abnormal storage (gargoylism); report of a case in an infant, age 5 months, and review of the literature, J. Mount Sinai Hosp. N. Y. **24:**1258, 1957.

510. Summerfeldt, P., and Brown, A.: Morquio's disease; report of two cases, Arch. Dis. Child. **11:**221, 1936.

511. Suzuki, K.: Cerebral G_{M1}-gangliosidosis; chemical pathology of visceral organs, Science **159:** 1471, 1968.

512. Svennerholm, L.: Gangliosidoses, Biochem. J. **111:**6p, 1969.

513. Swischuk, L. E.: The beaked, notched, or hooked vertebra; its significance in infants and young children, Radiology **95:**661, 1970.

514. Swoboda, W.: Anguläre dorsolumbale Kyphose als unbekanntes skelettzeichen beim konfenitalen Myxöedem, Fortschr. Röentgenstrahl. **73:**740, 1950.

515. Szabo, L., Polgar, J., Vass, Z., and Jozsa, L.: A Hurler's syndrome variant, Lancet **2:**1314, 1967.

516. Taketomi, T., and Yamakawa, T.: Glycolipids of the brain in gargoylism, Jap. J. Exp. Med. **37:**11, 1967.

517. Tayolr, H. E.: The role of mucopolysaccharides in the pathogenesis of intimal fibrosis and arteriosclerosis of the human aorta, Amer. J. Path. **24:**871, 1953.

518. Teller, W. M.: Urinary excretion patterns of individual acid mucopolysaccharides, Nature **213:**1132, 1967.

519. Teller, W. M., Rosevear, J. W., and Burke, E. C.: Identification of heterozygous carriers of gargoylism, Proc. Soc. Exp. Biol. Med. **108:**276, 1961.

520. Terry, K., and Linker, A.: Distinction among four forms of Hurler's syndrome, Proc. Soc. Exp. Biol. Med. **115:**394, 1964.

521. Thannhauser, S.: Lipoidoses; diseases of the cellular lipid metabolism, New York, 1950, Oxford University Press.

522. Thieffry, S., Lyon, G., and Maroteaux, P.: Encephalopathie métabolique associant une mucopolysaccharidose et une sulfatidose, Arch. Franç. Pédiat. **24:**425, 1967.

523. Thomas, G. H.: β-D-galactosidase in human urine; deficiency in generalized gangliosidosis, J. Lab. Clin. Med. **74:**725, 1969.

524. Thomas, J. E.: Gargoylism in the African; report of a case, Cent. Afr. J. Med. **4:**112, 1958.

525. Thomas, L.: Reversible collapse of rabbit ears after intravenous papain, and prevention of recovery by cortisone, J. Exp. Med. **104:**245, 1956.

526. Thomas, L., McCluskey, R. T., Potter, J. L., and Weissmann, G.: Comparison of the effects of papain and vitamin A on cartilage. I. The effects in rabbits, J. Exp. Med. 111:705, 1960.

527. Thompson, G. R., Nelson, N. A., Castor, C. W., and Grobelny, S. L.: A mucopolysaccharidosis with increased urinary excretion of chondroitin-4-sulfate, Ann. Intern. Med. 75:421, 1971.

528. Thompson, G. R., Nelson, N. A., and Grobelny, S. L.: A new mucopolysaccharidosis with increased urinary excretion of chondroitin sulfate A (abstract), Arthritis Rheum. 11:516, 1968.

529. Tondeur, M., and Loeb, H.: Étude ultrastructurelle du foie dans la maladie de Morquio, Pediat. Res. 3:19, 1969.

530. Turman, E. J.: Methods for controlling hereditary defects, Polled Hereford World, p. 10, Sept., 1960.

531. Tuthill, C. R.: Juvenile amaurotic idiocy, Arch. Neurol. Psychiat. 32:198, 1934.

532. Tyler, W. S., Gregory, P. W., and Meyer, K.: Sulfated mucopolysaccharides of urine from brachycephalic bovine dwarfs, Amer. J. Vet. Res. 23:96, 1962.

533. Ullrich, O.: Die Pfaundler-Hurlersche Krankheit; ein Beitrag zum Problem pleiotroper Genwirkung in der Erbpathologie des Menschen, Ergebn, Inn. Med. Kinderheilk. 63:929, 1943.

534. Ullrich, O., and Wiedemann, H. R.: Zur Frage der konstitutionellen Granulationanomalien der Leukocyten in ihrer Beziehung zu enchondralen Dysostosen, Klin. Wschr. 31:107, 1953.

535. Ultmann, J. E., Mutter, R. D., Tannenbaum, M., and Warner, R. R. P.: Clinical, cytologic and biochemical studies in systemic mast cell disease, Ann. Intern. Med. 61:326, 1964.

536. Uzman, L. L.: Chemical nature of the storage substance in gargoylism, Arch. Path. 60:308, 1955.

537. Uzman, L. L.: Personal communication, March 9, 1956.

538. Valentin, B.: Pleonosteosis familiaris (Léri). In Schwalbe-Gruber: Die Morphologie der Missbildungen des Menschen und der Tiere, Part 3, Jena, Gustav Fischer, p. 502.

539. Vanace, P. W., Friedman, S., and Wagner, B. M.: Mitral stenosis in an atypical case of gargoylism; a case report with pathologic and histochemical studies of the cardiac tissues, Circulation 21:80, 1960.

539a. Van Gemund, J. J., Daems, W. T., Vio, P. A. M., and Giesberts, M. A. H.: Electron microscopy of intestinal suction-biopsy specimens as an aid in the diagnosis of mucopolysaccharidoses and other lysosomal storage diseases, Maandschr. Kindergeneesk. 39:211, 1971.

540. Van Hoof, F., and Hers, H. G.: The abnormalities of lysosomal enzymes in mucopolysaccharidoses, Europ. J. Biochem. 7:34, 1968.

541. Van Hoof, F., and Hers, H. G.: Mucopolysaccharidosis by absence of α-fucosidase (letter), Lancet 1:1198, 1968.

542. Van Hoof, F., and Hers, H. G.: L'ultrastructure des cellules hépatiques dans la maladie de Hurler (gargoylisme), C. R. Acad. Sci. 259:1281, 1964.

543. Van Pelt, J. F.: Gargoylism, Thesis, Nijmegen University, 1960.

544. Van Pelt, J. F., and Huizinga, J.: Some observations on the genetics of gargoylism, Acta Genet. (Basel) 12:1, 1962.

545. Veasy, C. A.: Ocular findings associated with dysostosis multiplex and Morquio's disease, Arch. Ophthal. 25:557, 1941.

546. Voisin, J., and Voisin, R.: Un cas d'achondroplasie, Encephale (Paris) 4:221, 1909.

547. Von Alder, A.: Konstitutionell bedingte Granulationsveränderungen der Leucocyten und Knochenveränderungen, Schweiz. Med. Wschr. 80:1095, 1950.

548. Von Noorden, G. K., Zellweger, H., and Ponseti, I. V.: Ocular findings in Morquio-Ullrich's disease, Arch. Ophthal. 64:585, 1960.

549. Waardenburg, P. J., Franceschetti, A., and Klein, D.: Genetics and ophthalmology, vol. 1, Springfield, Ill., 1961, Charles C Thomas, Publisher.

550. Wagner, R.: Glycogen content of isolated white blood cells in glycogen storage disease, Amer. J. Dis. Child. 73:559, 1947.

551. Wallace, B. J., Kaplan, D., Adachi, M., Schneck, L., and Volk, B. W.: Mucopolysaccharidosis type III; morphologic and biochemical studies of two siblings with Sanfilippo syndrome, Arch. Path. 82:462, 1966.

552. Washington, J. A.: Lipochondrodystrophy. In Brennemann's practice of pediatrics, vol. 4, Hagerstown, Md., 1937, W. F. Prior Co., Inc., chap. 30.

553. Watson-Jones, R.: Léri's pleonosteosis, carpal tunnel compression of the median nerves and Morton's metatarsalgia, J. Bone Joint Surg. 31-B:560, 1949.

554. Watt, M. S., and Emery, A. E. H. (Edinburgh): Personal communication, 1971.

555. Weill, R., and Tassin, M. T.: Détection simultanée de polysaccharides acides et de certains protides, Ann. Histochim. 6:145, 1961.

555a. Weissmann, B., and Santiago, R.: α-L-iduronidase in lysosomal extracts, Biochem. Biophys. Res. Commun. 46:1430, 1972.

556. Whiteside, J. D., and Cholmeley, J. G.: Morquio's disease; review of literature with description of 4 cases, Arch. Dis. Child. 27:487, 1952.

557. Wiedemann, H. R.: Ausgedehnte und allgemeine erblich bedingte Bildungs- und Wachstumsfehler des Knochengerüstes, Mschr. Kinderheilk. 102:136, 1954.

558. Wiesmann, U., and Neufeld, E. F.: Scheie and Hurler syndromes: apparent identity of the biochemical defect, Science 169:72, 1970.

559. Wiesmann, U. N., Lightbody, J., Vassella, F., and Herschkowitz, N. N.: Multiple lysosomal enzyme deficiency due to enzyme leakage? (letter), New Eng. J. Med. 284:109, 1971.

560. Winchester, P. H.: Discussion. In Bergsma, D., editor: Clinical delineation of birth defects. IV. Skeletal dysplasias, New York, 1969, National Foundation—March of Dimes, p. 185.

561. Winchester, P. H., Grossman, H., Lim, W. N., and Danes, B. S.: A new acid mucopolysaccharidosis with skeletal deformities simulating rheumatoid arthritis, Amer. J. Roentgen. 106:121, 1969.

562. Wislocki, G. B., and Sognnaes, R. F.: Histochemical reactions of normal teeth, Amer. J. Anat. 87:239, 1950.

563. Wolf, H. G.: Zur Frage der Alder-Anomalie der Leukocyten, Z. Klinderheilk. 75:27, 1954.

564. Wolfe, H. J., Blennerhasset, J. B., and Young, G. F.: Hurler's syndrome; a histochemical study; new techniques for localization of very water-soluble acid mucopolysaccharides, Amer. J. Path. 45:1007, 1964.

565. Wolfe, L. S., Callahan, J., Fawcett, J. S., Andermann, F., and Scriver, C. R.: G_{M1}-gangliosidosis with chondrodystrophy or visceromegaly; β-galactosidase deficiency with gangliosidosis and the excessive excretion of keratan sulfate, Neurology 20:23, 1970.

566. Wolff, D.: Microscopic study of temporal bones in dysostosis multiplex (gargoylism), Laryngoscope 52:218, 1942.

567. Wood, G. C.: The formation of fibrils from collagen solutions. III. The effect of chondroitin sulphate and some other naturally occurring polyanions on the rate of formation, Biochem. J. 75:605, 1960.

568. Woodin, A. M.: The corneal mucopolysaccharide, Biochem. J. 51:319, 1952.

569. Worth, H. M.: The Hurler's syndrome; a study of radiologic appearances in the jaws, Oral Surg. 22:21, 1966.

570. Young, G. F., Wolfe, H. J., and Blennerhassett, J. B.: Mental subnormality in Hunter-Hurler syndrome (gargoylism); a suggested biochemical cause, Develop. Med. Child Neurol. 8:37, 1966.

571. Yuhl, E. T., and Schmitz, A. L.: The occipital emissary channel and increased intracranial pressure, Acta Radiol. [Diagn.] 9:124, 1969.

572. Zeeman, W. P. C.: Gargoylismus, Acta Ophthal. 20:40, 1942.

573. Zellweger, H., Giaccai, L., and Firzli, S.: Gargoylism and Morquio's disease, Amer. J. Dis. Child. 84:421, 1952.

574. Zellweger, H., Ponseti, I. V., Pedrini, V., Stamler, F. S., and von Noorden, G. K.: Morquio-Ullrich's disease, J. Pediat. 59:549, 1961.

575. Zelson, J., and Dekaban, A. S.: Biological behavior of lymphoctyes in Hunter-Hurler's disease, Arch. Neurol. 20:358, 1969.

576. Zierl, F.: Ueber Skelettveränderungen bei der juvenilen Form der amaurotischen Idiotie, Z. Ges. Neurol. Psychiat. 131:400, 1930.

577. Zimmer, J. G., McAllister, B. M., and Demis, D. J.: Mucopolysaccharides in mast cells and mastocytosis, J. Invest. Derm. 44:33, 1965.

578. Zugibe, F. T., Gilbert, E. F., and Gaziano, D.: Glycoprotein storage disease, a new entity, Amer. J. Med. 47:135, 1969.

12 · Other heritable and generalized disorders of connective tissue

In addition to the entities discussed in detail earlier in this book, a considerable number deserve at least brief mention. Some, e.g., fibrodysplasia ossificans progressiva and osteopoikilosis, may qualify as generalized heritable disorders of connective tissue. A large number of others have involvement apparently limited to the osseous skeleton.

FIBRODYSPLASIA OSSIFICANS PROGRESSIVA
Historical note

The name *myositis ossificans progressiva* is said[66] to have been assigned to this condition by von Dusch in 1868. The designation in which fibrositis is substituted for myositis has been used more frequently in recent decades,[25,52,79] since the primary change is in the connective tissues—specifically aponeuroses, fasciae, and tendons—and the muscles are only secondarily affected. (Rosenstirn[66] suggested "fibrocellulitis.") It is not entirely improper to refer to it as fibrositis, since the lesions may appear to be quite inflammatory during early stages. However, "fibrodysplasia," the term suggested by Bauer and Bode,[4] impresses me (as it has Falls[16]) as most valid. "FOP" is the abbreviation that will be used in this discussion. (Some[43] have referred to the condition as Münchmeyer's disease. This seems inappropriate in view of the fact that according to Rosenstirn,[66] Münchmeyer reported the fifteenth case, in 1869.)

In a review of the subject, to which little has since been added, Rosenstirn[66] in 1918 abstracted 119 cases and added his own. The first case may have been described in Guy Patin in 1692. Extraordinarily clear descriptions of the end stages of the disease were provided in the *Philosophical Transactions of the Royal Society of London* in the first half of the eighteenth century by John Freke and others. John Freke (1688-1756), a London surgeon and man of wide culture, was a friend of Fielding, who mentions him twice in *Tom Jones*. Freke saw his case of FOP at St. Bartholomew's Hospital[20]:

April 14, 1736, there came a Boy of a healthy Look and 14 Years of Age, to ask of us at the Hospital, what should be done to cure him of many large Swellings on his Back, which began about 3 Years since, and have continued to grow as large on many Parts as a Penny-loaf, particularly on the left side. They arise from all the *vertebre* of the Neck, and reach down to the *Os sacrum;* they likewise arise from every Rib of his Body, and joining together in all Parts of his Back, as the Ramifications of Coral do, they make, as it were, a fixed bony Pair of Bodice.*

Abernethy, Caesar Hawkins, Jonathan Hutchinson,[37] Volkmann, Kronecker, Virchow, Stephen Paget, Rolleston,[65] Garrod, F. Parkes Weber, Eugene L. Opie, and many others added cases. Since Rosenstirn, other reviews have appeared.[50,51,58] Lutwak estimated that about 260 cases had been reported up to 1963.

Helferich[32] is generally credited with having first described (in 1879) the important association of microdactyly with FOP. The distinctive type of deformity seen in these cases (monophalangy of the great toe) had been described as an isolated anomaly by Fränkel[18] in 1871.

In 1901 Rolleston[65] expressed the opinion that the disease is a defect of the mesoblast. This was probably one of the earliest statements of this idea. It has been stated by many others since that time. For example, Hirsch and Löw-Beer[35] called it an "exceedingly unusual anomaly of the mesenchyme."

Clinical manifestations

The onset of the process in the fasciae and tendons may be in fetal life[37,52,66] or rarely not until after the age of 20 years.[19,31,35] Chaco[9] noted clinical onset at 14 years of age in a boy who had typical microdactyly as well as fusion of some cervical vertebrae. Usually, however, evidences of the disorder appear in the early years of life, before the age of 10 years[53,84]

Typically, localized swellings appear first in the region of the neck and back and later in the limbs. They are sometimes painful. These lumps come and go in a matter of days. Sometimes injury appears to be involved in their inception. The lumps may or may not be attached to deep fascia. Sometimes the tumors are cystic and appear to contain blood. Discharge may occur. At times fever is associated with the development and/or absorption of the tumor. In fact, acute rheumatic fever may be simulated.[67] As the disorder progresses, wryneck deformity may develop. The masseter may also be affected, but the tongue, heart, larynx, diaphragm, and sphincters enjoy immunity from the process. The dorsal aspect of the trunk and the proximal (but usually only the proximal) portions of the extremities may be affected. The plantar and palmar fascia may be involved. At the attachments of fibrous structures to bones it is not uncommon for exostoses to develop—for instance, in the occipital area of the skull or as an anterior calcaneal spur.

Eventually, columns and plates (Fig. 12-2) of bone replace the tendons, fasciae, and ligaments. The spine may become completely rigid and the victims converted into pillars like Lot's wife at Sodom. Koontz' patient[40] "was completely unable to sit down . . . she either had to lie down or stand up. She had enough motion in one of her knee joints so that she could walk with a very halting, mincing step. She was of slight build, weighing very little, and it was simple to carry this plank-like girl around."[41] Fairbank[14] presents drawings of skeletons

---

*From Freke, J.: Philos. Trans. Roy. Soc., London, 1740.

showing extensive changes. Often a ridge of bone on the back appears like a handle by which the patient can literally be lifted.[76]

The skin is usually exempt, as are the muscles of the abdominal wall,* perineum, and eye. Fletcher and Moss[17] described involvement of some facial muscles and of sphincters in a long-standing case. The heart is not affected. Remissions and exacerbations are characteristic of the disease. Hernias may occur with increased frequency.[66]

In spite of marked involvement, patients have survived to fairly advanced years, e.g., 61 years in Case 73 described by Fairbank.[14] The patient who was 17½ years old when studied by Koontz[40] was still living and reasonably well, although severely disabled, at the age of 51 years.[41] She died at the age of 56 years.

Obviously, microdactyly can be a valuable diagnostic sign in the earlier stages of the process of ossification or before calcification has appeared. The great toe (Fig. 12-1) is affected in the great majority of cases, the thumb is affected less frequently (in less than half of cases), and at times other digits are affected. Hallux valgus frequently results and is often what impresses the observer rather than shortening of the digit (Fig. 12-2). Fairbank[14] states that all the fingers were shortened in 2 cases. The shortening is the result of change in the phalangeal bones, rarely in the metatarsals. The proximal phalanx may be completely suppressed. A synostosis of the phalanges of the great toe is perhaps the most typical change. Rosenstirn[66] believed that microdactyly is present in all true cases of FOP. Furthermore, the classic review of digital anomalies by Pol[63] indicates that the changes in FOP (Fig. 12-1) are in all likelihood unique to this condition and, for practical purposes, absolutely pathognomonic. Clinodactyly, radial curvature of the fifth finger, may occur in these cases.

The only other skeletal change that has been seen at all frequently is an abnormally broad neck of the femur[26,78] (Figs. 12-2 and 12-5). In children the epiphyseal ossification centers may be large for the patient's age (Fig. 12-5).

Occasionally there is tendency to bruise with negligible trauma.[26] No defect of coagulation is demonstrable in these instances, however.

Ludman and co-workers[49] described 3 cases of deafness with FOP. Two patients had been deaf from childhood. The possibility of ossifying involvement of the stapedius muscle was considered, but exploration of the middle ear in one showed no abnormality. Lutwak[50] noted partial deafness in 3 of 6 cases, and both of Letts's patients[44,45] had conductive hearing loss.

Review of cases

To my knowledge 12 patients with FOP have been seen in The Johns Hopkins Hospital during the past forty years.† All but 2 are still living. One was reported by Koontz.[40] Two were briefly referred to by Geschickter and Maseritz.[23] In none of these 12 families has another case of FOP been known. All the patients have deformity of the toes and/or fingers. One patient (Case 5) did not notice any abnormality until the age of 25 years, when lumps appeared above one knee. In another patient (Case 3) torticollis was noted at 1 month of age, and advanced

---

*Case 8 on p. 698 is an exception to this statement.
†Barker's case[2] was probably calcinosis universalis and not FOP.

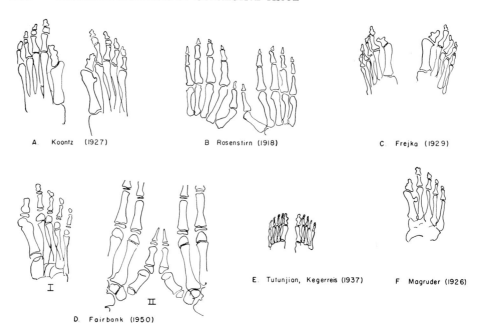

A. Koontz (1927) B. Rosenstirn (1918) C. Frejka (1929)

D. Fairbank (1950) E. Tutunjian, Kegerreis (1937) F. Magruder (1926)

Fig. 12-1. Tracings of x-ray films of hands and feet in selected reported cases (these are not reproduced to the same scale). **A,** Koontz[40]: Hands little affected. In feet, monophalangeal first digit and biphalangeal fifth digit. On the right the fourth toe is also biphalangeal. There are an exostosis on the first right metatarsal and a bone bridge between metatarsals on the left. **B,** Rosenstirn[66]: The short, pointed terminal phalanx of the thumb is typical. The first metacarpal on the left is abnormal in shape. (Frequently the first metacarpal and metatarsal have a disorganized trabecular pattern.) The terminal phalanges of the other digits, especially the second and third, are also short and pointed. **C,** Frejka[19]: The fingers were not commented on. The first toe is monophalangeal and the others are biphalangeal at the most. Typical hallux valgus is present. **D,** Fairbank[15]: **I,** 7 years of age. First metatarsal appears to have been lengthened by fusion with the proximal phalanx. The other toes are all biphalangeal. **II,** 10 years of age. The characteristic short, pointed terminal phalanx is seen. There was also microdactyly of the great toes. **E,** Tutunjian and Kegerreis[76]: No comment on the state of the hands. It is interesting to note that a monophalangeal first toe can be present without microdactyly or hallux valgus. **F,** Magruder[51]: Typical monophalangy of first toe and biphalangy of others. Note exostosis like that in Koontz's patient. **G,** Griffith[26]: Typically short, pointed terminal phalanx of thumbs and of other fingers. Clinically the fifth fingers were curved (clinodactylous). The great toes were monophalangeal. **H,** Michelsohn[56]: First toes are monophalangeal; fifth toes are biphalangeal. Typical thumbs. **I,** Vastine, Vastine, and Arango[78]: Identical twins. Monophalangy of first toes. Biphalangy of fourth and fifth toes. **J,** van Creveld and Soeters[77]: 5 years of age. Typical thumb. **K,** Mather[54]: Monophalangeal first toe. Biphalangeal fifth toe. It is noteworthy that in the feet of many of the patients in the illustrated cases of FOP, sesamoid bones have been conspicuous by their absence. In their place, projections similar to exostoses occur, particularly at the distal end of the first metatarsal. It is likely that these "exostoses" are synostoses of sesamoid bones with the metatarsal.

FOP was present when he was seen at the age of 16 months. In the literature there is a slight and nonsignificant predominance of males affected; 4 of the 11 are female. Serum alkaline phosphatase values have not been in excess of values anticipated on the basis of age.

Abstracts of these 12 cases follow:

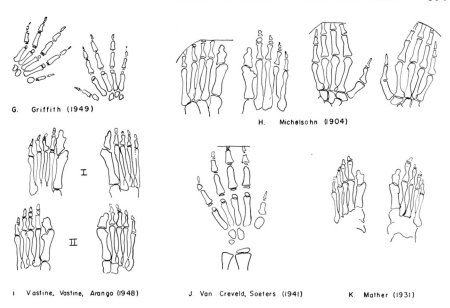

G.   Griffith (1949)

H.   Michelsohn (1904)

I

II

I Vastine, Vastine, Arango (1948)

J Van Creveld, Soeters (1941)

K. Mather (1931)

Fig. 12-1, cont'd. For legend see opposite page.

Case 1. The case of N. J., born in 1908, was reported by Koontz[40] in 1927, with excellent illustrations of the gross appearance and radiologic changes, including those of the thumbs and great toes. The maternal grandfather and his 2 brothers developed late in life what apparently were Dupuytren contractures. A cousin on the maternal side apparently had a deformity of the toes similar to the patient's. The patient's first symptom was stiffness at the age of 9 years. Menstruation never occurred. Both great toes and thumbs were short and malformed. Concentrations of calcium and phosphorus in the blood were normal. I examined the patient in April, 1956. She was then 48 years of age. The disease had progressed slowly but steadily. The jaw was partially fixed, she could not sit, and the arms were in an absolutely fixed position, with a minimum of wrist motion present. Using a long-handled fork and standing up, the patient was able to feed herself. This patient died in 1964 (at 56 years of age) of heart failure. Autopsy showed moderate coronary arteriosclerosis and pulmonary fibrosis. The mechanism of the heart failure was not entirely clear.

Case 2. B. W. (A85874), a 7½-year-old white girl, has a normal brother and sister. The father had stunting of the great toes similar to the patient's, but no other instance of FOP is known in the family. At 10 months, when the patient began to sit up, the head leaned to the left. At the age of 6½ years, she developed an exostosis on the right knee after trauma. However, she remained apparently well otherwise until the age of about 7 years, when she began to complain of pain in the left side of her neck, and firmness and tenderness were discovered there. Thereafter, swelling and induration developed on the back, abdomen, and shoulder. There was marked limitation of motion of the neck, arms, and spine, and the head was held to the left. Dermatomyositis was the initial diagnosis. See Fig. 12-2 for x-ray studies of this patient.

Follow-up (1971, 27 years old). After four years without a flare-up, the patient developed lesions at many sites and stiffness in both elbows, so that it became impossible for her to feed herself. An adrenal steroid (Medrol) has been administered for the last six months with apparent benefit. She is able to get about well and has no recognized hearing loss. Her jaw has limited motion. She is able to feed herself with a long-handled fork and drink with a long straw.

Case 3. R. W. (A62462) was found at birth to have hallux valgus and short thumbs. At 1 month the head was noted to be bent to the left and there was a firm mass in the sternocleidomastoid muscle. Thereafter asymmetry of the face developed. Lumps appeared in many areas over the back and scalp. These masses never appeared inflamed. There were, however, frequent bouts of unexplained fever. Examination revealed atrophy of the left side of the face. The sternocleidomastoid muscle on the left was converted into a stony hard mass. The ligamentum nuchae was similarly affected. Extensive involvement about the scapulae (which were attached to the ribs) and the trapezius muscle formed a yoke on the back.

Follow-up (1971, 24 years old). The disorder appeared to become quiescent at puberty. He was graduated from architectural school but encountered difficulty obtaining a job because of his disability. He walks without aids, dresses himself, and eats regular food, although jaw motion is moderately limited. He is unable to sit and must recline because of fixation of the pelvic girdle. Hearing is defective and he uses a hearing aid in the ear to which he is able to reach his hand.

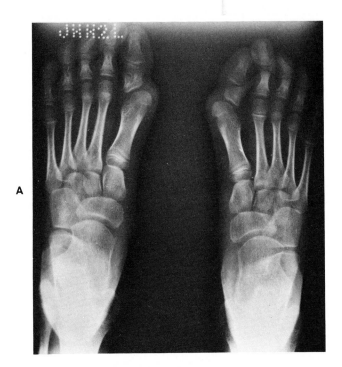

A

Fig. 12-2. X-ray studies in Case 2 of FOP (see text). As demonstrated in **A,** there was distortion of the contour of the distal tip of the first metatarsal and of the proximal phalanges, resulting in the hallux valgus deformity seen clinically. It is of note that in this case a normal number of phalangeal bones are present in all the toes. This is, as will be seen from inspection of Fig. 12-1, the exception; as a rule, monophalangy of the great toes at least is present. It will be interesting to see if synostosis occurs in the future, as was observed to occur in Michelsohn's patient.[56] The hands were normal. As demonstrated in **B,** the neck of the right femur is slightly widened and blunted; immediately adjacent to the epiphyseal line the left femur is normal. Anomalous bone is seen on each side of the lower lumbar spine, especially the left. The ossification in the axillary areas, **C,** has the appearance of cortical bone. In places, it resembled the ribs in contour. At least one false joint was identified. In the lateral view of the lumbar spine, **D,** plates of bone are clearly demonstrated on the back. **E** and **F,** Although all other features of Case 2 are typical of FOP, the hands do not show the usual changes. The thumbs are normal. Osteoporosis and unusually slender radius and ulna bones are demonstrated in the x-ray films taken at 19 years of age. (The x-ray films shown in **A** to **D** were made at the age of 8 years.) **G** and **H,** At 19 years of age, the patient shows relatively fixed position of the arms, involvement of the anterior abdominal musculature by ossification, and short great toes. (By the age of 19 years, fusion of the phalanges of the great toe was complete, creating monophalangy!)

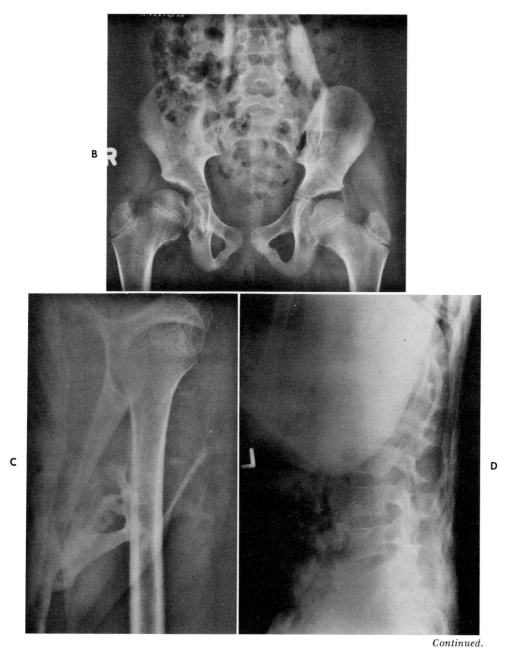

Continued.

Fig. 12-2, cont'd. For legend see opposite page.

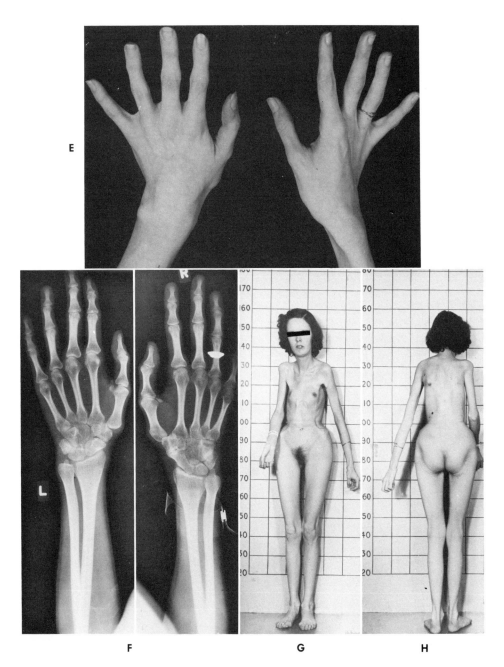

Fig. 12-2, cont'd. For legend see p. 692.

Case 4. V. W. (U52691) has 7 siblings, but none has either microdactyly or FOP. She was presumably well until the age of 6 years, when she fell from a swing, striking her back. Swelling and discoloration resulted. X-ray films at that time revealed "a spider's web on the spine." Thereafter, there was a steadily progressive increase in stiffness and limitation of motion of joints. The thumbs and toes had always been small. It is of note that the facial muscles were involved in this case. By the age of 25 years the jaws became locked and the upper teeth had to be removed to permit alimentation. (See Fig. 12-3 for drawings of this patient.)

Follow-up (1971). The patient died in 1965 at the age of 57 years after a severe respiratory infection.

Case 5. F. K. (U52689) was well until the age of 25 years, when he developed a "bump" above one knee after trauma. During the following year there were several episodes of soreness and swelling in the left side of the neck, with difficulty in swallowing. There are 6 siblings. No other members of the family had microdactyly or ossification. The patient's thumbs were small, with fusion of the interphalangeal and metacarpophalangeal joints (Fig. 12-4). All the terminal phalangeal joints of the second and fourth fingers were fused. Hearing was impaired bilaterally. As long as the patient could remember, he had had restriction of motion of the head, mandible, both shoulders, right elbow, both thumbs, both hips, left knee, left ankle, and toes of the left foot. Supposedly, poliomyelitis affecting mainly the left leg had occurred at 5 years of age, but suspicion is cast on the diagnosis by later developments. When restudied in 1963 this patient was found to be remarkably little changed from the state described and photographed thirty years previously. Review of the history indicated that in childhood he was never very active and that severe incapacitation probably began in his teens. As had been true thirty years earlier, he was rendered almost immobile by his disease and showed striking changes in the thumbs and great toes. The thumb was monophalangeal. The distal two phalanges of the index fingers were also fused, as were some of the proximal row of the carpal bones. In the feet a single blocklike bone replaced the first metatarsal and phalanges of the first toe. The second, third, and fourth metatarsals were fused with the proximal phalanges. The tarsal bones showed striking fusion with one another and with the metatarsals. The ankle joints were completely fused, as was also the spine, both the vertebral bodies and the apophyseal joints being affected. This is the most severe instance of bony fusions in this series. The deafness was of mixed conductive and nerve type. Although old otitis media was proposed as the cause, ossicle fusion seems possible.

Follow-up (1971, 63 years old). The patient's condition continues unchanged and on the whole he "gets along" remarkably well. Chronic constipation is a problem. Vomiting spells appear to be related to it. This man probably holds a record for survival with this disease.

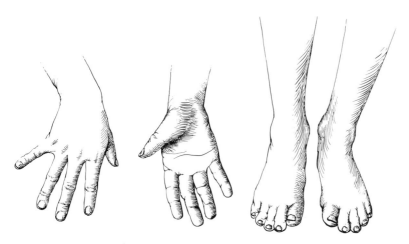

Fig. 12-3. Drawings of the hands and feet of patient described in Case 4 of the FOP series (see text). Microdactyly of the thumbs and toes is strikingly demonstrated.

Case 6. M. W. (422628) was seen at the age of 14 years, and a diagnosis of calcinosis of the muscles of both hips was rendered. However, on retrospect there can be no question that FOP was actually present. The boy had always been stiff, and after a blow on the back at the age of 5 years, a lump on the left scapula was noted. The mass was biopsied and called sarcoma. The boy was given only three months to live; he is still alive, although disabled, at the age of 27 years. Other lumps appeared, and flexion contracture of the hips and right knee gradually developed. The left great toe was short and deformed.

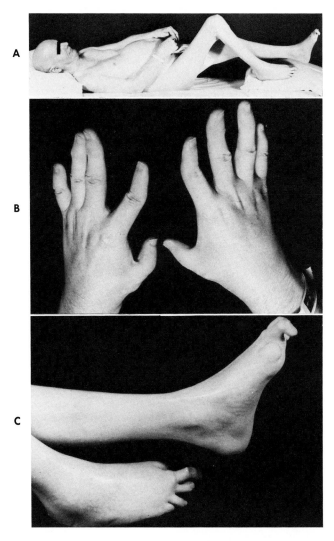

Fig. 12-4. Patient presented in Case 5 at the age of 55 years. He is almost immobile in the position shown, **A.** Short thumbs, **B,** and short great toes, **C,** are shown. The great toes never had a nail. As shown in **D,** the thumb has a single bone mass comprising fused metacarpal and phalanges. The two distal phalanges of the index and little fingers are also fused. In the foot, **E,** the great toe likewise has a single bone mass comprising fused metatarsal and phalanges. **F,** Bony bridges between lumbar vertebrae and the wing of the ilium and between the femur and pelvis are shown. These x-ray films were made in 1933. X-ray studies made in 1963 showed no change.

Case 7. P. H. (770577), born Oct. 4, 1951, had, as his first manifestation of FOP, the appearance (in 1954) of transient, nontender "bumps" in the posterior part of the scalp. A biopsy diagnosis of neurofibromatosis was made. The correct diagnosis was made in October, 1956, by which time typical ossifying changes in the aponeuroses of the back had developed. A striking feature at that time was local heat over the involved areas of the back. The thumbs and toes were characteristically short. Two older siblings, born in 1947 and 1949, are normal and no definite abnormality has been detected in members of the family. Other features of note include short, broad femoral necks and exostosis-like spurs on the upper end of each tibia at the site of muscle attachments. (See Fig. 12-5.) Steroid therapy undoubtedly suppresses acute inflammatory phases in this patient. It probably had no effect on the ossification process. (See Lutwak[50] for further details on this patient.)

Follow-up (1971). The patient is a prelaw student and does well academically. He is able

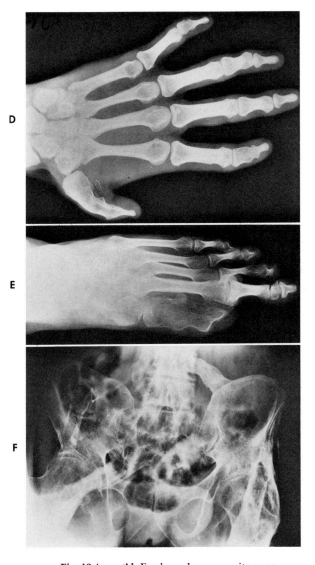

Fig. 12-4, cont'd. For legend see opposite page.

to care for himself completely, can sit in a chair, and lives in a dormitory. His hearing is unimpaired. Occasional small lumps appear on his back. He no longer takes cortisone but for several years has been on continuous tetracycline therapy.

Case 8. C. A. B. (1136294), born May 22, 1960, was noted at birth to have "bunions" on both feet. At approximately 2 weeks of age the mother noted that the infant's head could not be turned to one side. A physician rendered a diagnosis of wryneck. Heat, swelling, and firmness of the sternocleidomastoid and other neck muscles were progressive, and right sternocleidomastoid myomectomy was performed at the age of 1 year. Between 2 and 3 years of age she began to develop bony protuberances over the posterior chest wall. A characteristic evolution beginning with erythema, swelling, and warmth characterized the lesions. By 4½ years of age marked immobilization of the head and shoulder girdle with restriction of thoracic expansion had developed. As well as an extensive posterior truncal development of bone, the anterior abdominal wall contained firm lumps and plates. Mobility of the lower extremities was little if any reduced. The great toes were monophalangeal and short, with hallux valgus. The thumbs ap-

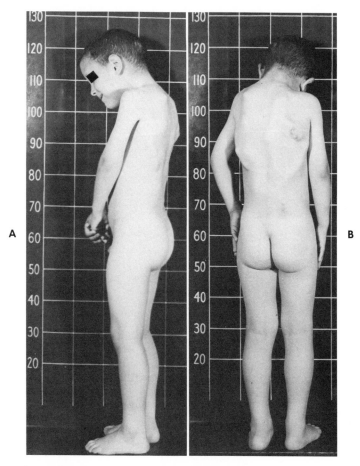

Fig. 12-5. Case 7. **A,** Lateral view (June, 1958). **B,** Rear view (June, 1958). **C,** Feet, showing microdactyly of great toes. **D,** X-ray film of feet (April, 1957). **E,** Occiput, showing ossified nodule. Note the ossification in the tissues of the posterior part of the neck. **F** and **G,** The neck of the femur is short and broad (1954 and 1957). **H,** Exostoses of the tibia at site of tendon attachment. **I,** Extensive ossification of nuchal ligament and adjacent ligaments. **J,** Short thumbs mainly because of short first metacarpals.

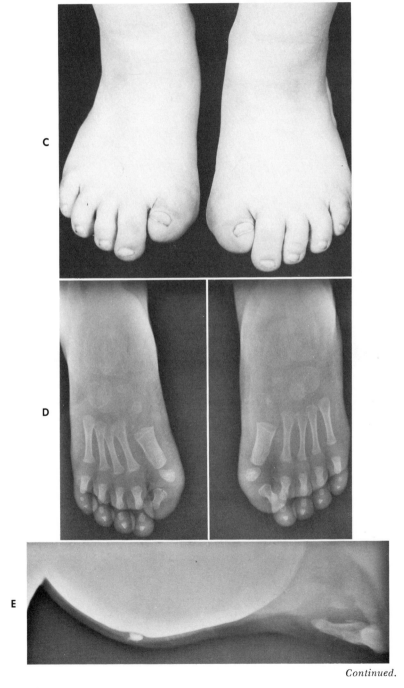

Continued.

Fig. 12-5, cont'd. For legend see opposite page.

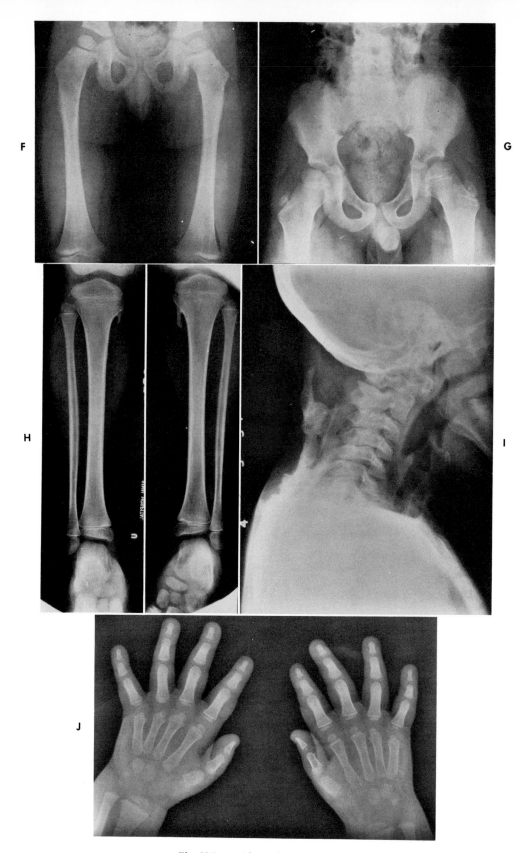

Fig. 12-5, cont'd. For legend see p. 698.

peared normal and were normal by x-ray study. As in Case 7, ossified tendinous insertions suggesting exostoses of diaphyseal aclasis were seen in the distal femur, radius, and ulna and the proximal humerus.

Follow-up (1971). The patient is severely incapacitated with involvement of the masseter, cervical, paraspinal, and abdominal muscles and ankylosis of the shoulders and hips. An ossific contracture of the right hip was accompanied by subluxation. Several teeth were removed to facilitate feeding. In 1969 exostoses were removed from the spine and both scapulae. Ulceration had developed over the bony prominences.

Case 9. J. U. (1011125), born December, 1959, first developed "lumps" in the scalp above the ears at 18 months of age. The thumbs and first toes were noted to be small at birth. Progressive involvement of the back, axillae, and arms led to complete immobility of the upper trunk, neck, shoulders, and elbows. At age 5½ years, he was still able to feed himself and, because of relatively little involvement of the legs, to play actively. The arms were small. The knees and ankles were prominent. No new lesions had appeared for over a year, the last one being on the bottom of the left foot. Lesions on the back had ulcerated with extrusion of calcific material but then healed satisfactorily. The patient is the youngest of 4 children of normal parents who were 41 (father) and 35 years old at the time of his birth. The oldest of the 4 children died of brain tumor at 6 years of age.

Follow-up (1971). The patient has marked shoulder-girdle limitation. Although surgical mobilization by excision of bony bridges was considered, no such procedures have been performed. He has a chronically ulcerated area over the left ankle.

Case 10. D. S. (1257571), a white male born June 6, 1967, was noted at birth to have short first toes. The thumbs were normal. At the age of 2 weeks a left sternomastoid tumor was noted, and at 1 month a hard, movable subcutaneous nodule about 3 cm. in diameter was seen over the sixth thoracic vertebra. By 3 months of age this nodule had begun to calcify. The diagnosis of FOP was made in October, 1967, when calcification of the sternocleidomastoid muscle was noted. By the age of 8 months motion of the head, especially to the left, was limited and nodules were present on the back of the head. At 5 months of age a fall resulted in right occipital skull fracture. Salaam-type seizures began about that time. The electroencephalogram was abnormal, evolving into a typical hypsarrhythmia pattern by February, 1968. Neurologic examination suggested left-sided hemiparesis. At this writing (1971) the disorder appears to be quiescent. The parents were 41 (father) and 36 years of age at the time of his birth.

Case 11. D. C. H. (1289606), a white male born Oct. 17, 1967, was noted at birth to have short first toes that turned inward and were loose-jointed. In the first week of life a nodule was noted on his back. This was removed at 6 weeks of age. Two more growths were removed from above the scar, and a larger mass, which extended almost to the crest of the ilium, was excised in February, 1968. Thereafter a generalized firm thickening over the entire back developed, with limitation of spinal motion. Excised masses were described as showing, microscopically, interlacing strands of "tumor cells" replacing muscle and dermis. The "tumor cells" were spindle-shaped and had central nuclei with a scanty amount of cytoplasm. A few scattered mitotic figures were seen. X-ray films showed an extensive plate of ossification extending from the sacral to the thoracic areas of the back. An exostosis was demonstrated on the medial aspect of the proximal tibial metaphysis at a site of muscle attachment. The parents were 32 (father) and 34 years of age at the time of his birth. On a diet low in calcium and vitamin D, the patient has grown normally and has shown no radiologic evidence of rickets, but the FOP process has continued to progress.

Case 12. S. E. (1430061), a white male, was born Nov. 20, 1969, to a 21-year-old mother and a 40-year-old father. The parents were unrelated. A child born in March, 1972, is normal. Bilateral hallux valgus was noted at birth. No trauma to the neck during delivery was recalled. At 3 months of age a pea-sized swelling appeared over the occiput. By 4½ months of age it was the size of a hen's egg. The second swelling noted was behind the left ear. Several swellings over the calvaria appeared and regressed spontaneously. Limitation of head motion due to restriction in the left side of the neck progressed to frank torticollis by the age of 4 months. Strabismus was first noted at about the same time but may have been present from birth. Facial asymmetry due to torticollis was evident from the age of 6 months. At the age of 8 months FOP was diagnosed on the basis of radiographically demonstrated ossification in the left sternocleidomastoid muscle, with associated phalangeal anomalies and hallux valgus. Fracture of the ossified sternomastoid occurred with a fall at the age of 18 months.

Examination (October, 1971) showed left torticollis, left facial hypoplasia, and left convergent strabismus due to left rectus palsy. The head was tilted to the left and forward with rotation of the face to the right. Well-circumscribed nodules were palpable over the parietal area of the skull and a rocky protuberance over the left mastoid area. Much of the left sternocleidomastoid was replaced by a bony mass. Both first toes were small with valgus deformity. The fifth fingers showed clinodactyly. The thumbs were biphalangeal but small, especially the left.

Radiologic studies showed no paraspinal ossification. The femoral necks were broad. Exostoses were seen at the site of muscle attachment at the lateral aspect of each tibia proximally.

Forced duction of the eye globes under anesthesia showed full movements, and the histology of the ocular muscles was normal, thus excluding FOP at that site.

The patient was treated with disodium editronate 20 mg./kg. b.w., and after 6 weeks the ossified mass of the left sternomastoid was excised. He was maintained in a halo cast for 8 weeks after operation. At ten weeks after operation, passive extension and left lateral flexion of the neck were measured as 20°, both having been 10° before operation.

Prevalence and inheritance

In 1918 Rosenstirn,[66] in reviewing this disorder, could find 119 cases in the literature. In later reviews[52,58] other cases have been added. Lutwak[50] found about 260 well-documented cases. As noted later, Geho and Whiteside,[22a] who have been supervising a drug trial, had treated 52 cases of FOP for a period of more than 6 months. The total group called to their attention or under treatment for a period shorter than 6 months is appreciably larger! The disease is appreciably more frequent in males, in a ratio of 4:1 according to some[67] but 3:2 by the statement of others. In Rosenstirn's collection of cases, 62% were male (68 males and 40 females, of cases clearly described as to diagnosis and sex). On the other hand, two thirds of the large series of patients on the treatment program of Geho and Whiteside were female.

Sympson[73] reported microdactyly in father and son, with FOP in the son, and Stonham[72] reported the same situation. Drago[10] observed the same situation in a mother and son. Koontz[40] described "contractures of two fingers" in 4 relatives of the patient. The anomaly apparently developed later in life, however, and may have been Dupuytren's contracture. Burton-Fanning and Vaughan[8] described FOP (the full syndrome) in both father and son. Gaster[22] observed the disorder, including phalangeal deformity, in 5 male members of three generations—3 brothers, the father, and the paternal grandfather. Vastine and co-workers[79] and Eaton and associates[12] each saw FOP in both of a pair of identical twins. It may be that this disease trait is dominant, with a particularly wide range of expressivity. Almost all cases are the result of new dominant mutation; very few of the patients have children to whom the disease can be transmitted. Laluque and colleagues[43] described FOP in a 16-year-old African girl in Douala, Cameroon, who gave birth to an apparently normal offspring. No comment was made on digital anomaly in either mother or child. All 23 patients studied by Becker and von Knorre[5] and by Tünte and associates[75] were sporadic.

There seems to be no increase in consanguineous marriages among the parents. Multiple affected sibs, except for identical twins, are rare. Viparelli[80] pointed out increased parental age in sporadic cases, suggesting that these represent new dominant mutations. Tünte and associates[75] confirmed the paternal age effect on the basis of 23 patients whose cases they collected anew and 16 found in the literature. The mean paternal age was 36.3 years, a value very similar to that which has been found in sporadic cases of the Marfan syndrome

(p. 150) and of achondroplasia (p. 757). The karyotype have been found normal in several patients,[44,75] including several in my series.

Pathology

The early histologic changes are not known. Obviously it is these changes which are of most significance in reference to the basic abnormality. It is clear[27] that the skeletal muscle is fundamentally normal. Geschickter and Maseritz[23] picture cartilage and also "young osteoid tissue surrounded by osteoblasts." The surgical pathologist may find it difficult to distinguish FOP from osteogenic sarcoma. In the case described by Paul[62] both were thought to have been present.

Localized ossifying tumors of soft tissue have been classified by some as myositis ossificans but are clearly a distinct entity that does not occasion confusion with FOP.[1]

The basic defect

Smith and co-workers[70] and Chaco[9] supported the view that FOP is primarily a myopathy. The conclusion was based on the findings of biopsy and of electromyography. Selye and associates[69] suggested that a useful model of FOP is the ossification that develops in the heart of the rat after a ligature is placed around the lower third of the ventricles.

That the fundamental disorder resides in connective tissue seems more likely, however. Isolated bone tissue may be found in the skin,[66] well removed from muscles. No aberration of calcium metabolism has been demonstrated. In one case (P. H., 770577) ossification began in the galea aponeurotica. The serum transaminase activity was normal during stages of activity of the disease, as manifested by fever, leukocytosis, and local heat. Because of the similarities of behavior to the calcification and ossification that occur after traumatic and other injury which involves necrosis of tissue, one suspects that this disorder is fundamentally a dystrophy of connective tissue, with secondary calcification. Rosenstirn[66] believed that the fundamental defect resides in the small blood vessel and that the initial lesion is a hemorrhage that is followed by organization and ossification.

The observations of Wilkins and associates[83] are important and point the way to an area of possibly productive investigation by other techniques, such as tissue culture of fibroblasts from these patients. Specifically they found a very high level of alkaline phosphatase activity in the areas of heterotopic cartilage and bone formation. The activity was, in fact, higher than in normal rib. Lins and Abath[47] also found high alkaline phosphatase activity in biopsy material, and by histochemical methods. Herrmann and colleagues[34] found high levels of alkaline phosphatase in cultured fibroblasts. On the other hand, Letts[45] could not show an increase in activity of alkaline phosphatase in tissue from an area of apparent activity.

Emphasizing that the proposal is merely hypothesis, Lutwak[50] cautiously suggested that a congenital deficiency of an inhibitor material or a relative excess of an inhibitor-destroying mechanism may be present in FOP. The hypothesis was based on the suggestion of the Neumans[57] and Glimcher.[24] Collagen everywhere in the body exists in a crystalline configuration conforming to that of calcium hydroxyapatite. Bone mineral crystallization occurs on collagen fibers, probably by a mechanism of epitaxy (crystal seeding). Calcium and phosphate are present in tissue fluids in concentrations adequate for crystallization. It has been postulated that normally a circulating inhibitor of crystallization is present, preventing mineral deposition. At sites of bone formation, the inhibitor is thought to be destroyed, permitting mineralization to occur.

An alternative hypothesis in FOP is the presence of an abnormal collagen capable of supporting ossification at abnormal sites.

An enigmatic feature of this syndrome has been the association of an anomaly of the conventional congenital type, microdactyly, with the other cardinal component, ectopic ossification, which behaves more like a hereditary weakness of some element of connective tissue. Previously, in discussing the explanation for the association of congenital anomalies of conventional types with hereditary disorders that behave more like abiotrophies, it was proposed that the presence of a basic tissue defect results in an abnormal environment for embryologic development, so that specific congenital defects occur predictably with increased incidence. Such may be the case with the microdactyly of FOP. Certainly, a disorder of normally ossified tissues is not too farfetched an association. However, a more straightforward explanation is possible. There is an intriguing set of observations reported by Michelsohn,[56] suggesting that in connection with the abnormality of growth of the first digits in FOP, there is no sharp distinction between antenatal and postnatal developments. The patient in question was a 17-year-old girl when seen. In the first months of life the mother noted pronounced shortening and stiffening of the great toes, with no morphologic or functional abnormality of the thumbs. At the age of 7 years, when the changes in the muscle were beginning, the thumbs became painfully swollen, later stiff, and then ankylosed. By definition the change in the great toes was synostosis and that in the thumbs, ankylosis. However, it may be that the same basic process was operating in both instances. The predominant and usually unique involvement of the first digit may be related to the difference in the growth pattern of the first digit as compared with the others.

The malformation of the digits appears to occur in the fairly regular manner of a Mendelian autosomal dominant trait; ossification occurs in less predictable fashion. The factors determining whether ossification will occur in a given case of microdactyly are entirely obscure. Rosenstirn[66] reported that both FOP and microdactyly occurred in a setter dog. Generalized myositis ossificans progressiva, apparently without digital abnormality, has been described in pigs[68] and is probably a dominant trait in that species: a boar and 34 of 115 pigs sired by it were affected.

Other considerations

In the differential diagnosis, calcinosis universalis, dermatomyositis, Weber-Christian disease, and other conditions must come under consideration. The picture suggests torticollis in the early stages.[52] Calcinosis universalis is probably basically a "collagen vascular" disease with secondary calcification.[82] It is certainly not a heritable disorder. The patient described by Barker,[2] a Negro male who was for many months on the wards of The Johns Hopkins Hospital, probably had calcinosis universalis and not FOP. FOP has been described in American Negroes and Africans.[13,43] Local myositis ossificans, a disorder fundamentally distinct from FOP, has been observed in many sites, including the larynx[60] and the muscles of mastication.[33,61,74]

The reported occurrence of FOP and XXXXY syndrome in brothers[34] was probably a coincidence. Frame and his associate[17a] described FOP and polystotic fibrous dysplasia in the same patient. Again, there is probably no connection between the two.

Beryllium has been used in the treatment of FOP.[76] Since beryllium suppresses alkaline phosphatase activity,[28,39] there might be some rationale for this therapy. This effect of beryllium was, however, unknown in 1937 when it was used; furthermore, its benefit was, at the most, doubtful. Adrenocortical hormones were used in Case 2 and in patients reported in the literature.[48,64] Again, benefit is, at the most, dubious. Somewhat encouraging results in an early and active case were described by Riley and Christie,[64] but no benefit was noted in an old, probably static case. In other instances[234] steroids did no good even when given early. X-ray therapy may aggravate the condition. Lutwak[50] found that the course of the disease was unaffected by treatment with hydrocortisone, dexamethasone, triiodothyronine, propylthiouracil, or disodium ethylenediaminetetraacetate (EDTA). Liberman and co-workers[46] thought that EDTA in a comparable situation—traumatic myositis ossificans with an unusually progressive course—was beneficial, causing disappearance of local inflammatory signs and normalization of alkaline phosphatase.

Bassett and colleagues[3] reported that diphosphonates (disodium-ethane-1-hydroxy-1, 1-diphosphate, or EHDP) had beneficial effects in early cases of FOP. The agent had previously been shown to prevent deposition of calcium *in vivo* and *in vitro*.

Weiss and associates[81] treated a severely disabled 21-year-old man with sodium etidronate and observed progressive increase in mobility of many joints, including the temporomandibular, increase in ability to ambulate, and a rise in the vital capacity from increased rib cage mobility. These improvements were accomplished, they felt, without demineralization of skeletal bone. By June, 1972, Geho and Whiteside[22a] had treated 52 cases of FOP for at least 6 months and for a mean time of 1½ years. The majority of these patients seemed to be "stabilized" or somewhat improved while on EHDP. Withdrawal of EHDP in several patients resulted in each case in exacerbation of the disease process. Reinstitution of EHDP therapy was accompanied by symptomatic relief.

A patient (Case 11, above) treated with a diet low in calcium and vitamin D experienced progression of his disease, probably at a pace unaffected by the treatment.

Surgical excision of bone bridges for mobilization of joints has been performed in some instances.[31] X-ray therapy to the area of operation may be helpful in preventing or delaying reossification. Harris[31] reported success in returning a man to work. The patient's affection was, however, milder than that in most patients (onset was at the age of 30 years), although the diagnosis is unquestioned.

Special nursing problems have been reviewed.[38]

Summary

The cardinal manifestations of fibrodysplasia ossificans progressiva are microdactyly and progressive ossification of fasciae, aponeuroses, and other fibrous structures related to muscles. Microdactyly is always most striking in the thumb and great toes. It probably represents fundamentally the same disorder occurring usually, although not exclusively, during antenatal development. There is usually a synostosis with resulting monophalangic great toe.

This disorder is probably inherited as a Mendelian dominant with irregular penetrance.

OSTEOPOIKILOSIS (OSTEO-DERMATO-POIKILOSIS)

Osteopoikilosis, like osteopetrosis, was first described in a definitive manner (earlier references[121] can be found) by the German radiologist H. Albers-Schönberg (1915).[85] It is sometimes referred to as "spotted bones," an appropriate designation, as seen from Fig. 12-6. "Osteopoikilosis" (variations: "osteopoecilia," "osteopecilia," "osteopoicilosis," "osteopoikilie") is derived from Greek words meaning "mottled bones." The bone lesion is also referred to as "osteitis condensans generalisata" or "osteosclerosis disseminata." Bauer and Bode[4] called it "osteodysplasia enostotica." The skin lesions were first described in 1928 by Buschke and Ollendorff[92] (and later by Curth[99]) as "dermatofibrosis lenticularis disseminata." Osteo-dermato-poikilosis might be a satisfactory designation for the entire syndrome.

Neither the osseous nor the cutaneous lesions have any known clinical significance whatever. They are usually discovered incidentally, since the bone lesions

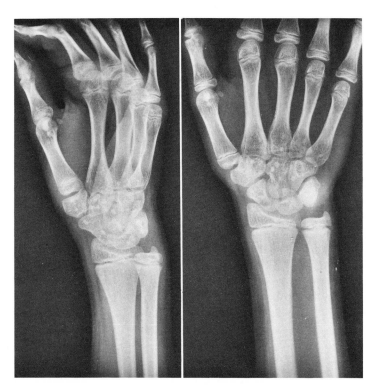

Fig. 12-6. Typical osteopoikilosis, discovered incidentally when radiologic studies for a wrist injury were performed (J.H.H. 644704) in a 13-year-old white boy.

are asymptomatic and the skin lesions inconspicuous. One reason why the clinician should be familiar with this condition is that he may avoid confusing the condition with osteoblastic metastases to the skeleton.[117]

The bone lesions are circumscribed, round areas of increased bone density, usually less than 1 cm. in diameter, situated particularly at the ends of the bones of the extremities (but not necessarily in the epiphyses) and in the small bones of the feet and wrists (Fig. 12-7). The lesions may or may not be bilaterally symmetric. At times the lesions are linear (striate) in distribution.[127] For example, Voorhoeve[125] found vertical striae parallel to the long axis of the bones and as a fan in the wings of the ilia, but no spots, in 2 children whose father had typical spots and no striae. (See Fig. 12-8 for a demonstration of the distribution of lesions.) The skull has been spared in most cases. Bistolfi[88] described involvement of the occipital bone. All 3 cases of Funstein and Kotschiew[103] had skull involvement, and indeed the calvarial lesions dominated the picture in Erbsen's[102] case. In the case of Martinčić[110] unusual involvement of the lumbar spine was present. Castellano and Piotti[94] described unusual costal and vertebral involvement.

As was nicely demonstrated by Funstein and Kotschiew[103] the islands tend, in pronounced cases, to be oriented along the "traction and pressure lines,"[110] especially at points of crossing of these lines.

The skin lesions, always inconspicuous, are most often located on the posterior aspect of the thighs and buttocks, occasionally on the arms and trunk, but never on the face. Their location bears no constant relation to that of the bone

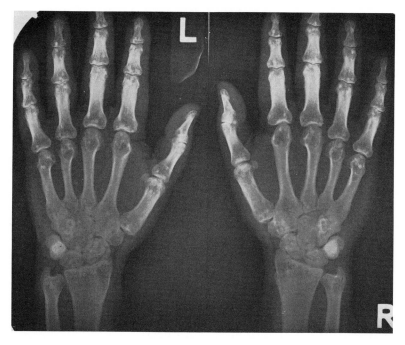

Fig. 12-7. Osteopoikilosis in M. M. (644555), 47 years of age. Asymptomatic. No skin manifestations. Family not available for study.

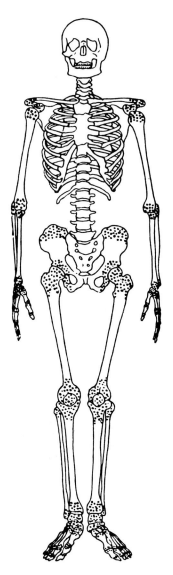

Fig. 12-8. Typical location of bone lesions in osteopoikilosis.[95]

lesions, although it is noteworthy that the head is usually affected neither by skin nor by bone lesions. The skin lesions are closely situated, slightly elevated, whitish yellow, and usually oblong or oval in outline. Like the bone lesions, they have been described as occurring in longitudinal streaks. They are usually about the size of a lentil or pea, from which the name of the skin lesions (dermatofibrosis lenticularis disseminata) is in part derived. Most of the cases of bone lesions that have been subjected to careful inspection have been found to show skin lesions as well. Busch[91] described skin changes in 6 of 14 members of one kindred who had osteopoikilosis, Buschke and Ollendorff[92] in 1 patient, and Šváb[122] and Windholz[127] in 2 patients each.

Information on the age of the patient at the appearance and evolution of both the osseous and cutaneous changes is meager. It is clear that lesions may be present at both sites in the first years of life. Furthermore, it appears that once formed, the bone lesions remain static for many years. The longest reported follow-up, seventeen years, was in a female first observed at the age of 14 years.[111]

Keloids may occur with increased frequency in these patients.[99] The only internal medical ramification that has even been suggested is that of fibrous nodules of the peritoneal lining, discovered at laparotomy in a 13-year-old patient who complained of severe abdominal pains.[120] It can fairly be stated that this was not a "clear case," however. Grossly the nodules suggested tubercles. Scleroderma beginning at the age of 7 months was described in association with osteopoikilosis by von Bernuth.[124] However, I doubt seriously that the bone condition described and pictured was the same as that under discussion here. In a case reported by Nichols and Shiflett[111] an obscure generalized skeletal disease was present in addition to osteopoikilosis; the authors thought there was no connection. There were exostoses in the cases of Albers-Schönberg,[85] Risseeuw,[116] and Albronda.[86] Copeman[96] saw osteopoikilosis in association with rheumatoid arthritis. In general, one seems justified in considering this situation as incapable of producing symptoms and as prognostically insignificant.

The bone lesions were examined histologically by Schmorl[118] in an 18-year-old boy who died of seemingly unrelated cause. He found that each "island" is a clump of osseous trabeculae that are thicker at the periphery than at the center. The trabeculae at the center form a complex network, with ordinary marrow in the space between. The skin lesions consist of collagenous fibrosis with preservation of the elastic fiber elements.[91,92] The skin lesion is a connective-tissue nevus[114] and in both clinical histology and appearance may be distinguished with difficulty from the connective-tissue nevus of tuberous sclerosis. Cairns[93] called the skin disorder "familial juvenile elastoma" on the basis of the histologic appearance in his cases. Although elastic tissue dominates the histologic picture in some cases, it seems likely that this is not a fundamental difference.[114]

Jonaseh[106a] found 12 cases among 211,000 radiographic cases in Germany.

From the point of view of inheritance, this disorder behaves as a Mendelian autosomal dominant. Busch[91] found 14 cases in three generations of one family, and the condition probably extended farther back in the ancestry, since there were 3 affected siblings in the first generation studied. Hinson[105] studied it in two generations. In x-ray films of the entire skeleton Bloom[89] found only a single spot in the sister of a patient with widespread involvement. Wilcox[126] saw the bone condition in father and daughter; Voorhoeve,[125] in father, son, and daughter. Risseeuw[116] saw the disorder in a man, 6 of his children, and a grandson. Albronda[86] saw the bone condition in a woman and 1 son and daughter; there was no skin change. Berlin and associates[87] observed two extensively affected kindreds. Many had osteopoikilosis without skin lesions. Some had dermatopoikilosis without bone lesions. Raque and Wood[114] described skin and bone lesions in a brother and sister and the son of the former. The combination of skin and bone lesions occurred in 2 or more family members in at least three other reports.[93,119,127] Marshall[109] described skin and bone changes in mother and son.

The basic defect appears to be a spotty hyperplasia of collagen in the corium and bone matrix. This is, however, little more than a restatement of the histologic findings. What is basically involved in this defect and why there is the peculiar spotty distribution are obscure. Voorhoeve[125] thought the bone lesions arise in cartilage. He based this theory on the fact that in 2 children he observed striated lesions extending a variable distance into the diaphysis from the epiphyseal line. The relative immunity of the skull and clavicle ("membranous bones") may be supporting evidence for endochondral origin.

MENKES KINKY HAIR SYNDROME*
Historical note

Like homocystinuria, the Menkes syndrome was described and elucidated within the last decade. Menkes and colleagues[259] observed a kindred in which 5 males in an X-linked recessive pedigree pattern (Fig. 12-9) were affected with the neurologic and hair changes that are now considered typical. Other clinical features were added on the basis of cases observed in various parts of the world.[249,250] The description of arteriographic and skeletal changes[265] was particularly noteworthy from the standpoint of delineating Menkes syndrome as a heritable disorder of connective tissue.

The elucidation of Menkes syndrome as a genetic defect in intestinal absorp-

---

*In this exposition, I have relied heavily on an unpublished manuscript by Danks and associates[252a] with their permission, which I acknowledge with thanks.

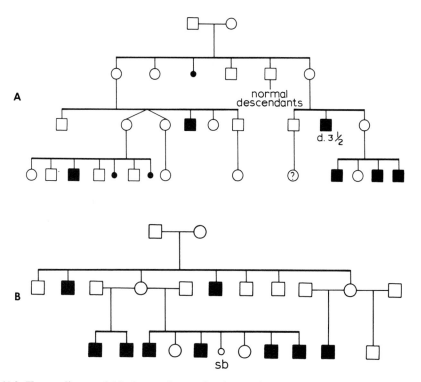

Fig. 12-9. Two pedigrees of Menkes syndrome showing typical X-linked recessive inheritance. **A,** Family of Menkes et al.,[259] restudied by French et al.[256] **B,** Family of Aguilar et al.[247]

tion of copper was an achievement of Danks and colleagues in Melbourne.[255] The work was first published in 1972, ten years after the first clinical report of the disorder.

Menkes and colleagues (1962) called their syndrome "a sex-linked recessive disorder with retardation of growth, peculiar hair and focal cerebral and cerebellar degeneration." O'Brien and colleagues then at Children's Hospital, Los Angeles, seem to have been responsible for calling it "kinky hair syndrome."[247,260a,265] O'Brien[260] suggested that "kinky hair syndrome" is a particularly useful designation for the detection of cases because the hair change thus becomes an easily remembered feature. On the other hand, Danks[252] points out that alopecia totalis, not kinky hair, may be the finding, and detection of cases may, he suggests, actually be hampered by the name. French and associates[256,257] referred to the disorder as trichopoliodystrophy, meaning dystrophy of the hair and gray matter. As in several other syndromes discussed here, the eponymic designation seems preferable for the present. A precise designation based on the defect in copper absorption may be possible in the near future.

Clinical manifestations

Premature birth is frequent, but birth weight is appropriate for the length of gestation. In the neonatal period the affected males often display instability of temperature, transient jaundice, and poor feeding but may seem to be progressing satisfactorily for the first several weeks. Lethargy and failure to feed well have their onset at 4 to 8 weeks of age. Hypothermia and peripheral circulatory failure (with or without septicemia) may divert attention from the serious brain disorder. Seizures develop early in some. Usually they are myoclonic in type and become difficult to control.

With the passage of time the evidence of brain disorder increases steadily, and the seizures become persistent. Muscle tone varies at different stages in the same patient. Severe spasticity is unusual. Hypothermia becomes a recurrent problem, as well as susceptibility to respiratory infection and septicemia. Subdural hematoma, a manifestation of the disorder of blood vessels, may be a presenting feature in the first 6 months of life or may be a terminal event. Survival in diagnosed cases has varied from 6 months to 3 years, but it is likely that some babies die at an earlier age without recognition of the specific disorder.

Danks and associates[253,255] suggest that the facial appearance is rather characteristic (Fig. 12-10A) and consists of "pallid skin, pudgy tissues, horizontal tangled eyebrows, and a 'cupid's bow' upper lip." The hair is usually normal in the neonate, but postnatal growth produces lackluster, hypopigmented hair that stands up in a tangled disarray on the vertex and breaks off to leave a palpable stubble in the occipital and temporal areas where it has rubbed on the bed. Microscopic examination of the hair shows pili torti (Fig. 12-10B) and clinches the diagnosis.

X-ray studies (Fig. 12-10C to H) of the skeleton show Wormian bones of the skull and metaphyseal spurs of the femurs and, less often, of the humerus and radius. Subperiosteal calcification may occur along the shafts of the long bones.

Arteriography (Fig. 12-11) shows widespread elongation, tortuosity, and luminal irregularity in all arteries of the body. Arterial occlusion can develop.

Notable negative findings include normal thyroid function studies, absence of

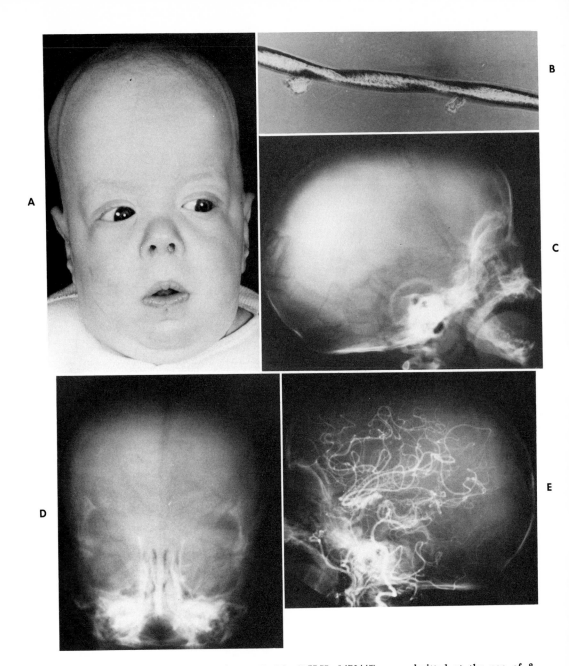

Fig. 12-10. Case of Menkes syndrome. P. M. (J.H.H. 1470445) was admitted at the age of 3 months for investigation of suspected visual loss. He was the product of a 37-week pregnancy. The parents were not related. Of 4 sibs, 1 had a lumbar meningocele and 1 had an unexplained convulsion at age 10 years. In the newborn nursery the baby showed persistent hypothermia and lethargy. In addition, unexplained hyperbilirubinemia occurred, with peaking of bilirubin level at 17 mg.% on the fifth day. At 6 weeks of age the parents noted that the infant did not smile or follow objects. His head control was poor and spontaneous movements diminished. Examination showed a prominent forehead and short, sparse, coarse hair of the scalp and eyebrows, **A.** A large right inguinal hernia was readily reducible. Several minor motor seizures occurred during the examination. Head control was poor. Although opticokinetic nystagmus was demonstrated, the patient did not follow bright objects consistently. The optic disks were dysplastic. The infant was generally hypotonic with hypoactive deep tendon reflexes.

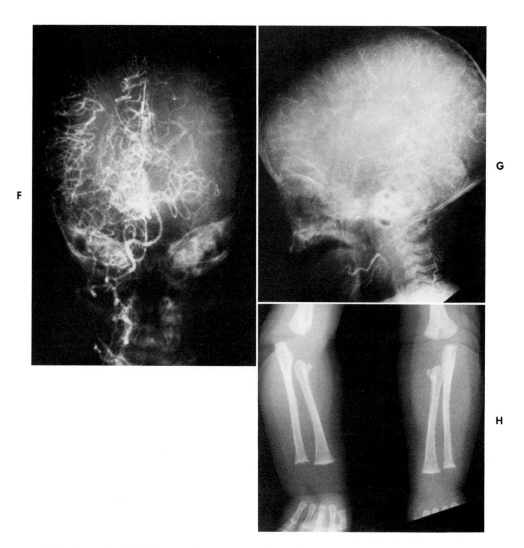

The diagnosis of Menkes syndrome was confirmed by microscopic demonstration of pili torti, **B,** and chemical finding of low serum ceruloplasmin (< 2 mg.%) and serum copper (10 μg.%). Furthermore, the findings of radiographic studies were entirely consistent. Skull x-ray films, **C** and **D,** showed multiple Wormian bones along the lambdoidal and squamosal sutures. Cerebral arteriograms, **E** to **G,** showed marked tortuous vessels with luminal irregularity of larger ones. Irregular bony fragments extended laterally from the proximal metaphyses of the radii, **H.** The distal ends of the radius, ulna, tibia, and fibula showed cupping bilaterally. Electroencephalogram showed multiple spike discharge consistent with a diffuse cerebral disturbance.

Patient seen through courtesy of Dr. Robert H. A. Haslum. Biochemical studies were done by Dr. N. A. Holtzman.

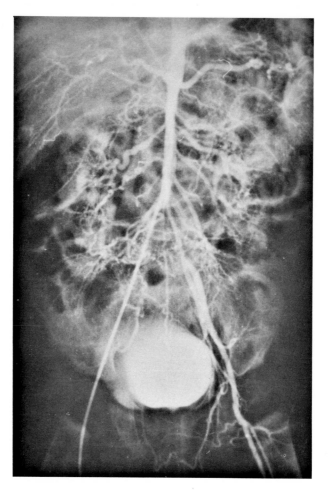

Fig. 12-11. Arteriogram in 4-month-old infant with Menkes syndrome showing widespread arterial changes. The right renal artery is narrowed proximally and dilated and tortuous distally. The left common iliac artery is narrowed. (Courtesy Dr. David M. Danks, Melbourne.)

anemia, normal white blood cell counts, and normal urinary excretion of amino acids.

Main findings of necropsy have been in the brain and blood vessels. The brain shows extensive neuronal degeneration, gliosis, and cystic degeneration. Indeed, the cerebral histopathology and the changes in the cerebral lipids were, until recently, focused on, excluding the important arterial changes.[247,257,263] The ocular histopathology has been described.[263] In arteries of all parts of the body, fragmentation and reduplication of the internal elastic lamina (Fig. 12-12) and even fragmentation of elastic fibers throughout the media are seen.

Incidence and genetics. X-linked recessive inheritance is well documented (Fig. 12-9). Some heterozygous females show mild pili torti. Serum copper levels are normal in heterozygotes, but intestinal absorption of copper and the level of copper in intestinal mucosa have not been studied.

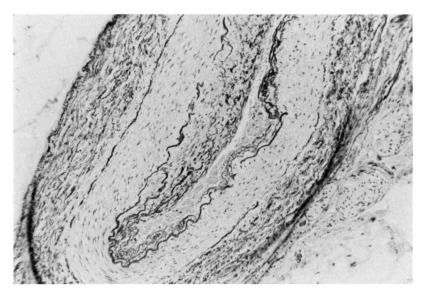

Fig. 12-12. Histopathology of large artery in Menkes syndrome. Disruption, fragmentation, and reduplication of the internal elastic lamina and thickening of the intima are demonstrated. (×130.) (Courtesy Dr. David M. Danks, Melbourne.)

Menkes syndrome is probably more frequent than the paucity of reported cases would suggest. Before Danks' work, such a high proportion of the few reported cases had affected relatives (Fig. 12-9) that I suspect many sporadic cases were missed. At least a third of all cases of a lethal X-linked recessive such as Menkes syndrome should be isolated (p. 15). Four out of five of Danks' families[253] had 2 or more cases. Danks and co-workers[252,253,255] suggested a frequency in Melbourne of about 1 in 35,000 live births.

Basic defect. Danks and associates[253,255] have shown a defect in copper metabolism, specifically a defect in intestinal absorption of copper, in Menkes syndrome. All patients studied have shown very low levels of serum copper, serum copper oxidase (ceruloplasmin), and liver copper. Red cell copper is normal. Oral administration of copper as copper sulfate, in dosage which is promptly effective in nutritional copper deficiency, has no effect on serum copper levels. Orally administered ^{64}Cu was very poorly absorbed. The copper content of suction biopsies of duodenal mucosa varied from 50 to 76 ppm in 4 biopsies from 2 patients with Menkes syndrome, compared with the normal value of 18.5 (S.D. 6.3).

The above findings point to a defect in the transport of copper from the intestinal mucosal cells into the bloodstream. Uptake by the mucosal cell from the intestinal content is probably normal. Since manifestations begin very early, perhaps even at birth, transport from the mother to the fetus may be defective. Normally the liver of the newborn has a high copper content,[262] most of the deposition having occurred in the last 6 weeks of gestation. Prematurity may aggravate the early onset of symptoms.

As the Melbourne group has pointed out, all features of Menkes syndrome, including those of connective tissues, are explicable on the basis of copper deficiency.[251,261] The lesions seen in the arterial wall are similar to those described in spontaneous or experimentally induced copper deficiency in animals. Cross-links of both elastin and collagen are formed from lysine residues (p. 41; Figs. 2-5 to 2-8) and require a copper-dependent amine oxidase for the first step. Bone changes are also known in copper-deficient babies and animals. The picture in animals is that of osteoporosis. Microscopic studies show deficient osteoid formation as in scurvy. Babies likewise show changes resembling scurvy. Al-Rashid and Spangler[248] suggested that deficient activity to the copper-dependent ascorbic acid oxidase is responsible for these changes.

Arterial insufficiency may account for much, perhaps even most, of the changes in the brain. Functional deficiency of cytochrome oxidase, a copper-containing enzyme, has, however, been involved as an explanation for the neurologic lesions of copper-deficient animals.[264] Deficiency of cytochrome oxidase may account for the hypothermia of Menkes syndrome.

Copper is required for the formation of disulfide cross-links in keratin. Excessive amounts of free sulfhydryl groups have been found in the wool of copper-deficient sheep[258] and in the hair in Menkes syndrome.[255] In both sheep and man, hypopigmentation of the hair has been attributed to deficient tyrosinase activity.

The reason for the normal levels of erythrocyte copper and the lack of anemia is unknown.

Other considerations

For treatment, parenteral administration of copper or some means of overcoming the presumed block at the intestinal mucosa will be necessary. To avoid irreversible damage, intrauterine diagnosis and treatment may be necessary.

Metachromasia of the cytoplasm of fibroblasts has been described in Menkes syndrome[254] as well as in several other heritable disorders of connective tissue, including the Marfan syndrome, and, of course, the mucopolysaccharidoses. Its significance is unclear.

LÉRI PLEONOSTEOSIS

In 1921 André Léri,[134] Parisian orthopedist, described a previously unrecognized condition in a 35-year-old man and his children by a second wife, a daughter 4 years of age and a son 3 weeks of age. The child by his first wife was normal. The disorder was not present at birth and became evident sooner or later in extrauterine life. The father was only 62 inches tall and had short, broad hands and feet with thickened palmar pads and accentuated creases, with limitation of motion in the wrists, elbows, hips, and knees. The toes, and presumably the thumbs as well, were broad and stiff. Fairly numerous cases have since been described in the French literature,[132,135,139,141,142] including one report from Russia,[132] and some in the German literature (see reference 136 for list of German reports); there have also been reports in journals of Brazil and Argentina (see reference 144), but there appears to be only one article in British journals[144] and none at all in the periodical American medical literature.

The term "pleonosteosis," suggested by Léri, and based on his impression, probably inaccurate, that the basic abnormality is one of excessive ossification.

The clinical characteristics of Léri pleonosteosis are broadening and deformity of the thumbs and great toes, flexion contractures of the interphalangeal joints, and limitation of motion in other joints, including even those of the spine. A form of "hammertoe" may develop. Mongoloid facies has been described[144] but is by no means an invariable feature (see Case 1 of reference 144). Furthermore, in the majority of cases of Mongoloid features, the patients are normally intelligent, e.g., Watson-Jones's[144] Patient 2, who was a university graduate. However, there are at least two reports of impairment of the intellect.[138,142]

There is usually semifixed internal rotation of the upper limbs and external rotation of the lower limbs. In general the limbs are short. The joints of the hands in particular may appear to be swollen. The hands are short, square, and thick. Changes in the lower extremities seem to be less striking, possibly because less intricate movements are required of the feet and ankles.

A complication of the fibrous hyperplasia in the hands and feet can be nerve compression: carpal tunnel syndrome involving the median nerves and Morton's metatarsalgia from involvement of the digital nerves of the feet.

Watson-Jones[144] described the dense fibrous tissue removed from the wrist and consisting essentially of a highly hyperplastic anterior carpal ligament. The specimen consisted of greatly increased, dense collagenous tissue which in portions was actually fibrocartilage. Elastic fibers were conspicuous in their absence. Mucinous material was present, and in tissue removed from the foot, numerous "tissue mast cells" were described.

The fundamental abnormality was thought by Léri to be one of excessive and perhaps precocious ossification of the epiphyses. It seemed more likely to Watson-Jones[144] that the joint deformities are due to capsular contractures, that in general the abnormality resides in the fibrous tissues, and that the "thickening of the bones may be due to periosteal traction at their metaphyseal attachments."

All evidence suggests that pleonosteosis is inherited as a Mendelian autosomal dominant trait.

Although uncommon, Léri pleonosteosis almost certainly occurs more frequently than the rarity of reports in American publications would suggest. In their monograph *Human Heredity,* Neel and Schull[138] describe a 34-year-old woman with progressive loss of joint mobility and moderately severe contractures beginning in adolescence. Movements of the hands in particular were awkward and clumsy. The mother, 58 years of age, was affected and by this time of life was unable to perform most fine movements of the hands and the rest of the body. A brother of the proposita and a half-brother of her mother were also affected. A feature of all affected persons was a broad thumb. The proposita sought information on whether her 2 sons would be affected. Since one of them already displayed broad thumbs, the inquirer was advised that a vocation requiring manual dexterity would be inadvisable. Rukavina and colleagues[143] have reported the family in full. Telephone follow-up in 1971 showed that III-1 committed suicide in 1956 about one month after divorce. His physical disorder contributed, he had felt, to his matrimonial difficulties. The proband and informant, III-2, now 55 years old, and her half-brother, III-3, seven years younger, have both developed glaucoma. Restricted motion in the neck in looking up or turning the head is a prominent feature in them. There are, it seems, no signs of carpal tunnel compression. The affected son of III-2 is unmarried; the unaffected son has 2 unaffected children.

The nosography of this disorder is far from fully established. Cocchi[128] includes this condition in the group of "polytopic enchondral dysostoses" in which he also includes the Morquio syndrome and the Hurler syndrome. In a detailed clinicopathologic study based on 2 brothers, Materna[136] described what he called Léri pleonosteosis, which differs radically from the condition in the 4 patients reported by Watson-Jones.[144] There was no mention of limitation of joint mobility. The entire skeleton revealed extensive changes with "innumerable microfractures," fish vertebrae, a wedge vertebra, and coarsening and widening of the tubular bone, among other changes. The father was thought to have the same disorder as his 2 sons. One of the sons died at the age of 42 years of heart failure; no autopsy was performed. In the other, heart disease believed to be rheumatic was discovered at autopsy. This brother had had repair of bilateral inguinal hernias at the age of 14 months. I have had no patient in whom the diagnosis of Léri pleonosteosis seemed justified. As noted on p. 637, some reported patients with this diagnostic label almost certainly had either MPS II or MPS I S.

In the differential diagnosis, a mucopolysaccharidosis (especially MPS I S, or the Scheie syndrome) and arthritis, either rheumatoid or degenerative, come in for consideration. One would be suspicious that the case thought by Rocher and Pesme[139] to be one of pleonosteosis with corneal opacification was, in fact, a mucopolysaccharidosis. Sometimes thoracic outlet syndrome (compression of components of the cervical plexus) is suspected.[144] A mucopolysaccharidosis is also the more likely diagnosis in Case 4 of Watson-Jones[144] (p. 553) and in some other reported cases reviewed by Rukavina and colleagues.[143] Other disorders with stiff joints and short stature include the Weill-Marchesani syndrome (Chapter 5), the "stiff-skin syndrome" reported by Esterly and McKusick[131] (p. 640), and the disorder described by Moore and Federman.[229]

The Moore-Federman syndrome is a dominantly inherited form of dwarfism with ocular and perhaps cardiac abnormality. The proband had retinal detachment, glaucoma, and hyperopia. Asthmatic bronchitis was frequent in the affected persons. Some had atrophy of the abductor pollicis brevis muscle, as in the carpal tunnel syndrome.[135a] Pronation and supernation were impressively limited. The skin of the forearms was taut and "bound down."

Another genetic disorder that is accompanied by the carpal tunnel syndrome is amyloid neuropathy II (Indiana, or Rukavina, type).[135b] Carpal tunnel compression was noted earlier as a feature of the Weill-Marchesani syndrome (Chapter 5) and of several of the mucopolysaccharidoses (Chapter 5).

PAGET'S DISEASE OF BONE

Is Paget's disease of bone a generalized disorder of connective tissue? The evidence that Paget's disease of bone can legitimately be considered a heritable abiotrophy, probably of the collagen matrix of bone, can be summarized in the way indicated below. None of the pieces of evidence is by itself conclusive, but taken together they make a rather convincing argument.

1. The hereditary nature of the process appears to be established. However, it is worthwhile to examine the evidence, since one review,[190] which is otherwise comprehensive, makes no mention of the genetic factor in discussing

etiology. In 1889 Paget[185] himself wrote: "I have tried in vain to trace any hereditary tendency to the disease. I have not found it twice in the same family." However, the observations of familial aggregation reported from even before that time (beginning with Pick[187] in 1883) are fairly numerous. (See Fig. 12-13.)

In 1946 Koller[173] could find in the literature twenty-eight families in which more than one case was described. Since then other reports[146,147,154,169,171,178,183, 193,199] of familial aggregation have appeared. Stemmermann[199] identified it in members of three successive generations. It appears to have occurred in four generations of a Jewish family known to me and also in two other kinships, as indicated in Fig. 12-13. Aschner and associates[146] described it in monozygous twin brothers and claimed that by 1952 a total of fifty-seven families with multiple cases had been described. Martin[177] and others (Fig. 12-13) also described the disease in both of identical twins. Galbraith[161] found seventy-seven reported families and added four. In 1968, Evens and Bartter[159] concluded that at least eighty-seven families with multiple affected members had been described. They added a kindred with affected members in three sibships related as cousins through the mothers, who were sisters.

When one undertakes to study the heredity of a condition such as Paget's disease, one encounters several difficulties. In the first place, the disease has some of the earmarks of an abiotrophy. That it is an abiotrophy remains, of course, to be established. At any rate the disease usually has its onset late in life, by which time the parents are likely to have died, the siblings may be widely scattered geographically, and the children will probably not yet be old enough to have developed the disease. In the second place, Paget's disease is often subtle in its manifestations. A very high proportion of affected persons are asymptomatic, and the change in bone is discovered only incidentally on radiologic examination made for unrelated purposes or possibly in search for an explanation of an otherwise obscure elevation of serum alkaline phosphatase activity. In the course of a detailed study of 7,941 individuals over 61 years of age, 85 cases of Paget's disease were found, but of these cases only 3 had complaints referable to the disorder of bone.[180] In connection with the last difficulty it may be that a study of families, using alkaline phosphatase determinations as a screening procedure, would be productive. The first type of difficulty—the age factor—would not, to be sure, be circumvented.

In general, the data accumulated are consistent with the view that the trait for Paget's disease is controlled by a simple autosomal Mendelian dominant gene. However, Ashley-Montagu[147] suggested that it is inherited "as an incompletely dominant gene, carried on an X-chromosome."

Considering how frequently Paget's disease occurs in at least mild form (3% of all persons over 40 years of age, according to Schmorl[192]), one might say that it would be extraordinary if thirty or forty families with more than one case could *not* be discovered. Along the same line it may be noted that Sabatini[191] found Paget's disease in two married couples in which the marital partners were unrelated. Actually I believe there is a significant familial aggregation of cases. Particularly in the pedigrees with more than 2 cases is the evidence convincing. The incidence of Paget's disease in the general population is roughly 0.013%.[173] It can be estimated that the chance of 2 or more cases occurring in the same family by random distribution alone is very slight indeed.

2. Angioid streaks of the retina are associated with only two conditions with

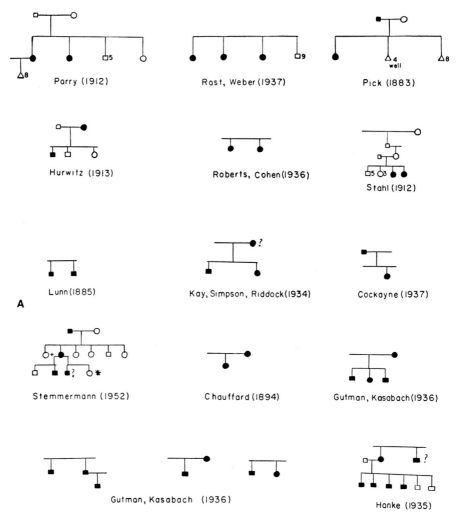

Fig. 12-13. Thirty-five pedigrees from the literature and two from the unpublished experience of Brayshaw and McKusick, showing familial aggregation of Paget's disease. Moehlig[178] and Ashley-Montagu[147] and probably others reported Jewish pedigrees. Concordance in identical twins was reported by Koller,[173] by Mozer,[182] and by Dickson and associates.[156] In the last instance there was a striking similarity of distribution in the twins, both having, for example, tibial involvement. In the twins observed by Mozer,[182] onset of the clinically evident abnormalities occurred at the age of 48 years in both. In Irvine's pedigree[169] the affected male died of a malignant osteoclastoma of the jaw, and both daughters had the onset of Paget's disease of the skull and jaw at the age of 18 years. In the pedigree of Brayshaw and McKusick, in this figure, the first individual in the second generation, a female (A. H., 511948), had so-called osteitis pubis and changes in the skull compatible with Paget's disease. The alkaline phosphatase, however, was always normal. The other 2 affected individuals (C. T., 502845; W. T., 620032) had Paget's disease in entirely typical form. These patients were discovered on study of the records of the hospital; if a more detailed study of the family were made, other members would probably be found to be affected.

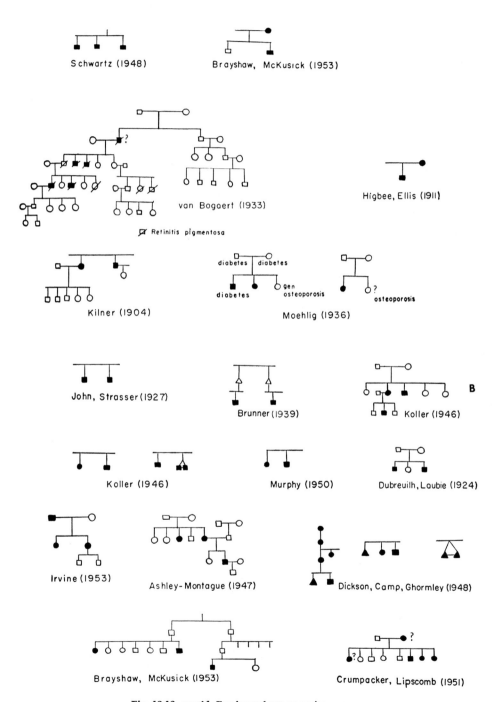

Fig. 12-13, cont'd. For legend see opposite page.

any regularity. These conditions are pseudoxanthoma elasticum and Paget's disease of bone.[181,201] Angioid streaks of the fundus of the eye, pseudoxanthoma elasticum in the skin, and Paget's disease in the bones have been observed in the same patient.[206] There may be reasons for believing that there is no fundamental relationship between Paget's disease and pseudoxanthoma elasticum: the first may be inherited as a Mendelian dominant and the second as a Mendelian recessive disorder; the first occurs more frequently in men and the second more frequently in women. (Paget's disease seems to occur more commonly in men but in more severe form in women.)

Although Paget's disease and pseudoxanthoma elasticum may be basically distinct entities, the fact that angioid streaks, which are an integral part of a definite disorder of connective tissue (PXE), occur also in Paget's disease suggests that Paget's disease may likewise be a disorder of connective tissue with abnormalities much more widespread than the bone lesions alone would suggest.

Also in Paget's disease, there occur other ocular abnormalities such as corneal degeneration,[203] cataract,[174] and choroiditis[152] independent of angioid streaks, which further raise the question of whether a generalized abiotrophy of connective tissue may be present.

3. A quality of reasonableness, although not constituting proof, makes it attractive to persons familiar with bone and with the clinical behavior of Paget's disease to speculate that the disease is fundamentally an abiotrophy of the collagen matrix of bone, which breaks down with the passage of years. Albright and Reifenstein[145] present evidence that Paget's disease is primarily a destruction or, perhaps it is permissible to say, a degeneration of bone with secondary reparative overproduction of bone.

In general, the involvement of the skeleton follows a pattern of localization consistent with the view that "wear-and-tear" is a contributing factor in the development of the lesions. Weight-bearing structures are usually involved primarily. The bones of the upper extremity are, for example, much less often involved than those of the legs. The victims of Paget's disease in severe form are often obese. The high incidence of obesity and tallness in the families of patients with Paget's disease was emphasized by Moehlig.[178,179]

The femur[192] is one of the most commonly affected bones (over 30% of cases), and the humerus, one of the least (less than 5%).* The most frequently affected bone is the sacrum (57% of cases). The vertebrae are affected in half of the cases, and the incidence of involvement in descending frequency is lumbar, thoracic, and cervical spine. In brief, beginning with the sacrum there is a progressive decrease in frequency of involvement as one progresses craniad. An amazing finding[192] is that the right femur is involved by Paget's disease over twice as often as the left femur (31% as against 15%). Undoubtedly, people are right-legged or left-legged just as they are right-handed or left-handed. In the skull Albright and Reifenstein[145] picture an instance of predominant involvement laterally at the attachment of the masseter and temporal muscles. Involvement of other areas of the skull, often a striking feature, is more difficult to explain on a "wear-and-tear" basis. However, it must be remembered that "wear-and-tear" is probably only a contributing factor in the development and localization of the disorder,

---

*The statistics cited here are derived from the classic necropsy study of Schmorl.[192]

the primary factor being perhaps a hereditary weakness. The situation with Paget's disease may be like that of pseudoxanthoma elasticum, in which "wear-and-tear" appears to be responsible for the site of principal localization of the skin changes. Schmorl[192] noted that changes tend to be most pronounced at the attachments of tendons and ligaments to bones. Kay and co-workers[171] made the important observation that in a brother and sister (Fig. 12-9A) with Paget's disease, both with unilateral involvement of the radius, the left radius was involved in the left-handed individual and the right radius in the right-handed one! This appears to be a nice demonstration of the cooperation of genetic and postnatal factors.

The significance of localized trauma preceding the onset of monostotic Paget's disease is difficult to evaluate (p. 332 of reference 198). The reported cases may represent coincidence.

4. Vascular disease has been thought to occur prematurely and with increased incidence in these patients[196] and to be independent of the "high output" heart failure, which may occur as a result of the vascular peculiarities that functionally resemble arteriovenous fistulae.[158,200] Medial sclerosis of the Mönckeberg type has been thought to occur especially often in these persons. Harrison and Lennox[165] found valvular calcification in 39% of their patients with Paget's disease, an incidence five times that in a control group of comparable age distribution. Vascular calcification may be related merely to the periodic hypercalcemia to which these persons are subjected. The elevation of circulating alkaline phosphatase may contribute. Extraskeletal calcification occurs commonly in these patients,[184,194,204] possibly for the reasons listed, possibly because of an abnormality of connective tissue. Urinary calculi, which are frequent, would seem to be explained by the high urinary excretion of calcium. Salivary calculi, which were identified in 20 of 111 cases,[190] may have a somewhat similar basis.

This fourth bit of evidence is by far the weakest of the points bearing on the possible nature of Paget's disease as an abiotrophy of the collagen matrix of bone.

Hitherto, a principal view of the pathogenesis of Paget's disease has implicated vascular changes. This view would consider that intimately related to the primary defect is the increased vascularity of the bones, which (1) may represent a significant and at times intolerable burden to the heart similar to that of arteriovenous fistulae,[196] (2) is a problem in hemostasis to surgeons, for instance the neurosurgeon performing craniotomy in instances of involvement of the skull,[155] and (3) results in the fact that the skin overlying bones severely affected by Paget's disease may be warmer than elsewhere. In the present state of ignorance it is probably at least equally valid to suspect that Paget's disease of bone may be an abiotrophy of the collagen matrix and that the vascular phenomena are secondary developments.

OTHER POSSIBLE HEREDITARY AND GENERALIZED DISORDERS OF CONNECTIVE TISSUE

A considerable number of distinct entities which are certainly or probably generalized hereditary disorders of connective tissue as defined here have been discussed in the differential diagnosis of the Marfan syndrome, the Ehlers-Danlos

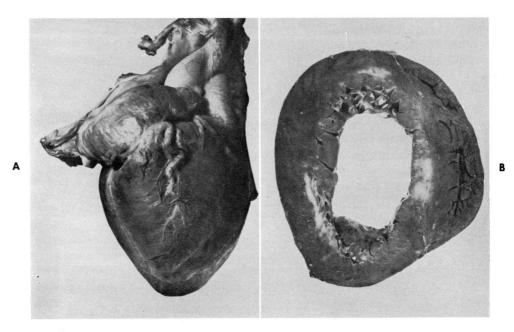

Fig. 12-14. Brothers with generalized arterial calcification of infancy. M. W. died of heart failure at the age of 4 months. Beginning at the age of 3 weeks he appeared to have a respiratory infection, with cough and dyspnea. He was pale and had episodes of sweating. On several occasions he had attacks in which he cried out suddenly and stiffened his body. Peripheral cyanosis, cardiac and hepatic enlargement, and ST segment and T-wave changes in the electrocardiogram were found. The striking feature was the presence of calcified, tortuous coronary arteries, **A.** When the heart was sectioned, evidence of old and recent myocardial infarction was discovered, **B.** Calcification was seen in small arteries of the omentum. Histologically many arteries, including the aorta and pulmonary artery, showed calcification around elastic laminae, which appeared fragmented, **C.** In the outer part of the pulmonary artery, granuloma formation was demonstrated in the area of interruption of the elastic fibers, **D.** The aorta, **E,** stained by the periodic acid–Schiff technique, showed deeply stained margins of abnormal elastic fibers contrasting with the weakly staining edges of normal fibers. In the coronary artery, **F,** after calcium was removed by dilute nitric acid, material staining with periodic acid–Schiff reagent was demonstrated surrounding the elastic lamellae. The association of the calcium deposition with abnormal elastic fibers was demonstrated in the stains of the aorta, **G,** with the von Kossa technique. The above histologic findings suggest that accumulation of mucopolysaccharide is a consequence of degenerative change in elastic fibers. Similar evidence is available in Erdheim's cystic medial necrosis, in the Marfan syndrome, and in experimental lathyrism. That alteration in the mucopolysaccharide of ground substance is followed by deposition of calcium salts is well recognized. In generalized arterial calcification of infants, the "basic defect" may reside in the elastic fibers. Accumulation of mucopolysaccharide and deposition of calcium may be secondary and tertiary phenomena. C. W., brother of M. W., died at the age of 7 months after an illness identical to that in M. W. Serum calcium concentration and alkaline phosphatase activity were normal. Autopsy revealed widespread arterial calcification and myocardial infarction. (Photographs and information courtesy Dr. Alan L. Williams, Melbourne, Australia.)

syndrome, osteogenesis imperfecta, and the mucopolysaccharidoses. These entities include the hypermobile Marfanoid syndrome (p. 177), the fragilitas oculi syndrome (pp. 340, 341, 433), the Larsen syndrome (p. 350), the Puretič syndrome (p. 637), and others.

Generalized arterial calcification of infancy has been noted in multiple sibs[221,227,245] (Fig. 12-14). The justification for mentioning it in a discussion of generalized heritable disorders of connective tissue is provided by the evidence suggesting that fundamentally the disorder is a degeneration of elastic fiber. The calcification shows a remarkable predilection for the internal elastic lamina. Considerable material with the staining properties of mucopolysaccharide accumu-

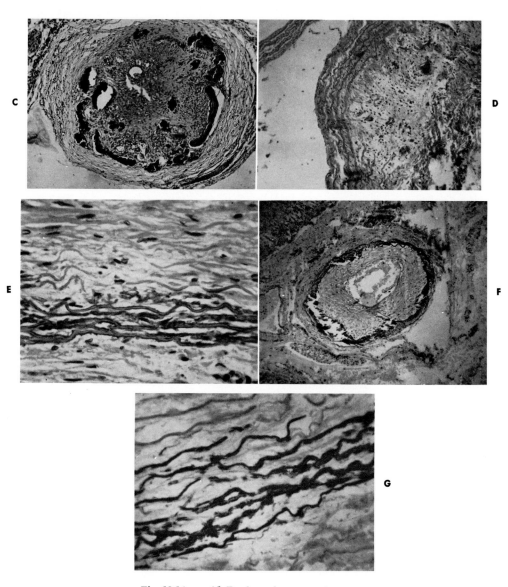

Fig. 12-14, cont'd. For legend see opposite page.

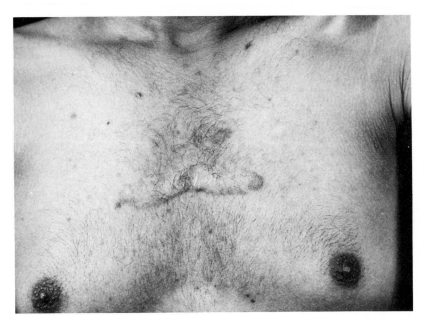

Fig. 12-15. Transverse keloid over sternum in mulatto male (D. C., 835228) whose father has an identical keloid. Trauma at this site preceding development of the keloid is not recalled.

lates around the elastic laminae.[246] Fine calcium incrustation of the lamina is the minimal lesion. Later the lamina is ruptured and occlusive changes of the tunica intima take place. Death from myocardial infarction usually occurs in the first six months after birth. The clinical diagnosis is suggested by the discovery of calcification in a peripheral vessel in an infant with electrocardiographic evidence of coronary artery disease. Idiopathic infantile hypercalcemia, of which there may be more than one etiologic variety, is probably unrelated; to my knowledge there is not yet evidence of a genetic variety of infantile hypercalcemia.

Clearly there are genetic differences in the tendency to *keloid* formation (Fig. 12-15). Negroes and some Caucasian families are notoriously susceptible.[207]

Certain hereditary syndromes display abnormalities of structures other than connective tissues. Such a syndrome is that which goes by Werner's name.[216,222, 233,237,240] The victim of the *Werner syndrome,* which is usually inherited as an autosomal recessive disorder, displays short stature, with slender limbs and stocky trunk; scleroderma-like changes, especially in the skin of the extremities, with the development of ulcers over the malleoli, Achilles tendons, heels, and toes and with atrophy of the corium, demonstrable microscopically; localized soft tissue calcifications; and, finally, premature arteriosclerosis with Mönckeberg calcification. However, the patients also display premature canities and balding, juvenile cataract,* weak, high-pitched voice, atrophy of the epidermis as well as

---

*The internist must keep the Werner syndrome[228] in mind in connection with patients who appear to have a more conventional, acquired variety of scleroderma. Cataracts can be the tip-off to the presence of this hereditary syndrome.

the corium, hypogonadism, osteoporosis, and increased incidence of diabetes mellitus. This disorder is intriguing, as far as definition of the basic defect is concerned. One is reminded of myotonia dystrophica, in which baldness, cataract, and hypogonadism cannot, in the present state of ignorance, be related to the disorder of muscle.

Connective tissues show changes also in progeria,[213a] for example, the scleroderma-like changes, but progeria can scarcely be called a heritable disorder of connective tissue. Indeed, a genetic basis for progeria is not proved. Sibs affected with the *bona fide* disorder have been reported in a few instances, and examples of parental consanguinity (3 out of 19 cases[213a]) are reported. However, there are far too few familial cases for this to be a simple recessive. Some of the instances of sibs with presumed progeria such as Hopkin Hopkin and his younger sister Joan, children of the Welch poet Lewis Hopkin, may have been instances of the Cockayne syndrome or some other progeroid disorder. Progeria is yet another condition in which multiple Wormian bones occur (see p. 438).

The editors of *Dermatology in Internal Medicine* placed pachydermoperiostosis[226a] with the heritable disorders of connective tissue. Although there are changes in connective tissue, this disorder also does not fit well with the other conditions discussed here. The main features are clubbing of the digits; periosteal new bone formation, especially at the distal ends of the long tubular bones; and coarsening of the facial features with thickening, furrowing, and oiliness of the skin of the face and forehead.[226a] The condition is probably inherited as an autosomal dominant with stronger manifestation in males than in females.[233a]

In *Dupuytren's contracture*[210,217,224,225,235,239] and in *Peyronie's disease*,[230,234] convincing evidence of a hereditary basis is available. Furthermore, the two conditions are probably associated more frequently than chance alone would dictate. The occurrence of knuckle pads[217,218,226,235,243,244] and plantar nodules[212] in association with Dupuytren's contracture, together with a possible relationship of the latter condition to epilepsy,[214,226,235] gives reason to think that Dupuytren's contracture is a common manifestation of a generalized disorder affecting connective tissue. Genetic investigation is hampered by its appearance late in life and the overall high frequency in older persons.[215]

Stickler and colleagues[71] described a "new" entity that appears to be a heritable disorder of connective tissue. Inherited as an autosomal dominant disorder, it is characterized by (1) progressive myopia, beginning in the first decade of life and leading to retinal detachment and blindness, and (2) premature degenerative changes in various joints. The designation suggested by the authors is "hereditary progressive arthro-ophthalmopathy." In a later publication Stickler and Pugh[238] noted the occurrence of vertebral changes and hearing deficit. They also pointed out that the family reported by David[213] probably had the same condition. It is possible, furthermore, that the syndrome of dwarfism, stiff joints, and ocular abnormalities reported by Moore and Federman[229] is the same disorder. However, the first two features were greater in their patients than in Stickler's, and the third aspect, although including detachment of the retina, also included hyperopia (not myopia), glaucoma, and cataract. Opitz and colleagues[231a] have extended the reaches of the Stickler syndrome to such an extent that it is not credible to me that one entity, or even allelic disorders, is being discussed.

There are a large number of members of the epiphysitis or *aseptic necrosis*

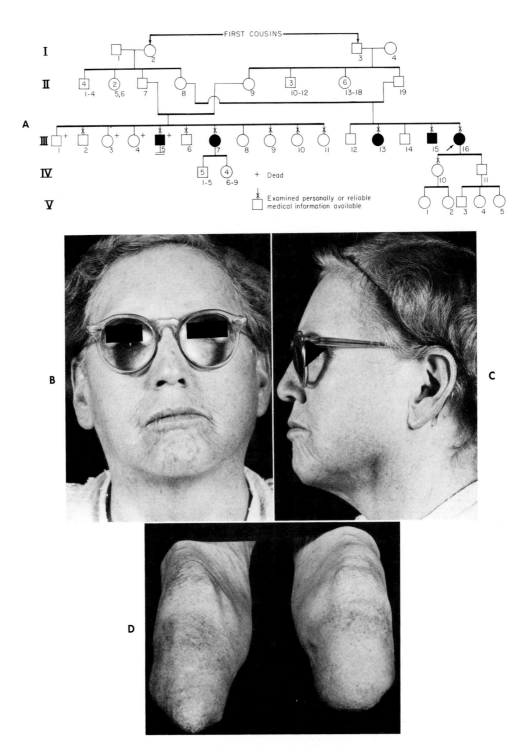

Fig. 12-16. For legend see opposite page.

Fig. 12-16. Werner syndrome. In two sibships of the kindred diagrammed in **A,** 5 cases of the Werner syndrome were observed. The two sibships are related to each other as double third cousins. The coefficient of relationship of the parents of the affected persons of both sibships is $\frac{1}{64}$, since they are second cousins. Briefly the characteristics of the patients with the Werner syndrome were as follows:

III-5, L. S. (J.H.H. 177405) had bilateral cataract extraction at 37 years of age. At 39 years of age he was noted to have premature graying of the hair, sclerodermatous changes of the extremities with extensive subcutaneous calcification and ulcers about the ankles, testicular atrophy, and short stature (60½ inches) with large torso. Tendons were also calcified, and there was striking crepitus on motion of most joints. It is noteworthy that macular degeneration resembling that usually considered senile in nature was observed at the age of 39 years. The patient died of sarcoma arising in the right thigh. Histologically the appearance of the tumor suggested nerve sheath origin.

III-7, M. S. K. was first discovered to have stigmata of the Werner syndrome when the kindred was restudied in 1962. Diminished vision began at the age of 11 years. Cataracts were removed at the age of 21 years and at 52 years. At the latter time mild diabetes was discovered. By 25 years of age she was strikingly gray-haired. She is 62 inches tall, with thin white hair and the characteristic facies of the Werner syndrome. The facial skin was tight and the nose beaked, but the extremities were spared. Three years previously, "central and disseminated patches of healed chorioretinitis" were described and interpreted as an aftermath of toxoplasmosis. However, in view of the retinal changes described in her brother, L. S., it seems possible that these changes were directly related to the Werner syndrome.

III-13, O. A. was reported by Boatwright, and associates.[208] Bilateral cataracts were discovered at 35 years of age. Scleroderma of the feet and legs with ulceration and subcutaneous calcification began at the age of 40 years. She was 59 inches tall, and the extremities were spindly, especially in comparison with the stocky trunk. The face was birdlike. After the time of the report she was demonstrated by barium swallow x-ray films to have esophageal changes suggesting scleroderma. Amputation of both legs was performed because of chronic ulcers, and osteogenic sarcoma was discovered in the right first metatarsal and cuneiform bones. The patient died seven months later. Because of the rarity of reported autopsies in the Werner syndrome, the findings in this case are of note. Death was the result of widespread metastases of osteogenic sarcoma arising in the leg. In addition, the aorta and coronary arteries showed extensive atherosclerosis. The mitral ring was extensively calcified.

III-15, E. L. R. was first reported by Boatwright and colleagues.[208] Bilateral cataracts were discovered at the age of 34 years. Soon afterward the hair became gray, and sclerodermatous changes developed in the feet and ankles, with painfully disabling callosities and ulcers. The voice was high pitched. The patient was found to have diabetes. The case was later reported in more detail, with autopsy findings, by Perloff and Phelps.[232] Autopsy revealed extensive atherosclerosis and vessel calcification but no abnormality of endocrine glands.

III-16, K. E. (459426), our proband, shown in **B** to **D,** was referred to also by Boatwright and colleagues and by Perloff and Phelps. Changes in the skin of the feet began at 20 years of age, and bilateral cataracts were discovered in her thirties. Below-knee amputations. **D,** were performed at the ages of 38 years and 45 years, after sympathectomy and skin grafts had failed. The chest had a barrel configuration and the extremities were spindly. The nose was beaked, **B** and **C.** Radiographic studies showed generalized osteoporosis and calcification at the root of the aorta, extending into the myocardium. A systolic ejection murmur in the aortic area was interpreted as indicative of aortic valve sclerosis with mild stenosis. Esophageal motility was normal. The chromosomes of this patient were found to be normal. X-ray films, e.g., of the hand, showed pronounced osteoporosis. There was subcutaneous calcification over the elbow.

Thus sarcoma occurred in at least 2 affected persons in this family. The increased frequency of neoplasia has been noted in the literature. The occurrence of aortic valve sclerosis is illustrated by K. E. (III-16). (Family studied by Dr. R. M. Goodman.)

group of disorders in which, more perhaps than in any other area of medicine, eponyms abound and confound. The following six entities are only a partial enumeration:

Phalangeal epiphyses . . . . .Thiemann[209]
Tubercle of tibia . . . . Osgood-Schlatter
Head of femur . . . . Legg-Calvé-Perthes[242]
Spine . . . . Scheuermann
Tarsal scaphoid . . . . Köhler
Semilunar . . . . Kienböck, etc.

All these disorders probably have a hereditary background, although the evidence in Legg-Perthes disease is most complete. Each form of aseptic necrosis seems to be a distinct genotypic entity. There is, for example, no evidence that more than one of these entities occurs in the same patient or that one member of an affected family has one variety whereas another member has a different variety. Interestingly, Legg-Perthes disease probably almost never occurs in *bona fide* form in the pure Negro, although a simulating condition occurs with sickle cell hemoglobin C disease.[236]

REFERENCES
Fibrodysplasia ossificans progressiva (FOP)

1. Angervall, L., Stener, B., Stener, I., and Åhrén, C.: Pseudomalignant osseous tumour of soft tissue; a clinical, radiological and pathological study of five cases, J. Bone Joint Surg. **51-B:** 654, 1969.
2. Barker, L. F.: Medical clinics, Philadelphia, 1922, W. B. Saunders Co.
3. Bassett, C. A., Donath, A., Macagno, F., Preisig, R., Fleisch, H., and Francis, M. D.: Diphosphonates in the treatment of myositis ossificans (letter), Lancet 2:845, 1969.
4. Bauer, K. H., and Bode, W.: Erbpathologie der Stützgewebe beim Menschen. Handbuch der Erbbiologie des Menschen, vol. 3, Berlin, 1940, Julius Springer, p. 105.
5. Becker, P. E., and von Knorre, G.: Myositis ossificans progressiva, Ergebn. Inn. Med. Kinderheilk. 27:1, 1968.
6. Bell, J.: On hereditary digital anomalies. Part I. On brachydactyly and symphalangism. The treasury of human inheritance, London, 1951, Cambridge University Press.
7. Brooks, W. D. W.: Calcinosis, Quart. J. Med. 3:293, 1934.
8. Burton-Fanning, F. W., and Vaughan, A. L.: A case of myositis ossificans, Lancet 2:849, 1901.
9. Chaco, J.: Myositis ossificans progressiva, Acta Rheum. Scand. 13:235, 1967.
10. Drago, A.: Contributo allo studio della moisite ossificente progressive multipla, Pediatria 27:715, 1919.
11. Dwivedi, R.: Myositis ossificans progressiva, J. Indian Med. Ass. 41:558, 1963.
12. Eaton, W. L., Conkling, W. S., and Daeschner, C. W.: Early myositis ossificans progressiva occurring in homozygotic twins; a clinical and pathologic study, J. Pediat. 50:591, 1957.
13. Ebrahim, G. J., Grech, P., and Slavin, G.: Myositis ossificans progressiva in an African child, Brit. J. Radiol. 39:952, 1966.
14. Fairbank, H. A. T.: An atlas of general affections of the skeleton, Baltimore, 1951, The Williams & Wilkins Co.
15. Fairbank, H. A. T.: Myositis ossificans progressiva, J. Bone Joint Surg. 32-B:108, 1950.
16. Falls, H. F.: Skeletal system, including joints. In Sorsby, A.: Clinical genetics, St. Louis, 1953, The C. V. Mosby Co., chap. 14.
17. Fletcher, E., and Moss, M. S.: Myositis ossificans progressiva, Ann. Rheum. Dis. 24:267, 1965.
17a. Frame, B., Azad, N., Reynolds, W. A., and Saled, S. M.: Polyostotic fibrous dysplasia and myositis ossificans progressiva, a report of coincidence, Amer. J. Dis. Child. 124:120, 1972.
18. Fränkel, B.: Ein Fall von erblicher Deformität, Berl. Klin. Wschr. 8:418, 1871.

19. Frejka, B.: Heterotopic ossification and myositis ossificans progressiva, J. Bone Joint Surg. **11**:157, 1929.
20. Freke, J.: Philos. Trans. Roy. Soc., London, 1740. Quoted by Ralph H. Major: Classic descriptions of disease, with biographical sketches of the authors, ed. 3, Springfield, Ill., 1945, Charles C Thomas, Publisher, p. 304.
21. Garrod, A. E.: The initial stage of myositis ossificans, St. Bartholomew's Hosp. Rep. **43**:43, 1907.
22. Gaster, A.: Discussion in meeting of West London Medico-Chirurgical Society, Oct. 7, 1904, West London Med. J. **10**:37, 1905.
22a. Geho, W. B., and Whiteside, J. A.: Experience with disodium etidronate on diseases of ectopic calcification. In Frame, B., editor: International Symposium on Clinical Metabolic Bone Diseases, Detroit, 1972, Henry Ford Hospital (in press).
23. Geschickter, C. F., and Maseritz, I. H.: Myositis ossificans, J. Bone Joint Surg. **20**:661, 1938.
24. Glimcher, M. J.: Specificity of the molecular structure of organic matrices in mineralization. In Sognnaes, R. F., editor: Calcification in biological systems, Washington, D. C., 1960, American Association for the Advancement of Science, p. 421.
25. Greig, D. M.: Clinical observations of the surgical pathology of bone, Edinburgh, 1931, Oliver & Boyd, p. 170.
26. Griffith, G.: Progressive myositis ossificans; report of a case, Arch. Dis. Child. **24**:71, 1949.
27. Gruber, G. B.: Anmerkungen zur Frage der Weichteilverknöcherung, besonders der Myopathia osteoplastica, Virchow Arch. **260**:457, 1926.
28. Gutman, A. B., and Yü, T. F.: A further consideration of the effects of beryllium salts on in vitro calcification of cartilage; metabolic interrelations, Trans. Josiah Macy Jr. Found. **3**:90, 1950.
29. Guyatt, B. L., Kay, H. D., and Branion, H. D.: Beryllium "rickets," J. Nutr. **6**:313, 1933.
30. Gwinn, J. L.: Radiological case of the month; progressive myositis ossificans, Amer. J. Dis. Child. **116**:655, 1968.
31. Harris, N. H.: Myositis ossificans progressiva, Proc. Roy. Soc. Med. **54**:70, 1961.
32. Helferich, H.: Ein Fall von sogenannter Myositis ossificans progressiva, Aerztl. Intelligenz-Blatl. **26**:485, 1879.
33. Hellinger, M. J.: Myositis ossificans of the muscles of mastication, Oral Surg. **19**:581, 1965.
34. Herrmann, J., Schuster, M., Walker, F. A., White, E. F., Opitz, J. M., and ZuRhein, G. M.: Fibrodysplasia ossificans progressiva and the XXXXY syndrome in the same sibship. In Bergsma, D., editor: Clinical delineation of birth defects. V. Phenotypic aspects of chromosomal aberrations, New York, 1969, National Foundation–March of Dimes.
35. Hirsch, F., and Löw-Beer, A.: Ueber einen Fall von Myositis ossificans progressiva, Med. Klin. **25**:1661, 1929.
36. Huggins, C. B.: The formation of bone under the influence of epithelium of the alimentary tract, Arch. Surg. **22**:377, 1931.
37. Hutchinson, J.: Reports of hospital practice, M. Times Gaz. **1**:March 31, 1860.
38. Jones, B., Love, B., and Crosbie, D.: The patient with myositis ossificans progressiva, Nurs. Clin. N. Amer. **4**:189, 1969.
39. Klemper, F. W., Miller, J. M., and Hill, C. J.: The inhibition of alkaline phosphatase by beryllium, J. Biol. Chem. **180**:281, 1949.
40. Koontz, A. R.: Myositis ossificans progressiva, Amer. J. Med. Sci. **174**:406, 1927.
41. Koontz, A. R.: Personal communication.
42. Kubler, E.: Neue Gesichtspunkte bei der Beurteilung der Verlaufsformen der Myositis ossificans progressiva, Fortschr. Roentgenstr. **81**:354, 1954.
43. Laluque, P., Fillaudeau, G., Tchuenbou, M., and Doo, H. M..: Réflexions à propos d'un cas de myosite ossifiante progressiva non traumatique ou maladie de Munchmeyer, Presse Méd. **71**:2098, 1963.
44. Letts, R. M.: Myositis ossificans progressiva, Canad. Med. Ass. J. **100**:133, 1969.
45. Letts, R. M.: Myositis ossificans progressiva; a report of two cases wth chromosome studies, Canad. Med. Ass. J. **99**:856, 1968.
46. Liberman, U. A., Barzel, U., and DeVries, A.: Myositis ossificans traumatica with unusual course; effect of EDTA on calcium, phosphorus and manganese excretion, Amer. J. Med. Sci. **254**:35, 1967.

47. Lins, F. M., and Abath, G. M.: Doenca ossificante progressiva, Pediat. Prát. **30**:131, 1959.
48. Lockhart, J. D., and Burke, F. G.: Myositis ossificans progressiva; report of a case treated with corticotropin (ACTH), Amer. J. Dis. Child. **87**:626, 1954.
49. Ludman, H., Hamilton, E. B., and Eade, A. W.: Deafness in myositis ossificans progressiva, J. Laryng. **82**:57, 1968.
50. Lutwak, L.: Myositis ossificans progressiva; mineral, metabolic and radioactive calcium studies of the effects of hormones, Amer. J. Med. **37**:269, 1964.
51. Magruder, L. F.: Myositis ossificans progressiva; case report and review of the literature, Amer. J. Roentgen. **15**:328, 1926.
52. Mair, W. F.: Myositis ossificans progressiva, Edinburgh Med. J. **39**:13, 69, 1932.
53. Maroteaux, P.: Myositis ossificans, Rev. Rhum. **32**:512, 1965.
54. Mather, J. H.: Progressive myositis ossificans, Brit. J. Radiol. **4**:207, 1931.
55. Maudsley, R. H.: Case of myositis ossificans progressiva, Brit. Med. J. **1**:954, 1952.
56. Michelsohn, J.: Ein Fall von Myositis ossificans progressiva, Z. Orthop. Chir. **12**:424, 1904.
57. Neuman, W. F., and Neuman, M. W.: Chemical dynamics of bone mineral, Chicago, 1958, The University of Chicago Press, p. 179.
58. Nutt, J. J.: Report of a case of myositis ossificans progressiva, with bibliography, J. Bone Joint Surg. **5**:344, 1923.
59. Pack, G. T., and Braund, R. R.: Development of sarcoma in myositis ossificans, J.A.M.A. **119**:776, 1942.
60. Pappas, D. G., and Johnson, L. A.: Laryngeal myositis ossificans; a case report, Arch. Otolaryng. **81**:227, 1965.
61. Parnes, E. I., and Hinds, E. C.: Traumatic myositis ossificans of the masseter muscle; report of case, J. Oral Surg. **23**:245, 1965.
62. Paul, J. R.: A study of an unusual case of myositis ossificans, Arch. Surg. **10**:185, 1925.
63. Pol: "Brachydaktylie," "Klinodaktylie," Hyperphalangie und ihre Grundlagen; Form und Entstehung der meist unter dem Bild der Brachydaktylie auftretenden Varietäten, Anomalien und Missbildungen der Hand und des Fusses, Virchow Arch. **299**:388, 1921.
64. Riley, H. D., Jr., and Christie, A.: Myositis ossificans progressiva, Pediatrics **8**:753, 1951.
65. Rolleston, H. D.: Progressive myositis ossificans, with references to other developmental diseases of the mesoblast, Clin. J. **17**:209, 1901.
66. Rosenstirn, J.: A contribution to the study of myositis ossificans progressiva, Ann. Surg. **68**:485, 591, 1918.
67. Ryan, K. J.: Myositis ossificans progressiva; review of the literature with report of a case, J. Pediat. **27**:348, 1945.
68. Seibold, H. R., and Davis, C. L.: Generalized myositis ossificans (familial) in pigs, Path. Vet. **4**:79, 1967.
69. Selye, H., Mahajan, S., and Mahajan, R. S.: Histogenesis of experimentally induced myositis ossificans in the heart, Amer. Heart J. **73**:195, 1967.
70. Smith, D. M., Zeman, W., and Johnston, C. C., Jr.: Myositis ossificans progressiva; case report with metabolic and histochemical studies, Metabolism **15**:521, 1966.
71. Stickler, G. B., Belau, P. G., Farrell, F. J., Jones, J. D., Pugh, D. G., Steinberg, A. G., and Ward, L. E.: Hereditary progressive arthro-ophthalmopathy, Mayo Clin. Proc. **40**:433, 1965.
72. Stonham, C.: Myositis ossificans, Lancet **2**:1481, 1892.
73. Sympson, T.: Case of myositis ossificans, Brit. Med. J. **2**:1026, 1886.
74. Trester, P. H., Markovitch, E., Zambito, R. F., and Stratigas, G. T.: Myositis ossificans, circumscripta and progressiva, with surgical correction of the masseter muscle; report of two cases, J. Oral Surg. **27**:201, 1969.
75. Tünte, W., Becker, P. E., and Knorre, G. V.: Zur Genetik der Myositis ossificans progressiva, Humangenetik **4**:320, 1967.
76. Tutunjian, K. H., and Kegerreis, R.: Myositis ossificans progressiva, with report of a case, J. Bone Joint Surg. **19**:503, 1937.
77. Van Creveld, S., and Soeters, J. M.: Progressive myositis ossificans, Amer. J. Dis. Child. **62**:1000, 1941.
78. Vastine, J. H., II, Vastine, M. F., and Arango, O.: Genetic influence on osseous development, with particular reference to the deposition of calcium in the costal cartilages, Amer. J. Roentgen. **59**:213, 1948.

79. Vastine, J. H., II, Vastine, M. F., and Arango, O.: Myositis ossificans progressiva in homozygotic twins, Amer. J. Roentgen. **59**:204, 1948.

80. Viparelli, V.: La miosite ossificante progressiva, Ann. Neuropsichiat. Psicoanal. **9**:297, 1962.

81. Weiss, I. W., Fisher, L., and Phang, J. M.: Diphosphonate therapy in a patient with myositis ossificans progressiva, Ann. Intern. Med. **74**:933, 1971.

82. Wheeler, C. E., Curtis, A. C., Cawley, E. P., Grekin, R. H., and Zheutlin, B.: Soft tissue calcification, with special reference to its occurrence in the "collagen diseases," Ann. Intern. Med. **36**:1050, 1952.

83. Wilkins, W. E., Reagan, E. M., and Carpenter, G. K.: Phosphatase studies on biopsy tissue in progressive myositis ossificans, Amer. J. Dis. Child. **49**:1219, 1935.

84. Woolley, M. M., Morgan, S., and Hays, D. M.: Heritable disorders of connective tissue; surgical and anesthetic problems, J. Pediat. Surg. **2**:325, 1967.

Osteopoikilosis

85. Albers-Schönberg, H.: Eine seltene bisher nicht bekannte Strukturanomalie des Skelettes, Fortschr. Roentgenstr. **23**:174, 1915.

86. Albronda, J.: Familiale osteopoikilie, Nederl. T. Geneesk. **100**:3533, 1956.

87. Berlin, R., Hedensio, B., and Lilja, B.: Osteopoikilosis; a clinical and genetic study, Acta Med. Scand. **181**:305, 1967.

88. Bistolfi: Cited by Curth.[90]

89. Bloom, A. R.: Osteopoecilia, Amer. J. Surg. **22**:239, 1933.

90. Briottet, J., Dechelotte, J., and Rivot, G.: Familial osteopoikilosis, J. Radiol. Electr. **47**:789, 1966.

91. Busch, K. F. B.: Familial disseminated osteosclerosis, Acta Radiol. Scand. **18**:693, 1937.

92. Buschke, A., and Ollendorff, H.: Ein Fall von Dermatofibrosis lenticularis disseminata und Osteopathia condensans disseminata, Derm. Wschr. **86**:257, 1928.

93. Carns, R. J.: Familial juvenile elastoma; osteopoikilosis (2 cases), Proc. Roy. Soc. Med. **60**:1267, 1967.

94. Castellano, E., and Piotti, F.: A case of spotty osteopecilia with unusual costal and vertebral localization, Minerva Med. **58**:4082, 1967.

95. Cocchi, U.: In Schinz, H. R., Baensch, W. E., Friedl, E., and Uehlinger, E.: Roentgen-diagnostics (J. T. Case, editor of American edition), New York, 1951, Grune & Stratton, Inc., p. 744.

96. Copeman, W. S. C., editor: Textbook of rheumatic diseases, Edinburgh and London, 1955, E. & S. Livingston, Ltd., p. 307.

97. Coughlin, E. J., Jr., Guare, H. F., and Moskovitz, A. J.: Chondrodystrophia calcificans congenita; case report with autopsy, J. Bone Joint Surg. **32-A**:938, 1950.

98. Crespo, D. I.: Osteopoikilosis, A.I.R. **4**:71, 1961.

99. Curth, H. O.: Dermatofibrosis lenticularis disseminata and osteopoikilosis, Arch. Derm. Syph. **30**:552, 1934.

100. Curth, H. O.: Follicular atrophoderma and pseudopelade associated with chondrodystrophia calcificans congenita, J. Invest. Derm. **13**:233, 1949.

101. Danielsen, L., Midtgaard, K., and Christensen, H. E.: Osteopoikilosis associated with dermatofibrosis lenticularis disseminata, Arch. Derm. **100**:465, 1969.

102. Erbsen, H.: Die Osteopoikilie (Osteopathia condensans disseminata), Ergebn. Med. Strahlenforsch. **7**:137, 1936.

103. Funstein, L., and Kotschiew, K.: Ueber die Osteopoikilie, Fortschr. Roentgenstr. **54**:595, 1936.

104. Green, A. E., Jr., Ellswood, W. H., and Collins, J. R.: Melorheostosis and osteopoikilosis; with a review of the literature, Amer. J. Roentgen. **87**:1096, 1962.

105. Hinson, A.: Familial osteopoikilosis, Amer. J. Surg. **45**:566, 1939.

106. Jeter, H., and McGehee, C. L.: Osteopoikilosis, J. Bone Joint Surg. **15**:990, 1933.

106a. Jonaseh, E.: 12 Fälle von Osteopoikilie, Fortschr. Roentgenstr. **82**:344, 1955.

107. Koch, J. C.: The laws of bone architecture, Amer. J. Anat. **21**:177, 1917.

108. Luzsa, G.: Osteopoikilia familiaris, Orv. Hetil. **103**:1267, 1962.

109. Marshall, J.: Osteopoikilosis and connective tissue naevi; a syndrome of hereditary polyfibromatosis, S. Afr. Med. J. **44**:775, 1970.

110. Martinčić, N.: Osteopoikilie (spotted bones), Brit. J. Radiol. **25:**612, 1952.
111. Nichols, B. H., and Shiflett, E. L.: Osteopoikilosis; report of an unusual case, Amer. J. Roentgen. **32:**52, 1934.
112. Osgood, E. C.: Polyostotic fibrous dysplasia and osteopathia condensans disseminata, Amer. J. Roentgen. **56:**174, 1946.
113. Pastinszky, J., and Csató, Z.: Über Hautveränderungen bei Osteopoikilie (Buschke-Ollendorff-Syndrom), Z. Haut. Geschlechtskr. **43:**313, 1968.
114. Raque, C. J., and Wood, M. G.: Connective-tissue nevus; dermatofibrosis lenticularis disseminata with osteopoikilosis, Arch. Derm. **102:**390, 1970.
115. Reilly, W. A., and Smith, F. S.: Stippled epiphyses with congenital hypothyroidism (cretinoid epiphyseal dysgenesis), Amer. J. Roentgen. **40:**675, 1938.
116. Risseeuw, J.: Familiäre osteopoikilie, Nederl. T. Geneesk. **80:**3827, 1936.
117. Ritterhoff, R. J., and Oscherwitz, D.: Osteopoikilosis associated with bronchogenic carcinoma and adenocarcinoma of stomach, Amer. J. Roentgen. **48:**341, 1942.
118. Schmorl, G.: Anatomische Befunde bei einem Fall von Osteopoikilie, Fortschr. Roentgenstr. **44:**1, 1931.
119. Smith, A. D., and Waisman, M.: Connective tissue nevi: familial occurrence and association with osteopoikilosis, Arch. Derm. **81:**249, 1960.
120. Steenhuis, D. J.: About a special case of osteitis condensans disseminata, Acta Radiol. **5:**373, 1926.
121. Stieda, A.: Ueber umschriebene Knochenverdichtungen im Bereich der Substantia spongiosa im Röntgenbilde, Beitr. Klin. Chir. **45:**700, 1905.
122. Sváb, d'Vaclav: A propos de l'ostéopoecilie héréditaire, J. Radiol. Electr. **16:**405, 1932.
123. Traub, E.: Epiphyseal necrosis in pituitary gigantism, Arch. Dis. Child. **14:**203, 1939.
124. Von Bernuth, F.: Ueber Sklerodermie, Osteopoikilie und Kalkgicht im Kindesalter, Z. Kinderheilk. **54:**103, 1932.
125. Voorhoeve, N.: A hitherto undescribed picture of abnormality of the skeleton, Acta Radiol. **3:**407, 1924.
126. Wilcox, L. R.: Osteopoikilosis (disseminated condensing osteopathy), Amer. J. Roentgen. **27:**580, 1932.
127. Windholz, F.: Ueber familiäre Osteopoikilie und Dermatofibrosis lenticularis disseminata, Fortschr. Roentgenstr. **45:**566, 1932.

Léri's pleonosteosis

128. Cocchi, U.: Hereditary diseases with bone changes. In Schinz, H. R., Baensch, W. E., Friedl, E., and Uehlinger, E.: Roentgen-diagnostics (J. T. Case, editor of American edition), New York, 1951, Grune & Stratton, Inc., vol. 1, pp. 720 ff.
129. Cohen and de Herdt: Pléonostéose familiale, J. Neurol. Psychiat. **28:**395, 1928.
130. Copeman, W. S. S., editor: Textbook of the rheumatic diseases, Edinburgh, 1955, E. & S. Livingstone, Ltd.
131. Esterly, N. B., and McKusick, V. A.: Stiff skin syndrome, Pediatrics **47:**360, 1971.
132. Feiguine, E., and Tikhodéeff, S.: Un cas rare d'osteopathie systematisée—un cas de pléonostéose en U. R. S. S., Arch. Méd. Enf. **35:**654, 1932.
133. Léri, A.: Dystrophie osseuse généralisée congénitale et heréditaire: la pléonostéose familiale, Presse Méd. **30:**13, 1922.
134. Léri, A.: Une maladie congénitale et heréditaire de l'ossification: la pléonostéose familiale, Bull. Soc. Méd. Hôp. Paris **45:**1228, 1921.
135. Léri, A.: Sur la pléonostéose familiale, Bull. Soc. Méd. Hôp. Paris **48:**216, 1924.
135a. Mahloudji, M., Teasdall, R. D., Adamkiewicz, J. J., Hartmann, W. H., Lambird, P. A., and McKusick, V. A.: The genetic amyloidoses with particular reference to hereditary neuropathic amyloidosis, type II (Indiana or Rukavina type), Medicine **48:**1, 1969.
136. Materna, A.: Zur Pathologie der Pléonosteose (Léri), Beitr. Path. Anat. **112:**112, 1952.
136a. McKusick, V. A. (Baltimore): Unpublished observations.
137. Moore, W. T., and Federman, D. D.: Familial dwarfism and "stiff joints"; report of a kindred, Arch. Intern. Med. **115:**398, 1965.
138. Neel, J. V., and Schull, W. J.: Human heredity, Chicago, 1954, The University of Chicago Press, p. 309.

139. Rocher, H. L., and Pesme, P.: Un cas de pléonostéose (maladie de Léri) avec cornées opal-escentes, J. Méd. Bordeaux **123**:121, 1946.

140. Rocher, H. L., and Roudil, G.: La pléonostéose (maladie de Léri), Bordeaux Chir. **4**:359, 1932.

141. Rothea, M.: La pléonostéose familiale (maladie d'André Léri), Theses, Paris and Nancy, No. 421.

142. Rouillard, J., and Barreau, P.: Un nouveau cas de pléonostéose heréditaire avec atteintes graves des grosses articulations, Bull. Soc. Méd. Hôp. Paris **51**:794, 1927.

143. Rukavina, J. G., Falls, H. F., Holt, J. F., and Block, W. G.: Léri's pleonosteosis; a study of a family with a review of the literature, J. Bone Joint Surg. **41-A**:397, 1959.

144. Watson-Jones, R.: Léri's pleonosteosis, carpal tunnel compression of the medial nerves and Morton's metatarsalgia, J. Bone Joint Surg. **31-B**:560, 1949.

Paget's disease

145. Albright, F., and Reifenstein, E. C., Jr.: The parathyroid glands and metabolic bone disease; selected studies, Baltimore, 1948, The Williams & Wilkins Co., pp. 284-301.

146. Aschner, B. M., Hurst, L. A., and Roizin, L.: Genetic study of Paget's disease in monozygotic twin brothers, Acta Genet. Med. **1**:67, 1952.

147. Ashley-Montagu, M. F.: Paget's disease (osteitis deformans) and heredity, Amer. J. Hum. Genet. **1**:94, 1947.

148. Barry, H. C.: Paget's disease of bone, Edinburgh and London, 1969, E. & S. Livingstone, Ltd.

149. Brunner, H.: Zur Pathologie der Ostitis deformans (Paget) des Schläfenbeins, Klin. Wschr. **2**:174, 1931.

150. Brunner, W.: Osteodystrophia deformans Paget unter besonderer Berücksichtigung unserer Erfahrungen der letzten 10 Jahre, Deutsch. Z. Chir. **52**:585, 1939.

151. Chauffard, A.: Discussion of paper by Gilles de la Tourette and Marinesco, Bull. Soc. Méd. Hôp. Paris **11** (ser. 3):426, 1894.

152. Clegg, J. T.: Paget's disease with mental symptoms and choroiditis, Lancet **2**:128, 1937.

153. Cockayne, E. A.: Quoted by Rast and Weber.[188]

154. Crumpacker, E. L., and Lipscomb, P. R.: The familial incidence of Paget's disease of bone (osteitis deformans); report of occurrence in three siblings, Med. Clin. N. Amer. **35**:1203, 1951.

155. Dandy, W. E.: Personal communication.

156. Dickson, D. D., Camp, J. D., and Ghormley, R. K.: Osteitis deformans (Paget's disease of bone), Radiology **44**:449, 1945.

157. Dubreuilh, W., and Laubie: Maladie osseuse de Paget chez deux frères, Bull. Soc. Franç. Derm. **3**:87, 1924.

158. Edholm, O. G., Howarth, S., and McMichael, J.: Heart failure and bone blood flow in osteitis deformans, Clin. Sci. **5**:249, 1945.

159. Evens, R. G., and Bartter, F. C.: The hereditary aspect of Paget's disease (osteitis deformans), J.A.M.A. **205**:900, 1968.

160. Faugeron, R.: Essai sur les rapports de la syphilis et de la maladie osseuse de Paget, Thèse de Paris, 1923.

161. Galbraith, H. J. B.: Familial Paget's disease of bone, Brit. Med. J. **2**:29, 1954.

162. Goldenberg, R. R.: The skeleton in Paget's disease, Bull. Hosp. Joint Dis. **12**:229, 1951.

163. Gutman, A. B., and Kasabach, H. H.: Paget's disease (osteitis deformans); analysis of 116 cases, Amer. J. Med. Sci. **191**:361, 1936.

164. Hanke, H.: Osteodystrophische Erkrankungen und ihre Begrenzung, Deutsch. Z. Chir. **245**:641, 1935.

165. Harrison, C. V., and Lennox, B.: Heart block in osteitis deformans, Brit. Heart J. **10**:167, 1948.

166. Higbee, W. S., and Ellis, A. G.: A case of osteitis deformans, J. Med. Res. **24**:43, 1911.

167. Hurwitz, S. H.: Osteitis deformans, Paget's disease; a report of six cases, Bull. Hopkins Hosp. **24**:263, 1913.

168. Hurwitz, S. H.: Osteitis deformans (Paget's disease), Bull Hopkins Hosp. **24**:266, 1913.

169. Irvine, R. E.: Familial Paget's disease with early onset, J. Bone Joint Surg. **35-B**:106, 1953.

170. John, E., and Strasser, U.: Zur Aetiologie, Klinik und Therapie der Ostitis fibrosa deformans (Paget), Deutsch. Z. Nervenheilk, **97:**81, 1927.

171. Kay, H. D., Simpson, S. L., and Riddock, G.: Osteitis deformans, Arch. Intern. Med. **53:**208, 1934.

172. Kilner, J.: Two cases of osteitis deformans in one family, Lancet **1:**221, 1904.

173. Koller, F.: Ueber die Heredität der Ostitis deformans Paget, Helv. Med. Acta **13:**389, 1946.

174. Laederich, L., Mamon, H., and Beuchesne, H.: Un cas de maladie osseuse de Paget avec cataracte de type endocrinien, Bull. Soc. Méd. Hôp. Paris **65:**529, 1938.

175. Lambert, R. K.: Paget's disease with angioid streaks of the retina, Arch. Ophthal. **22:**106, 1939.

176. Lunn, J. R.: Four cases of osteitis deformans, Trans. Clin. Soc. London **18:**272, 1885.

177. Martin, E.: Considérations sur la maladie de Paget, Helv. Med. Acta **14:**319, 1947.

178. Moehlig, R. C.: Osteitis deformans; familial constitutional hereditary background as etiological factors, J. Mich. Med. Soc. **51:**1004, 1027, 1952.

179. Moehlig, R. C.: Paget's disease (osteitis deformans) and osteoporosis; similarity of the 2 conditions as shown by familial background and glucose tolerance studies, Surg. Gynec. Obstet. **62:**815, 1936.

180. Monroe, R. T.: Diseases of old age, Cambridge, 1951, Harvard University Press, p. 304.

181. Morrison, W. H.: Osteitis deformans with angioid streaks; report of a case, Arch. Ophthal. **26:**79, 1941.

182. Mozer, J. J.: Discussion of Koller.[173]

183. Murphy, W.: Osteitis deformans in a brother and sister, Med. J. Aust. **1:**507, 1950.

184. Narins, L., and Oppenheimer, G. D.: Calcification of vas deferens associated with Paget's disease of bone, J. Urol. **67:**2118, 1952.

185. Paget, J.: Remarks on osteitis deformans, Illust. Med. News **2:**181, 1889.

186. Parry, T. W.: A case of osteitis deformans in which fracture of a femur took place as the result of stooping, Brit. Med. J. **1:**879, 1912.

187. Pick: Osteitis deformans, Lancet **2:**1125, 1883.

188. Rast, H., and Weber, F. P.: Paget's bone disease in three sisters, Brit. Med. J. **1:**918, 1937.

189. Roberts, R. E., and Cohen, M. J.: Osteitis deformans (Paget's disease of bone), Proc. Roy. Soc. Med. **19:**13, 1936.

190. Rosenkrantz, J. A., Wolf, J., and Kaicher, J.: Paget's disease (osteitis deformans); review of 111 cases, Arch. Intern. Med. **90:**610, 1952.

191. Sabatini, G.: Ostitis fibrosa di Paget in due coppie di coniugi, Minerva Med. **39:**607, 1948.

192. Schmorl, G.: Ueber Ostitis deformans Paget, Virchow Arch. **283:**694, 1932.

193. Schwartz, L. A.: Paget's disease in 3 male siblings; clinical report, J. Mich. Med. Soc. **47:**1244, 1948.

194. Seligman, B., and Nathanson, L.: Metastatic calcification in the soft tissues of the legs in osteitis deformans, Ann. Intern. Med. **23:**82, 1945.

195. Smith, S. M.: A case of osteitis deformans in which the disease is present in father and son, Trans. Med. Soc. London **28:**224, 1904-1905.

196. Sornberger, C. F., and Smedel, M. I.: Mechanism and incidence of cardiovascular changes in Paget's disease; critical review of literature with case studies, Circulation **6:**711, 1952.

197. Stahl, B. F.: Osteitis deformans, Paget's disease, with reports of two cases and autopsy in one, Amer. J. Med. Sci. **143:**525, 1912.

198. Stein, I., Stein, R. O., and Beller, M. L.: Living bone in health and disease, Philadelphia, 1955, J. B. Lippincott Co.

199. Stemmermann, W.: Die Ostitis deformans Paget unter Berücksichtigung ihrer Vererbung, Ergebn. Inn. Med. **3** (n.s.):185, 1952.

200. Storsteen, K. A., and Jones, N. J.: Arteriography and vascular studies in Paget's disease of bone, J.A.M.A. **154:**472, 1954.

201. Terry, T. L.: Angioid streaks and osteitis deformans, Trans. Amer. Ophthal. Soc. **32:**555, 1934.

202. Van Bogaert, L.: Ueber eine hereditäre und familiäre Form der Pagetschen Ostitis deformans mit Chorioretinitis pigmentosa, Z. Ges. Neur. **147:**327, 1933.

203. Von der Heydt, R.: Osteitis deformans with pigmented corneal degeneration, Amer. J. Ophthal. **20:**1139, 1937.

204. Wells, H. G., and Holley, S. W.: Metastatic calcification in osteitis deformans, Arch. Path. **34**:435, 1942.

205. Wilton, A.: On the genesis of osteitis deformans (Paget), Acta Orthop. Scand. **24**:30, 1954.

206. Woodcock, C. W.: Transactions of the Cleveland Dermatological Society, Arch. Derm. Syph. **65**:623, 1952.

Other possible hereditary and generalized disorders of connective tissue

207. Bloom, D.: Heredity of keloids, New York J. Med. **56**:511, 1956.

208. Boatwright, H., Wheeler, C. E., and Cawley, E. P.: Werner's syndrome, Arch. Intern. Med. **90**:243, 1952.

209. Böhme, A.: Kasuistischer Beitrag zur Thiemannschen Epiphysenerkrankung, Z. Ges. Inn. Med. **18**:491, 1963.

210. Bunnell, S.: Surgery of the hand, Philadelphia, 1948, J. B. Lippincott Co.

211. Cockayne, E. A.: Inherited abnormalities of the skin and its appendages, London, 1933, Oxford University Press, p. 310.

212. Conway, H.: Dupuytren's contracture, Amer. J. Surg. **87**:161, 1954.

213. David, B.: Über einen dominanten Erbgang bei eines polytopen enchondralen Dysostose Typ Pfändler-Hurler, Z. Orthop. **84**:657, 1953.

213a. DeBusk, F. L.: The Hutchinson-Gilford progeria syndrome, J. Pediat. **80**:697, 1972.

214. Early, P. F.: Dupuytren's contracture, J. Bone Joint Surg. **44-B**:602, 1962.

215. Early, P. F.: Genetics of Dupuytren's contracture, Brit. Med. J. **1**:908, 1964.

216. Epstein, C. J., Martin, G. M., Schultz, A. L., and Motulsky, A. G.: Werner's syndrome; a review of its symptomatology, natural history, pathologic features, genetics and relationship to the natural aging process, Medicine **45**:177, 1966.

217. Garrod, A. E.: Concerning pads upon the finger joints and their clinical relationship, Brit. Med. J. **2**:8, 1904.

218. Garrod, A. E.: On an unusual form of nodule upon the joints of the fingers, St. Bartholomew's Hosp. Rep. **29**:157, 1893.

219. Ghormley, R. K.: A case of congenital osteosclerosis, Bull. Hopkins Hosp. **33**:404, 1922.

220. Haverkamp Begemann, N., and van Lookeren Campagne, A.: Homozygous form of Pelger-Huët's nuclear anomaly in man, Acta Haemat. **7**:295, 1952.

221. Hunt, A. C., and Ley, D. G.: General arterial calcification of infancy, Brit. Med. J. **1**:385, 1957.

222. Irvin, G. W., and Ward, P. B.: Werner's syndrome, with a report of two cases, Amer. J. Med. **15**:266, 1953.

223. Klein, H.: Die Pelger-Anomalie der Leukocyten und die pathologische Anatomie des neugeborenen homozygoten Pelger-Kaninchens; ein Beitrag zum Formenkries der fetelen Chondrodystrophie, Z. Menschl. Vererb. Konstitutionsl. **29**:551, 1949.

224. Kostia, J.: A Dupuytren contracture family, Ann. Chir. Gynaec. Fenniae **46**:351, 1957.

225. Ling, R. S. M.: The genetic factor in Dupuytren's disease, J. Bone Joint Surg. **45-B**:709, 1963.

226. Lund, M.: Dupuytren's contracture and epilepsy, Acta Psychiat. Neurol. **16**:465, 1941.

226a. McKusick, V. A.: Pachydermoperiostosis. In Fitzpatrick, T. B., Arndt, K. A., Clark, W. H., Jr., Eisen, A. Z., Van Scott, E. J., and Vaughan, J. H., editors: Dermatology in internal medicine, New York, 1971, McGraw-Hill Book Co., pp. 1227-1228.

227. Menten, M. L., and Felteman, G. H.: Coronary sclerosis in infancy; report of three autopsied cases, two in siblings, Amer. J. Clin. Path. **18**:805, 1948.

228. Meyer, R. J.: The medical significance of lenticular opacities (cataract) before the age of fifty, with emphasis on their occurrence in systemic disorders, New Eng. J. Med. **252**:622, 665, 1955.

229. Moore, W. T., and Federman, D. D.: Familial dwarfism and "stiff joints," Arch. Intern. Med. **115**:398, 1965.

230. Murley, R. S.: Peyronie's disease, Brit. Med. J. **1**:908, 1964.

231. Nachtsheim, H.: Pelger anomaly in man and rabbit, J. Hered. **41**:131, 1950.

231a. Opitz, J. M.: Malformation syndromes (cont.). In Bergsma, D., editor: Clinical delineation of birth defects, Baltimore, 1973, The Williams & Wilkins Co.

232. Perloff, J. K., and Phelps, E. T.: A review of Werner's syndrome, with a report of the second autopsied case, Amer. Intern. Med. **48:**1205, 1958.

233. Reed, R., Seville, R. H., and Tattersall, R. N.: Werner's syndrome, Brit. J. Derm. **65:**165, 1953.

233a. Rimoin, D. L.: Pachydermoperiostosis (idiopathic clubbing and periostosis): genetic and physiologic considerations, New Eng. J. Med. **272:**923-931, 1965.

234. Schourup, K.: Plastic induration of the penis, Acta Radiol. **26:**313, 1945.

235. Skoog, T.: Dupuytren's contraction with special reference to etiology and improved surgical treatment; its occurrence in epileptics; note on knuckle pads, Acta Chir. Scand., supp. 138, 1948.

236. Smith, E. W., and Conley, C. L.: Genetic variants of sickle cell disease, Bull. Hopkins Hosp. **94:**289, 1954.

237. Smith, R. C., Winer, L. H., and Martel, S.: Werner's syndrome; report of two cases, Arch. Derm. **71:**197, 1955.

238. Stickler, G. B., and Pugh, D. G.: Hereditary progressive arthro-ophthalmopathy. II. Additional observations on vertebral abnormalities, a hearing defect, and a report of a similar case, Mayo Clin. Proc. **42:**495, 1967.

239. Teleky, L.: Dupuytren's contraction as occupational disease, J. Indust. Hyg. **21:**233, 1939.

240. Thannhauser, S. J.: Werner's syndrome (progeria of the adult) and Rothmund's syndrome; two types of closely related heredofamilial atrophic dermatoses with juvenile cataracts and endocrine features; a critical study with five new cases, Ann. Intern. Med. **23:**559, 1945.

241. Van der Sar, A.: The Pelger-Huët familial nuclear anomaly of the leucocytes, Amer. J. Clin. Path. **15:**544, 1944.

242. Wamoscher, Z., and Farhi, A.: Hereditary Legg-Calvé-Perthes disease, Amer. J. Dis. Child. **106:**97, 1963.

243. Weber, F. P.: A note on Dupuytren's contraction, camptodactylia and knuckle pads, Brit. J. Derm. Syph. **50:**26, 1938.

244. White, W. H.: On pads on the finger joints, Quart. J. Med. **1:**479, 1908.

245. Williams, A. L. (Melbourne): The pathology of cardiac failure in infancy, M.D. thesis, University of Melbourne, 1958.

246. Williams, A. L. (Melbourne): Personal communication, 1959.

Menkes syndrome

247. Aguilar, M. J., Chadwick, D. L., Okuyama, K., and Kamoshita, S.: Kinky-hair disease. I. Clinical and pathological features, J. Neuropath. Exp. Neurol. **25:**507, 1966.

248. Al-Rashid, R. A., and Spangler, J.: Neonatal copper deficiency, New Eng. J. Med. **285:**841, 1971.

249. Billings, D. M., and Degnan, M.: Kinky hair syndrome: a new case and a review, Amer. J. Dis. Child. **121:**447, 1971.

250. Bray, P. F.: Sex-linked neurodegenerative disease associated with monilethrix, Pediatrics **36:**417, 1965.

251. Carnes, W. H.: Role of copper in connective tissue metabolism, Fed. Proc. **30:**995, 1971.

252. Danks, D. M. (Melbourne, Australia): Personal communication, 1972.

253. Danks, D. M., Campbell, P. E., Stevens, B. J., Mayne, V., and Cartwright, E.: Menkes' kinky hair syndrome: an inherited defect in copper absorption with widespread effects, Pediatrics **50:**188, 1972.

254. Danks, D. M., Cartwright, E., Campbell, P. E., and Mayne, V.: Is Menkes' syndrome a heritable disorder of connective tissue? (letter), Lancet **2:**1089, 1971.

255. Danks, D. M., Stevens, B. J., Campbell, P. E., Gillespie, J. M., Walker-Smith, J., Blomfield, J., and Turner, B.: Menkes' kinky-hair syndrome: an inherited defect in intestinal absorption with widespread consequences, Lancet **1:**110, 1972.

256. French, J. H., Sherare, E. S., Lubell, H., Brotz, M., and Moore, C. L.: Trichopoliodystrophy. I. Report of a case and biochemical studies, Arch. Neurol. **26:**229, 1972.

257. Ghatak, N. R., Hirano, A., Poon, T. P., and French, J. H.: Trichopoliodystrophy. II. Pathological changes in skeletal muscle and nervous system, Arch. Neurol. **26:**60, 1972.

258. Gillespie, J. M.: The isolation and properties of some soluble proteins from wool. VIII. The proteins of copper-deficient wool, Aust. J. Biol. Sci. **17:**282, 1964.

259. Menkes, J. H., Alter, M., Steigleder, G. K., Weakley, D. R., and Sung, J. H.: A sex-linked recessive disorder with retardation of growth, peculiar hair and focal cerebral and cerebellar degeneration, Pediatrics **29**:764, 1962.

260. O'Brien, J. S. (Los Angeles, Calif.): Personal communication, 1968.

260a. O'Brien, J. S., and Sampson, E. L.: Kinky hair disease. II. Biochemical studies, J. Neuropath. Exp. Neurol. **25**:523, 1966.

261. O'Dell, B. L., Hardwick, B. C., Reynolds, G., and Savage, J. E.: Connective tissue defect in the chick resulting from copper deficiency, Proc. Soc. Exp. Biol. Med. **108**:402, 1961.

262. Ramage, H., Sheldon, J. H., and Sheldon, W.: A spectrographic investigation of the metallic content of the liver in childhood, Proc. Roy. Soc., London, (s.B.) **112**:308, 1933.

263. Seelenfreund, M. H., Gartner, S., and Vinger, P. F.: The ocular pathology of Menkes' disease (kinky hair disease), Arch. Ophthal. **80**:718, 1968.

264. Underwood, E. J.: Trace elements in human and animal nutrition, ed. 3, New York, 1971, Academic Press, pp. 79-115.

265. Wesenberg, R. L., Gwinn, J. L., and Barnes, G. R.: Radiological findings in the kinky-hair syndrome, Radiology **92**:500, 1969.

13 · Genetic disorders of the osseous skeleton

The osseous skeleton, the largest specialized connective tissue, participates in many of the generalized heritable disorders of connective tissue previously discussed in this book. In addition it is subject to a large number of gene-determined derangements, with primary effects apparently limited to bone and cartilage. A review of some of these disorders[31,38,72,113,154,258,333] may be helpful in completing the survey undertaken in this book.

The bone dysplasias represent a difficult category of hereditary disease because the types are legion; each is rare or fairly rare, so that most physicians, even specialists such as orthopedists and radiologists, encounter them rarely; almost nothing is known of the pathogenesis and, at least until recently, little even of the histopathology; no definitive therapy is available for most, and nomenclature is chaotic.

The principal method of nosologic study has been radiologic, complemented by observations of the clinical natural history and familial (i.e., genetic) characteristics. New methods are urgently needed.

Historical note and earlier publications

Important nosologic and genetic studies of skeletal dysplasias were published by Mørch of Copenhagen in 1941,[216] by Grebe of Frankenburg, Germany, in 1955,[97] and by Hobaek of Norway in 1961.[113] Lamy and Maroteaux,[154,155,201,202,204] in Paris, have contributed massively to this field. In 1964 Rubin[258] gave a relatively exhaustive survey of skeletal dysplasias, introducing a roentgenographic-anatomic system of classification that has proved useful as both a diagnostic and a pedagogic device. The contributions of Langer[158-165] of Minneapolis and Spranger[293-297] of Kiel, Germany, also deserve particular mention.

Mørch* recognized the occurrence of "different degrees of chondrodystrophy" but overlooked the heterogeneity in his series of cases. A survey of the cases illustrated in Mørch's monograph[216] indicates a number with a skeletal dysplasia distinct from achondroplasia. For example, patients 28[216, Fig. 11] and 58[216, Fig. 17] appear to have had pseudoachondroplastic spondyloepiphyseal dysplasia. Patient 99[216, Fig. 11] probably had hypochondroplasia. Patient 7[216, Fig. 17] prob-

---

*After World War II, E. Trier Mørch (1908-   ) came to Chicago and established a reputation in respiratory physiology and in anesthesiology. The Mørch respirator is his invention.

ably had spondyloepiphyseal dysplasia congenita. Multiple epiphyseal dysplasia comes to mind as a leading possibility in the cases of patients 100[216, Fig. 62] and 24.[216, Fig. 80] The father and son pictured in Fig. 52 (reference 216) clearly had some disorder other than achondroplasia. Mørch recognized some distinct entities such as osteogenesis imperfecta, gargoylism, chondrodystrophia calcificans congenita, and Ollier's disease. He pictured, as an example of phocomelia,[216, Fig. 33] a patient with mandibular hypoplasia and mesomelic dwarfism which may be Langer's mandibulomelic dysplasia[160] or perhaps the Nievergelt syndrome.[290]

Grebe[97] recognized heterogeneity in the broad group of skeletal dysplasias and divided the cases into "Mopstyp" (pug-dog-like) and "Dackeltyp" (dachshundlike). The former group consisted of cases of classic achondroplasia; the latter group, characterized by normal head and face, included mainly cases of pseudoachondroplastic spondyloepiphyseal dysplasia. A survey of the cases in Grebe's monograph permits identification of a number of distinct entities, some of which Grebe recognized as separate from either the Mopstyp or the Dackeltyp. Grebe's Fig. 16 (from Kaufmann[137]) illustrated a possible case of achondrogenesis (lethal chondrodystrophic type); Fig. 18 (from Dietrich) a case of metatropic dwarfism; Fig. 25a (from Schinz, Baensch, and Friedl) and Fig. 66a, b, and d, cases of thanatophoric dwarfism. The 2 brothers pictured in Grebe's Fig. 93 appear to have the Maroteaux-Lamy syndrome (MPS VI), even though the cornea was said to have been clear; the pelvic x-ray film shown in his Fig. 94 shows changes of mucopolysaccharidosis too severe to qualify as the Hunter syndrome (MPS II), which was the diagnosis suggested by Grebe. The brother and sister shown in Grebe's Fig. 96 and the individual with the isolated case pictured in his Fig. 81 clearly had diastrophic dwarfism. The sisters pictured in Fig. 100 were the original cases of Grebe's achondrogenesis (hypomelic type); Grebe introduced the term achondrogenesis. (As indicated on p. 759, the designation achondrogenesis has been used for two completely different disorders.)

In their monograph *Les chondrodystrophies génotypiques*,[154] Lamy and Maroteaux gave a useful synthesis of their own experience and that recorded to 1960. The brief historical sketches are useful. They pointed out that achondroplasia, then called fetal rickets, was recognized as a distinct entity by Depaul in 1851, although Parrot in 1878 made the distinction generally appreciated, perhaps because he introduced a new term: achondroplasia. Pierre Marie contributed to the nosography of achondroplasia in the adult (he pointed out the trident hand), and Porak also gave early descriptions, as well as pointing out the similarities but distinctness of achondroplasia and osteogenesis imperfecta congenita. Kaufmann[136,137] described the anatomicopathologic characteristics of achondroplasia, although his "chondrodystrophia foetalis hypertrophica" appears to have been metatropic dwarfism (p. 606).

The disorder described as "foetus achondroplase" by Lamy and Maroteaux [154, Fig. 5] was clearly an example of thanatophoric dwarfism, which they first delineated and named in a publication seven years later.[206] The X-linked spondyloepiphyseal dysplasia (SED) tarda was especially clearly delineated genetically and radiographically.[154] The authors recognized hypochondroplasia as an entity distinct from achondroplasia and concluded that inheritance is probably dominant.

The monograph by Hobaek[113] in 1961 presented a collection of forty-three families studied in detail from a clinical, genetic, and roentgenographic point of view. A large number of illustrations were provided. The genetics was often weak. It seems that Hobaek found a remarkably large number of families with recessive disorders. The fjord geography of Norway, with resulting inbreeding, was probably responsible. Hobaek's Family 11 is a good example of autosomal recessive SED tarda, and Family 13, of X-linked SED tarda. Families 7 and 9 appear from clinical and roentgenographic appearance to have had MPS IV. Family 19 is an example of spondylometaphyseal dysplasia.[113]

In his monograph[258] Rubin reviewed earlier classifications of bone dysplasias, namely, those of Brailsford,[31] Fairbank,[72,73] Jaffe (as communicated to Hirsch[112]), Jackson,[122] Sear,[273] Lamy and Maroteaux,[153] and Hobaek.[113]

Rubin[258] classed generalized hereditary dysplasias of the osseous skeleton according to whether the major site of abnormality is epiphyseal, physeal, metaphyseal, or diaphyseal (Fig. 13-1). (Rubin's proposal of the term *physis* and its adjective form *physeal* to refer to the growth zone seems both useful and logical.) Each class of dysplasia had, by this system, subclasses of hypoplasias and hyperplasias, and in most of the subclasses more than one genus of disorder was recognized. (See Table 13-1 and Fig. 13-2.) Several of the entities, e.g., cartilage-

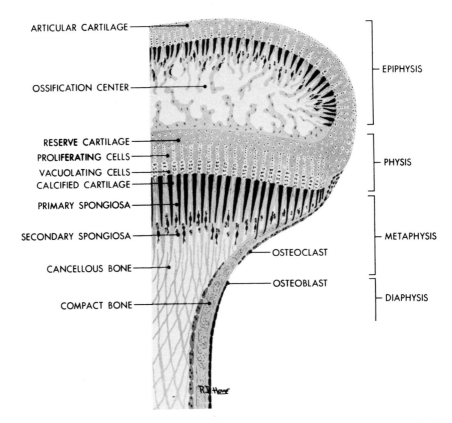

Fig. 13-1. Anatomicohistologic correlation of bone structure. (From Rubin, P.: Dynamic classification of bone dysplasias, Chicago, 1964, Year Book Medical Publishers, Inc.)

Table 13-1. Rubin's classification of bone disorders*

I. Epiphyseal dysplasias
  A. Epiphyseal hypoplasias
    1. Failure of articular cartilage: spondyloepiphyseal dysplasia
    2. Failure of ossification of center: multiple epiphyseal dysplasia
  B. Epiphyseal hyperplasia
    1. Excess of articular cartilage: dysplasia epiphysealis hemimelica
II. Physeal dysplasia
  A. Cartilage hypoplasia
    1. Failure of proliferating cartilage: achondroplasia
    2. Failure of hypertrophic cartilage: metaphyseal dysostosis; cartilage-hair hypoplasia
  B. Cartilage hyperplasias
    1. Excess of proliferating cartilage: hyperchondroplsia (the Marfan syndrome)
    2. Excess of hypertrophic cartilage: enchondromatosis
III. Metaphyseal dysplasias
  A. Metaphyseal hypoplasias
    1. Failure to form primary spongiosa: hypophosphatasia
    2. Failure to absorb primary spongiosa: osteopetrosis
    3. Failure to absorb secondary spongiosa: craniometaphyseal dysplasia
  B. Metaphyseal hyperplasia
    1. Excessive spongiosa: multiple exostoses
IV. Diaphyseal dysplasias
  A. Diaphyseal hypoplasias
    1. Failure of periosteal bone formation: osteogenesis imperfecta
    2. Failure of endosteal bone formation: idiopathic osteoporosis, congenita and tarda
  B. Diaphyseal hyperplasias
    1. Excessive periosteal bone formation: progressive diaphyseal dysplasia (Engelmann's disease)
    2. Excessive endosteal bone formation: hyperphosphatasemia (including juvenile Paget's disease and van Buchem's disease)

---

*Adapted from Rubin, P.: Dynamic classification of bone dysplasias, Chicago, 1964, Year Book Medical Publishers, Inc.

hair hypoplasia and the Ellis–van Creveld syndrome, have manifestations in non-osseous tissues as well.

Rubin[258] referred to the Morquio syndrome as spondyloepiphyseal dysplasia congenita, a doubtful appellation because, as he himself wrote, "The children are born normal and develop normally during the first year." Furthermore, it is preferable to reserve the term SED congenita for the specific disorder described on p. 601 in the differential diagnosis of the Morquio syndrome. He presented the pedigree and roentgenograms of a family with autosomal dominant spondyloepiphyseal dysplasia tarda, also reported by Moldauer and co-workers.[215] One of Rubin's cases of diastrophic dwarfism was in a 72-year-old man. In Fig. 8.3 of reference 258, labeled "severe achondroplasia, congenita, in newborn infant," is an obvious representation of thanatophoric dwarfism. Rubin reproduced Mac-Callum's histopathologic sections of a lethal case of "achondroplasia"—likewise almost certainly thanatophoric dwarfism (Fig. 8.4 of reference 258). In Rubin's Fig. 8.7 was shown a case of the Jansen type of metaphyseal chondrodysplasia observed by Dr. J. F. Holt, of Ann Arbor, Michigan. Holt[116] later presented useful neonatal films in this case. The patient had hypercalcemia, because of which surgical exploration was twice performed without finding a parathyroid tumor.

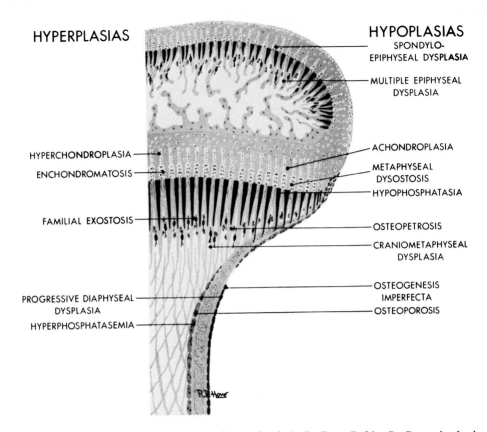

HYPERPLASIAS

HYPERCHONDROPLASIA

ENCHONDROMATOSIS

FAMILIAL EXOSTOSIS

PROGRESSIVE DIAPHYSEAL
DYSPLASIA

HYPERPHOSPHATASEMIA

HYPOPLASIAS

SPONDYLO-
EPIPHYSEAL DYSPLASIA

MULTIPLE EPIPHYSEAL
DYSPLASIA

ACHONDROPLASIA

METAPHYSEAL
DYSOSTOSIS

HYPOPHOSPHATASIA

OSTEOPETROSIS

CRANIOMETAPHYSEAL
DYSPLASIA

OSTEOGENESIS
IMPERFECTA

OSTEOPOROSIS

Fig. 13-2. Rubin's "dynamic classification of bone dysplasias." (From Rubin, P.: Dynamic classification of bone dysplasias, Chicago, 1964, Year Book Medical Publishers, Inc.)

The case of Gram and colleagues[96] was also illustrated by Rubin (Fig. 8.6 of reference 258). The facial and general appearance was remarkably like that in the patients of Lenz and Holt (Fig. 13-28). In Gram's case also, hypercalcemia prompted parathyroid exploration. The patient shown in Fig. 8.17 (reference 96), whose case was labeled gargoylism (one of Caffey's "intrauterine" or early onset cases[36]), almost certainly had I-cell disease. Contrast the cases illustrated in Rubin's Figs. 10.24 and 10.25 (reference 258), both labeled pyknodysostosis; they suggest the existence of two forms of this disorder, differing mainly in the presence or absence of osteosclerosis (p. 821).

Animal models of skeletal disorders of man

Animal models have potential usefulness in the elucidation of basic mechanisms in human skeletal abnormalities, although in the last analysis the "proper study of mankind is man."

Grüneberg[99] provided a useful review of inherited skeletal disorders in animals. Mice received main attention and appropriately so, because most information is available in this species which has been studied extensively by Grüneberg. Both systemic disorders of the skeleton and localized disorders, such as those of the appendicular skeleton ("limb anomalies"), were discussed, to a total of more than seventy.

Among the general principles pointed out by Grüneberg were the following: Spurious and genuine pleiotropism are distinguished, the latter being pleiotropism at the level of primary gene action.[99] Almost no instances of genuine pleiotropism are known. The principle of unitary primary gene action was reiterated. Gene effect can be remarkably modified by changes in the genetic background. For example, the brachyury gene in heterozygous mice (T/+) is usually distinguished from the same gene in the normal homozygote, +/+, by the short tail of the former and from the T/T homozygote by the lethality of the latter's condition; however, in some genetic backgrounds the heterozygote cannot be distinguished from the normal homozygote, the tail being normal in length.[99] Thus, the inheritance is dominant in the first instance and recessive in the second. Several examples are cited by Grüneberg to illustrate that in a pleiotropic syndrome the several manifestations are independently influenced by changes in the genetic background.

Some similarities between skeletal disorders in animals and man can be pointed out. Congenital hydrocephalus of mice (symbolized ch) is fundamentally a skeletal disorder[99]: "The hydrocephalus is due to a shortening of the chondrocranium and thus a secondary consequence of the underlying skeletal anomaly." The hydrocephalus of achondroplasia in man (p. 756) may have a similar basis. In ch as well as in others of the animal models (e.g., Danforth's short-tail heterozygote, Sd/+), absence or hypoplasia of the odontoid process of the axis occurs. This is a feature of the Morquio syndrome and several other forms of spondyloepiphyseal dysplasia in man. (In the dachs rabbit, the odontoid process has reverted to its phylogenic origin as the body of the atlas.) Furthermore, in ch the neural arches tend to remain open dorsally, as in chondrodysplasia punctata in man, and fusion of bones, equivalent to the carpal or tarsal bones of man, occur, as in the Ellis–van Creveld syndrome. With the "short-ear" mutation (symbolized se), hypoplasia or aplasia of the cartilaginous scapha of the ears is a hallmark of a generalized cartilaginous abnormality. "In the living mouse, the reduction in size of the ear does not become obvious until the animal is about three weeks old."[99] Ear involvement in diastrophic dwarfism is manifest some weeks after birth. Several of the disorders in animals, e.g., cartilage anomaly in the rat,[99] lead to death within a few days or weeks of birth from respiratory embarrassment secondary to involvement of the thoracic cage and perhaps the tracheal cartilages—analogous to the asphyxiating thoracic dysplasia of Jeune and co-workers[128], thanatophoric dwarfism, homozygous achondroplasia, and other conditions in man. In the rat disorder, abnormality involves not only the skeletal cartilages, which are mesodermal in origin, but also those of the larynx, which originate from the neural crest. The same phenomenon is observed in chondrodysplasia punctata. The gene-determined defect interferes with cartilage histiogenesis regardless of the germ layer from which the cartilage is derived. "Contrary to countless statements in the literature, there is very little evidence that genes ever act on a particular germ layer as a functional unit."[99] The dachs rabbit develops arthrosis in the hips and to a lesser extent in the shoulder, leading to increasing crippling.

The ancon or otter short-legged sheep first originated on the farm of Seth

Wight in Dover, Massachusetts, in 1791. For a time the strain enjoyed popularity in New England because the animals were unable to jump over stone walls, but progressive crippling of the feet was a disadvantage which eventually lead to extinction of the breed by the 1870's. A recessive mutation, probably identical, was detected in Norway in 1919 and studied in the late 1940's by Landauer and by Chang at Storrs, Connecticut.

Forehead bulging, parietal prominence, nasal depression, and maxillary recession with underbite are features of many of the animal skeletal dysplasias, e.g., the Dexter "bulldog calves" (Grüneberg[99]), as they are also of human achondroplasia. As in human achondroplasia, the heterozygous Dexter dwarf cattle are short-legged and brachycephalic, whereas the homozygous state is lethal, leading usually to abortion at four months or later, usually with hydramnios. Grüneberg[99] did not discuss the chondrodystrophies of cattle in detail. Studies date back to the investigations of the bulldog calf and Dexter cattle by Crew[49,50] in the early 1920's. A review and references are provided by Gregory.[98] He and Thompson and associates[312] presented evidence that the bovine chondrodystrophies are not homologous to the Hurler syndrome.

The recessive inheritance and disorganized enchondral ossification in rabbit "achondroplasia"[265a] suggest that this condition may be more analogous to thanatophoric dwarfism (p. 762) than to human achondroplasia. The English bulldog has many features suggesting achondroplasia, including well-organized, regular enchondral ossification. Short-limbed breeds such as the dachshund are difficult to relate to any skeletal dysplasia. In none of the breeds is it clear whether a one-gene difference is responsible for the cardinal characteristics. I have presently under study a dwarfed miniature poodle in which the radiographic changes are those of a spondyloepiphyseal dysplasia. This is probably the same entity as that described by Gardner[84a] and by Amlöf.[7a]

Snell's pituitary dwarf mouse has normal growth until a few weeks after birth; this is a recessive form of panhypopituitarism similar to that which has been described in several inbred groups such as the Hutterites and the inhabitants of the Island of Krk on the Dalmatian coast. Other forms of proportionate dwarfism have low birth weight and normal pituitary function.

The gray-lethal mouse[99] is an example of osteopetrosis. Since Grüneberg's publication in 1964, information on the role of thyrocalcitonin in its production has accumulated. Other osteopetrosis-like mutations include microphthalmia in the mouse and osteopetrosis in the rabbit. Brown and Dent[34a] reviewed the animal models of osteopetrosis in man.

Lane and Dickie[157] described three new recessive mutations of the mouse which produce a shortened, broad skull and disproportionate shortening of the limb bones. Thin epiphyseal plates, resulting from shortening of the columns of proliferating cartilage cells and a reduced number of hypertrophic cells, were described in all three mutations. The most severe was termed achondroplasia (symbolized cn). In the inbred mouse reciprocal transplantation of bone can be practiced between dwarfed and normal mice to determine whether the primary fault is in skeletal cells or elsewhere. Lane and Dickie[157] quoted Hungarian workers as concluding from such experiments that the defect in cn/cn homozygotes resides in chondrocytes but that products of the gene action circulate in the blood, producing further inhibiting effects on growth.

Table 13-2. The Paris nomenclature for constitutional disorders of bone

I. Constitutional diseases of bone with unknown pathogenesis: osteochondrodysplasias (abnormalities of cartilage and/or bone growth and development)
- A. Defects of growth of tubular bones and/or spine
    1. Manifest at birth
        a. Achondroplasia (p. 750)
        b. Achondrogenesis (p. 759)
        c. Thanatophoric dwarfism (p. 762)
        d. Chondrodysplasia punctata (formerly stippled epiphyses chondrodystrophia calcificans congenita), several forms (p. 767)
        e. Metatropic dwarfism (p. 771)
        f. Diastrophic dwarfism (p. 772)
        g. Chondroectodermal dysplasia (Ellis–van Creveld syndrome) (p. 775)
        h. Asphyxiating thoracic dysplasia (Jeune syndrome) (p. 775)
        i. Spondyloepiphyseal dysplasia congenita (p. 601)
        j. Mesomelic dwarfism
            (1) Nievergelt type[290]
            (2) Langer type [160]
        k. Cleidocranial dysplasia (formerly cleidocranial dysostosis) (p. 777)
    2. Manifest in later life
        a. Hypochondroplasia (p. 779)
        b. Dyschondrosteosis (p. 782)
        c. Metaphyseal chondrodysplasia (formerly metaphyseal dysostosis), Jansen type (p. 787)
        d. Metaphyseal chondrodysplasia (formerly metaphyseal dysostosis), Schmid type (p. 789)
        e. Metaphyseal chondrodysplasia, McKusick type (formerly cartilage-hair hypoplasia) (p. 789)
        f. Metaphyseal chondrodysplasia with malabsorption and neutropenia (p. 792)
        g. Metaphyseal chondrodysplasia with thymolymphopenia[85]
        h. Spondylometaphyseal dysplasia (Kozlowski type) [150]
        i. Multiple epiphyseal dysplasia (several forms) (p. 798)
        j. Hereditary arthro-ophthalmopathy (p. 727)
        k. Pseudoachondroplastic dysplasia (formerly pseudoachondroplastic type of spondyloepiphyseal dysplasia) (p. 798)
        l. Spondyloepiphyseal dysplasia tarda (p. 799)
        m. Acrodysplasia (formerly peripheral dysostosis)
            (1) Trichorhinophalangeal syndrome (Giedion syndrome)[89]
            (2) Epiphyseal type (Thiemann syndrome)[7,29]
            (3) Epiphysiometaphyseal type (Brailsford syndrome)[31]
- B. Disorganized development of cartilage and fibrous components of the skeleton
    1. Dysplasia epiphysealis hemimelica[258]
    2. Multiple cartilaginous exostoses (p. 807)
    3. Enchondromatosis (Ollier's disease) (p. 809)
    4. Enchondromatosis with hemangioma (Maffucci syndrome) (p. 809)
    5. Fibrous dysplasia (Jaffé-Lichtenstein syndrome)[38]
    6. Fibrous dysplasia with skin pigmentation and precocious puberty (McCune-Albright syndrome)[2]
    7. Cherubism[131]
    8. Multiple fibromatosis
- C. Abnormalities of density, of cortical diaphyseal structure, and/or of metaphyseal modeling
    1. Osteogenesis imperfecta congenita (Vrolik or Porak-Durante syndrome) (Chapter 8)
    2. Osteogenesis imperfecta tarda (Lobstein syndrome) (Chapter 8)
    3. Juvenile idiopathic osteoporosis[62]
    4. Osteopetrosis with precocious manifestations (p. 809)

Continued.

Table 13-2. The Paris nomenclature for constitutional disorders of bone—cont'd

C. Abnormalities of density of cortical diaphyseal structure, and/or of metaphyseal modeling—cont'd

    5. Osteopetrosis with delayed manifestations (p. 809)

    6. Pyknodysostosis (p. 820)

    7. Osteopoikilosis (Chapter 12)

    8. Melorheostosis[40]

    9. Diaphyseal dysplasia (Camurati-Engelmann syndrome) (p. 821)

   10. Craniodiaphyseal dysplasia[105]

   11. Endosteal hyperostosis (Van Buchem syndrome and other forms)[317]

   12. Tubular stenosis (Kenny-Caffey syndrome)[37]

   13. Osteodysplasty (Melnick-Needles syndrome)[212]

   14. Pachydermoperiostosis[249]

   15. Osteoectasia with hyperphosphatasia[14]

   16. Metaphyseal dysplasia (Pyle's disease)[95]

   17. Craniometaphyseal dysplasia (several forms)[95,117,214]

   18. Frontometaphyseal dysplasia[91]

   19. Oculo-dento-osseous dysplasia (formerly oculo-dento-digital syndrome)[92]

II. Constitutional diseases of bone with unknown pathogenesis: dysostoses (malformation of individual bones, singly or in combination)

  A. Dysostoses with cranial and facial involvement

    1. Craniosynostosis, several forms[51,276]

    2. Craniofacial dysostosis (Crouzon syndrome)[77]

    3. Acrocephalosyndactyly (Apert syndrome)[263]

    4. Acrocephalopolysyndactyly (Carpenter syndrome)[308]

    5. Mandibulofacial dysostosis (Treacher-Collins–Franceschetti syndrome)[257]

    6. Mandibular hypoplasia (includes Pierre Robin syndrome)[288]

    7. Oculomandibulofacial syndrome (Hallermann-Streiff-François syndrome)[74]

    8. Nevoid basal cell carcinoma syndrome[247]

  B. Dysostoses with predominant axial involvement

    1. Vertebral segmentation defects (including Klippel-Feil syndrome)[100]

    2. Cervico-oculo-acoustic syndrome (Wildervanck syndrome)[143]

    3. Sprengel's deformity[271]

    4. Spondylocostal dysostosis (several forms)[226,251]

    5. Oculovertebral syndrome (Weyers syndrome)[332]

    6. Osteo-onychodysostosis (formerly nail-patella syndrome) (p. 835)

  C. Dysostoses with predominant involvement of extremities[309]

    1. Amelia

    2. Hemimelia (several types)

    3. Acheiria

    4. Apodia

    5. Adactyly and oligodactyly

    6. Phocomelia

    7. Aglossia-adactylia syndrome[224]

    8. Congenital bowing of long bones (several types)[11]

    9. Familial radioulnar synostosis[106]

   10. Brachydactyly (several types)[309]

   11. Symphalangism[303]

   12. Polydactyly (several types)[309]

   13. Syndactyly (several types)[309]

   14. Polysyndactyly (several types)[309]

   15. Camptodactyly (p. 168)

   16. Clinodactyly[309]

   17. Biedl-Bardet syndrome[10,145]

   18. Popliteal pterygium syndrome[94]

   19. Pectoral aplasia–dysdactyly syndrome (Poland syndrome)[328]

Table 13-2. The Paris nomenclature for constitutional disorders of bone—cont'd

---

C. Dysostoses with predominant involvement of extremities—cont'd

    20. Rubinstein-Taybi syndrome[259]

    21. Pancytopenia-dysmelia syndrome (Fanconi syndrome)[133]

    22. Thrombocytopenia–radial-aplasia syndrome[103]

    23. Orofaciodigital (OFD) syndrome (Papillon-Léage syndrome)[93,250]

    24. Cardiomelic syndrome (Holt-Oram syndrome)[243]

III. Constitutional diseases of bone with unknown pathogenesis: idiopathic osteolyses

    A. Acro-osteolysis

        1. Phalangeal type[153]

        2. Tarsocarpal form, with or without nephropathy[316]

    B. Multicentric osteolysis[315]

IV. Primary disturbances of growth

    A. Primordial dwarfism (without associated malformations)[26,330]

    B. Cornelia de Lange syndrome[233]

    C. Bird-headed dwarfism (Virchow and Seckel forms)[194]

    D. Leprechaunism[304]

    E. Russell-Silver syndrome[115]

    F. Progeria[196]

    G. Cockayne syndrome[187]

    H. Bloom syndrome[27]

    I. Geroderma osteodysplastica[34]

    J. Spherophakia-brachymorphia syndorme (Weill-Marchesani syndrome) (Chapter 5)

    K. Marfan syndrome (Chapter 3)

  V. Constitutional diseases of bones with known pathogenesis: chromosomal aberrations

  VI. Constitutional diseases of bones with known pathogenesis: primary metabolic abnormalities

    A. Disorders of calcium/phosphorus metabolism

        1. Hypophosphatemic familial rickets (p. 835)

        2. Pseudodeficiency rickets (Royer or Prader syndrome) (p. 841)

        3. Late rickets (McCance syndrome)[184]

        4. Idiopathic hypercalciuria

        5. Hypophosphatasia (several forms) (p. 842)

        6. Idiopathic hypercalcemia[141]

        7. Pseudohypoparathyroidism (normo- and hypocalcemic forms)[198]

    B. Mucopolysaccharidoses (Chapter 11)

    See classification in Chapter 11.

    C. Mucolipidoses (p. 646) and lipidoses

        1. Mucolipidosis I (Spranger-Wiedemann syndrome; lipomucopolysaccharidosis)

        2. Mucolipidosis II (Leroy syndrome; I-cell disease)

        3. Mucolipidosis III (pseudo–Hurler polydystrophy)

        4. Fucosidosis (p. 662)

        5. Mannosidosis (p. 661)

        6. Generalized G_{M1} gangliosidosis (two forms)[227]

        7. Sulfatidosis with mucopolysacchariduria (Austin-Thieffry syndrome) (p. 661)

        8. Cerebrosidosis, including Gaucher's disease[30]

    D. Other metabolic extraosseous disorders

VII. Bone abnormalities secondary to disturbances of extraskeletal systems

    A. Endocrine disturbances, e.g., hypothyroidism

    B. Hematologic disturbances e.g., thalassemia

    C. Neurologic disturbances, e.g., sensory neuropathy

    D. Renal disturbances, e.g., cystinosis

    E. Gastrointestinal disturbances, e.g., celiac disease

    F. Cardiopulmonary disturbances, e.g., hypertrophic osteoarthropathy

The Pelger-Huët anomaly in man is a rare and harmless autosomal dominant variant of leukocyte nuclear morphology.[221] The nuclei of polymorphonuclear leukocytes have about two segments rather than the usual three to five. An apparently homologous disorder occurs in rabbits *(Pg/+)*. In the rabbit, *Pg/Pg* homozygotes have a severe disorder of the cartilaginous skeleton, a chondrodystrophy.[146] Although presumed homozygotes have been observed in man,[106a,299a] no skeletal abnormality accompanied the blood change. This suggests that the Pelger-Huët anomaly of man and that of the rabbit are not, in fact, homologous.

Classification and nomenclature

In November, 1969, a group met in Paris, under the auspices of the European Society of Pediatric Radiology, to consider questions of terminology of constitutional (i.e., generalized) skeletal disorders. The meeting, hereafter referred to as the Paris Conference, resulted in what we shall call the Paris Nomenclature, presented in Table 13-2. Pierre Maroteaux[200] served as rapporteur.

Inevitably classification was considered as well as nomenclature. A major dichotomy was made between osteochondrodysplasias (abnormalities in the growth and development of cartilage and/or bone) and dysostoses (malformations of bones, singly or in combination). In some instances classification was arbitrary because the disorder had features of both. Pyknodysostosis is an example; the mandibular abnormality is a dysostosis and the increased density of the skeleton, a dysplasia.

A special effort was made to avoid eponyms. Only those were retained which are in wide use for designating conditions that lack any other satisfactory denomination. In Table 13-2, proper names formerly used as eponyms have been placed in parentheses.

The introduction of new terms was also held to a minimum. One of the main innovations was the suggested substitution of *metaphyseal chondrodysplasia* for *metaphyseal dysostosis*. The new term is considered a more accurate reflection of the nature of the disorder.

Some personal preferences and Americanizations have been introduced in the listing as given in Table 13-2. At least one reference is given for most entries. Most of those conditions which are not discussed later in this chapter are briefly discussed with further references in my *Mendelian Inheritance in Man*.[189] Attention is also directed to the proceedings of the 1968 Conference on the Clinical Delineation of Birth Defects, devoted to skeletal dysplasias[23] and the proceedings of the 1972 Conference on the same subject.

OSTEOCHONDRODYSPLASIAS
Achondroplasia

Achondroplasia is the prototype chondrodystrophy or at least the prototype of short-limb dwarfism and the prototype of those forms evident at birth. The Morquio syndrome, on the other hand, is the prototype of short-trunk dwarfism and of forms of dwarfism which become apparent later in infancy or childhood. In the past many conditions have been called either achondroplasia or the Morquio syndrome. Even vitamin D–resistant rickets has at times been labeled achondroplasia.

Achondroplasia can be definitively diagnosed in the neonate (Fig. 13-3) be-

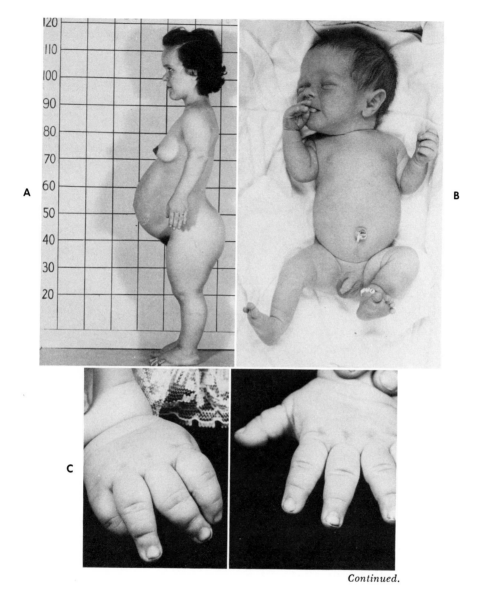

Continued.

Fig. 13-3. Achondroplasia in mother and in 2 of 3 children. **A,** Mother during third pregnancy. Unlike the patients affected by pseudoachondroplastic dysplasia, the bridge of the nose is scooped out and the forehead is bulging. **B,** Newborn achondroplastic son. **C,** Trident hands in 3-year-old daughter. The fingers, when apposed, do not touch in their entire length. **D,** 3-year-old achondroplastic daughter. **E,** X-ray film of newborn achondroplastic child showing characteristic changes: separation of vertebral ossification centers by excessive cartilage, caudad narrowing of the interpedunculate spaces in the lumbar spine, and small pelvic bones with notchlike sacroiliac groove, in addition to the shortening of the bones of the extremities. **F,** By way of contrast with **E,** the x-ray film of the unaffected sib, taken in the newborn period, is shown. **G,** The pedigree. The mother shown in **A** is in the second generation. Each of her 3 children, all delivered by cesarean section, was fathered by a different man. Achondroplasia has not been confirmed in the mother of the mother (I-2). (From McKusick, V. A., and colleagues: Medical genetics 1958-1960, St. Louis, 1961, The C. V. Mosby Co.)

cause of characteristic radiologic findings, especially in the spine and pelvis.[201] Excessive cartilage separates the ossification centers in the vertebral bodies. Furthermore, the interpedunculate intervals show caudad narrowing in the lumbar spine, rather than widening, as in the normal individual.[283] In achondroplasia the small spinal canal is evident on both frontal and lateral views and at all ages. The sacroiliac notch is reduced to a small size in the newborn with achondroplasia and remains small. The iliac wings are shortened. In the limbs the epiphyseal ossification centers, e.g., at the distal end of the femur, are set into the metaphysis, creating the circumflex (or chevron) sign or, at an earlier stage, a ball-in-socket appearance. From the ages of 1 month to about 7 months the femoral neck is relatively radiolucent due to flattening in the anteroposterior dimension.

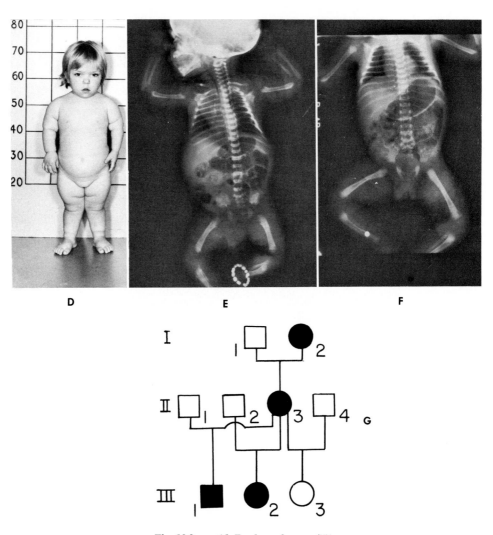

Fig. 13-3, cont'd. For legend see p. 751.

The achondroplastic child and adult have a characteristic facies and general appearance. Because of the defective development of the chondrocranium (Fig. 13-4), the nose is "scooped out" and the maxilla is hypoplastic. Because of relatively little change in those structures, the calvaria is bulging and the mandible is relatively prognathic.

Lumbar lordosis is exaggerated, with pelvic tilt such that the sacrum lies almost horizontal, and the buttocks are prominent. The gait is ducklike.

The shortness of the limbs is rhizomelic ("root of limb") as opposed to mesomelic: i.e., shortening is especially striking in the humerus and femur. In-

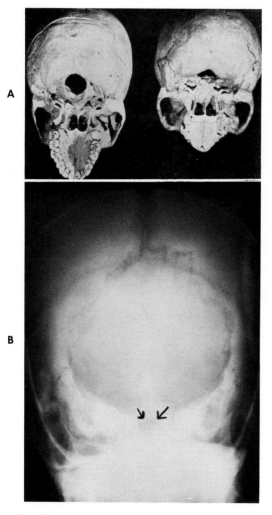

Fig. 13-4. Chondrocranium in achondroplasia. Many of the facial, cranial, and neurologic features of achondroplasia are the result of involvement of the chondrocranium but not of the calvaria, which is membrane bone. **A,** Comparison of the base of the skull in normal and achondroplastic persons. **B,** Towne's view of base of skull in 1-year-old child with achondroplasia, showing small misshapen foramen magnum. (A from Stockard, C. R.: The physical basis of personality, New York, 1931, W. W. Norton & Co., Inc.)

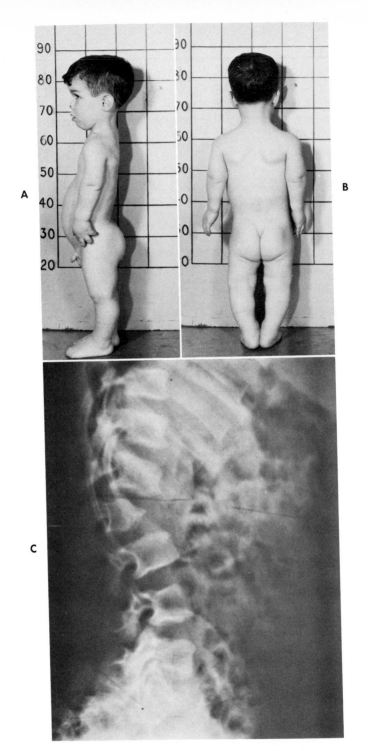

Fig. 13-5. Lumbar gibbus in achondroplasia. **A** to **C,** E. B. (J.H.H. 1320580), 4½ years old, was first noted to have lumbar gibbus at 3 months. (His father and mother were 48 and 41 years old, respectively, at his birth.) He has full extension at the elbows, an unusual finding in achondroplasia. Because of steady increase in the upper lumbar kyphos, a fusion operation was performed at 6 years of age. **A** and **B,** Side and rear views showing thoracolumbar kyphosis, as well as genu varum and other features of achondroplasia. **C,** Lateral x-ray view of lumbar spine showing marked scalloping of the posterior margin of the vertebral bodies, wedging of L-2, and subluxation of L-1 on L-2.

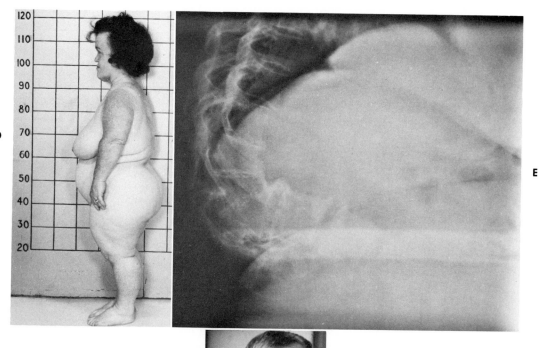

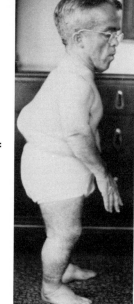

D and **E,** M. S. (J.H.H. 1382946), 46 years old, had typical features of achondroplasia. An unusually severe thoracolumbar kyphosis extended from T-11 to L-3 and formed almost a right angle. Spontaneous anterior fusion had developed between the bodies from T-12 to L-3. Neurologic examination was completely normal. She has successfully completed two pregnancies, producing each time an achondroplastic infant. **D,** Lateral view showing lumbar gibbus. **E,** X-ray view of severe lumbar gibbus, forming almost a right angle. The interspace between L-1 and L-2 can scarcely be identified, others are narrowed, and there is bony fusion between several vertebral bodies anteriorly.

F, E. A. H., 47 years old, is 44 inches tall. He works as a statistical clerk and is asymptomatic except for aching legs at night. As indicated, he has a severe lumbar gibbus.

complete extension and limitation in pronation and supination at the elbow are the rule. As pointed out by Pierre Marie and by other early writers, the hand is usually trident: a wedge-shaped gap between the third and fourth fingers creates this appearance, the three prongs of the trident being fingers 4 and 5, fingers 2 and 3, and the thumb (Fig. 13-3C is not entirely typical, as it shows the hand of a young child). The fingers usually cannot be placed in parallel apposition because of the large proximal segments (Fig. 13-3C).

The defective development of the chondrocranium (Fig. 13-4) is regularly reflected in a small "crumpled" foramen magnum, which can be visualized by appropriate roentgenographic views. This defect is probably in some way related to the development of hydrocephalus in achondroplasia, although I am not certain that the mechanism of this complication or its frequency in achondroplasia is known. I suspect that a great majority of achondroplasts have at least mild dilatation of the ventricles; some have striking hydrocephalus. I have observed a dozen or more patients in whom shunt procedures were performed and know of other achondroplasts in whom it probably should have been done, because, although the hydrocephalus always seems to arrest itself spontaneously, it may not do so before the child's intellect is significantly impaired. Most achondroplasts have intelligence in the normal range, but the mean is probably reduced. Occasional achondroplasts are found in institutions for mental deficiency. Although achondroplasia, of course, provides no immunity to any of the many other causes of mental retardation, and although, in the past at least, patients with various chondrodystrophies were often institutionalized apparently on an assumption that they must be retarded as well as dwarfed or because there was no other means to care for them, it is likely that the frequency of mental deficiency is increased in achondroplasia. True megalencephaly, presumably as a pleiotropic effect of the achondroplasia gene, has been claimed[60] but cannot be considered proved.

Matthews[209] suggests that dilatation of the ventricles is secondary, in large part, to the smallness of the spinal canal, which normally serves to vent cerebrospinal fluid pulsations transmitted from the arterial system. Other neurologic complications are clearly related to the small size of the spinal canal throughout its length. Even minor disc protrusion or spur formation can have serious neurologic effects.[70,268,319,320] Achondroplastic infants are hypotonic and as a result may have beaking of an upper lumbar vertebra like that in the Hurler syndrome (p. 533); beaking may progress to formation of wedge vertebra and striking lumbar gibbus, with further compromise of the spinal canal (Fig. 13-5). Usually the lumbar gibbus present in the young achondroplastic child when he begins to sit is corrected by the exaggerated lumbar lordosis that develops later.

Loose-jointedness is usually striking in the knees of the achondroplast and contributes to the bowlegs. (Valgus deformity of the knees is usually present in young children, as shown in Fig. 13-3D, and later converts to a varus deformity.) The fibula is relatively long proximally, contributing also to the deformity of the knees. Ponseti[241] removes the proximal end of the fibula, including the growth plate. Occasional achondroplasts have straight legs. Usually these patients are found to lack the ligamentous laxity found in patients with bowlegs.

Achondroplasia is an autosomal dominant disorder. About 80% of cases are sporadic,[216] presumably the result of new mutation occurring in the germ cell from one or the other parent. The average age of fathers of such sporadic cases of achondroplasia is about seven years in excess of the average age of fathers generally. Although the average age of the mothers tends to be increased also, the large body of data analyzed in this department[220] permitted analyses that showed paternal age to be the main factor.

Under the reasonable assumption of genetic equilibrium, the fact that about 80% of achondroplasts are sporadic cases should mean that the average reproductive fitness of achondroplasts is about 20%—and such seems to be the case. The reduced fitness (in the Darwinian sense) is largely due to reduced reproduction because of impediments in finding mates and difficulties of childbirth in the females. Survivorship is little reduced from the normal.[220] The young achondroplast seems to be a hardy organism. Impressions to the contrary[225] resulted from the confusion with achondroplasia of achondrogenesis, thanatophoric dwarfism, the Ellis–van Creveld syndrome,[139] asphyxiating thoracic dystrophy, and other forms of chondrodystrophy lethal early in life. It is true that the large head of the achondroplast places him in increased obstetric jeopardy. This was especially the case in the past, when rickets in the mother was more frequent, contributing to cephalopelvic disproportion, and obstetric practice was more primitive.

Compared with most autosomal dominant disorders, achondroplasia shows remarkably little variability. Practically never is the diagnosis in question. The mean adult heights of men (51.81 inches) and of women (48.62 inches) have small variances, 2.22 and 2.37 inches, respectively.[220] This small variability is expected with a disorder in which the sporadic cases constitute such a large proportion of cases: there is no opportunity for accumulation of modifier genes that mollify the phenotype. Little or no correlation between parental height and adult height of sporadic achondroplasts was found by Murdoch and co-workers.[220] I have a lingering clinical impression, however, that sporadic achondroplasts are taller when their parents are tall, and shorter when their parents are short. The question of correlation should be reinvestigated. Possibly the data on parental height obtained by Murdoch and co-workers were inexact because many of the parents, being older than the average (see above), had died at the time the data were collected. Inexact data may have blurred any correlation which in fact exists.

Past estimates of the frequency of achondroplasia are suspect because of diagnostic ambiguities. For the same reason estimates of mutation rate have almost certainly been too high. Improved knowledge of the diagnostic criteria of achondroplasia would make a study done today much more reliable. Indeed, achondroplasia should be a useful "sentinel" trait for the monitoring of mutation in defined populations.

Achondroplasts frequently marry other achondroplasts, thus creating the possibility of children homozygous for the achondroplasia gene. Such couples often give a history of offspring with a severe skeletal dysplasia and early death. We have firsthand observations on 2 infants who were born of achondroplastic couples and whose homozygous state would seem unquestionable. The findings in one of the couples are presented in Fig. 13-6.

Apparent exceptions to autosomal dominant inheritance are represented by the cases of achondroplasia in male and female first cousins (the mothers are

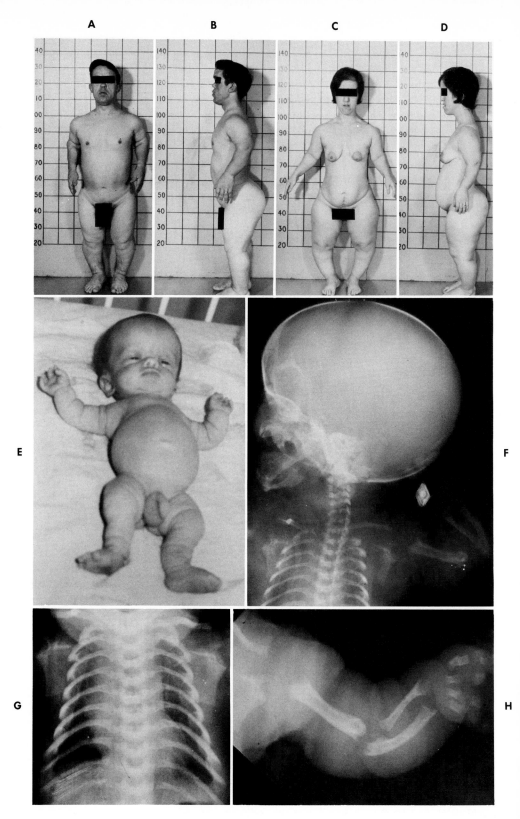

Fig. 13-6. For legend see opposite page.

sisters),[324] 3 distantly related achondroplasts in one kindred,[230] and a recessive achondroplasia-like condition reported by Nance and Sweeney.[222] Bowen[29a] has observed 2 sisters with unequivocal achondroplasia whose parents and 3 other sibs were normal. One affected sister had an affected child. Germinal mosaicism provides a possible explanation.

See p. 779 for a discussion of the possibility that the genes for achondroplasia and hypochondroplasia are allelic and for presentation of a patient who may be a genetic compound for these two mutant genes.

Nothing is known of the nature of the basic defect in achondroplasia. Even the "textbook" descriptions of the histopathology are in error because of confusion with forms of chondrodystrophy lethal in the neonatal period. Rimoin and colleagues[254] found well-organized endochondral ossification in rib and iliac crest biopsies; markedly disorganized endochondral ossification had been thought to characterize achondroplasia. In biopsies of fibular epiphyseal plates, Ponseti[241] described abnormally wide fibrous septa.

Achondrogenesis

This rare condition was first recognized as distinct by Parenti.[231] Fraccaro[80] also described cases, and Langer and colleagues[165] identified cases reported in the literature under various labels. It is a form of severe short-limb dwarfism that leads to stillbirth or neonatal death.[260] The trunk is also very short, being almost as wide as it is long (Fig. 13-7). The basis for this deformity is seen in a pathognomonic roentgenographic feature: marked underossification in the lumbar vertebrae, sacrum, pubis, and ischium. The wide pelvis is also characteristic (Fig. 13-7B). Histologically, endochondral ossification is strikingly disorganized and matrix is lacking between resting cartilage cells.

Achondrogenesis is an autosomal recessive disorder. Parental consanguinity and multiple affected sibs with normal parents are reported.[260]

A possible source of confusion is another quite different autosomal recessive disorder that is also called achondrogenesis. It was first reported by Grebe[97] and later described in Brazil by Quelce-Salgado[245] and by Scott.[272] The features are best described by referring the reader to Fig. 13-8. The two forms can be referred to as achondrogenesis type I (Parenti-Fraccaro, lethal, or osteochondrodysplastic type) and achondrogenesis type II (Grebe, Brazilian, or limb-malformation type).

The potential confusion does not stop with these two forms because there appear to be two or more different forms of achondrogenesis I. Although very

---

Fig. 13-6. Homozygous achondroplasia. **A** to **D,** The father and mother, with ordinary features of heterozygous achondroplasia. **E,** Their baby, homozygous for the achondroplasia gene, at the age of 4 weeks. The child died at age 11 weeks, of hydrocephalus and respiratory restriction. Note the large head and small thorax. **F** to **H,** X-ray views of homozygous infant. **F,** The large size of the head contrasts with the small size of the thorax. **G,** The scapulae are small. The ribs are short with cupped ends. The lung capacity is obviously limited. **H,** The changes are more severe than in heterozygous achondroplasia. Note the spinelike projections at the proximal and distal ends of the humerus. (From Hall, J. G., Dorst, J. P., Taybi, H., Scott, C. I., Langer, L. O., Jr., and McKusick, V. A.: Two probable cases of homozygosity for the achondroplasia gene. In Bergsma, D., editor: Clinical delineation of birth defects. IV. Skeletal dysplasias, New York, 1969, National Foundation–March of Dimes.)

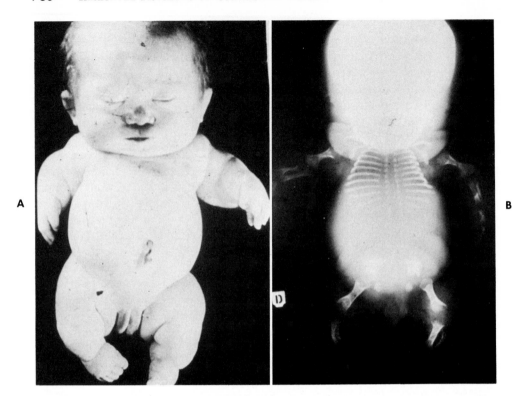

Fig. 13-7. Achondrogenesis, type I (the Parenti-Fraccaro, lethal, or osteochondrodysplastic type). **A,** Clinical appearance. **B,** Roentgenographic appearance. In addition to the short misshapen ribs, note the underossification in the lumbar vertebrae, lack of ossification in the sacrum, and wide pelvic curve. (From Langer, L. O., Jr., Spranger, J. W., Greinacher, I., and Herdman, R. C.: Radiology **92:**285, 1969.)

Fig. 13-8. Achondrogenesis, type II (the Grebe, Brazilian, or limb-malformation type). **A,** X-ray view of hands at the age of 4 years. The ulna is short and the radius bowed. No carpal or metacarpal bones are identified. Six digits, including an extra postaxial finger, are present. **B** and **C,** Hands and feet at the age of 5 years 4 months. The short forearms and legs and six fingers are shown. Each foot has six toes, and the great toes are broad, suggesting duplication. **D** to **F,** Front, lateral, and back views at the age of 8 years. The sixth fingers have been removed. **G** and **H,** Pelvis and legs at the age of 8 years. The pelvis and femora are relatively normal. The tibia is small and broad and the fibula is even smaller. Bones in the feet are severely deformed. Right and left arms, **I** and **J,** and feet, **K,** at the age of 10 years. The radii are short and bowed; the ulnae are very short because of a distal deficiency. The carpals, metacarpals, and phalanges, especially the proximal phalanges, are malformed but have developed remarkably since the age of 4 years. **A,** All the bones of the feet are likewise deformed, there being a complex polydactyly, with seven digits on the left foot. **L** and **M,** Appearance at 15 years of age; height is 42 inches. **N,** X-ray views of upper limbs at 15 years. Parental consanguinity was denied; the father and mother were 49 and 32 years old, respectively, at her birth. Two older brothers were normal and there had been no miscarriages. The patient completed high school and at the age of 25 years, when last examined, was earning her livelihood painting portraits and landscapes. Since childhood she has worn a stilt type of leg prosthesis. (Patient studied by Dr. Charles I. Scott.)

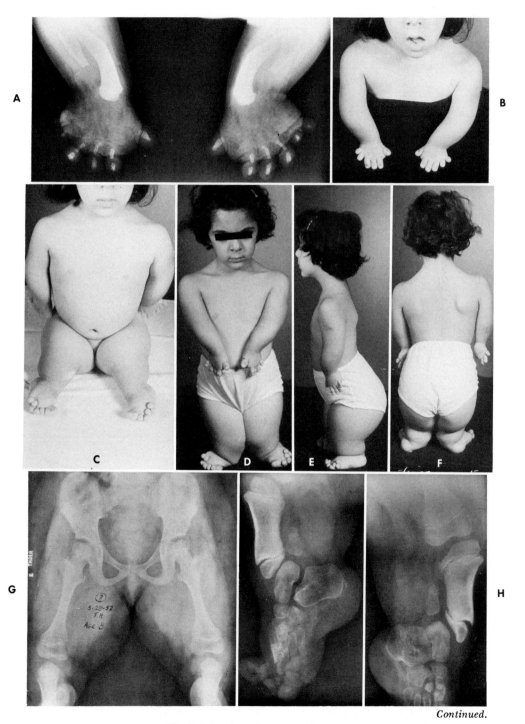

Continued.

Fig. 13-8. For legend see opposite page.

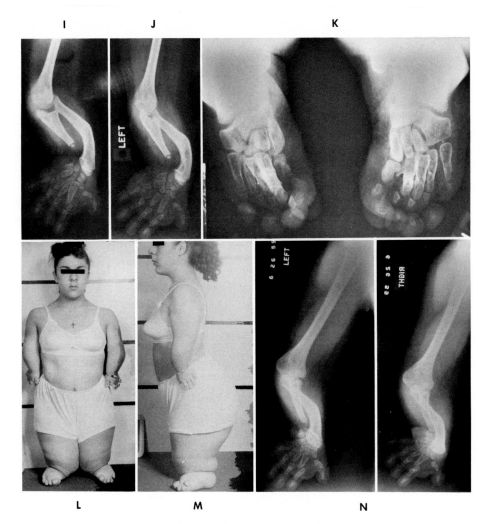

Fig. 13-8, cont'd. For legend see p. 760.

similar, the familial cases reported by Houston[118a] and the Doctors Urso[316a] are sufficiently different from earlier reported cases to be considered distinct.

Thanatophoric dwarfism

This disorder, taking its name from the Greek for "death-bearing," was delineated and named by Maroteaux and colleagues[206] in 1967. A fairly considerable literature on the condition has accumulated in the short span of time since then. A number of cases previously reported as achondroplasia can be recognized as examples of thanatophoric dwarfism.[225]

The head is large as a result of hydrocephalus, which sometimes requires decompression for delivery (Fig. 13-9A). Respiratory distress because of the severely restricted rib cage leads to early death, although survival of one patient for six months (D.A. McC., P11807) in continuous oxygen therapy is known

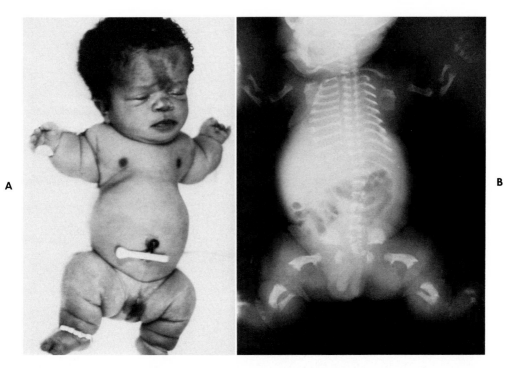

Fig. 13-9. Thanatophoric dwarfism. **A,** E. G. S. (J.H.H. 1344960) weighed 3060 grams at birth. Polyhydramnios, falling estriol levels, and meconium staining of fluid obtained by amniocentesis complicated late pregnancy. At birth the head circumference measured 32.5 cm. and the length was 42 cm. Prominent forehead, depressed nasal bridge, midline hemangioma, and small face with bulging eyes were noted. The chest was small and the abdomen protuberant. A low thoracic gibbus and short limbs with striking skin folds and limitation of elbow extension were noted. The infant died at 36 hours. **B,** On x-ray view, the chest was narrow with cupping of the short ribs at the costochondral junction. The vertebral bodies were markedly flattened and the disc space was increased, giving the classic appearance of thanatophoric dwarfism in the frontal view.

to me. Associated malformation of the brain and the cardiovascular system have been described.

The roentgenographic features are diagnostic. The ribs are very short, producing a small thorax. The scapulae are small and square. The vertebral bodies are very flat, and there are unusually wide intervertebral spaces. On the frontal view the lumbar vertebrae have the appearance of an inverted letter "U" or a letter "H" (Fig. 13-9B).

Thompson and Parmley[310] discussed the obstetric features of 7 cases seen in this hospital. Hydramnios and breech presentation were frequent.

Multiple affected sibs with normal parents and parental consanguinity have now been observed, making autosomal recessive inheritance very likely. Chemke et al.[41a] described 2 affected offspring of first-cousin parents. Langer and Gorlin[164a] agreed with the radiologic diagnosis of thanatophoric dwarfism.

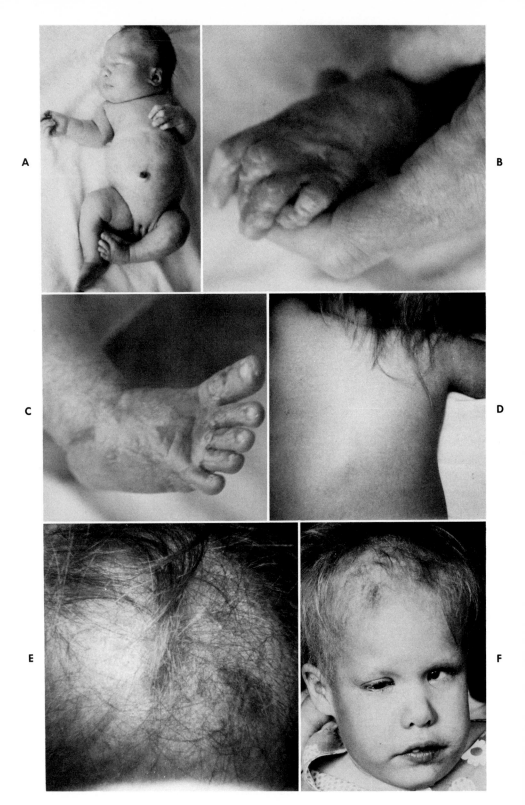

Fig. 13-10. For legend see p. 766.

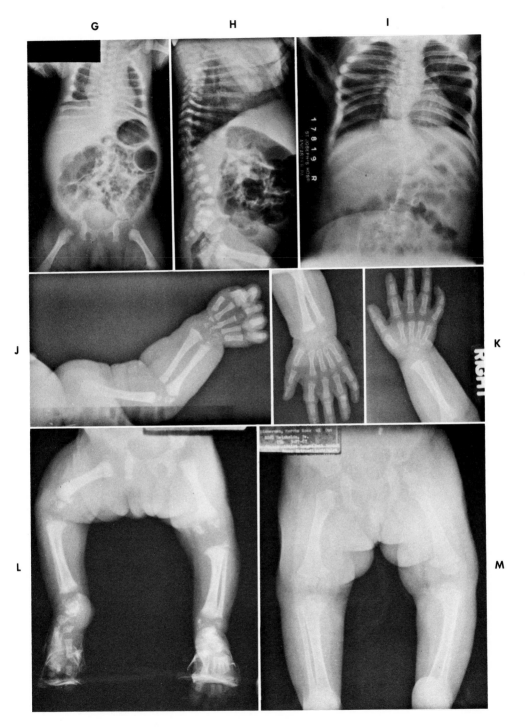

Fig. 13-10, cont'd. For legend see p. 766.

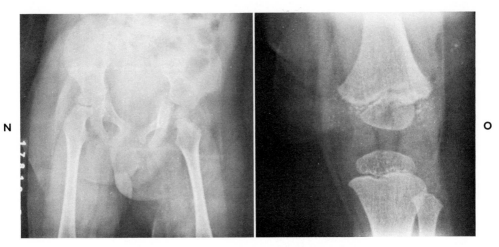

Fig. 13-10. Chondrodysplasia punctata, presumably the autosomal recessive form. M. Z., a white female, was noted at birth to have multiple abnormalities. The head was misshapen and the limbs were short, with scarring of the skin and contracture of the fingers. The skin was generally covered with dry, adherent, vernixlike material. Bilateral cataracts were present. On the basis of the radiographs, a diagnosis of chondrodysplasia punctata was made. When the patient was 3 months old, Dr. Harold G. Scheie found increased intraocular pressure in the right eye, which was much enlarged, with hazy cornea and iris bombé. This eye was enucleated. The histologic findings included dislocated cataractous lens, rubeosis iridis, posterior and anterior synechiae, atrophy of the retina and optic nerve, and thin sclera.

At the age of 2¾ years the child showed marked motor and mental retardation. She had just begun to sit on her own. The hair was sparse and spindly. All the skin was dry and scaly, and that of the scalp was especially so, with lesions resembling freckles. The fifth fingers were incurved. The right hip was dislocated and kyphoscoliosis was severe. The heel cords were very tight and the calf muscles wasted. The left eye showed searching nystagmoid movements and a hazy cornea.

The parents, in their twenties, were apparently unrelated but had a common background in a conservative Mennonite group.

A to **C**, Appearance at birth. Extensive skin lesions and contracture of the fingers are shown.

D and **E**, Appearance at the age of 2¾ years. Kyphoscoliosis and sparse, stringy hair with scaly skin of the scalp are shown.

F to **I**, Appearance at the age of 4¼ years. Spine and hips are shown at birth, **G** and **H**. The posterior portions of the ribs are spindly. Scoliosis is already present. Stippled calcification is seen in the region of the head of the femur and about the pedicles and spinous processes of the vertebrae, **H**. At 2¾ years of age, scoliosis is marked but no stippling remains and the ribs are no longer spindly, **I**.

The upper limbs at birth, **J**, showed striking stippling in the wrist and elbow and anterior dislocation of the radial head. By the age of 1 year, **K**, stippling had largely disappeared. The carpal ossification centers were delayed, especially on the left. The digits were short and the fifth was incurved.

L to **O**, X-ray views of lower limbs. **L**, Newborn. Striking stippling is evident at the hips, knees, and ankles. **M**, At the age of 1 year, the capital epiphysis of the right femur is poorly developed. **N** and **O**, At the age of 2¾ years, tilting of the pelvis and dysplasia of the hips are demonstrated. The right hip is dislocated. Impressive stippling was found only in the region of the left knee.

Parkington and colleagues[231a] described cloverleaf skull deformity with generalized skeletal changes like those of thanatophoric dwarfism. They observed, furthermore, 2 cases in sibs.

The histopathology[310] is one of disorganized endochondral ossification quite unlike that in achondroplasia.

Chondrodysplasia punctata

Chondrodysplasia punctata is the term suggested by the Paris Conference for the disorder that has been variously termed Conradi's disease,[5] chondrodystrophia calcificans congenita,[246] epiphyseal dysplasia punctata,[248] or stippled epiphyses, among other designations.[178] Two and perhaps more entities appear to be subsumed. To complicate the nosology further, stippled epiphyses occur with the cerebro-hepato-renal syndrome of Zellweger, the Smith-Lemli-Opitz syndrome, cretinism, trisomy 18, and other conditions.

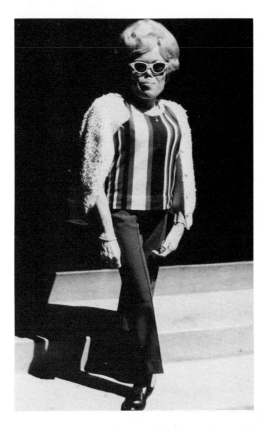

Fig. 13-11. Chondrodysplasia punctata in a 33-year-old woman. As an infant this patient was reported as having "calcinosis universalis with unusual features."[28] She showed a short left femur, unusual facies, lesions of the skin (described at birth as red, thick, and covered with cream-colored horny plaques), and cataracts. In the present picture the woman, who is of normal intelligence, is wearing a wig (the hair is sparse), is concealing her short left leg, and shows characteristic koala-bear facies. She has considerable scoliosis and generalized ichthyosiform skin lesions. This is presumably the autosomal dominant form of chondrodysplasia punctata. (Patient studied by Dr. Charles I. Scott, Jr.)

Both dominant and recessive forms of chondrodysplasia punctata probably exist.[296] The recessive type is characterized by rhizomelic dwarfism. Common findings include joint contractures, depression of the nasal bridge (leading to the designation "koala bear syndrome" by our Australian colleagues), cataracts, and an ichthyosiform dermatosis with alopecia (Fig. 13-10). Death often occurs in the first year of life. Survivors are usually retarded mentally. Roentgenographically, infants show, in addition to stippling of epiphyseal ossification centers, vertical clefting of the vertebral bodies on lateral projection, short humeri and femora, and changes in the metaphyses of tubular long bones.

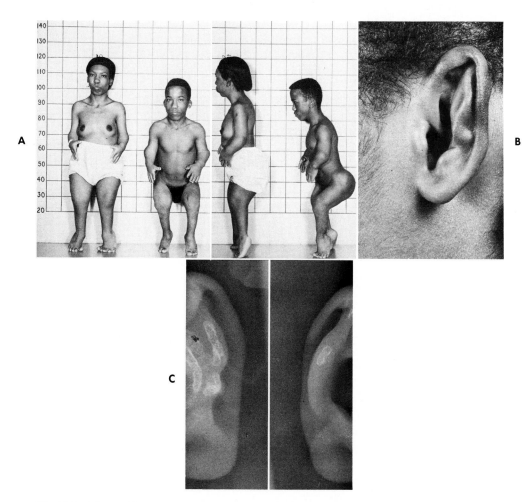

Fig. 13-12. Diastrophic dwarfism in sister and brother, 19 and 15 years old, respectively. Clubbed hands and feet and marked dwarfism are shown in **A.** The ears are rigid and deformed, **B,** and show ossification of pinnal cartilages, **C.** The severe deformity of the hands, **D,** and feet, **E,** is demonstrated. The position of the thumb—"hitchhiker thumb"—is characteristic. Its metacarpal is very short. Ankylosis of the proximal interphalangeal joints in the second, third, and fourth fingers of both hands is also demonstrated. Because of the stiff fingers the patient's method of writing, **F,** is awkward. In **G** are demonstrated severe derangement of the hip, scoliosis, and precocious ossification of costal cartilages.

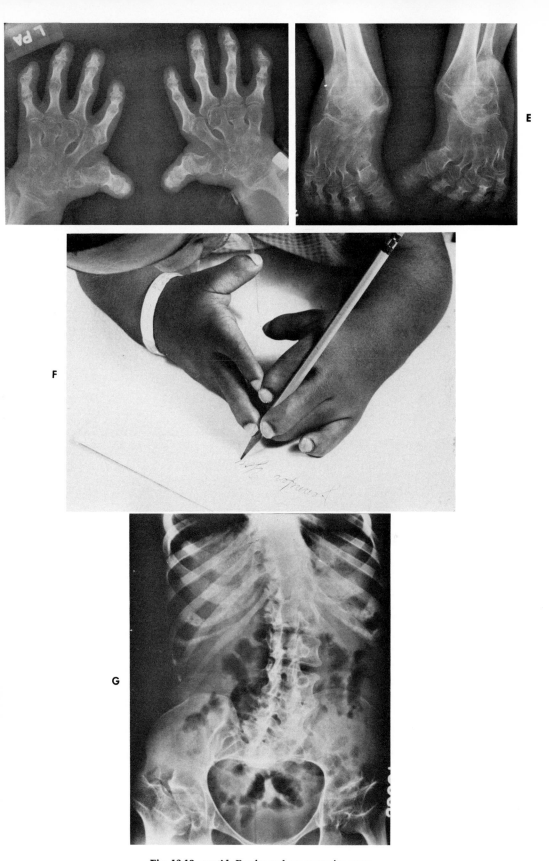

Fig. 13-12, cont'd. For legend see opposite page.

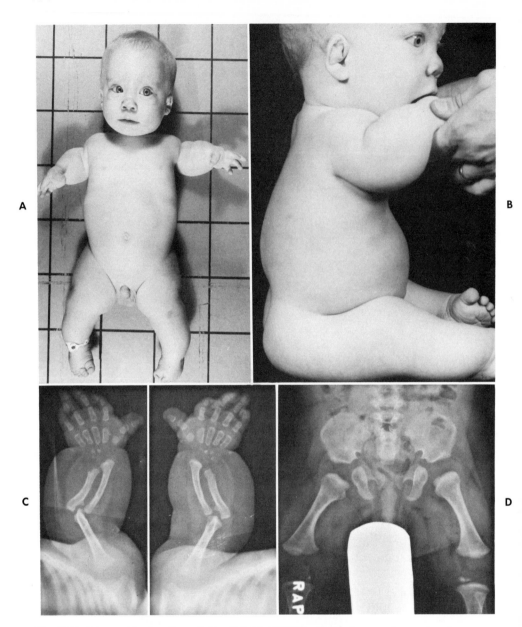

Fig. 13-13. Diastrophic dwarfism. B. D. (J.H.H. 1258051), shown here at 6 months of age, was born of apparently unrelated parents. At birth multiple skeletal abnormalities, including cleft palate and bilateral clubfoot, were noted. At 6 months he was also noted to have "hitchhiker" thumbs, capillary hemangiomas of the face, kyphoscoliosis, and thick, deformed pinnae. **A,** Overall view. **B,** The deformity of the spine and ears is evident. **C,** The upper limbs at 6 months of age. All bones are short. The radii and ulnae are bowed. The proximal end of each humerus is wide and flat. The radial heads are dislocated and the ulnae are relatively short distally. The first metacarpals are particularly short and the thumbs are everted. Clinodactyly of the second and fourth fingers is noted. **D,** Pelvis and femora at 6 months of age. The lower spinal canal is narrow, as is the sacrum. The greater sciatic notches are short and the acetabular roofs flat. The long bones are short and massive. **E,** The short, massive long bones and clubbed feet are demonstrated.

In Fig. 13-11 is illustrated chondrodysplasia punctata of presumed dominant type, the patient representing new mutation. Skin changes, cataract, dwarfism, and scoliosis can occur as in the recessive form. However, intelligence is unimpaired, and a particularly distinctive feature is unilateral shortening of the femur due to asymmetrical severity of the chondrodysplasia.

Another autosomal dominant form of chondrodysplasia punctata is a type of epiphyseal dysplasia. An example is the patient described by Rubin[258] as typical; this is Silverman's epiphyseal dysplasia punctata.[280] Another is probably the family of Raap,[246] who found the disorder in 4 sibs. Complete disappearance of x-ray changes had probably occurred in the affected parent. Patients with this form may escape associated abnormalities such as those of the skin, eye, and brain and achieve normal adult stature with little or no deformity and no radiographic residua.

Metatropic dwarfism

See the discussion of the differential diagnosis of the Morquio syndrome (p. 606). The Kniest disease is a variant of metatropic dwarfism.[294a]

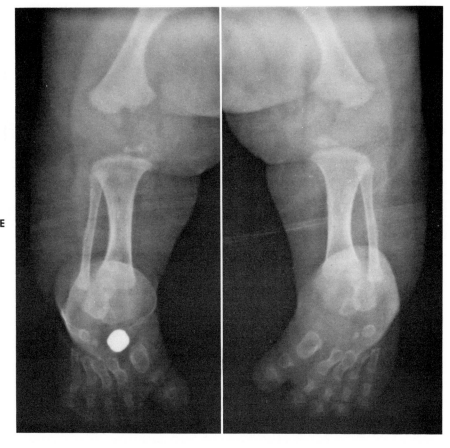

E

Fig. 13-13, cont'd. For legend see opposite page.

Diastrophic dwarfism

Diastrophic dwarfism[326] derives its name from the Greek word for "bent" or "twisted." (Diastrophism is a term used in geology to refer to the process of bending in the earth's crust by which mountains and ocean basins are formed.) The patients are usually diagnosed as having chondrodystrophy (or achondroplasia) with clubfoot or with arthrogryposis. As with so many of the other skeletal dysplasias, Lamy and Maroteaux[155] delineated the entity and assigned its name. We[326] were able to find 69 cases in the literature and assembled a personal series of 51 cases distributed in thirty-five kindreds.

The disorder is recognizable at birth by the clubfoot deformity and the "hitchhiker" thumb. In about 85% of the patients the pinna of the external ear becomes acutely inflamed and swollen in the first two or three weeks of life. The inflammation subsides in a few weeks, leaving the ears cauliflowered. Later calcification, indeed ossification, can be demonstrated.[195,305] We have been impressed with the precocious ossification of the costal cartilages. Cleft palate occurs in about a fourth of cases. In addition to the hitchhiker thumb, which results from deformity of the first metacarpal, the fingers develop symphalangism, i.e., fusion of the proximal interphalangeal joints.[301] The clubfoot deformity is notoriously difficult to treat, but acceptable results have been achieved with early and persistently applied therapy. These and other clinical features are demonstrated in Figs. 13-12 to 13-14.

Intelligence is normal. I know of an affected 50-year-old man who has 4 normal daughters and an affected sister, and of 2 women with diastrophic dwarfism,

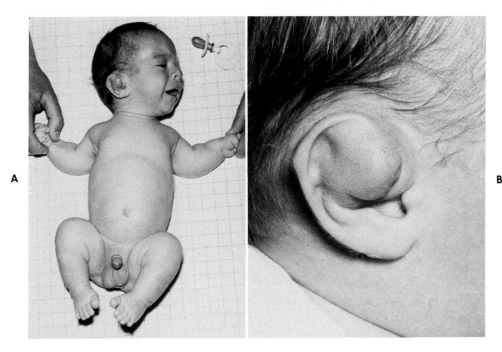

Fig. 13-14. Diastrophic dwarfism in infant (Jo. Mos., P 8843) at the stage of acute swelling of the ear. (Courtesy Dr. Dick Hoefnagel, Hanover, N. H.)

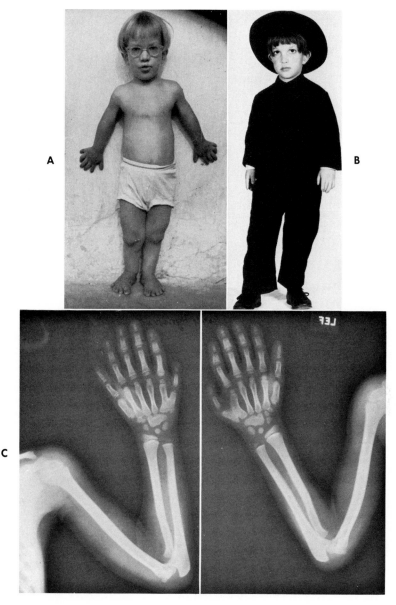

Fig. 13-15. Ellis–van Creveld syndrome. **A** and **B,** Amish boy, 5 and 9 years of age, respectively. Polydactyly, knock-knees, and short extremities are demonstrated in **A.** The extra digits have been amputated by age 9. Closure of an ostium secundum atrial septal defect was performed at that age. **C,** Negro female, 9 years old. The appearance of the extra finger and the fusion of the hamate and capitate bones are characteristic. (From McKusick, V. A., and colleagues: Trans. Ass. Amer. Phys. **77:**154, 1964.)

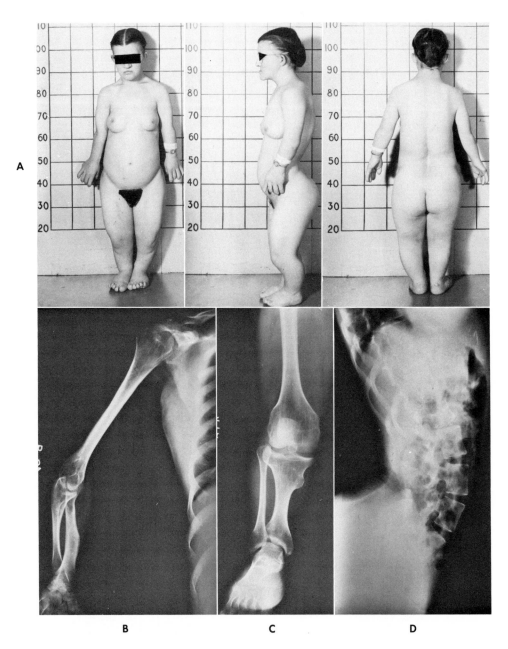

Fig. 13-16. Ellis–van Creveld syndrome. **A,** General appearance of 21-year-old female. The upper lip is retracted and sunken, in part due to early loss of teeth, in part due to "partial harelip." Signs of large atrial septal defect are present. The distal portion of the extremities is particularly short, **B** and **C.** X-ray examination showed short, wide long bones, especially in the forearm and leg. Deep cupping of the tibial condyles is characteristic, and the medial tibial exostosis is a common finding. **D,** Extreme spondylolisthesis is present. The fingernails are dystrophic, **E.** Extra fingers have been amputated. Normal hand for comparison.

each delivered of a normal infant by cesarean section. Rubin[258] pictured the x-ray findings of a 72-year-old man with diastrophic dwarfism. Inheritance is autosomal recessive.

Chondroectodermal dysplasia (Ellis–van Creveld syndrome)

The Ellis–van Creveld syndrome (chondroectodermal dysplasia) is manifested by dwarfism, polydactyly, dysplastic fingernails, and, in about half the cases, malformation of the heart, usually a single atrium,[36,139] or large ostium primum atrial septal defect (Fig. 13-18). An ostium secundum type of atrial septal defect was closed in the patient shown in Fig. 13-15*A*. Cases have been observed in persons of many nationalities, including Caucasians, Negroes, and Orientals. Many cases, about equaling the number reported in the literature, were observed[191,192] in a religious isolate, the Old Order Amish of Lancaster County, Pennsylvania. Inheritance is autosomal recessive. The clinical and roentgenographic features are shown in Figs. 13-15 to 13-21.

Asphyxiating thoracic dysplasia

This condition was originally dubbed "asphyxiating thoracic dystrophy of infancy" by Jeune and associates in 1955.[128] They described it in 2 sibs who died with respiratory distress in infancy. The Paris Conference recommended calling it asphyxiating thoracic dysplasia. Cases without respiratory problems and with survival at least to the teens have been described.

The central feature of this disorder is a thorax that is small in all dimensions. Some patients die from respiratory distress; others seem to "outgrow" the respiratory problems. Postaxial polydactyly of the hands and feet is present in some, but it rarely has the symmetrical malformation seen in the Ellis–van

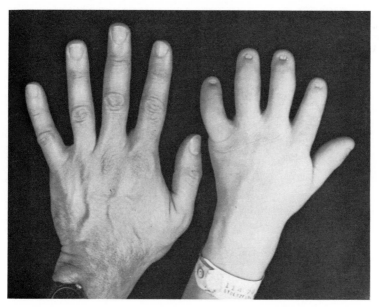

E

Fig. 13-16, cont'd. For legend see opposite page.

Creveld syndrome (EvC), and the feet are as likely to be affected as the hands, whereas in EvC the hands are always affected and the feet, in 10% or less of cases. Renal abnormality, with death from renal failure, has been observed in some patients.[108]

The roentgenographic features include, in the pelvis, retarded ossification of the triradiate cartilage, resulting in a double notch. This roentgenographic feature is found also in EvC. (See Fig. 13-20.) The pelvic, thoracic, and vertebral

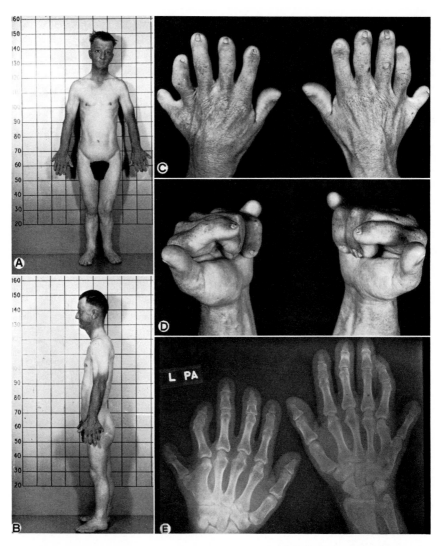

Fig. 13-17. Ellis–van Creveld syndrome in man 45 years old. **A** and **B,** Note the particular shortening of the distal portion of the extremities. **C,** In the hands note the polydactyly, brachydactyly, and dysplastic fingernails. **D,** The patient cannot make a tight first. The reason is shown in **E.** The proximal phalanges are long relative to the middle and distal phalanges. Note the partial fusion of the hamate and capitate bones of the wrist. (From McKusick, V. A., Egeland, J. A., Eldridge, R., and Krusen, D. E.: Bull. Hopkins Hosp. 115:306, 1964.)

x-ray findings are identical in this syndrome and in EvC, and in the hands the same cone-shaped epiphyses and other changes occur in both conditions (Fig. 13-22). Distinction usually can be made on the basis of knee roentgenograms, which show a characteristic deformity in EvC but not in asphyxiating thoracic dysplasia.

This disorder is autosomal recessive.

Spondyloepiphyseal dysplasia congenita

See the discussion of the differential diagnosis of the Morquio syndrome (p. 601).

Cleidocranial dysplasia

Cleidocranial dysplasia,[79,121,134] previously known as cleidocranial dysostosis, was renamed by the Paris Conference. Development is defective in the skull,

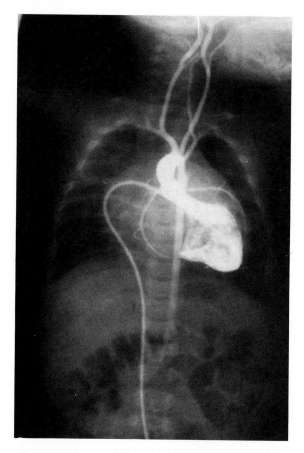

Fig. 13-18. Ellis–van Creveld syndrome with single atrium in a 4-month-old infant (L. E. B47024). The catheter introduced via a leg vein has passed into the left ventricle through the atrial septal defect which, from the roentgenographic appearance shown here, is judged to be of the ostium primum type from the single atrium. Ellis–van Creveld syndrome with single atrium in 4-month-old infant (L. E. B47024). Injection made in the left ventricle shows the "gooseneck" deformity of the left ventricular outflow tract characteristic of an endocardial cushion defect. (From Mc-Kusick, V. A., Egeland, J. A., Eldridge, R., and Krusen, D. E.: Bull. Hopkins Hosp. 115:306, 1964.)

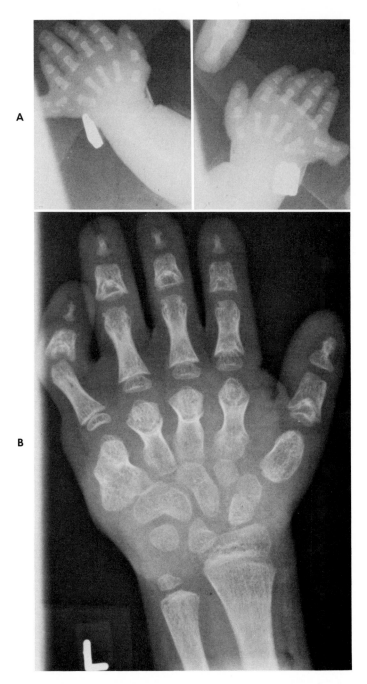

Fig. 13-19. Hands of children with the Ellis–van Creveld syndrome. **A,** G. S. at the age of 3 days. The extra postaxial digit has two components. **B,** Hand of boy shown in Fig. 13-15, at the age of 9 years. The terminal phalanges are hypoplastic. Many of the epiphyses are cone-shaped and set into "wine-bottle" metaphyses. The sixth digit has been amputated. The capitate and hamate are severely deformed.

which shows multiple Wormian bones and delay in the closure of sutures; in the clavicles, which are hypoplastic or absent; and in the pubic symphysis, which is wide. Spina bifida occulta in the lower cervical and upper thoracic spine and wide sacroiliac joints are frequent findings. The acetabulum may be hypoplastic, leading to dislocation of the hip. Changes occur in the phalangeal epiphyses. Acro-osteolysis-like dysplasia of the terminal phalanges, when considered in relation to the malformation of the skull, may suggest pyknodysostosis (p. 820). Dental anomalies are an almost invariable feature.

Cleidocranial dysplasia is an autosomal dominant disorder.

Hypochondroplasia

As noted earlier, achondroplasia is remarkably stereotypic, especially for a dominant disorder. Hypochondroplasia[325] resembles achondroplasia in many ways, but all the features are much milder.[18] It is also an autosomal dominant disorder and an entity in its own right. As might be expected of a milder disorder, a larger proportion of cases are familial than in achondroplasia. Within families the features are rather consistent; hypochondroplasia and achondroplasia, as presently defined, do not occur in the same family. A phenomenal case[189a] in which an offspring seems to have inherited the achondroplasia gene from her father and the hypochondroplasia gene from her mother is, of course, no exception to this statement. The fact that the child has a severe disorder of unique phenotype leads to the conclusion that the achondroplasia and hypochondroplasia genes are allelic, the child being a genetic compound comparable to SC

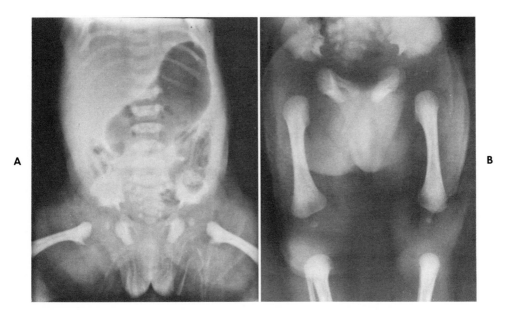

Fig. 13-20. Pelvis in infants with the Ellis–van Creveld syndrome. **A,** X-ray film made on day of birth. Unusual excrescences from the proximal femora may represent large lesser trochanters. The spinal canal lacks the caudad narrowing that is typical of achondroplasia. **B,** X-ray view of the pelvis and lower limbs in another infant, 19 days old. The acetabular roof is flat and characterized by a spicule at both the medial and lateral margins.

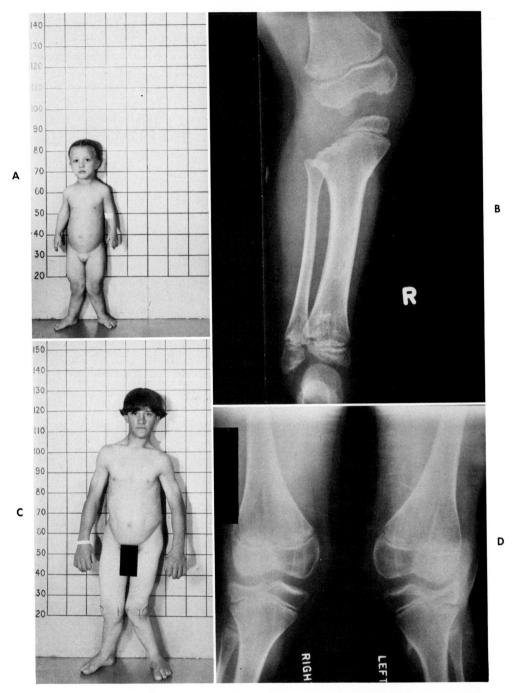

Fig. 13-21. Knees in the Ellis–van Creveld syndrome. **A** and **B,** Photograph and leg x-ray film of M. L. (1276980) at the age of 4 years. Genu valgum is striking. Hypoplasia of the lateral aspect of the proximal end of the tibia and fibula is demonstrated. **C** and **D,** Photograph and knee x-ray film of 14 year old. Severe genu valgum is again shown. The patellae are marked to show their far lateral displacement. The lateral aspect of the proximal tibial epiphysis is better developed than in the younger child; yet there is a depression of its surface, with genu valgum. A small exostosis is seen on the medial aspect of the left tibia.

disease among the hemoglobinopathies, which shows a phenotype distinct from both SS disease and CC disease.

Hypochondroplasia is probably fairly common, at least as common as achondroplasia, but the literature on the condition is remarkably scant. At birth, weight and length may be within the lower limit of normal; short stature is usually not recognized until the age of 2 or 3 years. The head and face are almost normal. Trident hand is not seen. Adult height ranges from 52 to 58 inches. Roentgenographically, the chevron sign at the knee and the caudad narrowing of the lumbar interpediculate distances are found but are much less marked than in achondroplasia. The pedicles may be particularly short. The diagnosis of hypochondroplasia is often difficult to make with confidence. It is entirely possible, indeed probable, that series of cases of hypochondroplasia, including my own, are made up of two or more fundamentally distinct entities. I suspect that more than one hypochondroplasia allele may exist at the achondroplasia locus. As expected of an autosomal dominant condition, parental age is advanced, on the average, in sporadic cases.

The clinical features are illustrated in Fig. 13-25. In the Paris nomenclature, hypochondroplasia was placed in the category of defects of tubular bones and/or spine not manifest at birth. I am not certain this is true; in many hypochondroplastic patients, dwarfism is recognized at birth. The new information suggesting

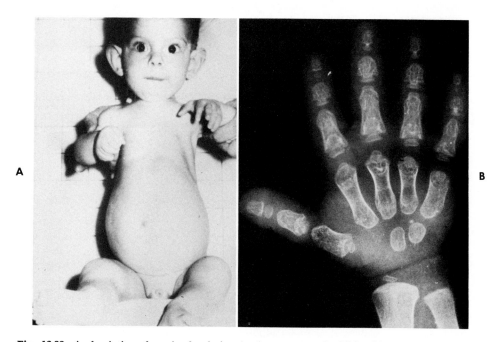

Fig. 13-22. Asphyxiating thoracic dysplasia. **A,** Appearance of child with severely restricted thoracic dysplasia. **B,** Hand of another child, 26 months old. Polydactyly was not present. Note similarity, otherwise, of x-ray view of hand to that in the Ellis–van Creveld syndrome (Fig. 13-19B). While the configuration of the pelvis in these cases is indistinguishable from that in the Ellis–van Creveld syndrome (Fig. 13-20), distinction is usually possible because the proximal tibia is normally formed.

allelism of the achondroplasia gene and the hypochondroplasia gene(s) gives further reason to put them together in the tabulation.

Dyschondrosteosis

The characteristics of dyschondrosteosis are mesomelic dwarfism and typical malformation of the distal radius and ulna, often referred to as Madelung's deformity.[12] The distal end of the ulna is hypoplastic and dorsally dislocated; the distal radius is bowed. The disorder was described and named by Léri and Weill in 1929.[176]

Langer[159] holds the view that most or all Madelung deformity is dyschondro-

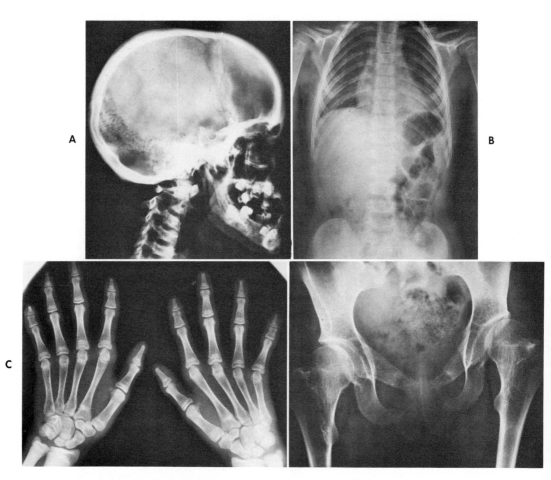

Fig. 13-23. Cleidocranial dysplasia has been observed in many members of at least three generations. **A,** Wide lambdoidal sutures with multiple Wormian bones are demonstrated in K. P., 25 years old. **B,** Hypoplasia of the clavicles, which are in two parts, is evident in D. S., 7 years old. Some affected members of the family have a severe anomaly of the lower cervical and upper thoracic spine. **C,** Note short middle phalanges in the second and fifth fingers and tapered terminal phalanges in N. S., 19 years of age. **D,** Note the hypoplasia of the pubis and ischium, with separation at the pubic symphysis, in R. S., 17 years old. The acetabula, especially the left, are shallow. Dislocation of the hip has occurred in several affected members of the family.

osteosis. Contrariwise, Felman and Kirkpatrick[75] concluded that patients with Madelung deformity who are above the 25th percentile for height probably do not have dyschondrosteosis, that isolated Madelung's deformity occurs as a distinct genetic trait, and that marked shortening of the tibia relative to the femur suggests dyschondrosteosis. The fibula was absent in the mother and son reported by Lamy and Bienenfeld.[152] Conductive hearing loss due to deformity of the middle ear was present in 2 of 5 affected sibs reported by Nassif and Harboyan.[223]

A short ulna, suggesting Madelung deformity, occurs sometimes with multiple exostoses (Fig. 13-41) and with many other skeletal dysplasias.

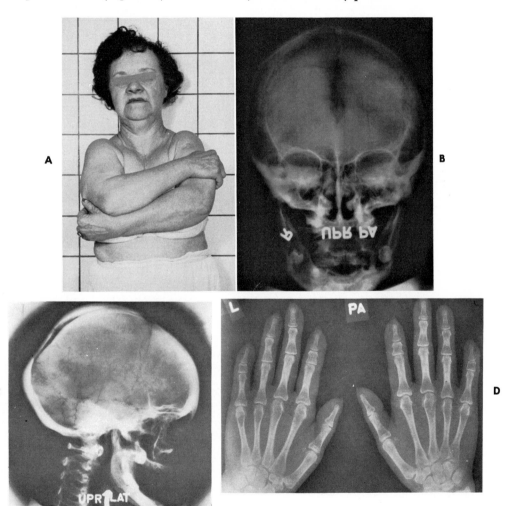

Fig. 13-24. Cleidocranial dysplasia in four generations of a kindred studied by Dr. Raymond Pearl and his colleagues in 1929 (unpublished). Demonstrated here are findings in E. S. (1058205) at the age of 58 years. **A,** Rather prominent forehead and ease of adduction of shoulders are shown. **B** and **C,** Note wide sutures, especially the sagittal, patent anterior fontanel and occipital Wormian bones. She is almost edentulous. **D,** Short second and fifth middle phalanges are shown, as in Fig. 13-23C. The mother of this woman, Pearl's proband, was affected, and she has an affected son and grandson. Affected members of this kindred are short of stature. The 2 members studied most extensively, both females, have adult heights of 59 and 56½ inches.

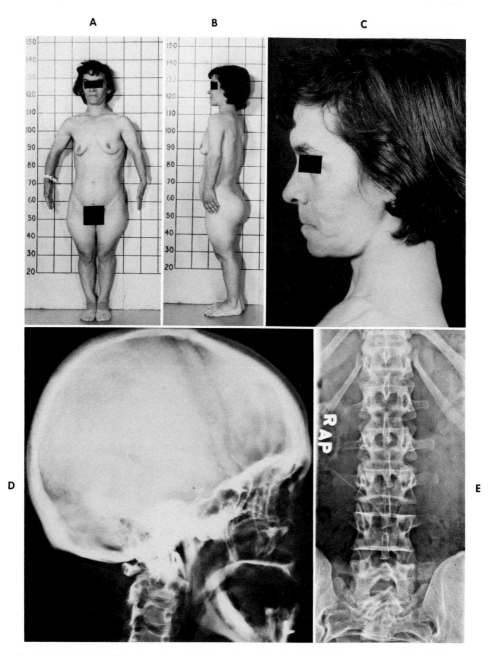

Fig. 13-25. Hypochondroplasia in mother and son. L. W. (1287010) was born of a 5-foot-tall woman and her 6-foot-tall husband. One of the 6 sibs, a brother, was only 5 feet tall. A speech impediment during childhood was apparently corrected by clipping the sublingual frenulum at the age of 10 years. L. W. had 2 sons, delivered by cesarean section; one (J. W.) inherited the mother's skeletal dysplasia. J. W. (1387009) was considered at birth to have a large head in relation to the body. During infancy he had numerous attacks of pneumonia. At 9 years of age a right inguinal hernia was repaired. Mental and motor development was slow. He walked at 3 years of age, was toilet-trained at 4 years, and spoke a few words by 7 years. When examined at the age of 11 years, he spoke in grunts but was able to obey commands. He attended an ungraded

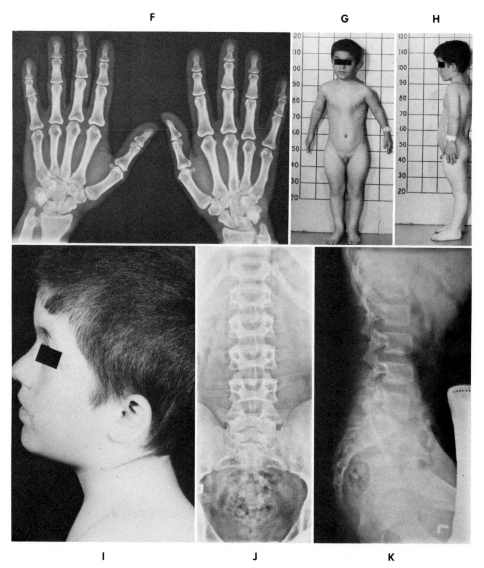

Continued.

school and was able to print his name and do simple arithmetic. He was sometimes difficult to manage because of hyperactivity. His I.Q. was estimated in the 50 to 60 range. Hearing and speech evaluation suggested a central communicative disorder with adequate hearing. **A** and **B,** Frontal and lateral views of L. W., the mother, at the age of 34 years. **C,** Normal profile in L. W. **D,** The skull shows minimal shortening of the base. **E,** Lower spine in L. W., showing narrow interpediculate distance and low articulation of the sacrum on the iliac bones. **F,** Hands in L. W., showing bones that are short but not as strikingly so as in achondroplasia. **G** and **H,** Frontal and lateral views of J. W., the 11-year-old son. Note the Harrison grooves. **I,** Normal profile of J. W. **J** and **K,** Frontal and lateral views of the spine in J. W., showing caudad narrowing of the spinal canal in both dimensions and increased space between the vertebral bodies. **L,** Pelvis in J. W., demonstrating the lack of the usual signs of achondroplasia. The calcified mass on the left is at an injection site. **M,** Bones of leg showing relatively long fibula distally. **N,** Hands of J. W., showing short bones and fifth finger clinodactyly.

Families with the dominant mode of transmission have been observed many times.[75,76,108,152,159] It is not completely certain whether inheritance is autosomal or X-linked. All series have appreciably more affected females than males. I have the impression that, in families, females are more severely affected than males. (The opposite is expected of an X-linked dominant.) If females are indeed more severely affected, the female preponderance in published series may be a result

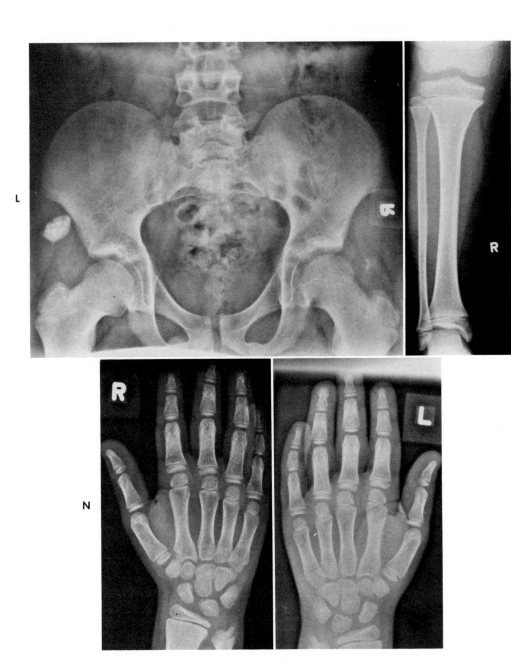

Fig. 13-25, cont'd. For legend see pp. 784-785.

of bias of ascertainment. Thus, this may be a sex-modified autosomal dominant disorder. However, until male-to-male transmission is well documented, the precise inheritance will remain in doubt. (See Fig. 13-26.)

Metaphyseal chondrodysplasias

This term is the Paris Conference recommendation for the group of disorders previously called metaphyseal dysostoses.

The very rare Jansen type[126] has severe abnormalities of all metaphyses, including those of the hands and feet. As demonstrated by x-ray studies, they are enlarged and have a spongy appearance. (The early radiographic changes as well as the later "textbook" appearance are shown in Fig. 13-27.) The patients are severely dwarfed and have enlarged joints. The arms are less shortened than the legs. A striking facial resemblance is shown by a comparison of cases reported

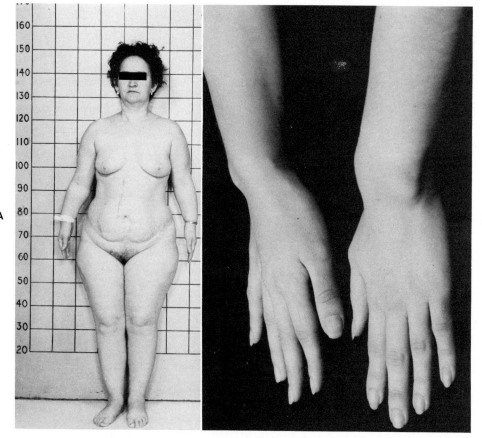

A   **B**

Fig. 13-26. Dyschondrosteosis in L. M. (J.H.H. 1381214), 42 years old. She is 58 inches tall and has Madelung's deformity of the distal forearms, **A.** Her mother, maternal grandmother, and 3 of her 5 daughters are likewise short and have Madelung's deformity. No males of the family are known to be affected. **B,** Arms of daughter, C. C. (1384650), 21 years old. Height is 62 inches. Madelung's deformity is demonstrated.

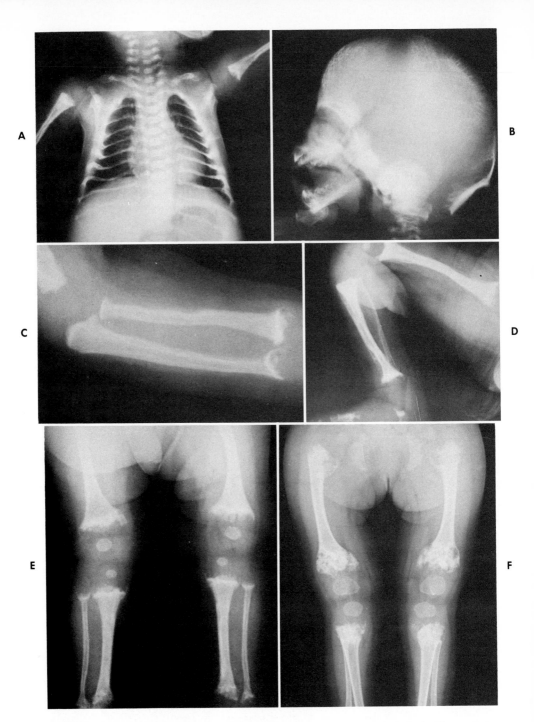

Fig. 13-27. Jansen type of metaphyseal chondrodysplasia in patient of Holt.[116] **A,** X-ray view at the age of 4 days. Irregularity of metaphyses, spindly, deformed ribs with fractures, and fetal demineralization are shown. **B,** At the age of 4 days, the calvaria shows a peculiar reticular pattern. **C** and **D,** At the age of 4 days, rachitiform changes and subperiosteal new bone formation and resorption are demonstrated. **E,** At 6 months the changes are suggestive of rickets except bone density is increased. **F,** At 5 years of age the gross changes in the metaphyses are typical of those described for this disorder.

This patient had hypercalcemia and was twice explored for parathyroid abnormality, with negative results. (Courtesy Dr. John F. Holt, Ann Arbor, Mich.)

by Gram and co-workers[96] and by Lenz and Holt.[175] (See Fig. 13-28.) As shown by restudy of Jansen's original case,[59] remarkable improvement occurs spontaneously. An unexplained feature is high serum calcium (13 to 15 mg./100 ml.) without symptoms. This feature often leads to surgical exploration of the parathyroid glands, with negative findings. Jansen's metaphyseal chondrodysplasia has been observed in mother and daughter[175] (Fig. 13-28). Remarkable improvement occurred in the mother by adulthood, although she was left severely dwarfed.

The Schmid type of metaphyseal chondrodysplasia[64] (Fig. 13-29) is an autosomal dominant disorder. Several kindreds with many affected members have been described, including the Mormon kindred with dwarfism reported by Stephens[298] as having achondroplasia. Short stature and bowlegs are the leading features. As demonstrated by x-ray studies, the metaphyseal changes, which are much less severe than in the Jansen type, vary from mild scalloping to gross irregularity, with widening of the metaphyses. Changes in the femoral necks are especially striking—more so than in cartilage-hair hypoplasia—and may lead to troublesome coxa vara. Roentgenographically and clinically, this type has been confused at times with vitamin D–resistant rickets. "Healing" of the metaphyseal lesions with bed rest and their reappearance with weight-bearing have been documented in the Schmid type.[64] This disorder is autosomal dominant. Advanced paternal age in sporadic cases has been noted.[256]

Cartilage-hair hypoplasia[193] (CHH) is another form of metaphyseal chondrodysplasia (Fig. 13-30). The patients have sparse, light-colored, fine hair as well as dwarfism. Adult height varies from 42 to 58 inches. The head and face are unaffected. The hands and feet are pudgy, with loose-jointedness and foreshortened fingernails. The elbows cannot be extended fully. Harrison's grooves are observed, and ankle deformity results from the fact that the fibula is excessively long distally relative to the tibia. (Just as some of the knee deformity can be avoided in achondroplasia by resection of the proximal end of the fibula, ankle deformity in CHH might be avoided by resection of the distal fibula.) Bowlegs are much less consistently present and involvement of the femoral necks is much milder than in the Schmid type. Features of CHH which I do not understand include intestinal malabsorption, with megacolon in some patients, a proneness to severe, sometimes fetal varicella, and a tendency to leukopenia and anemia.

As demonstrated by x-ray studies, the metaphyses, at the physeal surface, are scalloped and irregularly sclerotic, often with cystic areas. The ribs are flared and cupped at their junction with the costal cartilage.

This disorder is inherited as an autosomal recessive. It was first identified, because of its high frequency (about 2 per 1000 births), among the Old Order Amish.[193] However, it has been observed in non-Amish persons of European extraction.[47,104] I have recently seen it in 2 boys whose father is of Spanish–Puerto Rican lineage and whose mother, of Anglo-Saxon ancestry, was of unusually dark complexion. The light complexion of the 2 affected sons was a striking contrast with the dark complexion of the parents and a normal brother. The affected brothers have roentgenographic evidence of atlantoaxial instability, which was also present in 2 non-Amish cases in my series. I know, however, of no instance of neurologic complication related to this instability.

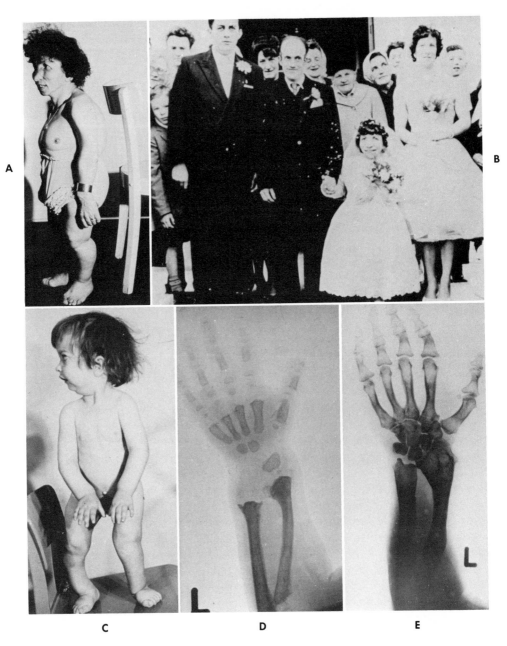

Fig. 13-28. Jansen type of metaphyseal chondrodysplasia in mother and daughter. **A,** General appearance of mother, with a height of 102 cm. **B,** Wedding picture showing mother with spouse of normal stature. **C,** Affected daughter. The small chin is characteristic. **D,** X-ray view of arm and hand of daughter. **E,** X-ray view of arm and hand of mother. **F,** X-ray view of femora of mother. **G,** X-ray view of legs of mother. Remarkable "healing" of metaphyseal lesions is demonstrated. The areas of bones that were previously the sites of striking lesions are now expanded and abnormally radiolucent. (From Lenz, W. D.: Discussion: Murk Jansen type of metaphyseal dyostosis. In Bergsma, D., editor: Clinical delineation of birth defects. IV. Skeletal dysplasias, New York, 1969, National Foundation–March of Dimes.)

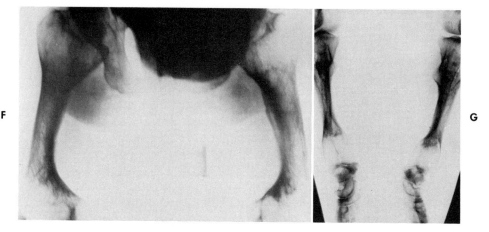

Fig. 13-28, cont'd. For legend see opposite page.

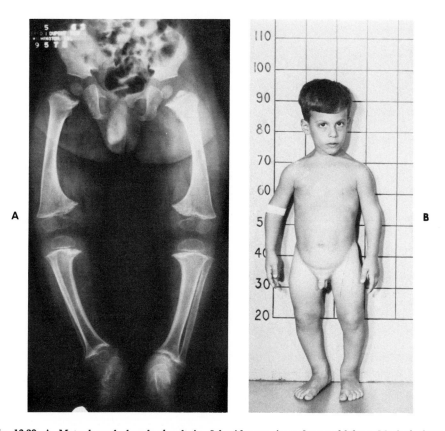

Fig. 13-29. A, Metaphyseal chondrodysplasia, Schmid type, in a 6-year-old boy. Marked changes are seen at both ends of the femora, tibiae, and fibulae. The epiphyseal ossification centers are well formed, however. Asymmetric wedgelike medial involvement of the distal femur and proximal tibia results in genu varum. B, Appearance of patient (R. C., 1257334) at the age of 6 years. Note the Harrison grooves. (A courtesy Dr. G. Dean MacEwen, Wilmington, Del.; from McKusick, V. A., Eldridge, R., Hostetler, J. A., Ruangwit, U., and Egeland, J. A.: Bull. Hopkins Hosp. 116:285, 1965.)

There may be an autosomal recessive form of metaphyseal chondrodysplasia that clinically resembles the Schmid type. In Fig. 13-31 is shown the pedigree of the kindred reported by Spahr and Spahr-Hartmann.[291]

The reader is referred elsewhere for information on the form of metaphyseal chondrodysplasia which is associated with malabsorption and neutropenia (the Shwachman syndrome[277,306]) and that associated with thymolymphopenia.[4,83-85]

Text continued on p. 798.

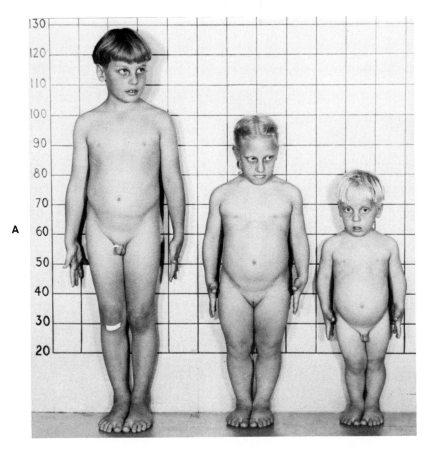

Fig. 13-30. Cartilage-hair hypoplasia (CHH). **A,** Three Amish children: (left to right), 7-year-old unaffected boy; 9-year-old affected girl; 5-year-old affected boy. The affected children have Harrison grooves of the chest resembling those of rickets and have thin hair which is lighter in color than that of unaffected sibs. **B,** X-ray changes in 2-year-old child with CHH. Note that the proximal femora are relatively spared. **C** and **D,** In rib biopsies, cartilage hypoplasia in a 5-year-old affected child, **D,** is contrasted with the normal findings in a 5-year-old child with congenital heart disease. **E,** Microscopic appearance of hair in 6 sibs ranging in age from 15 years (at the top) to 3 years (at the bottom). A hair from each of the 3 sibs in **A** is shown (third, fourth, and fifth from the top). Both small caliber of the hair and deficiency of pigment in the affected 9- and 5-year-old patients are demonstrated. **F,** Hair measurements of a group of CHH cases and unaffected parents and sibs. (**A** to **E** from McKusick, V. A., Eldridge, R., Hostetler, J. A., and Egeland, J. A.: Trans. Ass. Amer. Phys. 77:151, 1964; **F** from McKusick, V. A., Eldridge, R., Hostetler, J. A., Ruangwit, U., and Egeland, J. A.: Bull. Hopkins Hosp. 116:285, 1965.)

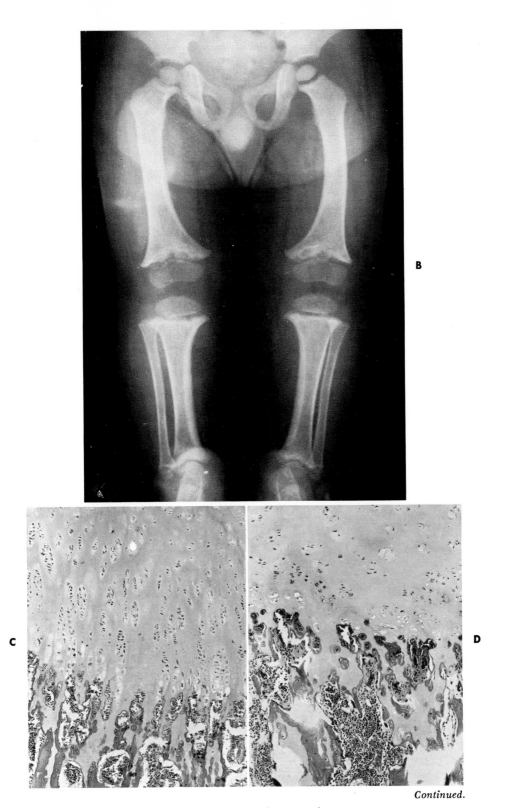

Continued.

Fig. 13-30, cont'd. For legend see opposite page.

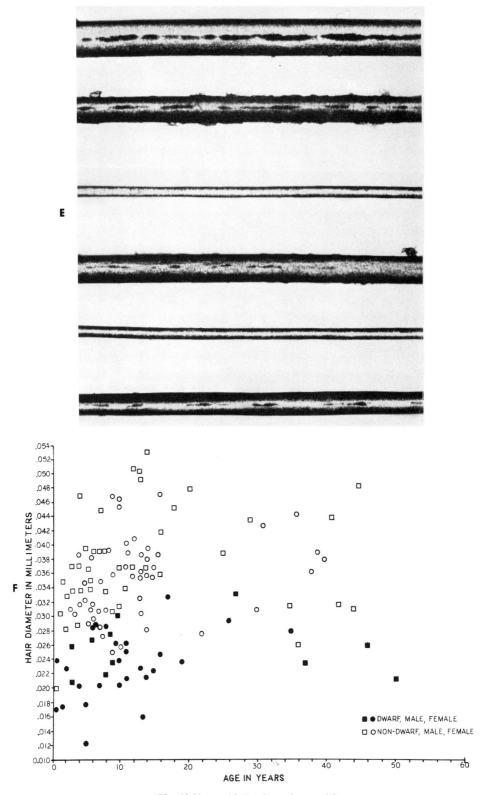

Fig. 13-30, cont'd. For legend see p. 792.

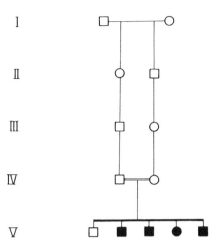

Fig. 13-31. Pedigree of metaphyseal chondrodysplasia, Spahr type, indicating autosomal recessive inheritance. (After Spahr and Spahr-Hartmann[201]; from McKusick, V. A., Eldridge, R., Hostetler, J. A., Ruangwit, U., and Egeland, J. A.: Bull. Hopkins Hosp. **116**:285, 1965.)

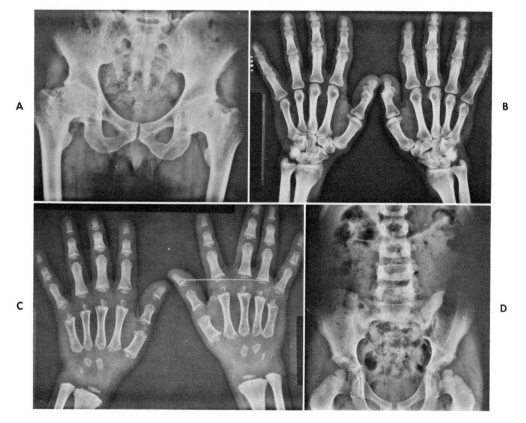

Fig. 13-32. Multiple epiphyseal dysplasia in father and son. The father, **A** and **B**, 40 years old, is moderately short of stature and has short fingers and severe osteoarthrosis of the hips. The son, **C** and **D**, 9 years old, shows the characteristic findings of multiple epiphyseal dysplasia, thus indicating the "cause" of the precocious osteoarthrosis in the father. His sister is also affected. Inheritance is autosomal dominant. The father's father, a brother, and several children of the brother are similarly affected.

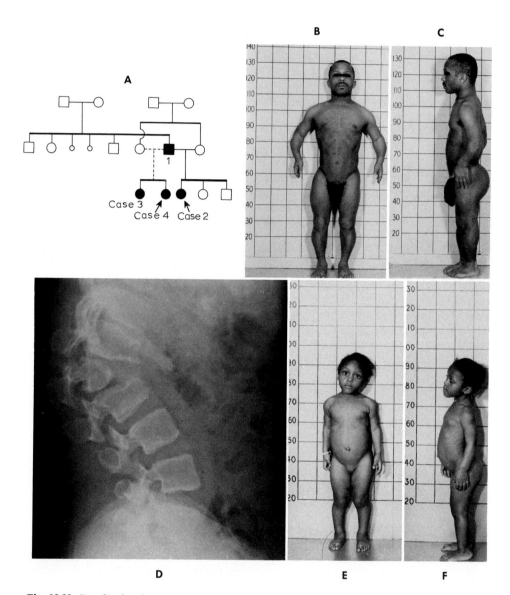

Fig. 13-33. Pseudoachondroplastic dysplasia, type I. The father and 3 children are affected, as shown in pedigree, **A**; the 2 mothers of the affected children are sisters. The father (Case 1, G. Q., 349115), **B** and **C**, was noted to have difficulty in standing and a waddling gait at the age of 2 years, and limitation in extension of the elbows and knees at 3 years. X-ray studies of the lumbar spine showed wedging of vertebral bodies T-12 to L-2, with absence of the anterior portion of L-1, resulting in gibbus, **D**.

The youngest daughter (Case 2, J. Q., 968463), **E** and **F**, was noted to limp at 2 years of age; x-ray films taken then were considered normal. By the age of 5 years, skeletal dysplasia was evident. The vertebral bodies, **G**, were short and oval, and the grooves of the apophyseal rings were unusually deep. In the legs, **H**, the epiphyses were flattened and metaphyseal ossification was irregular, especially in the periphery. In the hands, **I**, all bones were short. The carpal bones

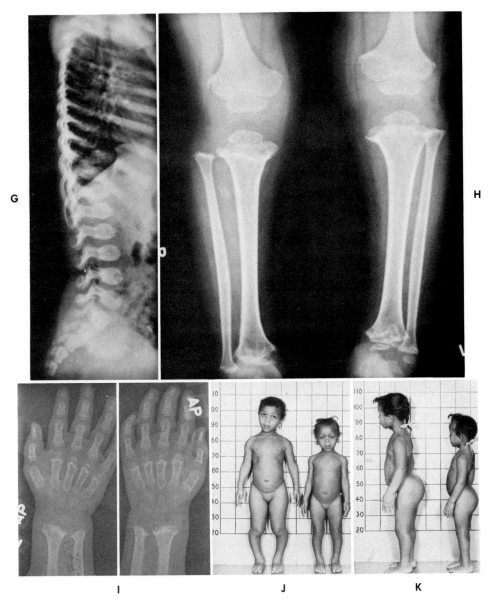

Continued.

showed delayed ossification and were small and irregular. The proximal ends of the metacarpals and the distal ends of the proximal phalanges formed blunt points.

The other 2 affected daughters (Cases 3 and 4) were 7½ and 5½ years of age at the time the pictures were made, **J** and **K.** Tibial bowing and Harrison grooves are more pronounced in the older child. The spinal x-ray views of the older child (Case 3) at 22 months, **L,** and at 7½ years, **M,** are shown. The oval shape, with anterior tonguing and increased intervertebral space, became less marked with age.

The knees of the older child (Case 3) at 7½ years, **N,** show both epiphyseal and metaphyseal changes. The lateral subluxation of the tibias with genu varum and deficient ossification in the medial portions of the proximal tibial metaphyses and epiphyses is similar to that in Blount's disease.

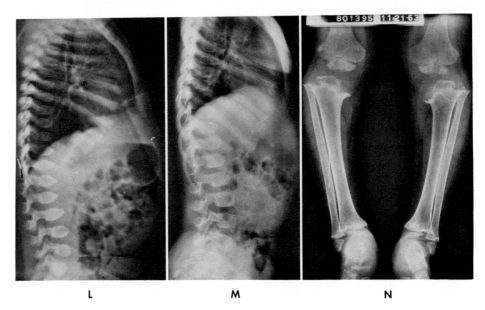

Fig. 13-33, cont'd. For legend see pp. 796-797.

Multiple epiphyseal dysplasia

This disorder, to which Fairbank's name is often assigned, may present between 5 and 10 years of age, when a waddling gait or difficulty in climbing stairs or running is noted. Joint pains and limitation of motion in various joints, e.g., knees, hips, and shoulders, are also common. In young patients a mistaken diagnosis of bilateral Legg-Perthes disease is often made, and older patients may be diagnosed as having precocious osteoarthritis of the hips. Dwarfing is generally not severe, adult heights usually being in the range of 54 to 60 inches; some affected persons are over 5 feet tall.

Roentgenographic findings (Fig. 13-32) consist of bilateral symmetric irregularity and underdevelopment of epiphyseal ossification centers. Changes in the hips, knees, and ankles are most severe, with milder changes in the upper limbs. Deficiency in the lateral part of the distal tibial epiphysis, demonstrable in children, is expressed in adults as a sloping distal tibial articular surface.[172] The patella may be bipartite. The proximal row of carpal bones is often short. Vertebral involvement is, at the most, mild.

Classically, multiple epiphyseal dysplasia displays autosomal dominant inheritance, but autosomal recessive inheritance of a clinically indistinguishable disorder has been observed in rare families.[132]

Pseudoachondroplastic dysplasias

Originally delineated by Maroteaux and Lamy[202] under the designation of pseudoachondroplastic spondyloepiphyseal dysplasia, this disorder is relatively frequent. Growth retardation is seldom recognized until the second year of life or later, at which time the body proportions resemble those of achondroplasia.[78]

The head and face are normal, however, and the fingers, although short, do not show the trident configuration typical of achondroplasia.

Roentgenographically, gross irregularities, with fragmentation of the epiphyses and hypertrophic mushroomlike metaphyses, are seen in the limbs. Prepubertally the lumbar vertebrae show, in lateral projection, a distinctive anterior tongue, resulting from delayed development of the anular cartilage (ring epiphyses).

Considerable heterogeneity exists in this category.[101] Clearly there are separable autosomal dominant and autosomal recessive types, and there appear to be two, or possibly more, distinct forms of each, making at least four types in all. This differentiation of four types of pseudoachondroplastic dysplasia is based on a study of 32 cases distributed in twelve families.

Type I is illustrated by the kindred described in Fig. 13-33. The radiographic changes are the mildest in this type. Inheritance is autosomal dominant. No chemical or cytologic abnormality has been found.

Type II, illustrated by the family presented in Fig. 13-34, is autosomal recessive. Brothers and sisters with normal parents have been affected, and in one family the parents were first cousins.

Type III, illustrated by the family presented in Fig. 13-35, is an autosomal dominant disorder. In cultured fibroblasts striking cytoplasmic metachromasia was demonstrated by Danes[55] and low levels of β-galactosidase by O'Brien.[228] This is the classic type, being present, it seems, in the patients on whom Maroteaux and Lamy[202] based their description. Also, this is probably the type in which Maynard and associates,[211] among others, have found, by electron microscopy, unusual inclusion material of the rough-surfaced endoplasmic reticulum.

Type IV (Fig. 13-36) is distinguished by its autosomal recessive inheritance and the marked severity of radiographic changes.

Spondyloepiphyseal dysplasia tarda

This condition went by a number of designations, including Morquio's disease,[124] before being correctly identified by Maroteaux and colleagues in 1957.[205] The shortness, which first becomes evident between the ages of 5 and 10 years, is primarily truncal. Pain in the back and hips and limitation of motion in these joints are frequent by the teen years. Adult height varies from 52 to 62 inches.[270] Disabling ankylosing polyarthrosis occurs by the fourth or fifth decade.

The roentgenographic features (Fig. 13-37) are distinctive,[161] especially those in the spine. Mild to moderate platyspondylisis is generalized, and there is both humping up centrally and posteriorly and eburnation of the end-plates of the vertebral bodies that at first glance suggests calcification of the intervertebral discs. Indeed, a casual similarity to the x-ray appearance of the ochronotic spine is created; in the latter condition, however, calcification occurs within the intervertebral discs. In SED tarda one sees a fish-mouth–shaped area in the anterior parts of the lumbar vertebrae on lateral view, this being the result of lack of the involvement seen centrally and posteriorly. The epiphyses in the bones of the limbs are dysplastic, especially those in proximal parts of the limbs, and the pelvis is small with deep acetabula. Precocious arthritis develops in the hips as well as in the spine.

Several large kindreds have been reported as showing the classic pattern of

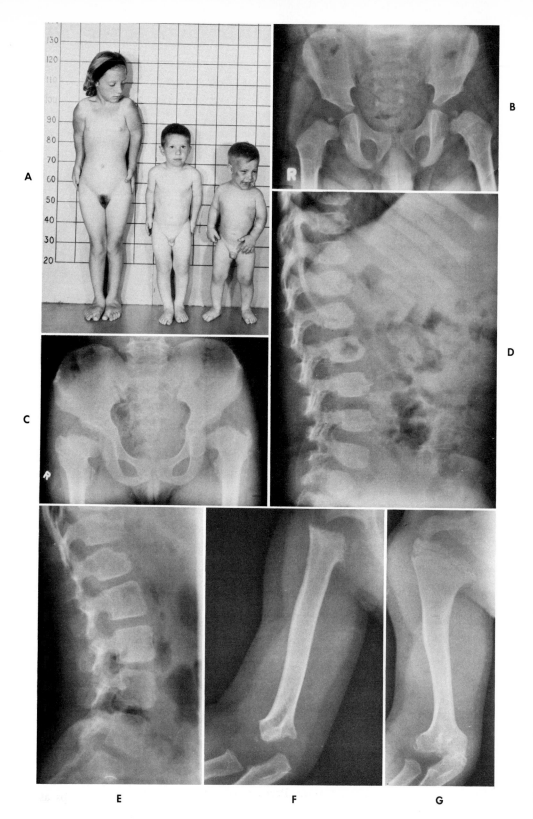

Fig. 13-34. For legend see opposite page.

X-linked recessive inheritance. The kindred reported by Jacobsen[124] was restudied by Bannerman,[15a] who could exclude close linkage with the Xg blood group locus.

The designation spondyloepiphyseal dysplasia tarda is customarily used for the X-linked recessive disorder with distinctive roentgenographic changes in the spine as just described. However, autosomal dominant forms[215] and autosomal recessive forms[208] of late spondyloepiphyseal dysplasia are well documented. They have roentgenographic changes in the spine distinct from those in the X-linked form but show, in addition to platyspondyly, the same tendency to precocious degenerative joint disease, especially in the hips.

Acrodysplasia: trichorhinophalangeal syndrome

Giedion[89] delineated this syndrome, which has abnormality of the hair (which is sparse and slow-growing on the head and entire body, with early balding and sparse lateral eyebrows), of the nose (which is pear-shaped, with a long philtrum) and of the fingers (which are crooked and show cone-shaped epiphyses). Giedion's patient had two supernumerary incisors. Giedion could

Text continued on p. 807.

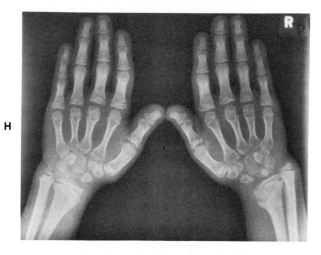

Fig. 13-34. Pseudoachondroplastic dysplasia, type II. These 3 sibs (B. H., 1249858; T. H., 1249863; M. H., 1249862) were 11, 3½, and 2 years of age, respectively, at the time these pictures were taken, **A.** They were considered normal at birth. Abnormally short arms were noted in the oldest child at 4 years, at which time x-ray studies were made and the parents were told that she had achondroplasia. All 3 children showed limitation of extension of the elbows and loose-jointed hands. **B** and **C,** Pelvis of M. H., 2 years old, and B. H., 11 years old. The femoral capital epiphyses are small at 2 years, and the femoral heads are flat and irregular in the 11-year-old. **D** and **E,** Lumbar vertebrae of M. H. at 2 years and of B. H. at 11 years. In the younger child, mild anterior tonguing is present. Irregularity and tonguing in the upper lumbar area are demonstrated in the 11-year-old child. **F** and **G,** Humerus of T. H. at 3 years and of M. H. at 11 years of age. The humeral capital epiphysis is poorly formed at 3 years, **F,** and the epiphysis and head are markedly flattened, with shortening of the humerus, at 11 years, **G. H,** The hand of B. H. at 11 years shows flattening of the epiphyses and small, irregular carpal bones. The terminal phalanges, especially in the thumbs, are stubby.

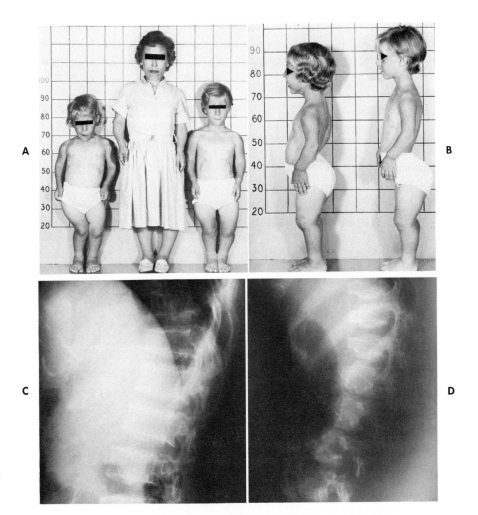

Fig. 13-35. Pseudoachondroplastic dysplasia, type III. **A,** The mother, 35 years old, and both children, 8 and 11 years old, are affected. (The mother's mother, 2 of her sisters, and 2 sons of one of the sisters are also affected. Inheritance is dominant and, although no male-to-male transmission has been observed in this kindred, probably autosomal.) Note the normal size and shape of the head. The skull is radiologically normal. **B,** Both girls show exaggerated lumbar lordosis. **C,** Lumbar spine in the mother, showing some flattening of vertebral bodies with irregularity of the end plates, which is, however, not diagnostic. **D,** Lumbar spine in the 11-year-old daughter, showing an anterior projection of the vertebral bodies, due to abnormally large notches for the annular cartilages, and striking irregularity of the end plates. The lumbar spine, as viewed in frontal projection, does not show caudad narrowing of the interpeduncular distance, as is characteristic of achondroplasia. **E,** Hips and pelvis of the mother. **F,** Drastic changes are shown in the hips and knees of the 11-year-old daughter. **G** to **I,** Hands of mother and older daughter. The mother, **G,** shows short fingers, bowed forearms, and prominence on the radial aspect of the right wrist. X-ray view, **H,** shows this prominence to be produced by displacement of the distal end of the radius past the first row of carpal bones. X-ray view, **I,** of the hand of the older daughter shows evidence of marked disturbance in ossification of the carpal bones as well as the metaphyses and epiphyses of all bones. **J,** Pedigree. The mother is indicated by the arrow. Since continuation of the pedigree she has had an unaffected child by her second husband.

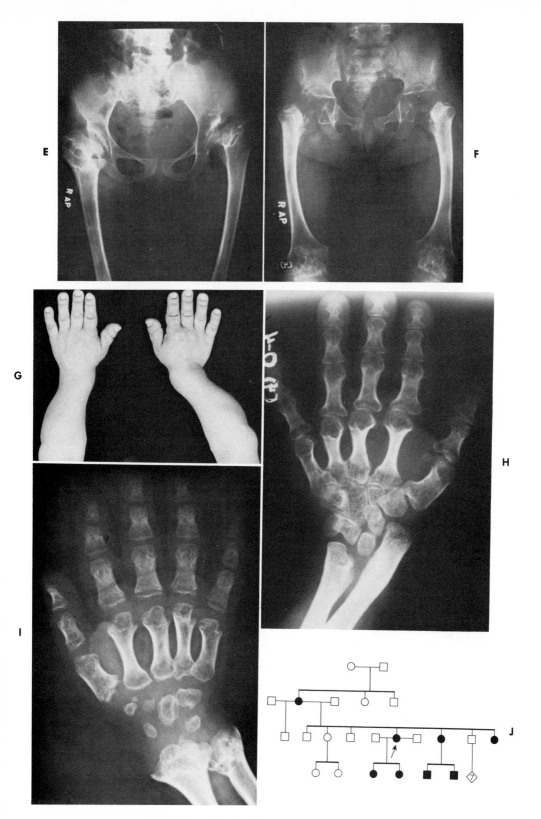

Fig. 13-35, cont'd. For legend see opposite page.

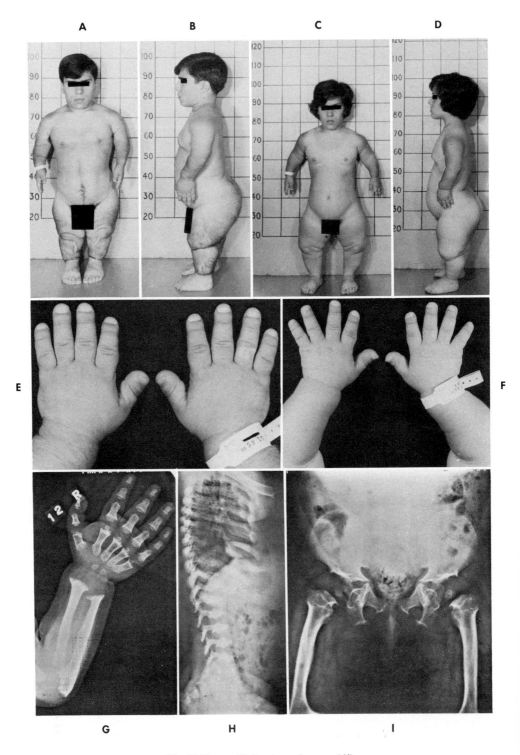

Fig. 13-36, cont'd. For legend see p. 807.

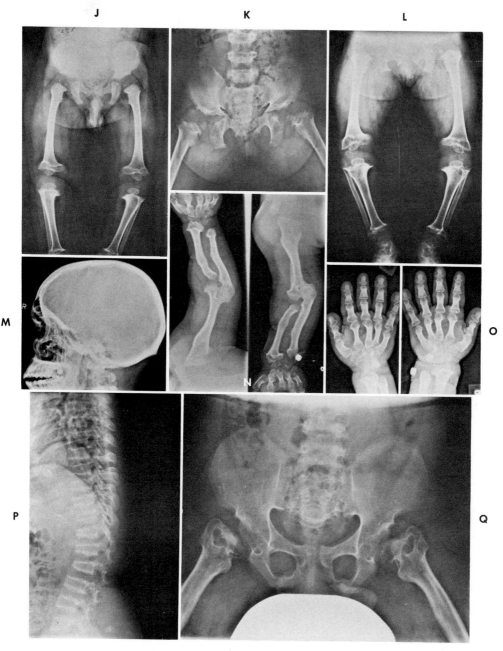

Fig. 13-36, cont'd. For legend see p. 807.

Continued.

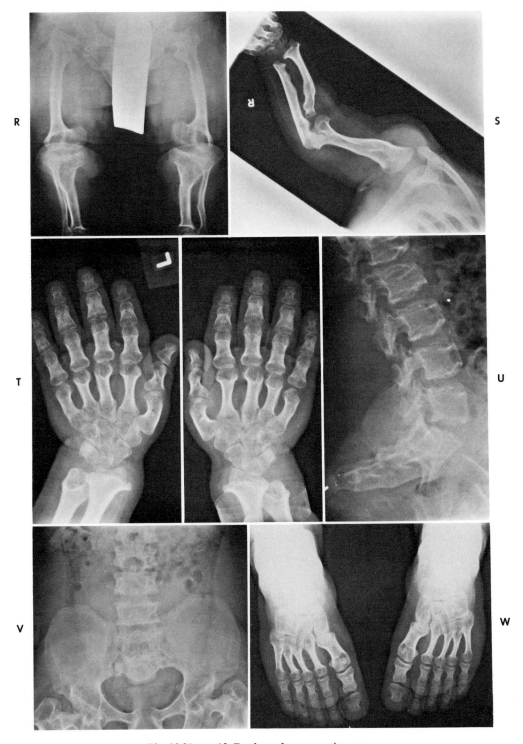

Fig. 13-36, cont'd. For legend see opposite page.

find two previous reports, in each of which 2 sibs were affected, and the parents were consanguineous in one case.

We have observed two affected families. In one, occurrence in grandfather, son, and grandson, with no consanguinity, seems to make autosomal dominant inheritance a certainty (Fig. 13-38). In the other,[120] a brother and sister are affected. The parents are nonconsanguineous and allegedly unaffected, but the father is not available for examination.

Multiple cartilaginous exostoses

Also known as diaphyseal aclasis, this disorder is manifested by cartilaginous excrescences near the ends of the diaphyses of bones of the extremities.[125,138,151,300] (See Fig. 13-40.) The ribs and scapulae may also be affected but the skull is not involved. Deformity of the legs, of the arms (resembling Madelung's deformity), and of the hands (e.g., short metacarpal) is frequent (Fig. 13-41). The patients are usually of reduced stature. Cutaneous osteomata have been described as an associated feature.[65] Sarcomatous transformation is rather frequent.[22,148,219] Inheritance is autosomal dominant. Neurologic complications occur in some from pressure on the spinal cord or peripheral nerves.[167,287] The same disorder has been observed in horses.[217]

Fig. 13-36. Pseudoachondroplastic dysplasia, type IV. S. R. (J.H.H. 1256145) and J. R. (J.H.H. 1256144) were 18 and 16 years old, respectively, at the time of the pictures shown in **A** to **F**. Another sib, unaffected, was 6 years old. There was no other known skeletal dysplasia in the family and no known parental consanguinity, although both parents were of Italian extraction. Unusual short and muscular limbs were noted in the boy at 9 months of age. At 1 year a diagnosis of Morquio syndrome was made on the basis of flattened vertebrae and short limb bones with irregular epiphyses. Bowing of the legs developed when he began to walk. Osteotomies for correction of bowlegs were performed at the age of 10 years in the brother and at 8 years in the sister. In both sibs the joints were hyperextensible and enlarged, especially the wrists.

A and **B**, S. R. at 18 years. **C** and **D**, J. R. at 16 years. **E** and **F**, Hands suggesting trident configuration in S. R. and J. R., respectively.

G to **J**, Early x-ray views of S. R. **G**, Hand at 2½ years. **H**, Spine at 7½ years. **I**, Pelvis at 7½ years. **J**, Pelvis and legs at 2½ years.

K and **L**, X-ray views of J. R. at 5½ years. **K**, Pelvis. **L**, Legs.

M to **R**, X-ray views of S. R. at 18 years. **M**, The skull is normal. **N**, The bones of the upper limbs are short and relatively wide, with considerable metaphyseal flaring. The humeral heads are flat, wide and deformed. **O**, The bones of the hands are all short and rather broad, whereas the carpal bones, although irregular, are disproportionately large. The ulnae are disproportionately short. **P**, All vertebral bodies are flattened, and those of the lower thoracic and upper lumbar segments are mildly wedge-shaped. **Q**, The femoral heads and necks and the acetabula are hypoplastic. **R**, The tibiae are shortened out of proportion to the femora, and the fibulae are too long for the tibiae. The metaphyses are severely flared at the knees.

S to **W**, X-ray views of J. R. at 16 years. **S** and **T**, The upper limbs are almost identical to those of S. R. **U**, Platyspondyly is less severe than in S. R., but the end plates are more irregular. Lumbosacral lordosis is severe, forming almost a right angle. **V**, Coxa vara is marked, with short thin femoral necks and hypoplastic femoral heads that project inferiorly from the necks like bird beaks. **W**, In the feet all the metatarsals and phalanges are short. The tarsal bones are relatively large and are more nearly normally formed than are the carpals.

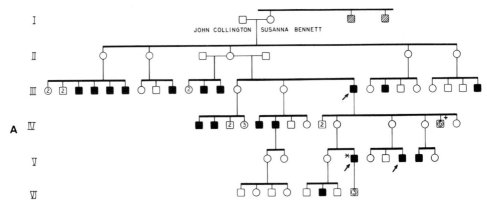

A

QUESTIONABLY AFFECTED
PICTURED BY JACOBSEN
+ DIED IN INFANCY OF CHOLERA INFANTUM
✳ RESTUDIED BY LANGER

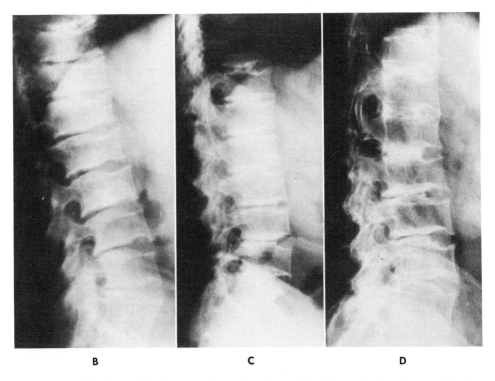

B   C   D

Fig. 13-37. X-linked spondyloepiphyseal dysplasia tarda. **A,** Partially updated pedigree of family reported by Jacobsen.[124] (See Bannerman[15a] for further pedigree data.) Radiographic findings shown in **B** to **E. B** to **D,** Graded changes in the lumbar spine. Heaping up of the posterior portion of the superior vertebral plate is pathognomonic, **B.** Progressive changes are shown in **C** and **D.** At first glance the late changes resemble those of alkaptonuria (cf. Fig. 9-4), where the intervertebral discs are calcified. However the changes are caused by severe eburnation of the humps on the superior and inferior vertebral end plates. **E,** Late degenerative "arthritis" of the hips. Note the deep acetabula. (Courtesy Dr. Leonard O. Langer, Jr., Minneapolis.)

Enchondromatosis

Known previously as dyschondroplasia and eponymically as Ollier's disease, enchondromatosis[44,242,262] is characterized by abnormal growth of unossified cartilage in the diaphyses of long bones. Involvement is usually asymmetric. The cartilaginous tumors cause expansion of the shaft of the involved bones and may impede longitudinal growth. In cases of severe involvement, all fingers may, for example, be remarkably enlarged (see illustrations in reference 44). No genetic basis for this disorder has been established. Specifically, no familial cases or chromosomal abnormality has been noted. The condition is mentioned here mainly because of the confusion—more of terms than of diagnosis—that has often existed with multiple exostoses.

Maffucci's syndrome[9,41] is enchondromatosis with hemangiomata. Brain tumor and malignant tumors of other organs occur rather frequently with this disorder, which, like Ollier's disease, has no known genetic basis. Maffucci's syndrome has been confused[19] with the *Klippel-Trénaunay-Weber syndrome,*[188] in which hemangioma is associated with asymmetric overgrowth of bones and related soft tissues. It is probably of the same nature as the *Sturge-Weber syndrome,* in which trigeminal hemangioma is associated with cerebral atrophy and calcification. Indeed, we and others have observed patients with both the Sturge-Weber syndrome and the Klippel-Trenaunay-Weber syndrome. Again, no genetic basis has been found.

Osteopetrosis

Osteopetrosis (likewise called marble bones, osteosclerosis fragilis generalisata, and Albers-Schönberg's* disease) occurs in at least two forms[1,3,140,180,339]: (1) an

---

*Albers-Schönberg[1] was one man; this is not a syndrome named for two persons, like the Ehlers-Danlos syndrome or the Grönblad-Stranberg syndrome. Care should be taken not to confuse osteopetrosis with osteopoikilosis, which was also first described in a definitive manner by Albers-Schönberg; some writers have evidenced this confusion.

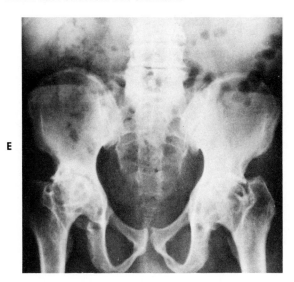

E

Fig. 13-37, cont'd. For legend see opposite page.

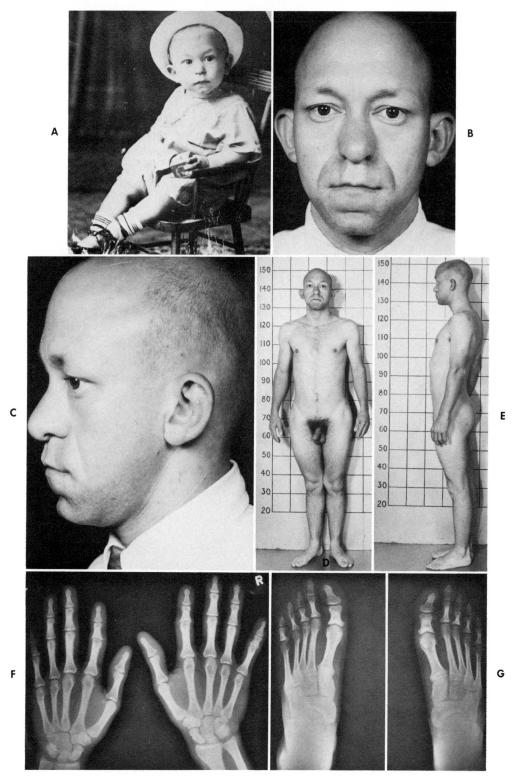

Fig. 13-38. For legend see opposite page.

autosomal recessive form,[186,314] which is also called the malignant form because of early death, and (2) a relatively benign, autosomal dominant form.[86,111,197] In addition, osteosclerosis, often incorrectly termed osteopetrosis, is a feature of several entities, including pyknodysostosis, van Buchem's disease (called endosteohyperostosis in the Paris Nomenclature), and others.[69,95,169,174,213,284]

The main clinical features of the autosomal dominant form of osteopetrosis are fractures and osteomyelitis, especially of the mandible. The bones show dra-

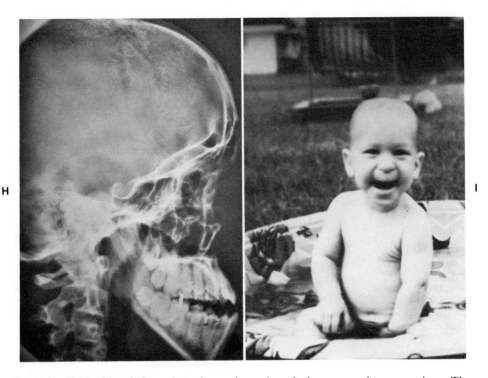

H   **I**

Fig. 13-38. Trichorhinophalangeal syndrome in males of three successive generations. The earliest affected person in this kindred was a man whose photographs as a small child, **A,** show sparse hair and the typical configuration of the nose with malar hypoplasia. He was 58½ inches tall and died at 43 years of age of a cerebrovascular accident. His wife has a form of dwarfism of uncertain type. Their only son, A. P. (J.H.H. 1256144), was always short of stature, with sparse hair. At 15 years of age, pattern balding began. **B** and **C,** Facial appearance of A. P. at the age of 19 years. The balding, malar hypoplasia, bulbous nose, and fleshy ears are noteworthy. He looks much older than his stated age. **D** and **E,** Except for short stature, the patient's habitus is not strikingly abnormal. However, the upper segment/lower segment ratio was 31:28, and the great toes are disproportionately short. **F** to **H,** X-ray findings in A. P. The hands, **F,** show shortening of the middle phalanges of the second and fifth fingers with irregularity of the proximal ends consistent with previous cone-shaped epiphyses. The feet, **G,** show short first toes and a short proximal phalanx of each third toe. The base of the proximal phalanx of each first toe is coned. The skull, **H,** shows hypoplasia of the mid-face.

A. P. married a woman with cartilage-hair hypoplasia and had a son who from birth has had sparse hair and the same nasal configuration as his father (see **I**). X-ray films made at birth and at 22 months of age showed delayed osseous development and small size, but no cone epiphyses had yet developed. (CHH, a recessive disorder, in the mother, is thought to be irrelevant to the condition occurring in the child.)

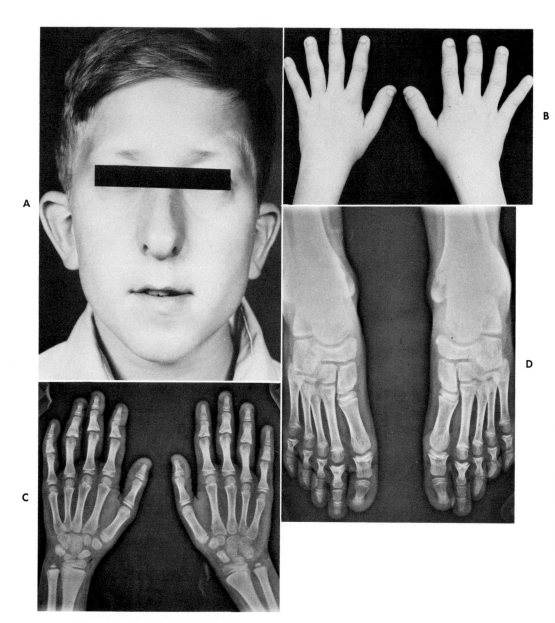

Fig. 13-39. Thichorhinophalangeal syndrome in a 14-year-old boy (K. R., 1348707). **A,** The face shows very sparse lateral eyebrows and characteristic nasal configuration. **B** and **C,** Photograph and x-ray view of hands. Cone-shaped epiphyses and crooked fingers are demonstrated. **D,** X-ray view of feet showing cone-shaped epiphyses.

matic changes radiologically and pathologically. The vertebral bodies have a characteristic "sandwich" appearance because of excessive sclerosis in upper and lower portions, with intervening less dense area. All bones, most often the short and round bones of the extremities, may have a "bone-within-bone" appearance. The bones are described by some as so hard as to turn the edge of a steel chisel, and by others are claimed to be more like chalk. Usually they are excessively brittle and susceptible to spontaneous fracture. The original patient of Albers-

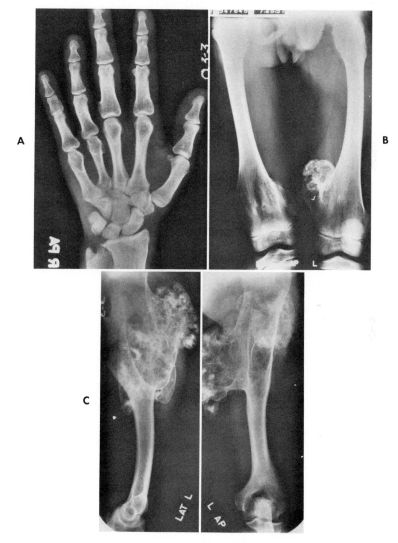

Fig. 13-40. Multiple cartilaginous exostoses. **A,** Small exostoses in 16-year-old girl whose father also has multiple exostoses. The shortening of the fourth metacarpal was probably caused by an exostosis, but the short middle phalanx of the little finger is an incidental abnormality. **B,** Exostoses of the femur in a 10-year-old boy. That on the right has been partially removed. **C,** Two views of enormous exostoses of left humerus in 40-year-old man.

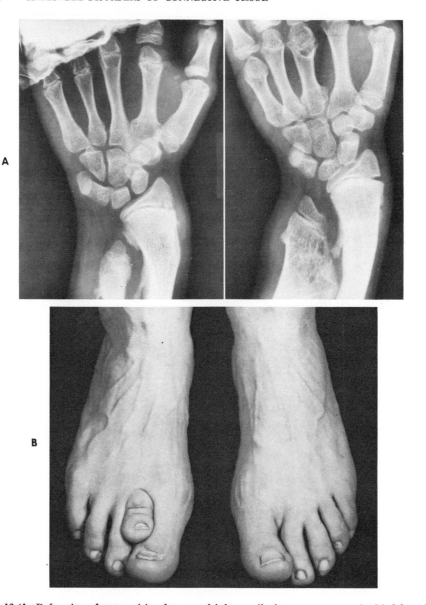

Fig. 13-41. Deformity of extremities from multiple cartilaginous exostoses. **A,** Madelung-like deformity of forearm. **B** and **C,** Short second metatarsal on right. **D,** Short fourth metatarsal.

Schönberg[1] was 26 years old and is said to have been living ten years later for re-examination by Reiche. Alexander's patient[3] was 43 years old. The patient illustrated in Fig. 13-42 died at the age of 45 years of a cause indirectly related to his skeletal disease.

The recessive, or malignant, form appears very early in life, like osteogenesis imperfecta may be detected *in utero*, involves the entire skeleton, and may result in such encroachment on the hematopoietic space of the bone marrow that pancytopenia is a leading clinical feature.[39,45,144,147,168,238,240,314] A disorder like that

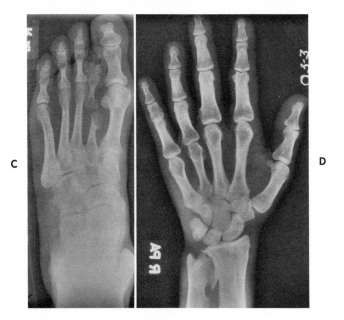

Fig. 13-41, cont'd. For legend see opposite page.

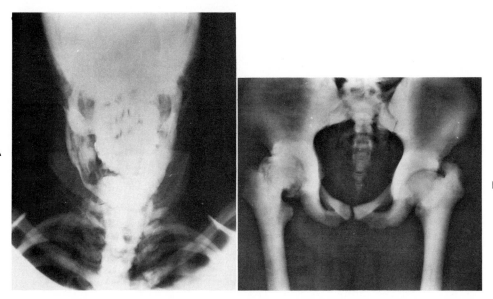

Fig. 13-42. Osteopetrosis, "benign" autosomal dominant type. In 1922 the late Dr. Ralph K. Ghormley[86] described "a case of congenital osteosclerosis" in a boy then 9 years old. The father and uncle were similarly affected. The uncle, who subsequently died in his seventies, had much trouble with osteomyelitis of the jaw. The father had a traumatic fracture. The proband sustained fractures whenever he engaged in rough sports. At 32 years of age he began to have trouble with osteomyelitis of the jaw and progressive stiffening of the hips. Despite his physical handicaps he became an international authority in the field of dielectrics. At the age of 45 years he developed symptoms of a temporal lobe abscess and died two days later. The abscess was presumably metastatic from the mandibular infection. **A,** Note the marked sclerotic change in all bones and the surgical defect in the mandible. **B,** Secondary osteoarthrosis of the hips is also demonstrated.

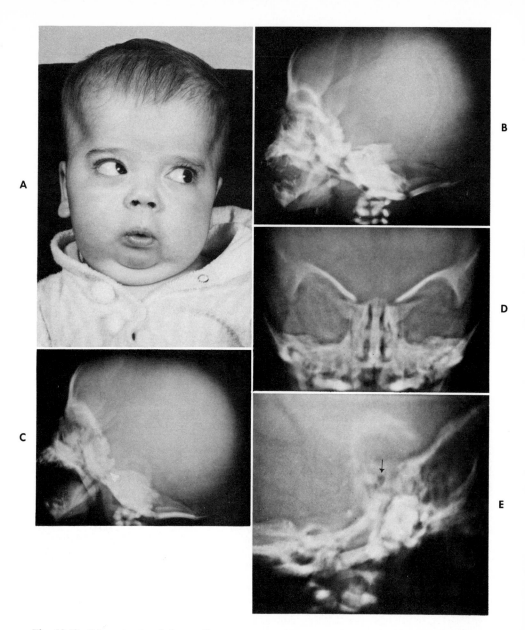

Fig. 13-43. Osteopetrosis of the malignant type. **A,** Appearance at 9 months of age, showing frontal bosselation. **B,** Skull in lateral view at 12 days of age. The sutures are abnormally wide, and the density of all bones is increased, most particularly in the face, orbital roofs, base of the skull, and cervical vertebrae. **C** and **D,** Skull at 5 weeks, showing the same changes in amplified form. The orbits are "harlequin-shaped," as in hypophosphatasia.[33] **E,** Special view, at 5 weeks, showing diminution in the caliber of the optic foramen by about 50% The infant subsequently was blind. **F** and **G,** Views of the trunk, taken at 4 months of age, showing greatly increased bone density. The oval radiodensities indicated by the arrows are sternal ossification centers. In the lateral view, **G,** the vertebral bodies show prominent anterior vascular notches. **H,** The hand and forearm at about 10 months of age show classic changes of osteopetrosis, including the "bone within bone" appearance in metacarpals and phalanges. **I,** At 10 months of age, the femur, like the distal radius and ulna, **H,** shows alternating zones of increased and decreased density. (From Avery, M. E., Dorst, J. P., and Walker, D. G.: Osteopetrosis. In Bergsma, D., editor: Clinical delineation of birth defects. IV. Skeletal dysplasias, New York, 1969, National Foundation–March of Dimes.)

in man has been observed in the rabbit,[235] in the mouse,[327] and in domestic fowl.[156] (See Fig. 13-43.)

The possible role of excessive thyrocalcitonin production in the pathogenesis of osteopetrosis has been investigated.[199] The evidence in man is inconclusive.

The following is an illustrative case of the malignant form of osteopetrosis*:

Case 1. K. A. (J.H.H. 12082333) was born in 1956 of parents of Swedish extraction but no known consanguinity. Persons of both sides of the child's family showed tooth decay in perhaps an unusual degree. At 6 days of age he was noted to be "a bit twitchy" and did not breast-nurse well. At the age of 11 days he was found to have a serum calcium of 7.8 and phosphorus of 7.4 mg./100 ml. The hematocrit was 50%. Skull x-ray studies showed changes that were interpreted as compatible with physiologic sclerosis, although in fact they were a bit too severe.

At about 5 weeks of age, he was noted to have a full fontanelle. Ventricular tap showed an elevated pressure. The hematocrit was now 26%, with 10% reticulocytes.

Over the subsequent months signs of optic atrophy developed, as well as splenomegaly. At 3 months of age the bone was noted to be abnormally soft on marrow aspiration, and on review of the roentgenograms, a diagnosis of osteopetrosis was made.

Prednisone was administered empirically for several months during the first year of life.

Surgical thyroidectomy was performed at the age of 8 months. Parathyroid glands were found and left in place. Histologically the thyroid gland showed no excess of perifollicular cells and thyrocalcitonin assays were interpreted as normal.

Growth and psychomotor development were retarded, but the head remained at about the 75th percentile in size. At the age of 2 years, height and weight were at about the fourth percentile, and the patient showed frontal bosselation (Fig. 13-43).

The x-ray findings are presented in Fig. 13-43.

At the age of 5 years the child is remarkably well. Treatment with prednisone seems, in retrospect, to have "tided him over" the difficult period in the first year of life, when he showed signs of hydrocephalus and marrow restriction. Møe[214a] concluded that adrenocorticosteroid is useful in management of this disorder. Furthermore, despite the absence of histologic or assay

---

*Reported by Avery and Dorst.[13a]

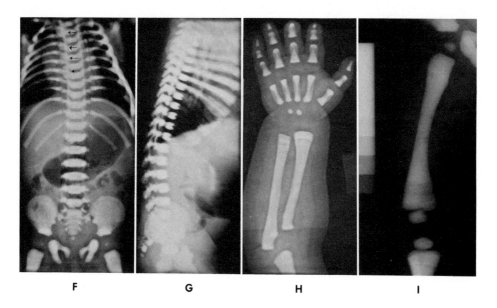

F   G   H   I

Fig. 13-43, cont'd. For legend see opposite page.

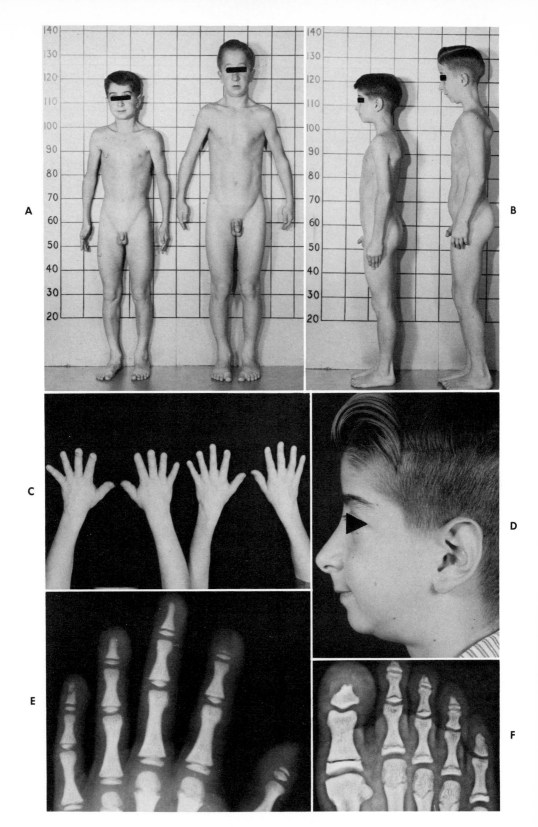

Fig. 13-44. For legend see opposite page.

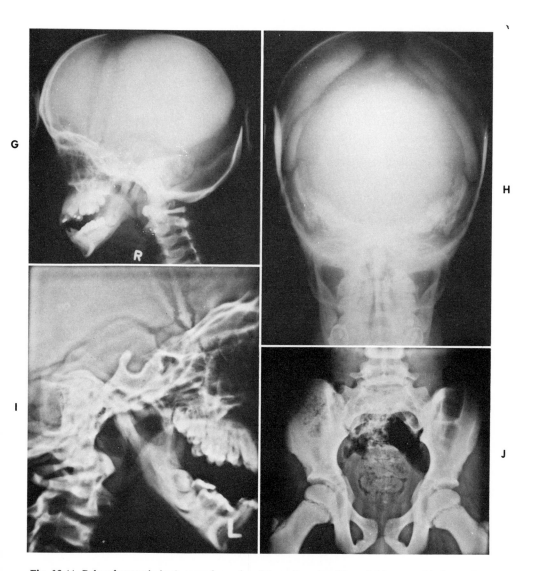

Fig. 13-44. Pyknodysostosis in 2 second cousins. These 2 males, 13 and 16 years old, have short stature, generalized osteosclerosis with bone fragility, multiple Wormian bones, delayed closure of the sutures and fontanelles of the skull, and hypoplasia of the terminal phalanges and of the distal ends of the clavicles. The mandible has no angle, and several teeth are missing or malpositioned. Neither set of parents is known to be consanguineous.

A and B, Cousins at the ages of 12 and 16 years. The short stature is evident. C, the terminal phalanges and fingernails are foreshortened, and several of the nails are spooned. Receding chin and lack of mandibular angle are demonstrated in the younger cousin. E and F, X-ray views of the fingers and toes show osteosclerosis and hypoplasia of the terminal phalanges, with fragmentation in the fifth finger. G to I, The skull of the younger cousin at the age of 13 years shows wide sutures that contain a few Wormian bones. The mandibular angle is nearly 180 degrees. The bones rival in density the teeth (exclusive of the fillings). The teeth, poorly detailed because of the sclerosis of the jawbones, are irregularly positioned. J, X-ray view of pelvis at the age of 13 years in the younger cousin, showing osteosclerosis and mild protrusion of the acetabulum.

evidence of increased thyrocalcitonin production, thyroidectomy seems to have been beneficial. Serum calcium and phosphorus levels are normal, and the patient shows no anemia and
no immature red cells. His only medication is replacement thyroid hormone.

Pyknodysostosis

In pyknodysostosis,*[190,204,275] as in cleidocranial dysplasia, both the cranium
and other parts of the skeleton are involved. Also as in cleidocranial dysplasia

---

*This term was spelled with a "c" in the original publication by Maroteaux and Lamy.[289] A
"k" (pyknodysostosis) is used interchangeably in the literature. I suppose that in the English
language, American writers would be expected to write "pyknodysostosis" and British writers
"pycnodysostosis" if they maintain conformity with the practice in regard to "leukocyte" and
"leucocyte."

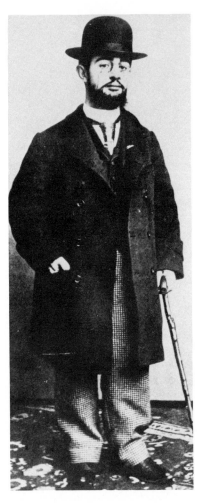

Fig. 13-45. Toulouse-Lautrec (1864-1901) was previously thought to have had osteogenesis imperfecta (p. 438). On review of the evidence in the light of the delineation of the "new"
skeletal dysplasia, pyknodysostosis, Maroteaux and Lamy[203] concluded that this was the condition
from which he suffered. Parental consanguinity, fragility of bones leading to fractures with
minor trauma, a receding chin, and possible open fontanelles, which prompted the artist to wear
a hat most of the time, are features pointed out as suggesting pyknodysostosis.

(with which pyknodysostosis was often confused in the past), multiple Wormian bones and delayed closure of the cranial sutures, particularly the lambdoid and sagittal sutures, are features. The ramus of the mandible is short and the angle lost, so that this bone is essentially straight and the jaw receding. All bones show increased density. As in osteopetrosis, the bones are more fragile than normal and fractures are frequent. Acro-osteolysis (actually, hypoplasia) of the terminal phalanges is a characteristic feature that is manifested clinically by short ends of the fingers. Inheritance is autosomal recessive. In addition to a mistaken diagnosis of cleidocranial dysplasia and of osteopetrosis,[274,313] one case was described as a *forme fruste* of gargoylism.[286] (See Fig. 13-44 for illustrative cases.)

As stated in Chapter 8, Henri de Toulouse-Lautrec may have suffered from pyknodysostosis (Fig. 13-45).

There are several entities that simulate pyknodysostosis. The case shown in Fig. 13-46, for example, shows changes in the bones which are rather different from those shown in Fig. 13-44, and although the view is inadequate, the ramus of the mandible seems well formed. The disorder in this patient may have been the Cheney syndrome.[42,66] This disorder, like pyknodysostosis, shows acro-osteolysis, multiple Wormian bones, and delayed closure of cranial sutures. Hypoplasia of the mandibular ramus is, at the most, mild. Generalized osteoporosis, with basilar impression and collapse of vertebral bodies in adulthood, is an important feature. Autosomal dominant inheritance distinguishes it from pyknodysostosis.

Young and co-workers[337] described 2 patients with a new syndrome tentatively termed mandibuloacral dysplasia and characterized by mandibular hypoplasia, acro-osteolysis, stiff joints, and atrophy of the skin. It is assumed to be a Mendelian disorder, but its mode of inheritance is unknown.

Diaphyseal dysplasia (Camurati-Engelmann syndrome)

This disorder is characterized by expansion and sclerosis of the diaphyses of the long bones, which lack the normal modeling, and by muscular hypoplasia leading to generalized weakness.[90] Pains in the legs are a conspicuous symptom. Involvement of the cranium occurs only to a minor degree, which is evident radiologically as a rule. Onset is often before the age of 10 years and always before 30 years of age. Nothing is known of the defect in bone and muscle, and even the histopathology is not fully described. This disorder is inherited as an autosomal dominant. Remarkable benefit from the administration of corticosteroids has been observed.[6] (See Fig. 13-47.)

Metaphyseal dysplasia (Pyle's disease)

Despite bizarre roentgenographic changes, this disorder has few clinical findings other than genu valgum. The craniofacial bones are at the most only mildly affected, thus distinguishing Pyle's disease from the craniometaphyseal dysplasias. (The designation Pyle's disease has been misused to refer to a variety of conditions. Spranger[293] reviewed the skull x-ray film of Pyle's original case and failed to find the changes characteristic of craniometaphyseal dysplasias.) The femora show an Erlenmeyer-flask deformity. The humerus is abnormally broad and "undermodeled" in its proximal two thirds, as are the ulna and radius in their distal two thirds. The metacarpals are broad in their distal portions, as are the phalanges in their proximal portions. The metaphyseal flaring is usually

Text continued on p. 826.

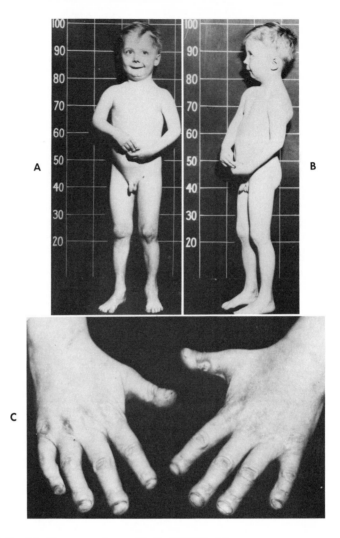

Fig. 13-46. Possible Cheney syndrome. M. F. (A19633). His appearance was unusual, particularly because of prominent forehead, receding chin, short stature, narrow shoulders, stubby clubbed-appearing terminal phalanges, and mottled rough skin over the chest and back down to the rib margin and over the legs and hands. X-ray films showed open cranial sutures with Wormian bones, increased bone density with longitudinal cortical streaks in the bones of the extremities, and areas of radiolucency in the proximal ends of the humeri, as well as some other bones. The outer end of the left clavicle and the distal phalanges of the fingers and toes showed fragmentation with some calcification in the soft tissues. **A** and **B,** General appearance, 4¾ years of age. **C,** Hands. The terminal phalanges are clubbed and stubby, with a short, spoonlike fingernail. **D** and **E,** There is a generalized osteoporosis, and the distal phalanges of all digits show fragmentation of the bone and soft tissue calcification. **F** and **G,** The skull shows widely open sutures and mosaics of multiple Wormian bones. **H,** The bones of the arms show variable density, generally decreased with dense longitudinal cortical streaks and osteolytic lesions, e.g., at the proximal metaphyses of the humeri. The patient died at home at the age of 8 years, of an infection, possibly influenza. He had hemiparalysis terminally, and the mother thinks he may have had meningitis. If this disorder is the Cheney syndrome (which has dominant inheritance), it may be relevant that the parents were not consanguineous; the case is probably a new mutant. (From McKusick, V. A., and colleagues: J. Chronic Dis. **17:**1077, 1964.)

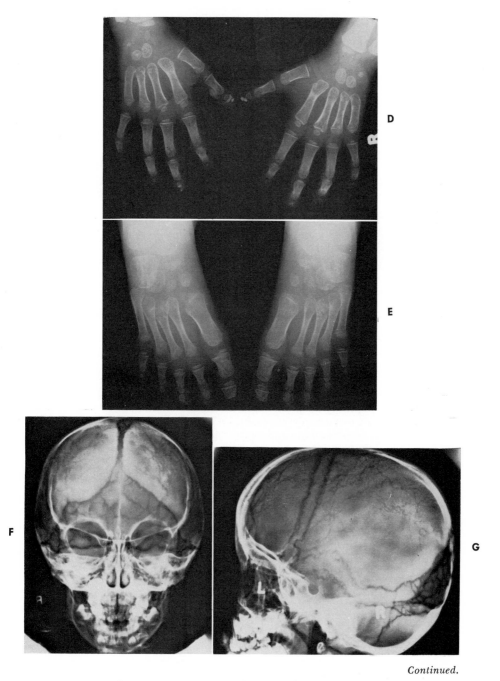

D

E

F

G

Continued.

Fig. 13-46, cont'd. For legend see opposite page.

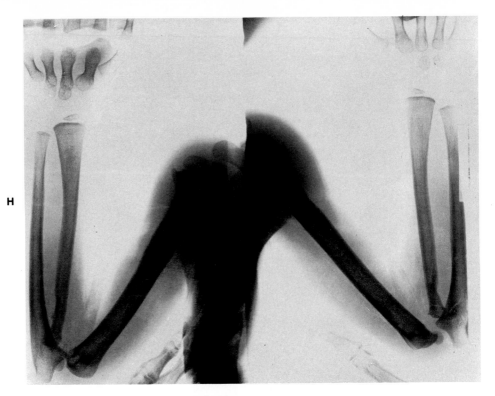

H

Fig. 13-46, cont'd. For legend see p. 822.

Fig. 13-47. Engelmann's disease (diaphyseal dysplasia). R. L. P. (877902) was considered normal at birth. During the first six months he had much feeding difficulty. Thickened formula and feeding in the upright position were necessary in order to prevent regurgitation. Although developmental landmarks were considered normal, he did not walk until 18 to 24 months of age. He never walked normally, tending to have an unsteady, waddling gait. He never ran and could not climb stairs without pulling himself up by his hands. He always fatigued easily, and from as early as he could communicate he complained of aching pains in the calves, thighs, and forearms. A diagnosis of Duchenne's muscular dystrophy was made at the age of 4 years. At the age of 8 years 8 months, gastrocnemius muscle biopsy showed diffuse muscle fiber atrophy with perivascular and focal endomysial collections of round cells. Skeletal x-ray studies established the diagnosis of Englemann's disease. Family history revealed no consanguinity or similar disorder.

A and **B,** The physical findings at the age of 12 years. Pathetic debility, generalized reduction in muscle mass, semiflexed position of the knees and hips, and lack of the normal tapering in the lower femora are evident. **C** to **E,** Skull x-ray views showing thickening and sclerosis of the chondrocranium, mandible, and orbits. **F** and **G,** X-ray views of upper limbs show swelling of the diaphyses of the long bones. The cortices are irregularly thickened and sclerotic. **H,** Modeling of the bones of the hands is less disturbed. Considerable sclerosis and cortical thickening is evident, however. The ribs, clavicles, vertebrae, and pelvis showed relatively little change. **I** and **J,** The lower limbs, like the upper limbs, show irregular internal and external cortical thickening, leading to irregular diaphyseal swelling. All these x-ray studies were made at the age of 12 years.

Follow-up (1972). In February, 1971 (16 years of age), the patient was almost constantly in pain, and the anterior thighs were painful to pressure. He could walk only one block at the most and required much aspirin for comfort. A course of prednisone was begun, giving 60 mg./day at first and tapering to 15 mg. on alternating days. Benefit was dramatic. He could walk up to two miles a day and no longer required analgesics. Side effects consisted of only mild Cushingoid facies.

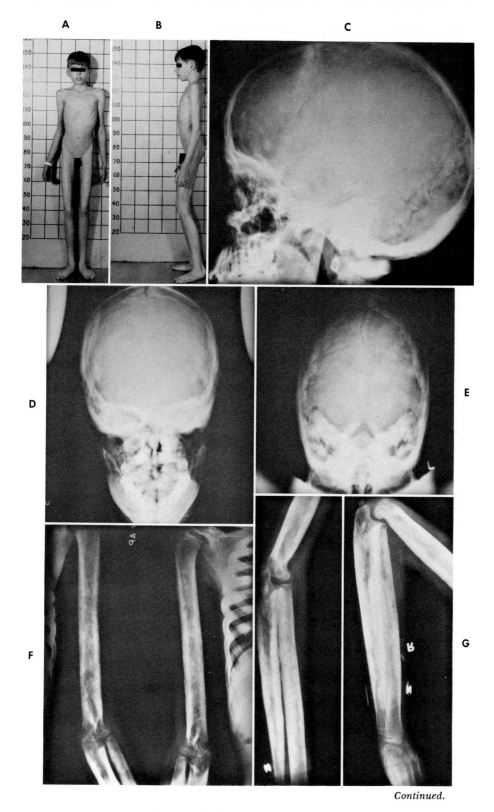

Continued.

Fig. 13-47. For legend see opposite page.

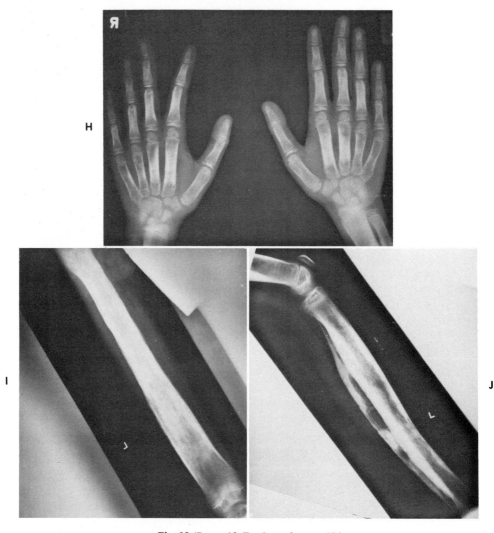

Fig. 13-47, cont'd. For legend see p. 824.

more abrupt and more marked in Pyle's disease than in the craniometaphyseal dysplasias.

Bakwin and Krida[15] restudied Pyle's original patient and on finding similar changes in the patient's sister, coined the term familial metaphyseal dysplasia. Others have also reported affected sibs, as well as parental consanguinity.[56a]

Craniometaphyseal dysplasias

Both autosomal dominant and autosomal recessive forms of the craniometaphyseal dysplasias[95] have been identified. In general the autosomal recessive form is more severe. Both are characterized by hyperostosis of the cranial and facial bones, with compression of cranial nerves at the foramina, and by changes in the metaphyses of the long bones.

In Fig. 13-48 is an illustration of the changes in a family with the dominant form of the disease. (Although this disorder was reported as an instance of Pyle's disease,[255] the designation is appropriately reserved for metaphyseal dysplasia with little or no craniofacial involvement and with autosomal recessive inheritance. Others[297] have reported, as Pyle's disease, cases that are better considered to be autosomal dominant craniometaphyseal dysplasia.) The diaphyseal flaring is less abrupt than in Pyle's disease, producing a clublike rather than an Erlenmeyer-flask deformity.

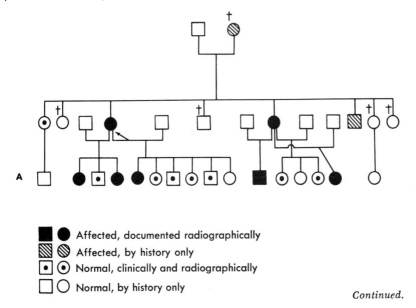

■ ● Affected, documented radiographically
▨ ◍ Affected, by history only
⊡ ⊙ Normal, clinically and radiographically
□ ○ Normal, by history only

Continued.

Fig. 13-48. Autosomal dominant craniometaphyseal dysplasia. The kindred diagrammed in the pedigree, **A,** contains 7 documented and 2 probable cases.

The proband (arrow) had left facial weakness from the age of 5 years. Progressive hearing loss was first noted at 9 years. Examination at 44 years, **B,** showed a broad nasal bridge with an elevated wing of bone extending to the zygoma bilaterally; left peripheral facial palsy; diminished hearing bilaterally; and weakness and hypoesthesia of the left side of the body. As demonstrated by x-ray examination, **C,** the calvaria was found to be markedly thickened, especially in the occipital area. The frontal and maxillary sinuses were opacified and the mastoid air cells were poorly aerated. Narrowing of the foramen magnum and internal auditory canals was thought to account for the left-side neurologic deficit and deafness, respectively. The long bones, especially the femora, **D,** were club-shaped as a result of metaphyseal flaring.

G. D., 12 years old, **E,** and one of the affected daughters of the proband, had noticeable decreased hearing and tinnitus in the right ear for one year, and several episodes of vertigo on awakening. The nasal bridge has an appearance very similar to that of her mother. In addition to x-ray changes like those seen in her mother, the bones of the hands showed defective modeling, **F.**

A sister of the proband (L. J.), 42 years old, had onset of progressive visual impairment at the age of 2 years. The findings of examination included, in addition to obvious craniofacial deformity, **G** and **H,** left total facial palsy, blindness, and deafness. X-ray changes in the skull were marked, **I.**

P. J., an 8-month-old daughter of L. J., **J,** already had typical facial features and typical x-ray findings of craniometaphyseal dysplasia in the skull, **K,** and long bones, **L.**

(From Rimoin, D. L., Woodruff, S. L., and Holman, B. L.: Craniometaphyseal dysplasia; autosomal dominant inheritance in a large kindred. In Bergsma, D., editor: Clinical delineation of birth defects. IV. Skeletal dysplasias, New York, 1969, National Foundation–March of Dimes.)

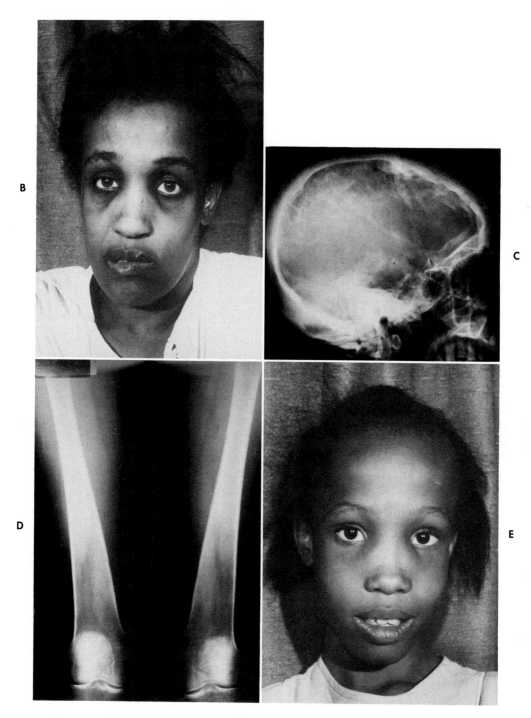

Fig. 13-48, cont'd. For legend see p. 827.

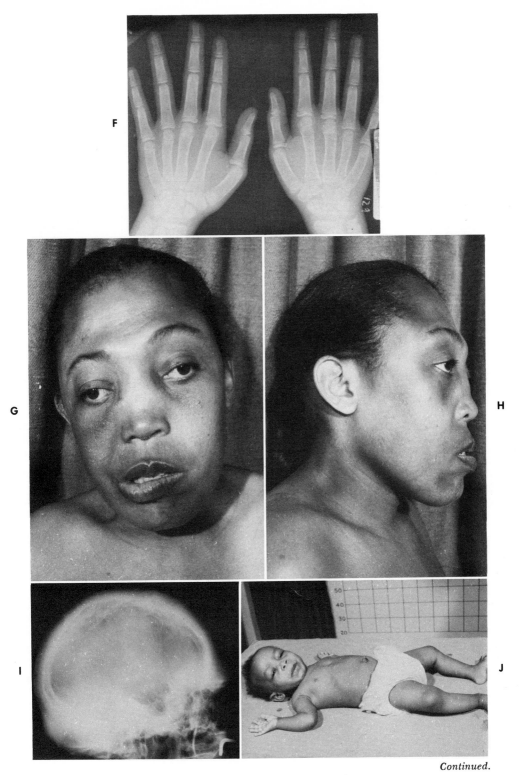

F

G

H

I

J

Continued.

Fig. 13-48, cont'd. For legend see p. 827.

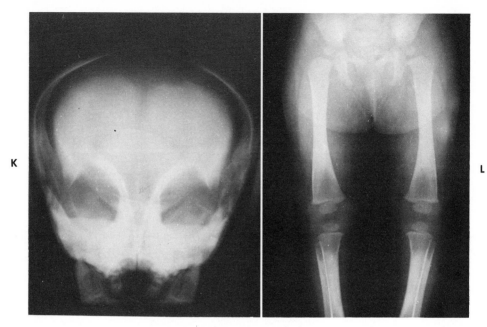

Fig. 13-48, cont'd. For legend see p. 827.

In the recessive form, nasal obstruction is usually complete,. and involvement of multiple cranial nerves is invariable. The patient described in Case 4 by Jackson and associates[123] was blind from optic atrophy at the age of 15 months. Deafness and facial paralysis are the rule. The facies is leonine in this disorder as well as in craniodiaphyseal dysplasia,[105] which is not discussed here; these disorders are "causes" of the old wastebasket diagnosis of "leontiasis ossea." Affected sibs were reported by Millard and colleagues[214] and by Lehmann,[173] and parental consanguinity was noted by Lièvre and Fischgold.[179]

DYSOSTOSES
Osteopathia striata

This form of sclerotic craniotubular osseous dysplasia takes its name from the longitudinal osteosclerotic streaks seen in the long bones by radiography. The functionally important feature of the disorder is the sclerotic hyperplasia of the craniofacial bones, which leads to disfigurement and disability from pressure on various cranial nerves. Voorhoeve[322] first described the condition in 1924. Cases have been reported by Hurt[119] and by Fairbank.[72] The patient shown in Fig. 13-49 had deafness and cataract. Jones and Mulcahy[130] reported a case with deafness. Rucker and Alfidi[260] seem to have reported the only familial occurrence: the father and paternal grandfather of his patient were said to have been affected. The father died of severe aortic stenosis. Taybi and Nurock[307] described a young child who probably had the disorder and who in the first year of life developed unexplained heart failure with murmur, cardiomegaly, and electrocardiographic changes, all of which cleared spontaneously. The patient

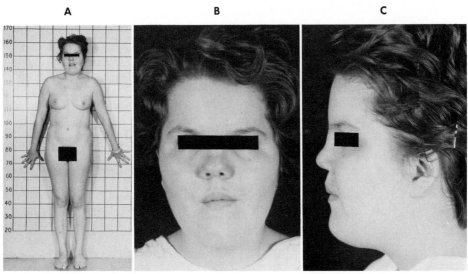

A   B   C

Continued.

Fig. 13-49. Osteopathia striata with cataracts and deafness. S. S. (J.H.H. 1129282), 20 years old at the time of study, had had deafness from at least 4 years of age and had worn a hearing aid from the age of 9 years. A heart murmur, noted early in life, disappeared by 6 years of age. Although the mother was aware of the misshapen head from the time the patient was a child and the anterior fontanelle was late in closing, bony abnormalities of the skull were first noted at 13 years of age, when some persistent deciduous teeth were extracted. Cataracts were first noted at 12 years. Stature and intelligence had always been at the lower limit of normal.

In addition to the features shown by the illustrations, examination at age 20 years showed slitlike stenosis of both external auditory canals.

A to C, Appearance at 20 years of age. The patient is less than 5 feet tall. The profile, C, is square. Fullness of the malar areas and jaw is greater on the left. D and E, X-ray views of the skull show dense sclerosis of the base and orbital roofs and focal sclerosis of the calvaria, with small orbits, obliteration of the paranasal sinuses, and airless, sclerotic mastoids.

F, Drawing of lens, showing appearance of cataracts. G, X-ray view of lower spine, showing moderate sclerosis. H, In the pelvis a wide band of sclerosis passes vertically along the medial portion of the ilium, through the full width of the acetabulum, and into the ischium bilaterally. Faint striations are present in the femoral heads and necks.

I, The lower femora and upper tibiae contain striking longitudinal streaking, which established the diagnosis in this case.

(F courtesy Dr. David L. Knox.)

shown in Fig. 13-49 had a heart murmur early in life that disappeared at about 6 years of age. Voorhoeve[322] observed affected brother and sister, 14 and 10 years old, respectively; the parents were presumably unaffected and were not related. No involvement of craniofacial bones was noted in his cases, however; thus his description may concern a different disorder from that shown in Fig. 13-49.

Spondylocostal dysostoses

At least two forms of spondylocostal dyostosis can be distinguished. One form is autosomal dominant and is represented by the family reported by Rimoin and

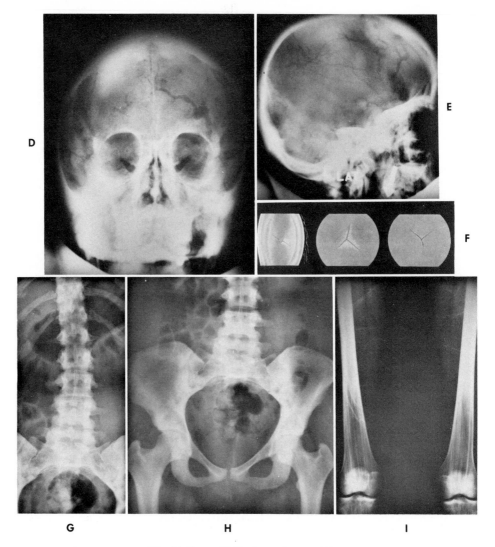

Fig. 13-49, cont'd. For legend see p. 831.

co-workers[251] and shown in Fig. 13-50. The patients have short-trunk dwarfism. The number of ribs is reduced to eleven, and several ribs are fused posteriorly. Hemivertebrae and vertebral fusion occur at multiple levels in the spine. To my knowledge, neurologic complications have not been observed, and survivorship seems to be unaffected.

A second variety is autosomal recessive. It is a more severe disorder than the autosomal dominant. Many of the affected infants die young of respiratory infection.[170] Block vertebrae, hemivertebrae, and rib anomalies occur as in the dominant form but tend to be more marked.[226] The family illustrated in Fig. 13-51 has the autosomal recessive form of the disorder.

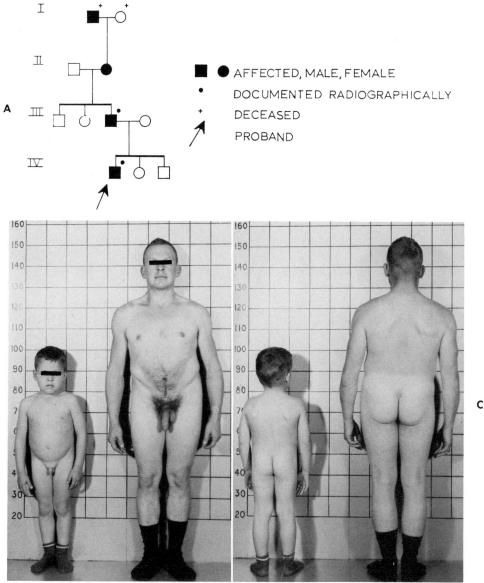

Continued.

Fig. 13-50. Spondylocostal dysostosis, autosomal dominant type, in four generations.[251] **A,** Pedigree. **B** and **C,** Affected father and son in the two most recent generations. The father (J.H.H. 1222178) had a height of 59 inches and an arm span of 67 inches. The son (J.H.H. 1222180), 5¾ years of age, was 40 inches tall (< 3rd percentile), with an armspan of 43 inches. In both, the chest was barrel-shaped, with increased anteroposterior diameter and flared lower ribs.

D to F, X-ray findings in the son at 3 months (**D**) and 5 years (**E** and **F**) of age. The dorsolumbar spine, **D,** shows hemivertebrae and "butterfly" vertebrae. The chest x-ray films (**D** and **E**) show fusion both of the fourth and fifth and of the ninth and tenth ribs on the left and of the fifth to the seventh ribs on the right. The sixth right rib is hypoplastic and the twelfth missing. The pelvic view, **F,** shows anomalies of the sacrum and absence of the coccyx.

G, In the father, the dorsolumbar spine, shows numerous hemivertebrae and "butterfly" vertebrae. The chest x-ray film shows bladelike fused ribs bilaterally. Only nine ribs were identified bilaterally.

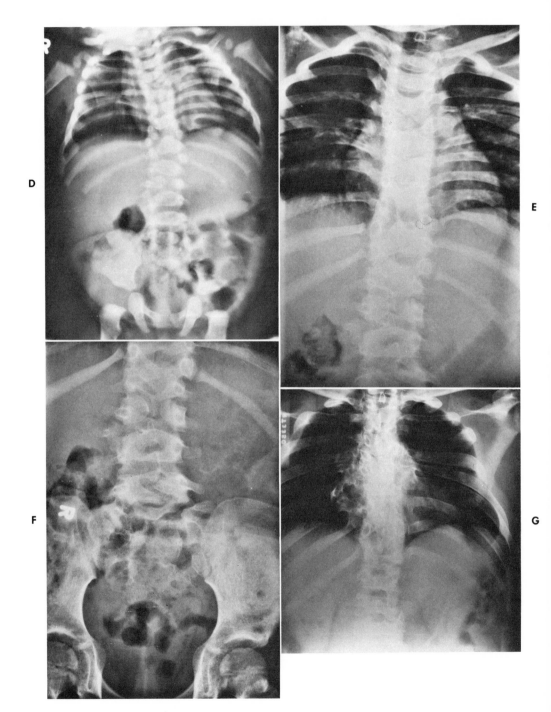

Fig. 13-50, cont'd. For legend see p. 833.

Osteo-onychodysostosis (formerly nail-patella syndrome)

This disorder is manifested by hypoplastic or absent fingernails and patellae, hornlike osseous posterior projections of the ilium ("iliac horns"), and anomaly of the elbows—usually hypoplasia of the head of the radius with dorsal dislocation and limitation of motion[67,275,311,321,334] (Fig. 13-52). Renal abnormality leading to uremia may be an integral feature, having been observed clinically in a number of instances.[267,282] Inheritance is autosomal dominant. The nail-patella syndrome enjoys the distinction of being caused by one of the few autosomal genes for which a genetic linkage has been identified. The nail-patella locus is on the same chromosome pair as the ABO blood group locus, from which it is separated by about ten recombination units. Furthermore, the nail-patella locus is very tightly linked with that which determines the enzyme adenylate kinase.[266] Which specific pair of autosomes carries these three loci is, however, unknown. The Ellis–van Creveld syndrome (p. 775) is another disorder in which skeletal and ectodermal abnormalities are associated.

PRIMARY METABOLIC ABNORMALITIES

Hypophosphatemic familial rickets (vitamin D–resistant rickets)

The skeleton shows changes typical of rickets (Fig. 13-53), but therapeutic response does not occur with the administration of vitamin D in reasonable dosage. Dwarfism is of the short-limbed variety, with much greater involvement of the lower than of the upper limbs and with genua varum and enlarged wrists and ankles. In the absence of treatment serum calcium is low and alkaline phosphatase high. The teeth show enlarged pulp chambers and elongated pulp horns extending to the dentinoenamel junction. Microorganisms invade the pulp through tubular defects in the dentin and cause periapical abscesses without caries.

Fig. 13-51. Autosomal recessive spondylocostal dysostosis. Four cases occurred in a kindred in eastern Kentucky (pedigree shown in **A**). The 3 affected sibs are pictured with their mother, **B**. The affected brother and sister are shown in **C** and **D**. Case 1, the older male in the pictures, was 14 years old at the time of the pictures. He measured 52¾ inches tall and had always been vigorous and healthy. The neck was short and webbed, with limited rotation and low posterior hairline. Multiple segmentation errors were demonstrated in the cervical and upper thoracic vertebrae, **E**. The ribs are irregularly spaced and some adjacent ribs are fused posteriorly. Hemivertebrae and sagittal clefts are evident in the lower thoracic and upper lumbar spine, **F**. Note the scoliosis and the fused ribs on the left. Segmentation is also abnormal in the sacrum and coccyx, **G**.

Case 2, the sister, was 9 years old and had likewise always been well. She was 45½ inches tall. Severe segmentation abnormalities of the vertebrae were shown in the cervical, **H**, thoracic, **I**, and lumbar, **J**, segments. The fusions of ribs, **K**, are more extensive than in her brother. The lower ribs almost touch the iliac crests, **K**.

Case 3, a 4-year-old child, was 39¼ inches tall (25th percentile). Movement of the head on the short, webbed neck was limited. As demonstrated by x-ray examination, **L** and **M**, changes are evident in the entire spine, including the sacrum, and are striking in the ribs.

Although we were not permitted to examine or radiograph Case 4, it was certain to us on meeting her that she has the same disorder as her cousins. (Cases studied with Dr. Robert A. Norum.)

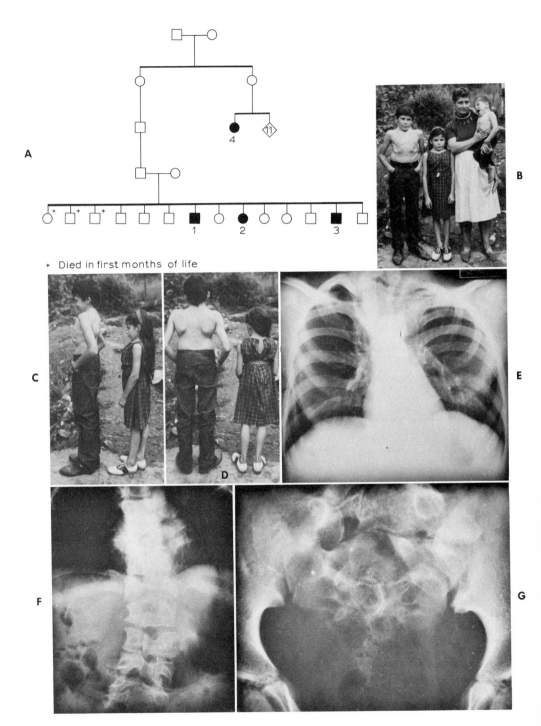

Fig. 13-51. For legend see p. 835.

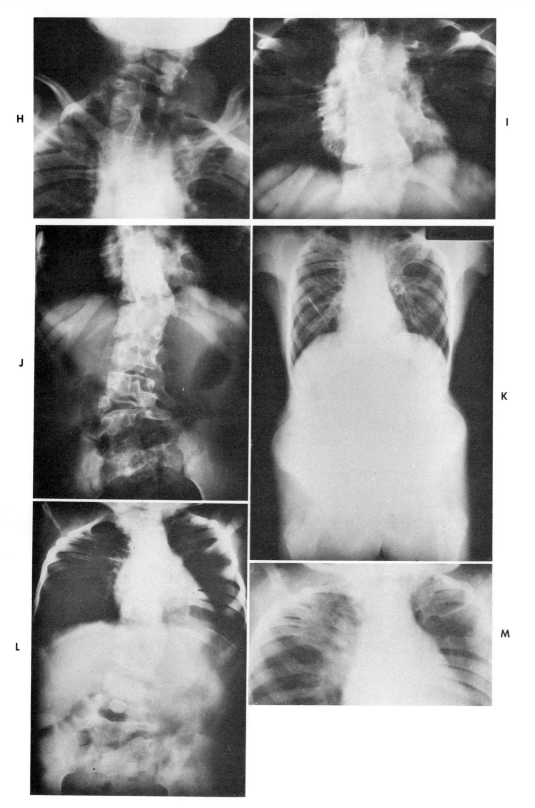

Fig. 13-51, cont'd. For legend see p. 835.

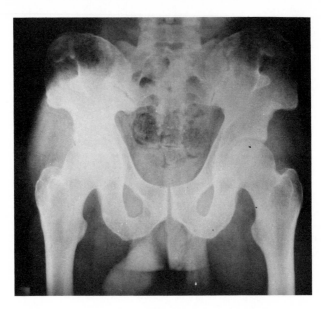

Fig. 13-52. Posterior iliac horns in a man with typical osteo-onychodysostosis (nail-patella syndrome). The horns should not be confused with the anterior superior iliac spines, which happen to appear rather hornlike on this roentgenogram.

Widened physes and radiolucent cupping and flaring of the metaphyseal ends are demonstrable by x-ray examination and are most severe in areas of most rapid growth.

Adults, especially males, with vitamin D–resistant rickets may suffer from ankylosing arthropathy (Fig. 13-54). Progressive reduction in mobility, especially in the axial skeleton, begins in the twenties. Cord compression may occur. By x-ray examination a "bamboo" spine may be demonstrated in severe cases. The ossification in paraspinous ligaments is paradoxically accompanied by generalized osteoporosis and by symmetric pseudo-fractures in the subtrochanteric area of the femora and elsewhere. Synostosis has been observed between the tibia and fibula, radius and ulna, and carpals and metacarpals.

Familial hypophosphatemia is an X-linked dominant disorder[335]; see Chapter 1 for a discussion of the pedigree characteristics of this form of inheritance. As is to be expected, heterozygous females are, on the average, less severely and more variably affected than are hemizygous males. Skipped generations—clinically unaffected heterozygous females—have been observed when skeletal deformity is used as the indication of involvement. When the concentration of serum phosphorus is used as the marker, essentially full penetrance is found. It has been suggested that the mutation-determined defect is deficiency in the conversion of vitamin D to its biologically active form, 25-hydroxycholecalciferol (25-HCC). However, treatment with 25-HCC has not been as dramatically effective as this hypothesis would demand.

The treatment of vitamin D–resistant rickets, as presently practiced, consists of the administration of vitamin D in high dosage (50,000 units) combined with phosphate supplementation.[90a]

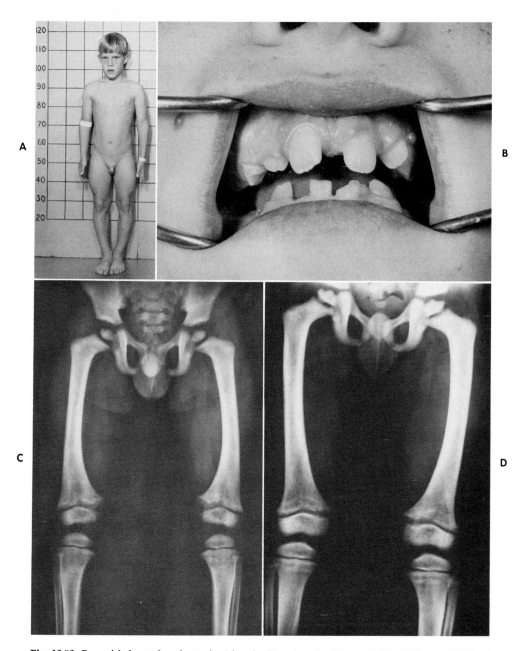

Fig. 13-53. Boy with hypophosphatemic (vitamin D–resistant) rickets. A. W. (J.H.H. 1364620), 8 years old, was first noted to have bowing of the femora and tibiae at 1 year of age. Treatment with vitamin D was initiated at 6 years 4 months. At 8 years serum phosphorus was 2.8 mg./100 ml.; calcium, 10.3 mg./100 ml.; and alkaline phosphatase, 575 mIU. (The mother was of normal stature and without deformities, but the serum phosphorus level was 2.9 mg./100 ml.) The boy, **A,** showed short stature, bowed legs, and frontal and occipital bosselation. Although the teeth showed no caries, several deciduous teeth had been lost because of abscess formation, and the boy showed a fistula in the gingiva above the maxillary left deciduous canine, **B.** By x-ray examination this tooth showed an apical abscess, and most of the teeth had large pulp chambers. **C** and **D,** X-ray views of the legs at the ages of 2 and 4½ years, respectively. Widening of the physeal plates is evident at the distal femora at 2 years (**C**) and at both ends of the femora and tibiae at 4½ years (**D**). All bones were abnormally dense, which is consistent with therapy with vitamin D. Supplemental phosphate was administered with improved healing of the rickets. (Patient studied with Dr. W. King Smith.)

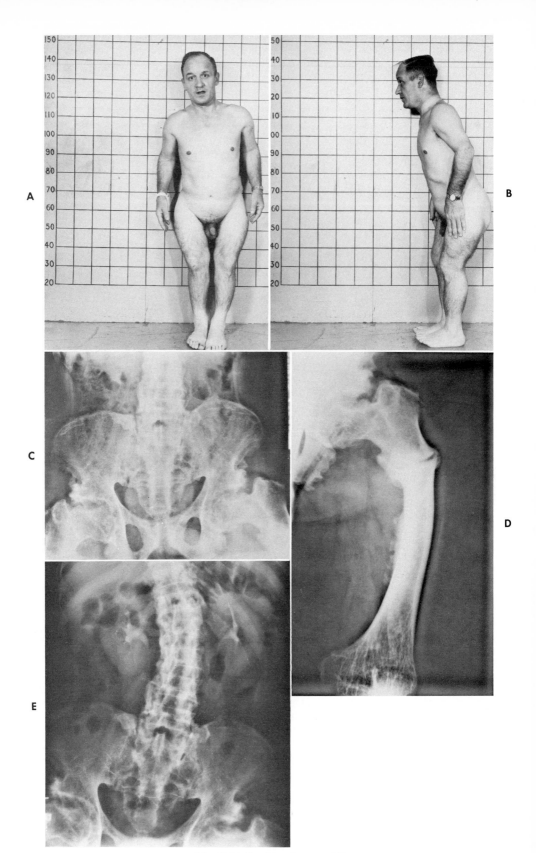

Fig. 13-54. For legend see p. 842.

Bianchine and colleagues[25] have observed a kindred with an autosomal dominant form of hypophosphatemia indistinguishable, except for the finding of male-to-male transmission, from the X-linked form.

Pseudo-deficiency rickets (vitamin D–dependency rickets)

The clinical picture in this disorder more nearly resembles that of deficiency rickets, and therapeutic response is more satisfactory to lower dosages of vitamin

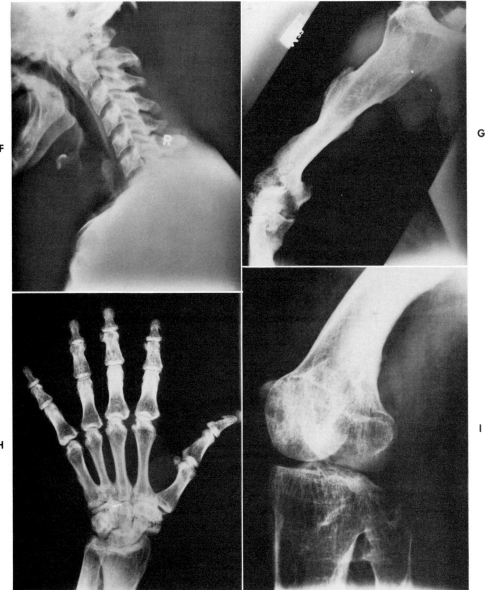

Fig. 13-54, cont'd. For legend see p. 842.

Fig. 13-54. Adult male with hypophosphatemic (vitamin D–resistant) rickets. C. E. (J.H.H. 1223061), 41 years old, was first seen for short stature and arthritis. His mother, 61 inches tall, is probably also affected. C. E. did not walk until the age of 2 years and was considered to have rickets as a child. However, he never received specific therapy and never had orthopedic surgery. Pain and stiffness began in his spine and hips in his early twenties and progressed gradually to involve all joints. At 41 years of age, he was a stiff, bent-over man with marked limitation in all joints. Serum phosphorus varied between 1.7 and 2.1 mg./100 ml.; alkaline phosphatase was 97 ImU (normal < 80); renal phosphorus resorption was 52% (normal, 80%); and tests for the rheumatoid factor were negative.

A and **B,** Appearance at 43 years of age. The neck, back, and hips are severely restricted in motion. Coxa vara is evident. **C,** X-ray view of pelvis showing ossification of paraspinous ligaments in lower lumbar spine, grossly abnormal trabecular pattern of bones, marked hypertrophic changes above the acetabula, advanced changes in the hip joints, and coxa vara. **D,** X-ray view of left femur showing unossified fracture line in the subtrochanteric zone. Note the irregular hyperostotic changes on the medial aspect of the femur and on the ischial tuberosity. The right femur was almost identically affected.

E, Normal pyelogram showing scoliosis and "bamboo vertebrae" as a result of ossification in the paraspinous ligaments. **F,** X-ray view of cervical spine showing bizarre occipital exostosis and ectopic ossification around the joints of the cervical vertebrae which produced fixation. **G,** X-ray view showing short humerus with large and broad exostoses at sites of muscle attachment. Changes at the elbow limit extension. **H,** X-ray view of hand showing abnormal trabecular pattern of bones, spurs at tendon attachments, and short carpus with the distal row of bones being small and in part fused. **I,** X-ray of the knee, showing abnormal trabecular pattern of the bones and proximal fusion of the tibia and fibula.

D, than in hypophosphatemic rickets. Furthermore, inheritance is autosomal recessive, not X-linked. The affected children show muscular hypotonia and may have tetany.

Hypophosphatasia

Hypophosphatasia[52,185,265] is one of the few hereditary generalized disorders of the osseous skeleton in which an enzyme defect has been identified. A rickets-like clinical picture and craniostenosis are leading features. Premature shedding of teeth may be the only overt manifestation.[237] Blue sclerae and, as demonstrated by x-ray examination, "harlequin orbits" are often features in the early onset form.[33] Inheritance is autosomal recessive. The diagnosis is suspected on the basis of characteristic radiologic changes and is confirmed by demonstration of low alkaline phosphatase in the serum. The leukocytes lack alkaline phosphatase activity,[21] and phosphorylethanolamine is excreted in the urine in excess. Heterozygotes, e.g., parents of affected children, demonstrate reduced leukocytic alkaline phosphatase. Fraser[81] recognized the following four types, categorized according to the age of onset and the severity of manifestations: (1) present at birth or before the age of 6 months, (2) onset in children after 6 months of age, (3) onset in adulthood,[20,24] and (4) an atypical group. The genetic relationship of these four types is uncertain. A form with autosomal dominant inheritance was suggested by Silverman.[281] A father and 2 sons and perhaps the paternal grandmother were affected. Clinical features were early loss of teeth, bowed legs requiring osteotomy, and a beaten-copper appearance of the skull by x-ray examination. The proband had served in the United States Air Force.

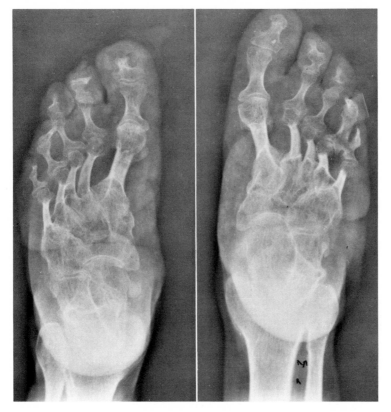

Fig. 13-55. Results of foot-binding in early life. X-ray view of a Canton-reared Chinese woman showing short bones with broad ends and possible fusion of the right fourth and fifth proximal phalanges at their bases.

The disorder in the family reported by Danovitch and co-workers[58] may also have been dominant. Jardon and associates[127] described a woman with hypophosphatasia who was asymptomatic until the age of 50 years. She showed pseudofractures of the proximal femora and calcification of the paraspinous ligaments similar to those in adults with hypophosphatemic rickets (Fig. 13-54).

CONCLUDING REMARK

The wide variety of skeletal dysplasias that result from gene mutation does not permit summarization. Present knowledge is mainly descriptive, i.e., at the phenotypic level. We can look forward, however, to a time when the understanding of each disorder at a molecular level will be sufficiently advanced to allow logical classification and a synthesis which is now impossible.

Fortunately from the viewpoint of entity-delineation, phenocopies (exogenously induced mimics of genetic disorders) are rare among the skeletal dysplasias. Thus one source of confusion in a highly heterogeneous category of disease is eliminated. Fig. 13-55 presents x-ray films of the feet, which *per se* might be thought to represent some genetic skeletal dysplasia and thus are a phenocopy.

REFERENCES

1. Albers-Schönberg, H.: Eine bisher nicth beschriebene Allgemeinerkrankung des Skelettes im Röntgenbilde, Fortsch. Roentgenstr. **11:**261, 1907.
2. Albright, F., Butler, A. M., Hampton, A. O., and Smith, P.: Syndrome characterized by osteitis fibrosa disseminata, areas of pigmentation and endocrine dysfunction, with precocious puberty in females; report of five cases, New Eng. J. Med. **216:**727, 1937.
3. Alexander, W. G.: Report of a case of so-called "marble-bones" with a review of the literature and a translation of article, Amer. J. Roentgen. **10:**280, 1923.
4. Alexander, W. J., and Dunbar, J. S.: Unusual bone changes in thymic alymphoplasia, Ann. Radiol. **11:**389, 1968.
5. Allansmith, M., and Senz, E.: Chondrodystrophia congenita punctata (Conradi's disease): review of literature and report of case with unusual features, Amer. J. Dis. Child. **100:**109, 1960.
6. Allen, D. T., Saunders, A. M., Northway, W. H., Jr., Williams, G. F., and Schafer, I. A.: Corticosteroids in the treatment of Engelmann's disease (progressive diaphyseal dysplasia), Pediatrics **46:**523, 1970.
7. Allison, A. C., and Blumberg, B. S.: Familial osteoarthropathy of the fingers, J. Bone Joint Surg. **40-B:**538, 1958.
7a. Amlöf, J.: On achondroplasia in the dog, Zbl. Veterinaermed. **8:**43, 1961.
8. Amman, F.: Investigations cliniques et génétiques sur le syndrome de Bardet-Biedl en Suisse, J. Genet. Hum. **18** (supp.):1, 1970.
9. Anderson, I. F.: Maffucci's syndrome; report of a case, with a review of the literature, S. Afr. Med. J. **39:**1066, 1965.
10. Andrén, L., Dymling, J. F., Hogeman, K. E., and Wendeberg, B.: Osteopetrosis acro-osteolytica; a syndrome of osteopetrosis, acro-osteolysis and open sutures of the skull, Acta Chir. Scand. **124:**496, 1962.
11. Angle, C. R.: Congenital bowing and angulation in long bones, Pediatrics **13:**257, 1954.
12. Anton, J. I., Reitz, G. B., and Spiegel, M. B.: Madelung's deformity, Ann. Surg. **108:**411, 1938.
13. Austin, J. H.: Mental retardation; metachromatic leucodystrophy. In Carter, C. C., editor: Medical aspects of mental retardation, Springfield, Ill., 1965, Charles C Thomas, Publisher.
13a. Avery, M. E., Dorst, J. P., and Walker, D. G.: Osteopetrosis. In Bergsma, D., editor: Clinical delineation of birth defects. IV. Skeletal dysplasia, New York, 1969, National Foundation–March of Dimes, pp. 305-311.
14. Bakwin, H., Golden, A., and Fox, S.: Familial osteoectasia with macrocranium, Amer. J. Roentgen. **91:**609, 1964.
15. Bakwin, H., and Krida, A.: Familial metaphyseal dysplasia, Amer. J. Dis. Child. **53:**1521, 1937.
15a. Bannerman, R. M.: X-linked spondyloepiphyseal dysplasia tarda (SDT). In Bergsma, D., editor: Clinical delineation of birth defects. IV. Skeletal dysplasias, New York, 1969, National Foundation–March of Dimes.
16. Barrie, H., Carter, C., and Sutcliffe, J.: Multiple epiphyseal dysplasia, Brit. Med. J. **2:**133, 1958.
17. Bartter, F. C.: Hypophosphatasia. In Stanbury, J. B., Wyngaarden, J. B., and Fredrickson, D. S., editor: The metabolic basis of inherited disease, ed. 2, New York, 1966, McGraw-Hill Book Co., pp. 1015-1023.
18. Beals, R. K.: Hypochondroplasia; report of five kindreds, J. Bone Joint Surg. **51-A:**728, 1969.
19. Bean, W. B.: Dyschondroplasia and hemangiomata (Maffucci's syndrome), Arch. Intern. Med. **95:**767, 1955.
20. Beisel, W. R., Austen, K. F., Rosen, H., and Herndon, E. G., Jr.: Metabolic observations in adult hypophosphatasia, Amer. J. Med. **29:**369, 1960.
21. Beisel, W. R., Benjamin, N., and Austen, K. F.: Absence of leucocyte alkaline phosphatase activity in hypophosphatasia, Blood **14:**975, 1959.
22. Bennett, G. E., and Berkheimer, G. A.: Malignant degeneration in a case of multiple benign exostoses; with a brief review of the literature, Surgery **10:**781, 1941.
23. Bergsma, D., editor: Clinical delineation of birth defects. IV. Skeletal dysplasias, New York, 1969, National Foundation–March of Dimes.

24. Bethune, J. E., and Dent, C. E.: Hypophosphatasia in the adult, Amer. J. Med. **28:**615, 1960.

25. Bianchine, J. W., Stambler, A. A., and Harrison, H. E.: Familial hypophosphatemic rickets showing autosomal dominant inheritance, In Bergsma, D., editor: Clinical delineation of birth defects. X. Endocrine system. Baltimore, 1971, The Williams & Wilkins Co.

26. Black, J.: Low birth weight dwarfism, Arch. Dis. Child. **36:**633, 1961.

27. Bloom, D.: The syndrome of congenital telangiectatic erythema and stunted growth, J. Pediat. **68:**103, 1966.

28. Bloxsom, A., and Johnston, R. A.: Calcinosis universalis with unusual features, Amer. J. Dis. Child. **56:**103, 1938.

29. Böhme, A.: Kasuistischer Beitrag zur Thiemannschen Epiphysenerkrankung, Z. Ges. Inn. Med. **18:**491, 1963.

29a. Bowen, P.: In Bergsma, D., editor: Clinical delineation of birth defects. XIX. Skeletal dysplasias (cont.), Baltimore, 1973, The Williams & Wilkins Co.

30. Brady, R. O.: The sphingolipidoses, New Eng. J. Med. **275:**312, 1966.

31. Brailsford, J. F.: Radiology of bones and joints, ed. 5, Baltimore, 1953, The Williams & Wilkins Co.

32. Brandner, M.: Normal values of the vertebral body and intervertebral disc index during growth, Amer. J. Roentgen. **110:**618, 1970.

33. Brenner, R. L., Smith, J. L., Cleveland, W. W., Bejar, R. L., and Lockhart, W. S., Jr.: Eye signs of hypophosphatasia, Arch. Ophthal. **81:**614, 1969.

34. Brocher, J. E. W., Klein, D., Bamatter, F., Franceschett, A., and Boreux, G.: Röntgenologisch Befunde bei Geroderma osteodysplastica hereditaria, Fortsch. Roentgenstr. **109:**185, 1968.

34a. Brown, D. M., and Dent, P. B.: Pathogenesis of osteopetrosis: a comparison of human and animal spectra, Pediat. Res. **5:**181, 1971.

35. Bruland, H.: Pseudo-chondrodystrophia rheumatica (rheumatic dwarfism): review and discussion of two cases, Acta Rheum. Scand. **6:**209, 1960.

36. Caffey, J.: Chondroectodermal dysplasia (Ellis–van Creveld disease), report of three cases, Amer. J. Roentgen. **68:**875, 1952.

37. Caffey, J.: Congenital stenosis of medullary space in tubular bones and calvaria in two proportionate dwarfs—mother and son—coupled with transitory hypocalcemic tetany, Amer. J. Roentgen. **100:**1, 1967.

38. Caffey, J.: Pediatric x-ray diagnosis, ed. 5, Chicago, 1967, Year Book Medical Publishers, Inc.

39. Callender, G. R., Jr., and Miyakawa, G.: Osteopetrosis in adult; case report, J. Bone Joint Surg. **35-A:**204, 1953.

40. Campbell, C. J., Papademetriou, T., and Bonfiglio, M.: Melorheostosis; a report of the clinical, roentgenographic and pathological findings in fourteen cases, J. Bone Joint Surg. **50-A:**1281, 1968.

41. Carleton, A., Elkington, J. S. C., Greenfield, J. G., and Robb-Smith, A. H. T.: Maffucci's syndrome (dyschondroplasia with haemangiomata), Quart. J. Med. **11:**203, 1942.

41a. Chemke, J., Graff, G., and Lancet, M.: Familial thanatophoric dwarfism (letter), Lancet **1:**1358, 1971.

42. Cheney, W. D.: Acro-osteolysis, Amer. J. Roentgen. **94:**595, 1965.

43. Christensen, W. R., Lin, R. K., and Berghout, J.: Dysplasia epiphysalis multiplex, Amer. J. Roentgen. **74:**1059, 1955.

44. Cleveland, M., and Fielding, J. W.: Chondrodysplasia (Ollier's disease); report of a case with a thirty-eight year follow-up, J. Bone Joint Surg. **41-A:**1341, 1959.

45. Cohen, J.: Osteopetrosis; case report, autopsy findings and pathologic interpretation; failure of treatment with vitamin A, J. Bone Joint Surg. **33-A:**923, 1951.

46. Cohen, M. E., Rosenthal, A. D., and Matson, D. D.: Neurological abnormalities in achondroplastic children, J. Pediat. **71:**367, 1967.

47. Coupe, R. L., and Lowry, R. B.: Abnormality of the hair in cartilage-hair hypoplasia, Dermatologica **141:**329, 1970.

48. Cowan, D. J.: Multiple epiphysial dysplasia, Brit. Med. J. **2:**1629, 1963.

49. Crew, F. A. E.: The bulldog calf; a contribution to the study of achondroplasia, Proc. Roy. Soc. Med. **17:**39, 1924.

50. Crew, F. A. E.: The significance of an achondroplasia-like condition met with in cattle, Proc. Roy Soc. [Biol.] **95**:228, 1923.

51. Cross, H. E., and Opitz, J.: Craniosynostosis in the Amish, J. Pediat. **75**:1037, 1969.

52. Currarino, G., Neuhauser, E. B. D., Reyesbcak,, G. C., and Sobel, E. H.: Hypophosphatasia, Amer. J. Roentgen. **78**:392, 1957.

53. Daeschner, C. W., Singleton, E. B., Hill, L. L., and Dodge, W. F.: Metaphyseal dysostosis, J. Pediat. **57**:844, 1960.

54. Dandy, W. E.: Hydrocephalus in chondrodystrophy, Bull. Johns Hopkins Hosp. **32**:5, 1921.

55. Danes, B. S. (New York City): Personal communication, 1969.

56. Danes, B. S., and Bearn, A. G.: Hurler's syndrome; demonstration of an inherited disorder of connective tissue in cell culture, Science **149**:987, 1965.

56a. Daniel, A.: Pyle's disease, Indian J. Radiol. **14**:126, 1960.

57. Danks, D. M. (Melbourne, Australia): Personal communication, 1970.

58. Danovitch, S. H., Baer, P. N., and Laster, L.: Intestinal alkaline phosphatase activity in familial hypophosphatasia, New Eng. J. Med. **278**:1253, 1968.

59. DeHaas, W. H. D., DeBoer, W., and Griffionene, F.: Metaphysial dysostosis; a late follow-up of the first reported case, J. Bone Joint Surg. **51-B**:290, 1969.

60. Dennis, J. P., Rosenberg, H. S., and Alvord, E. C., Jr.: Megalencephaly, internal hydrocephalus, and other neurological aspects of achondroplasia, Brain **84**:427, 1961

61. Dent, C. E. (London): Personal communication, 1964.

62. Dent, C. E., and Friedman, M.: Idiopathic juvenile osteoporosis, Quart. J. Med. **34**:177, 1965.

63. Dent, C. E., Friedman, M., and Watson, L.: Hereditary pseudo vitamin D–deficiency rickets ("hereditäre Pseudomangelrächitis"), J. Bone Joint Surg. **50-B**:708, 1968.

64. Dent, C. E., and Normand, I. C. S.: Metaphysial dysostosis, type Schmid, Arch. Dis. Child. **39**:444, 1964.

65. Donaldson, E. M., and Summerly, R.: Primary osteoma cutis and diaphyseal aclasis, Acta Derm. **85**:261, 1962.

66. Dorst, J. P., and McKusick, V. A.: Acro-osteolysis (Cheney syndrome). In Bergsma, D., editor: Clinical delineation of birth defects. III. Limb malformations, New York, 1969, National Foundation–March of Dimes.

67. Elliott, K. A., Elliott, G. B., and Kindrachuk, W. H.: The "radial subluxation—fingernail defect—absent patella" syndrome: observations on its nature, Amer. J. Roentgen. **87**:1067, 1962.

68. Elsbach, L.: Bilateral hereditary micro-epiphysial dysplasia of the hips, J. Bone Joint Surg. **41-B**:514, 1959.

69. Engelmann, G.: Osteopathia hyperostotica sclerotisans multiplex infantilis, Fortschr. Roentgenstr. **39**:1101, 1929.

70. Epstein, J. A., and Malis, L. J.: Compression of spinal cord and cauda equina in achondroplastic dwarfs, Neurology **5**:875, 1955.

71. Evans, R., and Caffey, J.: Metaphyseal dysostosis resembling vitamin D–refractory rickets, Amer. J. Dis. Child. **95**:640, 1958.

72. Fairbank, H. A. T.: An atlas of general affections of the skeleton, Edinburgh, 1951, E. & S. Livingstone, Ltd.

73. Fairbank, T.: Dysplasia epiphysialis multiplex, Brit. J. Surg. **34**:225, 1947.

74. Falls, H. F., and Schull, W. J.: Hallermann-Streiff syndrome; a dyscephaly with congenital cataracts and hypotrichosis, Arch. Ophthal. **63**:409, 1960.

75. Felman, A. H., and Kirkpatrick, J. A., Jr.: Madelung's deformity; observations in 17 patients, Radiology **93**:1037, 1969.

76. Felman, A. H., and Kirkpatrick, J. A., Jr.: Dyschondrosteose; mesomelic dwarfism of Léri and Weill, Amer. J. Dis. Child. **120**:329, 1970.

77. Flippen, J. H., Jr.: Cranio-facial dysostosis of Crouzon; report of a case in which the malformation occurred in four generations, Pediatrics **5**:90, 1950.

78. Ford, N., Silverman, F. N., and Kozlowski, K.: Spondylo-epiphyseal dysplasia (pseudo-achondroplasia type), Amer. J. Roentgen. **86**:462, 1961.

79. Forland, M.: Cleidocranial dysostosis; a review of the syndrome and report of a sporadic case with hereditary transmission, Amer. J. Med. **33**:792, 1962.

80. Fraccaro, M.: Contributo allo studio delle malattie del mesenchima osteopoietico; l'acondrogenesi, Folia Hered. Path. 1:190, 1952.

81. Fraser, D.: Hypophosphatasia, Amer. J. Med. **22**:730, 1957.

82. Freiberger, R. H.: Multiple epiphyseal dysplasia; a report of three cases, Radiology **70**:379, 1958.

83. Fulginiti, V. A., Hathaway, W. E., Pearlman, D. S., Blackburn, W. R., Reiquam, C. W., Githens, J. H., Claman, H. N., and Kempe, C. H.: Dissociation of delayed-hypersensitivity and antibody synthesizing capacities in man; report of two sibships with thymic dysplasia, lymphoid tissue depletion, and normal immunoglobulins, Lancet **2**:5, 1967.

84. Fulginiti, V. A., Hathaway, W. E., Pearlman, D. S., and Kempe, C. H.: Agammaglobulinaemia and achondroplasia (letter), Brit. Med. J. **2**:242, 1967.

84a. Gardner, D. L.: Familial canine chondrodystrophia foetalis (achondroplasia), J. Path. Bact. **77**:243, 1959.

85. Gatti, R. A., Platt, N., Pomerance, H. H., Hong, R., Langer, L. O., Kay, H. E. M., and Good, R. A.: Hereditary lymphopenic agammaglobulinemia associated with a distinctive form of short-limbed dwarfism and ectodermal dysplasia, J. Pediat. **75**:675, 1969.

86. Ghormley, R. K.: A case of congenital osteosclerosis, Bull. Hopkins Hosp. **33**:444, 1922.

87. Gibson, R.: A case of the Smith-Lemli-Opitz syndrome of multiple congenital anomalies in association with dysplasia epiphysealis punctata, Canad. Med. Ass. J. **92**:574, 1965.

88. Giedion, A.: Thanatophoric dwarfism, Helv. Paediat. Acta **23**:175, 1968.

89. Giedion, A.: Das tricho-rhino-phalangeale Syndrome, Helv. Paediat. Acta **21**:475, 1966.

90. Girdany, B. R.: Engelmann's disease (progressive diaphyseal dysplasia)—a nonprogressive familial form of muscular dystrophy with characteristic bone changes, Clin. Orthop. **14**: 102, 1959.

90a. Glorieux, F. H., Scriver, C. R., Reade, T. M., Goldman, H., and Roseborough, A.: Use of phosphate and vitamin D to prevent dwarfism and rickets in X-linked hypophosphatemia, New Eng. J. Med. **287**:481, 1972.

91. Gorlin, R. J., and Cohen, M. M., Jr.: Frontometaphyseal dysplasia; a new syndrome, Amer. J. Dis. Child. **118**:487, 1969.

92. Gorlin, R. J., Meskin, L. H., and St. Geme, J. W.: Oculodentodigital dysplasia, J. Pediat. **63**:69, 1963.

93. Gorlin, R. J., and Pindborg, J. J.: Orodigitofacial dysostosis. In Gorlin, R. J., and Pindborg, J. J., editor: Syndromes of the head and neck, New York, 1964, McGraw-Hill Book Co., pp. 438-446.

94. Gorlin, R. J., Sedano, H. O., and Červenka, J.: Popliteal pterygium syndrome, Pediatrics **41**: 503, 1968.

95. Gorlin, R. J., Spranger, J., and Koszalka, M. F.: Genetic craniotubular bone dysplasias and hyperostoses; a critical analyses. In Bergsma, D., editor: Clinical delineation of birth defects. IV. Skeletal dysplasias, New York, 1969, National Foundation—March of Dimes, pp. 79-95.

96. Gram, P. B., Fleming, J. L., Frame, B., and Fine, G.: Metaphyseal chondrodysplasia of Jansen, J. Bone Joint Surg. **41-A**:951, 1959.

97. Grebe, H.: Chondrodysplasie, Rome, 1955, Gregor Mendel Institute.

98. Gregory, P. W.: Genetic interrelationships of bovine chondrodystrophies. In Bergsma, D., editor: Clinical delineation of birth defects. IV. Skeletal dysplasias, New York, 1969, National Foundation—March of Dimes, pp. 207-213.

99. Grüneberg, H.: The pathology of development: a study of inherited skeletal disorders in animals, New York, 1964, John Wiley & Sons, Inc.

100. Gunderson, C. H., Greenspan, R. H., Glaser, G. H., and Lubs, H. A., Jr.: The Klippel-Feil syndrome; genetic and clinical reevaluation of cervical fusion, Medicine **46**:491, 1967.

101. Hall, J. G., and Dorst, J. P.: Four types of pseudo-achondroplastic spondyloepiphyseal dysplasia (SED). In Bergsma, D., editor: Clinical delineation of birth defects. Part IV. Dysplasias, New York, 1969, National Foundation—March of Dimes, pp. 242-259.

102. Hall, J. G., Dorst, J. P., Taybi, H., Scott, C. I., Langer, L. O., Jr., and McKusick, V. A.: Two probable cases of homozygosity for the achondroplasia gene. In Bergsma, D., editor: Clinical delineation of birth defects. IV. Skeletal dysplasias, New York, 1969, National Foundation—March of Dimes, p. 24.

103. Hall, J. G., Levin, J., Kuhn, J. P., Offenheimer, E. J., Van Berkum, K. A. P., and McKusick, V. A.: Thrombocytopenia with absent radius (TAR), Medicine **48**:411, 1969.

104. Halle, M. A., Collipp, P. J., and Roginsky, M.: Cartilage-hair hypoplasia in childhood, New York J. Med. **70:**2705, 1970.

105. Halliday, J. A.: Rare case of bony dystrophy, Brit. J. Surg. **37:**52, 1949.

106. Hansen, O. H., and Andersen, N. O.: Congenital radio-ulnar synostosis; report of 37 cases, Acta Orthop. Scand. **41:**225, 1970.

106a. Haverkamp Begemann, N., and van Lookeren Campagne, A.: Homozygous form of Pelger-Huët's anomaly in man, Acta Haemat. **7:**295, 1952.

107. Herdman, R. C., and Langer, L. O.: The thoracic asphyxiant dystrophy and renal disease, Amer. J. Dis. Child. **116:**192, 1968.

108. Herdman, R. C., Langer, L. O., and Good, R. A.: Dyschondrosteosis, the most common cause of Madelung's deformity, J Pedita. **68:**432, 1966.

109. Herndon, C. N.: Cleidocranial dysostosis, Amer. J. Hum. Genet. **3:**314, 1954.

110. Hink, V. S., Clark, W. M., Jr., and Hopkins, C.: Normal interpedicular distances (minimum and maximum) in children and adults, Amer. J. Roentgen. **97:**141, 1966.

111. Hinkel, C. L., and Beiler, D. D.: Osteopetrosis in adults, Amer. J. Roentgen. **74:**46, 1955.

112. Hirsch, S.: Generalized osteochondrodystrophy, J. Bone Joint Surg. **19:**297, 1937.

113. Hoback, A.: Problems of hereditary chondrodysplasias, Oslo, 1961, Oslo University Press.

114. Hodgkinson, H. M.: Double patellae in multiple epiphysial dysplasia, J. Bone Joint Surg. **44-B:**569, 1962.

115. Holden, J. D.: The Russell-Silver's dwarf, Develop. Med. Child. Neurol. **9:**457, 1967.

116. Holt, J. F.: Discussion (of Jansen's metaphyseal dysostosis). In Bergsma, D., editor: Clinical delineation of birth defects. IV. Skeletal dysplasias, New York, 1969, National Foundation–March of Dimes, pp. 73-75.

117. Holt, J. F.: The evolution of cranio-metaphyseal dysplasia, Ann. Radiol. **9:**209, 1966.

118. Horwitz, A. L., and Dorfman, A.: The growth of cartilage cells in soft agar and liquid suspension, J. Cell. Biol. **45:**434, 1970.

118a. Houston, C. S., Awen, C. F., and Kent, H. P.: Fatal neonatal dwarfism, J. Canad. Assoc. Radiol. **23:**45, 1972.

119. Hurt, R. L.: Osteopathia striata—Voorhoeve's disease; report of case presenting features of osteopathia striata and osteopetrosis, J. Bone Joint Surg. **35-B:**89, 1953.

120. Hussels, I. E.: Trichorhinophalangeal syndrome in two sibs. In Bergsma, D., editor: Clinical delineation of birth defects. XI. Orofacial structures, Baltimore, 1971, The Williams & Wilkins Co., pp. 301-303.

121. Iversen, J.: Cleidocranial dysostosis, Acta Obstet. Gynec. Scand. **41:**93, 1962.

122. Jackson, W. P. U.: An irregular, familial chondro-osseous defects, J. Bone Joint Surg. **33-B:**420, 1951.

123. Jackson, W. P. U., Hanelin, J., and Albright, F.: Metaphyseal dysplasia, epiphyseal dysplasias, diaphyseal dysplasia, and related conditions; familial metaphyseal dysplasia and craniometaphyseal dysplasia: their relation to leontiasis ossea and osteopetrosis: disorders of "bone remodeling," Arch. Intern. Med. **94:**871, 1954.

124. Jacobsen, A. W.: Hereditary osteochondrodystrophia deformans; a family with 20 members affected in five generations, J.A.M.A. **113**121, 1939.

125. Jaffe, H. L.: Hereditary multiple exostoses, Arch. Path. **36:**335, 1943.

126. Jansen, M.: Über atypische Chondrodystrophie (Achondroplasie) und über eine noch nicht beschriebene angeborene Wachstumsstörung des Knochensystems: metaphysäre Dysostosis, Z. Orthop. Chir. **61:**253, 1934.

127. Jardon, O. M., Burney, D. W., and Fink, R. L.: Hypophosphatasia in an adult, J. Bone Joint Surg. **52A:**1477, 1970.

128. Jeune, M., Beraud, C., and Carron, R.: Dystrophie thoracique asphyxiante de caractère familial, Arch. Franç Pedit. **12:**886, 1955.

129. Johnston, C. C., Jr., Lavy, N., Lord, T., Vellios, F., Merritt, A. D., and Deiss, W. P., Jr.: Osteopetrosis; a clinical, genetic, metabolic, and morphologic study of the dominantly inherited, benign form, Medicine **47:**149, 1968.

130. Jones, M. D., and Mulcahy, N. D.: Osteopathia striata, osteopetrosis, and impaired hearing; a case report, Arch. Otolaryng. **87:**116, 1968.

131. Jones, W. A.: Cherubism; a thumbnail sketch of its diagnosis and a conservative method of treatment, Oral Surg. **20:**648, 1965.

132. Juberg, R. C., and Holt, J. F.: Inheritance of multiple epiphyseal dysplasia, tarda, Amer. J. Hum. Genet. **20**:549, 1968.

133. Juhl, J. H., Wesenberg, R. L., and Gwinn, J. L.: Roentgenographic findings in Fanconi's anemia, Radiology **89**:646, 1967.

134. Kalliala, E., and Taskinen, P. J.: Cleidocranial dysostosis; report of six typical cases and one atypical case, Oral Surg. **15**:808, 1962.

135. Kaufman, R. L., Rimoin, D. L., McAlister, W. H., and Kissane, J. M.: Thanatophoric dwarfism, Amer. J. Dis. Child. **120**:53, 1970.

136. Kaufmann, E.: Die Chondrodystrophia hyperplastica; ein Beitrag zu den fötalen Skeleterkrankungen, Beitr. Path. Anat. **13**:32, 1893.

137. Kaufmann, E.: Untersuchungen über die sogenannten fötale Rachitis (Chondrodystrophia foetalis), Berlin, 1892, Reimer.

138. Keith, Sir A.: The nature of the structural alteration in the disorder known as multiple exostoses, J. Anat. **54**:101, 1919-1920.

139. Keizer, D. R. R., and Schilder, J. H.: Ectodermal dysplasia, achondroplasia, and congenital morbus cordis, Amer. J. Dis. Child. **82**:345, 1951.

140. Kelley, C., and Lawlah, J. W.: Albers-Schönberg disease; a family survey, Radiology **47**:507, 1946.

141. Kenny, F. M., Aceto, T., Jr., Purisch, M., Harrison, H. E., Harrison, H. C., and Blizzard, R.. M.: Metabolic studies in a patient with idiopathic hypercalcemia of infancy, J. Pediat. **62**:531, 1963.

142. Khoo, F. Y., Chang, P. Y., Lee, C. T., and Fan, K. S.: Multiple cartilaginous exostoses (hereditary deforming chondrodysplasia), Chinese Med. J. **66**:252, 1948.

143. Kirkham, T. H.: Cervico-oculo-acusticus syndrome with pseudopapilloedema, Arch. Dis. Child. **44**:504, 1969.

144. Klein, A.: Zur Frage der Erblichkeit der Marmorknochenkrankheit, Fortschr. Roentgenstr. **76**:366, 1952.

145. Klen, D., and Ammann, F.: The syndrome of Laurence-Moon-Bardet-Biedl and allied diseases in Switzerland; clinical, genetic and epidemiological studies, J. Neurol. Sci. **9**:479, 1969.

146. Klein, H.: Die Pelger-Anomalie der Leukocyten und die pathologische Anatomie des neugeborenen homozygoten Pelger-Kaninchens; ein Beitrag zum Formenkreis der fetalen Chondrodystrophie, Z. Menschl. Vererb. Konstitutional. **29**:551, 1949.

147. Kneal, E., and Sante, L. R.: Osteopetrosis (marble bones); report of a case with special reference to early roentgenologic and pathologic findings, Amer. J. Dis. Child. **81**:693, 1951.

148. Knight, J. D. S.: Sarcomatous change in three brothers with diaphysial aclasis, Brit. Med. J. **1**:1013, 1960.

149. Komins, C.: Familial metaphyseal dysplasia (Pyle's disease), Brit. J. Radiol. **27**:670, 1954.

150. Kozlowski, K., Maroteaux, P., and Sprager, J.: La dysostose spondyle-métaphysaire, Presse Méd. **75**:2769, 1967.

151. Krooth, R. S., Macklin, M. A. P., and Hillbish, T. F.: Diaphysial aclasis (multiple exostoses) on Guam, Amer. J. Hum. Genet. **13**:340, 1961.

152. Lamy, M., and Bienenfeld, C.: La dyschondrosteose. In Gedda, L., editor: De genetica medica, Rome, 1954, Gregor Mendel Institute.

153. Lamy, M., and Maroteaux, P.: Acro-osteolyse dominante, Arch. Franç. Pédiat. **18**:693, 1961.

154. Lamy, M., and Maroteaux, P.: Les chondrodystrophies génotypiques, L'Expansion Scientifique Française, Paris, 1960.

155. Lamy, M., and Maroteaux, P.: Le nanisme diastrophique, Presse Méd. **68**:1977, 1960.

156. Landauer, W.: Studies on the creeper fowl. XII. Size of body, organs and long bone of late homozygous creeper embryos, Storrs Agric. Exper. Station, University of Connecticut Bull. No. 232, 1939; also: Studies on fowl paralysis. III. A condition resembling osteopetrosis (mable bone) in the common fowl, Bull. No. 222, 1938.

157. Lane, P. W., and Dickie, M. M.: Three recessive mutations producing disproportionate dwarfing in mice: achondroplasia, branchymorphic, and stubby, J. Hered. **59**:300, 1968.

158. Langer, L. O., Jr.: Diastrophic dwarfism in early infancy, Amer. J. Roentgen. **93**:399, 1965.

159. Langer, L. O., Jr.: Dyschondrosteosis: a heritable bone dysplasia with characteristic roentgenographic features, Amer. J. Roentgen. **95**:178, 1965.

160. Langer, L. O. Jr.: Mesomelic dwarfism of the hypoplastic ulna, fibula, mandible type, Radiology **89**:654, 1967.

161. Langer, L. O., Jr.: Spondyloepiphyseal dysplasia tarda; hereditary chondrodysplasia with characteristic vertebral configuration in an adult, Radiology **82**:833, 1964.

162. Langer, L. O., Jr.: Thoracic-pelvic-phalangeal dystrophy, asphyxiating thoracic dystrophy of the newborn, infantile thoracic dystrophy, Radiology **91**:447, 1968.

163. Langer, L. O., Jr., Baumann, P. A., and Gorlin, R. J.: Achondroplasia, Amer. J. Roentgen. **100**:12, 1967.

164. Langer, L. O., Jr., Baumann, P. A., and Gorlin, R. J.: Achondroplasia; clinical radiologic features with comments on genetic implications, Clin. Pediat. **7**:474, 1968.

164a. Langer, L. O., Jr., and Gorlin, R. J. (Minneapolis): Personal communication, 1971.

165. Langer, L. O., Jr., Spranger, J. W., Greinacher, I., and Herdman, R. C.: Thanatophoric dwarfism; a condition confused with achondroplasia in the neonate, with brief comments on achondrogenesis and homozygous achondroplasia, Radiology **92**:285, 1969.

166. Larose, J. H., and Gay, B. B., Jr.: Metatropic dwarfism, Amer. J. Roentgen. **106**:156, 1969.

167. Larson, N. E., Dodge, H. W., Rushton, J. B., and Dahlin, D. C.: Hereditary multiple exostoses with compression of the spinal cord, Proc. Mayo Clin. **32**:728, 1957.

168. Laubmann, W.: Ueber die Knochenstruktur bei Marmorknochenkrankheit, Virchow Arch. **296**:343, 1935.

169. Lavine, L. S., and Koven, M. T.: Engelmann's disease (progressive diaphyseal dysplasia), J. Pediat. **40**:235, 1952.

170. Lavy, N. W., Palmer, C. G., and Merritt, A. D.: A syndrome of bizarre vertebral anomalies, J. Pediat. **69**:1121, 1967.

171. Leahy, M. S.: The hereditary nephropathy of osteo-onychodysplasia (nail-patella syndrome), Amer. J. Dis. Child. **112**:237, 1966.

172. Leeds, N. E.: Epiphyseal dysplasia multiplex, Amer. J. Roentgen. **84**:506, 1960.

173. Lehmann, E. C. H.: Familial osteodystrophy of the skull and face, J. Bone Joint Surg. **39-B:**313, 1957.

174. Lennan, E. A., Schechter, M. M., and Hornabrook, R. W.: Engelmann's disease; report of a case with a review of the literature, J. Bone Joint Surg. **43-B:**273, 1961.

175. Lenz, W. D., and Holt, J. F.: Discussion: Murk Jansen type of metaphyseal dysostosis. In Bergsma, D., editor: Clinical delineation of birth defects. IV. Skeletal dysplasias, New York, 1969, National Foundation–March of Dimes, pp. 71-75.

176. Léri, A., and Weill, J.: Une affection congenitale et symétrijue du développement osseux; la dyschondrostéose, Bull. Soc. Méd. Hôp. Paris **53**:1491, 1929.

177. Leroy, J. G., DeMars, R. I., and Opitz, J. M.: I-cell disease. In Bergsma, D., editor: Clinical delineation of birth defects. V. Birth defects; skeletal dysplasias, New York, 1969, National Foundation–March of Dimes, pp. 174-185.

178. Licht, J., and Jesiotr, M.: Chondroangiopathia calcarea seu punctata (chondrodystrophia calcificans congenita); an atypical, stationary form of the disease, Amer. J. Roentgen. **78**492, 1957.

179. Lièvre, J. A., and Fischgold, H.: Leontiasis ossea chez l'enfant (osteopétrose partielle probable), Presse Méd. **64**:763, 1956.

180. Lorey and Reye: Ueber Marmorknochenkrankheit, Fortschr. Roentgenstr. **30**:35, 1923.

181. Lucas, G. L., and Opitz, J. M.: The nail-patella syndrome; clinical and genetic aspects of 5 kindreds with 38 affected family members, J. Pediat. **68**:273, 1966.

182. Lux, S. E., Johnston, R. B., Jr., August, C. S., Say, B., Penchaszadeh, V. B., Rosen, F. S., and McKusick, V. A.: Neutropenia and abnormal cellular immunity in cartilage-hair hypoplasia, New Eng. J. Med. **282**:234, 1970.

183. MacCallum, W. G.: Chondrodystrophia foetalis; notes on the pathological changes in four cases, Bull. Hopkins Hosp. **26**:182, 1915.

184. McCance, R. A.: Osteomalacia with Looser's nodes (milkman's syndrome) due to a raised resistance to vitamin D acquired about the age of 15 years, Quart. J. Med. **16**:33-46, 1947.

185. McCance, R. A., Fairweather, D. V. I., Barrett, A. M., and Morrison, A. B.: Genetic, clinical, biochemical and pathologic features of hypophosphatasia, Quart. J. Med. **25**:523, 1956.

186. McCune, D. J., and Bradley, C.: Osteopetrosis (marble bones) in an infant; review of the literature and report of a case, Amer. J. Dis. Child. **48**:949, 1934.

187. MacDonald, W. B., Fitch, K. D., and Lewis, I. C.: Cockayne's syndrome; an heredo-familial disorder of growth and development, Pediatrics **25**:997, 1960.

188. McKusick, V. A.: Frederick Parkes Weber—1863-1962, J.A.M.A. **183**:45, 1963.

189. McKusick, V. A.: Mendelian inheritance in man; catalogs of autosomal dominant, autosomal recessive and X-linked phenotypes, ed. 3, Baltimore, 1971, The Johns Hopkins Press.

189a. McKusick, V. A.: Unpublished observations, 1972.

190. McKusick, V. A., and colleagues: Medical genetics 1963, J. Chronic Dis. **17**:1077, 1964.

191. McKusick, V. A., Egeland, J. A., Eldridge, R., and Krusen, D. E.: Dwarfism in the Amish. I. The Ellis–van Creveld syndrome, Bull. Hopkins Hosp. **115**:306, 1964.

192. McKusick, V. A., Eldridge, R., Hostetler, J. A., and Egeland, J. A.: Dwarfism in the Amish, Trans. Ass. Amer. Physicians **77**:151, 1964.

193. McKusick, V. A., Eldridge, R., Hostetler, J. A., Ruangwit, U., and Egeland, J. A.: Dwarfism in the Amish. II. Cartilage-hair hypoplasia, Bull. Hopkins Hosp. **116**:285, 1965.

194. McKusick, V. A., Mahloudji, M., Abbott, M. H., Lindenberg, R., and Kepas, D.: Seckel's bird-headed dwarfism, New Eng. J. Med. **277**:279, 1967.

195. McKusick, V. A., and Milch, R. A.: The clinical behavior of genetic disease; selected aspects, Clin. Orthop. **33**:22, 1964.

196. Macleod, W.: Progeria, Brit. J. Radiol. **39**:224, 1966.

197. McPeak, C. N.: Osteopetrosis; report of eight cases occurring in three generations of one family, Amer. J. Roentgen. **37**:816, 1936.

198. Mann, J. B., Alterman, S., and Hills, A. G.: Albright's hereditary osteodystrophy comprising pseudohypoparathyroidism and pseudo-pseudohypoparathyroidism, with a report of two cases representing the complete syndrome occurring in successive generations, Ann. Intern. Med. **56**:315, 1962.

199. Marks, S. C., Jr., and Walker, D. G.: The role of the parafollicular cell of the thyroid gland in the pathogenesis of congenital osteopetrosis in mice, Am. J. Anat. **126**:299, 1969.

200. Maroteaux, P.: Nomenclature internationale des maladies osseuses constitutionnelles, Ann. Radiol. **13**:455, 1970.

201. Maroteaux, P., and Lamy, M.: Achondroplasia in man and animals, Clin. Orthop. **33**:91, 1964.

202. Maroteaux, P., and Lamy, M.: Les formes pseudo-achondroplastiques des dysplasies spondylo-epiphysaires, Presse Méd. **67**:383, 1959.

203. Maroteaux, P., and Lamy, M.: The malady of Toulouse-Lautrec, J.A.M.A. **191**:715, 1965.

204. Maroteaux, P., and Lamy, M.: La pycnodysostose, Presse Méd. **70**:999, 1962.

205. Maroteaux, P., Lamy, M., and Bernard, J.: La dysplasie spondyloépiphysaire tardive, **Presse** Mé. **65**:1205, 1957.

206. Maroteaux, P., Lamy, M., and Robert, J.-M.: Le nanisme thanatophore, Presse Méd. **75**: 2519, 1967.

207. Maroteaux, P., and Savart, P.: La dystrophie thoracique asphyxiante; étude radiologique et rapports avec le syndrome d'Ellis et van Creveld, Ann. Radiol. **7**:332, 1964.

208. Martin, J. R., Macewan, D. W., Blais, J. A, Metrakos, J., Gold, P., Langer, F., and Hill, R. O.: Platyspondyly, polyarticular osteoarthritis, and absent β_2-globulin in two brothers, Arthritis Rheum. **13**:53, 1970.

209. Mathews, E. S. (Baltimore): Personal communication, 1971.

210. Maudsley, R. H.: Dysplasia epiphysealis multiplex, J. Bone Joint Surg. **37-B**:228, 1955.

211. Maynard, J. A., Cooper, R. R., and Ponseti, I. V.: An unusual rough-surfaced endoplasmic reticulum inclusion found in pseudoachondroplasia, Lab. Invest. **26**:40, 1972.

212. Melnick, J. C., and Needles, C. F.: An undiagnosed bone dysplasia; a 2-family study of 4 generations and 3 generations, Amer. J. Roentgen. **97**:39, 1966.

213. Mikity, V. G., and Jacobson, G.: Progressive diaphyseal dysplasia (Engelmann's disease), J. Bone Joint Surg. **40-A**:206, 1958.

214. Millard, D. R., Jr., Maisels, D. O., Batstone, J. H. F., and Yates, B. W.: Craniofacial surgery in craniometaphyseal dysplasia, Amer. J. Surg. **113**:615, 1967.

214a. Møe, P. J., and Skjaeveland, A.: Therapeutic studies in osteopetrosis, Report of 4 cases, Acta Paediat. Scand. **58**:593, 1969.

215. Moldauer, M., Hanelin, J., and Bauer, W.: Familial precocious degenerative arthritis and the natural history of osteochondrodystrophy. In Blumenthal, Herman T., editor: Medical and clinical aspects of aging, New York, 1962, Columbia University Press, pp. 226-233.

216. Mørch, E. T.: Chondrodystrophic dwarfs in Denmark, Opera ex Domo Biol. Hered. Hum., Univ. Hafn., vol. 3, 1941.

217. Morgan, J. P., Carlson, W. D., and Adams, O. R.: Hereditary multiple exostosis in the horse, J. Amer. Vet. Med. Ass. 140:1320, 1962.

218. Mori, P. A., and Holt, J. F.: Cranial manifestations of familial metaphyseal dysplasia, Radiology 66:335, 1956.

219. Munro, R. S., and Goldring, J. S. R.: Chondrosarcoma of the ilium complicating hereditary multiple exostoses, Brit. J. Surg. 39:73, 1951-52.

220. Murdoch, J. L., Walker, B. A., Hall, J. G., Abbey, H., Smith, K. K., and McKusick, V. A.: Achondroplasia—a genetic and statistical survey, Ann. Hum. Genet. 33:227, 1970.

221. Nachtsheim, H.: The Pelger anomaly in man and rabbit; a Mendelian character of the nuclei of the leukocytes, J. Hered. 41:131, 1950.

222. Nance, W. E., and Sweeney, A. J.: A recessive inherited chondrodystrophy, Birth Defects Orig. Art. Ser. 6(no. 4):25, 1970.

223. Nassif, R., and Harboyan, G.: Madelung's deformity with conductive hearing loss, Arch. Otolaryng. 91:175, 1970.

224. Nevin, N. C., Dodge, J. A., and Kernohan, D. C.: Aglossia-adactylia syndrome, Oral Surg. 29:443, 1970.

225. Noonan, C.: Antenatal diagnosis of achondroplasia with comment on Deuel's "halo" sign, Amer. J. Obstet. Gynec. 101:929, 1968.

226. Norum, R. A.: Costovertebral anomalies with apparent recessive inheritance. In Bergsma, D., editor: Clinical delineation of birth defects, IV. Skeletal dysplasias, New York, 1969, National Foundation—March of Dimes, pp. 326-329.

227. O'Brien, J.: Generalized gangliosidosis, J. Pediat. 75:167, 1969.

228. O'Brien, J. S. (LaJolla, Calif.): Personal communication, 1970.

229. O'Duffy, J. D.: Hypophosphatasia associated with calcium pyrophosphate dihydrate deposits in cartilage; report of a case, Arthritis Rheum. 13:381, 1970.

230. Opitz, J. M.: Delayed mutation in achondroplasia? In Bergsma, D., editor: Clinical delineation of birth defects. IV. Skeletal dysplasias, New York, 1969, National Foundation—March of Dimes, pp. 20-23.

231. Parenti, G. C.: La anosteogenesi (una varieta della osteogenesi imperfetta), Pathologica 28:447, 1936.

231a. Parkington, M. W., Gonzales-Crussi, F., Khakee, S. G., and Wollin, D. G.: Cloverleaf skull and thanatophoric dwarfism. Report of four cases, two in the same sibship, Arch. Dis. Child. 46:656, 1971.

232. Parrot, J.: Sur la malformation achondroplasique et le Dieu Ptah, Bull. Soc. Athrop. 1: 296, 1878.

233. Pashayan, H., Whelan, D., Guttman, S., and Fraser, F. C.: Variability of the deLange syndrome; report of 3 cases and genetic analysis of 54 families, J. Pediat. 75:853, 1969.

234. Patton, J. T.: Skeletal changes in hypophosphatemic osteomalacia. In Jelliffe, A. M., and Strickland, B., editors: Symposium ossium, Edinburgh and London, 1970, E. & S. Livingstone, Ltd., p. 299.

235. Pearce, L., and Brown, W. H.: Hereditary osteopetrosis in the rabbit, J. Exp. Med. 88:579, 597, 1928.

236. Peterson, J. C.: Metaphyseal dysotosis; questionably a form of vitamin D–resistant rickets, J. Pediat. 60:656, 1962.

237. Pintsone, B., Eisenberg, E., and Silverman, S.: Hypophosphatasia; genetic and dental studies, Ann. Intern. Med. 65:722, 1966.

238. Pirie, A. H.: The development of marble bone, Amer. J. Roentgen. 24:147, 1930; Marble bones, Amer. J. Roentgen. 30:618, 1933.

239. Pirnar, T., and Neuhauser, E. B. D.: Asphyxiating thoracic dystrophy of the newborn, Amer. J. Roentgen. 98:358, 1966.

240. Plotz, M., and Chakales, H. J.: Osteopetrosis (Albers-Schönberg disease; marble bone disease), New York J. Med. 53:445, 1953.

241. Ponseti, I. V.: Skeletal growth in achondroplasia, J. Bone Joint Surg. 52-A:701, 1970.

242. Potterfield, T. C., and Gonzalez, I.: Ollier's dyschondroplasia, J. Pediat. 33:705, 1948.

243. Poznanski, A. K., Gall, J. C., Jr., and Stern, A. M.: Skeletal manifestations of the Holt-Oram syndrome, Radiology 94:45, 1970.

244. Pyle, E.: A case of unusual bone development, J. Bone Joint Surg. 13:874, 1931.

245. Quelce-Salgado, A.: A new type of dwarfism with various bone aplasias and hypoplasias of the extremities, Acta Genet. 14:63, 1964.

246. Raap, G.: Chondrodystrophia calcificans congenita, Amer. J. Roentgen. 49:77, 1943.

247. Rater, C. J., Selke, A. C., and Van Epps, E. F.: Basal cell nevus syndrome, Amer. J. Roentgen. 103:589, 1968.

248. Resnick, E.: Epiphyseal dysplasia punctata in a mother and identical male twins, J. Bone Joint Surg. 25:461, 1943.

249. Rimoin, D. L.: Pachydermoperiostosis (idiopathic clubbing and periostosis); genetic and physiologic considerations, New Eng. J. Med. 272:923, 1965.

250. Rimoin, D. L., and Edgerton, M. T.: Genetic and clinical heterogeneity in the oral-facial-digital syndromes, J. Pediat. 71:94, 1967.

251. Rimoin, D. L., Fletcher, B. D., and McKusick, V. A.: Spondylocostal dysplasia; a dominantly inherited form of short-trunked dwarfism, Amer. J. Med. 45:948, 1968.

252. Rimoin, D. L., Hughes, G. N. F., and Kaufman, R. L.: Metatropic dwarfism; morphological and biochemical evidence of heterogeneity (abstract), Clin. Res. 17:317, 1969.

253. Rimoin, D. L., Hughes, G. N. F., Kaufman, R. L., Rosenthal, R. E., McAlister, W. H., and Silberberg, R.: Enchondral ossification in achondroplastic dwarfism, New Eng. J. Med. 283:728, 1970.

254. Rimoin, D. L., McAlister, W. H., Saldino, R. M., and Hall, J. G.: Cartilage histology in selected types of congenital dwarfism, Progr. Pediat. Radiol. (In press.)

255. Rimoin, D. L., Woodruff, S. L., and Holman, B. L.: Craniometaphyseal dysplasia (Pyle's disease); autosomal dominant inheritance in a large kindred. In Bergsma, D., editor: Clinical delineation of birth defects. IV. Skeletal dysplasias, New York, 1969, National Foundation–March of Dimes, pp. 96-104.

256. Rosenbloom, A. L., and Smith, D. W.: The natural history of metaphyseal dysostosis, J. Pediat. 66:857, 1965.

257. Rovin, S., Dachi, S. F., Borenstein, D. B., and Cotter, W. B.: Mandibulofacial dysostosis, a familial study of five generations, J. Pediat. 65:215, 1964.

258. Rubin, P.: Dynamic classification of bone dysplasias, Chicago, 1964, Year Book Medical Publishers, Inc.

259. Rubinstein, J. H.: The broad-thumbs syndrome; progress report. In Bergsma, D., editor: Clinical delineation of birth defects. II. Malformation syndromes, New York, 1968, National Foundation–March of Dimes, pp. 25-41.

260. Rucker, T. N., and Alfidi, R. J.: A rare familial systemic affection of the skeleton; Fairbank's disease, Radiology 82:63, 1964.

261. Saldino, R. M.: Lethal short-limbed dwarfism; achondrogenesis and thanatophoric dwarfism, Amer. J. Roentgen. 112:185, 1971.

262. Sanderson, G. H., and Smith, F. S.: Chondrodysplasia (Ollier's disease), J. Bone Joint Surg. 20:61, 1938.

263. Schauerte, E. W., and St. Aubin, P. M.: Progressive synosteosis in Apert's syndrome (acrocephalosyndactyly), with a description of roentgenographic changes in the feet, Amer. J. Roentgen. 97:67, 1966.

264. Schiemann, H.: Über Chondrodystrophie (Achondroplasie, Chondrodysplasie), Akad. der Wissenschaften und Lit., Abhandlungen der aoth.-naturwissenschaft, Klasse Nr. 5, 1966.

265. Schlesinger, B., Luder, J., and Bodian, M.: Rickets with alkaline phosphatase deficiency; an osteoblastic dysplasia, Arch. Dis. Child. 30:265, 1955.

266. Schleuterman, D. A., Bias, W. B., Murdoch, J. L., and McKusick, V. A.: Linkage of the loci for the nail-patella syndrome and adenylate kinase, Amer. J. Hum. Genet. 21:606, 1969.

267. Schoeder, G.: Osteo-onychodysplasia hereditaria (albuminurica). Literaturbericht und Einordnung einer Sippe in dieses Missbildungssyndrom, Z. Menschl. Vererb. Konstitutionsl. 36:42, 1961.

268. Schreiber, F., and Rosenthal, H.: Paraplegia from ruptured lumbar discs in achondroplastic dwarfs, J. Neurosurg. 9:648, 1952.

269. Schwarz, E.: Craniometaphyseal dysplasia, Amer. J. Roentgen. 84:461, 1960.

270. Schwarz, E., and Fish, A.: Roentgenographic features of a new congenital dysplasia, Amer. J. Roentgen. 84:511, 1960.

271. Schwarzweller, F.: Der angeborene Schulterblätthochstät den Wirbelsaule, Z. Menschl. Vererb. Konstitutionsl. **20**:341, 1937.
272. Scott, C. I.: Discussion [of achondrogenesis]. In Bergsma, D., editor: Clinical delineation of birth defects. IV. Skeletal dysplasias, New York, 1969, National Foundation–March of Dimes, p. 14.
272a. Scott, C. I., Jr.: The genetics of short stature, Prog. Med. Gen. **7**:243, 1972.
273. Sear, W. R.: The congenital bone dystrophies and their co-relation, J. Fac. Radiologists **4**:221; **5**:140, 1953.
274. Seigman, E. L., and Kilby, W. L.: Osteopetrosis; report of a case and review of recent literature, Amer. J. Roentgen. **63**:865, 1950.
275. Senturia, H. R., and Senturia, B. D.: Congenital absence of patellae associated with arthrodysplasia of elbows and dystrophy of nails, Amer. J. Roentgen. **51**:352, 1944.
275a. Shepard, T. H., Fry, L. R., and Moffett, B. C., Jr.: Microscopic studies of achondroplastic rabbit cartilage, Teratology **2**:13, 1969.
276. Shillito, J., Jr., and Matson, D. D.: Craniosynostosis; a review of 519 surgical patients, Pediatrics **41**:829, 1968.
277. Shmerling, D. H., Prader, A., Hitzig, W. H., Giedion, A., Hadorn, B., and Kühni, M.: The syndrome of exocrine pancreatic insufficiency, neutropenia, metaphyseal dysostosis and dwarfism, Helv. Paediat. Acta **24**:547, 1969.
278. Shnitka, T. K., Asp, D. M., and Horner, R. N.: Congenital generalized fibromatosis, Cancer **11**:627, 1958.
279. Shuler, S. E.: Pycnodysostosis, Arch. Dis. Child. **38**:620, 1963.
280. Silverman, F. N.: Dysplasies epiphysaires; entité proteiforme, Ann. Radiol. **4**:833, 1961.
281. Silverman, J. L.: Apparent dominant inheritance of hypophosphatasia, Arch. Intern. Med. **110**:191, 1962.
282. Simila, S., Vesa, L., and Wasz-Hockert, O.: Hereditary onycho-osteodysplasia (the nail-patella syndrome) with nephrosis-like renal disease in a newborn boy, Pediatrics **46**:61, 1970.
283. Simril, W. A., and Thurston, D.: Normal interpediculate space in spines of infants and children, Radiology **64**:340, 1955.
284. Singleton, E. B., Daeschner, C. W., and Teng, C. T.: Peripheral dysostosis, Amer. J. Roentgen. **84**:499, 1960.
285. Singleton, E. B., Thomas, J. R., Worthington, W. W., and Hild, J. R.: Progressive diaphyseal dysplasia (Engelmann's disease), Radiology **67**:233, 1956.
286. Sjölin, K. E.: Gargoylism, forme fruste, Acta Paediat. **40**:165, 1951.
287. Slepian, A., and Hamby, W. B.: Neurologic complications associated with hereditary deforming chondrodysplasia; review of the literature and a report on two cases occurring in the same family, J. Neurosurg. **8**:529, 1951.
288. Smith, J. L., and Stowe, F. R.: The Pierre Robin syndrome (glossoptosis, micrognathia, cleft palate); a review of 39 cases with emphasis on associated ocular lesions, Pediatrics **27**:128, 1961.
289. Solomon, L.: Hereditary multiple exostosis, J. Bone Joint Surg. **45-B**:292, 1963.
290. Solonen, K. A., and Sulamaa, M.: Nievergelt syndrome and its treatment; a case report, Ann. Chir. Gynaec. Fenn. **47**:142, 1958.
291. Spahr, A., and Spahr-Hartmann, I.: Dysostose metaphysaire familiale; étude de 4 cas dans une fratrie, Helv. Paediat. Acta **16**:836, 1961.
292. Spillane, J. D.: Three cases of achondroplasia with neurological complications, J. Neurol. Neurosurg. Psychiat. **15**:246, 1952.
293. Spranger, J.: Familial metaphyseal dysplasia? (letter), Lancet **2**:475, 1970.
294. Spranger, J., and Langer, L. O., Jr.: Spondyloepiphyseal dysplasia congenita, Radiology **94**:313, 1970.
294a. Spranger, J. W., and Maroteaux, P.: Kniest disease. In Bergsma, D., editor: Clinical delineation of birth defects. XIX. Skeletal dysplasias (cont.), Baltimore, 1973, The Williams & Wilkins Co.
295. Spranger, J., Paulsen, K., and Lehmann, W.: Die kraniometaphysäre Dysplasie (Pyle), Z. Kinderheilk. **93**:64, 1965.
296. Spranger, J. W., Opitz, J. M., and Bidder, U.: Heterogeneity of chondrodysplasia punctata, Humangenetik **11**:190, 1971.

297. Spranger, J. W., Opitz, J. M., and Bidder, U.: Heterogeneity of chondrodysplasia punctata. In Bergsma, D., editor: Clinical delineation of birth defects. XII. Birth defects; skin, hair and nails, Baltimore, 1971, The Williams & Wilkins Co.

298. Stephens, F. E.: An achondroplastic mutation and the nature of its inheritance, J. Hered. **34:**229, 1943.

299. Stickler, G. B., Maher, F. T., Hunt, J. C., Burke, E. C., and Rosevear, J. W.: Familial bone disease resembling rickets (hereditary metaphysial dysostosis), Pediatrics **29:**996, 1962.

299a. Stobbe, H., and Jorke, D.: Befjnde an homozygoten Pelger-merkmalstragern, Schweiz. Med. Wschr. **95:**1524, 1965.

300. Stocks, P., and Barrington, A.: Hereditary disorders of bone development. Treasury of human inheritance, vol. 3, part 1, Diaphysial aclasia (multiple exostoses), multiple enchondromatosis, cleidocranial dysostosis, London, 1925, Cambridge University Press.

301. Stoner, C. N., Hayes, J. T., and Holt, J. F.: Diastrophic dwarfism, Amer. J. Roentgen. **89:** 914, 1963.

302. Stout, A. P.: Juvenile fibromatoses, Cancer **7:**953, 1954.

303. Strasburger, A. K., Hawkins, M. R., Eldridge, R., Hargrave, R. L., and McKusick, V. A.: Symphalangism; genetic and clinical aspects, Bull. Hopkins Hosp. **117:**108, 1965.

304. Summitt, R. L., and Favara, B. E.: Leprechaunism (Donohue's syndrome); a case report, J. Pediat. **74:**601, 1969.

305. Taybi, H.: Diastrophic dwarfism, Radiology **80:**1, 1963.

306. Taybi, H., Mitchell, A. D., and Friedman, G. D.: Metaphyseal dysostosis and the associated syndrome of pancreatic insufficiency and blood disorders, Radiology **93:**563, 1969.

307. Taybi, H., and Nurock, A. B.: Discussion of osteopathia striata. In Bergsma, D., editor: Clinical delineation of birth defects. IV. Skeletal dysplasias, New York, 1969, National Foundation–March of Dimes.

308. Temtamy, S. A.: Carpenter's syndrome; acrocephalopolysyndactyly; an autosomal recessive syndrome, J. Pediat. **69:**111, 1966.

309. Temtamy, S. A., and McKusick, V. A.: A synopsis of hand malformations, with emphasis on genetic factors. In Bergsma, D., editor: Clinical delineation of birth defects. III. Limb malformations, New York, 1969, National Foundation–March of Dimes.

310. Thompson, B. H., and Parmley, T. H.: Obstetric features of thanatophoric dwarfism, Amer. J. Obstet. Gynec. **109:**396, 1971.

311. Thompson, E. A., Walker, E. T., and Wiens, H. T.: Iliac horns, osseous manifestation of hereditary arthrodysplasia associated with dystrophy of fingernails, Radiology **53:**88, 1949.

312. Thompson, J. N., Palmer, C. G., and Christian, J. C.: The absence of metachromasia in brachycephalic bovine dwarf cell cultures. In Bergsma, D., editor: Clinical delineation of birth defects. IV. Skeletal dysplasias, New York, 1969, National Foundation–March of Dimes, pp. 214-215.

313. Thomsen, G., and Guttadauro, M.: Cleidocranial dysostosis associated with osteosclerosis and bone fragility, Acta Radiol. **37:**559, 1952.

314. Tips, R. L., and Lynch, H. T.: Malignant congenital osteopetrosis resulting from a consanguineous marriage, Acta Paediat. **51:**585, 1962.

315. Torg, J. S., DiGeorge, A. M., Kirkpatrick, J. A., Jr., and Trujillo, M. M.: Hereditary multicentric osteolysis with recessive transmission; a new syndrome, J. Pediat. **75:**243, 1969.

316. Torg, J. S., and Steel, H. H.: Essential osteolysis with nephropathy; a review of the literature and case report of an unusual syndrome, J. Bone Joint Surg. **50-A:**1629, 1968.

316a. Urso, F. P., and Urso, M. J.: Achondrogenesis in two sibs. In Bergsma, D., editor: Clinical delineation of birth defects. XIX. Skeletal dysplasias (cont.), Baltimore, 1973, The Williams & Wilkins Co.

317. Van Buchem, F. S. P., Hadders, H. N., Hansen, J. F., and Woldring, M. G.: Hyperostosis corticalis generalisata; report of seven cases, Amer. J. Med. **33:**387, 1962.

318. Virchow, R.: Das normale Knochenwachstum und die rachitische Störung desselben, Virchow Arch. Path. Anat. **5:**409, 1853.

319. Vogl, A.: The fate of the achondroplastic drawf (neurologic complications of achondroplasia), Exp. Med. Surg. **20:**108, 1962.

320. Vogl, A., and Osborne, R.: Lesions of the spinal cord (transverse myelopathy) in achondroplasia, Arch. Neurol. Psychiat. **61:**644, 1949.

321. Von Knorre, G.: Ueber die hereditare Arthro-osteo-onycho-dysplasie (Turner-Kieser-Syndrome), Menschl. Vererb. Konstitutionsl. **36:**118, 1961.

322. Voorhoeve, N.: L'image radiologique non encore décrité d'une anomalie du squelette; ses rapports avec la dyschondroplasie et l'osteopathia condensans disseminata, Acta Radiol. **3:**407, 1924.

323. Vulliamy, D. G., and Normandale, P. A.: Cranio-facial dysostosis in a Dorset family, Arch. Dis. Child. **41:**375, 1966.

324. Wadia, R.: Achondroplasia in two first cousins (mothers were sisters); all four parents normal and neither parental pair related. In Bergsma, D., editor; Clinical delineation of birth defects. IV. Skeletal dysplasias, New York, 1969, National Foundation–March of Dimes, pp. 227-230.

325. Walker, B. A., Murdoch, J. L., McKusick, V. A., Langer, L. O., and Beals, R. K.: Hypochondroplasia, Amer. J. Dis. Child. **122:**95, 1971.

326. Walker, B. A., Scott, C. I., Hall, J. G., Murdoch, J. L., and McKusick, V. A.: Diastrophic dwarfism, Medicine **51:**1, 1972.

327. Walker, D. G.: Osteopetrosis. In Bergsma, D., editor: Clinical delineation of birth defects. IV. Skeletal dysplasias, New York, 1969, National Foundation–March of Dimes, pp. 308-311.

328. Walker, J. C., Jr., Meijer, R., and Aranda, D.: Syndactylism with deformity of the pectoralis muscle—Poland's syndrome, J. Pediat. Surg. **4:**569, 1969.

329. Walter, H.: Der diastrophische Zwergwuchs (Fortschritte des algemeinen und klinishen Humangenetik, vol. II), Stuttgart, 1970, G. Thieme.

330. Warkany, J., Monroe, B. B., and Sutherland, B. S.: Intrauterine growth retardation, Amer. J. Dis. Child. **102:**249, 1961.

331. Weinberg, H., Frankel, M., and Makin, M.: Familial epiphysial dysplasia of the lower limbs, J. Bone Joint Surg. **42-B:**313, 1960.

332. Weyers, H., and Thier, C. J.: Malformations mandibulofaciales et délimitation d'un syndrome oculo-vertebrale, J. Genet. Hum. **7:**143, 1958.

333. Wiedemann, H.-R.: Die grossen Konstitutions-Krankheiten des Skeletts, Stuttgart, 1960, Gustav Fischer Verlag.

334. Wildervanck, L. S.: Hereditary congenital abnormality of elbows, knees and nails in five generations, Acta Radiol. **33:**41, 1950.

335. Williams, T. F., Winters, R. W., and Burnett, C. H.: A genetic study of familial hypophosphatemia and vitamin D–resistant rickets. In Stanbury, J. B., Wyngaarden, J. B., and Fredrickson, D. S., editors: The metabolic basis of inherited disease, ed. 2, New York, 1966, McGraw-Hill Book Co., pp. 1179-1199.

336. Witkop, C. J., Jr.: Genetics and dentistry, Eugen. Quart. **5:**15, 1958. Also in Pruzansky, S., editor: Congenital anomalies of the face and associated structures, Springfield, Ill., 1961, Charles C Thomas, Publisher.

337. Young, L. W., Radebaugh, J. F., Rubin, P., Sensenbrenner, J. A., and Fiorelli, G.: Mandibular hypoplasia, acro-osteolysis, stiff joints and cutaneous atrophy. In Bergsma, D., editor: Clinical delineation of birth defects. XI. Orofacial structures, Baltimore, 1971, The Williams & Wilkins Co.

338. Zimmer, E. A.: Heinrich Albers-Schönberg, Schweiz. Med. Wschr. **95:**140, 1965.

339. Zwerg, H. G., and Laubmann, W.: Die Albers-Schönbergsche Marmorkrankheit, Ergebn. Med. Strahlenforsch. **7:**95, 1936.

14 · The future in the study of heritable disorders of connective tissue

O'Brien* has usefully indicated the existence of five levels of sophistication, or five stages, in the understanding of a genetic disorder:

1. *Description of the phenotype* includes not only clinical signs and symptoms but also the natural history (age of onset, rate of progression, age at death) and the signs elicited by special means such as the roentgenographic and the gross histologic and cellular morphology.

2. *Delineation of the Mendelian nature of the condition* involves establishing the precise mode of inheritance.

3. *Discovery of the general biochemical nature of the disorder,* by identification of substance(s) excreted in the urine or stored in tissues in excess or of other chemical alterations, is usually the next step.

4. *Identification of a defect in a specific enzyme or other protein gene product* is the penultimate level of sophistication.

5. *Determination of the precise nature of the genic change* involves questions of whether the defect concerns a structural gene or a controller gene, whether the protein gene product is inducible by some means, whether an apparent enzyme defect is in fact a defect in a cofactor, etc. On the answer to these questions may depend useful modes of therapy or even definitive manipulations that fall under the general category of genetic engineering.

Most of the major conditions discussed here can be said to have passed through the first three levels. The mucopolysaccharidoses are at the fourth level since a defect has been demonstrated in a specific substance which, when replaced, leads to correction of the metabolic defect. Trial of therapy in this group of disorders based on the *in vitro* observations of the "correction factor" will be a leading development of the near future. Understanding of homocystinuria is likewise at the fourth level.

It is presumed that in the dominantly inherited disorders, e.g., the Marfan syndrome, the Ehlers-Danlos syndrome, and osteogenesis imperfecta, substitution

---

*O'Brien, J. S.: Ganglioside storage diseases. In Hirschhorn, K., and Harris, H., editors: Advances in human genetics, vol. 3, New York, 1971, Plenum Publishing Corp.

of a single amino acid may have occurred in a defective tissue protein such as collagen. Identification of such is likely to come along in the next few years. The precedent here is, of course, the change in sickle cell hemoglobin. Therapy for these conditions may be difficult to establish, just as effective therapy for sickle cell anemia is not available despite extensive information about the nature of the abnormality at the molecular level.

The prediction of the fruitfulness of cell culture methods in the study of heritable disorders of connective tissue, made in the first edition of this book, 1956 (p. 210), has been fulfilled in the case of the mucopolysaccharidoses. Similar methods are being applied to other disorders, such as the Marfan and Ehlers-Danlos syndromes, with promising results. Important advances are likely in the skeletal dysplasias, somewhat loosely referred to as osteochondrodystrophies. In the next decade, tissue culture of chondrocytes from these disorders will probably permit detection of the enzymatic or other biochemical defect in a considerable number of these conditions.

Rich opportunity for further study of heritable disorders of connective tissue at the clinical level also remains: separation of the entities that presently are thought to be one, i.e., demonstration of genetic heretogeneity; improvement in methods for recognizing mild affection; analysis of the factors, particularly the environmental ones, which are involved in the variability in clinical severity; further nosologic study of all these conditions, particularly the genetic disorders of the osseous skeleton; further exploration of surgical procedures for correcting the structural effects, such as the aortic aneurysm and the scoliosis of the Marfan syndrome; and therapeutic trials in the Marfan syndrome, osteogenesis imperfecta, and the mucopolysaccharidoses (as discussed elsewhere).

15 · General summary and conclusions

The clinical and other features of the principal heritable disorders of connective tissue discussed in this monograph are summarized in Table 15-1. In general, the clinical picture of each of the heritable disorders of connective tissue is as specific and predictable as that of other clinical entities, e.g., infectious diseases. There is, of course, a certain amount of variability in clinical expression, as the physician learns to expect.

The heritable disorders of connective tissue are not congenital malformations in the conventional sense. Osteogenesis imperfecta, cutis laxa, the Ehlers-Danlos syndrome, and the Marfan syndrome appear to be primary disorders of the fibrous elements of connective tissue. Homocystinuria and alkaptonuria have been demonstrated to be secondary disorders of the fibrous elements of connective tissue, which is damaged by metabolites that accumulate in these Garrodian inborn errors of metabolism. They behave as abiotrophies (as does the aortic involvement of the Marfan syndrome). The recessive inheritance and abiotrophic behavior of pseudoxanthoma elasticum suggests that it also may be a secondary disorder of connective tissue.

The mucopolysaccharidoses partake of the characteristics of thesauroses ("storage diseases"), or in the most specific and recent parlance, lysosomal diseases.

The intimate interrelationships of the several elements of connective tissue are indicated by the difficulties in identifying the specific element of connective tissue that is defective in several of these syndromes.

The heritable disorders of connective tissue are ripe for major advances in identification of the fundamental molecular defect, involving either an enzymic or a nonenzymic protein. An enzyme defect can be expected in those conditions with recessive inheritance; a defect in a nonenzymic protein, e.g., collagen, should be sought in those disorders which have a dominant mode of inheritance. The basic defect is now known in at least one form of the Ehlers-Danlos syndrome and in several mucopolysaccharidoses.

Many principles of heredity are illustrated by these disorders. Examples of autosomal dominant, autosomal recessive, and X-linked inheritance are provided. The three most important principles of clinical genetics, repeatedly illustrated by the heritable disorders of connective tissue, are genetic hetero-

859

Table 15-1. Heritable disorders of connective tissue—a synopsis*

Disorder	Skin	Joints	Eye	Bone	Cardiovascular system	Fascia	Inheritance	Fundamental defect
Marfan syndrome	Striae distensae	Hyperextensibility	*Ectopia lentis,* suspensory ligament of lens	Excessive length of long bones: *dolichostenomelia*	*Aortic aneurysm*	Hernia	Autosomal dominant	Defect of collagen?
Weill-Marchesani syndrome	Thickened	Limitation of motion	Microspherophakia; ectopia lentis	Short stature			Autosomal recessive	
Homocystinuria	Malar flush	Somewhat stiff	*Ectopia lentis*	*Dolichostenomelia;* osteoporosis; fracture	*Arterial and venous thromboses*		Autosomal recessive	Defect in cystathionine synthetase
Ehlers-Danlos syndrome	*Fragility; hyperelasticity; bruisability*	*Hyperextensibility*	Ectopia lentis; microhemorrhages of retina		Rupture of aorta and large arteries	Eventration of diaphragm; hernia	Autosomal dominant	Defect of collagen
Cutis laxa	*Lax, pendulous*				Cor pulmonale	Hernia	Autosomal dominant and recessive forms	?
Osteogenesis imperfecta	Thin; abnormal scar formation	Hyperextensibility	Sclera, thinning of: *blue sclerae*	Brittle bones; otosclerosis (deafness)	Rare aortic or mitral change	Hernia	Autosomal dominant	Defect of collagen?
Alkaptonuria	*Ochronotic pigmentation*	*Arthritis*	Ochronotic pigmentation		Valvular sclerosis; accelerated arteriosclerosis?		Autosomal recessive	Defect of homogentisic acid oxidase
Pseudoxanthoma elasticum	*Dystrophy* in wear-and-tear areas		Bruch's membrane, crazing of: *angioid streaks*		Peripheral arteries, medial sclerosis of; *hemorrhages*		Autosomal recessive	Degeneration of elastic fibers
Hurler syndrome (prototype mucopolysaccharidosis)	Roughening; nodular thickening; hirsutism	*Limitation of mobility*	*Clouding of cornea*	Dwarfism; *dysostosis multiplex*	Intimal deposits in coronary arteries; valvular lesions	Hernia	Autosomal recessive	Defect in degradation of mucopolysaccharides

*Italicized items indicate predominant manifestations in the case of each syndrome.

geneity (p. 23ff.), pleiotropism (pp. 2 and 13), and variability (on which the phenomena of expressivity and penetrance depend). Other genetic principles illustrated here include paternal age effect in mutation, consequences of homozygosity for dominant genes, role of consanguinity in autosomal recessive traits, the Lyon principle, and recessive inheritance of enzymopathies.

The recognition of the more easily detectable external expressions of the basic defect of connective tissue provides clinical clues to the nature of internal disturbances that are less accessible for study. Most dramatic among the illustrations of this time-honored principle are (1) the association of ectopia lentis with aortic regurgitation in the Marfan syndrome and (2) the association of angioid streaks of the fundus oculi and characteristic skin changes with massive gastrointestinal hemorrhage in pseudoxanthoma elasticum. The basis for these diagnostically useful associations is the pleiotropic effect of a single mutant gene.

Genetic heterogeneity is illustrated by the Marfan syndrome and homocystinuria and by the multiple forms of the Ehlers-Danlos syndrome and the mucopolysaccharidoses.

Phenotypic variability dependent on the genetic background against which the specific mutant gene operates is illustrated by the Marfan syndrome and other disorders.

The heritable disorders of connective tissue can be useful tools for the study of the normal biology of connective tissue. Further confirmation is provided for the principle enunciated by Sir Archibald Garrod and quoted at the outset: clinical and other investigations of hereditary disorders will shed light on normal developmental and biochemical mechanisms.

Index